Pain Management

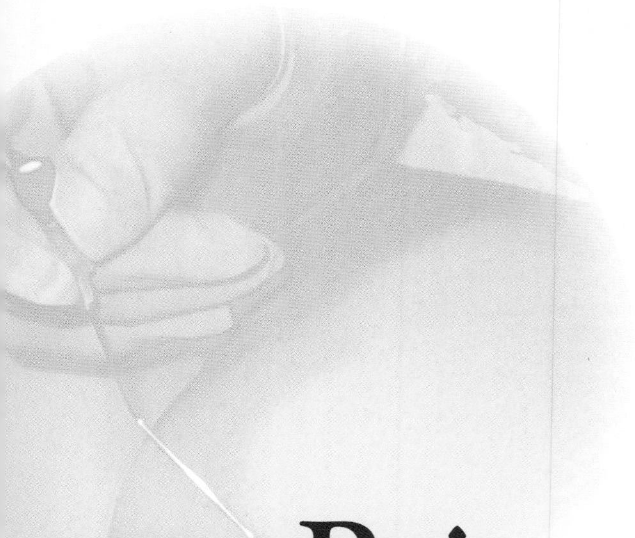

Pain Management

Steven D. Waldman, MD, JD

Clinical Professor, Department of Anesthesiology
University of Missouri–Kansas City School of Medicine
Kansas City, Missouri
Medical Director, Headache and Pain Center
Leawood, Kansas

Color drawings by Joseph I. Bloch, CMI, Graphic World, and Electronic Publishing Services

Volume 2

SAUNDERS
ELSEVIER

SAUNDERS
ELSEVIER

1600 John F. Kennedy Blvd.
Ste 1800
Philadelphia, PA 19103-2899

PAIN MANAGEMENT

ISBN-13: 978-0-7216-0334-6
ISBN-10: 0-7216-0334-3
Vol 1 PN: 9997627075
Vol 2 PN: 9997627083

Notice

Knowledge and best practice in this field are constantly changing. As new research and experience broaden our knowledge, changes in practice, treatment, and drug therapy may become necessary or appropriate. Readers are advised to check the most current information provided (i) on procedures featured or (ii) by the manufacturer of each product to be administered, to verify the recommended dose or formula, the method and duration of administration, and contraindications. It is the responsibility of the practitioner, relying on his or her own experience and knowledge of the patient, to make diagnoses, to determine dosages and the best treatment for each individual patient, and to take all appropriate safety precautions. To the fullest extent of the law, neither the publisher nor the author assumes any liability for any injury and/or damage to persons or property arising out of or related to any use of the material contained in this book.

Library of Congress Cataloging-in-Publication Data
Pain management/edited by Steven D. Waldman.—1st ed.
p. ; cm.
Includes bibliographical references and index.
ISBN 0-7216-0334-3
1. Pain—Treatment. I. Waldman, Steven D.
[DNLM: 1. Pain—therapy. WL 704 P14654 2007]
RB127.P332284 2007
616′.0472—dc22 2006026880

Executive Publisher: Natasha Andjelkovic
Editorial Assistant: Katie Davenport
Publishing Services Manager: Tina Rebane
Project Manager: Mary Anne Folcher
Design Direction: Ellen Zanolle
Cover Designer: Ellen Zanolle

Printed in China

Last digit is the print number: 9 8 7 6 5 4 3 2 1

To my children: David for his caring nature and amazing work ethic, Corey for his integrity and determination, Jennifer for her intellect and compassion, and Reid for his ambition and unabashed joie de vie.

Steven D. Waldman, MD

Summer 2006

Contributors

Ahmed N. Abdelhalim, MD
Assistant Professor, Department of Radiology, State University of New York at Buffalo School of Medicine and Biomedical Sciences; Staff Neuroradiologist, Department of Diagnostic Imaging, Roswell Park Cancer Institute, Buffalo, New York

Salahadin Abdi, MD, PhD
Professor and Chief, Department of Anesthesiology, Perioperative Medicine and Pain Management, University of Miami; Chief of Pain Medicine, Jackson Memorial Hospital, Miami, Florida

Bernard M. Abrams, MD
Clinical Professor of Neurology, University of Missouri-Kansas City School of Medicine, Kansas City, Missouri; Neurologist, Menorah Medical Center, Overland Park, Kansas

Vimal Akhouri, MD, MB
Instructor, Department of Anesthesiology and Critical Care, Harvard Medical School, Beth Israel Deaconess Medical Center, Boston, Massachusetts

Ronald A. Alberico, MD
Associate Professor of Radiology and Assistant Clinical Professor of Neurosurgery, State University of New York at Buffalo School of Medicine; Director of Neuroradiology/Head and Neck Imaging, and Director of Pediatric Neuroradiology, Roswell Park Cancer Institute, Buffalo, New York

J. Antonio Aldrete, MD, MS
Professor, Department of Anesthesiology, University of Alabama at Birmingham; Aldrete Pain Care Center, Birmingham, Alabama

Frank Andrasik, PhD
Professor of Psychology, University of West Florida; Senior Research Scientist, Institute for Human and Machine Cognition, Pensacola, Florida

Sairam Atluri, MD
TriState Pain Management Institute, Loveland, Ohio

Shelley Wiechman Askay, PhD
Assistant Professor, Department of Rehabilitation Medicine, University of Washington; Attending Psychologist, Harborview Medical Center, Seattle, Washington

Zahid H. Bajwa, MD
Assistant Professor of Anesthesia and Neurology, Harvard Medical School; Director, Education and Clinical Pain Research, Beth Israel Deaconess Medical Center, Boston, Massachusetts

David P. Bankston, MD
Consultant in Pain Management, The Headache and Pain Center, Leawood, Kansas

Ralf Baron, MD
Professor of Neurology, Chair, Department of Neurological Pain Research and Therapy, Vice Chair, Neurological Clinic, Christian-Albrechts-Universität Kiel, Kiel, Germany

Jonathan Barry
Department of Anesthesiology and Pain Management, Texas Tech University Health Sciences Center, Lubbock, Texas

Andreas Binder, MD
Consultant, Department of Neurological Pain Research and Therapy, Neurological Clinic, Christian-Albrechts-Universität Kiel, Kiel, Germany

Donna Bloodworth, MD
Associate Professor, Baylor College of Medicine; Outpatient Director, Physical Medicine, Harris County Hospital District, Houston, Texas

Nikolai Bogduk, MD
Professor of Pain Medicine, Department of Clinical Research, Royal Newcastle Hospital, Newcastle, Australia

David Borenstein, MD
Clinical Professor of Medicine, The George Washington University Medical Center; Arthritis and Rheumatism Associates, Washington, DC

Mark V. Boswell, MD, PhD
Associate Professor of Anesthesiology, Chief of the Anesthesiology Pain Service, Case Western Reserve University School of Medicine, University Hospitals of Cleveland, Cleveland, Ohio

Geoffrey Bove, DC, PhD
Department of Anesthesia, Critical Care, and Pain Management, Beth Israel Deaconess Medical Center, Boston, Massachusetts

Fadi Braiteh, MD
Medical Oncology Fellow, The University of Texas MD Anderson Cancer Center, Houston, Texas

David L. Brown, MD
Edward Rotan Distinguished Professor and Chairman, Department of Anesthesiology and Pain Medicine, The University of Texas MD Anderson Cancer Center, Houston, Texas

Eduardo Bruera, MD
Professor and Chair, Department of Palliative Care and Rehabilitation Medicine, The University of Texas MD Anderson Cancer Center, Houston, Texas

Allen W. Burton, MD
Associate Professor and Section Chief, Pain Management, University of Texas MD Anderson Cancer Center, Houston, Texas

Roger K. Cady, MD
Headache Care Center, Springfield, Missouri

Kenneth D. Candido, MD
Professor of Anesthesiology, Chief, Division of Pain Management, Loyola University School of Medicine, Maywood, Illinois

John A. Carrino, MD, MPH
Assistant Professor of Radiology, Harvard Medical School; Clinical Director of Magnetic Resonance Therapy, and Co-Director of Spine Intervention Service, Brigham and Women's Hospital, Boston, Massachusetts; Visiting Associate Professor of Radiology, Russell H. Morgan Department of Radiology and Radiological Science, and Chief, Musculoskeletal Radiology Division, Johns Hopkins Outpatient Center, Johns Hopkins University School of Medicine, Baltimore, Maryland

Joseph S. Chiang, MD
Professor, Department of Anesthesiology, The University of Texas MD Anderson Cancer Center, Houston, Texas

Martin K. Childers, DO, PhD
Associate Professor, University of Missouri-Columbia, Columbia, Missouri

Eric T. Chou, MD
Department of Radiology, Brigham and Women's Hospital, Harvard Medical School, Boston, Massachusetts

Philip G. Conaghan, MB, BS, PhD, FRACP, FRCP
Professor, Academic Unit of Musculoskeletal Disease, Department of Rheumatology, Faculty of Medicine and Health, University of Leeds, Leeds, United Kingdom

Darin J. Correll, MD
Instructor of Anesthesia, Harvard Medical School; Director, Acute Postoperative Pain Service, Department of Anesthesiology, Perioperative and Pain Medicine, Brigham and Women's Hospital, Boston, Massachusetts

Scott C. Cozad, DDS, MD
Therapeutic Radiologist Inc., Kansas City, Missouri

Edward V. Craig, MD
Clinical Professor of Orthopaedic Surgery, Weil Medical College of Cornell University; Attending Orthopaedic Surgeon, The Hospital for Special Surgery, New York, New York

Paul Creamer, MD, FRCP
Consultant Rheumatologist, Southmead Hospital, Bristol, United Kingdom

Miles R. Day, MD, FIPP, DABPM
Associate Professor, Department of Anesthesiology and Pain Management, Southwestern Medical School, McDermott Center for Pain Management, Dallas, Texas

Debra A. DeAngelo, DO
Active Staff, Hanover Hospital, Hanover, Pennsylvania

Seymour Diamond, MD
Adjunct Professor, Department of Cellular and Molecular Pharmacology, and Clinical Professor, Department of Family Medicine, Chicago Medical School at Rosalind Franklin, University of Medicine and Science, North Chicago; Director, Diamond Inpatient Headache Unit, Saint Joseph Hospital, and Director and Founder, Diamond Headache Clinic, Chicago, Illinois

Paul Dieppe, MB BS, MD, FRCP, FFPH
Director, Medical Research Council Health Services Research Collaboration, Department of Social Medicine, University of Bristol, Bristol, United Kingdom

Charles D. Donohoe, MD
Associate Clinical Professor, University of Missouri-Kansas City, School of Medicine, Kansas City, Missouri

James Evans, MD
Assistant Professor, Department of Neurosurgery, Medical College of Thomas Jefferson University, Philadelphia, Pennsylvania

Adel G. Fam, MD, FRCP, MRCP(UK), FACP
Professor Emeritus of Medicine (Rheumatology), Division of Rheumatology, University of Toronto; Staff Consultant Rheumatologist (Retired), Sunnybrook Health Sciences Centre, Toronto, Ontario, Canada

Kathleen U. Farmer, PsyD
Headache Care Center, Springfield, Missouri

Frederick G. Freitag, DO
Clinical Assistant Professor, Department of Family Medicine, The Chicago Medical School at Rosalind Franklin, University of Medicine and Science, North Chicago; Associate Director, Diamond Headache Clinic, Chicago, Illinois

M. Kay Garcia, RN, LAc, DrPH
Adjunct Associate Professor, American College of Acupuncture and Oriental Medicine; Advanced Practice Nurse/Acupuncturist, Department of Anesthesiology and Pain Medicine, MD Anderson Cancer Center, Houston, Texas

Scott Goodman, MD
Consultant in Neurology, Headache and Pain Center, Leawood, Kansas

Vitaly Gordin, DM
Associate Professor and Director, Pain Medicine Fellowship Program, Pennsylvania State University College of Medicine, Hershey, Pennsylvania

Martin Grabois, MD
Professor and Chair, Department of Physical Medicine and Rehabilitation, Baylor College of Medicine, Houston, Texas

Douglas R. Gracey, MD, FACP, FCCP
Professor of Medicine, Mayo Clinic College of Medicine; Emeritus Chair, Division of Pulmonary and Critical Care Medicine, Mayo Clinic, Rochester, Minnesota

Mark A. Greenfield, MD
Consultant in Pain Management, Headache and Pain Center, Leawood, Kansas

Rakesh Gupta, MD
Advanced Pain Consultants, Voorhees, New Jersey

Brian Hainline, MD
Clinical Associate Professor, Department of Neurology, New York University School of Medicine, New York

Howard R. Hall, PhD, PsyD
Division of Behavioral Pediatrics, Case Western Reserve University and Rainbow Babies and Children's Hospital, Cleveland, Ohio

Samuel J. Hassenbusch III, MD, PhD
Professor, Department of Neurosurgery, The University of Texas MD Anderson Cancer Center, Houston, Texas

Brian L. Hazleman, MA, MB, FRCP
Consultant Rheumatologist and Director of the Rheumatology Research Unit, Addenbrooke's Hospital; Associate Lecturer, Department of Medicine, University of Cambridge, and Fellow, Corpus Christi College, Cambridge, United Kingdom

James E. Heavner, DVM, PhD
Professor, Anesthesiology and Physiology, Texas Tech University Health Science Center, Lubbock, Texas

D. Ross Henshaw, MD
Orthopaedic Surgeon and Director of Sports Medicine, Danbury Hospital, Danbury, Connecticut

David Dai-Fu Hou, MD
Clinical Fellow, Department of Radiology, Brigham and Women's Hospital, Harvard Medical School, Boston, Massachusetts

Subhash Jain, MD
Centers for Pain Management, New York, New York

Jeffrey W. Janata, PhD
Associate Professor, Department of Psychiatry, Case Western Reserve School of Medicine; Director, Behavioral Medicine Program, University Hospitals of Cleveland, Cleveland, Ohio

Joel Katz, MD
Professor and Canada Research Chair in Health Psychology, Department of Psychology and School of Kinesiology and Health Science, York University; Director, Acute Pain Research Unit, Department of Anesthesia and Pain Management, Toronto General Hospital and Mount Sinai Hospital, Toronto, Ontario, Canada

Bruce L. Kidd, MD
Reader in Rheumatology, University of London, Bone & Joint Research Unit, Queen Mary's School of Medicine, London, United Kingdom

Matthew T. Kline, MD
Private Practice, Philadelphia, Pennsylvania

Dan J. Kopacz, MD
Staff Anesthesiologist, Southern Colorado Anesthesia Associates, Colorado Springs, Colorado

Dhanalakshmi Koyyalagunta, MD
Associate Professor, The University of Texas MD Anderson Cancer Center, Houston, Texas

Lawrence Kropp, MD
Interventional Pain Consultants of Alaska, LLC, Anchorage, Alaska

Milton H. Landers, DO, PhD
Assistant Clinical Professor, Department of Anesthesiology, University of Kansas School of Medicine; Pain Management Associates, Wichita, Kansas

Mark J. Lema, MD, PhD
Professor and Chair, Department of Anesthesiology, State University of New York at Buffalo School of Medicine and Biomedical Sciences; Chair, Department of Anesthesiology and Pain Medicine, Roswell Park Cancer Institute, Buffalo, New York

Jennifer B. Levin, PhD
Assistant Professor, Department of Psychiatry, Case Western Reserve School of Medicine; Clinical Psychologist, University Hospitals of Cleveland, Cleveland, Ohio

Mirjana Lovrincevic, MD
Clinical Assistant Professor of Anesthesiology, State University of New York at Buffalo School of Medicine and Biomedical Sciences; Staff Anesthesiologist/Pain Physician, Roswell Park Cancer Institute, Buffalo, New York

Z. David Luo, MD, PhD
Assistant Professor, Departments of Anesthesiology and Pharmacology, University of California Irvine Medical Center, Orange, California

Laxmaiah Manchikanti, MD
Pain Management Center of Paducah, Paducah, Kentucky

Chad Markert, PhD
Postdoctoral Fellow, University of Missouri-Columbia, Columbia, Missouri

Brian McGuirk, MD
Department of Clinical Research, Royal Newcastle Hospital, Newcastle, Australia

Ronald Melzack, PhD
Professor Emeritus, Department of Psychology, McGill University, Montreal, Quebec, Canada

Jose L. Mendez, MD
Formerly Fellow, Pulmonary and Critical Care Medicine, and Currently Fellow, Sleep Medicine, Mayo Clinic and Mayo College of Medicine, Rochester, Minnesota

Jeffrey P. Meyer
Midwest Pain Consultants, PC, Midwest City, Oklahoma

Michael Munz, MD, FACS, FRCS
Staff Neurosurgeon, Fort Wayne Neurological Center, Fort Wayne, Indiana

David P. Myers, MD, CAP, FASAM
President, HealthCare Connection of Tampa, Inc., Tampa, Florida

Joel A. Nielsen, DO
Private Practice, Weston, Wisconsin

George R. Nissan, DO
Clinical Assistant Professor of Medicine, The Chicago Medical School at Rosalind Franklin University of Medicine and Science; North Chicago; Staff Physician and Director of Research, Diamond Headache Clinic, Chicago, Illinois

Son Truong Nguyen, DO
Senior Anesthesiologist, St. Luke's Hospital, San Francisco, California

Kathleen A. O'Leary, MD
Associate Professor, Department of Anesthesiology, School of Medicine and Biomedical Sciences, State University of New York at Buffalo; Operating Room Director, Department of Anesthesiology and Pain Medicine, Roswell Park Cancer Institute, Buffalo, New York

Robert H. Overbaugh, MD
Chief Fellow, Pain Medicine, Pennsylvania State University College of Medicine, Hershey, Pennsylvania

John L. Pappas, MD
Vice Chief, Anesthesiology, and Director, Interventional Pain Center, William Beaumont Hospital, Troy, Michigan

Winston C. V. Parris, MD
Professor, Department of Anesthesiology, Duke University, and Chief, Division of Pain Management, Duke University Medical Center, Durham, North Carolina

Divya Patel, MD
Private Practice, East Hanover, New Jersey

Richard B. Patt, MD
The Patt Center for Cancer Pain and Wellness P.A., Houston, Texas

David R. Patterson, PhD, ABPP, ABPH
Professor, Department of Rehabilitation Medicine, University of Washington; Attending Psychologist, Harborview Medical Center, Seattle, Washington

Brett T. Quave, MD
Pain Management Fellow, Loma Linda University Medical Center, Loma Linda, California

Gabor B. Racz, MD, ChB, DABPM
Grover E. Murray Professor and Chairman Emeritus, Director of Pain Services, Texas Tech University Health Sciences Center, Lubbock, Texas

P. Prithvi Raj, MD, FIPP
Professor Emeritus, Texas Tech Health Sciences Center, Lubbock, Texas

Somayaji Ramamurthy, MD
Professor, University of Texas Health Science Center; Attending Physician and Director of the Pain Clinic, University Hospital, San Antonio, Texas

K. Dean Reeves, MD, FAAPM&R
Clinical Associate Professor, Department of Physical Medicine and Rehabilitation, University of Kansas School of Medicine, Kansas City, Kansas

Lowell W. Reynolds, MD
Professor of Anesthesiology, Loma Linda University School of Medicine, and Medical Director and Fellowship Director, Loma Linda University Medical Center, Loma Linda, California

Carla Rime, BA (Psychology)
University of West Florida, Pensacola, Florida

Steven Rosen, MD
Medical Director, Fox Chase Pain Management Associates, Jenkintown, Pennsylvania

Matthew P. Rupert, MD, MS
Total Pain Care LLC, Meridian, Mississippi

Lloyd R. Saberski, MD
Medical Director, The Institute for Therapeutic Discovery, Delanson, New York

Jörn Schattschneider, MD
Consultant, Department of Neurological Pain Research and Therapy, Neurological Clinic, Christian-Albrechts-Universität Kiel, Kiel, Germany

Thomas F. Schrattenholzer, MD
Pain Management Fellow, Loma Linda University Medical Center, Loma Linda, California

Curtis P. Schreiber, MD
Headache Care Center, Springfield, Missouri

David M. Schultz, MD
Medical Director, Medical Advanced Pain Specialists, Minneapolis, Minnesota

Sam R. Sharar, MD
Professor, Department of Anesthesiology, University of Washington; Director, Harborview Anesthesiology Research Center, and Attending Anesthesiologist, Harborview Medical Center, Seattle, Washington

Shawn M. Sills
Pain Management Fellow, Loma Linda University Medical Center, Loma Linda, California

Khuram A. Sial, MD
Temecula Pain Management Center, Temecula, California

Steven Simon, MD, RPH
Assistant Clinical Professor, Department of Physical Medicine and Rehabilitation, University of Kansas Medical Center; Director, the Pain Management Institute, Overland Park, Kansas

Thomas T. Simopoulos, MD, MA
Clinical Instructor of Anesthesia and Pain Management, Harvard Medical School; Director of Acute and Interventional Pain Services, Beth Israel Deaconess Medical Center, Boston, Massachusetts

Vijay Singh, MD
Medical Director, Pain Diagnostics Associates, Niagara, Wisconsin

Kimberley Smith-Martin, MD, FAAPMR
Interventional Physiatrist, Pain Management Specialist, Premier Orthopaedics Associate, Vineland, New Jersey

Daneshvari R. Solanki, MD, FRCA
Professor of Anesthesiology, University of Texas Medical Branch, Galveston, Texas

David A. Soto-Quijano, MD
Department of Physical Medicine and Rehabilitation, Veterans Affairs Medical Center, Houston, Texas

Michael D. Stanton-Hicks, MD BS
Vice Chairman, Division of Anesthesiology, Pain Management and Research, The Cleveland Clinic Foundation, Cleveland, Ohio

M. Alan Stiles, DMD
Clinical Instructor, Department of Oral and Maxillofacial Surgery, Thomas Jefferson University and Medical School, Philadelphia, Pennsylvania

Robert B. Supernaw, PharmD
Professor and Dean, School of Pharmacy, Wingate University, Wingate, North Carolina

Rand S. Swenson, DC, MD, PhD
Assistant Professor, Section of Neurology, Dartmouth-Hitchcock Medical Center, Lebanon, New Hampshire

Gale E. Thompson, MD
Staff Anesthesiologist, Department of Anesthesiology, Virginia Mason Medical Center, Seattle, Washington

Kavin D. Treffer, DO
Associate Professor, Department of Family Medicine, and Osteopathic Manipulative Medicine Coordinator, Kansas City University of Medicine and Biosciences, College of Osteopathic Medicine; Chair, Osteopathic Principles and Utilization Committee, Kansas City, Missouri

Robert Trout, MD
Consultant in Physical Medicine and Rehabilitation, The Headache and Pain Center, Leawood, Kansas

George Urban, MD
Clinical Instructor, Department of Medicine, The Chicago Medical School at Rosalind Franklin University of Medicine and Science, North Chicago, Illinois; Associate Director, Diamond Headache Clinic, Chicago, Illinois

Luminita Vladutu, MD
Department of Anesthesiology and Pain Management, Texas Tech University Health Sciences Center, Lubbock, Texas

Howard J. Waldman, MD, DO
Consultant in Physical Medicine and Rehabilitation, The Headache and Pain Center, Leawood, Kansas; Director of Neurophysiology Laboratory, Doctors Hospital, Leawood, Kansas

Katherine A. Waldman, OTR
Headache and Pain Center, Leawood, Kansas

Steven D. Waldman, MD, JD
Clinical Professor, Department of Anesthesiology, University of Missouri–Kansas City School of Medicine, Kansas City, Missouri; Medical Director, Headache and Pain Center, Leawood, Kansas

Carol A. Warfield, MD
Lowenstein Professor of Anesthesia, Harvard Medical School; Chair, Department of Anesthesia, Critical Care, and Pain Medicine, Beth Israel Deaconess Medical Center, Boston, Massachusetts

Michael L. Whitworth, MD
President, Advanced Pain Management Surgery, Columbus, Indiana

Alon P. Winnie, MD
Professor, Department of Anesthesiology, Northwestern University Medical School, Chicago, Illinois

Gilbert Y. Wong
Assistant Professor, Department of Anesthesiology, Mayo Clinic College of Medicine; Consultant, Department of Anesthesiology, Division of Pain Medicine, Mayo Clinic, Rochester, Minnesota

Tony L. Yaksh, PhD
Professor of Anesthesiology and Pharmacology, and Vice Chair for Research in Anesthesiology, University of California, San Diego, La Jolla, California

Anthony T. Yarussi
Department of Anesthesiology and Pain Medicine, Roswell Park Cancer Institute, Buffalo, New York

Way Yin, MD
Medical Director, Interventional Medical Associates of Billingham, P.C., Billingham, Washington

Michael S. Yoon, MD
Clinical Assistant Professor, Temple University Hospital, Philadelphia; Assistant Surgeon, Abington Memorial Hospital, Abington, Pennsylvania

Preface

Pain management is a young medical specialty compared to its brethren. Its birth in the early 1950s has been attributed to Dr. John Bonica. His seminal book, *The Management of Pain,* guided the specialty though its infancy by providing those few early pain management physicians with the first comprehensive pain management text. Our specialty's toddler years were nurtured by the many excellent pain management texts edited by Dr. Prithvi Raj. Raj's *Practical Management of Pain* was the first comprehensive pain management text to truly emphasize the practical clinical aspects of the specialty. Subsequent editions of *Practical Management of Pain* have further refined this emphasis on practicality and set a high standard for pain management literature in general. As our specialty reached adolescence, it began to change as the increased subspecialization spawned a need for more topic-focused literature. Dr. Richard Patt's excellent text *Cancer Pain* and my own first attempt at textbook editing, *Interventional Pain Management,* are examples of such topic-focused literature. The teenage years of the specialty yielded a demand for more targeted how-to texts. This emphasis on how rather than why spawned the new type of book, the how-to-do-it atlas. The *Atlas of Interventional Pain Management,* first published by Saunders in 1998, was the first of this kind and its subsequent editions and many other text-atlases published since continued this practical emphasis. With early adulthood, our specialty has begun to mature. Many of us practicing the specialty of pain management have come to realize that just knowing why or just knowing how is simply not enough and this realization led me to the desire to edit this text.

This book was first conceived during my collaboration with Allan Ross, then a senior editor for anesthesiology and pain management at WB Saunders, who realized that the push toward more specialized texts and atlases had left a void in the comprehensive pain management literature. Thus, *Pain Management* was born. This two-volume text was designed to be a worthy successor to the texts that have come before it and to provide the pain management specialists with a comprehensive single-source reference for the specialty of pain management.

It should be emphasized that this treatise is the result of many dedicated pain management specialists selflessly giving up their time (often late at night or on weekends as their clinical responsibilities allowed) to contribute chapters to it. As the book's editor, I am deeply indebted to them for their contributions, encouragement, and support. All shared my desire to produce the most clinically useful text that we could to help those practitioners dedicated to the treatment of pain. I would also like to acknowledge the tireless efforts of the editorial and production staff at Elsevier led by Executive Publisher Natasha Andjelkovic and Publishing Services Manager Tina Rebane to turn the myriad chapters, revisions, and hundreds of figures, tables, and radiographs into an accurate and infinitely readable text. I can only hope that you find *Pain Management* a worthwhile addition to your reference library and enjoy reading and using it as much as I enjoyed editing and writing for it.

Steven D. Waldman, M.D.

Contents

Volume 1

Volume 2

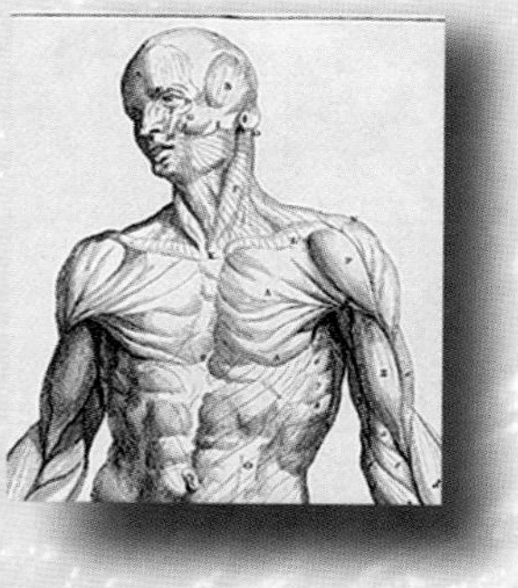

Part H

Pain Syndromes of the Lumbar Spine and Sacroiliac Joint

chapter 82

Low Back Pain

David Borenstein

Low back pain is defined as an acute, subacute, or chronic discomfort localized to the anatomic area below the posterior ribs and above the lower margins of the buttock. Low back pain is second only to the common cold as the most common affliction of humans. The lifetime prevalence of back pain is greater than 70% in most industrialized countries.[1] National statistics from the United States indicate a 1-year prevalence of 15% to 20%.[2] Low back pain is the fifth most common reason for visiting a physician, according to a U.S. National Ambulatory Care survey.[3]

Low back pain is a symptom that is associated with a wide range of clinical disorders.[4] Most patients with back pain have the symptom on a mechanical basis. Nachemson[5] suggested that 90% of individuals have a mechanical reason for their back pain. Mechanical low back pain may be defined as pain secondary to overuse of a normal anatomic structure (e.g., muscle strain) or pain secondary to trauma or deformity of an anatomic structure (e.g., herniated nucleus pulposus). Characteristically, mechanical disorders are exacerbated by physical activities, such as lifting, and are relieved by other activities, such as assuming a supine position. The remaining 10% of adults with back pain have the symptom as a manifestation of a systemic illness. In some systemic illnesses (i.e., nonmechanical), back pain is noted in almost every individual who has the disorder (e.g., ankylosing spondylitis). In other illnesses, back pain is a rare complaint (e.g., infective endocarditis). Mechanical and systemic disorders associated with low back pain are listed in Table 82–1.

The natural history of low back pain is one of improvement. More than 50% of all patients improve after 1 week, and 90% are better at 8 weeks. Recurrence of spinal pain occurs in 75% of individuals, however, over the next year. Back pain persists for 1 year or longer in 10% of spinal pain patients.[6]

The challenge for the practicing physician is to separate individuals with mechanical disorders from patients with systemic illnesses. The patient's symptoms and signs help differentiate mechanical from systemic causes of localized axial pain. In addition, these clinical findings, along with radiographic and laboratory data, designate specific disorders in these two major groups. This chapter focuses on the process of identifying the factors that define the most likely cause of the symptom of low back pain.

Another symptom frequently associated with low back pain is sciatica or radicular pain. Individuals who have

Table 82–1

Disorders Associated with Low Back Pain

Mechanical	**Miscellaneous**	**Infectious**
Muscle strain	Paget disease	Vertebral osteomyelitis
Herniated disk	Vertebral sarcoidosis	Diskitis
Osteoarthritis	Infective endocarditis	Pyogenic sacroiliitis
Spinal stenosis	Retroperitoneal fibrosis	Herpes zoster
Spondylolysis	**Neoplastic/Infiltrative**	Lyme disease
Adult scoliosis	Benign tumors	**Referred Pain**
Rheumatologic	Osteoid osteoma	***Vascular***
Ankylosing spondylitis	Osteoblastoma	Abdominal aorta
Reactive arthritis	Osteochondroma	***Gastrointestinal***
Psoriatic arthritis	Giant cell tumor	Pancreas
Enteropathic arthritis	Hemangioma	Gallbladder
DISH syndrome	Eosinophilic granuloma	Intestine
Vertebral osteochondritis	Aneurysmal bone cyst	***Genitourinary***
Polymyalgia rheumatica	Gaucher disease	Kidney
Fibromyalgia	Sacroiliac lipoma	Ureter
Behçet disease	Malignant tumors	Bladder
Whipple disease	Skeletal metastases	Uterus
Hidradenitis suppurativa	Multiple myeloma	Ovary
Hematologic	Chondrosarcoma	Prostate
Hemoglobinopathies	Chordoma	**Neurologic/Psychiatric**
Myelofibrosis	Lymphoma	Neuropathic arthropathy
Mastocytosis	Intraspinal lesions	Neuropathies
Endocrinologic	Metastases	Tumors
Osteoporosis	Meningioma	Vasculitis
Osteomalacia	Gliomas	Compression
Parathyroid disease	Vascular malformations	Psychogenic rheumatism
Microcrystalline disease	Syringomyelia	Malingering
Ochronosis		
Fluorosis		
Heritable genetic disorders		

radicular pain to the lower extremity have disorders associated with neural impingement (e.g., herniated intervertebral disk, spinal stenosis) or referred pain (e.g., facet syndrome). These illnesses with pain affecting structures beyond the lumbosacral spine are subjects of other chapters in this book.

INITIAL EVALUATION

The initial diagnostic evaluation for low back pain includes a history and physical examination. The history concentrates on the onset of pain. Was the onset associated with a specific trauma or an unusual period of strenuous physical activity? What are the duration and frequency of the pain? Systemic disorders cause chronic pain that is more persistent than episodic. Location and radiation help identify the structures that are possible pain generators. Aggravating and alleviating factors characterize the mechanical quality of the disorder. Mechanical and systemic disorders may be worsened or improved with a change of activity. Pain improvement with immobility helps define specific disorders (e.g., muscle injury, vertebral compression fracture) in either group. The time of day associated with the maximum degree of pain also is characteristic of certain disorders. Inflammatory arthritis of the lumbar spine causes most symptoms in the morning, whereas mechanical disorders are most problematic at the end of the day. The quality of the pain helps separate musculoskeletal pain (aching) sources from sources associated with neural injuries (burning). The intensity of pain is important to document to determine patients' improvement, but does not discriminate between mechanical and systemic disorders.

Physical examination includes a complete evaluation of the musculoskeletal system, including palpation of the axial skeleton and assessment of range of motion and alignment of the spine. Neurologic examination to detect evidence of spinal cord, spinal root, or peripheral nerve dysfunction is essential. In most patients, radiographic and laboratory tests are not indicated. Erythrocyte sedimentation rate and plain radiographs are most informative in patients who are 50 years old or older, who have a previous history of cancer, or who have constitutional symptoms.

The initial evaluation should eliminate the presence of cauda equina syndrome, a rare condition that requires emergency intervention. Cauda equina compression is characterized by low back pain, bilateral motor weakness of the lower extremities, bilateral sciatica, saddle anesthesia, and bladder or bowel incontinence. Common causes of cauda equina compression include central herniation of an intervertebral disk, epidural abscess or hematoma, and tumor masses. If cauda equina syndrome is suspected, immediate radiographic evaluation is required. MRI is the most sensitive radiographic technique for visualizing the spine. Surgical decompression must be completed within 48 hours for the best opportunity to recover neurologic function.[7]

NONMECHANICAL DISORDERS

Most individuals with spinal pain and nonmechanical illnesses can be identified by the presence of one or more of the following: fever or weight loss, pain with recumbency, prolonged morning stiffness, localized bone pain, or visceral pain.

Fever or Weight Loss

Patients with a history of fever or weight loss are likely to have an infection as the cause of low back pain. Patients with vertebral osteomyelitis may have pain that develops gradually over time. In a review of 142 patients with vertebral osteomyelitis, 66% had symptoms for 3 months or longer before diagnosis.[8] The pain becomes constant, is present at rest, and is exacerbated by motion. Physical findings include a decreased range of spinal motion, muscle spasm, and percussion tenderness over the vertebral column. Fever is present in 58% of patients. Approximately 40% of patients with vertebral osteomyelitis have an unequivocal extraspinal primary source of infection, including the skin, lungs, or urinary tract.[9]

Plain radiographs should be reviewed for localized areas of osteopenia. Early abnormalities that appear after 1 to 2 months of infection in pyogenic vertebral osteomyelitis include subchondral bone loss, narrowing of disk space, and loss of definition of the vertebral body (Fig. 82–1). If radiographs are normal, a bone scintiscan is indicated because abnormalities appear at an earlier stage of disease.[10] Bone scintiscan is a sensitive but not specific test for bone lesions. CT may show bone changes before their appearance on routine radiographs; however, alterations of bony architecture are not specific for osteomyelitis and may be confused with severe degenerative disk disease or vertebral malignancy. MRI is the most useful radiographic technique for identifying osteomyelitis.[11] The involvement of the vertebral bodies, the intervening disk, and the extent of the extraosseous infection into the surrounding soft tissues can be determined.

The definitive diagnosis of osteomyelitis is based on the recovery and identification of the causative organism from aspirated material, biopsy of the bony lesion, or blood cultures. Blood cultures may be positive in 50% of patients with osteomyelitis and obviate the need for bone biopsy. *Staphylococcus aureus* is the bacterium associated with vertebral osteomyelitis in 60% of patients.[12] Gram-negative organisms *(Escherichia coli, Proteus, Pseudomonas)* are often grown from parenteral drug abusers and elderly patients with urinary tract infections. Cultures from peripheral sources of infection should be obtained from patients suspected to have vertebral infection.

Therapy of vertebral osteomyelitis includes antibiotics, bed rest, and immobilization. The choice of antibiotic therapy is based on the organism causing the infection and its sensitivity to specific agents. Patients are treated with 4 to 6 weeks of parenteral antibiotics followed by a course of oral antibiotics that may have a duration of 6 months. Bed rest is useful in decreasing pain by limiting motion. Some patients require braces when spinal instability is present.

Pain with Recumbency

Tumors of the spinal column are the prime concern in patients with nocturnal pain or pain with recumbency. The mechanism of increased nocturnal pain with benign or malignant tumors is unknown. Increased pressure associated with increased blood flow at night has been suggested as one possible mechanism of nocturnal pain.[13] An example of a benign bone tumor associated with nocturnal pain is an osteoid osteoma. The nocturnal pain with an osteoid osteoma is slowly progressive over months. The pain may be responsive to nonsteroidal anti-inflammatory drugs (NSAIDs), but recurs with discontinuance of the medication. Stretching of spinal nerves over an expanding mass is a potential mechanism that mediates increased pain with recumbency.

Metastatic lesions in the skeleton are the most common neoplastic lesion of bone with a 25:1 ratio of metastatic to primary tumor.[14] Metastases occur more commonly in the axial skeleton than in the appendicular skeleton. The lumbar and thoracic spines are affected in approximately 46% and 49%, with the remainder affecting the cervical spine. Suspicion for the presence of metastasis is increased in individuals older than age 50 with back pain unassociated with a trauma. These patients have progressive back pain that increases in intensity over time. Radicular pain may increase at night as the spine lengthens with recumbency. Pain with recumbency is a symptom associated with spinal tumors. Examples of benign and malignant vertebral column tumors are listed in Table 82–1.

Physical examination shows localized tenderness over the vertebral column and neurologic dysfunction if the spinal cord is compressed by benign or malignant lesions. Radiographic evaluation of the lumbosacral spine is useful in identifying characteristic changes in the bony and soft tissue areas of the spine associated with neoplastic lesions. The finding of a lucent nidus, a lesion about 1.5 cm in diameter with a surrounding well-defined area of dense sclerotic bone, is virtually pathognomonic of osteoid osteoma. Osteomas arise in the posterior elements of a vertebra. The size and location of these lesions make them difficult to detect with plain radiographs. Bone scintiscans are useful in localizing the lesion if plain radiographs are negative. CT is the most useful test for precise localization of the lesion and differentiating it from other bone lesions. MRI adds little in regard to clarifying bone architecture and is not used routinely in the evaluation of this primary bone tumor.

Radiographic abnormalities of metastatic lesions include osteolytic, osteoblastic, and mixed lytic and blastic lesions. Osteolytic lesions are associated with carcinomas of the lung, kidney, breast, and thyroid. Multiple osteoblastic lesions are associated with prostate, breast, and colon carcinomas and bronchial carcinoid (Fig. 82–2). Vertebral lesions that contain lytic and blastic metastases are associated with carcinoma of the breast, lung, prostate, or bladder. Vertebral body destruction is not associated with alterations in the intervertebral disk. The presence of vertebral body and intervertebral disk destruction is more closely associated with infection. Early in the course of a metastatic lesion, plain radiographs are unremarkable because 30% to 50% of bone must be destroyed before a lesion is evident on plain radiographs.[15] Bone scintiscan is more sensitive than plain radiographs and is able to detect areas of bone involvement in 85% of patients with

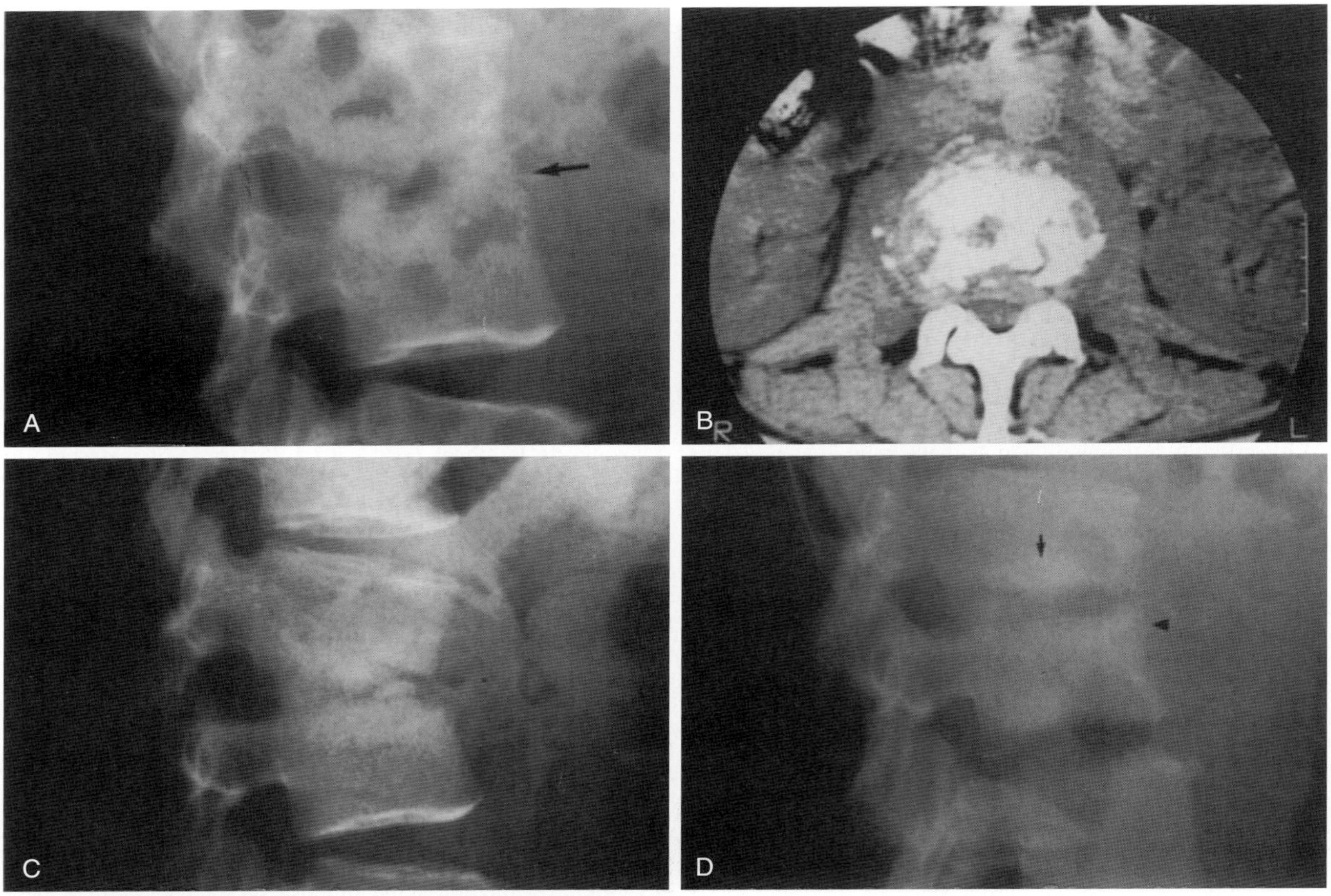

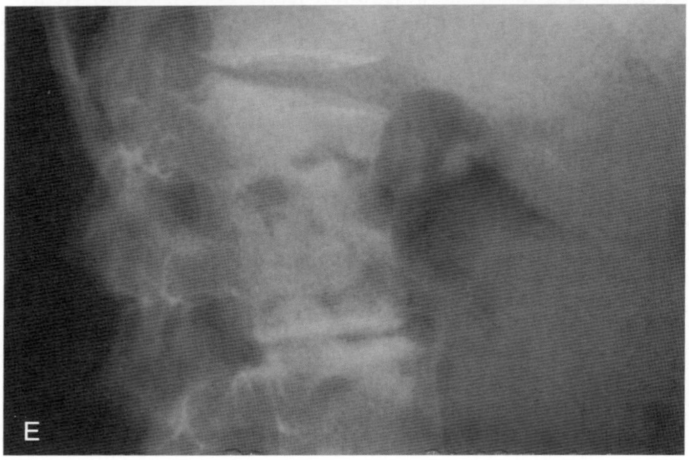

FIGURE 82–1 ■ Serial radiographs of a 41-year-old man with staphylococcal osteomyelitis of the lumbar spine. **A,** Radiograph obtained November 8, 1985. Erosion of the L2 and L3 end plates is associated with destruction of the intervertebral disk *(arrow)*. **B,** CT scan obtained November 20, 1985. CT scan reveals marked bony destruction associated with soft tissue extension of the infection. **C,** Radiograph obtained November 27, 1985. Further collapse of the L2 vertebral body is seen with reactive sclerosis. **D,** Radiograph obtained November 4, 1986. Reactive sclerosis is noted in the vertebral body *(arrow)*, and osteophytes are forming *(arrowhead)* at the body margin. **E,** Radiograph obtained January 13, 1987. Total fusion of the L2 and L3 vertebral bodies has occurred. The duration of infection from onset to total fusion was 12 to 14 months. (From Borenstein D, Wiesel S, Boden S: Low Back and Neck Pain: Comprehensive Diagnosis and Management, 3rd ed. Philadelphia, WB Saunders, 2004, p 416.)

metastases. Bone scintiscan may be the more useful diagnostic test in differentiating pain caused by metastatic disease from pain caused by a benign lesion. CT normally is reserved for assessment of patients with positive scans but negative radiographs. CT differentiates among bony metastases, benign lesions, and no abnormality.[16] CT is particularly useful in showing small areas of bone destruction and of bone and tumor impingement on the spinal canal. CT should not be used as a screening procedure because of the exposure to high levels of radiation. MRI is better at showing the extent of tumor inside the spinal canal, the size of extraosseous extension, and bone marrow invasion, whereas CT is better at showing the degree of cortical bone loss.[17] A study of 40 patients with metastatic disease revealed that patients with breast, kidney, or prostatic cancer or multiple myeloma had abnormal MRI, but normal CT and bone scintiscan.[18] Gadolinium diethylenetriaminepentaacetic acid, an MRI contrast agent, enhances the capability of MRI to differentiate the size, location, configuration, and characteristics of spinal tumors from normal tissues.[19]

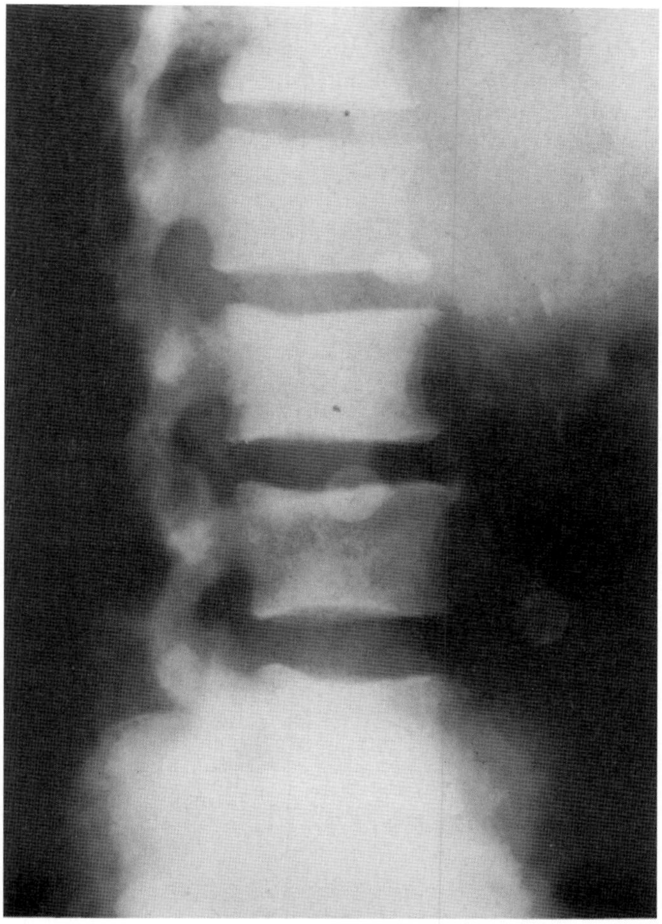

FIGURE 82–2 ■ Lateral view of the lumbosacral spine and pelvis in a 66-year-old man with a 3-month history of back pain reveals multiple, discrete osteoblastic lesions that proved to be metastatic prostatic carcinoma on biopsy. (From Borenstein D, Wiesel S, Boden S: Low Back and Neck Pain: Comprehensive Diagnosis and Management, 3rd ed. Philadelphia, WB Saunders, 2004, p 534.)

The diagnosis of a primary tumor of the lumbosacral spine requires biopsy of the lesion. The diagnosis is confirmed by histologic examination of biopsy material. For patients with metastatic disease with no known primary neoplasm, biopsy of the lesion for tissue diagnosis is required. Closed needle biopsy of the lesions in the lumbar spine can yield definitive information safely. The therapy for benign lesions is excisional biopsy completed for histologic examination of the lesion. Benign lesions that are not entirely removed may grow and cause recurrent pain. Treatment of metastatic disease of the spine is directed toward palliation of pain. Cure is not possible because most solitary metastatic lesions are accompanied by asymptomatic deposits that become evident over time. Surgical intervention to prevent progression of structural instability can result in a mean survival time of 26 months after operation.[20]

Local Vertebral Column Pain

Patients with pain over the vertebral column have fractures of the vertebral body or expansion of the bone marrow space. Any systemic process that increases mineral loss from bone (e.g., osteoporosis, hyperparathyroidism, Paget disease) or hypertrophy or replacement of bone marrow cells with inflammatory or neoplastic cells (multiple myeloma, hemoglobinopathy) weakens vertebral bone to the degree that fracture may occur spontaneously or with minimal impact. Although many patients with these disorders develop acute bone pain, patients with osteoporosis may experience microfractures that cause chronic pain. Severe pain usually lasts 3 to 4 months and then resolves; however, some patients are left with persistent, dull spinal pain without any evidence of vertebral fracture. The source of pain may be microfractures too small to be detected by radiographs or biomechanical effects of the deformity on the lumbar spine below. Recurrent pain, increased deformity, and loss of height suggest new fractures. With hemoglobinopathies, marrow hyperplasia causes loss of bone trabeculae in the axial skeleton. Acute crises associated with bone infarctions cause acute pain. Between crises, back pain may persist secondary to alterations of bony architecture.

Physical examination is remarkable for pain with palpation localized to the affected area of the lumbar spine. If present, muscle spasm tends to surround the area of bony tenderness. This phenomenon is particularly noticeable in the setting of sacral fractures.

Radiographic evaluation concentrates on the area of the spine that is tender with palpation. Plain radiographs may pinpoint skeletal abnormalities, but may be normal because greater than 30% of the bone calcium must be lost before decreased bone content is recognized (Fig. 82–3).[21] Microfractures may not be detected with plain radiographs. Bone scintiscans are useful to detect increased bone activity soon after a fracture occurs. CT scans also may identify the location of a fracture or area of bone that has been replaced with hypertrophied or inflammatory tissue. MRI is helpful in identifying the disease processes that complicate the course of patients with hemoglobinopathies, such as infections.[22]

Laboratory evaluation is helpful for differentiating the myriad of systemic illnesses that cause localized vertebral bone pain. Screening tests that heighten the physician's suspicion of a systemic illness include an elevated erythrocyte sedimentation rate or decreased hematocrit. Abnormalities of complete blood count may indicate a primary hemoglobinopathy or replacement of bone marrow elements with neoplastic cells. Serum chemistries may detect abnormalities of calcium metabolism associated with elevated parathyroid hormone levels (hyperparathyroidism). The diagnosis of osteoporosis should be considered in an individual with normal laboratory values and decreased bone mineral content. A variety of radiographic techniques are available to quantify vertebral bone mineral.[23]

The treatment for patients with local vertebral column pain is specific for the underlying disorder causing alterations in bone calcium or vertebral bone marrow. Most of these patients require analgesic therapy for extended periods to diminish the degree of spinal pain they experience.

Prolonged Morning Stiffness

Morning stiffness of the lumbosacral spine is a frequent symptom of patients with mechanical and nonmechanical low

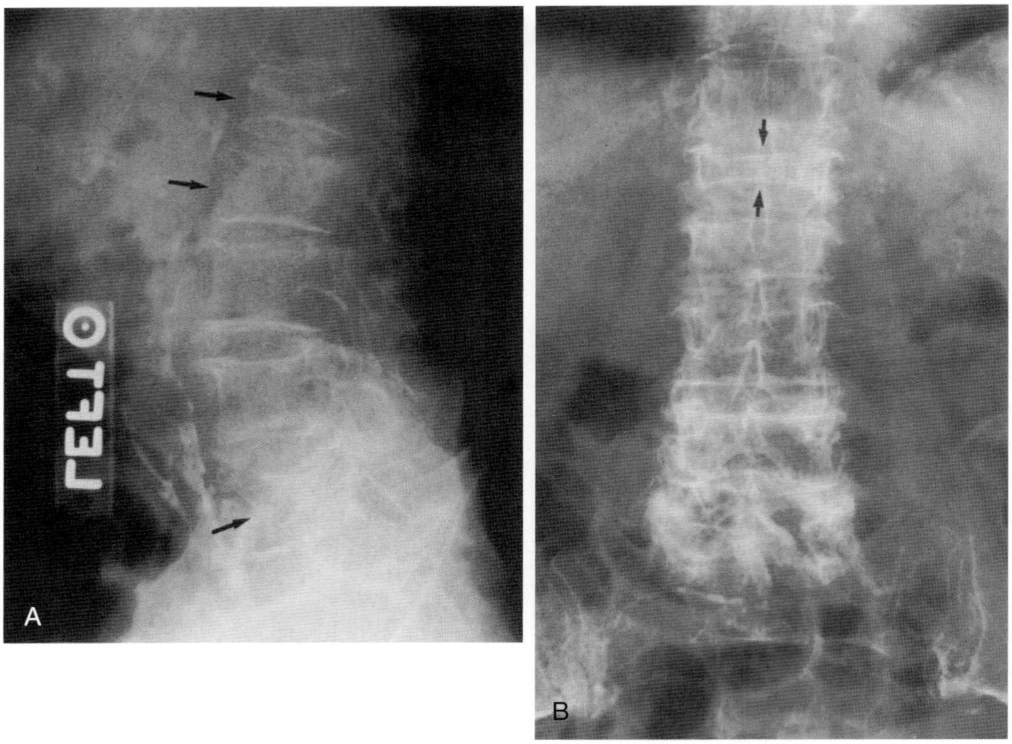

FIGURE 82–3 ■ An 83-year-old woman presented with a history of acute low back pain localized to the thoracolumbar junction. **A,** Lateral view reveals generalized osteoporosis with diminished height of L1, L2, and L5 *(arrows)*. **B,** Anteroposterior view reveals marked loss of height of the L1 vertebral body *(arrows)*. (From Borenstein D, Wiesel S, Boden S: Low Back and Neck Pain: Comprehensive Diagnosis and Management, 3rd ed. Philadelphia, WB Saunders, 2004, p 575.)

back pain. Mechanical back pain is associated with morning stiffness of short duration (≤1 hour). Morning stiffness lasting more than 1 hour is a common symptom of spondyloarthropathy. The spondyloarthropathies include ankylosing spondylitis, reactive arthritis, psoriatic arthritis, and enteropathic arthritis. Patients with a spondyloarthropathy may have a history of bilateral sacroiliac joint pain associated with morning stiffness that may be present for years without a specific diagnosis.[24] Patients with reactive arthritis and psoriatic spondylitis may develop unilateral sacroiliac disease associated with low back pain that is lateralized to the affected side. Patients with reactive arthritis and psoriatic spondylitis also may develop spondylitis (lumbar spine inflammation) without sacroiliitis.

Physical examination of patients with spondyloarthropathy shows various degrees of decreased motion in the lumbosacral spine corresponding to the extent and severity of disease. Plain radiographs of the lumbosacral spine are helpful for identifying early changes of spondyloarthropathy. Radiographic abnormalities include loss of lumbar lordosis, joint erosions in the lower one third of the sacroiliac joints, and squaring of the vertebral bodies (Fig. 82–4). CT of the sacroiliac joints is more sensitive for recognition of sacroiliitis than conventional radiographs. The test should be reserved for patients with normal or equivocal radiographs in whom a diagnosis of spondyloarthropathy is suspected. MRI also may be able to detect alterations of sacroiliac joints that are not shown with conventional radiographs, but incurs a greater expense.

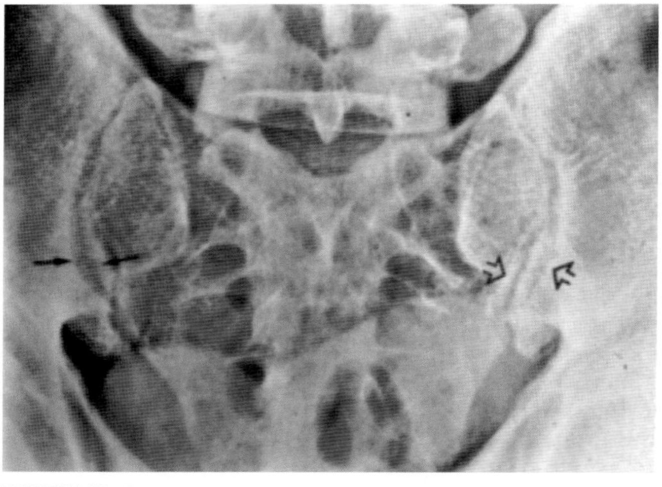

FIGURE 82–4 ■ A 35-year-old man had a 5-year history of low back pain and morning stiffness. He previously had not sought medical care for back pain. Posteroanterior view of the sacroiliac joints reveals early joint margin erosions on both sides of the joints *(black arrows)* and sclerosis *(open arrows)*. Bilateral sacroiliac joint disease was compatible with a diagnosis of ankylosing spondylitis. (From Borenstein D, Wiesel S, Boden S: Low Back and Neck Pain: Comprehensive Diagnosis and Management, 3rd ed. Philadelphia, WB Saunders, 2004, p 200.)

Treatment of spondyloarthropathy includes a combination of NSAIDs with physical therapy to maximize the motion of the spine. A class of therapy for ankylosing spondylitis includes tumor necrosis factor inhibitors. These drugs represent a major advance for the treatment of ankylosing spondylitis.

Visceral Pain

Disorders of the vascular, genitourinary, and gastrointestinal systems can cause stimulation of sensory nerves that results in the perception of pain in the damaged area and in superficial tissues supplied by the same segments of the spinal cord. The duration and sequence of visceral pain follows the periodicity of the involved organ. Colicky pain occurs in peristaltic waves and is associated with a hollow viscus, such as the colon, gallbladder, uterus, or ureter. Throbbing pain is associated with vascular structures. Somatic pain frequently is exacerbated by activity and improved by rest. Patients with viscerogenic pain get little relief from bed rest. Many patients prefer to be moving in an attempt to achieve a comfortable position.

Back pain is rarely the only symptom of visceral disease. Kidney pain is felt in the costovertebral angle. Ureteral pain from nephrolithiasis may cause dull flank pain with chronic distention or colic if obstruction occurs at the ureteropelvic junction. Patients with bladder infections may develop diffuse low back pain centered over the sacrum. Pain from genital organs may occur locally or in a referred pattern. Endometriosis causes recurrent low back pain on a monthly basis corresponding to menstrual periods. The severity of endometrial pain is not particularly modified by changes in position. Pain may be related to pancreatitis, peptic ulcer disease, or colon or rectal disorders. The diagnosis of an aortic aneurysm should be suspected in an elderly individual with chronic nondescript back pain that does not improve with rest or is not exacerbated with activity. Vascular lesions cause dull, steady abdominal pain that is unrelated to activity. Throbbing or tearing back pain also may be associated with vascular abnormalities, including an expanding abdominal aneurysm. Any change in the frequency, intensity, or location of the pain suggests expansion in the size of the aneurysm. Patients with an abdominal aneurysm are usually older individuals who have had a history of lower extremity claudication. Irritation of retroperitoneal structures causes back pain associated with epigastric discomfort that may radiate to the hips or thighs. Rupture or acute expansion of the aneurysm is associated with tearing pain and circulatory collapse.

Physical examination of the abdomen may be able to identify the source of maximal pain. Tenderness with palpation of the abdomen may localize over the epigastrium (aorta) or lower quadrant (uterus). Physical examination has adequate sensitivity to identify individuals with a large enough aneurysm to warrant elective intervention.[25] Ovarian tenderness and enlargement also may be palpated. Range of motion of the lumbar spine is unaffected. Palpation of the lumbar spine is painless.

Ultrasonography and CT of the abdomen readily identifies aortic aneurysms. Abdominal ultrasound detects aneurysms with sensitivity that approaches 100%.[26] The longitudinal and transverse diameters can be determined without radiation or contrast medium. The effectiveness of ultrasound is diminished by excessive bowel gas that obscures the infrarenal abdominal aorta and by the pancreas, which hides the suprarenal aorta. Ultrasound is inadequate to plan vascular surgery. CT is highly sensitive and specific for identification of aneurysms. In contrast to ultrasound, CT visualizes aortic anomalies, horseshoe kidney, and involvement of the iliac and hypogastric arteries. CT is a most effective test for planning surgery.

MRI is the radiographic technique best able to identify endometriosis. MRI is 98% sensitive for the identification of endometriosis. MRI may find deposits in the pouch of Douglas, ureterosacral ligaments, ovaries, uterine surface, retrovaginal septum, fallopian tubes, bowel, or appendix.

Therapy for visceral disorders causing back pain is directed toward the organ system associated with the disorder. The therapy of abdominal aneurysm is surgical. Improved survival is documented for individuals with elective surgery for intact aneurysms. If an aneurysm is smaller that 5.5 cm in diameter, elective repair has a 30-day operative mortality of 5.4%. At 3 years, surgery has no better advantage than surveillance does with regard to survival.[27] At 8 years, patients who undergo surgery have lower mortality than patients monitored with ultrasound every 6 months.[28]

MECHANICAL LOW BACK PAIN

Most individuals with mechanical low back pain have symptoms localized to the lumbar region demarcated from the 12th rib to the crease of the buttock. In general, mechanical pain is relieved by certain motions and exacerbated by opposite actions.

Lumbosacral Strain

Many individuals with pain in the lumbar spine have back strain. The cause of back strain is unclear. Possible causes of pain associated with back strain include muscular or ligamentous injuries, continuous mechanical stress from poor posture, or a small tear in an annulus fibrosus.

Damage may occur in lumbar spine structures if the force generated in a task does not match the stress placed on the spine.[29] If the force is too great or too little, paraspinous muscles are at risk of being damaged, resulting in muscle contraction and pain. Excess fatigability and paraspinal weakness occur in patients with low back pain. Muscle wasting and weakness arises rapidly as a result of reduced motor unit recruitment because of fear of pain or reflex inhibition of motion.[30]

Patients with muscle strain have pain limited to a local area. In others, the distribution of pain may follow the referred pattern of muscles of the same mesenchymal origin. These individuals have myofascial pain. Most individuals experience pain simultaneously with an injury. Subsequently, increased pain occurs with tissue edema and associated reflex contraction of the surrounding muscles and limitation of motion. Exacerbation of pain occurs with motion that contracts the injured muscle. Certain motions may be painless, whereas others cause incapacitating pain.

On physical examination, any active motion of the involved muscle against resistance causes pain. The damaged muscle may be tender on palpation. The muscle may have increased contraction and firmness compared with the surrounding muscles under normal tension. Neurologic examination is normal.

Therapy for back strain includes controlled physical activity, NSAIDs, and muscle relaxants. The recommendation to maintain activity as tolerated is an important component of muscle strain therapy.[31] A short period of 2 days has been shown to be effective in relieving back pain. Cherkin and colleagues[32] conducted a longitudinal observational study of the efficacy of medications at 7 days for the treatment of acute low back pain in 219 patients. Patients receiving a muscle relaxant and NSAIDs had the best self-reported outcomes. Muscle relaxants have a beneficial role in relieving pain associated with muscle spasm in the absence of sedation.[33]

Lumbar Spondylosis (Osteoarthritis)

Osteoarthritis affects the apophyseal joints of the lumbar spine. The same pathology that affects the appendicular joints, such as the knees, also can damage the axial joints. Major changes occur in the lumbar spine between the third and fifth decades of life. The first manifestations of aging develop in the intervertebral disks. The nucleus loses its turgor, and the annulus fissures and degenerates. Disk degeneration itself may not be a painful process. Patients with disk degeneration may be asymptomatic until alterations in facet joint alignment result in the onset of articular pain. In response to disk degeneration, the apophyseal joints narrow, resulting in osteoarthritis.[34] The resulting biomechanical insufficiency results in transfer of stresses posteriorly to the facet joints.[35] Capsular strains, hypermobility, and degenerative changes develop. Traction spurs, and redundancy of the ligamentum flavum manifest these changes radiographically. Progression of this process results in spinal stenosis.

Patients with osteoarthritis of the facet joints have pain over the lower lumbar spine. Any body movements that compress the joints (extension) exacerbate symptoms of dull, aching pain. Stiffness of the lumbar spine is another common symptom.

Radiographs of the lumbar spine reveal loss of disk height, traction osteophytes, decreased interpedicular distance, and facet degeneration (Fig. 82–5). CT scan is able to identify the irregularity of articular surfaces and alterations in positional orientation of the facet joints.

The therapy of osteoarthritis, whether in the knee or lumbar spine, consists of analgesics, NSAIDs, and exercises. The choice of these therapies is a trial-and-error process. Ideal therapies may not be tolerated by patients. Maximum doses of medications may be ineffective. An ongoing dialogue between the patient and physician is the best method to identify the ideal regimen for an individual patient.

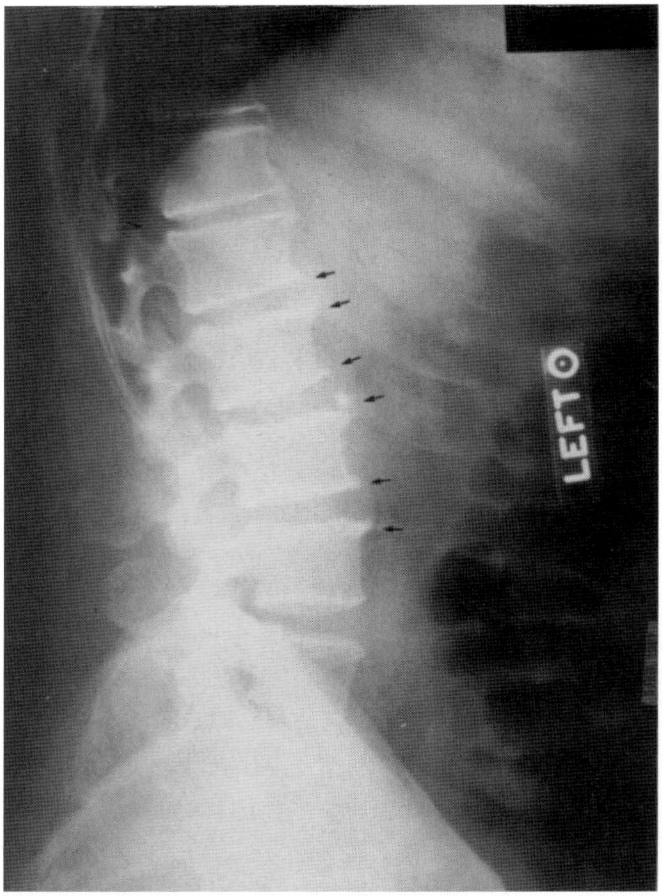

FIGURE 82–5 ■ Lateral view illustrating traction osteophytes *(arrows)* at multiple levels associated with disk degeneration. The osteophytes are horizontally oriented and emerge slightly above or below the disk space. A claw osteophyte is noted at the fourth arrow from the top; a traction osteophyte is located at the fifth arrow from the top. (From Borenstein D, Wiesel S, Boden S: Low Back and Neck Pain: Comprehensive Diagnosis and Management, 3rd ed. Philadelphia, WB Saunders, 2004, p 262.)

■ CONCLUSION

The evaluation of a patient with pain localized to the lumbar spine is a daunting task. The disease possibilities are numerous. The diagnostic options are complicated and expensive. Therapies have the potential to relieve significant amounts of suffering when chosen appropriately. Inappropriate therapies may be ineffective at best, and harmful at worst. The prognosis ranges from total recovery to life-threatening illness. This chapter clarifies the evaluation and treatment of the low back pain patient. Disorders of the lumbar spine have characteristic symptoms and signs that help categorize the illnesses into specific categories. Appropriate therapies can be selected when these specific categories are identified. A successful outcome is most likely when these basic rules are followed.

References

1. Damkot DK, Pope MH, Lord J, Frymoyer JW: The relationship between work history, work environment, and low back pain in men. Spine 9:395, 1984.
2. Deyo RA, Tsui-Wu Y-J: Descriptive epidemiology of low-back pain and its related medical care in the United States. Spine 12:264, 1987.
3. Hart LG, Deyo RA, Cherkin DC: Physician office visits for low back pain: Frequency, clinical evaluation, and treatment. Spine 20:11, 1995.
4. Borenstein DG, Wiesel SW, Boden SD: Low Back and Neck Pain: Comprehensive Diagnosis and Management, 3rd ed. Philadelphia, WB Saunders, 2004.
5. Nachemson A: The lumbar spine: An orthopedic challenge. Spine 1:59, 1976.
6. van den Hoogen HJM, Koes BW, Deville W, et al: The prognosis of low back pain in general practice. Spine 22:1515, 1997.

7. Shapiro S: Medical realities of cauda equina syndrome secondary to lumbar disc herniation. Spine 25:348, 2000.
8. Zimmermann B, Lally EV: Infectious diseases of the spine. Semin Spine Surg 7:177, 1995.
9. Ross PM, Fleming JL: Vertebral body osteomyelitis: Spectrum and natural history: A retrospective analysis of 37 cases. Clin Orthop 118:190, 1976.
10. Jensen AG, Espersen F, Skinhoj P, et al: Bacteremic *Staphylococcus aureus* spondylitis. Arch Intern Med 158:509, 1998.
11. Dagirmanjian A, Schils J, McHenry M, et al: MR imaging of vertebral osteomyelitis revisited. AJR Am J Roentgenol 167:1539, 1996.
12. Schwartz ST, Spiegel M, Ho G Jr: Bacterial vertebral osteomyelitis and epidural abscess. Semin Spine Surg 2:95, 1990.
13. Sherman MS, McFarland G: Mechanism of pain in osteoid osteomas. South Med J 58:163, 1965.
14. Fornasier VL, Horne JG: Metastases to the vertebral column. Cancer 36:590, 1975.
15. Edelstyn GA, Gillespie PG, Grebbel FS: The radiological demonstration of skeletal metastases: Experimental observations. Clin Radiol 18:158, 1967.
16. Redmond J, Spring DB, Munderloh SH, et al: Spinal computed tomography scanning in the evaluation of metastatic disease. Cancer 54:253, 1984.
17. Zimmer WD, Berquist THE, McLeod RA, et al: Bone tumors: Magnetic resonance imaging versus computed tomography. Radiology 155:709, 1985.
18. Avrahami E, Tadmor R, Dally O, et al: Early MR demonstration of spinal metastases in patients with normal radiographs and CT and radionuclide bone scans. J Comput Assist Tomogr 13:598, 1989.
19. Sze G, Stimac GK, Bartlett C, et al: Multicenter study of gadopentetate dimeglumine as a MR contrast agent: Evaluation in patients with spinal tumors. AJNR Am J Neuroradiol 11:967, 1990.
20. Wise JJ, Fischgrund JS, Herkowitz HN, et al: Complication, survival rates, and risk factors of surgery for metastatic disease of the spine. Spine 24:1943, 1999.
21. Ardan GM: Bone destruction not demonstrable by radiography. Br J Radiol 24:107, 1951.
22. Modic MT, Pflanze W, Fieglin DH, Belhobek G: Magnetic resonance imaging of musculoskeletal infections. Radiol Clin North Am 24:247, 1986.
23. U.S. Preventive Services Task Force: Screening osteoporosis in postmenopausal women: Recommendations and rationale. Ann Intern Med 137:526, 2002.
24. Kidd BL, Cawley MID: Delay in diagnosis of spondarthritis. Br J Rheumatol 27:230, 1988.
25. Fink HA, Lederle FA, Roth CS, et al: The accuracy of physical examination to detect abdominal aortic aneurysm. Arch Intern Med 160:833, 2000.
26. LaRoy LL, Cormier PJ, Matalon TAS, et al: Misdiagnosis of ruptured abdominal aneurysms. AJR Am J Roentgenol 152:785, 1989.
27. Lederle FA, Wilson SE, Johnson GR, et al: Immediate repair compared with surveillance of small abdominal aortic aneurysms. N Engl J Med 346:1437, 2002.
28. The United Kingdom Small Aneurysm Trial participants: Long-term outcomes of immediate repair compared with surveillance of small abdominal aortic aneurysms. N Engl J Med 346:1445, 2002.
29. Cooper RG: Understanding paraspinal muscle dysfunction in low back pain: A way forward. Ann Rheum Dis 52:413, 1993.
30. Hides JA, Stokes MJ, Saide M, et al: Evidence of lumbar multifidus muscle wasting ipsilateral to symptoms in patients with acute/subacute low back pain. Spine 19:165, 1994.
31. Malmivarra A, Hakkinen U, Aro T, et al: The treatment of acute low back pain: Bed rest, exercises, or ordinary activity. N Engl J Med 332:351, 1995.
32. Cherkin DC, Wheeler KJ, Barlow W, et al: Medication use for low back pain in primary care. Spine 23:607, 1998.
33. Borenstein D, Korn S: Efficacy of a low-dose regimen of cyclobenzaprine hydrochloride in acute skeletal muscle spasm: Results of two placebo-controlled trials. Clin Ther 25:1056, 2003.
34. Butler D, Trafimow JH, Andersson GB, et al: Disc degenerate before facets. Spine 15:111, 1990.
35. Borenstein D: Does osteoarthritis of the lumbar spine cause chronic low back pain? Curr Rheumatol Rep 6:14, 2004.

chapter 83

Lumbar Radiculopathy

Laxmaiah Manchikanti, Vijay Singh, and Mark V. Boswell

HISTORICAL CONSIDERATIONS

Solid descriptions of lumbar radiculopathy date back to the Hippocratic collection described as sciatica (Fig. 83–1).[1] Sciatica was described as, "hipache at the end of the sacrum and the buttocks with radiation into the thigh." In 1543, Andreas Vesalius[2,3] provided a detailed account of the anatomy of the disk. In 1764, Cortugno,[4] an Italian physician, implicated the sciatic nerve as the cause and described sciatica as follows: "for it seems to be an acrid and irritating matter, which lying on the nerve, preys on the stamina, and gives rise to pain." Cortugno's description distinguished sciatica from generalized low back pain. In 1824, Bell[5] provided a model description of posttraumatic disk herniation. In 1841, Valleix[3,6] described the gross and microscopic details of the intervertebral disk in autopsy findings of a patient who died after a severe injury with a fractured disk. In 1858, Von Luschka[7] provided the first descriptions of a posterior protrusion of a disk, although he attached no clinical significance to this finding and had made no correlation to sciatica. Brissaud[3,8] coined the term *sciatic scoliosis*.

History of the first diskectomy dates back to 1908 by Krause.[9] In 1911, Middleton and Teacher,[10,11] a practicing physician and a pathologist at Glasgow University, described classic disk extrusion in a man after a lifting incident with the "feeling of a crack" in the small of his back. Goldthwait,[12] commonly known for his description of facet joint arthropathy, in 1911 showed that the anulus fibrosus with pulpi nucleus may produce paralysis by loosening and backward projection. Since then, multiple physicians from all over the world described their experiences with various types of disk surgery.[3,13-18] As a result of mistakes in the semantics and descriptions, the final credit for disk herniation went to Mixter and Barr[19] in 1934 (Figs. 83–2 and 83–3). In their classic publication, they described a herniated lumbar disk as the cause of radiculopathy. In 1948, Hirsch[20] confirmed the disk as the cause of sciatica by injecting procaine into a patient's disk, which resulted in sciatica. Spinal fusion for disk disease was first attempted in 1891 by Hadra.[21]

In 1880, the Lasègue test was described by Forst (Fig. 83–4).[22,23] In 1885, Roentgen,[24] a Holland-born physicist of German ancestry, discovered the x-ray, for which he received a Nobel prize (Fig. 83–5). The myelogram was introduced in 1918 by Dandy.[25] The importance of spinal myelography was discovered by Sicard.[26] Diskography was first reported by Lindblom in 1948.[27] In 1961, Oldendorf,[28] a neurologist at UCLA, envisioned CT (Fig. 83–6) with rapid developments by others.[29,30] CT was followed by the development of MRI.[3]

Following the descriptions of Mixter and Barr,[19] it was assumed that the mechanical deformation of the nerve root induced by the displaced disk material was the primary cause of the symptoms, and the surgical removal of the herniated mass was the preferred treatment. Since then, however, a multitude of experimental studies have indicated the complex mechanism of pathogenesis of sciatica or lumbar radiculopathy.[31-34] Now it is recognized that radicular pain is evoked by stimulation of the sensory (dorsal) root of a spinal nerve, or its dorsal root ganglion.[31-41] Radicular pain is not synonymous with radiculopathy, however.[42] In contrast to radicular pain, radiculopathy pertains to a pathologic state in which a disorder affects the function of nerve roots.[33,42]

CLINICAL SYNDROME

Etiology

Radicular pain is a single and subjective clinical feature.[42] It can be a feature of radiculopathy, along with numbness or weakness or both, but it can occur alone. Radiculopathy is separate from radicular pain, with a combination of numbness, motor loss, and pain, depending on which fibers in the nerve roots are affected and how they are affected.[33,42] Any lesion that affects the lumbosacral nerve roots may cause radiculopathy, radicular pain, or both.[42] The most common lesion causing the radiculopathy or radicular pain is lumbar disk herniation, accounting for 98% of the causes of radicular pain or radiculopathy. Multiple other causes accounting for approximately 2% of cases of radiculopathy or radicular pain include vertebral causes (e.g., spinal stenosis, spondylolisthesis, osteophytosis, vertebral subluxation); neuromeningeal causes (e.g., meningeal cysts, ossification of dura, nerve root anomalies); neoplastic causes of radicular pain (e.g., benign and malignant tumors); and infectious, vascular, cystic, and miscellaneous causes.

Experimental studies indicated that the epidural presence of the herniated part of the disk, the nucleus pulposus, may induce structural and functional changes in the adjacent nerve roots and sensitize the nerve root to produce pain when deformed mechanically.[35-40] The intervertebral disk and posterior longitudinal ligament have been shown to contain free nerve endings.[42-47] The outer third of the anulus is richly

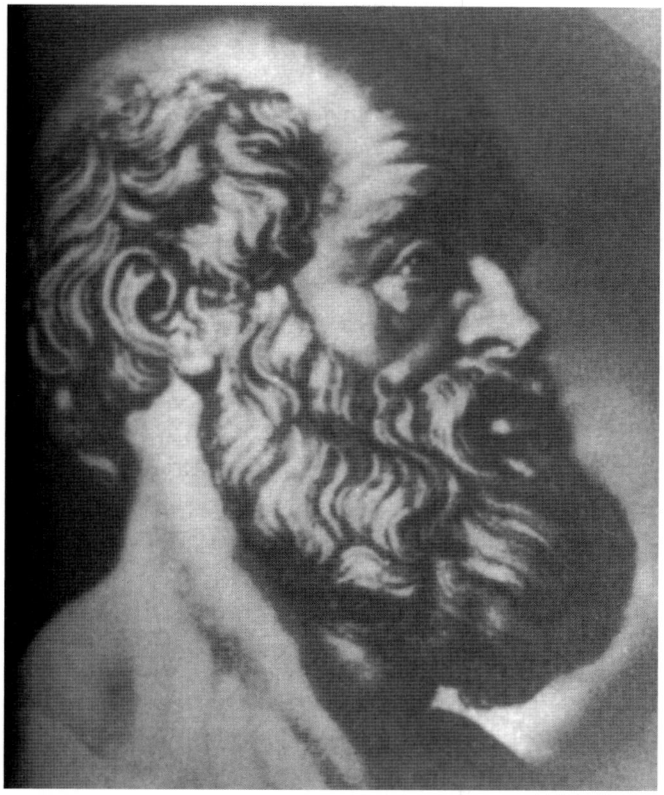

FIGURE 83–1 ■ Hippocrates (1460-1375 BC).

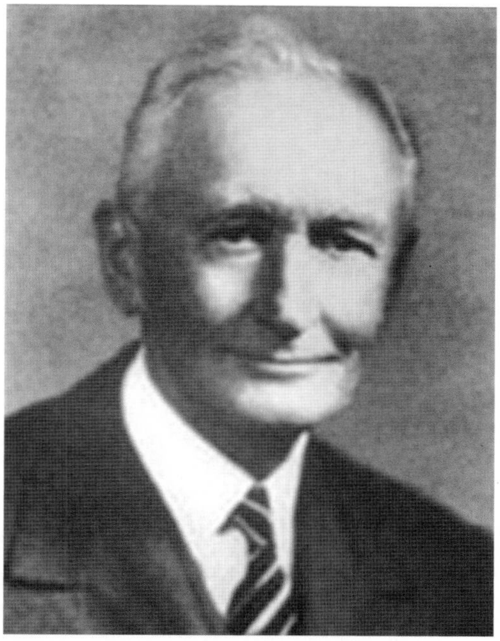

FIGURE 83–2 ■ William Jason Mixter (1880-1958), Boston.

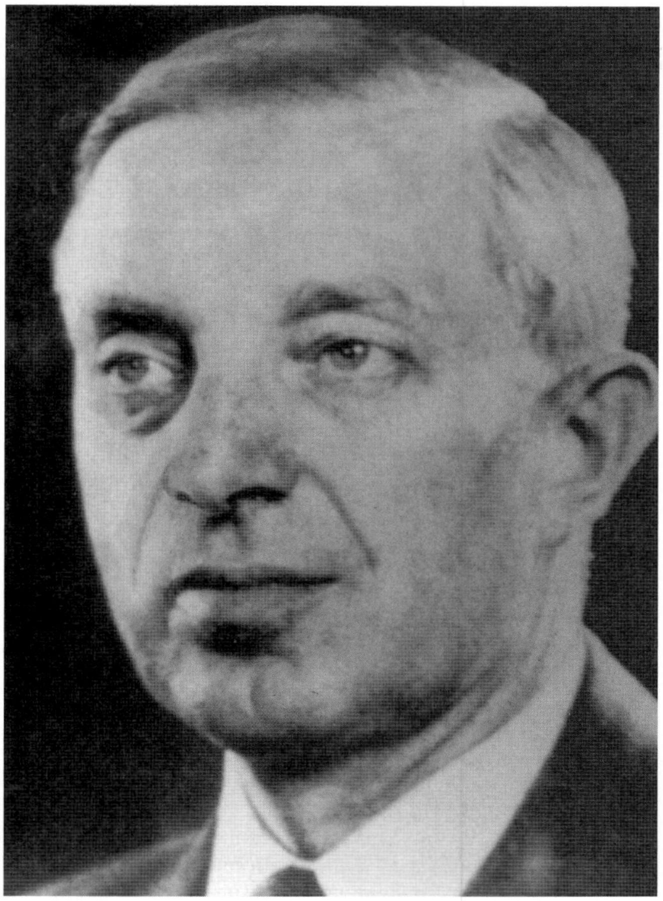

FIGURE 83–3 ■ Joseph Seaton Barr (1901-1964), Boston.

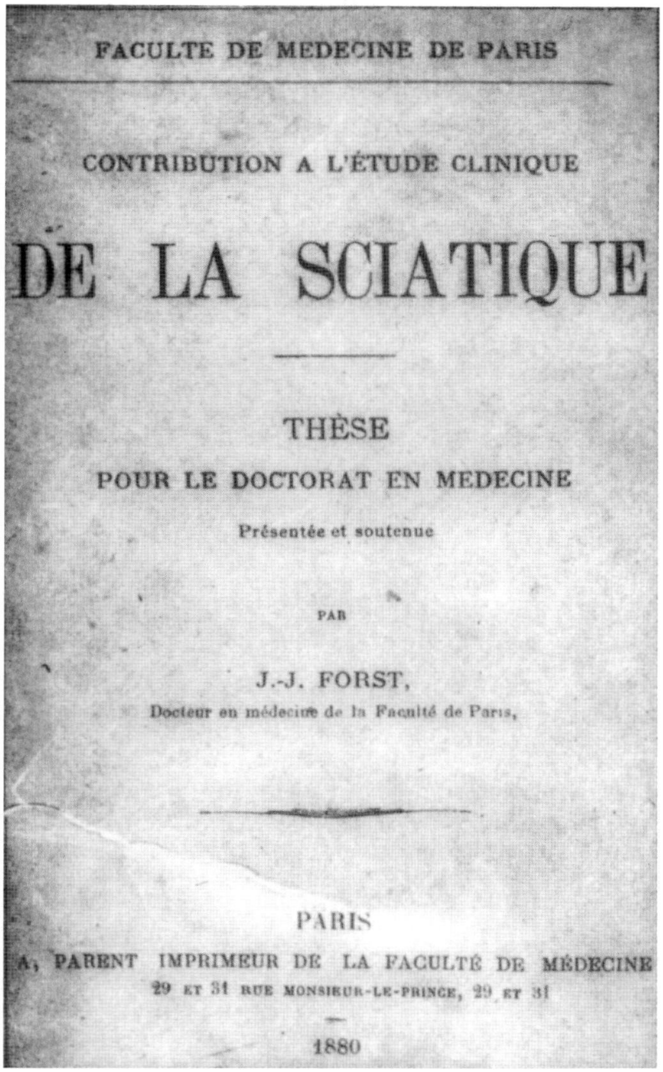

FACULTE DE MEDECINE DE PARIS

CONTRIBUTION A L'ÉTUDE CLINIQUE

DE LA SCIATIQUE

THÈSE

POUR LE DOCTORAT EN MEDECINE

Présentée et soutenue

PAR

J.-J. FORST,

Docteur en médecine de la Faculté de Paris,

PARIS

A. PARENT IMPRIMEUR DE LA FACULTÉ DE MÉDECINE

29 ET 31 RUE MONSIEUR-LE-PRINCE, 29 ET 31

1880

FIGURE 83–4 ■ Title page of Forst's thesis on the "Lasègue" test.

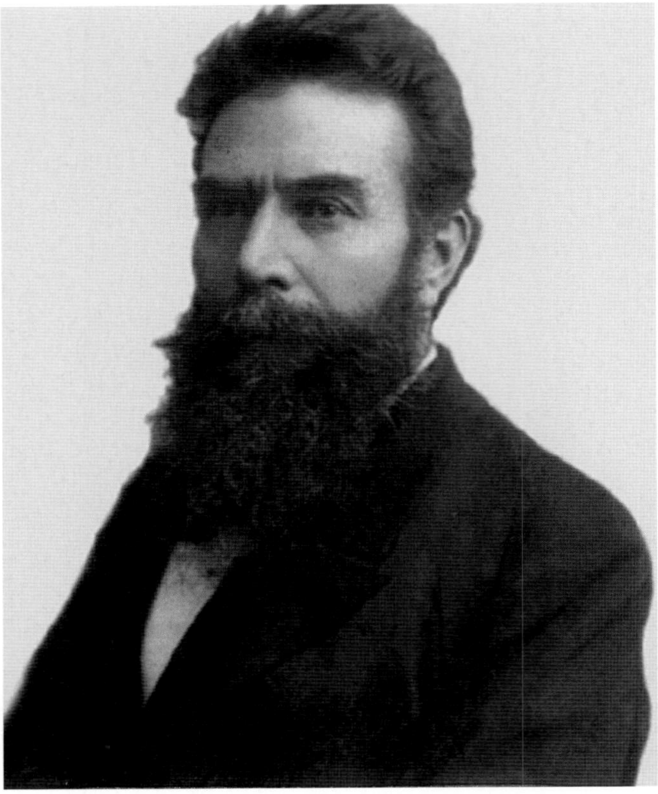

FIGURE 83–5 ■ William Conrad Roentgen (1845-1923).

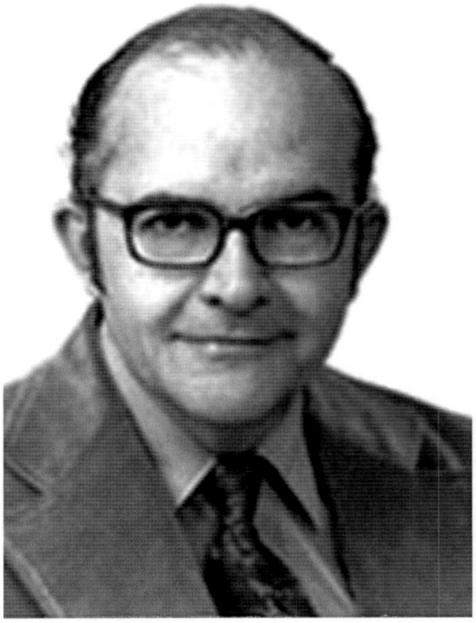

FIGURE 83–6 ■ William Oldendorf (born 1925), Professor of Neurology and Psychiatry, University of California at Los Angeles.

innervated,[44-46] and nerve fibers may extend as deeply as the middle third of the anulus. In patients with chronic low back pain and abnormal disks, however, the nerve supply may extend even more deeply into the anulus and nucleus.[47-49]

Pain from disk herniation can arise from nerve root compression and stimulation of nociceptors in the anulus or posterior longitudinal ligament. A simple compression or mass effect cannot be the mechanism of pain, however, resulting from disk disease. Several studies evaluating progressive disk herniation showed that even though the resolution of symptoms tends to be associated with diminution of the size of the disk herniations, it is not always the case because compression may continue despite the resolution of symptoms.[51-55] In 1935 Mixter and Ayers,[56] only a year after the hallmark description of Mixter and Barr,[19] showed that radicular pain can occur without disk herniation. The pathophysiology of lumbar radicular pain is a subject of not only ongoing research, but also of controversy.

Proposed etiologies include neural compression with dysfunction, vascular compromise, inflammation, and biochemical influences.[31] Spinal nerve roots have unique properties that may explain their proclivity to produce symptoms.[57] Spinal nerve roots, in contrast to peripheral nerves, lack a well-developed intraneural blood-nerve barrier, which probably makes them more susceptible to symptomatic compression injury than peripheral nerves, making them more vulnerable to endoneural edema formation.[58-60] Endoneural edema can be induced by increased vascular permeability, which is caused by mechanical nerve root compression.[58,59] Elevated endoneural fluid pressure, caused by intraneural edema, also can impede capillary blood flow and may cause intraneural fibrosis[58]; this may play a crucial role in lumbar radiculopathy because spinal nerve roots receive approximately 58% of their nutrition from the surrounding CSF.[57-60] Perineural fibrosis, by interfering with CSF-mediated nutrition, may render nerve roots hyperesthetic and hypersensitive to compressive forces.[57-59] In addition, it has been reported that venous and capillary stasis with congestion also may contribute to symptomatic nerve root syndromes.[58,59] Consequently, nerve root ischemia or venous stasis, or both, may generate pathologic biochemical changes, which cause radicular pain.[58]

Another complicating factor has been that the occlusion pressure for radicular arterioles is significantly higher in experimentally induced ischemia through nerve root compression, whereas compensatory nutrition from CSF diffusion during low-pressure radicular compression is probably inadequate in the presence of either epidural inflammation or fibrosis.[57,59] It also was shown that rapid onset of neural and vascular compromise is more likely to produce symptomatic radiculopathy than gradual mechanical deformity.[59-63] Inflammation has taken a central role in recent years since the description by McCarron and colleagues[64] of nucleus pulposus producing a marked epidural inflammatory reaction in dogs. Since then, many investigators have shown the inflammatogenic properties of the nucleus pulposus and its role in producing spinal pain.[36-38,40,41,65-74] Studies after exposure to autologous nucleus pulposus have shown myelin and axonal injury to the nerve roots and reduced nerve conduction velocities.[38,59] Some of these descriptions are contradicted, however, with more recent studies suggesting that normal frozen and hyaluronidase-digested nucleus pulposus in experimentally degenerated nucleus pulposus failing to produce similar changes in nerve root function.[75,76] An autoimmune or chemical basis for lumbar radicular pain was postulated in 1977.[77,78] Extensive literature has been published focusing attention on multiple agents, such as phospholipase A_2, metalloproteinase, interleukin-6, prostaglandin E_2, and tumor necrosis factor.[79]

Signs and Symptoms

Bogduk and Govind[80] stated that it is difficult to find a comprehensive definition of the clinical features of radicular pain in the literature. Classically, radicular pain has been described as following a dermatomal distribution. Research has shown, however, that radicular pain, whether caused by disk herniation or spinal stenosis, may not follow a dermatomal distribution.[80-82] Typical radicular pain is described with a distribution pattern of the entire length of the lower extremity, specifically below the knee; with a pattern describing a narrow band, traveling quasisegmentally but not dermatomally, and not distinguishable by segment; with a shooting, lancinating quality, perhaps like an electric shock; and with a depth described as deep and superficial.[80] The distinguishing features of lumbar radicular pain and somatic referred pain are shown in Table 83–1. Haldeman and colleagues[83] showed that pain below the knee is neither a valid indicator of radiculopathy, nor of abnormalities on electrodiagnostic studies and findings of nerve root compression on CT.

Lumbosacral radicular pain is felt in the lower extremity when L4, L5, S1, or S2 nerve roots are involved radiating typically along the back of the thigh, into the leg and into the foot. In contrast, radicular pain from L1, L2, and L3 is felt in the lower abdominal wall, groin, and anterior thigh. The pain may not follow the corresponding dermatomes, however, and it may not be distinguishable on the basis of the distribution.[81] Lumbar radicular pain has been described as radiating into the lower extremity along a narrow band not more than 5 to 8 cm wide.[84] This narrow band is one of the more distinguishing characteristics to separate it from somatic referred pain. In contrast to radicular pain, somatic pain is felt in a wide region described in the patterns of a patch or a region rather than a band.[85] Experimental studies have shown that radicular pain is shooting or lancinating in character,[84-86] rather than dull or aching.[80] While somatic pain may be felt deeply, radicular pain is the only pain felt superficially in the skin (see Table 83–1).[85,87] Although radicular pain is most likely to travel below the knee, and somatic referred pain is most often limited to above the knee, radicular pain may be restricted to the thigh or posterior hip, and somatic pain may radiate below the knee.[88,89] Symptoms may be confusing because radicular and somatic pain may coexist.

Deyo and associates[90] analyzed the sensitivity and specificity of the patient's history for the diagnosis of tumors, spinal stenosis, spinal osteomyelitis, herniated disks, and compression fractures. They showed that a previous history of malignancy was the most specific information for tumor

Table 83–1

Features of Somatic and Radicular Pain

	Somatic or Referred Pain	*Radicular Pain*
Segment Causes	Posterior segment or element	Anterior segment
	Facet joint pain	Disk herniation
	Sacroiliac joint pain	Annular tear
	Myofascial syndrome	Spinal stenosis
	Internal disk disruption	
Symptoms		
Quality	Dull, aching, deep	Sharp, shooting, superficial, lancinating
	Like an expanding pressure	Like an electrical shock
	Poorly localized	
	Back worse than leg	Leg worse than back
	No paresthesia	Paresthesia present
	Covers a wide area	Well defined and localized
	No radicular or shooting pain	Radicular distribution
Modification	Worse with extension	Worse with flexion
	Better with flexion	Better with extension
	No radicular pattern	Radicular pattern
Radiation	Low back to hip, thigh, groin	Follows nerve root distribution
	Radiation below knee unusual	Radiation below knee common
	Quasisegmental	Radicular pattern
Signs		
Sensory Alteration	Uncommon	Probable
Motor Changes	Only subjective weakness	Objective weakness
	Atrophy rare	Atrophy possibly present
Reflex Changes	None	Commonly described, but seen only occasionally
Straight Leg Raises	Only low back pain	Reproduction of leg pain
	No root tension signs	Positive root tension signs

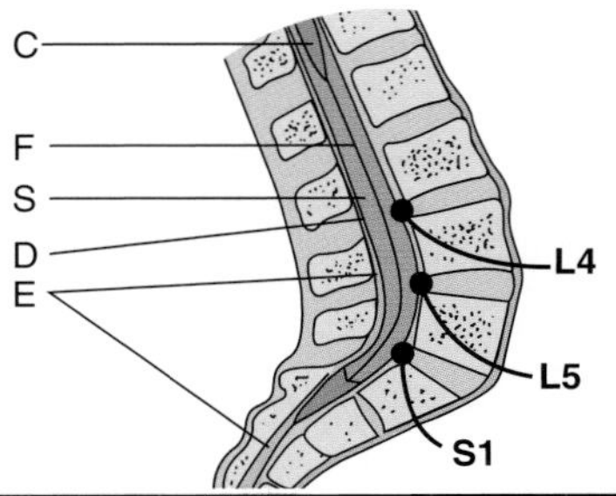

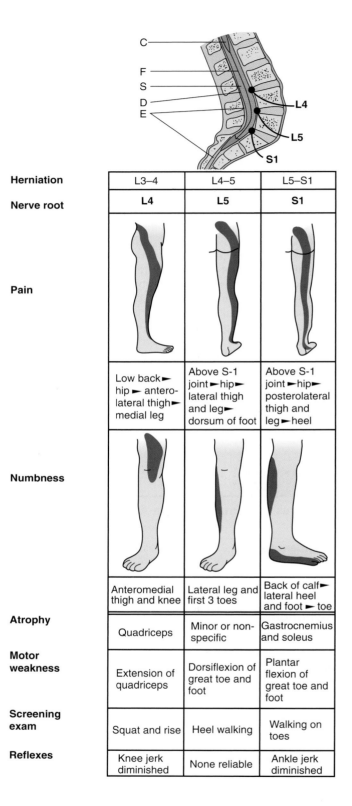

Herniation	L3–4	L4–5	L5–S1
Nerve root	L4	L5	S1
Pain	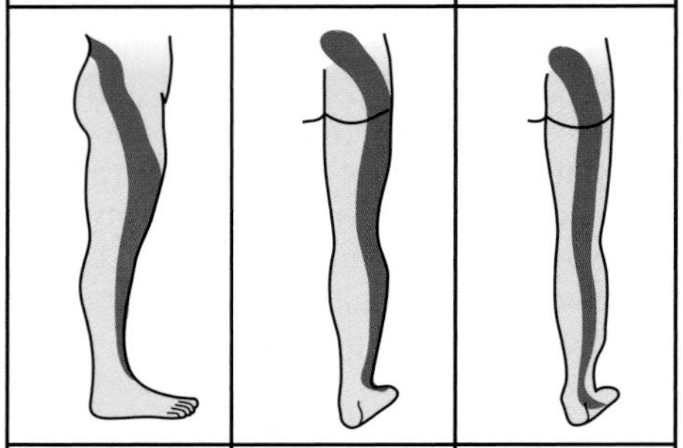		
	Low back ► hip ► antero-lateral thigh ► medial leg	Above S-1 joint ► hip ► lateral thigh and leg ► dorsum of foot	Above S-1 joint ► hip ► posterolateral thigh and leg ► heel
Numbness	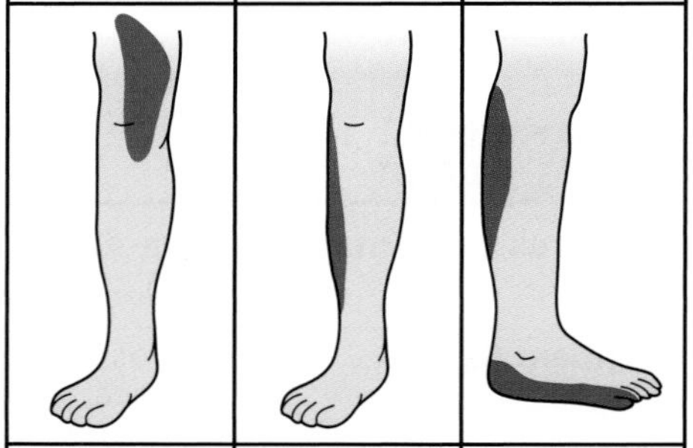		
	Anteromedial thigh and knee	Lateral leg and first 3 toes	Back of calf ► lateral heel and foot ► toe
Atrophy	Quadriceps	Minor or non-specific	Gastrocnemius and soleus
Motor weakness	Extension of quadriceps	Dorsiflexion of great toe and foot	Plantar flexion of great toe and foot
Screening exam	Squat and rise	Heel walking	Walking on toes
Reflexes	Knee jerk diminished	None reliable	Ankle jerk diminished

FIGURE 83–7 ■ Clinical features of a posterolateral lumbar intervertebral disk herniation. C, conus medullaris; D, dural tube; E, epidural space; F, filum terminale; S, subarachnoid space. (Modified from Wilkinson JL: Neuroanatomy for Medical Students. Bristol, John Wright & Sons, 1986, p. 46; Keim HA, Kirkaldy-Willis WH: Low back pain. Clin Symp 39:18, 1987; and Bigos S, Bowyer O, Braen G, et al: Acute Low Back Problems in Adults. Practice Guideline, Quick Reference Guide Number 14. AHCPR Pub. No. 95-0643. Rockville, MD, U.S. Department of Health and Human Services, Public Health Service, Agency for Health Care Policy and Research, 1994. Adapted from Giles LG: Diagnosis of mechanical low back pain with or without referred leg pain. In: Clinical Anatomy and Management of Low Back Pain, vol 1. Oxford, Butterworth-Heinemann, 1997, p 322.)

(0.98), but had comparatively low sensitivity, whereas pain when resting in bed had high sensitivity (0.90) and low specificity. Sciatica was highly sensitive for a clinically important herniated disk, as was old age for spinal stenosis and compression fractures.

Subjective complaint of numbness is considered reasonably sensitive (0.76), but not specific (0.33), as a sign of radiculopathy.[83] The objective sensory loss may indicate the segment involved more appropriately, however, if the radicular pain is accompanied by sensory loss. Objective signs of numbness are reasonably sensitive, although numbness is not specific as a sign of radiculopathy.

Physical findings involving straight leg raising are reasonably specific for radicular pain secondary to disk herniation.[90] Cross-leg straight leg raising is superior to ipsilateral straight leg raising. Straight leg raising and objective sensory loss correlate well with positive findings on electrodiagnostic tests and compressive features on CT.[83] Deyo and associates[90] showed that in the older age groups, spinal stenosis becomes a more significant problem. Identification of neurologic impairment is important to diagnosis and treatment. Ipsilateral imitation of straight leg raising is common, but nonspecific. In contrast, cross-leg straight leg raising is less sensitive, but more specific. Other neurologic signs include impairment of ankle dorsiflexor weakness, with a sensitivity of 0.9 and specificity of 0.54; great toe extensor weakness, with a sensitivity of 0.2 to 0.57 and specificity of 0.71 to 0.82; ankle reflex, with a sensitivity of 0.52 and specificity of 0.62; patellar reflex, with a sensitivity of 0.04 and specificity of 0.93 to 0.97; quadriceps weakness, with a sensitivity of approximately 0.5 and specificity of 0.99; and ankle plantar flexor weakness with a sensitivity of 0.06 and specificity of 0.95.

Physical Examination

A neurologic and musculoskeletal examination is carried out in evaluating a patient with symptoms of radiculopathy or radicular pain. Figure 83–7 illustrates clinical features of disk herniation at various levels.[91] Objective neurologic signs of radiculopathy, with dermatomal abnormalities, myotomal weakness, reflex inhibition, and positive straight leg raising, indicate radiculopathy. The clinical examination does not differentiate, however, among a multitude of causes in disk herniation even though a few of the causes were described earlier from all the tests; straight leg raising has the best sensitivity, but low specificity.[92] The other clinical tests have modest to poor sensitivities and specificities. Combinations of multiple tests considered together also have not been shown to improve likelihood ratios.[92] On the history and physical examination, the following three elements are important in the diagnosis of lumbar disk herniation:

1. Predominant leg or radicular pain below the knee in a dermatomal distribution
2. Nerve root tension signs with straight leg raising between 30 and 70 degrees or a positive cross-leg straight-leg raising
3. Corroborating neurologic signs with muscle weakness and wasting, sensory impairment, and reflex suppression

The physical findings may be corroborated with imaging or electrophysiologic studies.

DIAGNOSTIC TESTS

Imaging

The objective of imaging is to show the cause of the pain and its location.[93] Although plain radiography is the most common imaging technique, it does not satisfy the objective of identifying the cause of the pain. The major utility of plain films is to exclude systemic pathology. The value of plain radiography, if any, is limited to the demonstration of foraminal stenosis, tumors, and infections.

In contrast to plain radiography, CT and MRI are powerful and reliable tools for the investigation of the lumbar radicular pain. Both tests are reasonably reliable and valid. Because of its greater resolution of soft tissues and intraosseous tissues, however, MRI is considered superior to CT for the demonstration of conditions such as nerve tumors, cysts, infection, and other disorders. In contrast, CT is superior to MRI in the demonstration of bone and is the preferred modality for diagnosis of complex fractures or deformities. Studies show, however, that sensitivity and specificity for plain CT, CT myelography, and MRI are the same, with an approximate sensitivity of 0.90 and specificity of 0.70. A positive and negative predictive value of 0.82 is also the same for all three modalities.[94,95] Compared with surgical findings, CT has an accuracy of 77% to 92%, and MRI has an accuracy of 76% to 90%.[96-99] Studies in asymptomatic volunteers also have shown a high prevalence of disk abnormalities.

On CT, a herniated nucleus pulposus was evident in 20% of individuals younger than age 40 and in 27% of individuals older than age 40.[95] On MRI, disk bulges and disk herniations occurred with increasing frequency with age, with a high prevalence of asymptomatic disk herniations.[100,101] A positive relationship with symptoms and disk herniation has been shown in some cases, but not all.[52,54,96,102-104] Symptoms secondary to large disk herniations tend to improve better than symptoms secondary to small herniations, and resolution of symptoms correlates with reduction in size of the large herniations. Large herniations are reduced in size to a greater extent than smaller herniations.

Contrast-enhanced MRI apparently shows inflammatory changes surrounding affected nerve roots. There is no consistent relationship, however, between enhancement and the presence or severity of clinical symptoms or signs.[93,96] Although there are no major differences between CT and MRI, the use of CT myelography has been attractive for spinal stenosis even though it has not been presented in sufficient detail in the literature to allow calculation of sensitivity and specificity.

Neurophysiologic Studies

Electromyography is designed to identify signs of denervation and muscles innervated by the affected nerve root. The utility of electrophysiologic studies has been based on the ability to objectify abnormalities of nerve conduction resulting from radiculopathy and to identify the particular segment. Andersson and colleagues,[105] in a consensus summary on the diagnosis and treatment of lumbar disk herniation, concluded that "although neurophysiological testing is frequently used to diagnose patients with radiculopathy associated with disk herniation, these tests are not clinically necessary to confirm the presence of radiculopathy." These investigators added that neurophysiologic testing can determine the chronicity and severity of spinal nerve root lesions and differentiate the nervous system level of involvement (i.e., cord, peripheral nerve, and muscle). Neurophysiologic testing may be appropriate when the clinical situation is less clearly delineated and to differentiate a disk herniation from other neurologic disorders, such as neuropathy or peripheral nerve entrapment.

DIFFERENTIAL DIAGNOSIS

An important differential diagnosis to consider in radiculopathy is compression or irritation of the nerve root by sources other than disk herniation, spinal stenosis, and diskogenic pain with disk herniation. Although prevalence of all these conditions is extremely low, the list is long, and the exercise is tedious. The list is detailed in a monograph by Bogduk and Govind.[32]

Kirkaldy-Willis and Hill[106] described five nerve entrapment sites as follows:

1. Anterior to the dura and nerve sleeves—the sinuvertebral and spinal nerves from the disk
2. In the medial part of the nerve canal—the spinal nerves
3. In the posterolateral part of the main spinal canal—the cauda equina from enlarged posterior joints
4. In the lateral part of the nerve canal—spinal and sinuvertebral nerves from subluxed and enlarged superior articular processes
5. At the posterior joints—the medial branches of the posterior primary rami

The five frequently seen syndromes are:

1. Herniation of nucleus pulposus
2. Central spinal stenosis
3. Nerve entrapment in the lateral recess
4. Sacroiliac and piriformis syndromes
5. Facet joint pain

Although facet joint pain may be the easiest to identify based on somatic and radicular pain and diagnostic blocks, sacroiliac and piriformis syndromes, herniated disk, spinal stenosis, and lateral recess entrapment have similar features and warrant differential diagnosis.

Sacroiliac and piriformis syndromes may manifest with lower extremity pain, but without low back pain. The usual presentation is buttock, trochanteric, and posterior thigh pain, which rarely may radiate as far as the ankle.[106] Sensory changes are rarely described.

Central spinal stenosis resulting in lumbar radiculopathy is differentiated by pain on walking that is relieved by rest, the feeling that the legs are going to give way, a feeling of cold or numbness in the legs, a feeling that the legs are made of rubber and do not belong to the patient, and night pain that is relieved by walking. Radiologic evaluation often differentiates this from disk herniation.[106]

Lateral recess stenosis with nerve entrapment mostly resembles facet joint pain or sacroiliac syndrome. Low back pain is often absent, and muscle weakness is rare. The pain may radiate all the way into the ankle and occasionally into toes. Radiologic examination often differentiates it from lumbar radiculopathy secondary to disk herniation.

Disk herniation has a typical presentation as described earlier. Atypical presentations have been described in which the herniation is central and does not entrap the L5 or S1 nerves; L3-4 herniation produces anterior thigh pain, quadriceps weakness, and loss of feel of legs; and a higher lesion produces lower abdominal and scrotal pain, occasionally confused with renal or ureteric disorders, and with lateral herniation. Table 83–2 illustrates the diagnostic features for various levels of nerve root involvement.

TREATMENT

Lumbar radicular pain or radiculopathy may be treated with conservative management, interventional management, or surgical management.

Conservative Management

Conservative treatments include back school, exercises to teach spinal stabilization, strengthening exercises, flexibility exercises, and drug therapy. In managing acute and subacute radicular pain, there is limited evidence that nonsteroidal anti-inflammatory drugs (NSAIDs) do not provide effective pain relief for nerve root pain.[107] There is also strong evidence that different types of NSAIDs are equally effective. NSAIDs can have serious adverse effects, particularly at high doses and in elderly patients.

Muscle relaxants have not been studied in radicular pain. There is strong evidence, however, that muscle relaxants effectively reduce acute low back pain, although the different types of muscle relaxants are equally effective. Muscle relaxants also have significant adverse effects, including drowsiness, and carry a significant risk of habituation and dependency, even after relatively short courses. *Systemic steroids* have been shown to have the same effectiveness as a placebo in managing radicular pain.[108]

Only limited evidence indicates *bed rest* is effective in managing acute disk prolapse or nerve root pain.[109] There is limited evidence that bed rest with traction is not effective. Traction essentially may add complications to immobilization with deleterious effects, in particular, joint stiffness, muscle wasting, loss of bone mass, pressure sores, and thromboembolism.[110]

There is strong evidence that most types of specific *back exercises* (e.g., flexion, extension, aerobics, or strengthening exercises) are not more effective than alternative treatments for acute low back pain with which they have been compared, including no intervention.[107] There is conflicting evidence, however, that McKenzie exercises may produce some short-term symptomatic improvement in acute low back pain.[107] *Back schools* have been shown to have conflicting evidence on their effectiveness in managing low back pain.

Manipulation has been shown to have moderate evidence that it is more effective than a placebo treatment for short-term pain relief of acute low back pain.[107] *Transcutaneous electrical nerve stimulation (TENS)* was shown to have conflicting evidence regarding its effectiveness in the treatment of acute low back pain.[107] *Other modalities,* including ice, heat, short-wave diathermy, massage, and ultrasound, for the treatment of acute low back pain have been shown to be ineffective.[107]

For chronic low back pain, the following modalities have been studied:

1. *Exercise therapy:* There is strong evidence that exercise therapy is effective, and there is moderate evidence that various exercises are equally effective.[111]

Table 83–2

Diagnostic Features for Various Levels of Nerve Root Involvement

Herniation	*Nerve Root*	*Pain*	*Numbness*	*Atrophy*	*Motor Weakness*	*Screening Examination*	*Reflexes*
L3-4	L4	Low back; hip; anterolateral thigh; medial leg	Anteromedial thigh and knee	Quadriceps	Extension of quadriceps	Squat and rise	Knee jerk diminished
L4-5	L5	Above S1 joint; hip; lateral thigh and leg; dorsum of foot	Lateral leg and first 3 toes	Minor or nonspecific	Dorsiflexion of great toe and foot	Heel walking	None reliable
L5-S1	S1	Above S1 joint; hip; posterolateral and thigh leg; heel	Back of calf; lateral heel and foot; toe	Gastrocnemius and soleus	Plantar flexion of great toe and foot	Walking on toes	Ankle jerk diminished

2. *Back schools:* There is limited evidence that an intensive back school program in an occupational setting in Scandinavia is more effective than no actual treatment. There is conflicting evidence on the effectiveness of back schools in nonoccupational settings and outside Scandinavia.
3. *Behavioral therapy:* Multidimensional programs that include cognitive behavioral therapy programs are statistically and clinically superior to control groups on key outcome variables. Compared with active treatment, however, cognitive behavioral treatment has a small to moderate effect on outcome variables. Cognitive behavioral treatment programs seem to have their largest effects on psychological function, pain, physical function, and medication intake.[112]
4. *Multidisciplinary pain treatment programs:* There is strong evidence that a multidisciplinary treatment program aimed at functional restoration is useful for patients with long-lasting, severe, chronic low back pain.[111]
3. *Manual therapy:* There is moderate evidence that manual therapy is more effective than usual care by the general practitioner, bed rest, analgesics, and massage for short-term pain relief. There is limited and conflicting evidence of any long-term effect.[111]
4. *Traction:* There is strong evidence that traction has no effect in treating chronic low back pain.[111]
5. *Arthrosis:* There is limited evidence that a lumbar corset with support may produce some subjective improvement.[111]
6. *TENS:* There is inconsistent evidence that TENS is effective.[111]
7. *Acupuncture:* There is inconsistent evidence that acupuncture is effective.

Interventional Techniques

Epidural steroids in the lumbar spine are administered transforaminally, caudally, or by interlaminar route. Synthesis of evidence on epidural steroid injections by Manchikanti and colleagues[79] and Boswell and coworkers[113] was most comprehensive. Evidence from other reviews was conflicting, however.[114-118] Manchikanti and colleagues[79] and Boswell and coworkers[113] evaluated the evidence based on short-term relief (<3 months) or long-term relief (≥3 months). The results were as follows:

1. For caudal epidural steroid injections, the evidence was strong for short-term relief and moderate for long-term relief.
2. For interlaminar epidural steroid injections, the evidence was moderate for short-term relief and limited for long-term relief.
3. For transforaminal epidural steroid injections, the evidence was strong for short-term relief and long-term relief.

Surgical Treatment

Surgical techniques include minimally invasive surgical procedures, such as percutaneous disk decompression, laser diskectomy, and endoscopic diskectomy, and open surgical procedures, such as diskectomy and laminectomy.

Surgery for Lumbar Disk Prolapse

Evidence regarding surgery for lumbar disk prolapse is as follows:

1. There is limited direct evidence on the efficacy of surgical diskectomy for lumbar disk prolapse.[119,120]
2. There is strong indirect evidence from randomized controlled trials of chemonucleolysis that diskectomy is more effective than chemonucleolysis, which is more effective than placebo.[119] Diskectomy provides faster relief from the acute attack, although any positive or negative effects on the lifetime natural history of disk problems are unclear.[119]
3. There is strong evidence that chemonucleolysis with chymopapain produces better clinical outcomes than placebo.[119]
4. There is strong evidence that microdiskectomy and standard diskectomy give broadly comparable clinical outcomes.[119]
5. There is no acceptable evidence on laser diskectomy.[119]
6. There is limited evidence that fusion to supplement decompression for degenerative spinal stenosis produced better clinical outcomes.[119]

SIDE EFFECTS AND COMPLICATIONS

Apart from long-lasting disability, complications of disk herniation include nerve damage and cauda equina syndrome. Other complications are related to treatment; conservative management and surgical management alike have multiple side effects. All types of narcotic and non-narcotic analgesics have a multitude of side effects. Acetaminophen is associated with hepatic toxicity. NSAIDs can have serious side effects, particularly at high doses and in elderly patients. Opioids cause dizziness, respiratory depression, central nervous system dysfunction, and dependency and addiction. Significant adverse effects of muscle relaxants include drowsiness and a significant risk of habituation and dependency. Bed rest is associated with deconditioning; traction adds to other complications of immobilization, including muscle wasting, loss of bone density, pressure sores, and thromboembolism. Although risks of manipulation are low, serious complications could occur, resulting in severe or progressive neurologic deficit. Manipulation under anesthesia also is associated with an increased risk of serious neurologic damage.[111]

Interventional techniques also are associated with multiple complications.[79] The most common and worrisome complications of caudal, interlaminar, and transforaminal epidural injections are related to needle placement and drug administration. Complications include dural puncture, spinal cord trauma, infection, hematoma formation, abscess formation, subdural injection, intracranial air injection, epidural lipomatosis, pneumothorax, nerve damage, headache, death, brain damage, increased intracranial pressure, intravascular injection, vascular injury, cerebrovascular pulmonary embolus, and effects of steroids. Complications of surgical techniques include infection, nerve damage, spinal cord trauma, death, epidural fibrosis, and post–lumbar laminectomy syndrome.

CONCLUSION

Descriptions of lumbar radiculopathy date back to the Hippocratic collection describing sciatica. Since the early descriptions of sciatica, a multitude of experimental studies have indicated the complex mechanism of pathogenesis of sciatica or lumbar radiculopathy. Radicular pain is a subjective clinical feature; however, it can be a feature of radiculopathy, along with neurologic symptoms and signs.

Lumbar disk herniation is reliably diagnosed with three elements of history examination, including predominant leg or radicular pain below the knee in a dermatomal distribution, nerve root tension signs, and corroborating neurologic signs. Imaging with CT and MRI seems to be equally beneficial. Neurophysiologic studies are indicated to differentiate a disk herniation from other neurologic disorders, such as neuropathy or peripheral nerve entrapment.

Among the numerous modalities of treatments available in managing lumbar radiculopathy, the effectiveness of physical modalities, manipulation, and traction in patients with lumbar disk herniation is inadequately studied and controversial. Similarly, the effectiveness of different types of exercise programs for the treatment of patients with lumbar disk herniation has not been determined. There is moderate evidence that caudal epidural steroids are effective in disk herniation and radiculopathy, whereas there is strong evidence that transforaminal epidural steroids are effective. Microdiskectomy and open diskectomy are effective modalities in managing radiculopathy secondary to disk herniation.

KEY POINTS

- Radicular pain is evoked by the stimulation of the sensory (dorsal) root of the spinal nerve, or its dorsal root ganglion. It is not synonymous with radiculopathy.
- Radiculopathy is associated with radicular pain and any combination of numbness or motor loss.
- Radicular and somatic referred pain may differ in distribution, pattern, quality, and depth, along with causation.
- Nerve root or radicular pain, root irritation signs, and root compression signs are important in the diagnosis of radiculopathy.
- Imaging should be undertaken only if warranted by the patient's clinical condition. In the absence of clinical indicators of a "red flag" condition, medical imaging is neither indicated nor warranted.
- Neurophysiologic testing is used to differentiate a disk herniation from other neurologic disorders, such as neuropathy or peripheral nerve entrapment.
- The efficacy of physical modalities, manipulation, and traction in patients with lumbar disk herniation is inadequately studied and controversial.
- The efficacy of different types of exercise programs for the treatment of patients with lumbar disk herniation has not been determined.
- There is moderate evidence that caudal epidural steroids are effective in disk herniation and radiculopathy; there is strong evidence that transforaminal epidural steroids are effective.
- Microdiskectomy and open diskectomy are effective modalities of treatment in managing radiculopathy secondary to disk herniation.

References

1. Adams F: The Genuine Works of Hippocrates. Baltimore, Williams & Wilkins, 1939.
2. Thurwold J: The Century of the Surgeon. New York, Pantheon Books, 1957.
3. Wiltse LL: The history of spinal disorders. In Frymoyer JW, Ducker TB, Hadler NM, et al (eds): The Adult Spine: Principles and Practice, 2nd ed. Philadelphia, Lippincott-Raven, 1997, p 3.
4. Cortugno D: De Ischiade Nervosa Canmentarius. L. Naples, Simonocos Brothers, 1764.
5. Bell C: Observations on Injuries of the Spine and of the Thigh Bone. London, Thomas Tegg, 1824.
6. Valleix: Quoted in Reynolds F, Katz S: Herniated Lumbar Intervertebral Disc. American Academy of Orthopaedic Surgeons Symposium on the Spine. St. Louis, CV Mosby, 1969.
7. Von Luschka H: Die Hagelenke des menschilichen Korpers. IV. Berlin, G. Remier, 1858.
8. Brissaud: Quoted in Reynolds F, Katz S: Herniated Lumbar Intervertebral Disc. American Academy of Orthopaedic Surgeons Symposium on the Spine. St. Louis, CV Mosby, 1969.
9. Oppenheim H, Krause F: Ueber Einklemmung bzw. Strangulation der cauda equina. Dtsche Med Wochenschr 35:697, 1909.
10. Middleton GS, Teacher JH: Extruded disc at the T12-L1 level: Microscopic exam showed it to be nucleus pulposus. Glasgow Med J I(A):vlxxvi, 1911.
11. Middleton GS, Teacher JH: Injury of the spinal cord due to rupture of an intervertebral disc during muscular effort. Glasgow Med J 76:1, 1911.
12. Goldthwait JE: The lumbosacral articulation. Boston Med Surg J 164:365, 1911.
13. Magnusson PB: Differential diagnosis of causes of back pain accompanied by sciatica. Ann Surg 119:878, 1944.
14. Dandy WE: Loose cartilage from the intervertebral disc simulating tumor of the spinal cord. Arch Surg 19:660, 1929.
15. Hedtmann A: Das sog. Postdiskotomiesyndrom: Fehlschläge der Bandscheiben-Operation? Z Orthop 130:456, 1992.
16. Loew F, Caspar W: Surgical approach to lumbar disc herniations. Adv Standards Neurosurg 5:153, 1978.
17. Caspar W: A new surgical procedure for lumbar disc herniation causing less tissue damage through a miscrosurgical approach. Adv Neurosurg 4:74, 1977.
18. Williams RW: Microlumbar discectomy: A conservative surgical approach to the virgin herniated lumbar disc. Spine 3:175, 1978.
19. Mixter WJ, Barr JS: Ruptures of the intervertebral disc with involvement of the spinal canal. N Engl J Med 211:210, 1934.
20. Hirsch C: An attempt to diagnose level of disc lesion clinically by disc puncture. Acta Orthop Scand 18:131, 1948.
21. Hadra BE: Wiring of the spinous processes in Pott's disease. Trans Am Orthop Assoc 4:206, 1891.
22. Forst JJ: Contribution a l'étude clinique de la sciatique. Doctoral thesis. Paris, 1880.
23. Lasegue C: Considerations sur la sciatique. Arch Gen Med 4:558, 1864.
24. Roentgen C: In Tablott J (ed): A Biographical History of Medicine. Orlando, Grune & Stratton, 1970.
25. Dandy WE: Ventriculography following the injection of air into the cerebral ventricles. Ann Surg 68:5, 1918.
26. Sicard JA, Forestier J: Methode radiographique d'exploration de la cavité epidurale par le lipiodol. Rev Neurol 37:1264, 1921.
27. Lindblom K: Diagnostic puncture of intervertebral discs in sciatica. Acta Orthop Scand 17:231, 1948.
28. Oldendorf WH: Displaying the internal structural pattern of a complex object. Trans Biomed Elect (BME) 8:68, 1961.
29. Hounsfield G: Quoted by Oldendorf WH: The Quest for an Image of the Brain. New York, Raven Press, 1980.
30. Cormack: Quoted by Oldendorf WH: The Quest for an Image of the Brain. New York, Raven Press, 1980.
31. Wheeler AH, Murrey DB: Chronic lumbar spine and radicular pain: Pathophysiology and treatment. Curr Pain Headache Rep 6:97, 2002.
32. Bogduk N, Govind J: Definition. In: Medical Management of Acute Lumbar Radicular Pain: An Evidence-Based Approach. University of Newcastle, Australia, Newcastle Bone and Joint Institute, 1999, p 5.

33. Merskey H, Bogduk N: Classification of Chronic Pain: Descriptions of Chronic Pain Syndromes and Definitions of Pain Terms, 2nd ed. Seattle, IASP Press, 1994.
34. Olmarker K, Størkson R, Berge OG: Pathogenesis of sciatic pain: A study of spontaneous behavior in rats exposed to experimental disc herniation. Spine 27:1312, 2002.
35. Kawakami M, Tamaki T, Weinstein JN, et al: Pathomechanism of pain-related behavior produced by allografts of intervertebral disc in the rat. Spine 21:2101, 1996.
36. Kayama S, Konno S, Olmarker K, et al: Incision of the anulus fibrosus induces nerve root morphologic, vascular, and functional changes: An experimental study. Spine 21:2539, 1996.
37. Olmarker K, Myers RR: Pathogenesis of sciatic pain: Role of herniated nucleus pulposus and deformation of spinal nerve root and dorsal root ganglion. Pain 78:99, 1998.
38. Olmarker K, Rydevik B, Nordborg C: Autologous nucleus pulposus induces neurophysiologic and histologic changes in porcine cauda equina nerve roots. Spine 18:1425, 1993.
39. Otani K, Arai I, Mao GP, et al: Experimental disc herniation: Evaluation of the natural course using assessment of changes in nerve conduction of the spinal nerve roots and MRI changes of the intervertebral discs. Spine 22:2894, 1997.
40. Yabuki S, Kikuchi S, Olmarker K, et al: Acute effects of nucleus pulposus on blood flow and endoneurial fluid pressure in rate dorsal root ganglia. Spine 23:2517, 1998.
41. Manchikanti L, Boswell MV, Rivera JJ, et al: A randomized, controlled trial of spinal endoscopic adhesiolysis in chronic refractory low back and lower extremity pain. BMC Anesthesiol 5:10, 2005.
42. Jackson HC, Winkelmann RK, Bickel WH: Nerve endings in the human lumbar spinal column and related structures. J Bone Joint Surg Am 48:1272, 1966.
43. Roofe PG: Innervation of annulus fibrosus and posterior longitudinal ligament. Arch Neurol 44:100, 1940.
44. Malinsky J: The ontogenetic development of nerve trigeminations in the intervertebral discs of man. Acta Anat 38:96, 1959.
45. Yoshizawa H, O'Brien JP, Smith WT, et al: The neuropathology of intervertebral discs removed for low back pain. J Pathol 132:95, 1980.
46. Bogduk N, Tynan W, Wilson AS: The innervation of the human lumbar intervertebral discs. J Anat 132:39, 1981.
47. Nakamura S, Takahashi K, Takahashi Y, et al: Origin of nerves supplying the posterior portion of lumbar intervertebral discs in rats. Spine 21:917, 1996.
48. Coppes MH, Marani E, Thomeer RT, et al: Innervation of annulus fibrosus in low back pain. Lancet 336:189, 1990.
49. Coppes MH, Marani E, Thomeer RT, et al: Innervation of "painful" lumbar discs. Spine 22:2342, 1997.
50. Freemont AJ, Peacock TE, Goupille P, et al: Nerve ingrowth into diseased intervertebral disc in chronic back pain. Lancet 350:178, 1997.
51. Saal JA, Saal JS, Herzog RJ: The natural history of lumbar intervertebral disc extrusions treated nonoperatively. Spine 15:683, 1990.
52. Bush K, Cowan N, Katz DE, et al: The natural history of sciatica associated with disc pathology: A prospective study with clinical and independent radiologic follow-up. Spine 17:1205, 1992.
53. Bush K, Chaudhuri R, Hillier S, et al: The pathomorphologic changes that accompany the resolution of cervical radiculopathy: A prospective study with repeat magnetic resonance imaging. Spine 22:183, 1997.
54. Delauche-Cavallier MC, Budet C, Laredo JD, et al: Lumbar disc herniation: Computed tomography scan changes after conservative treatment of nerve root compression. Spine 17:927, 1992.
55. Saal JS, Saal JA, Yurth EF: Nonoperative management of herniated cervical intervertebral disc with radiculopathy. Spine 21:1877, 1996.
56. Mixter WJ, Ayers JB: Herniation or rupture of the intervertebral disc into the spinal canal. N Engl J Med 213:385, 1935.
57. Mooney V: Where is the pain coming from? Spine 12:754, 1987.
58. Rydevik BL: The effects of compression on the physiology of nerve roots. J Manip Physiol Ther 1:62, 1992.
59. Olmarker K, Rydevik B: Pathophysiology of spinal nerve roots as related to sciatica and disc herniation. In Herkowitz HN, Garfin SR, Balderston R, et al (eds): Rothman-Simeone Studies: The Spine. Philadelphia, WB Saunders, 1999, p 159.
60. Olmarker K, Rydevik B, Holm S: Edema formation in spinal nerve roots induced by experimental, graded compression: An experimental study on the pig cauda equina with special reference to differences in effects between rapid and slow onset of compression. Spine 14:569, 1989.
61. Olmarker K, Rydevik B, Holm B, et al: Effects of experimental graded compression on blood flow in spinal nerve roots: A vital microscopic study on the porcine cauda equina. J Orthop Res 7:817, 1989.
62. Olmarker K, Holm S, Rydevik B: Importance of compression onset rate for the degree of impairment of impulse propagation in experimental compression injury of the porcine cauda equina. Spine 35:416, 1990.
63. Olmarker K, Holm S, Rosenqvist AL, et al: Experimental nerve root compression: Presentation of a model for acute, graded compression of the porcine cauda equina, with analysis of neural and vascular anatomy. Spine 16:61, 1992.
64. McCarron RF, Wimpee MW, Hudkins PG, et al: The inflammatory effects of nucleus pulposus: A possible element in the pathogenesis of low back pain. Spine 12:760, 1987.
65. Olmarker K, Blomquist J, Stromberg J, et al: Inflammatogenic properties of nucleus pulposus. Spine 20:665, 1995.
66. Kawakami M, Tamaki T, Hashizume H, et al: The role of phospholipase A_2 and nitric oxide in pain-related behavior produced by an allograft of intervertebral disc material to the sciatic nerve of the rat. Spine 22:1074, 1997.
67. Saal JS, Franson RC, Dobrow R, et al: High levels of inflammatory phospholipase A_2 activity in lumbar disc herniations. Spine 15:674, 1990.
68. Chaoyang C, Cavanaugh JM, Ozaktay C, et al: Effects of phospholipase A_2 on lumbar nerve root structure and function. Spine 22:1057, 1997.
69. Nygaard OP, Mellgren SI, Osterud B: The inflammatory properties of contained and noncontained lumbar disc herniation. Spine 22:2484, 1997.
70. Kanerva A, Kommonen B, Gronbald M, et al: Inflammatory cells in experimental intervertebral disc injury. Spine 22:2711, 1997.
71. Franson RC, Saal JS, Saal JA: Human disc phospholipase A_2 is inflammatory. Spine 17:129, 1992.
72. Goupille P, Jayson MI, Valat JP, et al: The role of inflammation in disc herniation-associated radiculopathy. Semin Arthritis Rheum 28:60, 1998.
73. Piperno M, le Graverand MPH, Reboul P, et al: Phospholipase A_2 activity in herniated lumbar discs. Spine 22:2061, 1997.
74. Yabuki S, Igarashi T, Kikuchi S: Application of nucleus pulposus to the nerve root simultaneously reduces blood flow in dorsal root ganglion and corresponding hindpaw in the rat. Spine 25:1471, 2000.
75. Olmarker K, Brisby H, Yabuki S, et al: The effects of normal, frozen and hyaluronidase digested nucleus pulposus on nerve root structure and function. Spine 24:471, 1997.
76. Iwabuchi M, Rydevik B, Kikychi S, et al: Effects of annulus fibrosus and experimentally degenerated nucleus pulposus on nerve root conduction velocity. Spine 26:1651, 2001.
77. Gertzbein SD: Degenerative disc disease of the lumbar spine: Immunological implications. Clin Orthop 190:68, 1977.
78. Marshall LL, Trethewie ER, Curtain CC: Chemical radiculitis: A clinical, physiological, and immunological study. Clin Orthop 190:61, 1977.
79. Manchikanti L, Staats P, Singh V, et al: Evidence-based practice guidelines for interventional techniques in the management of chronic spinal pain. Pain Physician 6:3, 2003.
80. Bogduk N, Govind J: Clinical features. In: Medical Management of Acute Lumbar Radicular Pain: An Evidence-Based Approach. University of Newcastle, Australia, Newcastle Bone and Joint Institute, 1999, p 21.
81. Norlen G: On the value of the neurological symptoms in sciatica for the localization of a lumbar disc herniation. Acta Chir Scand 95:1, 1944.
82. van Akkerveeken PF: Lateral stenosis of the lumbar spine: A new diagnostic test and its influence on management of patients with pain only. Thesis, Rijksuniversitet te Utrecht, 1989.
83. Haldeman S, Shouka M, Robboy S: Computed tomography, electrodiagnostic and clinical findings in chronic workers' compensation patients with back and leg pain. Spine 13:345, 1988.
84. Smyth MJ, Wright V: Sciatica and the intervertebral disc: An experimental study. J Bone Joint Surg Am 40:1401, 1959.
85. Kellgren JH: On the distribution of pain arising from deep somatic structures with charts of segmental pain areas. Clin Sci 4:35, 1939.
86. McCulloch JA, Waddell G: Variation of the lumbosacral myotomes with bony segmental anomalies. J Bone Joint Surg Br 62:475, 1980.

87. Feinstein B, Langton JNK, Jameson RM, et al: Experiments on pain referred from deep somatic tissues. J Bone Joint Surg Am 35:981, 1954.
88. Mooney V, Robertson J: The facet syndrome. Clin Orthop 115:149, 1976.
89. Fairbank JCT, Park WM, McCall IW, et al: Apophyseal injections of local anaesthetic as a diagnostic aid in primary low back pain syndromes. Spine 6:598, 1981.
90. Deyo RA, Rainville J, Kent DL: What can the history and physical examination tell us about low back pain? JAMA 268:760, 1992.
91. Giles LG: Diagnosis of mechanical low back pain with or without referred leg pain. In: Clinical Anatomy and Management of Low Back Pain, vol 1. Oxford, Butterworth-Heinemann, 1997, p 322.
92. Bogduk N, Govind J: Examination. In: Medical Management of Acute Lumbar Radicular Pain: An Evidence-Based Approach. University of Newcastle, Australia, Newcastle Bone and Joint Institute, 1999, p 33.
93. Bogduk N, Govind J: Imaging. In: Medical Management of Acute Lumbar Radicular Pain: An Evidence-Based Approach. University of Newcastle, Australia, Newcastle Bone and Joint Institute, 1999, p 43.
94. Thornbury JR, Fryback DG, Turski PA, et al: Disk-caused nerve compression in patients with acute low-back pain: Diagnosis with MR, CT myelography, and plain CT. Radiology 186:731, 1993.
95. Wiesel SW, Tsourmas N, Feffer HL, et al: A study of computer-assisted tomography: I. The incidence of positive CAT scans in an asymptomatic group of patients. Spine 9:549, 1984.
96. Herzog RJ: The radiologic assessment for a lumbar disc herniation. Spine 21:19S, 1996.
97. Forristal RM, Marsh HO, Pay NT: Magnetic resonance imaging and contrast CT of the lumbar spine: Comparison of diagnostic methods and correlation with surgical findings. Spine 13:1049, 1988.
98. Fries JW, Abodeely DA, Vijungco JG, et al: Computed tomography of herniated and extruded nucleus pulposus. J Comput Assist Tomogr 6:874, 1982.
99. Albeck MJ, Hilden J, Kjaer L, et al: A controlled comparison of myelography, computed tomography, and magnetic resonance imaging in clinically suspected lumbar disc herniation. Spine 20:443, 1995.
100. Boden SD, Davis DO, Dina TS, et al: Abnormal magnetic resonance scans of the lumbar spine in asymptomatic subjects. J Bone Joint Surg Am 72:403, 1990.
101. Jensen MC, Bran-Zawadzki MN, Obuchowski N, et al: Magnetic resonance imaging of the lumbar spine in people without back pain. N Engl J Med 331:69, 1994.
102. Thelander U, Fagerlund M, Friberg S, et al: Describing the size of lumbar disc herniations using computed tomography. Spine 19:1979, 1994.
103. Bozzao A, Galluci M, Masciocchi C, et al: Lumbar disc herniation: MR imaging assessment of natural history in patients treated without surgery. Radiology 185:135, 1992.
104. Matsubara Y, Kato F, Mimatsu K, et al: Serial changes on MRI in lumbar disc herniations treated conservatively. Neuroradiology 37:378, 1995.
105. Andersson GBJ, Brown MD, Dvorak J, et al: Consensus summary on the diagnosis and treatment of lumbar disc herniation. Spine 21:75S, 1996.
106. Kirkaldy-Willis WH, Hill RJ: A more precise diagnosis for low back pain. Spine 4:102, 1979.
107. van Tulder MW, Waddell G: Conservative treatment of acute and subacute low back pain. In Nachemson AL, Jonsson E (eds): Neck and Back Pain: The Scientific Evidence of Causes, Diagnosis, and Treatment. Philadelphia, Lippincott Williams & Wilkins, 2000, p 241.
108. Haimovic IC, Beresford HR: Dexamethasone is not superior to placebo for treating lumbosacral radicular pain. Neurology 36:1593, 1986.
109. de Craen AJM, Di Giulio G, Lampe-Schoenmaeckers AJ, et al: Analgesic efficacy and safety of paracetamol-codeine combinations versus paracetamol alone: A systematic review. BMJ 313:321, 1996.
110. Pal P, Mangion P, Hossian MA, et al: A controlled trial of continuous lumbar traction in the treatment of back pain and sciatica. Br J Rheumatol 25:1181, 1986.
111. van Tulder MW, Goossens M, Waddell G, et al: Conservative treatment of chronic low back pain. In Nachemson AL, Jonsson E (eds): Neck and Back Pain: The Scientific Evidence of Causes, Diagnosis, and Treatment. Philadelphia, Lippincott Williams & Wilkins, 2000, p 271.
112. Linton SJ: Utility of cognitive-behavioral psychological treatments. In Nachemson AL, Jonsson E (eds): Neck and Back Pain. The Scientific Evidence of Causes, Diagnosis, and Treatment. Philadelphia, Lippincott Williams & Wilkins, 2000, p 361.
113. Boswell MV, Hansen HC, Trescot AM, et al: Epidural steroids in the management of chronic spinal pain and radiculopathy. Pain Physician 6:319, 2003.
114. Kepes ER, Duncalf D: Treatment of backache with spinal injections of local anesthetics, spinal and systemic steroids. Pain 22:33, 1985.
115. Bogduk N, Christophidis N, Cherry D, et al: Epidural Use of Steroids in the Management of Back Pain: Report of Working Party on Epidural Use of Steroids in the Management of Back Pain. Commonwealth of Canberra, Australia, National Health and Medical Research Council, 1994.
116. Benzon HT: Epidural steroid injections for low back pain and lumbosacral radiculography. Pain 24:277, 1986.
117. Koes BW, Scholten R, Mens JMA, et al: Epidural steroid injections for low back pain and sciatica: An updated systematic review of randomized clinical trials. Pain Digest 9:241, 1999.
118. Watts RW, Silagy CA: A meta-analysis on the efficacy of epidural corticosteroids in the treatment of sciatica. Anaesth Intensive Care 23:564, 1995.
119. Waddell G, Gibson JN, Grant I: Surgical treatment of lumbar disc prolapse and degenerative lumbar disc disease. In Nachemson AL, Jonsson E (eds): Neck and Back Pain: The Scientific Evidence of Causes, Diagnosis, and Treatment. Philadelphia, Lippincott Williams & Wilkins, 2000, p 305.
120. Weber H: Lumbar disc herniation: Controlled, prospective study with ten years of observation. Spine 8:131, 1983.

chapter 84

Lumbar Facet Syndrome

Nikolai Bogduk

There is no lumbar facet syndrome. A syndrome is a clinical entity defined, and recognized, by a specific constellation of clinical features. Reiter's syndrome is defined by the combination of urethritis, uveitis, and spondylarthropathy. Tolosa-Hunt syndrome is headache combined with palsy of one or more of the third, fourth, and sixth cranial nerves.

No combination of clinical features defines lumbar facet syndrome. Although some proponents had submitted that aggravation of pain by certain movements of the back is indicative of facet syndrome,[1,2] this has been refuted by studies using controlled diagnostic blocks.[3-5] Even the most recent study of Revel and associates[6] does not define a facet syndrome. Rather, the clinical tests used by these investigators serve to identify patients who do not have facet pain.

There is no syndrome. What patients have is lumbar zygapophyseal joint pain. This is an entity defined, not by clinical features, but by a specific source of pain. In many circles it is a diagnosis that is rejected or disdained, but ironically it is one of the best studied, and most strongly validated, entities in the specialty of pain medicine. Those who deny it either simply do not want to know or are unaware of the literature and its strength.

Few, if any, other conditions in pain medicine satisfy the following theoretical and practical criteria:

- The pain has an anatomic basis.
- The pain has been produced experimentally in normal volunteers.
- The pain can be diagnosed by a test that has been validated.
- The test used to diagnose the condition protects normal volunteers from experimentally induced versions of the condition.
- When tested, patients with the condition obtain complete relief of their pain.
- When diagnosed with the condition, patients can be treated.
- When treated, patients obtain complete relief of pain.
- When pain recurs, it can again be completely relieved.

ANATOMY

The lumbar zygapophyseal joints are formed by the superior and inferior articular processes of consecutive lumbar vertebra (Fig. 84–1). Each joint is named according to the segmental numbers of the vertebrae that form it. The joint between L5 and the sacrum is known as the lumbosacral or L5-S1 zygapophyseal joint. Each has the typical structure of a synovial joint.

The joints are innervated by the medial branches of the lumbar dorsal rami. Each joint receives articular branches from the ipsisegmental medial branch and from the medial branch above (see Fig. 84–1).[7,8] The joints, therefore, are endowed with the necessary neurologic apparatus potentially to be a source of pain.

A source of confusion arises in naming the nerves that innervate each joint. The segmental numbers of the nerves are one segment less than the name of the joint. Thus, the L4-5 joint is innervated by the L3,4 medial branches, and the L5-S1 joint is innervated by the L4,5 nerves. As a matter of discipline, for clarity in communication, practitioners should take care, when referring to a segment, whether they are referring to the joint or to the nerves that innervate it. One device is to use a hyphen (L4-5) when naming a joint, but a comma (L4,5) when naming its nerves. A hyphen indicates conjunction and, therefore, a joint; a comma indicates consecutive and, therefore, a pair of nerves.

EXPERIMENTALLY STIMULATED PAIN IN NORMAL VOLUNTEERS

When lumbar zygapophyseal joints are stimulated experimentally with a noxious stimulus, normal volunteers suffer and describe pain that resembles that reported in patients with low back pain. The experimental stimuli that have been used include injections of hypertonic saline into the joints,[9,10] injections of contrast medium to distend the capsules of the joints,[11] and electrical stimulation of the nerves that innervate the joints.[11,12]

In all studies that have been conducted, noxious stimulation of the zygapophyseal joints has produced low back pain and some degree of referred pain. Studies have differed on with respect to the distribution of referred pain (Fig. 84–2). As a rule, the referred pain tends to radiate inferolaterally from the site of stimulation. Pain from upper lumbar zygapophyseal joints extends into the loin or toward the posterior iliac crest from above. Pain from lower lumbar joints extends across the iliac crest into the buttock.

The pattern of referred pain is segmental in nature, in so far as pain from higher levels tends to be perceived in more cephalad regions than is pain from lower levels, but the pattern is not distinctive. Within and between studies, the distribution of pain from particular segments overlaps with the distribution of pain from adjacent and lower segments. Consequently, the location of referred pain cannot be used reliably to infer the exact location of its source. Although not quantified, it has been noted qualitatively that the distance of referral appears to be proportional to the intensity of stimulation. When stronger, noxious stimuli are applied the referred pain spreads further.[9]

Also not rigorously studied, but noted in one study, experimentally induced referred pain from the lumbar zygapophyseal joints can be associated with increased electromyographic activity in the hamstring muscles.[9] This is in accord with the more general observation that pain from structures innervated by the lumbar dorsal rami can be accompanied by involuntary activity in muscles of the lower limb.[13]

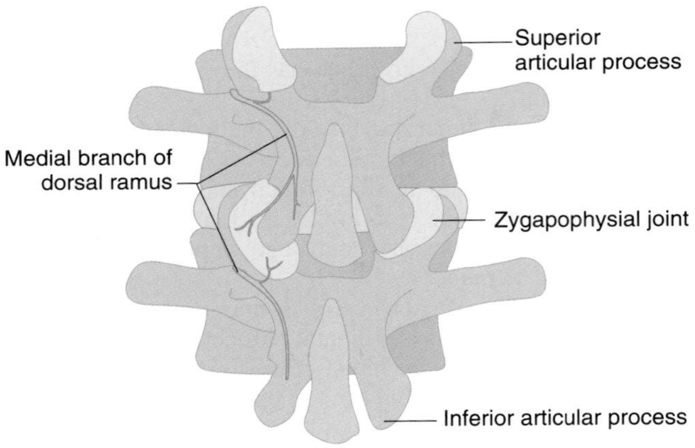

FIGURE 84–1 ■ Diagram of posterior view of lumbar segment showing the structure and innervation of the zygapophyseal joints. The zygapophyseal joint is formed by the adjacent superior articular process and inferior articular process. Each is innervated by articular branches from the medial branch (mb) of the same segment and the one above.

DIAGNOSTIC BLOCKS

Pain from a lumbar zygapophyseal joint can be relieved temporarily by anesthetizing the joint. This can be done by injecting local anesthetic into the cavity of the joint or by anesthetizing the medial branches that innervate the joint.

Intraarticular blocks constitute a direct test of zygapophyseal joint pain and were originally promoted in orthopedic and radiologic circles.[14-30] Intraarticular blocks have face validity, in that it can be shown, by injecting contrast medium into the joint, that the local anesthetic accurately and exclusively targets the joint. However, although still used, intraarticular blocks have not been validated further. In particular, they have not been subjected to controls and have not been shown to have predictive validity or therapeutic utility. Provocation of pain during injection of a joint is not diagnostic of the joint being painful. Provocation is not associated with subsequent relief when the joint is anesthetized.[31]

In contrast, medial branch blocks have been extensively tested. They involve injecting a tiny amount of local anesthetic (0.3 mL), under fluoroscopic control, onto each of the medial branches that innervate the target joint. The blocks require a preliminary test dose of contrast medium, because in about 8% of cases the injection can be into the vena comitans of the medial branch. Venous uptake is not a complication, given the small volume of local anesthetic injected, but it risks obtaining a false-negative response.

The face-validity of lumbar medial branch blocks has been established. Provided that correct target points are used,

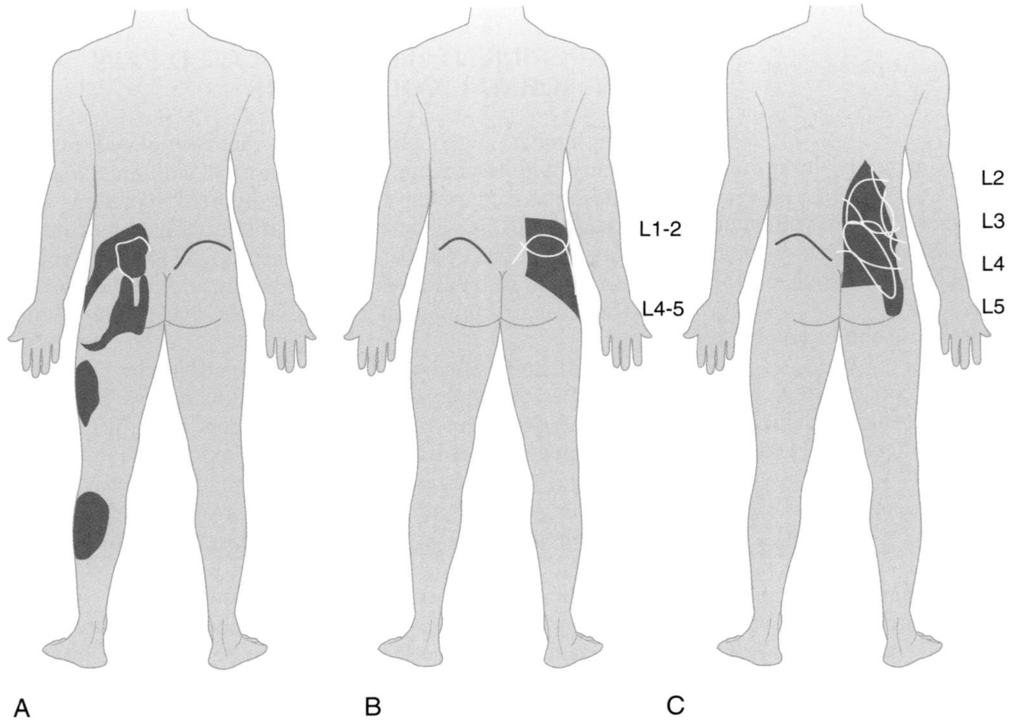

FIGURE 84–2 ■ Maps of referred pain patterns elicited from the lumbar zygapophyseal joints in normal volunteers. **A,** After injection of hypertonic saline into the lower lumbar joints, segments not specified. **B,** After injection of hypertonic saline into the L1-2 and L4-5 joints. **C,** After electrical stimulation of the medial branches at the segments indicated.

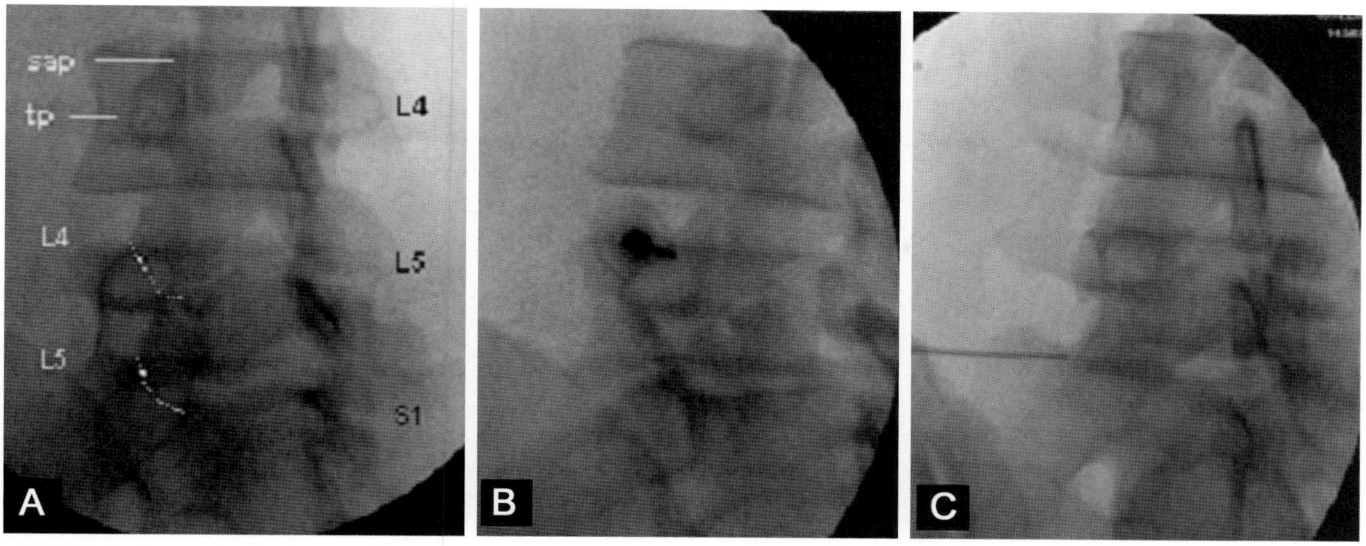

FIGURE 84–3 ■ Lumbar medial branch blocks. **A,** At typical segmental levels (L1-L5), the target point lies on the nerve midway between the notch between the superior articular process (sap) and the transverse process (tp), and where the nerve hooks medially under the mammilloaccessory ligament. At L5, a homologous point applies lateral to the superior articular process. The numbering of the nerves *(white)* is one less than their respective vertebrae *(black).* **B,** Oblique view of a needle in position on for an L4 medial branch block. **C,** Anteroposterior view of a needle in position for an L5 dorsal ramus block.

the local anesthetic covers the target nerve and does not spread to affect other structures that might be alternative sources of pain. The correct target point lies midway between two points[32]: the notch between the superior articular process and the transverse process, where the medial branch enters the posterior compartment of the spine, and the mammilloaccessory notch, where it hooks medially beneath the mammilloaccessory ligament (Fig. 84–3).[33] If deposited here, local anesthetic surrounds the nerve reliably. It may spread dorsally into the cleavage plane between the multifidus and longissimus lumborum or between fascicles of the multifidus at lower lumbar levels, but it does not indiscriminately anesthetize the back muscles. Target points more rostral on the transverse process risk some of the local anesthetic spreading to the intervertebral foramen where, theoretically, it might affect the spinal nerve and compromise the specificity of the block. Pointing the bevel of the needle caudad guards against this direction of spread.

The L5 medial branch cannot be selectively anesthetized. At this segmental level the target nerve is the L5 dorsal ramus itself, which runs over the ala of the sacrum. The target point is nevertheless analogous to that at typical lumbar levels. It lies opposite the middle of the base of the superior articular process of S1. Placing the needle further rostrad risks flow of injectate to the L5-S1 intervertebral foramen. Placing it more caudad risks flow to the S1 posterior foramen.

The face validity of medial branch blocks was established by stimulating the lumbar zygapophyseal joints, in normal volunteers, with injections of hypertonic saline, before and after medial branch blocks of the target joint. Medial branch blocks protect volunteers from experimentally induced zygapophyseal joint pain.[34]

Single, uncontrolled blocks of lumbar medial branches are not valid. They have a false-positive rate of between 25% and 41%.[35-37] This means that if the prevalence of lumbar zygapophyseal joint pain is 15% (see later), for every three blocks that appear to be positive, two will be false positive. If the prevalence is 40%, three of every five blocks will be false positive. Such yields of false-positive results are unacceptable and underscore the necessity for every block to be subjected to controls. Two types of controls are available: placebo controls and comparative blocks.

Placebo controls provide the highest order of validity, but they are difficult to implement in practice. Blocks would need to be performed on three separate occasions. A first block is required to establish that the target joint is, indeed, symptomatic. Thereafter, the second block cannot automatically be a placebo, because mischievous patients would know that the second agent is the sham. For the second block, the patient must randomly receive either an active agent or a placebo. For the third block, the patient receives the complementary agent.

Less discriminating, but more practical are comparative local anesthetic blocks.[38,39] On each of two occasions the patient receives an active agent, but the agents are varied. When a short-acting agent is used, the patient should obtain short-lasting relief. When a long-acting agent is used, the patient should obtain longer-lasting relief. When tested against placebo, this protocol has a sensitivity of 54% and a specificity of 88%.[39] That means that when comparative blocks are positive, the patient is very likely to have genuine zygapophyseal joint pain but the protocol fails to detect all genuine patients. If the criteria are relaxed to count as positive all patients who obtain complete relief of their pain, irrespective of duration of relief, the sensitivity rises to 80% but the specificity drops to 55%. This means that more patients who have zygapophyseal joint pain will be detected but not all positive responses will be truly positive.

Some practitioners, and some insurers, object to controlled blocks. Mistaken, or misguided, they believe that they can diagnose zygapophyseal joint pain with a single block and that controlled blocks simply increase costs. This attitude overlooks the cost of false-positive responses. If only single blocks are used, the diagnosis will be false in over 60% of cases and all subsequent decisions about these patients will be founded on a false premise. Cost-saving pays for diagnostic noise and therapeutic failure. Meanwhile an economics study has shown that, even at modest rates of reimbursement, controlled blocks are cost effective.[40]

CLINICAL PRESENTATION

There are no diagnostic clinical features of lumbar zygapophyseal joint pain. The patient has lumbar spinal pain and may have somatic referred pain into the lower limb. Most often the pain is referred only to the region of the buttock or proximal thigh, but it can extend beyond the knee and even into the foot. It is not true that pain below the knee is always sciatica. Pain distal to the knee has successfully been relieved, in some patients, by anesthetizing lower lumbar zygapophyseal joints.[9,21]

No associated features, however, are unique to lumbar zygapophyseal joint pain. Aggravation of pain by any movements or by any applied, clinical maneuver does not distinguish lumbar zygapophyseal joint pain from pain stemming from other sources.[3-5,41]

This should not be surprising. All the elements of the lumbar spine share a similar segmental innervation. Therefore, the symptoms that they produce should be similar. No movement selectively stresses just the zygapophyseal joints. The disk will also be stressed by movement, along with ligaments and muscles. Therefore, all sources of pain should be aggravated in a similar manner by movement.

Yet, this lack of distinctive clinical features is not an indictment of the condition. Demands for there to be a distinctive clinical syndrome are based on the cynical and artificial expectation that all disorders in the specialty of pain medicine must have distinctive features and that if they do not they cannot exist. Elsewhere in other medicine specialties conditions abound that do not constitute distinctive clinical syndromes. Most causes of chest pain cannot be diagnosed unless and until investigations such as radiography are performed. Most causes of abdominal pain are not distinctive until imaging, laboratory tests, ultrasound, or endoscopy is performed. For lumbar zygapophyseal joint pain, the definitive test is the use of controlled, diagnostic blocks.

Revel and colleagues[6] identified five features that were significantly associated with zygapophyseal joint pain: (1) pain not worsened when rising from forward flexion; (2) pain well relieved by recumbency; (3) pain not exacerbated by coughing; (4) pain not worsened by extension-rotation; and (5) pain not worsened by hyperextension. Four of these five features are negative in nature. They refer to pain not being aggravated. In practice, these features serve more to identify patients who do not have zygapophyseal joint pain than to diagnose those who do.

Patients with zygapophyseal joint pain are typically positive to all five of the features that Revel and colleagues describe,[6] but so, too, are 34% of patients who do not have zygapophyseal joint pain. As long as patients who do not have zygapophyseal joint pain outnumber those who do, the diagnostic value of Revel's tests is limited.[42] If the pretest prevalence of zygapophyseal joint pain is 10%, the posttest diagnostic confidence rises only 25%.[42] If the pretest prevalence is 40%, the posttest diagnostic confidence increases to only 66%. Thus, Revel's features do not provide for a definite diagnosis. By eliminating those patients who are unlikely to have zygapophyseal joint pain, they serve to increase the chances that those who remain do have zygapophyseal joint pain, but the low prevalence of zygapophyseal joint pain means that many or most of those who are positive to the tests will, nevertheless, still not have zygapophyseal joint pain.

PREVALENCE

By using controlled diagnostic blocks, multiple studies have established that lumbar zygapophyseal joint pain is common. Its actual prevalence varies according to the population studied but is not negligible.

Among injured workers, with a median age of 38 years, the prevalence was found to be 15% (95% confidence interval [CI]: 10% to 20%).[4] In an older population, without a history of trauma, it was found to be 40% (CI: 27% to 53%).[5] A similar prevalence (45%; CI: 39% to 54%) was found in a heterogeneous population attending a pain clinic.[36]

These figures, however, may constitute an overestimate, because the studies often used a generous criterion for a positive response to blocks. They considered positive anyone who had greater than 50% relief of pain. This falls short of 100% relief, which would be more compelling evidence that the zygapophyseal joint tested was the sole source of pain. Nevertheless, one study did provide data in this regard. When the criterion was 50% relief of pain, the prevalence of zygapophyseal joint pain was 40%. When the criterion was 90% relief, the prevalence decreased to 32%.[5] Thus, although the prevalence decreases when the diagnostic criteria are more stringent, the prevalence does not evaporate. It remains substantial.

PATHOLOGY

The pathology that causes lumbar zygapophyseal joints to be painful is not known. Lumbar zygapophyseal joint pain is an entity whose source can be established but whose pathology remains elusive.

Although evident as a pathology of the lumbar zygapophyseal joints,[43,44] osteoarthrosis cannot be blamed. The radiologic features of osteoarthrosis, as seen radiographically,[45,46] or on computed tomography,[47] do not correlate with whether the affected joint is painful or not. Osteoarthrosis is a normal age change and does not constitute a basis for zygapophyseal joint pain.

At post-mortem examination, it has been shown that the lumbar zygapophyseal joints can sustain small fractures that are not evident in radiographs.[48,49] In principle, such lesions could be construed as likely causes of pain. Such lesions have been detected in living individuals, using stereoradiography,[50] but they have not been pursued with CT or other imaging tests and have not been correlated with zygapophyseal joint pain.

Rare disorders that can affect the lumbar zygapophyseal joints are rheumatoid arthritis,[51] infection,[52-55] and pigmented villonodular synovitis.[56,57] These conditions, however, do not explain the large numbers of patients whose pain is relieved when their zygapophyseal joints are anesthetized.

TREATMENT

Although readily diagnosed, lumbar zygapophyseal joint pain is not easily treated. Few treatments explicitly for diagnosed lumbar zygapophyseal joint pain have been tested let alone validated. There is no evidence that conservative therapies of any kind relieve zygapophyseal joint pain. There is no evidence that fusing a segment relieves zygapophyseal joint pain. The tested treatments are limited to minimally invasive procedures.

Intraarticular Corticosteroids

Perhaps the most prolific treatment for lumbar zygapophyseal joint is intraarticular injection of corticosteroids.[14-18,23-30] This treatment has a chequered past and a vexatious future.

There is no rationale for the intraarticular use of corticosteroids. There is no evidence that lumbar zygapophyseal joint pain is caused by inflammation. Corticosteroids were adopted for zygapophyseal joint pain simply on the strength that they appeared to be effective when used for osteoarthritis in joints of the limbs.

An abundance of descriptive and observational studies underlies the use of intraarticular corticosteroids for lumbar zygapophyseal joint pain.[14-18,23-30] In none of these studies was injection of corticosteroids tested in patients with proven zygapophyseal joint pain. Corticosteroids were injected presumptively and without controls. The reported success rates are, therefore, meaningless.

If a diagnosis of zygapophyseal joint pain has not been made, the injection of corticosteroids into a joint is indiscriminate. If corticosteroids do have a specific therapeutic effect, they will work, under those circumstances, only in those patients who happen to have zygapophyseal joint pain and in whom the correct joint was fortuitously injected. Thus, the success rate would be a measure of the prevalence of zygapophyseal joint pain in the sample studied. If this is low, the success rate will appear to be low. Conversely, given the low prevalence of zygapophyseal joint pain, success rates of 80% are patently absurd, for they mean that patients had a therapeutic response when they were treated for a source of pain that they did not have.

Both of these arguments are confounded by the lack of controls. Without controls, consumers cannot know if the reported efficacy of intraarticular corticosteroids represents a genuine attributable effect or a placebo effect.

Lumbar intraarticular corticosteroids have not been subjected to a proper controlled trial. All trials, to date, that have used controls have carried fatal flaws.

Laudably, the studies of Lilius and associates[58-60] compared the efficacy of corticosteroids with that of normal saline. Those studies, however, treated unselected patients. Diagnostic blocks were not performed. No steps were taken to ensure that the patients had zygapophyseal joint pain. Therefore, the studies are not a test of the efficacy of intraarticular corticosteroids for zygapophyseal joint pain. What they do prove, however, is that indiscriminate injection of corticosteroids in patients with back pain is patently ineffective.

The most rigorous study to date has been that of Carette and colleagues,[61] who found that corticosteroids had no attributable effect beyond that of injection of normal saline. They did preselect their patients, but they used liberal diagnostic criteria. They enrolled patients who obtained at least 50% relief of pain after a single diagnostic block. Under these conditions, it is highly likely that patients were enrolled who did not have zygapophyseal joint pain or whose pain did not exclusively arise in their zygapophyseal joints.

Proponents of intraarticular corticosteroids have seized on this flaw and have argued that the Carette and colleagues' study did not discredit intraarticular corticosteroids, that in patients who really do have zygapophyseal joint pain, corticosteroids work better than demonstrated by Carette and colleagues.[61] Indeed, this study does not disprove this contention, but critics have not revealed whether their practice is more disciplined than that of Carette and colleagues.[61] No advocates of intraarticular corticosteroids have demonstrated that patients were selected by controlled diagnostic blocks and thereafter obtained good outcomes when corticosteroids were injected.[18,23-26] They simply proselytize that corticosteroids work. Unless diagnostic blocks are used, the results of Lilius and associates apply.[58-60] When injected simply for back pain, intraarticular corticosteroids do not work.

Radiofrequency Neurotomy

Radiofrequency neurotomy is a procedure in which pain from a zygapophyseal joint can be relieved by coagulating, percutaneously, the nerves that innervate the joint. It, too, is a treatment with a checkered past.

It was originally described as facet denervation,[62-66] and astounding results were claimed for it.[67-82] But anatomic studies showed that there were no nerves where the electrode was placed.[83,84] Yet, this did not dissuade some operators who continued to use the discredited technique,[85,86] even in controlled trials.[87]

Anatomic studies showed that the articular branches to the zygapophyseal joints could not be selectively coagulated, but their parent nerves, the medial branches of the dorsal rami, could be.[83,84] Because these nerves ran a constant course across the root of the transverse process at each segmental level, electrodes placed on that bony landmark could be relied on to incur the target nerve. These realizations converted the procedure from facet denervation to lumbar medial branch neurotomy.[83,84]

By using the modified surgical anatomy, some studies claimed good success.[88,89] But even that technique was flawed. A laboratory study showed that electrodes do not coagulate distally from their tip.[90] Therefore, an electrode placed perpendicular to the course of the nerve would not reliably coagulate it. The electrodes coagulate circumferentially, that is, sideways. Therefore, to coagulate the nerve, the electrode must be placed parallel to it.

This explanation has not been heeded. Operators still insist on placing electrodes perpendicular or semiperpendicular to the target nerve, in the manner in which block needles are introduced onto the nerve.[91-94] Doing so limits the chances of coagulating the nerve thoroughly. If the nerve is incompletely coagulated, relief of pain may not occur. If only a short length of nerve is coagulated, relief of pain may be only brief in duration. Accurate technique is paramount.

One controlled study used an invalid technique.[91] It found that active treatment was not more effective than sham treatment. Indeed, the results of active treatment were worse than

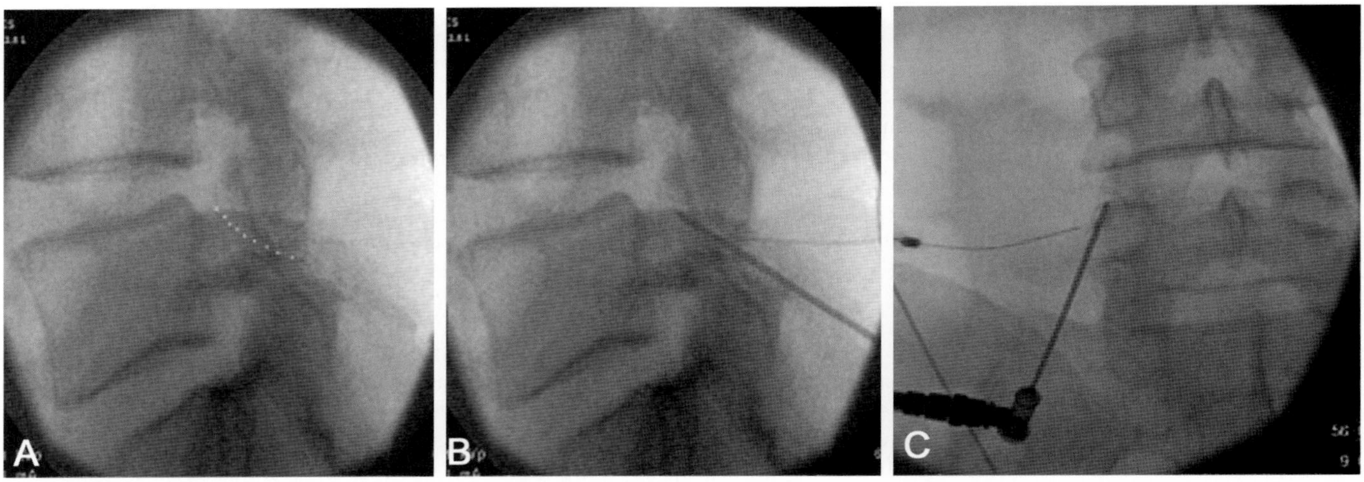

FIGURE 84–4 ■ Lumbar radiofrequency neurotomy. **A,** Lateral view of the target zone, on which the course of the medial branch has been depicted. **B,** Lateral view of the electrode in place, parallel to and on the nerve. **C,** Anteroposterior view of the electrode, inserted obliquely from below, in order to lie parallel to the nerve.

those of sham treatment. More significantly, however, no patient obtained any appreciable relief. This result is not surprising given the operative technique used. In effect, this study compared one sham against another and did not constitute a valid test of lumbar medial branch neurotomy.

Another controlled study used a suboptimal technique but fortuitously was able to obtain short-lasting results.[95] It was not a proper test of how well medial branch neurotomy works or can work, but it did show convincingly that the effects were not due to placebo.

Only one published study has used an anatomically correct technique in correctly selected patients (Fig. 84–4).[96] It establishes the benchmark of how effective lumbar medial branch neurotomy can be. All patients had to have near-complete relief of pain after diagnostic blocks on two occasions. All were treated with the electrode placed parallel to the target nerve. Postoperative electromyography proved that the nerves had been coagulated. At 12 months follow-up some 80% of patients still had at least 60% relief of their pain and some 60% of patients still had 80% relief.

For lumbar medial branch neurotomy to work, the patients must have zygapophyseal joint pain. The procedure is not indicated simply for undiagnosed back pain. Patients must obtain complete, or near complete, relief of their pain when the medial branches of the target joint are anesthetized. Moreover, the diagnostic blocks must be controlled.

For lumbar medial branch neurotomy to work, correct technique must be used. Placing electrodes perpendicular to the target nerves risks not coagulating the nerve or coagulating it only partially. If the nerve is missed, no relief will occur. If the nerve is only partially coagulated, partial relief will occur. If only a limited length of nerve is coagulated, the duration of relief will be limited. For optimal and lasting results, the electrode must be placed parallel to the nerve.

Medial branch neurotomy is not a permanent cure. The nerve coagulated will regenerate. Pain will recur. In that event, however, the procedure can be repeated and relief restored. A study reported in 2004 by Schoffrman and Kine[97] shows that, in patients whose pain recurs after an initially successful neurotomy, repeating the treatment restores relief and that two, three, and even four repetitions continue to provide relief. The median duration of relief after each repetition is just short of a calendar year.

■ CONCLUSION

An irony applies. Lumbar zygapophyseal joint pain is one of the best-studied and best-validated entities in the specialty of pain medicine. At the same time it is one of the most abused. Few other conditions have an established anatomic basis, have a validated diagnostic test, and have a treatment that can abolish the pain. Yet, so few practitioners practice according to the evidence. They do not use diagnostic blocks. They do not use controlled blocks to ensure that their diagnosis is valid. They use treatments that do not work, yet ignore treatments that do. They claim to use a procedure that has been proven to work but use the wrong technique. It is hard to find another realm of medicine in which there is so much dissonance between science and practice.

It is no wonder, therefore, that insurers and others are so opposed to lumbar facet syndrome and its management. They are justified in being opposed to what is practiced, but they are not justified in opposing the science. Unfortunately, those who follow the science responsibly are compromised by those who ignore it. Lack of recognition of lumbar facet syndrome is not a scientific issue; it is a social one, in which the lack of responsibility and discipline by medical practitioners is to blame.

References

1. Helbig T, Lee CK: The lumbar facet syndrome. Spine 13:61, 1988.
2. Revel ME, Listrat VM, Chevalier XJ, et al: Facet joint block for low back pain: Identifying prediction of a good response. Arch Phys Med Rehabil 73:824, 1992.
3. Schwarzer AC, Derby R, Aprill CN, et al: Pain from the lumbar zygapophyseal joints: A test of two models. J Spinal Disord 7:331, 1994.
4. Schwarzer AC, Aprill CN, Derby R, et al: Clinical features of patients with pain stemming from the lumbar zygapophyseal joints. Is the lumbar facet syndrome a clinical entity? Spine 19:1132-1137, 1994.

5. Schwarzer AC, Wang S, Bogduk N, et al: Prevalence and clinical features of lumbar zygapophyseal joint pain: A study in an Australian population with chronic low back pain. Ann Rheum Dis 54:100, 1995.
6. Revel M, Poiraudeau S, Auleley GR, et al: Capacity of the clinical picture to characterize low back pain relieved by facet joint anesthesia: Proposed criteria to identify patients with painful facet joints. Spine 23:1972, 1998.
7. Bogduk N, Wilson AS, Tynan W: The human lumbar dorsal rami. J Anat 134:383, 1982.
8. Bogduk N: The innervation of the lumbar spine. Spine 8:286, 1983.
9. Mooney V, Robertson J: The facet syndrome. Clin Orthop 115:149, 1976.
10. McCall IW, Park WM, O'Brien JP: Induced pain referral from posterior elements in normal subjects. Spine 4:441, 1979.
11. Fukui S, Ohseto K, Shiotani M, et al: Distribution of referred pain from the lumbar zygapophyseal joints and dorsal rami. Clin J Pain 13:303, 1997.
12. Windsor RE, King FJ, Roman SJ, et al: Electrical stimulation induced lumbar medial branch referral patterns. Pain Physician 5:347, 2002.
13. Bogduk N: Lumbar dorsal ramus syndrome. Med J Aust 2:537, 1980.
14. Carrera GF: Lumbar facet arthrography and injection in low back pain. Wisc Med J 78:35, 1979.
15. Carrera GF: Lumbar facet joint injection in low back pain and sciatica: Preliminary results. Radiology 137:665, 1980.
16. Carrera GF: Lumbar facet joint injection in low back pain and sciatica: Description of technique. Radiology 137:661, 1980.
17. Carrera GF, Williams AL: Current concepts in evaluation of the lumbar facet joints. CRC Crit Rev Diagn Imag 21:85, 1984.
18. Destouet JM, Gilula LA, Murphy WA, Monsees B: Lumbar facet joint injection: Indication, technique, clinical correlation, and preliminary results. Radiology 145:321, 1982.
19. Dory MA: Arthrography of the lumbar facet joints. Radiology 140:23, 1981.
20. Drevet JG, Chirossel JP, Phelip X: Lombalgies-lomboradiculalgies et articulations vertebrales posterieures. Lyon Med 245:781, 1981.
21. Fairbank JCT, Park WM, McCall IW, O'Brien JP: Apophyseal injection of local anesthetic as a diagnostic aid in primary low-back pain syndromes. Spine 6:598, 1981.
22. Glover JR: Arthrography of the joints of the lumbar vertebral arches. Orthop Clin North Am 8:37, 1977.
23. Lau LSW, Littlejohn GO, Miller MH: Clinical evaluation of intra-articular injections for lumbar facet joint pain. Med J Aust 143:563, 1985.
24. Lewinnek GE, Warfield CA: Facet joint degeneration as a cause of low back pain. Clin Orthop 213:216, 1986.
25. Lippit AB: The facet joint and its role in spine pain: Management with facet joint injections. Spine 9:746, 1984.
26. Lynch MC, Taylor JF: Facet joint injection for low back pain. J Bone Joint Surg Br 68:138, 1986.
27. Moran R, O'Connell D, Walsh MG: The diagnostic value of facet joint injections. Spine 12:1407, 1986.
28. Murtagh FR: Computed tomography and fluoroscopy guided anaesthesia and steroid injection in facet syndrome. Spine 13:686, 1988.
29. Raymond J, Dumas J-M: Intra-articular facet block: Diagnostic test or therapeutic procedure? Radiology 151:333, 1984.
30. Raymond J Dumas J-M, Lisbona R: Nuclear imaging as a screening test for patients referred for intra-articular facet block. J Can Assist Radiol 35:291, 1984.
31. Schwarzer AC, Derby R, Aprill CN, et al: The value of the provocation response in lumbar zygapophyseal joint injections. Clin J Pain 10:309, 1994.
32. Dreyfuss P, Schwarzer AC, Lau P, Bogduk N: Specificity of lumbar medial branch and L5 dorsal ramus blocks: A computed tomographic study. Spine 22:895, 1997.
33. Bogduk N: The lumbar mamilloaccessory ligament: Its anatomical and neurosurgical significance. Spine 6:162, 1981.
34. Kaplan M, Dreyfuss P, Halbrook B, Bogduk N: The ability of lumbar medial branch blocks to anesthetize the zygapophyseal joint. Spine 23:1847, 1998.
35. Schwarzer AC, Aprill CN, Derby R, et al: The false-positive rate of uncontrolled diagnostic blocks of the lumbar zygapophyseal joints. Pain 58:195, 1994.
36. Manchikanti L, Pampati V, Fellows B, Bakhit CE: Prevalence of lumbar facet joint pain in chronic low back pain. Pain Physician 2:59, 1999.
37. Manchikanti L, Pampati V, Fellows B, Bakhit CE: The diagnostic validity and therapeutic value of lumbar facet joint nerve blocks with or without adjuvant agents. Curr Rev Pain 4:337, 2000.
38. Barnsley L, Lord S, Bogduk N: Comparative local anaesthetic blocks in the diagnosis of cervical zygapophyseal joint pain. Pain 55:99, 1993.
39. Lord SM, Barnsley L, Bogduk N: The utility of comparative local anaesthetic blocks versus placebo-controlled blocks for the diagnosis of cervical zygapophyseal joint pain. Clin J Pain 11:208, 1995.
40. Bogduk N, Holmes S: Controlled zygapophyseal joint blocks: The travesty of cost-effectiveness. Pain Med 1:25, 2000.
41. Manchikanti L, Pampati V, Fellows B, Baha AG: The inability of the clinical picture to characterize pain from facet joints. Pain Physician 3:158, 2000.
42. Bogduk N: Commentary on the capacity of the clinical picture to characterize low back pain relieved by facet joint anesthesia. Pain Med J Club J 4:221, 1998.
43. Eisenstein SM, Parry CR: The lumbar facet arthrosis syndrome. J Bone Joint Surg Br 69:3, 1987.
44. Bough B, Thakore J, Davies M, Dowling F: Degeneration of the lumbar facet joints: Arthrography and pathology. J Bone Joint Surg Br 72:275, 1990.
45. Lawrence JS, Bremner JM, Bier F: Osteoarthrosis: Prevalence in the population and relationship between symptoms and x-ray changes. Ann Rheum Dis 25:1, 1966.
46. Magora A, Schwartz A: Relation between the low back pain syndrome and x-ray findings: I. Degenerative osteoarthritis. Scand J Rehab Med 8:115, 1976.
47. Schwarzer AC, Wang S, O'Driscoll D, et al: The ability of computed tomography to identify a painful zygapophyseal joint in patients with chronic low back pain. Spine 20:907, 1995.
48. Taylor JR, Twomey LT, Corker M: Bone and soft tissue injuries in postmortem lumbar spines. Paraplegia 28:119, 1990.
49. Twomey LT, Taylor JR, Taylor MM: Unsuspected damage to lumbar zygapophyseal (facet) joints after motor vehicle accidents. Med J Aust 151:210, 1989.
50. Sims-Williams H, Jayson MIV, Baddely H: Small spinal fractures in back patients. Ann Rheum Dis 37:262, 1978.
51. Lawrence JS, Sharp J, Ball J, Bier F: Rheumatoid arthritis of the lumbar spine. Ann Rheum Dis 23:205, 1964.
52. Roberts WA: Pyogenic vertebral osteomyelitis of a lumbar facet joint with associated epidural abscess. Spine 12:948, 1988.
53. Rush J, Griffiths J: Suppurative arthritis of a lumbar facet joint. J Bone Joint Surg Br 71:161, 1989.
54. Chevalier X, Marty M, Larget-Piet B: *Klebsiella pneumoniae* septic arthritis of a lumbar facet joint. J Rheumatol 19:1817, 1992.
55. Rousselin B, Gires F, Vallee C, Chevrot A: Case report 617. Skeletal Radiol 19:453, 1990.
56. Campbell AJ, Wells IP: Pigmented villonodular synovitis of a lumbar vertebral facet joint. J Bone Joint Surg Am 64:145, 1982.
57. Titelbaum DS, Rhodes CH, Brooks JSJ, Goldberg HI: Pigmented villonodular synovitis of a lumbar facet joint. Am J Nucl Rad 13:164, 1992.
58. Lilius G, Harilainen A, Laasonen EM, Myllynen P: Chronic unilateral back pain: Predictors of outcome of facet joint injections. Spine 15:780, 1990.
59. Lilius G, Laasonen EM, Myllynen P, et al: Lumbar facet joint syndrome: A randomised clinical trial. J Bone Joint Surg Br 71:681, 1989.
60. Lilius G, Laasonen EM, Myllynen P, et al: Lumbar facet joint syndrome: Significance of non-organic signs: A randomized placebo-controlled clinical study. Rev Chir Orthop Reparatric Appar Mot 75:493, 1989.
61. Carette S, Marcoux S, Truchon R, et al: A controlled trial of corticosteroid injections into facet joints for chronic low back pain. N Engl J Med 325:1002, 1991.
62. Shealy CN: Facets in back and sciatic pain. Minn Med 57:199, 1974.
63. Shealy CN: The role of the spinal facets in back and sciatic pain. Headache 14:101, 1974.
64. Shealy CN: Technique for Percutaneous Spinal Facet Rhizotomy. Burlington, MA, Radionics, 1974.
65. Shealy CN: Percutaneous radiofrequency denervation of spinal facets. J Neurosurg 43:448, 1975.
66. Shealy CN: Facet denervation in the management of back sciatic pain. Clin Orthop 115:157, 1976.
67. Banerjee T, Pittman HH: Facet rhizotomy: Another armamentarium for treatment of low backache. N C Med J 37:354, 1976.
68. Burton CV: Percutaneous radiofrequency facet denervation. Appl Neurophysiol 39:80, 1976/1977.
69. Fassio B, Bouvier JP, Ginestie JF: Denervation articulaire posterieure percutanée et chirurgicale: Sa place dans le traitement des lombalgies. Rev Chir Orthop 67(Suppl II):131, 1980.

70. Florez G, Erias J, Ucar S: Percutaneous rhizotomy of the articular nerve of Luschka for low back and sciatic pain. Acta Neurochir Suppl 24:67, 1977.
71. Fuentes E: La neurotomia apofisaria transcutanea en el tratamento de la lumbalgia cronica. Rev Med Chile 106:440, 1978.
72. McCulloch JA: Percutaneous radiofrequency lumbar rhizolysis (rhizotomy). Appl Neurophysiol 39:87, 1976/1977.
73. McCulloch JA, Organ LW: Percutaneous radiofrequency lumbar rhizolysis (rhizotomy). Can Med Assoc J 116:30, 1977.
74. Mehta M, Sluijter ME: The treatment of chronic back pain. Anaesthesia 34:768, 1979.
75. Oudenhoven RC: Articular rhizotomy. Surg Neurol 2:275, 1974.
76. Oudenhoven RC: Paraspinal electromyography following facet rhizotomy. Spine 2:299, 1977.
77. Oudenhoven RC: The role of laminectomy, facet rhizotomy and epidural steroids. Spine 4:145, 1979.
78. Pawl RP: Results in the treatment of low back syndrome from sensory neurolysis of lumbar facets (facet rhizotomy) by thermal coagulation. Proc Inst Med Chgo 30:150, 1974.
79. Schaerer JP: Radiofrequency facet rhizotomy in the treatment of chronic neck and low back pain. Int Surg 63:53, 1978.
80. Sluijter ME: Percutaneous Thermal Lesions in the Treatment of Back and Neck Pain. Radionics Procedure Technique Series. Burlington, MA, Radionics, 1981.
81. Sluijter ME, Mehta M: Treatment of chronic back and neck pain by percutaneous thermal lesions. In Lipton S, Miles J (eds): Persistent Pain: Modern Methods of Treatment. London, Academic Press, 1981, vol 3, pp 141-179.
82. Uyttendaele D, Verhamme J, Vercauteren M: Local block of lumbar facet joints and percutaneous radiofrequency denervation: Preliminary results. Acta Orthop Belg 47:135, 1981.
83. Bogduk N, Long DM: The anatomy of the so-called "articular nerves" and their relationship to facet denervation in the treatment of low back pain. J Neurosurg 51:172, 1979.
84. Bogduk N, Long DM: Percutaneous lumbar medial branch neurotomy: A modification of facet denervation. Spine 5:193, 1980.
85. Andersen KH, Mosdal C, Vaernet K: Percutaneous radiofrequency facet denervation in low-back and extremity pain. Acta Neurochir 87:48, 1987.
86. Cho J, Parl Y, Chung SS: Percutaneous radiofrequency lumbar facet rhizotomy in mechanical low back pain syndrome. Stereotact Funct Neurosurg 68:212, 1997.
87. Gallagher J, Petriccione di Valdo PL, Wedley JR, et al: Radiofrequency facet joint denervation in the treatment of low back pain: A prospective controlled double-blind study to assess its efficacy. Pain Clinic 7:193, 1994.
88. Ogsbury JS, Simon RH, Lehman RAW: Facet denervation in the treatment of low back syndrome. Pain 3:257, 1977.
89. Rashbaum RF: Radiofrequency facet denervation: A treatment alternative in refractory low back pain with or without leg pain. Orthop Clin North Am 14:569, 1983.
90. Bogduk N, Macintosh J, Marsland A: Technical limitations to the efficacy of radiofrequency neurotomy for spinal pain. Neurosurgery 20:529, 1987.
91. Leclaire R, Fortin L, Lambert R, et al: Radiofrequency facet joint denervation in the treatment of low back pain: A placebo-controlled clinical trial to assess efficacy. Spine 26:1411, 2001.
92. Jerosch J, Castro WHM, Liljenqvist U: Percutaneous facet coagulation: Indication technique, results, and complications. Neurosurg Clin North Am 7:119, 1996.
93. Wenger CC: Radiofrequency lesions for the treatment of spinal pain. Pain Digest 8:1, 1998.
94. Deen HG, Fenton DF, Lamer TJ: Minimally invasive procedures for disorders of the lumbar spine. Mayo Clin Proc 78:1249-1256, 2003.
95. van Kleef M, Barendse GAM, Kessels A, et al: Randomized trial of radiofrequency lumbar facet denervation for chronic low back pain. Spine 24:1937, 1999.
96. Dreyfuss P, Halbrook B, Pauza K, et al: Efficacy and validity of radiofrequency neurotomy for chronic lumbar zygapophyseal joint pain. Spine 25:1270, 2000.
97. Schofferman J, Kine G: Effectiveness of repeated radiofrequency neurotomy for lumbar facet pain. Spine 29:2471, 2004.

chapter 85

Occupational Back Pain

Brian McGuirk and Nikolai Bogduk

There is an abundant literature on back pain. Most of it, however, is descriptive or anecdotal. Only a small proportion of it constitutes evidence. Occupational back pain may be considered as a particular subset of back pain, defined by its context. It is back pain sustained at work or attributed to injury at work. It is perhaps the largest subset of back pain. It, too, is served by an abundant literature, but ironically an even smaller proportion of that literature constitutes evidence than for back pain in general.

It is not possible to compose a chapter on occupational back pain that is based exclusively on evidence. Too many issues that apply to occupational back pain have simply not been studied scientifically. Therefore, to address this problem we have combined the resources of an occupational physician of some 30 years' standing with those of an academician. We base the chapter on $(EBM)^2$ which is (Experienced-Based Medicine) × (Evidence-Based Medicine).

■ OVERVIEW

Occupational back pain differs from back pain in the general community because it is confounded by extraneous influences (Fig. 85–1). In the occupational setting, the progression of acute back pain to chronic back pain (and preventing the progression) is governed by how it is managed medically, but it is also affected by issues of certification, attribution, and compensation. Indeed, it is a common prejudice that pursuit of financial compensation is the critical driving factor that causes acute back pain to persist and become chronic. An analysis of the literature shows that this is not typically the case.[1-3]

The factors that most affect the outcome of acute occupational back pain are how it is managed medically and how it is certified. When the pain becomes chronic, medical management remains a factor but attribution and compensation arise as confounding issues.

Another perception is that occupational back pain is a growing problem (Fig. 85–2). The number of patients with chronic pain continues to increase. This can be attributed to inadequate or incorrect management of acute back pain. Patients present with fears and misunderstandings that are not properly addressed. Once it becomes chronic, back pain persists because there is no effective treatment or because available treatments that can work are not applied. Meanwhile, authorities battle to suppress the growth of chronic back pain, not by medical means, but by legislating against it or by bringing false witness to bear when disputes reach legal circles.

■ MEDICAL MANAGEMENT

The medical management of occupational back pain should be no different from that of back pain in general. From a biologic perspective, back pain occurring at work should, by and large, be no different from back pain sustained in the general community. Therefore, in the first instance, the literature on back pain in general can be applied to the management of occupational back pain specifically. Care needs to be taken, however, to distinguish acute from chronic back pain. The two differ in their biology; the evidence concerning each is distinctly different, and the treatment of each is different.

Acute Low Back Pain

For the management of acute low back pain, multiple evidence-based guidelines are available.[4,5] Some have been formulated specifically in the context of occupational back pain.[6-8] These guidelines are uniform in their recommendations. They emphasize that patients should be assessed foremost for possible, but rare serious causes of back pain, the so-called red flag conditions. To this end, we have devised a compact checklist (Fig. 85–3) that addresses all the possible indicators for red flag conditions.[9] If the patient answers "no" to all of the questions, the practitioner can be more than reasonably assured that the patient does not have a serious cause for the back pain and no further investigations are required. Answering "yes" does not necessarily imply a serious cause but invites the practitioner to explore what is suggested by the positive response. The checklist has been tested and found to be effective and efficient in clinical practice.[10]

In particular, routine medical imaging, especially plain radiography, is not indicated. The indications for medical imaging are specific and explicit. Plain radiographs are indicated only in patients at risk of having had a fracture. These risks are severe trauma and the possibility of pathologic fracture because of either metastases or osteoporosis in the elderly or in patients taking corticosteroids.[11] For other conditions plain radiography is not indicated. As a screening test for tumors or infections, the investigation of choice is magnetic resonance imaging (MRI) because of its high sensitivity and specificity for these conditions.[11] However, MRI is indicated only if the red flag assessment reveals clinical indicators of a possible serious disorder. For patients with acute low back pain, MRI is not indicated "just in case."

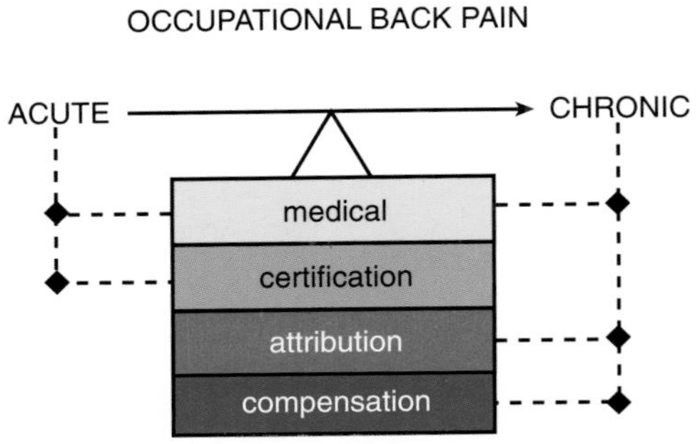

FIGURE 85–1 ■ Extraneous factors that confound assessment for occupational back pain. The links show where particular factors are most influential.

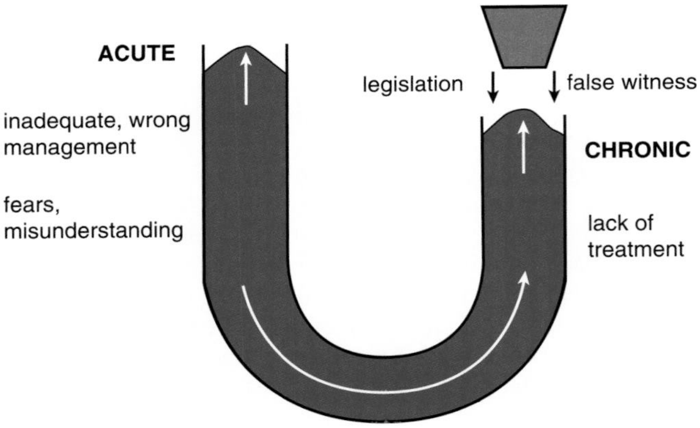

FIGURE 85–2 ■ The U-tube of occupational back pain. Patients with acute back pain present with fears and misunderstandings but are subjected to inadequate or wrong management. Like an increased pressure, an increased number of poorly managed patients with acute pain drives an increase in the number with chronic pain. Treatment for those patients is lacking. Meanwhile, authorities try to stem the rise in chronic pain by legislative measures and by false witness.

Once red flags have been excluded, the guidelines emphasize that medical assessment should be thorough. This requires exploration of the patient's beliefs and fears about the pain. Those fears and beliefs need to be addressed as much as, if not more than, the more conventional medical aspects of the problem. Unfortunately, this domain of the patient's problem is commonly neglected. In one audit of workers' compensation patients, only 28% of reports made any mention of psychosocial factors; the assessments were poor, and in fewer than half of the cases was any action taken.[12]

In the context of occupational back pain, those fears and beliefs may pertain to work. Patients who have been injured at work may blame work at large, rather than the specific accident, for their problem. They may fear a recurrence of the accident. They may fear that continuing to work will make their condition worse. Because of their propensity to impede full rehabilitation, these fears and beliefs need to be addressed.

For management, the guidelines recommend explanation, assurance, and activation as the key components of management. Passive interventions are discouraged. Bed rest is to be avoided, and it can be explained to patients that it has been shown that bed rest is less effective than remaining active and that those who retire to bed have pain for longer periods and are less likely to recover than those who remain active.[13,14]

Simple analgesics may be used for pain relief. Nonsteroidal antiinflammatory drugs are not indicated. For the relief of pain they are no more effective than placebo.[15] Simple exercises may be used to encourage and maintain movement, but formal or named exercises are not required.[16]

Several studies have now shown that such measures are effective. Indahl and colleagues[17,18] showed that a single, prolonged consultation, focusing on fears and activation, was enough to double the return-to-work rate. Others[19] confirmed this. Our own study showed that complete recovery could be achieved in over 70% of patients simply by providing explanation, assurance, and support.[10]

A comprehensive plan of management, and instructions on how to pursue one, cannot be explained in a single chapter in a textbook. Readers interested in descriptions, explana-

Name:						**Low Back Pain**		
D.O.B						M.R.N.		
Presence of			**Cardiovascular**			**Endocrine**		
Trauma	Y	N	Risk factors?	Y	N	Corticosteroids?	Y	N
Night sweats	Y	N	**Respiratory**			**Musculoskeletal**		
Recent surgery	Y	N	Cough?	Y	N	Pain elsewhere?	Y	N
Catheterization	Y	N	**Urinary**			**Neurological**		
Venipuncture	Y	N	UTI?	Y	N	Symptoms/signs	Y	N
Occupational	Y	N	Hematuria?	Y	N	**Skin**		
Hobby exposure	Y	N	Retention?	Y	N	Infections?	Y	N
Sporting exposure	Y	N	Stream problems?	Y	N	Rashes?	Y	N
(Overseas) travel	Y	N	**Reproductive**			**G.I.T.**		
Illicit drug use	Y	N	Menstrual	Y	N	Diarrhea?	Y	N
Weight loss	Y	N	**Hematopoietic**			**Signature:**		
History of cancer	Y	N	Problems?	Y	N			
Comments						**Date:**		

FIGURE 85–3 ■ A checklist for red flag clinical indicators, suitable for inclusion in medical records used in general practice. (From Bogduk N, McGuirk B: Medical Management of Acute and Chronic Low Back Pain: An Evidence-Based Approach. Elsevier, Amsterdam, 2002, with permission.)

tions, and justifications of an evidence-based algorithm or in instructions as to how to implement a management plan should consult sources where this is described.[20]

Prompt return to work is an imperative. It has been shown that patients who return to work, or remain at work, recover sooner and have fewer recurrences.[7,8] The longer patients spend off work the less chance they have of recovering.[7] This can, and should, be explained to patients as part of their management. Most patients are able to return to work.[7,8] Most will comply with advice to return to work and will remain at work.[7,21]

But return to work is not simply a matter of ordering the patient to do so. *Return to work is achieved by identifying barriers and helping the patient overcome them.*

Pertinent in this regard is workplace intervention. It has been shown that adding a worksite visit to the management improves outcomes.[22] It results in reduced absence from work, faster return to work, less disability, less sickness impact, and reduced pain. The effects are greater, and statistically significant, when clinical intervention is combined with occupational intervention than when occupational intervention or clinical intervention is used in isolation.

Significantly, workplace intervention is not tantamount to ergonomic intervention. By and large, formal ergonomic intervention has not been vindicated by research studies. Rather, worksite intervention is a psychosocial intervention.

Not every patient who presents with acute low back pain will have a problem with work. Once the patient has been properly assessed, has had the condition explained, and has been empowered with a plan of management, some patients can resume their normal work. Others may do so tentatively and be surprised, yet relieved, that they can successfully resume work.

For other patients, matters pertaining to work may be important factors in delaying or preventing rehabilitation. The possible problems can range from inappropriate beliefs and fears on the part of the patient to clearly unsafe and even outrageous work practices that oppressively are imposed on the patient. Whether or not serious workplace issues obtain in a particular case is a matter of judgment on the part of the practitioner and the patient but *can only be determined if work is examined* in a concerted manner during the consultations with the patient.

In assessing work matters, a practitioner may be at a significant disadvantage if he or she does not really understand what is involved in a particular job. Without a knowledge of the workplace, the practitioner may appear foolish or elitist to the patient and, therefore, unconvincing when giving advice (e.g., "what would you know?"). Uninformed advice just to be careful tends to promote fear, avoidance, and invalidism. Specific ergonomic instruction is probably neither required nor valid. Instead, the practitioner could ask what the job involves and learn from the patient. With the patient he or she could reconstruct the workstation and mimic the worker's activities. It would be better still if the practitioner was actually familiar with the work practices by having visited the workplace, if not having experienced the work practices. With some insight into what the worker does, the practitioner can assist by explaining how the worker can be sensible in executing tasks.

Rural practitioners may well be better able to engage in workplace intervention. If they are faced with large or regular numbers of patients with back pain, it would be profitable for them to become familiar with the various worksites of their patients. Not only does this provide them with familiarity with the sites and their practices, but it also establishes social contact with management, which can be of advantage should the need arise for the practitioner to intervene on behalf of a patient. When advocacy is required, it is potentially impressive and reassuring to the patient when it emerges, in the course of a consultation, that the practitioner knows not only what the job entails but also the key personnel.

For urban practitioners this may not be practicable. Their patients may work far afield, and the practitioner may not be able to have visited and experienced all the possible worksites of their patients. Beyond learning what they can about the job from the patient, the urban practitioner may need to collaborate with a colleague or specialist practitioner trained in occupational medicine, if concerted workplace intervention is required.

The workplace intervention should not be misrepresented or misconstrued as an adversarial occupational health and safety visit. Rather, it involves several overt and subtle dimensions.

Foremost, the patient's practitioner, or a surrogate representative (e.g., rehabilitation provider, occupational therapist), should become familiar with the patient's work and work environment, so that he or she can help the patient return to work in an informed and insightful manner.

Second, on behalf of the worker, the practitioner can negotiate with the employer:

- Any amendments to the workplace specifically to prevent recurrences of accidents of the type in which the worker may have been injured
- Modifications to the workplace otherwise to prevent or avoid recurrences of back pain problems
- Mutually acceptable modified duties that allow the worker to return to work and therein feel welcome

Guidelines for the management of occupational back pain emphasize that communication and cooperation between workers, supervisors, managers, and the primary care provider are fundamental to successful outcome.[7]

Third, the practitioner can be seen to have been the patient's advocate. In this regard, it is not so much what the practitioner does in terms of actual ergonomic changes but that he or she is seen to have done something. While the full implications of this dimension have never been evaluated, its power should not be underestimated, given the extent to which fear of work and dissatisfaction with the workplace are prognostic of poor outcome.

A pragmatic review[23] has emphasized the virtue and importance of modified duties (as opposed to so-called light duties). Such duties consist of appropriately modified work according to the injured worker's physical capacity, developed in the context of sympathetic communication with the worker, and nonadversarial handling of the claim from workers' compensation. A critical issue in this regard is to return the worker to his or her preinjury job, as far as possible, with restrictions if required, rather than assigning the patient to different and usually more menial duties. Moreover, it is recommended that a supportive workplace response to injury needs to start when the pain is first reported and that an individualized and accommodative approach to return to work should follow promptly.[23] Such measures can reduce both the incidence and the duration of disability resulting in time lost from work by up to 50%.[23]

Understated in the literature is the significance of return to work for the dignity of the patient. By not returning to work, not only does the patient risk becoming a chronic invalid but he or she loses personal dignity and the social recognition of peers. Off work, the patient is alone and isolated and risks becoming a victim of an impersonal and impassionate system that controls his or her life. As an object, the patient is directed from assessment to assessment, from treatment to treatment, and no longer has control of his or her destiny. Some patients come to feel that they are treated like criminals who are required to prove their innocence. All of these factors sow the seeds for depression and resentment.

Equally important in this respect is the type of work that is provided. When a patient is physically unable to return to preinjury duties, it is nevertheless important that he or she feels that they are contributing. Being given what is obvious to the patient and others, especially work colleagues, as being nothing more than a "made-up" job (e.g., counting paper clips) is demeaning, particularly when the reason for such an approach is purely to minimize workers' compensation costs and/or to keep some specious safety record intact. Doing so is almost certainly guaranteed to result in the patient's taking time off work.

Guidelines and reviews recommend that if acute pain persists and becomes subacute (i.e., lasting longer than 7 weeks), the patient should be referred to a multidisciplinary rehabilitation program that can provide workplace intervention.[7,8] Indeed, the evidence shows that such programs are not indicated and are not effective for patients with acute back pain[24] but are demonstrably effective for patients with subacute pain.[25,26] This line of action, however, is not the only one, for it has been shown that the same outcomes can be achieved by a single practitioner, provided that the practitioner provides good treatment.[17-19] The key factor is that the intervention must be closely related to the workplace or be tied explicitly to the specific goal of return to work.[23]

Euphemistic Back Pain

Patients with occupational back pain are often misrepresented, with accusations or suspicions of being malingerers. Malingering is rare, probably less than 5%.[27] But some patients present ostensibly with back pain but for other reasons. They are not actually malingering; they are not being fraudulent. Euphemistic back pain is a considerate neologism without prejudice that can be applied to such patients.

These patients do, indeed, have back pain, but their back pain is not the true reason that they present. Under other circumstances, their pain would not be of sufficient gravity to seek medical care. Rather, these patients have another agenda, and use their back pain euphemistically to seek attention. They may be dissatisfied with their employer or supervisor, or they may be dissatisfied with their job. They may have a social problem at work that they feel that they are unable to solve. They use a complaint of back pain as a potential means of escaping their dissatisfaction. Viewed another way, they are calling for intervention on matters that they are not directly espousing.

Rather than simply asking a series of questions purporting to address these issues, the "secret" is to LISTEN to the patient. Why did the patient present? What are his or her expectations? For the back pain, most are looking for reassurance that nothing is seriously wrong and having received that advice they seek a "quick fix." They usually have their own perceptions as to what constitutes appropriate management, often obtained, in this day and age, from information available on the Internet. Their interpretation of this information varies widely and often necessitates further appropriate explanation and advice.

Unfortunately, but in reality, this takes TIME. It is most unlikely that patients will volunteer any of the so-called psychosocial issues at the first consultation unless they are relaxed and comfortable and are presenting to their own general practitioner. They perceive these issues to be of a personal nature and (usually) do not realize their implications. When the general practitioner is harassed and unable or unwilling to spend time with the patient, these issues are rarely discussed, and thus the seeds of chronicity are sown at an early stage.

All is not lost, however. Often certain key words or points are volunteered that can be acted on by an alert physician. In this regard they might be considered as the equivalent, at the history stage of the consultation, to the Waddell signs (see later). They all invite consideration and management of what amounts to the parallel or hidden agenda. Examples include:

- An unsupportive work environment (e.g., " I came to see you because my supervisor didn't believe me when I told him/her that I had developed back pain and wouldn't consider giving me some less strenuous activities.")
- A perception/belief that work is harmful or that all pain must be abolished before attempting to return to work (e.g., "I need time off work because until my pain has settled if I try to continue working I can only make things worse.")
- Catastrophizing usually associated with fear-avoidance and other behaviors (e.g., "I told them at work that the job was too heavy, but they wouldn't listen. Now my back is so bad I won't be able to work again. I can't do anything because the pain is so bad, and when I try it only makes the pain worse. I've been to the pharmacy and the painkillers don't help. All I do is lie around, but this doesn't help either. I can't sleep unless I have several beers.")
- Personal issues (e.g., "Doctor, is it serious? My mother developed back pain and eventually they diagnosed cancer and she only lasted 3 months.")
- Overprotective spouse/avoidance of normal activity (e.g., "I brought my partner along so he/she could help me. I don't know what I would do without him/her. He/she does everything for me so I can rest.")

By no means is this list intended to be complete, but it represents some of the issues that can become evident in the course of a consultation where the patient has the opportunity to voice these concerns.

Very significant can be the patient who says very little, responds to direct questions in monosyllables, and often is disheveled, with lack of personal grooming. Almost invariably these patients are severely depressed and may indicate an unrelated (and often undiagnosed) psychiatric disorder, which has been heightened by the back injury.

If these patients are recognized, medical management can be channeled toward dealing with the psychosocial problems that the patient harbors and, one hopes, reveals upon inquiry. Doing so addresses the real problem instead of mistakenly trusting that treating the back pain will solve the problem. Whether the psychosocial problem can be resolved depends on the individual circumstances. But failing to recognize these problems, or ignoring them, eliminates any chance of resolving the problem in those cases where it is solvable. Furthermore, not recognizing these patients and channeling them into conventional management simply adds to the population of medicalized patients who will not, and do not, recover.

CERTIFICATION

Certification is the earliest of several processes that distinguish occupational back pain from back pain in the general community. Although specific requirements differ in different countries, states, and provinces, some form of certification is usually required for a patient who presents with occupational back pain.

The most innocuous form of paperwork is certification required simply to record the case, essentially for archival or administrative purposes. Recording an event should not interfere with medical management or with prognosis. The practitioner remains free to implement a plan of management as he or she would for a patient for whom no paperwork is required.

Yet even this seemingly innocuous exercise can be hazardous. Practitioners need to take care how they label the patient. Certain diagnostic labels are not only incorrect but they also can be disturbing to patients.[28,29] "Disk degeneration" may seem an accepted rubric to fellow practitioners, but to some patients it evokes images of inexorable deterioration. This is not compatible with assurances of prompt recovery. "Instability" conveys connotations of fragility and possible catastrophe. It is not compatible with encouragement to resume normal activities. "Arthritis" implies an incurable chronic condition. It is not compatible with rapid recovery. Although used with impunity within the medical profession, these terms are potentially alarming to patients and may compromise a rehabilitation plan. Moreover, they should not be used because none is a legitimate diagnosis. There is no merit in using false terms whose only effect is the potential to engender or reinforce fears.

No universally accepted, alternative labels have been developed for a diagnosis of nonspecific back pain. Even that term potentially conveys an impression that the doctor does not know the cause and, therefore, might not be competent or sufficiently interested. As an offer in this regard, we have proposed a unique and challenging set of terms. We propose "red back pain" for conditions associated with red flag indicators. We use "yellow back pain" for pain associated with evident psychosocial features. We use "green back pain" for back pain about which the patient should have no concerns and through which they can proceed with confidence. We have explained and justified these terms elsewhere and demonstrate how they can be explained to patients.[29]

Under some administrations, certification can mean providing a management plan. Completing the paperwork may be tedious but should not interfere with good medical management. The report should simply state what the plan of management is going to be. Efficient practitioners might prepare a generic plan on a word processor, which saves time in preparing plans or reports individually for each new patient (see Appendix 85–1). Due consideration, however, must be given to any relevant restrictions required by privacy legislation.

The most vexatious form of certification, however, is the certificate for time off work or for light duties. If these are used injudiciously they can compromise the patient's prognosis and outcome.

Simply giving patients time off work, reflexly, routinely, or because the patient expects it, can be deleterious to prognosis. Practitioners cannot expect, and cannot rely on the presumption, that the passage of time, while the patient is idle, alone, and unsupervised, will cure back pain or solve the patient's problems. Indeed, such a passive intervention is contrary to established evidence concerning the management of back pain and can be outrightly deleterious. Certificates, therefore, should be viewed as potentially toxic to the patient.

All patients should be encouraged and helped to return to work. In most instances they will not require time off work. If time off work is required it should be for explicit and specifiable purposes. Giving patients time off work should be treated in the same manner as admitting a patient to hospital. It is done for a therapeutic purpose. Something that the practitioner prescribes must be done during the time off work, and the patient should be constantly monitored for progress. It becomes an irresponsible, and dangerous, practice when practitioners give patients a certificate for time off work just to get them out of their office; and if this is rationalized on the basis of a perceived need of the patient to rest, it reflects an ignorance of the evidence base.

Related to the writing of certificates is the absurdity of so-called light duties. This concept is absurd on three counts. First, there is no formula available to medicine by which what a patient can and cannot do can be calculated. It is not a professional concept. Anyone who prescribes light duties is inventing them as a layperson. Second, it is a dismissive, not a therapeutic, intervention. Instead of assisting patients to return to work, they are relegated to menial tasks that offend their dignity. In some jurisdictions, workers are returned to the workplace simply to enhance workers' compensation performance data. Yet at the workplace, the worker does nothing and is treated with resentment. The third absurdity is perhaps the most crucial. Most employers simply cannot accommodate employees on light duties. There are no light duties available. Compelling employers to take on such workers breeds resentment and, in practice, often means that the employer sends the patient home.

Not to be confused with light duties is modification of work practices. By negotiation with the employer injured workers can be returned to useful employment if practices can be modified. This might entail retaining the worker in his or her accustomed role but having the worker perform the duties in another way. It might entail reassigning the worker temporarily to other duties while he or she recovers from the episode of back pain. An important and often underestimated facet of this is that by keeping an employee in the preinjury work environment he or she continues to have access to colleagues at work. Reassignment, however, should prospectively be temporary. Progress and recovery should be monitored assiduously, and the worker should return to the former role as soon as able to do so. Not monitoring patients is tantamount to neglect, and the abandoned patient is unlikely to return to his or her former role. Prescribing and monitoring modified activities should be part of the concerted medical intervention. It cannot be left to its own devices. When this intervention appears to fail it is not because it does not intrinsically work. It fails when the patient is not assiduously monitored. It fails when practitioners forget that they put the patient on modified duties and fail to bring them up to conventional duties. It fails when practitioners neglect to titrate and monitor their intervention.

Certification is susceptible to confounding, competing, and interfering influences. A proper and concerted medical plan can be confounded when other doctors, who are less responsible, disagree and provide the patient with certificates for time off work. They can be confounded by friends of the patient providing incorrect and deleterious lay advice. They can be confounded by management, or insurance doctors, not understanding the merits of a proper rehabilitation plan and demanding instant fixes. Under those circumstances it is important that a single physician be responsible for, and in charge of, the patient's management and certification. Some jurisdictions, recognizing the importance of this view, have legislated to include this requirement.[30]

Even so, this may not always be practical. Management by the individual practitioner can be unduly complicated by legislation whereby others (e.g., rehabilitation providers) are given a legal responsibility to be involved in the development of return-to-work plans. The single recourse in this regard is for the practitioner to lead by example. By persevering, the prospect arises that successes will be noticed and that others will support what the practitioner is doing. They can enlist the cooperation of employers by explaining to them the merits of their plan of management. Unfortunately, until that occurs, the practitioner and the patient risk being continually frustrated by interference from other doctors, allied healthcare professionals, insurers, and managers, who do not understand the evidence concerning the management of back pain and prefer to impose their own primitive notions onto the process.

CHRONIC BACK PAIN

When a patient's pain persists, despite good medical management, there is no point persevering with the same interventions. Continuing to ply analgesics and exercises will not suddenly abolish the pain when these measures have not worked to date. Continuing to explore and attempt to modify the patient's fears and beliefs will not suddenly change these attitudes.

On the other hand, if the patient has not been managed well, there is a prospect that implementing good management, albeit late, might still help the patient. It is unfortunate that most patients do not initially receive good management. Much of medical practice for patients with chronic back pain, therefore, amounts to salvaging the patient from the efforts of others.

Nevertheless, even under good management, not all patients recover. Ten to 30% can be expected to have persistent pain.[10] Some of these patients may have only minor pain and no disabilities (e.g., a pain score of only 15 out of 100). They may not require further intervention. Some, however, remain in pain and become disabled by it.

The foremost question is whether the persistence is due to an unrecognized lesion or to psychosocial factors. The tendency, to date, has been to attribute all chronic back pain to psychosocial factors and to neglect medical factors.

The belief in psychosocial factors is founded on epidemiologic data that show that psychosocial factors are poor prognostic factors. It has been a fashion, therefore, to commit patients with chronic back pain to behavioral therapy. However, at the outset, it should be recognized that the epidemiologic data, themselves, account for no more than 30% of the variance between patients who "remain chronic" and those who recover. Some 70% of the variance remains unexplained.[6,7] Psychosocial factors are not the cardinal determinant of chronicity. They are simply the most publicized.

Psychosocial Treatment

Despite, or contrary to, the predictions of psychosocial theories about back pain, psychological treatment has not proved to be the answer. As a sole intervention, behavioral therapy has not proved to be effective.[31] It may have a place as a component in multidisciplinary pain therapy, but even multidisciplinary pain therapy, focusing on education, cognitive therapy, and exercises has not become the solution for chronic back pain. It might be what is currently promoted as the preferred intervention, but it does not produce results.

A recent systematic review[32] found that:

- There is strong evidence that intensive multidisciplinary biopsychosocial rehabilitation with functional restoration improves function when compared with inpatient or outpatient non-multidisciplinary rehabilitation.[33-35]
- There is moderate evidence that intensive multidisciplinary biopsychosocial rehabilitation with functional restoration reduces pain when compared with outpatient non-multidisciplinary rehabilitation or usual care.[33-35]
- There is contradictory evidence regarding vocational outcomes of intensive multidisciplinary biopsychosocial rehabilitation; whereas Bendix and associates[33] reported improvements in "work-readiness," Alaranta and colleagues[35] and Mitchell and coworkers[36] showed no benefit on sickness leave.
- Regarding less intensive multidisciplinary biopsychosocial rehabilitation, five trials could not show improvements in pain, function, or vocational outcomes when compared with non-multidisciplinary outpatient rehabilitation or usual care.[33,37-40]

With respect to the major two of these conclusions, an inspection of the published data provides an insight into the effect size. In the first study of Bendix and associates,[33] the intensive functional restoration program reduced disability from 15.5 on a 30-point scale to 8.5, at 4 months and reduced back pain from 5.3, on a scale of 0 to 10, to 2.7. These would seem to be reasonable improvements, although few patients were rendered pain free or fully rehabilitated.

The second study of Bendix and associates[34] reported more modest gains. Function improved from 16.9 to only 12.1, and pain was reduced from 6.1 to 5.7. Alaranta and colleagues[35] achieved an average reduction in pain of only 17 points on a 100-point scale. With respect to functional capacity, the significant gain reported by these researchers[35] was that a smaller proportion of their index patients suffered back problems during light activities or at rest but there were no differences from control patients with respect to the proportion of patients being pain free or having problems only during moderate activities.

Bendix and associates[33,34] achieved significantly greater reductions in sick leave and contacts with the healthcare system. However, this was not the experience of Alaranta and colleagues[35] or of Mitchell and associates.[36]

Of the studies not covered by systematic reviews, one[41] showed that multidisciplinary management achieved no greater reduction in pain than an untreated control group; the major gains were reduction in use of medication and a 48% return to work. Another[42] found no consistent advantages of multidisciplinary treatment over usual care with respect to pain, but the index patients were slightly more satisfied with their jobs and were slightly less distressed psychologically. However, return-to-work rates were not better.

Practitioners, insurers, and employers should understand what these data show:

- Multidisciplinary, behavioral therapy does not eliminate back pain and does not achieve greater return to work than usual care.
- Psychologically based programs are not effective. They achieve palliative effects in that they may reduce distress and prevent deterioration, but there is no evidence that they restore patients to normal activities, including work. In this regard, they may be appropriate when complete restoration and return to work is not a goal or is considered unachievable.
- Intensive programs focused on exercises are more effective than less intensive programs or programs that focus on behavior. Yet even so, the improvements achieved are limited. Patients can expect to have *less pain* and be able to function *somewhat better,* but their problems are not eliminated. In essence, multidisciplinary treatment is tantamount to palliative care.

Medical and Physical Treatment

Medical treatments, in the form of drug therapies, and physical treatments, in the form of physical therapy, exercises, or manual therapy, are abjectly unsuccessful for the resolution of chronic low back pain.[43,44] Persisting with such interventions when they fail to resolve the patient's problems is intellectually and professionally irresponsible. The only justification for continuing with these interventions might be that they constitute some form of palliative care, but that is not the same as representing them as desirable treatments.

Investigations

Conventional investigations, such as radiography and computed tomography, are inappropriate for chronic low back pain. There is nothing known to cause back pain that such investigations can reveal. The one useful test is MRI.[45]

The foremost role that MRI serves is as a screening test to rule out serious disorders. Of all investigations, MRI is best able to detect or exclude conditions such as occult tumors or indolent infections that have not declared any clinical features by which they might be suspected.

To some extent MRI also has a positive role. It is able to reveal high-intensity zones in the posterior annulus fibrosus of lumbar disks. This sign is uncommon. It occurs in only about 30% of patients with chronic low back pain, but it is highly specific.[45] It is indicative that the affected disk is internally disrupted and painful. Its likelihood ratio in this regard is 6. On average, this likelihood ratio allows practitioners to be 80% certain that the affected disk is the source of the patient's pain.

Invasive Investigations

Although conventional medical imaging cannot reveal the source or cause of pain in most patients with chronic low back pain, other tests can. They are all tests performed with an injection of some form.

Zygapophyseal joint pain can be pursued using controlled diagnostic blocks.[46] Diskogenic pain can be pursued using disk stimulation and diskography.[46] Sacroiliac joint pain can be pursued using intraarticular blocks.[46]

Given the availability of these tests, patients can be investigated to establish the source of their chronic back pain. Pinpointing a diagnosis, at the very least serves to establish that they do, indeed, have a genuine source of pain and refutes the accusation that they are malingering or suffering from psychogenic pain. Pinpointing the source of pain can also serve to direct treatment to that source.

Contrary to the prevailing, but unsubstantiated, notion that 80% of chronic back pain cannot be diagnosed, the opposite holds true. Among patients with chronic low back pain, zygapophyseal joint pain accounts for 10% to 40% (depending on the population); sacroiliac joint pain accounts for some 20%; and internal disk disruption accounts for at least 39%.[46] These sources of pain, however, cannot be determined other than by invasive investigations. Not investigating patients by these means leaves them with an undetermined diagnosis and at the mercy of a system that does not want them to exist.

Precision Treatment

Lumbar zygapophyseal joint pain can be treated with percutaneous lumbar medial branch neurotomy (see Chapter 84).[47] Diskogenic pain can be treated with disk excision and arthrodesis, or perhaps by a variety of percutaneous procedures, such as intradiskal electrothermal therapy (see Chapter 84).[47] Of the known sources of chronic low back pain, the sacroiliac joint is the most difficult to treat. No means of relieving sacroiliac joint pain has been validated. Emerging, however, are various ways of denervating this joint.[47]

ATTRIBUTION

In some jurisdictions, a patient who cannot return to work because of back pain may be entitled to compensation in the form of income replacement or some other financial benefit. In other jurisdictions such provisions do not apply, and patients continue to suffer their pain and are unable to work.

Pivotal to any claim for compensation is attribution. It has to be shown that work was responsible for the patient's problem. In different countries, states, and provinces, the laws differ. In some, all that is required is for the patient to have developed the problem at work. In others, work has to be shown to have been a substantial contributory factor. Much of the process in establishing attribution is legal and is determined by the laws and practices where the case is conducted. From a medical perspective, however, two issues arise: medical opinion that work was the cause and medical opinion that it was not.

In a given case, there is no absolute way in which work can be proved to have been the cause of injury and subsequent back pain. At the time of alleged injury, medical witnesses were not present to perform real-time fluoroscopy, which could demonstrate the biomechanics of injury. Patients are not monitored with regular MRI, which might have demonstrated that a lesion was not present before injury but developed soon after injury.

From a positivist perspective all to which an expert witness could testify is that the patient's clinical features are consistent with an injury having occurred. If the source of pain has been pinpointed by MRI, or by invasive investigations, an expert can testify that the source of pain, or lesion found, is consistent with having been injured at work.

Epidemiologic data can support, but not confirm, such testimony. Epidemiologic studies can demonstrate, in populations, if certain activities or work practices are significantly associated with increased risk of injury or increased incidence of back pain. In this regard, there is an extensive literature (beyond the scope of this chapter). That literature has been reviewed by the Occupational Safety and Health Administration of the U.S. Department of Labor,[48] which found that, overall, many occupations and several occupational activities are significantly associated with a genuine, increased risk of back pain.

A problem with epidemiologic data, however, is that these data cannot be directly applied to individual cases. The fact that there is, on average, an increased risk, does not per se prove that work was responsible for an individual patient's back pain. At best, when the epidemiologic data are positive, they only provide a background of likelihood that work was responsible. On the other hand, if correlations are absent in the epidemiologic data, it becomes harder to sustain the argument that work was responsible. A more direct line of evidence, or argument, is required.

Thus, if heavy lifting, or twisting, has been established as a risk factor for back pain, and if the patient's work has involved sustained heavy lifting or twisting, it can be argued that those activities are likely to have been responsible for the patient's complaint. In this regard, the cardinal occupational risk factors for back pain are[48] heavy physical work (notably in healthcare, manufacturing, or construction), prolonged exposure to heavy work and forward bending, lifting and forceful movements, bending and twisting, and working in a bent position.

Conversely, epidemiologic evidence can be used to refute assertions made pejoratively to discredit patients. In this regard, the legal system has been slow to catch up with scientific evidence. Sometimes, it even prefers to shun that evidence because it disturbs the way in which lawyers and the courts have been accustomed to dealing with claims. Two examples arise.

By word of mouth, spondylolysis and spondylolisthesis are regarded, in some circles, as causes of back pain. Indeed, the AMA Guidelines to evaluation of impairment reward patients with an automatic increase in total person impairment if their radiographs demonstrate spondylolysis or spondylolisthesis.[49] Yet this practice flies in the face of the available evidence. A systematic review of the literature established that, in adults, these conditions are not associated with back pain.[50]

Similar arguments apply to spondylosis. A retort, common from witnesses for insurers, is that work was not responsible for the patient's pain; rather, the person's pain is due to preexisting degenerative joint disease. Such witness is false and is contrived simply to deny claims.

Multiple studies have demonstrated that there is minimal to no association between back pain and spondylosis (Table 85–1).[51-62] The data from individual studies, and the pooled data, yield likelihood ratios barely greater than 1.0 and odds ratios less than 2.0, both of which are neither statistically nor clinically significant. In colloquial terms, one could say that a patient with back pain is only 5% more likely to have degenerative changes than by chance alone. Degenerative changes are normal age changes and do not constitute a diagnosis of the cause of back pain.

Under those conditions, the argument cannot be sustained that a worker's back pain was simply due to preexisting degenerative changes. This argument flies in the face of the available scientific data yet is still, so often, used to deny claims.

COMPENSATION

In different jurisdictions, different entitlements are available to injured workers. Those entitlements may be adjudicated in different ways: by tribunals, judges, or juries. It is neither possible nor appropriate, therefore, to provide an internationally relevant synopsis of these administrative and legal provisions. Nevertheless, certain principles and phenomena are common to all systems.

Compensation was originally devised to support genuinely injured workers who were no longer able to work. The compensation served to replace the income that they had lost so that that they could maintain a livelihood. In a sense, it was a charitable and compassionate benefaction but not a reward for having been injured.

For genuinely injured workers who are permanently disabled, compensation is a reasonable recourse. If society cannot solve their medical problem, it might at least ensure that the worker is not left destitute because he or she cannot work. However, compensation can be abused. Individuals may pursue compensation for reasons other than its intended purpose.

Claimants may be under the misapprehension that compensation is an easy means of securing a cash sum, like winning the lottery, that otherwise in their life they could never expect. Such a sum amounts to a means of escape from the working class. (This can be magnified in rural areas, where often there are limited options for employment and high unemployment rates.) This misapprehension might be reinforced by peers who share that perception.

Claimants may feel aggrieved because they believe that they were innocently injured, and the pursuit of compensation

Table 85–1

Validity of Degenerative Changes on Plain Radiographs as a Diagnosis of Low Back Pain

Degenerative Changes	*Back Pain*		*Sensitivity/Specificity*	*Odds Ratio*	*Likelihood Ratio*	*Ref. No.*
	Present	*Absent*				
Present Absent	130 106	92 142	0.55/1.9	0.61	1.4	51,52
Present Absent	170 66	135 106	0.72/2.0	0.44	1.3	51,52
Present Absent	90 105	61 127	0.46/1.8	0.68	1.4	53
Present Absent	45 151	19 77	0.23/1.2	0.80	1.2	54
Present Absent	115 243	71 237	0.32/1.6	0.77	1.4	55
Present Absent	39 28	42 100	0.58/3.3	0.70	1.9	56
Present Absent	462 320	360 390	0.59/1.6	0.52	1.1	57
Present Absent	55 18	77 45	0.75/1.8	0.37	1.2	58
Present Absent	139 35	51 41	0.80/3.2	0.45	1.5	59
Present Absent	177 41	35 20	0.81/2.5	0.36	1.3	60
Present Absent	217 155	164 53	0.58/0.5	0.24	0.8	61
Present Absent	208 179	102 115	0.54/1.3	0.53	1.2	62
Present Absent	1847 1447	1209 1453	0.56/1.5	0.55	1.2	Pooled

is tantamount to the pursuit of justice. They may feel aggrieved because the system has not fixed their problem. Under those conditions, compensation amounts to a penalty against the system for having failed the worker.

Lawyers may be responsible. Perhaps with the best of intentions, lawyers advise clients of what they are entitled to and encourage them to pursue their maximum entitlements. (Particularly relevant in this respect is where employees in the older age groups, usually those with more menial jobs, who perceive such an approach as a means of supplementing their superannuation entitlements, as well as an "early" retirement.) When lawyers work on commission, questions can be raised about the motivation of lawyers who influence clients to maximize claims.

Each of these factors may be counterproductive to recovery. Workers seeking a windfall will not be motivated to recover; without their pain they cannot lay claim to compensation. Aggrieved workers will not recover, or will deny recovery, until they feel justice has been served. Overtly or indirectly, lawyers may direct their clients to retain their complaint so as to maximize the entitlement.

Unfortunately, no one has determined the extent to which any or all of these factors operate, either to prolong the compensation process or to discourage recovery. Unfortunately as well, each of the cynical reasons for pursuing compensation disenfranchises honest injured workers who have a genuine disability. They find themselves caught in a cynical system that deals with every claim as potentially fraudulent. The genuinely injured worker is then treated as a criminal, with the burden of proof placed on him or her.

It is almost pointless to appeal that more research needs to be conducted in this arena, to determine how often patients are honest or misguided and the extent to which their recovery is impeded by confounding influences. The problem is obvious, but means for its solution are not readily available. We have no test for honesty. The courts are not a substitute, because the outcome of a court case may be as much dependent on successful rhetoric as it is on objective evidence.

There is, however, an avenue that is immediately available. If legal matters, or personal issues such as vengeance, are counterproductive to recovery, they become part of the patient's medical problems. It is possible, and appropriate, therefore, for the treating physician to explore these issues with the patient. Just as they can have mistaken and inappropriate beliefs about the biology of their pain, they may have inappropriate beliefs about compensation. These can be addressed. That is not to say that patients should be dissuaded from seeking compensation. Rather, the patient needs to understand what is involved and to what he or she will be subjected as the claim is pursued. The patient needs to reconcile the extent to which recovery is compromised by the pursuit of a claim. It is with this that the treating doctor can assist. There is no guarantee that addressing these issues will improve the patient's condition, but unless they are explored there is no hope that it will improve.

Unfortunately, many doctors do not appear to be any more aware of these issues and potential implications than are their patients, and it reflects a need for further training. Alternatively, there are some practitioners who choose, based on their own political and social biases, to act as surrogate lawyers not only supporting such approaches but even going as far as to provide obviously biased reports to the legal fraternity in support of their perception of their patient's entitlement. What they fail to recognize, or refuse to acknowledge, are the full ramifications of their actions. In most jurisdictions the "acceptance" of a compensation claim by the courts is no longer the "pot of gold" it may once have been; and once the claim has been settled, and all outstanding accounts (including the lawyer's fees) have been paid, the patient may end up in a parlous state over the long term, with little money, no job, and no prospects.

INNUENDOS

Certain myths pervade the medicolegal system. They are the notions of secondary gain and malingering and the belief that Waddell's tests can detect patients with so-called nonorganic back pain.

Purportedly, patients eligible for compensation fabricate or maintain their back pain to obtain financial gain. Variably, this behavior has been described as secondary gain or malingering. Technically, secondary gain is a reward that the patient obtains as a result of being ill but nevertheless the illness is basically genuine. What cynics argue is that they would not be as ill as claimed if secondary gain was not available. Malingering differs in that the patient is not genuinely ill but invents a false complaint of illness to obtain financial reward.

As applied in clinical practice at large, not by experts, both of these concepts are essentially colloquial and abused. They are terms used to describe patients in a pejorative manner, usually to deny their compensation claims. The scientific literature about them is extremely sobering.

A systematic review showed that evidence is lacking of secondary gain being a determinant of behavior by injured workers with back pain.[63] Indeed, when looked for, secondary gain has proved difficult to detect. Lawyers, insurers, and employers, therefore, should be advised that this phenomenon lacks scientific evidence and when used pejoratively is essentially only a lay point of view.

Similarly for malingering, a systematic review of the literature was particularly convincing.[27] Although commonly referred to, malingering has proved to be rare when looked for. Moreover, it is not a medical diagnosis. There are no valid diagnostic criteria. A medical practitioner might believe that a patient is malingering, but there is no medical test that can prove that he or she is. Malingering is a social or legal diagnosis and requires lay techniques, such video surveillance, to support it.

When Waddell developed his nonorganic signs, they were designed to alert physicians to patients who were communicating something more than the simple signs of back injury.[64] The objective was to cue physicians into pursuing something more than conventional medical management. Positive Waddell's signs constituted an invitation to the physician to explore the patient's fears, beliefs, and attitudes about the pain and about the circumstances. The tests were introduced to enrich medical practice. They did not.

Many practitioners abused the tests. They interpreted, portrayed, and applied them as tests of malingering or of psychogenic pain. For having positive Waddell's signs, patients were abused in medicolegal reports and had legitimate claims denied. Discourteously and conveniently, those who abused the tests did not commit themselves to print. Therefore, there is no conveniently citable evidence of their behavior. However, the improper practice became sufficiently commonplace, widespread, and evident, that Waddell was prompted to publish again, deprecating the practice and restating what the tests were legitimately for.[65]

Waddell's tests are not for detecting malingerers; they do not detect nonorganic pain. If used in this way they should not be accepted by fellow practitioners or by courts. The tests echo the pivotal principles concerning the management of back pain. Patients are often distressed by their pain. They harbor fears and may behave in strange ways when in strange circumstances—such as being interrogated by an independent medical examiner. Positive responses to Waddell's tests do not render the patient as being less than genuine in his or her beliefs. They are only signs that something more than simply back pain is occurring with the patient and that those other factors should be addressed.

A structured review of all the literature on Waddell's signs provided illuminating conclusions.[66] There was consistent evidence for Waddell's signs being associated with decreased functional performance, poor nonsurgical treatment outcome, and greater levels of pain. There was generally consistent evidence for Waddell's signs NOT being associated with psychological distress, abnormal illness behavior, or secondary gain. There was also generally consistent evidence that Waddell's signs are an organic phenomenon and that they cannot be used to discriminate organic from nonorganic problems.

PREVENTION

A final distinguishing feature of occupational back pain is the notion of primary prevention. In the past, experts or consultants optimistically believed that the incidence of occupational back pain could be reduced if ergonomic, and related, measures were taken to prevent it. As a result, campaigns were initiated to teach workers safe lifting techniques and otherwise to educate them about back pain.

Reviews of the literature have shown that classic measures have not succeeded in preventing occupational back pain.[7,67-69] Safe handling does not prevent it. Education does not prevent it. Exercises have a positive but modest effect. Back pain occurs nonetheless.

Intriguingly to some, but obvious to those intimately involved with industry, studies have shown gains in another domain. If management (i.e., the employer) is made responsible for the welfare of patients and if management expresses compassion and encouragement to the worker, the incidence of back pain comes down and the duration of sick leave decreases.[70] There seems to be more power in an employer's checking a patient and inviting him or her back to work than in a doctor telling the patient that he or she should go back to work.

The same can be achieved if management is engaged, from day 1, and cooperates with a sensible rehabilitation plan. In a mining company in Australia, dramatic decreases in compensation claims were achieved by two measures, each reflecting an important sociologic dimension.[71] First, a physiotherapist cooperated with the worksite nurse to develop an efficient system of triage and first aid. At the coalface (literally and figuratively) the nurse and the physiotherapists treated injured workers on site but encouraged and supported them not to stop work. Only patients with ostensibly serious injuries were referred to an orthopedic surgeon, who saw them promptly. Meanwhile, at another social level, it was the orthopedic surgeon who met prospectively with management, peer to peer as it were, to engage management's cooperation and support. With that secured, the nurse and physiotherapist could continue their medical management unhindered.

A somewhat similar approach has been applied by one of the authors (BMcG) as occupational physician to a large health service in Australia. What has become evident from his discussions with management is the lack of training (and perhaps empathy) of many immediate supervisors in managing such patients at a worksite level. Often their personal attitudes toward the patient, which can be reflective of interpersonal prejudices, delay recovery.

TEN CONFOUNDERS

Occupational back pain does not deserve to be any more difficult than back pain in the general community. The prognosis should be good. Yet it continues to be a problem. The reasons are multiple.

Back pain cannot be assessed and treated in 5 or even 25 minutes. Good initial assessment may take 50 minutes. General practitioners, however, are typically not geared for such consultations or are unaccustomed to providing them. Incomplete and inadequate early management becomes the *first* confounder.

Early assessment and early management requires focus on psychosocial factors. General practitioners are not accustomed, or are not prepared, to pursue this. It appears too time consuming to talk to patients, to discover what they do and do not understand and what they fear. It is too time consuming to explain to them what is wrong with their back and why they need not be afraid. It is too time consuming to explore vocational issues. It is not conventional to visit the workplace and to be the patient's trusted advocate. It seems that medical practitioners believe, or expect, that back pain should be something that has a simple "quick fix." The irony is that it does not. The management of acute back pain is time consuming. If that time is provided, the management is eminently successful.[10,17-19] If the time is denied, management becomes suboptimal. That becomes the *second* confounder.

Occupational back pain requires certification. That can be tedious if seen as an imposition; but it can become expeditious if based on a regular, sensible plan of management that is evidence based. But certification can be abused. "Time off work" and "light duties" can be expedient entries by which to complete certificates rapidly, but neither is justified by the evidence. To the contrary, certificates should be used as an integral part of the management plan. What they describe should be treated as a prescription, with all the responsibilities that follow. Misuse of certificates becomes the *third* confounder.

Return to work and workplace intervention are paramount components of the management of occupational back pain. Both provide for better outcomes. But both are demanding of aptitude, inclination, and time. Failure to become engaged with the workplace becomes the *fourth* confounder.

Whereas the majority of patients with back pain should recover, provided that they are managed well, some will have suffered a genuine and substantial injury, from which they do not recover. They will not recover if treatments are prescribed that are known not to work. Practitioners should be aware of what works and what does not work. Continuing to prescribe treatments destined to fail, and blaming the patient when they do, becomes the *fifth* confounder.

Conventional investigations do not provide for a diagnosis of chronic back pain. If a diagnosis is required, invasive tests need to be undertaken. Denying patients these tests, and leaving them without a diagnosis, becomes the *sixth* confounder.

Even if a diagnosis can be made, proven treatments are the exception rather than the rule. Entrenched and socially accepted interventions do not cure these patients. Innovative treatments have unknown efficacy. Lack of proven treatments for chronic back pain becomes the *seventh* confounder.

Left with no treatment for persisting pain, the patient with occupational back pain will lodge a claim for compensation in those countries where legislation allows for such entitlements. This will be accompanied by others who lodge claims for specious reasons. Fraudulent or dishonest claims pervert the compensation system, so that all claims are met with suspicion. Genuine claimants become victims of this suspicion. This becomes the *eighth* confounder.

Pursuit of a claim may dominate over pursuit of recovery. Tension may develop between doctors and lawyers, with each claiming to act in the interests of the worker. The lawyer's imperative is to maximize the entitlement. This requires maximizing disability. The doctor's imperative is to eliminate or reduce disability. This conflict becomes the *ninth* confounder.

Claims will be resisted, if not denied. Statements, although not evidence, will be brought to bear that their complaint and claim are not true. Lack of integrity and dishonesty on the part of expert witnesses becomes the *tenth* confounder.

The system does not want these patients to exist. It blames the patient for presenting in the first instance and for persisting if his or her pain persists. Against the background of 10 confounders, the blame lies not with the patient but with the system.

References

1. Mendelson G: Not "cured by a verdict": Effect of legal settlement on compensation claimants. Med J Aust 2:132, 1982.
2. Mendelson G: Follow-up studies of personal injury litigants. Int J Law Psychiatry 7:179, 1984.

3. Mendelson G: Compensation and chronic pain. Pain 48:121, 1992.
4. Koes BW, van Tulder M, Ostelo R, et al: Clinical guidelines for the management of low back pain in primary care: An international comparison. Spine 26:2504, 2001.
5. Australian Acute Musculoskeletal Pain Guidelines Group: Evidence-Based Management of Acute Musculoskeletal Pain. Brisbane, Australian Academic Press, 2003. Available at http://www.nhmrc.gov.au
6. Carter JT, Birrell LN (eds): Occupational Health Guidelines for the Management of Low Back Pain at Work—Principal Recommendations. London, Faculty of Occupational Medicine, 2000.
7. Waddell G, Burton AK: Occupational health guidelines for the management of low back pain at work: Evidence review. Occup Med 51:124, 2001.
8. Staal JB, Hlobil H, van Tulder MW, et al: Occupational health guidelines for the management of low back pain: An international comparison. Occup Environ Med 60:618, 2003.
9. Bogduk N, McGuirk B: History. In Bogduk N, McGuirk B: Medical Management of Acute and Chronic Low Back Pain: An Evidence-Based Approach. Amsterdam, Elsevier, 2002, pp 27-40.
10. McGuirk B, King W, Govind J, et al: The safety, efficacy, and cost-effectiveness of evidence-based guidelines for the management of acute low back pain in primary care. Spine 26:2615, 2001.
11. Bogduk N, McGuirk B: Imaging. In Bogduk N, McGuirk B: Medical Management of Acute and Chronic Low Back Pain: An Evidence-Based Approach. Amsterdam, Elsevier, 2002, pp 49-63.
12. Cohen M, Nicholas M, Blanch A: Medical assessment and management of work-related low back or neck/arm pain. J Occup Health Safety Aust NZ 16:307, 2000.
13. Koes BW, van den Hoogen HMM: Efficacy of bed rest and orthoses on low back pain: A review of randomized clinical trials. Eur J Phys Med Rehabil 4:96, 1994.
14. Waddell G, Feder G, Lewis M: Systematic reviews of bed rest and advice to stay active for acute low back pain. Br J Gen Pract 47:647, 1997.
15. van Tulder MW, Scholten RJPM, Koes BW, Deyo RA: Nonsteroidal antiinflammatory drugs for low back pain: A systematic review within the framework of the Cochrane Collaboration Back Review Group. Spine 25:2501, 2000.
16. van Tulder M, Malmivaara A, Esmail R, Koes B: Exercise therapy for low back pain: A systematic review within the framework of the Cochrane Collaboration Back Review Group. Spine 21:2784, 2000.
17. Indahl A, Velund L, Reikeraas O: Good prognosis for low back pain when left untampered: A randomized clinical trial. Spine 20:473, 1995.
18. Indahl A, Haldorsen EH, Holm S, et al: Five-year follow-up study of a controlled clinical trial using light mobilization and an informative approach to low back pain. Spine 23:2625, 1998.
19. Hagen EM, Eriksen HR, Ursin H: Does early intervention with a light mobilization program reduce long-term sick leave for low back pain? Spine 25:1973, 2000.
20. Bogduk N, McGuirk B: Algorithm for acute low back pain. In Bogduk N, McGuirk B: Medical Management of Acute and Chronic Low Back Pain: An Evidence-Based Approach. Amsterdam, Elsevier, 2002, pp 71-81.
21. Hall H, McIntosh G, Melles T, et al: Effect of discharge recommendations on outcome. Spine 19:2033, 1994.
22. Loisel P, Abenhaim L, Durand P, et al: A population-based, randomized clinical trial on back pain management. Spine 22:2911, 1997.
23. Frank J, Sinclair S, Hogg-Johnson S, et al: Preventing disability from work-related low-back pain: New evidence gives new hope—if we can just get all the players onside. Can Med Assoc J 158:1625, 1998.
24. Sinclair SJ, Hogg-Johnson S, Mondloch MV, Shields SA: The effectiveness of an early active intervention program for workers with soft-tissue injuries: The early claimant cohort study. Spine 22:919, 1997.
25. Lindstrom I, Ohlund C, Eek C, et al: Mobility, strength, and fitness after a graded activity program for patients with subacute low back pain: A randomized prospective clinical study with a behavioural therapy approach. Spine 17:641, 1992.
26. Lindstrom I, Ohlund C, Nachemson A: Physical performance, pain, pain behavior and subjective disability in patients with subacute low back pain. Scand J Rehab Med 27:153, 1995.
27. Fishbain DA, Cutler R, Rosomoff HL, Rosomoff RS: Chronic pain disability exaggeration/malingering and submaximal effort research. Clin J Pain 15:244, 1999.
28. Bogduk N: What's in a name? The labelling of back pain. Med J Aust 173:400, 2000.
29. Bogduk N, McGuirk B: Appendix 2: How to label acute back pain. In Bogduk N, McGuirk B: Medical Management of Acute and Chronic Low Back Pain: An Evidence-Based Approach. Amsterdam, Elsevier, 2002, pp 215-218.
30. NSW Injury Management & Workers Compensation Act 1998. Sydney, Australia, New South Wales Government, 1998.
31. van Tulder MW, Ostelo R, Vlaeyen JWS, et al: Behavioral treatment for chronic back pain: A systematic review within the framework of the Cochrane Back Review Group. Spine 25:2688, 2000.
32. Guzman J, Esmail R, Karjalainen K, et al: Multidisciplinary rehabilitation for chronic back pain: Systematic review. BMJ 322:1511, 2001.
33. Bendix AF, Bendix T, Ostenfeld S, et al: Active treatment programs for patients with chronic low back pain: A prospective, randomized, observer-blinded study. Eur Spine J 4:148, 1995.
34. Bendix AF, Bendix T, Vaegter K, et al: Multidisciplinary intensive treatment for chronic low back pain: A randomized, prospective study. Cleve Clin J Med 63:62, 1996.
35. Alaranta H, Rytokoski U, Rissanen A, et al: Intensive physical and psychosocial training program for patients with chronic low back pain: A controlled clinical trial. Spine 19:1339, 1994.
36. Mitchell RI, Carmen GM: The functional restoration approach to the treatment of chronic pain in patients with soft tissue and back injuries. Spine 19:633, 1994.
37. Harkapaa K, Jarvikoski A, Mellin G, Hurri H: A controlled study on the outcome of inpatient and outpatient treatment of low-back pain: I. Pain, disability, compliance, and reported treatment benefits three months after treatment. Scand J Rehab Med 21:81, 1989.
38. Basler H, Jakle C, Kroner-Herwig B: Incorporation of cognitive-behavioral treatment into the medical care of chronic low back patients: A controlled randomized study in German pain treatment centers. Patient Ed Counsel 31:113, 1997.
39. Nicholas MK, Wilson PH, Goyen J: Operant-behavioural and cognitive-behavioural treatment for chronic low back pain. Behav Res Ther 29:225, 1991.
40. Nicholas MK, Wilson PH, Goyen J: Comparison of cognitive-behavioral group treatment and an alternative non-psychological treatment for chronic low back pain. Pain 48:339, 1992.
41. Deardorff WW, Rubin HS, Scott DW: Comprehensive multidisciplinary treatment of chronic pain: A follow-up study of treated and non-treated groups. Pain 45:35, 1991.
42. Haldorsen EMH, Kronholm K, Skouen JS, Ursin H: Multimodal cognitive behavioural treatment of patients sicklisted for musculoskeletal pain: A randomised controlled study. Scand J Rheumatol 27:16, 1998.
43. Bogduk N, McGuirk B: Monotherapy. In Bogduk N, McGuirk B: Medical Management of Acute and Chronic Low Back Pain: An Evidence-Based Approach. Amsterdam, Elsevier, 2002, pp 144-161.
44. Bogduk N: Management of chronic low back pain. Med J Aust 180:79, 2004.
45. Bogduk N, McGuirk B: Assessment. In Bogduk N, McGuirk B: Medical Management of Acute and Chronic Low Back Pain: An Evidence-Based Approach. Amsterdam, Elsevier, 2002, pp 127-138.
46. Bogduk N, McGuirk B: Precision diagnosis. In Bogduk N, McGuirk B: Medical Management of Acute and Chronic Low Back Pain: An Evidence-Based Approach. Amsterdam, Elsevier, 2002, pp 169-176.
47. Bogduk N, McGuirk B: Precision treatment. In Bogduk N, McGuirk B: Medical Management of Acute and Chronic Low Back Pain: An Evidence-Based Approach. Amsterdam, Elsevier, 2002, pp 187-197.
48. Occupational Safety and Health Administration. Department of Labor. 29 CFR Part 1910. Ergonomics Program; Final Rule. Federal Register 65(220):68469, 2000.
49. Cocchiarella L, Andersson GBJ (eds): American Medical Association Guides to the Evaluation of Permanent Impairment, 5th ed. Chicago, AMA Press, 2001, p 404.
50. van Tulder MW, Assendelft WJJ, Koes BW, Bouter LM: Spinal radiographic findings and nonspecific low back pain: A systematic review of observational studies. Spine 22:427, 1997.
51. Symmons DPM, van Hemert AM, Vandenbroucke JP, Valkenburg HA: A longitudinal study of back pain and radiological changes in the lumbar spines of middle aged women: I. Clinical findings. Ann Rheum Dis 50:158, 1991.
52. Symmons DPM, van Hemert AM, Vandenbroucke JP, Valkenburg HA: A longitudinal study of back pain and radiological changes in the lumbar

spines of middle-aged women: II. Radiographic findings. Ann Rheum Dis 50:162, 1991.
53. Horal J: The clinical appearance of low back disorders in the city of Gothenburg, Sweden: Comparison of incapacitated probands with matched controls. Acta Orthop Scand Suppl 118:1, 1969.
54. Frymoyer JW, Newberg A, Pope MH, et al: Spine radiographs in patients with low-back pain. J Bone Joint Surg 66A:1048, 1984.
55. Biering-Sorensen F, Hansen FR, Schroll M, Runeborg O: The relation of spinal x-ray to low-back pain and physical activity among 60-year-old men and women. Spine 10:445, 1985.
56. Wiikeri M, Nummi J, Riihimaki H, Wickstrom G: Radiologically detectable lumbar disc degeneration in concrete reinforcement workers. Scand J Work Environ Health 1(Suppl):47, 1978.
57. Lawrence JS: Disc degeneration: Its frequency and relationship to symptoms. Ann Rheum Dis 28:121, 1969.
58. Kellgren JH, Lawrence JS: Rheumatism in miners: II. X-ray study. Br J Ind Med 9:197, 1952.
59. Sairanen E, Brushhaber L, Kaskinen M: Felling work, low back pain and osteoarthritis. Scand J Work Environ Health 7:18, 1981.
60. Hult L: The Munkfors investigation. Acta Orthop Scand Suppl 16:1, 1954.
61. Magora A, Schwartz A: Relation between the low back pain syndrome and x-ray findings: I. Degenerative osteoarthritis. Scand J Rehab Med 8:115, 1976.
62. Torgerson WR, Dotter WE: Comparative roentgenographic study of the asymptomatic and symptomatic lumbar spine. J Bone Joint Surg 58A: 850, 1976.
63. Fishbain DA, Rosomoff HL, Cutler RB, Rosomoff RS: Secondary gain concept: A review of the scientific evidence. Clin J Pain 11:6, 1995.
64. Waddell G, McCulloch JA, Kummel E, Venner RM: Nonorganic physical signs in low-back pain. Spine 5:117, 1980.
65. Main CJ, Waddell G: Behavioral responses to examination: A reappraisal of the interpretation of "nonorganic signs." Spine 23:2367, 1998.
66. Fishbain DA, Cole B, Cutler RB, et al: A structured evidence-based review on the meaning of nonorganic physical signs: Waddell signs. Pain Med 4:141, 2003.
67. Volin E: Do workplace interventions prevent low-back disorders? If so, why? A methodological commentary. Ergonomics 42:258, 1999.
68. Linton SJ, van Tulder MW: Preventive interventions for back and neck pain problems: What is the evidence? Spine 26:778, 2001.
69. van Poppel MNM, Koes BW, Smid T, Bouter LM: A systematic review of controlled clinical trials on the prevention of back pain in industry. Occup Environ Med 54:841, 1997.
70. Wood DJ: Design and evaluation of a back injury prevention program within a geriatric hospital. Spine 12:77, 1987.
71. Ryan WE, Krishna MK, Swanson CE: A prospective study evaluating early rehabilitation in preventing back pain chronicity in mine workers. Spine 20:489, 1995.

Appendix 85–1

A Matrix for Preparing a Succinct Medical Report from a General Practitioner

PRINCIPLES

For administrative purposes, a medical report from the treating doctor does not need to be lengthy. It is not a report from an expert witness that defends or contests the cause of pain, its prognosis, or its attribution. It needs only to communicate succinctly the facts as you found them, and what is happening to the patient. Those who use the report, in the first instance, want to know only what to expect:

- A short or protracted course?
- Requiring few or multiple services?
- Return to work or not?

All this information can be compiled into a short report (1 to 2 pages) that outlines the typical algorithm for management of acute low back pain.[3]

COMPONENTS

[Enter your letterhead]
[Enter address of insurer]
[Enter date of report]
Dear [Insurer]

[Title and name of patient] presented to me on [date of consultation] with a complaint of low back pain the [he/she] attributed to [circumstances of onset] on [date of incident].

Assessment

I obtained a history and performed a physical examination.

[EITHER]

The history, supplemented by a red flag checklist, revealed no evidence of a serious cause for the pain.

[OR]

The history revealed that [patient's name]...[stipulate any red flags]. Accordingly, I have arranged for [patient's name] to undergo [state investigations ordered], and I am awaiting the results of these investigations before adjusting my plan of management. In the meantime I [proceed to plan of management, as outlined below].

Physical examination revealed tenderness in/at [briefly state the location of any tenderness]. [List movements] were restricted by pain to about [75%, 50%, 25%] expected normal range for age.

[EITHER]

In taking the history, I found no suggestion of any psychosocial problems.

[OR]

In taking the history, I found the [patient's name] expressed certain psychosocial, yellow flag, risk factors for chronicity, which I will address in my management plan.

[OPTION]

For the purposes of completing the certificate I recognize the problems associated with how to label low back pain.[1,2] Accordingly I have not entered on the certificate any specious or counterproductive labels. Instead, in accordance with recent suggestions,[3] I have provided a diagnosis of

[EITHER]

Red Back Pain

in order to indicate that [patient's name] exhibits certain features that need to be taken seriously.

[OR]

Yellow Back Pain

in order to indicate that I have found no evidence of any serious physical cause for the pain but that [patient's name] exhibits certain fears, beliefs, and behaviors that would constitute poor prognostic factors if left unattended and which I propose to address.

[OR]

Green Back Pain

in order to indicate that I have found no evidence of any serious physical cause for the pain, and no psychosocial impediments to recovery. Wherefore, there is no reason why [patient's name] should not proceed promptly and confidently to resume normal activities while the back pain recovers naturally.

1. Schonstein E, Kenny DT: Diagnoses and treatment recommendations on workers compensation medical certificates. Med J Aust 173:419, 2000.
2. Bogduk N: What's in a name? The labeling of back pain. Med J Aust 173:400, 2000.
3. Bogduk N, McGuirk B: Medical Management of Acute and Chronic Low Back Pain: An Evidence-Based Approach. London, Elsevier, 2002, pp 215-218.

Management

For pain management, I have explained to [patient's name] what the likely causes are of [his/her] pain, and have reassured [him/her] that this is nothing to worry about. I have explained the natural history of this condition and how we can expect a good outcome. I have prescribed [name drug] on a time-contingent basis, providing analgesia while natural recovery takes its course.

In order to restore movement, I have mobilized [his/her] back muscles with some soft tissue techniques [if done] and have instructed [patient's name] in some simple exercises. I have explained how resuming normal activities and remaining active provide for a good prognosis. I will continue to assist [patient's name] to regain normal activities of daily. [if relevant] I have set modest goals in the first instance that I expect [patient's name] can achieve over [insert time: day or two, few days].

I plan to review [patient's name] in [2 days/1 week] to assess [his/her progress], at which time I shall check [his/her] compliance with my suggested interventions. I will then have the opportunity to correct any misunderstandings and reinforce what I have done already. If required, I can implement other interventions that are not immediately indicated at this stage. Should there be a change in the management plan at that time, I will inform you of those changes if they significantly alter the prognosis and anticipated return to work.

[EITHER]

[patient's name] has no inappropriate beliefs or fears about [his/her] pain and requires no intervention in this regard.

[OR]

Because [patient's name] has certain fears and inappropriate beliefs about [his/her] pain, I will seek to engage [him/her] about these, with every prospect of allaying these fears and promoting an appropriate optimistic outlook.

With respect to work,

[EITHER]

[patient's name] feels able and encouraged to return to work. Accordingly, I have completed the certificate for administrative purposes but have not provided any time off.

[OR]

[patient's name] should be able to return to work promptly, and I have encouraged [him/her] to do so. Therefore, I have completed the certificate only to allow for time off work to obtain this medical consultation.

[OR]

I have explained to [patient's name] the benefits of returning to work promptly, and I will assist [him/her] to do so. This will not require restricted duties but should entail modified duties. These I have explained to [patient's name]. I [have negotiated/will negotiate] these modifications on [his/her] behalf with [patient's name]'s employer. I expect [patient's name] should be able to embark on this return to work plan within [stipulate time]. I have provided [him/her] with a certificate for the intervening period, during which time I expect [patient's name]'s pain to settle, and [he/she] will improve movements and activities with a brief course of home rehabilitation.

[OR]

We may have some problems returning to work, because [list reasons]. Accordingly I propose to

[EITHER]

outline personal plan of intervention [e.g., discussion, explanation]

[OR]

engage the assistance of [stipulate assistance, e.g., occupational medicine consultant or occupational therapist]. However, I will remain pivotal to the management of [patient's name], and will keep you informed of any plan that we devise and how it progresses.

I have issued a certificate for a period of [insert duration] that should allow for the additional assessment and consultations required.

My account for this report is enclosed.

Yours truly,

[signature]

chapter 86

Arachnoiditis and Related Conditions

J. Antonio Aldrete

Although by definition the term *arachnoiditis* implies inflammation of the arachnoid, this entity is by far a more complex disease than the meaning of the word indicates. The most common location of the disease is in the lumbosacral region, because this is where most of the procedures invading the spine (spinal and epidural anesthesia, spinal taps, laminectomies, and fusions) are performed. Arachnoiditis can also occur in the thoracic and cervical regions as well as in specific locations in the dependent areas of the skull.

The most common causes of arachnoiditis include the following:

- Myelography may be causative, mostly from nonionic oil-soluble dyes (e.g., Pantopaque).[1] Currently used Iopamidol 200 (Isovue) and Iohexol 240 (Omnipaque) are water soluble and safer, but bloody taps, paresthesias, and doses exceeding 10 mL or concentrations higher than 240 mg of iodine/mL of bound iodine predispose to the occurrence of arachnoiditis.[2] Ionic contrast media should not be used in or around the spine.[3]
- Infections of the spine can be caused by common bacteria such as *Neisseria meningitides, Haemophilus influenzae, Streptococcus viridans, Enterococcus fecalis, Klebsiella,* and so on. However, infections from interventional procedures are more common and are caused by organisms such as *Staphylococcus aureus, Pseudomonas aeruginosa,*[4] and, in ambulatory patients, *Staphylococcus epidermidis.*[5] Mycosis are caused by *Coccidioides;* parasitoses include malaria, trichinosis, and cysticercosis; and viral infections include those caused by herpes zoster, adenovirus, human immunodeficiency virus, and West Nile virus.
- During neuraxial anesthesia, injuries may occur from direct needle or catheter trauma and from chemical substances that may irritate the spinal cord and/or the nerve roots, such as local anesthetics (5% lidocaine) and additives such as bicarbonate and preservatives (sodium bisulfate), blood (traumatic taps or epidural blood patches whenever the intradural compartment is breached). Under certain circumstances, paresthesias from needle trauma may allow the passage of otherwise innocuous concentrations of local anesthetics (2% lidocaine or 1% tetracaine) to come into contact with the endoneurium, resulting in axon demyelination.[6] Similarly, certain neurolytic substances such as phenol and alcohol may cross the dural barrier and enter the subarachnoid space.
- Interventional procedures for pain relief such as incidental subarachnoid injection of corticosteroids, all of which contain preservatives (polyethylene glycol, benzilic alcohol, or benzalkonium), can be causative. Misguided radiofrequency electrode application, diskography,[7] intradiskal electrotherapy probes,[8] failed attempts to inject neurolytic substances near sympathetic chains, methylmethacrylate in the vertebral body, epidural neurolysis, and 10% saline solution may have grave consequences if they end up intradural.
- Surgical interventions, chiefly laminectomies and spinal fusions with or without hardware, are the most common cause of arachnoiditis. The mechanism for causing arachnoiditis is related to the entry of blood into the subarachnoid space, because patients are usually in the prone position and the dural sac is at the bottom of the wound; incidental durotomies, especially when they are not recognized and not repaired, are ominous events,[9] leading to significant CSF leaks and pseudomeningoceles,[10] as well as to the possible initiation of a severe inflammatory reaction of the arachnoid.[11] A second alternative occurs in cases in which large hematomas accumulate extradurally; the degradation of old blood may liberate cytokines and leukotrienes that cross the dural barrier, resulting in the same end product.
- Similar pathophysiologic processes can be considered as the cause of arachnoiditis when blood enters the subarachnoid or the epidural space, such as when neuraxial anesthesia is performed in anticoagulated patients or in those who receive antithrombin preparations[12]; in addition, large volumes of blood injected to seal dural tears may, by a pressure gradient, permit the entry of blood into the CSF compartment. Furthermore, extradural hematomas and granulomas may compress the spinal cord and nerve roots to the point of leaving permanent neurologic deficits (cauda equina) coexisting with arachnoiditis only when blood gains access to the CSF.
- Intrathecal therapies done with antibiotics or chemotherapeutic agents (e.g., amphotericin, methotrexate) or the antimetabolites (cytarabine), depending on the dose, concentration and state of hydration of the patient, may cause arachnoiditis.

- Arachnoiditis caused by chronic sinus infection penetrating the floor of the skull may appear in the dependent areas of the cranium around the optic chiasm and the mastoid region.

As far as the extent of spinal arachnoiditis, it may affect the nerve roots and the meningeal layers; the spinal cord is involved whenever direct trauma (from needles or catheters) or blunt trauma occurs.[13]

PAIN MECHANISMS

Undoubtedly, patients with arachnoiditis experience severe constant pain with typical features of neuropathic type. The actual anatomicopathologic mechanisms responsible for the pain and related symptoms are initiated by peripheral nociceptive afferent fibers that terminate in the dorsal horn of the spinal cord. Because the thinly laminated A-δ fibers end in lamina I and lamina V, the unmyelinated C fibers enter the outer lamina I and II, activating a large number of second-order interneurons within the dorsal horn,[14] including two main groups of dorsal horn cells: (1) the nociceptive-specific cells that respond mostly to noxious stimuli and to innocuous stimuli[15] and (2) the multireceptive convergent cells that are usually activated by innocuous stimuli.

Some networks communicating with various types of spinal cord neurons modulate nociceptive information and transmit it to neurons that project to the brain. Certain stimuli sensitize these projecting neurons, increasing nociceptive transmission, whereas others produce inhibition. This relationship between the excitatory and the inhibitory processes has confirmed the "gate theory" of pain transmission.[16]

When temporal summation of postsynaptic, excitatory potentials exceeds the action potential threshold, it produces another phenomenon represented in neuropathic pain, the so-called "central sensitization." After an injurious event, the arachnoid usually responds with an acute inflammatory reaction in which repetitive C-fiber input evokes a state of spinal facilitation similar to what has been labeled as "wind up," characterized by repeated stimuli evoking progressively greater responses in dorsal horn neurons, as well as a gradual increase in extension of the size of their receptive fields.[14]

In addition, various receptors and transmitters intervene in this phenomena:

- Calcitonin gene-related peptide
- *N*-methyl-D-aspartate (NMDA) (participates in the wind-up phenomenon and in central sensitization)
- Nerve growth factor
- Substance P of the neurokinin type
- Neurokinin A
- Nitric oxide (especially contributing to hyperalgesia and allodynia)
- Eicosanoids including prostaglandins, thromboxanes, and leukotrienes

In neuropathic pain, C fibers and large A-β fibers mediate the information from low-threshold mechanoreceptors interacting with dynamic range neurons. It appears that histologic changes that occur in posttraumatic total or partial section of peripheral nerves differ from injuries on nerve roots caused by irritant chemical agents. For example, preliminary observations conducted by Romero-Figueroa and associates[17] after intrathecal injection of 22% phenol in rats resulted in almost complete demyelinization of some nerve roots; intravascular thrombosis was a consistent feature, whereas nonaffected nerve roots had their vessels patent (Fig. 86–1). Sprouting was noted within 2 weeks after phenol administration, and by 2 months a near-complete recovery had occurred, although there was an obviously abnormal pattern of myelin distribution in the axons.

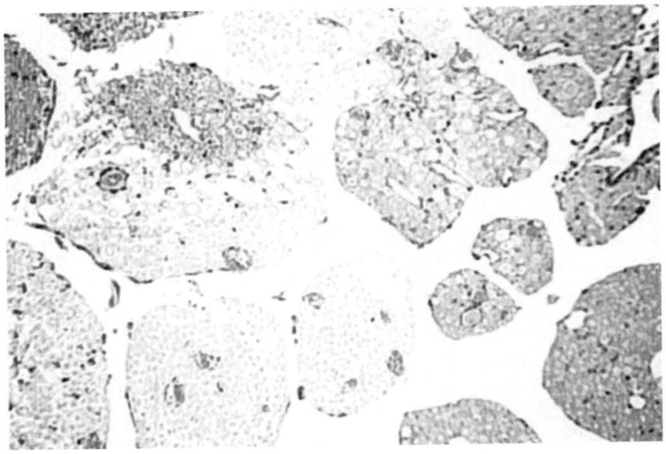

FIGURE 86–1 ■ Lesions on nerve roots produced by the intrathecal injection of 22% phenol in rats. Two days after injection there is marked demyelinization of axons in nerve roots with thrombosed vessels. Normal myelination of the axons is evident in nerve roots with patent vessels (Hematoxylin-eosin stain ×30). (From Romero-Figueroa S, Aldrete JA, Martinez-Cruz A, Guizar-Sahgun G: Ischemic axon degeneration in nerve roots after intrathecal phenol with evidence of atypical regeneration. Submitted for publication.)

DIAGNOSIS

Laboratory Diagnosis

Efforts to identify a laboratory test that would indicate the presence or the progress of arachnoiditis have been unsuccessful. Exceptions may be certain infections in which immune reactivity to certain microorganisms has been determined within the meningeal layers using specific antibody synthesis.[18,19]

Although CSF leukocytosis and hyperproteinemia have been noted[20] in the early stage, pleocytosis, high levels of proteins, and a reduced amount of β-endorphin (in monkeys) have been found in the late stages of arachnoiditis.[21] Other observations suggest that plasma and CSF C-reactive protein values are elevated in the inflammatory phase of this disease with elevations during flare-ups. In another study researchers are looking at the changes of plasma homocysteine in these cases, although findings remain preliminary.

Electrodiagnostic Studies

Nerve conduction, electromyographic, and somatosensory evoked potential studies have been considered helpful in the diagnosis of radiculitis and in cases of radiculopathy and

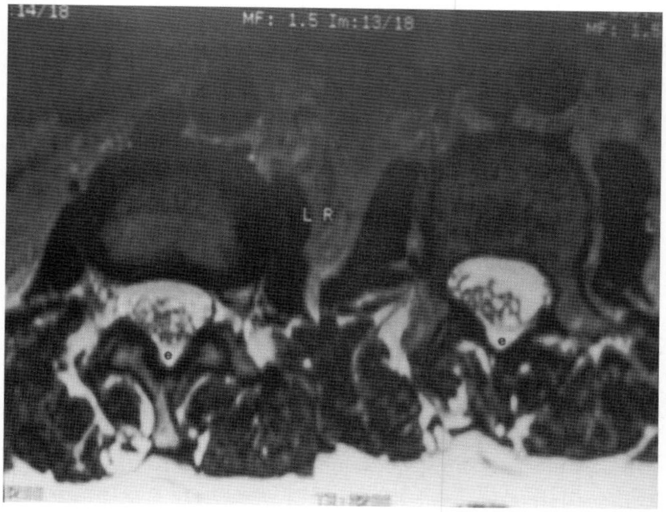

FIGURE 86–2 ■ Two axial MRI views of the lumbar spine with clumped nerve roots mostly on the right side of the dural sac at the L3-L4 level. Epidural spaces are patent (e).

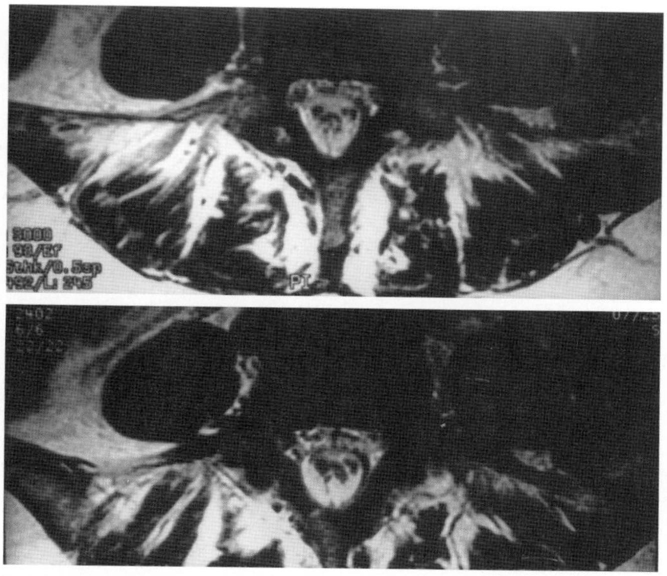

FIGURE 86–3 ■ Two axial MRI views of lumbar spine at the L2 level. The nerve roots are clumped mostly at the upper half of the dural sac. No epidural space is observed. Note considerable atrophy of paravertebral muscles.

peripheral neuropathy; however, neither in the early nor in the late stage of arachnoiditis has a specific pattern been identified. No specific findings have been noted in the various modalities.

Epiduroscopy and Myeloscopy

The information obtained from epidural endoscopy is limited as far as the extent of the disease (several levels) and the ability to diagnose intrathecal pathology with an extradurally located scope; besides, the presence of other abnormalities such as facet joint arthropathy, peridural scarring at L2 or L3, dural sac deformities, and disk pathology (i.e., or synovial cysts[22]) cannot be identified by this technique. In cases of myeloscopy the large dural orifice left can become a serious problem as to CSF leaks. Claims of diagnosis of arachnoiditis by myeloscopy that have been missed by MRI remain unsubstantiated.[23]

Radiologic Diagnosis

For spinal arachnoiditis, MRI has been recognized as the gold standard.[24] It requires the administration of the intravenous enhancing agent gadolinium[25] to best identify the presence of nerve root edema and clumping of nerve roots in all its varieties (Figs. 86–2 and 86–3) and intradural fibrosis and has the specific feature of being able to differentiate between scar tissue and nerve roots.[26]

"Enhanced" nerve roots are usually found in the inflammatory stage of arachnoiditis and noted as swollen, thicker, and, in the axial views, sometimes to have a stellar appearance. This feature has also been shown in patients with the so-called transient nerve root irritation syndrome, which in fact represents an inflammatory response[27] manifested as radicular edema (Fig. 86–4). In cases of myelopathic syringomyelia from a needle puncture (Fig. 86–5), the extent (several intervertebral levels) and communication with the subarachnoid compartment might be identified.[13]

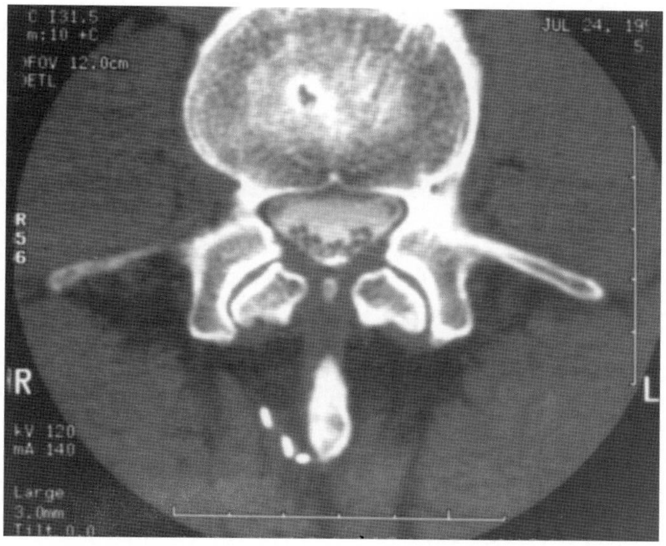

FIGURE 86–4 ■ CT scan after myelogram at the L3-L4 level demonstrating "enhanced" nerve roots mostly on the posterior half of the dural sac. They are edematous and "stellar" in aspect seen in the posterior half of the dural sac.

In some instances, when patients have metal objects (e.g., surgical staples, screws, plates), MRI is contraindicated (except when the object is made of titanium); second best is a myelogram performed with a water-soluble dye, followed by CT that allows the visualization of intrathecal pathology. Plain films are helpful to identify intrathecal calcifications or added pathology (spondylolisthesis). Although water-soluble dyes are currently used, excessive volumes, paresthesias, or bloody taps may exacerbate arachnoiditis by igniting another inflammatory reaction.[28,29]

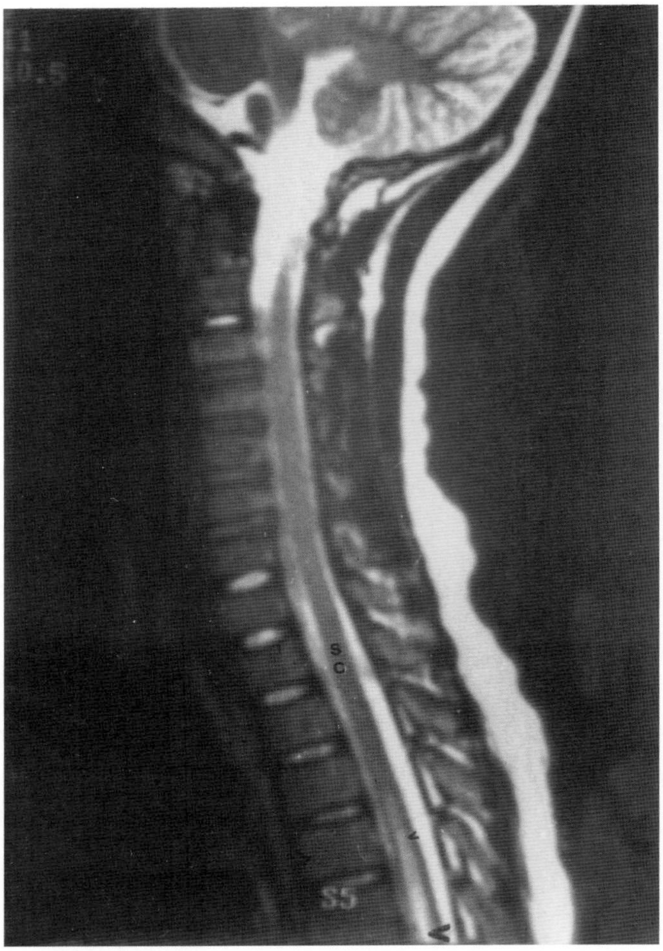

FIGURE 86–5 ■ Sagittal MR image of the cervical and thoracic spines showing syringomyelia (*arrows*) in the spinal cord (sc) from T6 down.

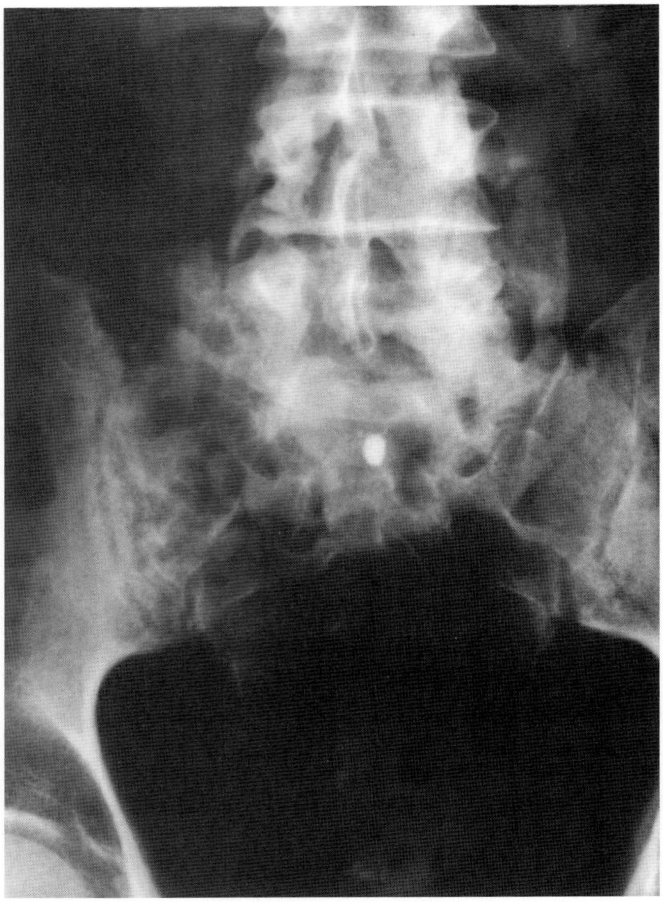

FIGURE 86–6 ■ Anteroposterior radiograph of lumbosacral spine. Large droplet of Pantopaque is present at the distal portion of the dural sac (S1) 11 years after a myelogram.

In addition to having a limited view, epidurography may reveal only dural sac deformities and peridural scarring; intrathecal pathology cannot be visualized. Pantopaque droplets and intrathecal calcifications can be seen by CT or on plain radiographs (Fig. 86–6).

Clinical Diagnosis

No one single symptom identifies arachnoiditis clinically; nevertheless, from the examination of patients with radiologically confirmed arachnoiditis it is apparent that the predominant type of symptoms are related to neuropathic pain, although the distribution is not classically "in dermatome" as it may be expected to be in sciatica.[30]

Burning pain is indeed the characteristic manifestation on one or both lower extremities with or without hyperalgesia and allodynia, usually accompanied by sensory disturbances including hypoesthesia, dysesthesia, and tingling sensation. Hyperreflexia may be present, although it depends on other lesions being present. Muscle spasms are common. Peculiarly enough most patients also have some kind of autonomic nervous system manifestations, such as low-grade fever, frequent diaphoresis and nocturnal sweating, and chronic fatigue. Most patients with lumbosacral nerve root involvement have considerable bladder dysfunction, with incontinence and incomplete emptying being more common in females whereas dysuria, frequency, and residual urine after micturition occurs in men. Rectal dysfunction was more commonly manifested as constipation with or without rectal incontinence and present in both genders in about 40% of the patients.

In most clinical settings, seldom are patients asked about changes in sexual function after the onset of arachnoiditis. In this same group of patients it was found that loss of libido and difficulty in arousing were the most frequent dysfunction in both men and women, with impotence, penal pain at erection, with low back pain during intercourse in men and pain during and after intercourse in women.[30]

Needless to say considerable depression is present in most patients with arachnoiditis; some of them also have anxiety and feelings of loss, guilt, and despair because no cure is available. These symptoms contribute to intramarital and interfamily conflicts and dysfunction, leading to separation or divorce in about one third of the patients. Cigarette smoking was prevalent as well as divorce and disability. This perspective implies a population group that has several disabling clinical manifestations that impair these patients' ability to maintain a functional family and be involved in social interactions. This can prevent them from supporting themselves and their families and they thus become dependent on the healthcare system and their close relatives and often have a sense of permanent loss.

Correlative Diagnosis

In attempts to identify suggestive features that would indicate the apparent injurious event that produced arachnoiditis in a group of 322 patients with a confirmed diagnosis, a certain pattern of radiologic lesions could be identified in most of the cases caused purely by injection of irritant substances (e.g., neurolytics, dyes, local anesthetics, and/or corticosteroids containing preservatives or enzymes), which resulted mostly in clumping of nerve roots, with adhesion of some nerve roots to the dural sac wall. Usually localization of symptoms to one or both sides, as well as the intervertebral level affected, corresponded to the clinical symptomatology present and the findings of the neurologic examination. There are a number of patterns of nerve root clumping without necessarily one of them being the typical representation of arachnoiditis; nevertheless, it is important to determine the location of the clumping as well as the intervertebral levels where it is apparent.[24,26,31] In cases of arachnoiditis caused by surgical interventions, in addition to finding lesions at the level of the operated intervertebral space(s), there was peridural scarring and fibrosis along with dural sac deformities and/or deviation (Fig. 86–7). Not uncommonly, distal ectasia or pseudomeningocele may be present (Fig. 86–8). However, because the same patient may have undergone myelographies, laminectomies, and a variety of invasive procedures, in these cases it is not clearly evident which intervention caused the lesions, unless it can be identified by a sudden appearance of clumped nerve roots (see Fig. 86–2) at MRI corresponding to related clinical neurologic findings and the level at which the intervention was done.

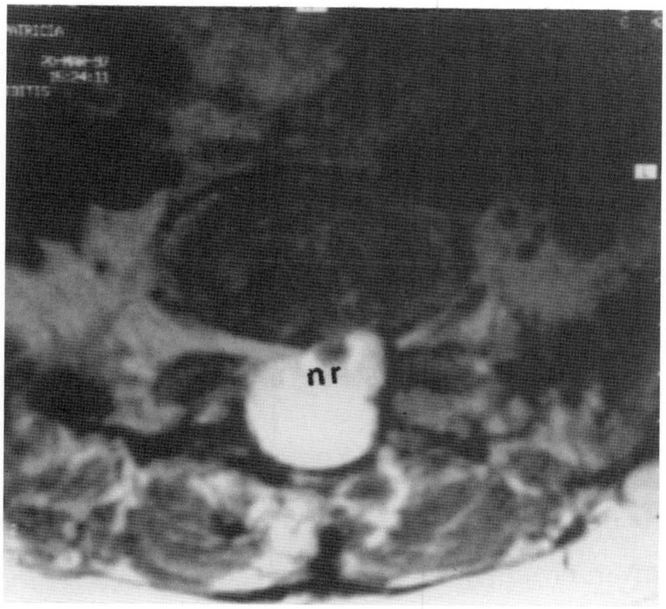

FIGURE 86–7 ■ Axial MR image of the lumbar spine at the L4-L5 level showing a deformity of the dural sac expanding the dural cuff (left) and the nerve roots (nr) clumped anteriorly.

■ PREVENTION

Because there is no definitive treatment, prevention is a primordial concern that would reduce the number of cases of arachnoiditis; this includes a number of recommendations that although appear to be simple are crucial.

In the case of infections, associated symptoms or findings may be of help to define the cause and an MRI would confirm the diagnosis of peridural or intrathecal location. Although the rationale for spinal taps to sample CSF appears reasonable, the chances for post-dural puncture headache would make it problematic, especially with the present availability of MRI.

In the case of interventional procedures of the spine, paresthesias may be a reason for discontinuing them because a perforation of the dura and arachnoid is implied as well as penetration of the perineural layer of a nerve root; furthermore, the injection of local anesthetics, even at usual concentrations, may, under these circumstances, irritate the endoneurial structures, initiating an inflammatory response.[6] Because there are no nerve trunks in the posterior epidural space, eliciting paresthesias implies that the tip of the needle was in the subarachnoid space.

■ TREATMENT

Because in the two phases of arachnoiditis different disease mechanisms are involved, the therapeutic approach needs to be different for each of these stages.

Another warning sign is the presence of blood or serosanguineous CSF, implying the puncture of a vessel within the intrathecal compartment. The injection of any chemical substances, including local anesthetics or dyes,[1,2,28] may, under these circumstances, appear to increase the likelihood of arachnoidal response. Similarly, the concomitant peridural administration of certain additives such as sodium bicarbonate, vasoconstrictors (epinephrine or phenylephrine), or therapeutic agents such as corticosteroids or blood in the presence of an incidental penetration of the dura may initiate intrathecal inflammation, even when small volumes of these substances have been applied.

The decision to postpone these procedures is not easy, and it needs to be practical; but if it is feasible, delay may be considered before proceeding, in view of the added risk versus doing it another day. As alternatives, one may consider proceeding but using an extraspinal (paravertebral or transforaminal) technique or a peripheral nerve block, if indicated.

Treatment of the Acute Phase of Arachnoiditis

Because there is a certain critical interval when proper diagnosis and treatment may stop the inflammatory process, a certain urgency is in order. If a neurologic deficit, uncontrollable severe burning pain, or loss of bladder or bowel control occurs after an invasive or surgical procedure, the following are recommended:

- Perform a complete neurologic examination.
- Obtain a neurology consultation.
- Perform an MRI in a search for specific lesions that may need to be treated promptly (e.g., intrathecal or extradural hematoma, dural leaks).

Once the clinical diagnosis of arachnoiditis, cauda equina syndrome, pseudomeningocele, or any other neurologic deficit is made and confirmed by the typical appearance of "enhanced nerve roots" and if the patient is considered to be in the inflammatory stage of the disease (estimated to last 8 to 10 weeks after the injurious event) (Fig. 86–4), treatment is indicated to prevent it from evolving into the permanent proliferative phase. For this, it is recommended to institute the following protocol:

- Limit physical activities.
- Administer 7 to 15 mg/kg of methylprednisolone, intravenously daily for 5 days.
- Administer magnesium oxide, 400 mg, four times a day for 30 days.
- Use antiinflammatory agents such as indomethacin, 25 mg, or celecoxib, 200 mg, twice daily with meals for 30 days.
- Use gabapentin, 400 mg, three times a day for 30 days.
- Monitor improvement by repeating the neurologic examination every 3 days and the MRI every 3 to 4 weeks.
- In the event that radiologic confirmation is inconclusive but the clinical manifestations are evident, treating physicians may consider proceeding with the just-listed protocol, anyhow.
- For information, consult www.arachnoiditis.com.

If the symptoms return 1 week from the end of the intravenous corticosteroid treatment, another series of the agent has been helpful in reducing the recurrent manifestations. Preliminary observations have indicated that the sooner this protocol is initiated, the better the chances for having the symptoms subside completely or partially. This study, which is still in progress, appears to suggest that procrastination is not helpful whereas prompt treatment may offer the possibility of reversing the neurologic deficits and burning pain. Once the third month passes, usually the symptoms are permanent. Interventional procedures during this phase of arachnoiditis are best avoided.

Treatment of Chronic Arachnoiditis

Most patients with the diagnosis of arachnoiditis have features of neurogenic pain; therefore, the concepts already described in Chapters 2 to 6 and 32 to 38 apply to its mechanisms, pathophysiology, and the treatment proposed for it. There are, however, some special characteristics in this disease that merit mention.[32] Considering that the intensity of burning pain, hyperalgesia, and allodynia is severe and continuous, the initiation of opioid medications is not one to be undertaken lightly; because tolerance to this group of medications and the dependency syndrome most likely will develop, it is preferable to initiate treatment with schedule III agents.[33] Apparent increases in pain intensity, usually accompanied by requests to increase the dosage, usually imply a reduction of the efficacy, owing to tachyphylaxis rather than to progression of the disease, because arachnoiditis tends to evolve very slowly. Moreover, the development of hyperalgesia with progressive dosages of narcotics[34] has been recognized as a detractor to indiscriminate use of these medications. Naturally, other associated conditions such as spondylolisthesis, spondylosis, recurrent herniated nucleus pulposus, and so on, need to be ruled out because their symptoms may superimpose on those of arachnoiditis that will manifest with similar symptoms but will require a different type of treatment.

Whenever possible and as early as feasible one can prescribe one of the anticonvulsant medications. Gabapentin has been the most effective in "taming" the pain, with topiramate and phenytoin as possible alternatives if side effects develop.[35]

Psychological counseling is usually required in the majority of the patients to help patients to cope with the sense of loss and specifically the depression, which can become severe; psychiatric consultation is required in severe cases and to selectively define the type of antidepressant best for each of these patients, as well as to determine the need for anxiolytic medications, hypnotics, and so on.

Muscle relaxants are indicated if severe muscle spasms appear; the usual physical therapy modalities may actually increase their pain; however, because it is crucial to maintain some type of fitness, it is preferred to institute a program of isometric exercises, together with hydrotherapy and stationary bike program for cardiovascular fitness. Selectively, other treatments are designed for each patient; in cases of neurogenic bladder, patients are taught to reduce fluids at certain times (evening) to prevent sleep disturbances. If necessary, in females with marked sphincter dysfunction they may be taught self-catheterization as well as how to prevent urinary tract infections. Medications indicated for erectile dysfunction may be tried, although their effectiveness is usually meager.

Other measures have been proposed to help with some of the autonomic nervous system symptoms, such as anticholinergic medications to reduce the profuse diaphoresis experienced by these patients. Because of its effective relaxing action on striated muscle, magnesium oxide assists with the treatment of muscle spasms and also appears to be effective in the treatment of constipation occurring from the ingestion of opiates or rectal neurogenic malfunction. In cases of impairment of CSF ascending return from either surgical interventions resulting in dural sac ectasia or massive clumping of nerve roots, propranolol, 40 to 80 mg/day, has been shown to reduce the pressure sensation experienced by some patients in the most dependent region of the spine. Similarly, the concurrent administration of acetazolamide, 250 to 500 mg/day, appears to tame the pain, presumably by changing the CSF pH; in both instances the effects on the heart rate from the former and on plasma potassium concentration from the latter have to be monitored.

Acupuncture, in its various modalities, has had limited use and ambiguous results; nevertheless it is worth trying, although its efficacy appears to depend greatly on the experience and expertise of the practitioner.

Interventionism

It most be recognized that the majority of the invasive procedures have no application in cases of arachnoiditis because most of them are aimed at extradural structures; nevertheless, most of them have been tried. Undoubtedly, they may provide partial and short-lasting pain relief because in many cases procedures such as epidural corticosteroid, facet, or sacroiliac joint injections may address concomitant disease(s) but would have little significant and longer-lasting effect on arachnoiditis; the same commentary applies to diagnostic procedures such as differential spinal procedures, diskograms, and so on.

Spinal Cord Stimulation

Two other modalities appear to have a more realistic indication, one of which is spinal cord stimulation, which supposedly acts by one or more of the following mechanisms:

- Interruption of stimuli traveling through spinothalamic fibers
- Expand descending DLF pathways
- Supraspinal gating mechanisms
- Alteration of spinal neurotransmitter pools via disinhibition at supraspinal sites

Undoubtedly, the technologic advances have improved since Shealy first proposed the concept and introduced the first prototype; although a few authors have specifically applied this to patients with arachnoiditis,[36,37] most other publications have included patients with various diagnoses, some of them including subgroups of patients with arachnoiditis.[38-40] However, their results are varied, and one concept seems to come out of it: after 6 months from implantation, only 50% of the patients had 50% of pain relief; the rest had either unsatisfactory results or had left the study. Problems with infection, fibrosis around the tip of the electrode, and lead migration still plague this technique.[40,41] These commentaries apply solely to their indications for arachnoiditis, but it seems that spinal cord stimulation has better results in mononeuronal conditions, complex regional pain syndrome,[39] angina pectoris,[42] pain from vascular origin,[43] and postherpetic neuralgia and diabetic neuropathy.[44] Of late, Carter[45] assessed the evidence from the published articles on spinal cord stimulation by meta-analysis, finding significant problems with the methodology of most studies, including patient selection, no comparative methods of treatment, lack of randomization, and blinding. He concluded that the absence of quality evidence in the literature prevents its recommendation for other specific diseases such as arachnoiditis.

Nonimplantable and Implantable Pumps

Although initially proposed for patients with terminal cancer, the application of these devices to patients with chronic nononcologic pain has become customary.[46] Specially designed catheters that had to be surgically implanted were used for epidural infusions of opiates; later on, common epidural catheters were implanted for ambulatory patients[47] for periods varying from 1 week to 7 months, with average stay of about 29 days and a rate of infection of 0.6%.[5] Although these infusions temporarily reduce the pain in most patients, their effect was palliative because they did nothing to improve the arachnoiditis. The patients were provided a vacation from pain, which many patients felt was worth it. The concern about infection plus the frequent occurrence of epidural fibrosis made this location and the limited period of implantation an alternative only for short-lasting therapy.[48,49]

Implantable infusion pumps that would deliver smaller dosages of opiates into the subarachnoid space appear to provide more effective pain relief. This therapeutic approach seems to be especially indicated in patients with chronic arachnoiditis, requiring refills every 6 to 8 weeks.[50] Undoubtedly it produced analgesia, allowing for physical activities that otherwise would have been impossible to conduct. Infusates combining morphine with baclofen, bupivacaine, clonidine, or ketamine allowed for reduction in the dosage of the opiate or another narcotic such as hydromorphone is chosen. Infections are rare after the initial implantation; however, dependency develops gradually, with patients believing that their disease is advancing, whereas they are developing a tolerance that is necessitating increases in the dosage.[51] Larger doses of morphine approaching 20 mg/day produce significant sexual dysfunction in both men[52] and women[53] with hyperalgesia, allodynia, and hyperreactivity in various species that is not reversible with naloxone, possible related to the formation of morphine-3-glucuronide.[34,51] Lower-extremity edema has been reported in about 20% of the patients receiving intrathecal infusions of opiates, purportedly due to the sympathetic blockade from these medications[54,55]; most patients with this problem have had varicose veins or pedal edema before implantation, which becomes a relative contraindication for this therapeutic modality.

However, the greatest concern has been the reports of granulomas forming at the tip of the catheter that seem to occur mostly with opiate infusions,[51,56] starting within 6 months and from dosages above 10 mg/day. As the catheter tip becomes gradually obstructed, the tendency has been to increase the dosage or the concentration, which in fact accelerates granuloma formation. Multifocal accumulation of neutrophils, monocytes, macrophages, and plasma cells is characterized by high protein and normal glucose levels in the CSF.[57,58] Opiates have been shown to initiate release of nitric oxide in human endothelial cells; the continued exposure of inmunocytes to morphine may lead to exaggerated response of monocytes to other proinflammatory stimuli activating nitric oxide synthase in the arachnoid vasculature and increasing local capillary permeability.[59] Absence of positive stains for bacteria, failure to obtain CSF or infusate cultures, and normal CSF glucose levels imply the presence of granuloma, which is confirmed by the finding of a soft mass with a necrotic center at surgery.[59,60] Because of possible liability and lack of therapeutic evidence,[61] these complications have cast a serious doubt on the apparent benefits of these devices.

Nonconventional Treatment of Chronic Arachnoiditis

In addition to propranolol, indomethacin, and acetazolamide, it appears prudent to continue a sensible strategy that, although not specific, is tangibly applicable to this disease. Medications that have been approved by the U.S. Food and Drug Administration have been re-evaluated for different indications; and when studies have suggested an apparent beneficial effect on one of the pathologic processes included in patients with arachnoiditis, it seems logical and justified to assess their value, because they appear to have minimal risk. Some of the medications include probenecid, a medication used to treat gout that has been shown to facilitate the transfer of certain medications across the dural barrier[61]; the cholesterol-lowering simvastatin, which has revealed itself as a notable antiinflammatory drug; the chelating agent penicillamine[62]; and even the antioxidant lipoidic acid, which is already known and available in the "alternative" medicine armamentarium. This sensible approach of giving a "second look" to medications that may be considered "off label" has been legitimized by the use of the erythropoietin as a protector of neural tissue in stroke,[63,64] diabetic neuropathy,[65] and other neurologic conditions.[64] Similarly, antioxidants such as *N*-acetylcysteine, neurotrophic peptides such as nerve growth factor and prosaposin, as well as the neurotransmitter memantine[44] are being tried in multiple sclerosis, amyotrophic lateral sclerosis, and diabetic neuropathy because they seem to offer potential benefit to patients with diseases that have, in the past, been considered incurable.

References

1. Hoffman GS, Ellsworth CA, Wells EE, et al: Spinal arachnoiditis—what is the clinical spectrum: II Arachnoiditis induced by Pantopaque and autologous blood, a possible model for human disease. Spine 8:541, 1983.
2. Aldrete JA: Myelography. In Aldrete JA (ed): Arachnoiditis: The Silent Epidemic. Denver, Futuremed, 2000, p 49.-
3. Bohn HP, Reich L, Suljaga-Retchel K: Inadvertent intrathecal use of ionic contrast media for myelography. AJNR Am J Neuroradiol 13:1515, 1992.
4. Gastmeier K, Gastmeier P: The risk of infections with long-term epidural catheters. Anesteziol Ranimation 16:267, 1991.
5. Aldrete JA, Williams SK: Infections from extended epidural catheterization in ambulatory patients. Reg Anesth Pain Med 23:491, 1998.
6. Aldrete JA: Neurologic deficit and arachnoiditis from neuraxial anesthesia. Acta Anaesthesiol Scand 47:3, 2003.
7. Epstein NE: Surgically confirmed cauda equina and nerve root injury following percutaneous discectomy at an outside institution: A case report. J Spinal Disord 3:380, 1990.
8. Ackerman WE: Cauda equina syndrome after intradiscal electrothermal therapy. Reg Anesth Pain Med 27:622, 2002.
9. Goodkin R, Laska LL: Unintended "incidental" durotomy during surgery of the lumbar spine: Medico-legal implications. Surg Neurol 43:4, 1995.
10. Aldrete JA, Ghaly RF: Postlaminectomy pseudomeningocele: An unexpected cause of low back pain. Reg Anesth 20:75, 1995.
11. Matsui H, Tsuji H, Kanamori M, et al: Laminectomy induced arachnoradiculitis: A postoperative serial MRI study. Neuroradiology 37:660, 1995.
12. Rabito SF, Ahmed S, Feinstein L, Winnie AP: Intrathecal bleeding after the intraoperative use of heparin and urokinase during continuous spinal anesthesia. Anesth Analg 82:409, 1996.
13. Aldrete JA, Ferrari H: Myelopathy with syringomyelia following thoracic epidural anaesthesia. Anaesth Intensive Care 32:100, 2004.
14. Woolf CJ, King AE: Physiology and morphology of multireceptive neurons with C-afferent fiber inputs in the deep dorsal horn of the rat lumbar spinal cord. J Neurophysiol 58:460, 1987.
15. Stamford JA: Descending control of pain. Br J Anaesth 75:217, 1995.
16. Melzac R, Wall PD: Pain mechanisms: A new theory. Science 150:971, 1965.
17. Romero-Figueroa S, Aldrete JA, Martinez-Cruz A, Guizar-Sahgun G: Ischemic axon degeneration in nerve roots after intrathecal phenol with evidence of atypical regeneration. Submitted for publication.
18. Makarova TT: Changes in the immune reactivity of the body in cerebral arachnoiditis. Vrach Delo 9:991, 1989.
19. Blagoveshenskaia NS, Mukhamedzhanov NZ, Siminova AV: Diagnostic value of immunologic methods in rhinosinusogenic cerebral arachnoiditis. Vestn Otorrhinolaringol 5:3, 1988.
20. Nakajima T, Eno N, Watanabe N, et al: Analysis of various proteins of CSF on central nervous diseases. Nippon Ganka Gakkai Zasshi 82:778, 1978.
21. Lipman BT, Haughton VM: Diminished CSF beta-endorphin concentration in monkeys with arachnoiditis. Invest Radiol 23:190, 1988.
22. Peek RD, Thomas JC, Wilse L: Diagnosis of lumbar arachnoiditis by myeloscopy. Spine18:2286, 1993.
23. Tobita T, Okamoto M, Tomita M, et al: Diagnosis of spinal disease with ultrafine flexible fiberscopes in patients with chronic pain. Spine 28:2006, 2003.
24. Ross JS, Masaryk TJ, Modic MT: MRI imaging of lumbar arachnoiditis. AJNR Am J Neuroradiol 149:1025, 1987.
25. Boden SD, Davis DO, Dina TS, et al: Contrast-enhanced MR imaging performed after successful lumbar disc surgery: Prospective study. Radiology 182:59, 1992.
26. Delamarter RB, Ross JS, Masaryk TJ, et al: Diagnosis of lumbar arachnoiditis by magnetic resonance imaging. Spine 15:304, 1990.
27. Avidan A, Gomori M, Davidson E: Nerve root inflammation demonstrated by magnetic resonance imaging in a patient with transient neurologic symptoms after intrathecal injection of lidocaine. Anesthesiology 97:257, 2002.
28. Howland WJ, Curry JL, Butler AK; Pantopaque arachnoiditis: Experimental study of blood as potentiating agent. Radiology 80:371, 1963.
29. Jourdan C, Arthur F, Convert J, et al: A rare and severe complication of meningeal hemorrhage: Spinal arachnoiditis with paraplegia. Aggressologie 31:413, 1990.
30. Aldrete JA: Clinical diagnosis. In Aldrete JA (ed): Arachnoiditis: The Silent Epidemic. Denver, Futuremed, 2000, pp 201-219.
31. Aldrete JA, Brown TL, Ghaly RF, et al: Correlaci6n de hallazgos radiologicos con los eventos adversos que posiblemente hallam causado aracnoiditis. Rev Soc Esp Dolor 63:269-276, 2005.
32. Rowbotham MC, Twilling L, Davies PS, et al: Oral opioid therapy for chronic peripheral and central neuropathic pain. N Engl J Med 348:1223, 2003.
33. Acker JC: Creating the American Junkie: Addiction Research in the Classic Era of Narcotic Control. Baltimore, Johns Hopkins University Press, 2002, pp 32-49.
34. Mercadante S, Ferrera P, Villari P, Arcuri E: Hyperalgesia: An emerging iatrogenic syndrome. J Pain Symptom Manage 26:769, 2003.
35. Aldrete JA: Reduction of neuropathic pain in patients with arachnoiditis: Crossover study of gabapentin vs phenytoin. Pain Digest 9:136, 1998.
36. De la Porte C, Siegfried J: Spinal cord stimulation in lumbosacral spinal fibrosis. Spine 8:593, 1983.
37. Fascio B, Sportes J, Romain M, et al: Chronic medullary neurostimulation in lumbosacral spinal arachnoiditis. Rev Chir Orthop 74:473, 1988.
38. Kumar K, Malik S, Demaria D: Treatment of chronic pain with spinal cord stimulation versus alternate therapies: Cost-effectiveness analysis. Neurosurgery 51:106, 2002.
39. Racz GB, McCarron RF, Talboys P: Percutaneous dorsal column stimulator for chronic pain control. Spine 14:1, 1989.
40. North RD, Wetzel FT: Spinal cord stimulation for chronic pain of spinal origin: A valuable long term solution. Spine 27:2584, 2002.
41. Aguilar JL, Samper D, Domingo F: Tecnicas de neuroestimulacion. In Aldrete JA (ed): Tratado de Algiologia. Mexico City, Ciencia y Cultura Latinoamericana, 1999, pp 1139-1162.
42. Hatvaust RW, De Jongste MJ, Staal MJ, et al: Spinal cord stimulation in chronic intractable angina pectoris: A randomized, controlled, efficacy study. Am Heart J 136:1114, 1998.
43. Ghajar AW, Miles JB: The differential effect of the level of spinal cord stimulation on patients with advance peripheral vascular disease in the lower limbs. Br J Neurosurg 12:402, 1998.
44. Sang CN, Booher S, Gilton I, et al: Dextromethorphan and memantine in painful diabetic neuropathy and post-herpetic neuralgia: Efficacy and dose response trials. Anesthesiology 96:1053-1061, 2002.
45. Carter ML: Spinal cord stimulation in chronic pain: A review of the evidence. Anaesth Intensive Care 32:11, 2004.
46. Plummer JL, Cherry DA, Cousins MJ, et al: Long term spinal administration of morphine in cancer and non-cancer pain: A retrospective study. Pain 44:215, 1991.
47. Aldrete JA: Extended epidural catheter infusions with analgesics in patients with non-cancer pain at their homes. Reg Anesth 22:35, 1997.
48. Aldrete JA: Epidural fibrosis after permanent catheter insertion and infusion. J Pain Symptom Manage 10:624, 1995.
49. Aldrete JA; Infections in permanently implanted epidural catheter lifeport units. Pain Clinic 9:151, 1996.
50. Krames ES: Intraspinal opioid therapy for chronic nonmalignant pain: Current practice and clinical guidelines [Review]. J Pain Symptom Manage 11:333, 1996.

51. Yaksh T, Harty G, Onofrio B: High doses of spinal morphine produce a non-opiate receptor mediated hyperesthesia: Clinical and theoretic implications. Anesthesiology 64:590, 1986.
52. Paice JA, Penn RD, Ryan WG: Altered sexual function and decreased testosterone in patients receiving intraspinal opioids. J Pain Symptom Manage 9:126, 1994.
53. Paice JA, Penn RD: Amenorrhea associated with intraspinal morphine. J Pain Symptom Manage 10:582, 1995.
54. Aldrete JA, Couto da Silva JM: Leg edema from intrathecal opioid infusions. Eur J Pain 4:361, 2000.
55. Couto da Silva JM, Couto da Silva JM Jr, Aldrete JA: Body temperature and diaphoresis disturbances in a patient with arachnoiditis. Anesth Analg 93:1578, 2001.
56. Bidlack J, Hemmick L: Morphine enhancement of mitogen-induced T-cell proliferation. Prog Clin Biol Res 328:405, 1990.
57. Yaksh TL, Tozier NA, Allen JW, et al: Chronically infused intrathecal morphine in dogs. Anesthesiology 99:174, 2003.
58. Gradert TL, Baze WB, Satterfield WC, et al: Safety of chronic intrathecal morphine infusion in a sheep model. Anesthesiology 99:188, 2003.
59. Bennett G, Serafini M, Burchiel KJ, et al: Evidence-based review of the literature in intrathecal delivery of pain medication. J Pain Symptom Manage 20:12, 2000.
60. Coffey RJ, Burchiel KJ: Inflammatory mass lesions associated with intrathecal drug infusion catheters: Report and observations in 41 patients. Neurosurgery 50:433, 2002.
61. Artru AA: Spinal cerebrospinal fluid chemistry and physiology. In Yaksh TL (ed): Spinal Drug Delivery. Amsterdam, Elsevier Science BV, 1999, pp 177-237.
62. Graham R, Clark B, Waton M, et al: Toward a rational, therapeutic strategy for arachnoiditis: A possible role of D-penicillamine. Spine 16:172, 1991.
63. Ehrenreich H, Hassellatt M, Dembowski C, et al: Erythropoietin therapy for acute stroke is both safe and beneficial. Molec Med 8:495, 2002.
64. Bianchi R, Buyukakilli B, Brines M, et al: Erythropoietin both protects from and reverses experimental diabetic neuropathy. Proc Natl Acad Sci U S A 101:823, 2004.
65. Lipton SA: Erythropoietin for neurological protection and diabetic neuropathy. N Engl J Med 350:2516, 2004.

chapter 87

Spondylolysis and Spondylolisthesis

Nikolai Bogduk

Fundamental to the stability of the lumbar spine is the architecture of the posterior elements of the lumbar vertebrae. The inferior articular processes project downward and act like hooks to engage the superior articular processes of the vertebra below (Fig. 87–1A). This arrangement provides for stability against anterior translation. If the upper vertebra in a segment attempts to translate forward (see Fig. 87–1B), its inferior articular processes impact the superior articular processes of the lower vertebra, which prevents translation.

The inferior articular processes are suspended from the lamina on each side (Fig. 87–2A). The superolateral portion of the lamina can be perceived as lying between the superior articular process and the inferior articular process of the parent vertebra. Accordingly, it is known as the pars interarticularis: the part between the joints. Defects can occur in the pars interarticularis whereupon the inferior articular process becomes disconnected from the rest of its parent vertebra (see Fig. 87–2B). Traditionally, this condition is known as spondylolysis, because it was originally likened to dissolution of the pars interarticularis.

The perceived threat to the stability of the lumbar spine is that when a pars defect develops the vertebra is denied the restraining function of the inferior articular processes, and it can dislocate into forward translation (Fig. 87–3). The resultant dislocation is known as spondylolisthesis: slipping of the vertebra.

These abnormalities may have some relevance in the assessment of instability and deformity in children, but they have little relevance in the practice of adult pain medicine. Arcane is the belief that radiographic abnormalities of the lumbar spine constitute or provide a diagnosis of low back pain. Yet spondylolysis and spondylolisthesis are still promoted as causes of low back pain in some medical circles. They are also still promoted as causes of pain in medicolegal circles. Indeed, according to the AMA Guides for assessment of impairment,[1] patients are rewarded with higher total person impairment scores if they exhibit spondylolysis. Nothing could be so undeserving. Nothing could be so dissonant with the scientific evidence.

■ SPONDYLOLYSIS

An early belief concerning spondylolysis was that it constituted a congenital defect, produced by failure of ossification centers in the lamina to fuse with those of the pedicle and vertebral body. This belief is incompatible with the embryology of the lumbar spine. There is no separate ossification center that arises in the lamina.[2] Consequently, there is no ossification center that can fail to fuse with that of the pedicle body and produce a defect. The pars interarticularis develops from a single ossification center that produces the lamina, pedicle, and articular processes on each side. The possibility of failure to fuse applies only to the midline posteriorly, where the ossification centers of each side can fail to meet (spina bifida), or to the neurocentral junction, between the pedicles and the vertebral centrum. Furthermore, it has been shown that pars defects do not occur in infants[2] and they do not occur in individuals paralyzed from birth, who have never used their lumbar spine in weight bearing.[3]

Spondylolysis has also been viewed as a genetic problem, largely because it was found to have an inordinately high prevalence among Eskimos.[4] Later studies, however, showed that this prevalence was not due to race. Not all Eskimos exhibit the high prevalence. Rather, its prevalence is related to differences in lifestyle, which render the defect an acquired abnormality.[4] In all races, the prevalence increases with age[5] and is related to repeated activities that involve hyperextension, rotation, or flexion of the lumbar spine.[5]

Anatomic studies have shown that the pars interarticularis is the weakest region of bone in a lumbar vertebra.[6] Yet, ironically, it is subject to enormous stresses during activities of daily living. Whereas most individuals are endowed with a pars interarticularis that is thick enough to withstand the stress put upon it, others are endowed with a less than adequate pars. They become susceptible to acquired injuries.

Biomechanics studies have shown that the pars interarticularis is susceptible to stress failure. This can occur if the vertebra is loaded in repeated torsion or repeated extension.[7-10] In all of these movements, impaction of the inferior articular process, as it resists movement, causes it to bend backward, which stresses the pars. Under repeated loading, the pars will fracture.

These biomechanics data correlate with the available epidemiologic data. Pars fractures are more common in people who participate in sports, particularly, although not exclusively, those whose sports involve twisting of the lumbar spine or forced extension (Table 87–1).[11-15] Among Eskimos, they are more common in individuals who live on ice and who use kayaks.[4] However and nevertheless, pars fractures are not

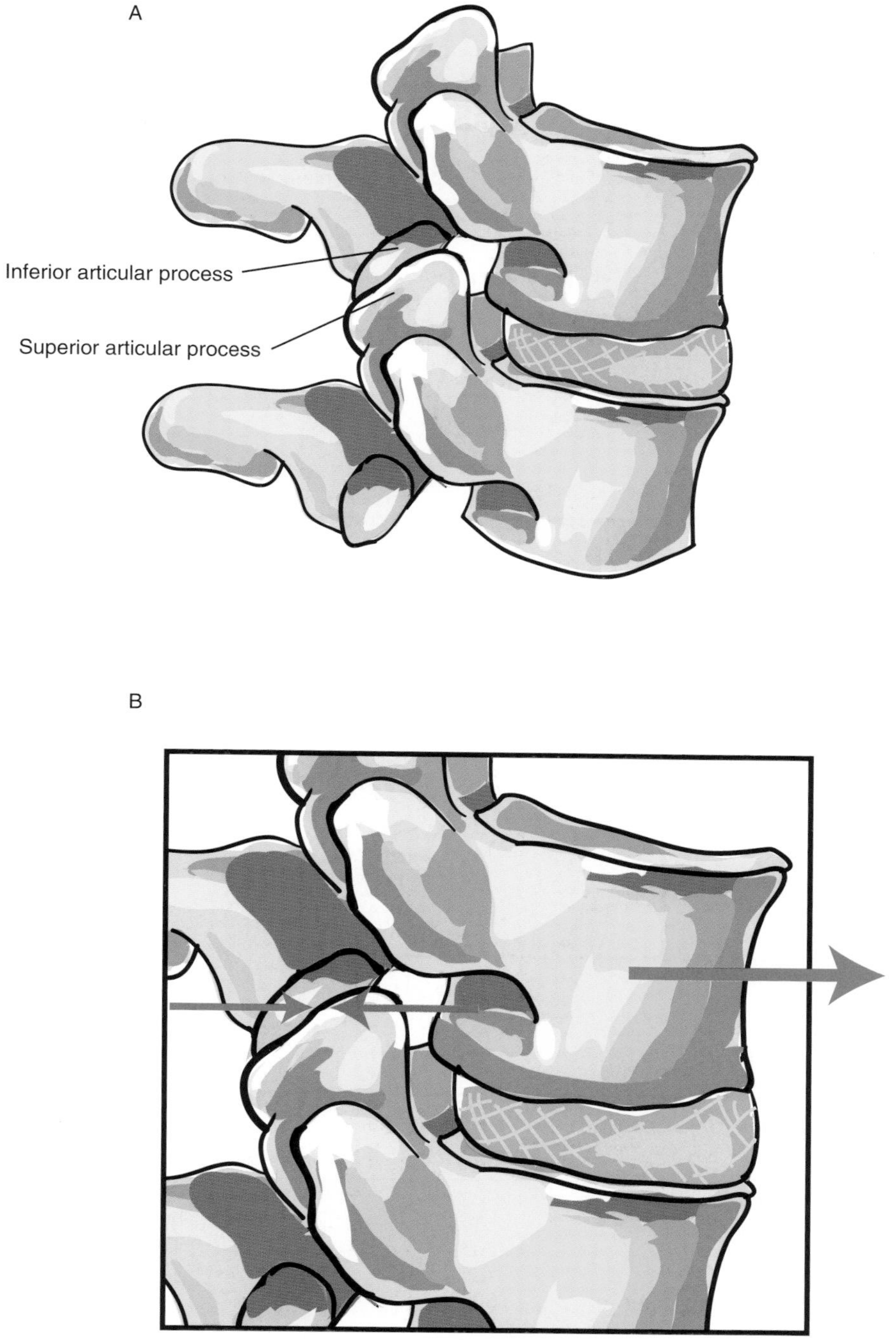

FIGURE 87–1 ■ Structure and function of the inferior articular processes of lumbar vertebrae. **A,** In a lateral view, the inferior articular processes hang down like hooks to engage the superior articular processes of the vertebra below. **B,** If the upper vertebra attempts to translate forward, its inferior articular processes impact the superior articular processes of the vertebra below, whereby translation is prevented.

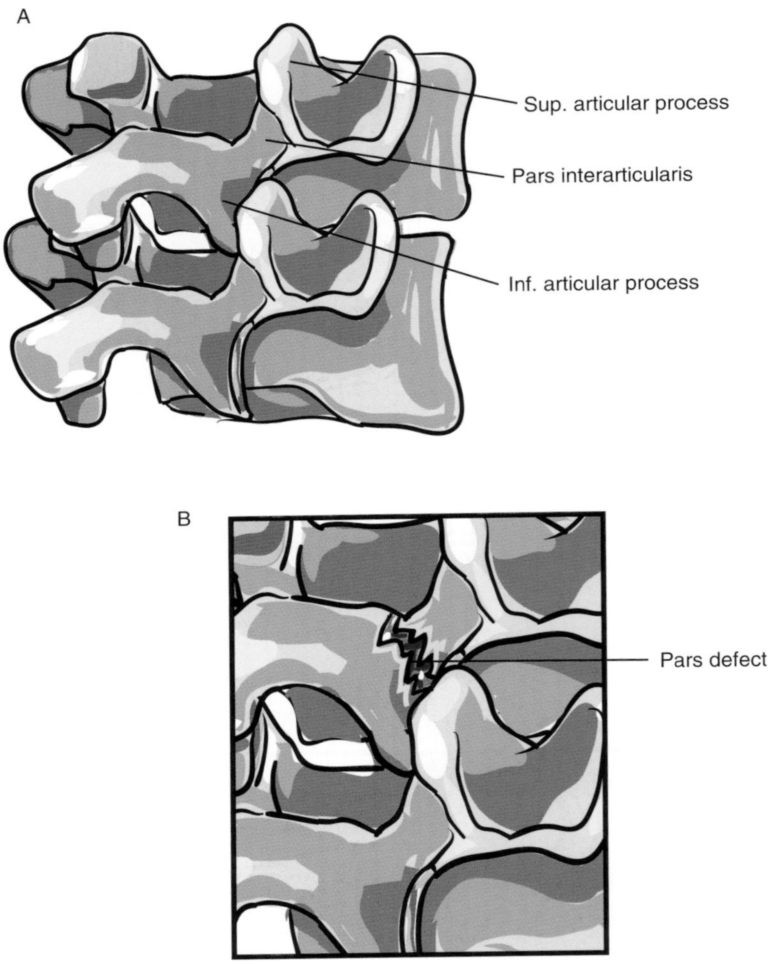

FIGURE 87–2 ■ Defect in the pars interarticularis. **A,** An oblique view showing the superior articular process, the inferior articular process of a lumbar vertebra, and the pars interarticularis. **B,** The same view showing a pars defect.

Table 87–1

Prevalence of Spondylolysis in Athletes

Category	*Prevalence*	*Ref. No.*
Contact sports	>20%	11
Gymnasts	11%	12
Various sports	>20%	13
Football	13%	14
Fast bowlers in cricket	50%	15

restricted to such individuals. Some 7% of the asymptomatic, adult population have spondylolysis.[16] The prevalence is higher (7.7%) in men than in women (4.6%) but varies by geographic region and by nature of work and number of pregnancies.[17]

Pathology

Overwhelmingly, the epidemiologic and biomechanical evidence indicates that pars defects are a type of stress fracture. This is consonant with their morphology.

If studied early, spondylolysis has all the features of an acute fracture: hyperemia and a jagged fracture line. If the fracture does not heal, the appearance of the defect is that of a pseudarthrosis. The bony margins are eburnated and smooth. The defect is filled with fibrous tissue, forming a syndesmosis.[18] The fibrous tissue may contain fragments of bone,[19] which underscores the traumatic origin of the defect. The defect may undercut the capsules of one or both of the adjacent zygapophyseal joints.[18] Under those conditions it can communicate with the cavities of those joints, which may become evident on arthrography of the joints.[20]

When pars fractures are bilateral, the entire lamina and its inferior articular processes are effectively disconnected from the pedicles and vertebral body. The lamina becomes flail, for which reason it has been described as the "rattler." The multifidus muscle still acts on the spinous process of the lamina, drawing it into extension. However, only the fibrous tissue of the defect resists this motion. Consequently, the flail lamina can exhibit excessive motion during normal movements of the lumbar spine.

Diagnosis

The traditional means of diagnosing a pars fracture has been plain radiography. The fractures can be difficult to see on

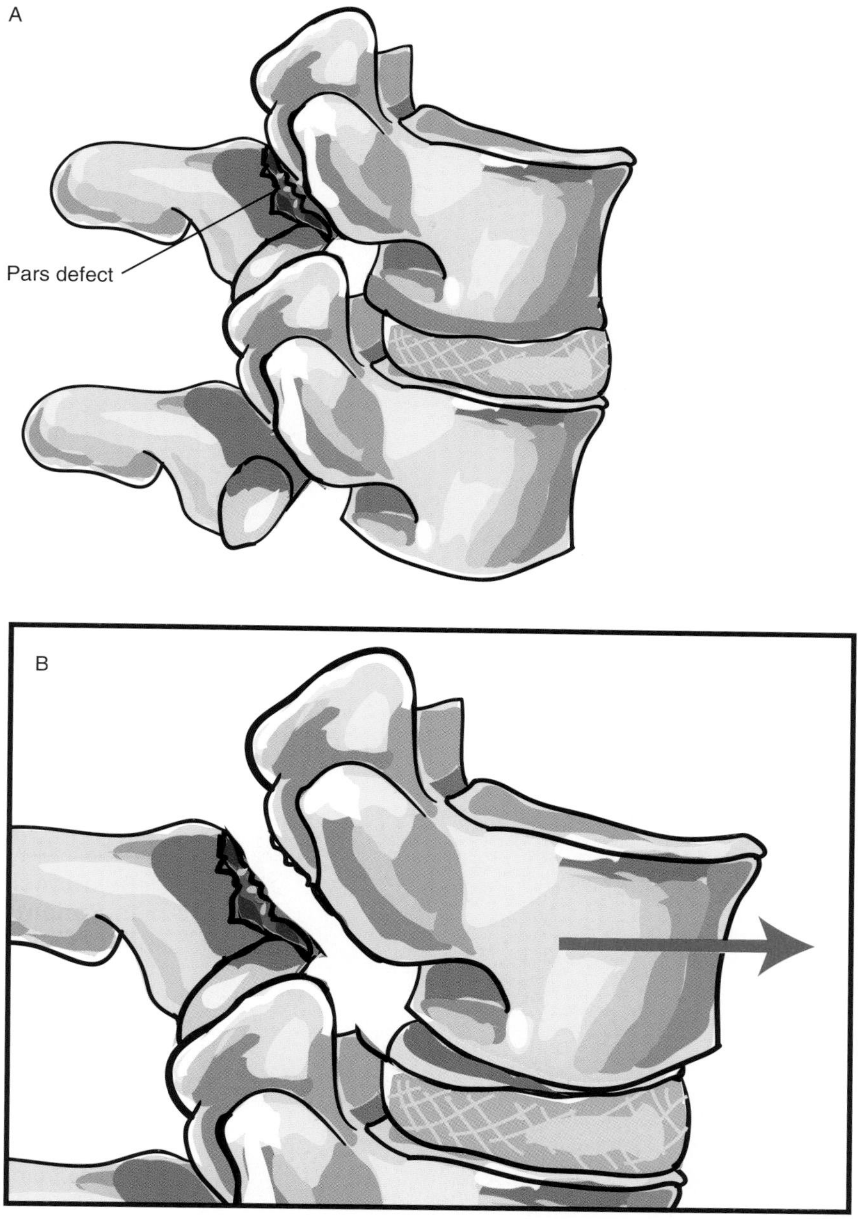

FIGURE 87–3 ■ Spondylolisthesis. **A,** A defect appears in the pars interarticularis, which prevents the inferior articular process from protecting the vertebra from forward translation. **B,** Disconnected from its posterior elements by the defect, the vertebral body is able to translate forward, leaving its inferior articular processes, laminae, and spinous processes behind.

anteroposterior or lateral films, and for that reason the oblique view of the lumbar spine was introduced. In an oblique view, the posterior elements of a lumbar vertebra assume the appearance of a "Scottie dog" (Fig. 87–4). The pars interarticularis corresponds to the neck of the dog. In a patient with a pars fracture, the fracture appears as a necklace around the dog's neck (Fig. 87–5).

Radiography, however, can detect only an established fracture. A greater imperative is to detect abnormalities that precede actual fracture, so that fracture can be averted. This is possible with bone scanning.

Bone scans show hyperemia and so will be positive for stress reactions, recent fracture, or a healing fracture.[3,21] Typically, they are not positive in chronic pars fractures, the hyperemia having settled.

Once a pars fracture has occurred, however, the role and utility of bone scan is questionable, because the relationship between clinical features and bone scans is imperfect (Table 87–2). Pars defects are not positive on bone scan in asymptomatic individuals. They may be positive in patients with chronic back pain or in patients with a history of repeated minor trauma; and they are more likely to be positive in patients with a history of a traumatic incident, but not reliably so.[22]

In athletes with back pain who are suspected of having a pars fracture, the correlations between bone scan and radiography are various and differ from study to study (Table 87–3).[23-26] Most are negative to both investigations. Only a minority are positive to both. Some have a positive bone scan but a negative radiograph, which is consistent with a stress

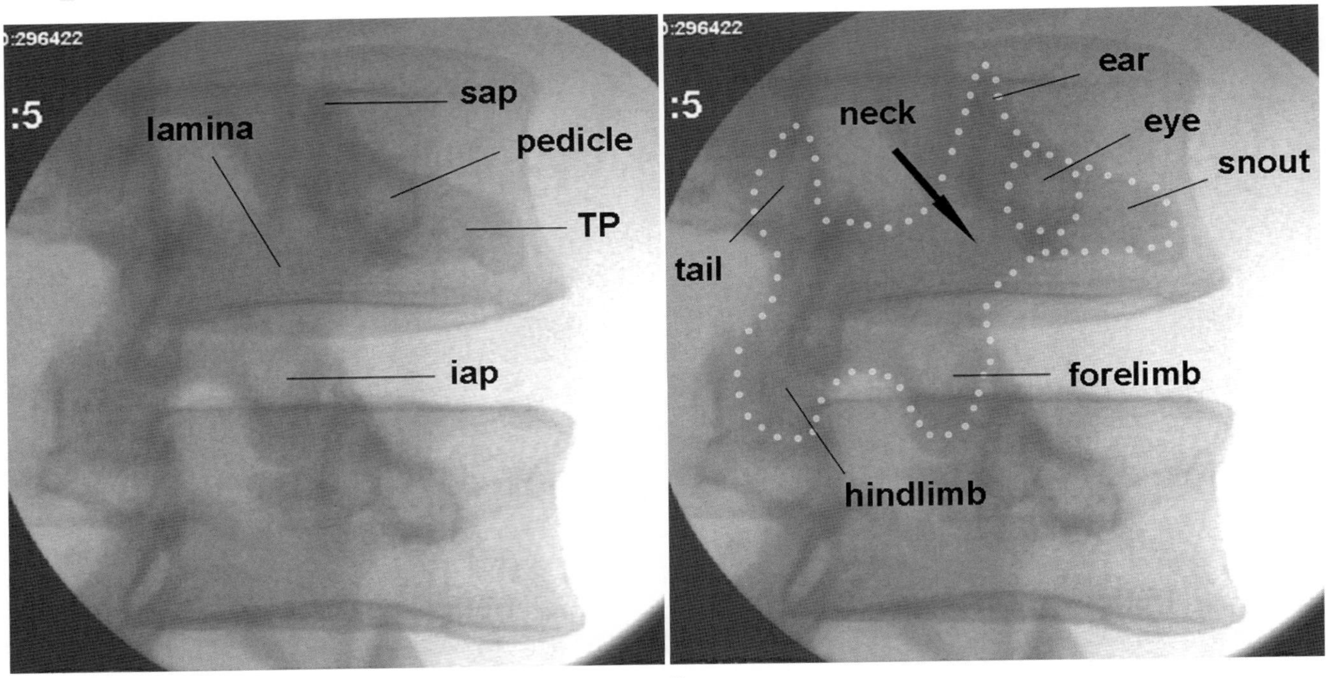

A B

FIGURE 87–4 ■ Radiographic appearance of the pars interarticularis. **A,** An oblique view with the posterior elements labeled: sap, superior articular process; TP, transverse process; iap, inferior articular process. **B,** How the posterior elements can be likened to the appearance of a Scottie dog.

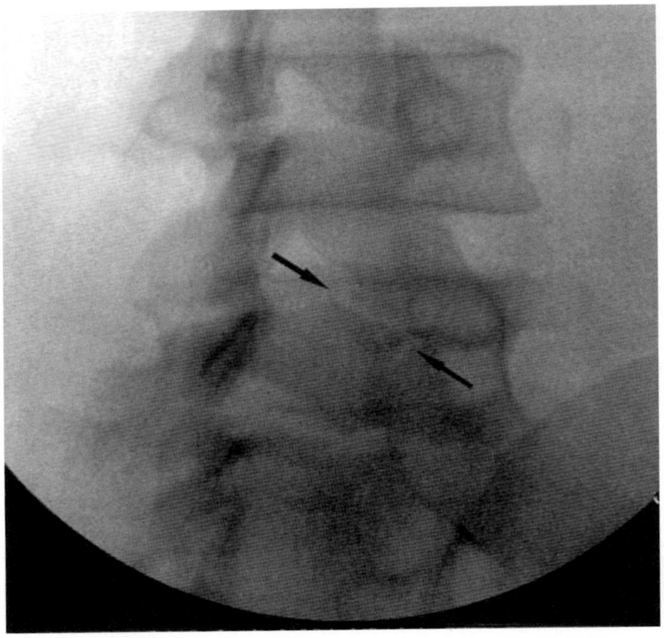

FIGURE 87–5 ■ Oblique radiograph of a pars interarticularis fracture. The fracture appears as a *white line,* across the neck of the "Scottie dog," between the *arrows.*

Table 87–2

Relationship Between History and Bone Scan in Patients with a Radiographically Evident Pars Defect

History	***Bone Scan***	
	Positive	*Negative*
Trauma within 1 year	9	4
Repeated minor trauma	9	20
Chronic back pain	5	35
No pain	0	14

Data from Lowe J, Schachner E, Hirschberg E, et al: Significance of bone scintigraphy in symptomatic spondylolysis. Spine 9:654, 1984.

Table 87–3

Correlation between Bone Scan and Radiography in the Detection of Pars Fractures

Bone Scan	***Radiography***		***Ref. No.***
	Positive	*Negative*	
Positive	9	4	23
Negative	9	16	
Positive	18	5	24,25
Negative	7	7	
Positive	5	1	26
Negative	22	38	

reaction without actual fracture. Some have a positive radiograph but a negative bone scan, which is consistent with an old fracture.

The virtue of the bone scan lies in being able to detect stress reactions before fracture occurs. It has been found that athletes with positive bone scans but negative radiographs were able to return to their sport and follow-up radiographs revealed no defects.[25] In those with both tests positive, bone scans resolved but radiographs revealed persisting defects.

MRI is a suitable, and perhaps preferable, alternative to bone scan. On MRI, five grades of abnormality can be detected, ranging from completely normal through stress reactions without fracture, incipient or partial fracture, overt fracture, and fracture without reactive edema.[27] In this regard, MRI has the advantage over bone scan that it can simultaneously show bone marrow reaction as well as fracture. Its cost-effectiveness has not been calculated, but the cost of a single MRI would seem competitive with that of a bone scan plus plain radiography.

The data suggest that in individuals at risk of a stress fracture, bone scan or MRI is the investigation of choice to screen for stress reactions before fracture. However, only a minority of patients suspected of fracture will actually have a fracture. There is no role for plain radiography as the initial test. If bone scan is used, it is the critical test. Radiography is indicated only if the bone scan is positive. If MRI is used, plain radiography becomes superfluous.

These guidelines, however, apply to individuals at risk of a pars fracture. They do not apply to patients in general with back pain. In those patients, pars fractures are an uncommon, and unlikely, source of pain.

Relationship to Pain

Most vexatious is the relationship of spondylolysis to pain. Whereas there is merit in detecting stress reactions to avert fracture and to preserve the integrity of the lumbar spine, this does not amount to establishing a diagnosis for the cause of pain.

Detecting a pars fracture does not constitute making a diagnosis. The confounding factor is that pars fractures are very common in individuals with no pain. Overton[16] reviewed the radiographs of 32,600 asymptomatic individuals and found pars fractures in 7.2%. Consequently, pars fractures can be expected to occur as an incidental finding in 7% of patients presenting with back pain. Their pain arises from sources other than the pars defect. Other studies have directly compared symptomatic and asymptomatic individuals and found no difference in the prevalence of spondylolysis (Table 87–4).[28,29]

Finding a pars fracture in a patient has no diagnostic validity. The positive likelihood ratio is essentially 1.0, which means the test contributes nothing to diagnosis. The data of Magora and Schwartz[29] actually indicate that pars fractures are more common in asymptomatic individuals. The likelihood ratio of 0.14, being less than 1.0, means that finding a pars fracture actually detracts from making a diagnosis.

These conclusions have been reinforced by a systematic review.[30] Multiple studies have confirmed an equivalent prevalence of spondylolysis in symptomatic and asymptomatic individuals. The odds ratios for spondylolysis as a risk factor for pain are nonsignificant.

Nevertheless, it is possible for a pars fracture to become symptomatic. The fibrous tissue of the defect contains nerve endings[31] ostensibly derived from the dorsal rami that innervate the affected segment and thus this tissue has the necessary apparatus to be a source of pain. What is required is the application of a means, other than radiography, by which to incriminate the fracture as a source of pain.

The definitive test is to anesthetize the defect.[32] Pars blocks are the only means available by which to determine whether a radiographically evident defect is a symptomatic or an asymptomatic one. Such a test is imperative in view of the high prevalence of defects in asymptomatic individuals. Relief of pain implies that the defect is actually the source of pain and predicts surgical success.[32] Patients who do not respond to blocks preoperatively are less likely to respond to fusion of the defect, even if the fusion is technically satisfactory.[32]

Unfortunately, there have been no systematic population studies to establish just how often pars fractures are responsible for back pain, either in general patients or in athletes. Too many practitioners are satisfied, despite the scientific evidence, that finding a fracture by radiography is sufficient to establish a diagnosis.

Also untested is the contention that the pain could arise not from the fracture but from the zygapophyseal joints of the flail lamina. Medial branch blocks of the suspected joint would be a valid test for this contention, but no study has reported the prevalence of pain from the zygapophyseal joints in patients with pars fractures.

Table 87–4

Validity of Radiography in the Diagnosis of Painful Spondylolysis

Pars Fracture	*Pain*	*No Pain*	*Sensitivity/Specificity*	*Likelihood Ratio*	*Ref. No.*
Unilateral	2	26	0.03/0.97	1.08	28
None	660	910			
Bilateral	62	65	0.09/0.93	1.3	
None	600	871			
Any	64	91	0.10/0.90	1.0	
None	598	845			
Any	44	64	0.07/0.83	0.14	29
None	604	312			

Treatment

The ideal opportunity for treatment is before fracture occurs. Finding a stress reaction allows the affected part to be rested. Athletes can modify their training regimens. If that is done the prospect obtains that fracture can be avoided. Bone scan is the only means by which an early diagnosis can be established.

In principle, if and once a fracture has occurred, healing and complete resolution can occur. Radiographic union can be expected in some 37% of patients, especially if the fracture is unilateral.[33]

In practice, most pars fractures pass unnoticed and are undetected at inception. They do not need to be detected because most remain asymptomatic, and thus they become incidental radiographic findings. If and when symptomatic, however, their optimal management has not been established. Bracing is recommended, supplemented by hamstring stretching, pelvic tilts, and abdominal strengthening, as the patient becomes pain free during activities of daily living[33]; however, this regimen has not been controlled for natural history.

Local anesthetic blocks of the pars fracture may be diagnostic, but they have not been established as therapeutic. In principle, radiofrequency neurotomy of the medial branches of the lumbar dorsal rami of the affected segment should relieve the pain of a pars fracture, but this treatment has not been formally tested for this condition.

For persistent pain, the mainstay of treatment has been arthrodesis of the pars fracture, by various means.[34-36] For some procedures, success rates of 80% have been reported. However, the efficacy of surgery, at large, is elusive because the treatment of pars fractures has often been confounded by, or confused with, the treatment of spondylolisthesis.

SPONDYLOLISTHESIS

Spondylolisthesis is an obvious structural abnormality of the lumbar spine, typically affecting the fifth or fourth lumbar vertebra. It is characterized by anterior displacement of the affected vertebra in relation to the one below (Fig. 87–6). The displacement implies that the vertebra has slipped forward.

Formally, spondylolisthesis is classified according to etiology (Table 87–5).[37] Of the various forms, isthmic, lytic spondylolisthesis is the most common and constitutes the archetypical form.

Although other methods have been used to quantify the magnitude of vertebral slippage,[38] the most commonly used are variants of the method of Taillard.[39] Spondylolisthesis is graded according to the extent to which the affected vertebra has moved across the superior surface of the vertebra below (Fig. 87–7). Four grades are recognized (I to IV) according to whether the posterior corner of the affected vertebra lies opposite one, two, three, or four quarters of the way across the supporting vertebra.

A perception is that segments affected by spondylolisthesis are unstable and that the slippage will progress. Longitudinal studies deny this as a rule. In a study of 27 children followed into adulthood, no female patient exhibited an increase in slip of greater than 10%, and only four males exhibited progression, which ranged in magnitude from 10% to 28%.[5] That study concluded that slippage occurs largely at the time of acquisition of bilateral pars fractures. No patient exhibited progression after the age of 18 years. These conclusions were echoed by another study of 311 adolescents.[40] Only 3% exhibited progression greater than 20%.

Another study[41] confirms some but disputes some of these findings. During follow-up of 272 adolescent patients, the mean progression of slip was only 3.5%, which indicates that, as a rule, spondylolisthesis does not progress appreciably. However, 23% of patients exhibited progression by 10% or more. (The proportion who exhibited progression by more than 20% was not reported.) Greater amounts of progression occurred in patients who had larger slips at presentation. However, in all cases, the greatest amount of slipping (90%)

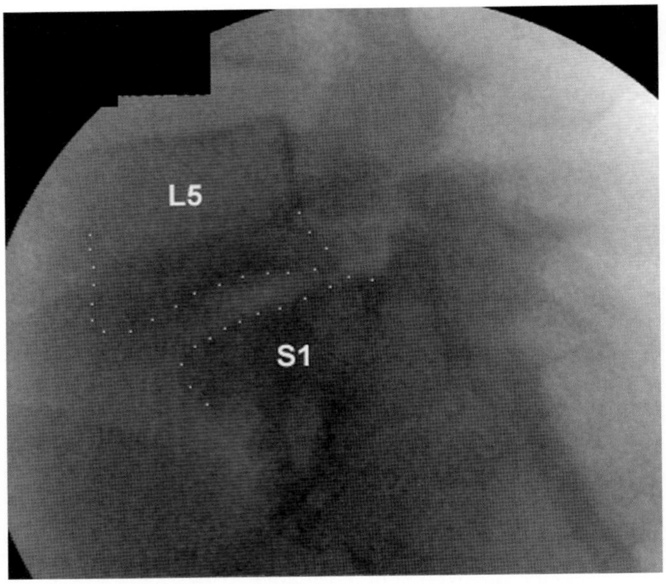

FIGURE 87–6 ■ Lateral radiograph of an L5 vertebra that exhibits spondylolisthesis. For clarity, the inferior margin of L5 and the superior margin of S1 have been traced with *dots*.

Table 87–5

Classification of Spondylolisthesis by Etiology

Type	*Cause*
Dysplastic	Congenital abnormality of upper sacrum
Isthmic	
Lytic	Fatigue fracture of pars interarticularis
Elongated pars	Congenital
Acute fracture	Acute trauma
Degenerative	Loss of cartilage and/or progressive deformation of zygapophyseal joints
Traumatic	Fracture in posterior elements other than pars
Pathologic	Intrinsic bone disease

Data from Wiltse LL, Newman PH, MacNab I: Classification of spondylolysis and spondylolisthesis. Clin Orthop 117:23, 1976.

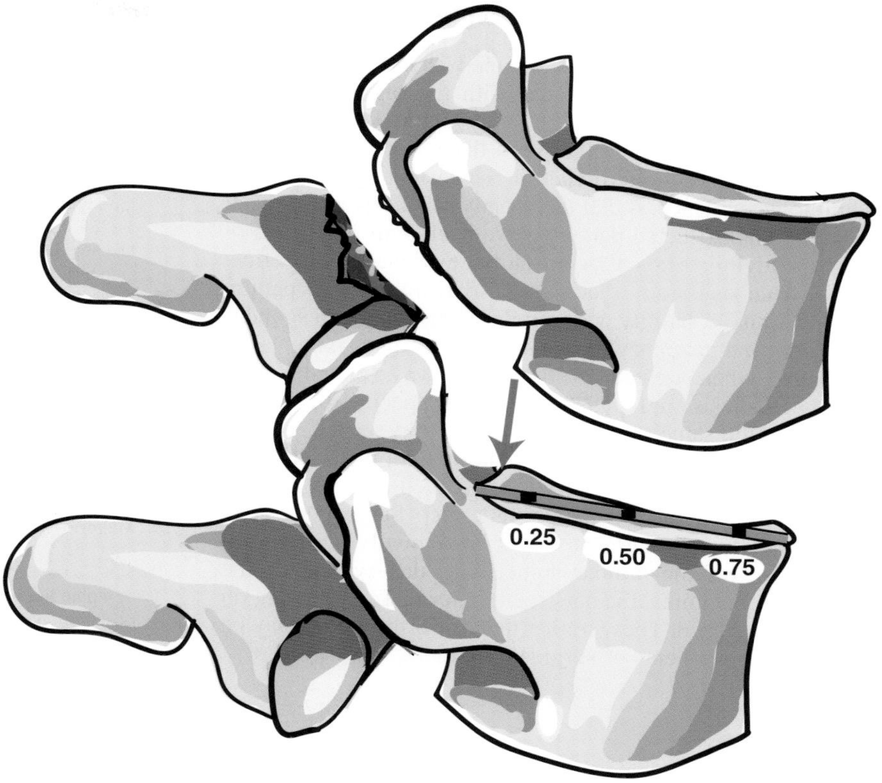

FIGURE 87–7 ■ The grading of spondylolisthesis. The grade is expressed in terms of whether the posterior corner of the affected vertebra lies opposite the first, second, third, or fourth quarter of the anteroposterior width of the supporting vertebra.

had already occurred at the time of presentation. Subsequent progression accounted for only 10% of the final slip, on the average. This calculation reinforces the rule that most of the slip occurs when the pars fracture is acquired.

Relationship to Pain

Spondylolisthesis is not related to back pain. This has been resoundingly established in a systematic review.[30] For an association with back pain, the odds ratios range between 1 and 2 for half the studies conducted and are less than 1 for the remainder. These values preclude any diagnostic significance of finding spondylolisthesis. One study[42] found that women with spondylolisthesis were more likely to report pain during the previous day, but there was no association with pain during the previous year, previous month, or previous week. No association at all was found for men. Pain intensity was not related to the magnitude of slip.

Treatment

It is somewhat ironic that for a condition known not to be associated with back pain there is such an abundance of literature for its treatment. Proponents of conservative therapy advocate flexion exercises, other exercises,[43-45] traction,[43] braces,[43,46] casts,[43] corsets,[43] and manipulation.[47,48] However, arthrodesis is the longest-established treatment, with success rates of 70% to 80% being claimed.[49-60] The one randomized study established that operative treatment was more effective than exercises.[61]

While the literature celebrates the success of treatment, it is not consistently clear from that literature what was being treated. Investigators treated patients for low back pain only,[47] low back pain or back pain with radiculopathy,[55] low back pain with or without radiculopathy,[56] low back pain and sciatica,[53,58] low back pain or leg pain,[59] low back pain and leg pain,[52] low back pain with or without nerve root irritation,[53] or radicular pain only.[49] Some did not specify the clinical features of their patients and, so, ostensibly treated patients for the lesion.[43,46,48]

Mechanisms of Pain

The literature on treatment fails to provide evidence on the mechanism by which spondylolisthesis might cause pain. Indeed, it seems to have paid no attention to this issue, with patients having been treated without regard to differing symptoms or their cause. It is the lesion, rather than symptoms, that has attracted treatment.

On the one hand, it is credible that spondylolisthesis could cause radicular pain, by stretching nerve roots, by narrowing the intervertebral foramen, or by the flail lamina impinging on the nerve roots. The one study that explicitly addressed the latter phenomenon showed that radicular pain could be relieved simply by removing the loose lamina.[49]

On the other hand, the mechanisms by which spondylolisthesis might cause back pain are no more than speculative. It is conceivable that the patient may have back pain stemming from the disk of the affected segment or that there may be pain from the pars fracture or from the zygapophyseal joints of the flail lamina. None of these contentions, however, has been formally tested, let alone proven.

The one piece of circumstantial evidence stems from a small retrospective study. It claimed that progression of spondylolisthesis was associated with the onset of marked degeneration of the disk.[62] The study implied that the pain which the patients suffered arose in the affected disk.

An alternative interpretation, consistent with the epidemiologic evidence, is that the spondylolisthesis is irrelevant to symptoms. Affected patients have back pain regardless of their spondylolisthesis. Circumstantial evidence to this effect comes from one study that showed that the clinical pattern and functional disability were similar in patients with spondylolisthesis and patients with nonspecific low back pain.[63] Furthermore, when treated in the same way, patients with spondylolisthesis and patients with nonspecific back pain respond in the same way.[47]

If this is the case, spondylolisthesis is immaterial to the diagnosis and immaterial to outcome. Even surgery may be having a nonspecific, serendipitous effect. Surgery not only fuses the affected segment but it also involves extensive débridement of the lumbar spine, with denervation of the zygapophyseal joints, the pars fracture, or disk, depending on the technique used. These, rather than the arthrodesis, may be the active components of surgical treatment.

References

1. Cocchiarella L, Andersson GBJ (eds): American Medical Association Guides to the Evaluation of Permanent Impairment, 5th ed. Chicago, AMA Press, 2001, p 404.
2. Rowe GG, Roche MB: The etiology of separate neural arch. J Bone Joint Surg Am 35:102, 1953.
3. Hensinger RN: Spondylolysis and spondylolisthesis in children and adolescents. J Bone Joint Surg Am 71:1089, 1989.
4. Stewart TD: The age incidence of neural-arch defects in Alaskan natives, considered from the standpoint of etiology. J Bone Joint Surg Am 35:937, 1953.
5. Fredrickson BE, Baker D, McHolick WJ, et al: The natural history of spondylolysis and spondylolisthesis. J Bone Joint Surg Am 66:699, 1984.
6. Cyron BM, Hutton WC: Variations in the amount and distribution of cortical bone across the partes interarticulares of L5: A predisposing factor in spondylolysis? Spine 4:163, 1979.
7. Cyron BM, Hutton WC: The fatigue strength of the lumbar neural arch in spondylolysis. J Bone Joint Surg Br 60:234, 1978.
8. Farfan HF, Osteria V, Lamy C: The mechanical etiology of spondylolysis and spondylolisthesis. Clin Orthop 117:40, 1979.
9. Green TP, Allvey JC, Adams MA: Spondylolysis: Bending of the inferior articular processes of lumbar vertebrae during simulated spinal movements. Spine 19:2683, 1994.
10. Farfan HF, Cossette JW, Robertson GH, et al: The effects of torsion on the lumbar intervertebral joints: The role of torsion in the production of disc degeneration. J Bone Joint Surg Am 52:468, 1970.
11. Ichikawa N, Ohara Y, Morishita T, et al: An aetiological study on spondylolysis from a biomechanical aspect. Br J Sports Med 16:135, 1982.
12. Jackson DE, Wiltse LL, Cirincione RJ: Spondylolysis in the female gymnast. Clin Orthop 117:68, 1976.
13. Hoshina I: Spondylolysis in athletes. Physician Sportsmed 8:75, 1980.
14. McCarroll JR, Miller JM, Ritter MA: Lumbar spondylolysis and spondylolisthesis in college football players. Am J Sports Med 14:404, 1986.
15. Foster D, John D, Elliot B, et al: Back injuries to fast bowlers in cricket: A prospective study. Br J Sports Med 23:150, 1989.
16. Overton RD: Spondylolysis. JAMA 195:671, 1966.
17. Virta L, Ronnemaa T, Osterman K, et al: Prevalence of isthmic lumbar spondylolisthesis in middle-aged subjects from eastern and western Finland. J Clin Epidemiol 45:917, 1992.
18. Roche MB: The pathology of neural-arch defects. J Bone Joint Surg Am 31:529, 1949.
19. Eisenstein SM, Ashton IK, Roberts S, et al: Innervation of the spondylolysis "ligament." Spine 19:912, 1994.
20. Ghelman B, Doherty JH: Demonstration of spondylolysis by arthrography of the apophyseal joint. AJR Am J Roentgenol 130:986, 1978.
21. Papanicolaou N, Wilkinson RH, Emans JB, et al: Bone scintigraphy and radiography in young athletes with low back pain. AJR Am J Roentgenol 145:1039, 1985.
22. Lowe J, Schachner E, Hirschberg E, et al: Significance of bone scintigraphy in symptomatic spondylolysis. Spine 9:654, 1984.
23. Elliot S, Huitson A, Wastie ML: Bone scintigraphy in the assessment of spondylolysis in patients attending a sports injury clinic. Clin Radiol 39:269, 1988.
24. Jackson DE, Wiltse LL, Cirincione RJ: Spondylolysis in the female gymnast. Clin Orthop 117:68, 1976.
25. Jackson DW, Wiltse LL, Dingeman RD, Hayes M: Stress reactions involving the pars interarticularis in young athletes. Am J Sports Med 9:304, 1981.
26. Van den Oever M, Merrick MV, Scott JHS: Bone scintigraphy in symptomatic spondylolysis. J Bone Joint Surg Br 69:453, 1987.
27. Hollenberg GM, Beattie PF, Meyers SP, et al: Stress reactions of the lumbar pars interarticularis: The development of a new MRI classification system. Spine 27:181, 2002.
28. Libson E, Bloom RA, Dinari G: Symptomatic and asymptomatic spondylolysis and spondylolisthesis in young adults. Int Orthop 6:259, 1982.
29. Magora A, Schwartz A: Relation between low back pain and x-ray changes: IV. Lysis and olisthesis. Scand J Rehab Med 12:47, 1980.
30. van Tulder MW, Assendelft WJJ, Koes BW, Bouter LM: Spinal radiographic findings and nonspecific low back pain: A systematic review of observational studies. Spine 22:427, 1997.
31. Schneiderman GA, McLain RF, Hambly MF, Nielsen SL: The pars defect as a pain source: A histological study. Spine 20:1761, 1995.
32. Suh PB, Esses SI, Kostuik JP: Repair of a pars interarticularis defect—the prognostic value of pars infiltration. Spine 16(Suppl 8):S445, 1991.
33. Blanda J, Bethem D, Moats W, Lew M: Defects of pars interarticularis in athletes: A protocol for nonoperative treatment. J Spinal Disord 6:406, 1993.
34. Buck JE: Direct repair of the defect in spondylolisthesis. J Bone Joint Surg Br 52:432, 1970.
35. Pedersen AK, Hagen R: Spondylolysis and spondylolisthesis: Treatment by internal fixation and bone-grafting of the defect. J Bone Joint Surg Am 70:15, 1988.
36. Bradford DS, Iza J: Repair of the defect in spondylolysis or minimal degrees of spondylolisthesis by segmental wire fixation and bone grafting. Spine 10:673, 1985.
37. Wiltse LL, Newman PH, Macnab I: Classification of spondylolysis and spondylolisthesis. Clin Orthop 117:23, 1976.
38. Meschan I: A radiographic study of spondylolisthesis with special reference to stability determination. Radiology 47:249, 1946.
39. Taillard W: Le spondylolisthesis chez l'enfant et l'adolescent. Acta Orthop Scand 24:115, 1854.
40. Danielson BI, Frennered AK, Irstam LKH: Radiologic progression of isthmic lumbar spondylolisthesis in young patients. Spine 16:422, 1991.
41. Seitsalo S, Osterman K, Hyvarinen H, et al: Progression of spondylolisthesis in children and adolescents: A long-term follow-up of 272 patients. Spine 16:417, 1991.
42. Virta L, Ronnemaa T: The association of mild-moderate isthmic lumbar spondylolisthesis and low back pain in middle-aged patients is weak and it only occurs in women. Spine 18:1496, 1993.
43. Pizzutillo PD, Hummer CD: Nonoperative treatment for painful adolescent spondylolysis or spondylolisthesis.
44. Gramse RR, Sinaki M, Ilstrup D: Lumbar spondylolisthesis: A rational approach to conservative treatment. Mayo Clin Proc 55:681, 1980.
45. Sinaki M, Lutness MP, Ilstrup DM, et al: Lumbar spondylolisthesis: Retrospective comparison and three-year follow-up of two conservative treatment programs. Arch Phys Med Rehabil 70:594, 1989.
46. Steiner ME, Micheli LJ: Treatment of symptomatic spondylolysis and spondylolisthesis with the modified Boston brace. Spine 10:937, 1985.
47. Mierau D, Cassidy JD, McGregor M, Kirkaldy-Willis WH: A comparison of the effectiveness of spinal manipulative therapy for low back pain patients with and without spondylolisthesis. J Manip Physiol Ther 10:49, 1987.
48. Cassidy JD, Potter GE, Kirkaldy-Willis WH: Manipulative management of back pain in patients with spondylolisthesis. J Can Chir Assoc 22:15, 1978.

49. Gill GG, Manning JG, White HL: Surgical treatment of spondylolisthesis without fusion: Excision of the loose lamina with decompression of the nerve roots. J Bone Joint Surg Am 37:493, 1955.
50. Klenerman L: Posterior spinal fusion in spondylolisthesis. J Bone Joint Surg Br 44:637, 1962.
51. Wiltse LL, Hutchinson RH: Surgical treatment of spondylolisthesis. Clin Orthop 35:116, 1964.
52. Rombold C: Treatment of spondylolisthesis by posterolateral fusion, resection of the pars interarticularis, and prompt mobilization of the patient: An end-result study of seventy-three patients. J Bone Joint Surg Am 48:1282, 1966.
53. Laurent LE, Osterman K: Operative treatment of spondylolisthesis in young patients. Clin Orthop 117:85, 1976.
54. Kaneda K, Stoh S, Nohara Y, Oguma T: Distraction rod instrumentation with posterolateral fusion in isthmic spondylolisthesis: 53 cases followed for 18-89 months. Spine 10:383, 1985.
55. Hanley EN, Levy JA: Surgical treatment of isthmic lumbosacral spondylolisthesis: Analysis of variables influencing results. Spine 14:48, 1989.
56. Johnson LP, Nasca RJ, Dunham WK: Surgical management of isthmic spondylolisthesis. Spine 13:93, 1988.
57. Seitsalo S: Operative and conservative treatment of moderate spondylolisthesis in young patients. J Bone Joint Surg 72B:908, 1990.
58. Frennered AK, Danielsson BI, Nachemson AL, Nordwall AB: Midterm follow-up of young patients fused in situ for spondylolisthesis. Spine 16:409, 1991.
59. Lenke LJ, Bridwell KH, Bullis D, et al: Results of in situ fusion for isthmic spondylolisthesis. J Spinal Disord 5:433, 1992.
60. Suk SI, Lee CK, Kim WJ, et al: Adding posterior lumbar interbody fusion to pedicle screw fixation and posterolateral fusion after decompression in spondylolytic spondylolisthesis. Spine 22:210, 1997.
61. Moller H, Hedlund R: Surgery versus conservative management in adult isthmic spondylolisthesis: A prospective randomised study: I. Spine 25:1711, 2000.
62. Floman Y: Progression of lumbosacral isthmic spondylolisthesis in adults. Spine 25:342, 2000.
63. Moller H, Sundin A, Hedlund R: Symptoms, signs, and functional disability in adult spondylolisthesis. Spine 25:683, 2000.

chapter 88

Sacroiliac Joint Pain and Related Disorders

Steven Simon

The sacroiliac (SI) joint has been a source of pain to both sufferers of low back pain and those who refuse to recognize its contribution to this common problem.[1] Many of the frustrations experienced by those who hurt but continually have "negative" examinations and studies can be traced to this overlooked synovial joint and its unrecognized maladies. In this chapter I explore the anatomy, motion, pain generators, evaluation, and treatment of the SI joint and its relation to low back pain.

ANATOMY

The axial spine rests on the sacrum, a triangular fusion of vertebrae arranged in a kyphotic curve and ending with the attached coccyx in the upper buttock. Iliac wings (innominate bones) attach on either side, forming a bowl with a high back and a shallow front. Three joints result from this union: the pubic symphysis in the anterior midline and the left and right SI joints in the back (Fig. 88–1). Multiple ligaments and fascia attach across these joint spaces, limiting motion and providing stability (Figs. 88–2 and 88–3).[2] The hip joints are formed by the femoral heads and the acetabular sockets deep within the innominate bones. The hips create a direct link between the lower extremities and the spine, to relay ground reaction forces from weight bearing and motion. A physiologic balance between lumbar lordosis and sacral curvature exists both at rest and in motion. Changes of pelvic tilt and lumbar lordosis occur in the anteroposterior (AP) plane, relying on attached muscles and fascia, but do not have significant effect on the SI joints owing to a self-bracing mechanism. The sacrum positioned between the innominate bones functions as a keystone in an arch, allowing only cephalocaudad (CC) and AP motion.[3] Innervation is varied and extensive owing to the size of this joint, which includes outflow from anterior and posterior rami of L3-S1.[4]

The SI is a synovial (diarthrodial) joint that is more mobile in youth than later in life. The upper two thirds of the joint becomes more fibrotic in adulthood. The female pelvis is also more mobile to accommodate pregnancy and parturition. Ligament and muscle attachments help to maintain stability of the pelvic ring latissimus allowing movement within limits. Further motion is also limited by the irregular shape of the joint articulation, in which ridges and grooves increase resistance friction and add to the keystone arch structure. Prolonged loading (such as standing or sitting for long periods) and alterations of the sacral base (leg asymmetry or ligamentous injury) are associated with joint hypermobility and resultant low back pain.[3,5,6]

Multiple muscle attachments cross the SI joints and contribute to pelvic stability and force transfer.[3] The thoracolumbar fascia includes attachments to the 12th rib, lumbar spinous and lateral processes, and pelvic brim. Fascial and muscle attachments expand to include erector spinae, internal obliques, serratus posterior inferior, sacrotuberous ligament, dorsal SI ligament, iliolumbar ligament, posterior iliac spine, and sacral crest. Major muscles attached to the SI include the gluteus maximus, gluteus medius, latissimus dorsi, multifidus, biceps femoris, psoas, piriformis, obliquus, and transversus abdominis. Vleeming and coworkers concluded that the purpose of these muscles is not for motion but to confer stability for loading and unloading forces produced by walking and running.[7]

MOTION

Ligaments also limit mobility of the SI joint and functionally comprise the distal two thirds of the joint.[8] Motion is described in three dimensions: AP, CC, and left-right (LR). The major ligaments and their actions are listed next (see Figs. 88–2 and 88–3).

1. The interosseous ligament resists joint separation and motion in the cephalad and AP directions.
2. The dorsal sacroiliac ligament covers and assists the interosseous ligament.
3. The anterior SI ligament, a thickening of the anterior inferior joint capsule, resists CC and LR motion.
4. The sacrospinous ligament resists rotational motion of the pelvis around the axial spine.
5. The iliolumbar ligaments resist motion between the distal lumbar segments and the sacrum and help to stabilize the sacral position between the iliac wings.

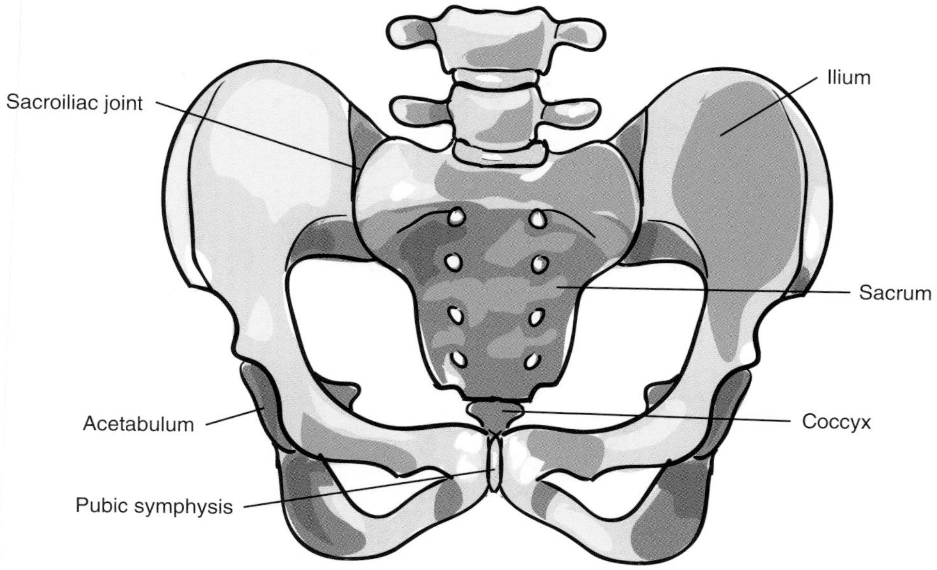

FIGURE 88–1 ■ Anatomy of the bony pelvis.

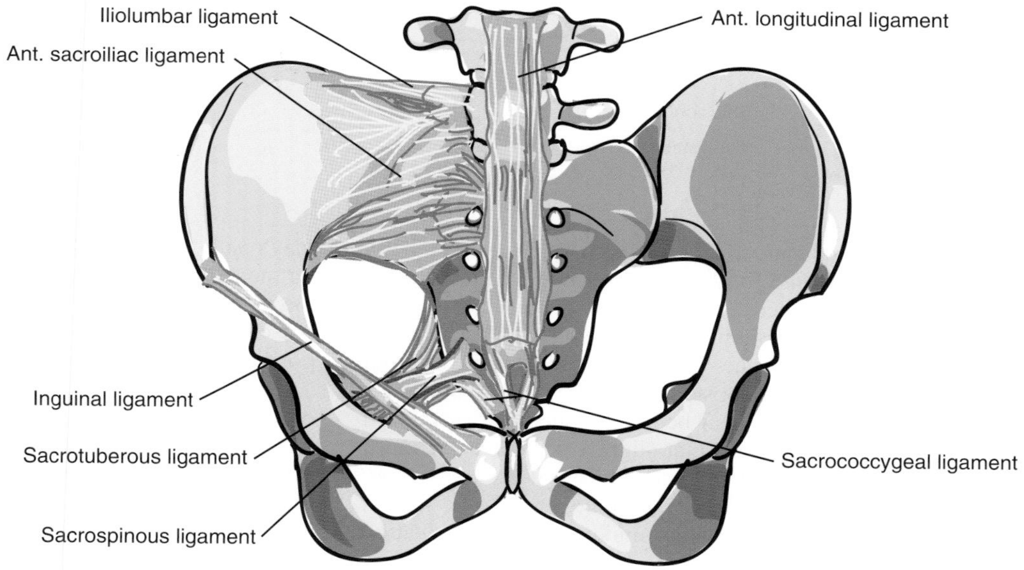

FIGURE 88–2 ■ The anterior ligaments of the pelvis.

6. The sacrotuberous ligament resists flexion of the iliacs on the axial spine.
7. The pubic symphysis resists AP motion of the innominates, shear, and LR forces.

Next, actual movement of the pelvis and SI joints and their functions will be reviewed. We have already established that ground reaction forces from weight bearing pass through the legs and pelvis to the spine. The point in the body where these forces are in balance is termed the *center of gravity* and has been determined to be about 2 cm below the navel. Gravity can also be considered a force line that produces different effects on the pelvic girdle as it shifts from anterior to posterior relative to the center of the acetabular fossae.[9] Body posture and positioning, muscle strength, and weight distribution determine alterations in the force lines. An anterior force line produces anterior (downward) rotation of the pelvis, decreasing tension in the sacrotuberous ligament and maintaining tension in the posterior interosseous ligaments. As the line of gravity moves posterior to the acetabula, the pelvis rotates posterior (i.e., the anterior rim tilts upward), and the sacrotuberous and posterior interosseous ligaments tighten. This is easier to visualize if we imagine a line between the femoral heads on which the pelvis rotates. The vertical distance of motion is about 2.5 cm in each direction at L3.[10] The pelvis also rotates in relation to the spine during walking. As the legs alternately move forward, the pelvic innominate bones rotate forward and toward midline, but the spine and sacrum counter-rotate, although to a lesser degree.[11] The SI joint lies between these moving planes and forces; central to

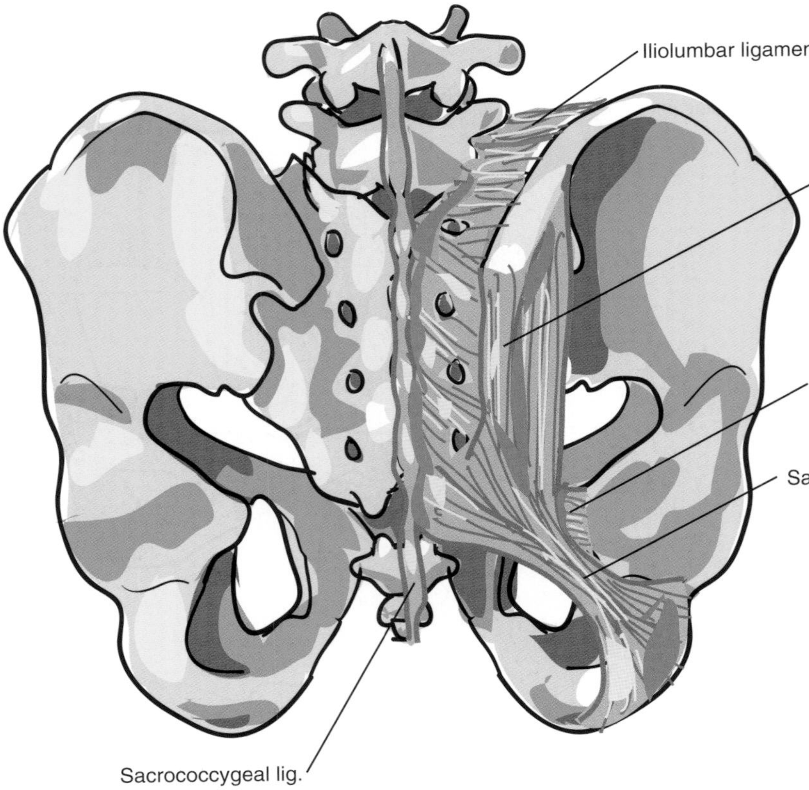

FIGURE 88–3 ■ The posterior ligaments of the pelvis.

vertical, horizontal, and rotational activity. Hula and belly dancers have perfected rhythmic pelvic motion, much to the delight of their audiences.

Dysfunction of the joint without direct trauma commonly arises from an imbalance in the anterior pelvis without adequate stabilization of posterior (sacrotuberous and interosseous) ligaments. Lifting or bending while leaning forward produces anterior pelvic tilt that slightly separates the innominates from the sacrum, making unilateral AP shift more likely, especially if proper ergonomic technique is not used.[12,13] The net effect of such a unilateral anterior rotation on the ipsilateral side would be to raise the pelvic brim and posterior superior iliac spine (PSIS) and cause "apparent" leg lengthening in supine positions and shortening in long sitting. (By *apparent* means that the affected leg is not necessarily longer, but appears to be owing to its attachment to the hip socket, which is rotated forward, or caudad in a supine position. Long sitting in this situation positions the acetabulum posterior to the SI joint, resulting in apparent shortening.) Bilateral anterior SI rotation would not produce leg length asymmetry but would stretch the iliopsoas, simulating tight and tender hip flexors. Posterior unilateral rotation would produce ipsilateral PSIS and brim drop as well as a shortening of the supine leg and lengthening with long sitting.

■ PAIN GENERATORS

The net effect of this type of sustained unilateral force is to create an imbalance of attached myofascial insertions. Pain may result from periosteal irritation or circulatory congestion on the shortened side and loss of strength and tenderness on the elongated side. The joint line is stressed by the combined muscle and ligament pull, resisting resolution and normal positioning.

The SI joint line is densely innervated by several levels of spinal nerves (L3-S1) and may produce lumbar disk-like symptoms when stimulated.[4] Muscle insertions near the area, such as the gluteus maximus and hamstrings, refer pain to the hip and ischial area, respectively, when stressed. Fortin and associates have examined normal and symptomatic patients to generate a pain map of SI symptoms. The most common discomfort was described as aching or hypersensitivity along the joint line to the ipsilateral hip and trochanter (Fig. 88–4).[1,14]

Other pains, reported less frequently, occur about 2 inches lateral to the umbilicus on a line between the navel and anterior superior iliac spine (ASIS) or referred into the groins and testicles. Sitting can be painful when anterior rotation of the pelvis changes the relationship of acetabulum to femoral head. Because the ischial tuberosity cannot move while the subject is seated, balanced support for the pelvic "bowl" is lost, an effect aggravated by the tendency to sit lopsided. The resultant forces produce AP or LR torque on the SI joint. Standing decreases this pain because the femoral heads are repositioned and can, in this fashion, buttress the pelvis. Sciatic nerve stretch may also be relieved by allowing the pelvis to rotate, thereby shifting weight to the opposite leg.

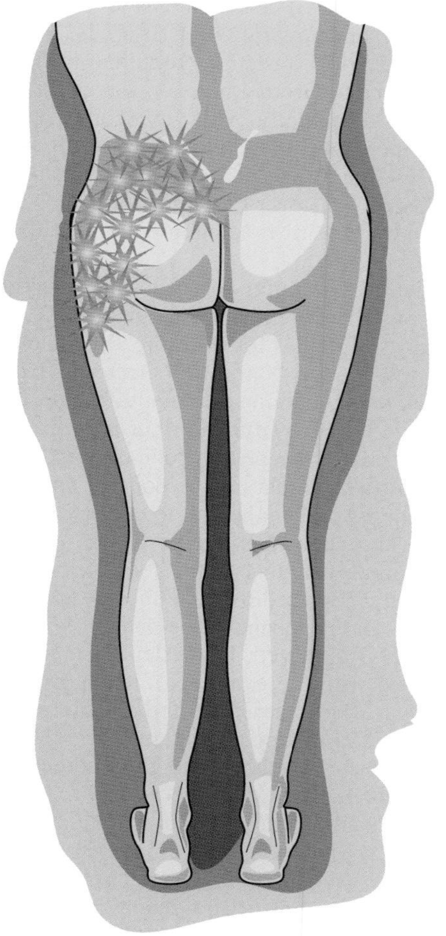

FIGURE 88–4 ■ Distribution of pain emanating from the sacroiliac joint.

■ EVALUATION

A thorough history must be taken to seek preexisting disease or injury, or new trauma, and to evaluate the patient's general health. Bladder, bowel, or sexual dysfunction or numbness often suggests an emergency that requires immediate care. The pain history should also include how long the problem has been present and treatments, including medications, injection, modalities, bracing, or manipulations and their outcomes. Provocative and palliative positions or activity can be guides to aid in treatment planning. Functional loss is significant because it can be an indication of suffering and a measure of treatment success as the patient begins to resume activities.

Radiography is indicated to investigate fractures or lumbosacral lesions. Inflammatory changes in the SI joint are characteristic of rheumatoid spondylitis (Marie-Strümpell spondylitis) and can be verified with blood tests for HLA-B27. Males in their 20s to 30s generally present with atraumatic low back pain and stiffness. Although films may be negative on initial view, and fuzziness over the SI region and stiffness in the lumbar spine may be the only early signs of this progressive disease, many of the tests listed later will still have positive results. Quantitative radionuclide bone scanning has also been helpful in early diagnosis.[15]

How the patient walks reveals important information on antalgic gait, weight shifting, and asymmetry of the pelvic brim or of shoulder height. Spinal examination for range of motion, scoliosis, myospasm, and ligamentous irritation will localize pain generators. Familiarity with the anatomy in this region (i.e., of muscle insertions and actions) is essential to understanding mechanical relationships to pelvic girdle positioning and the necessity of balancing forces to cure, rather than just palliate, an SI syndrome. Various tests have been developed to detect SI dysfunction. Most can be performed simply during the regular examination and verified by provocation.

1. *Fortin finger test:* The patient points to the area of pain with one finger. The result is positive if the site is within 1 cm of the PSIS, and generally inferomedial.
2. *Fabere maneuver* (*f*lexion, *ab*duction, *e*xternal *r*otation, and *e*xtension of hip, also known as *Patrick's test*): The patient lies supine. One heel is placed on the opposite knee and the elevated leg is guided toward the examining table. Result is positive if pain is elicited along the SI joint. (This also stresses the hip joint and may result in trochanteric pain.)
3. *Gaenslen test:* The patient is supine. The hip and knee are maximally flexed toward the trunk, and the opposite leg is extended. Some examiners perform this with the extended leg off the examining table to force the SI joint through maximal range of motion. Finding is positive if pain is felt across the SI joint. This also stresses the hip joint, producing trochanteric pain.
4. *Compression test:* The patient lies on one side. The examiner applies pressure on one pelvic brim in the direction of the other. A positive result is pain across the SI joint.
5. *Compression test at SI joint:* The patient is prone. The examiner places a palm along the SI joint or on the sacrum and makes a vertical downward thrust. Discomfort along the joint line is positive.
6. *Pubic symphysis test:* The patient is supine. Pressure is applied with the examining finger at the left or right pubic bone adjacent to the symphysis. The result is positive if pain is felt at the site. (Most patients are not aware of this tenderness before it is elicited. The examiner should ask permission before applying pressure and might consider having a witness in the room to avoid the misconception of inappropriate sexual contact.)
7. *Distraction test:* The patient is supine. The examiner alternately presses each ASIS in a posterolateral direction. Result is positive if it produces pain or if movement is asymmetrical.
8. *Fade test:* The patient is supine. The hip is flexed and adducted to midline. The examiner applies pressure to the long axis of the femur to push the ilium posterior. A positive result is pain.
9. *Passive straight leg raising:* The patient is supine. The examiner grasps the heel and lifts the leg vertically from the examining table with the knee extended. The patient is asked to hold the leg elevated and then to slowly lower it. A positive result is ipsilateral pain, which suggests anterior rotation.
10. *One-legged stork test:* The patient stands with examiner behind. The examiner's thumbs are placed on one PSIS and on the sacrum at S2. The patient then flexes the pal-

pated hip to 90 degrees. If the examiner's thumb moves upward instead of inferolaterally, as would be expected, the result is positive.

11. *Van Durson standing flexion test:* The patient stands with examiner behind. The examiner's thumbs are placed just below each PSIS. The patient flexes the trunk forward without bending the knees. A positive sign is asymmetrical motion (i.e., upward motion on the involved side).
12. *Piedallu or seated flexion test:* The patient is seated with the examiner behind. The examiner's thumbs are placed just below each PSIS. The patient flexes the trunk forward. A positive result is asymmetry of motion (i.e., upward motion on the involved side).
13. *Rectal examination:* Although it is not specific for SI involvement, a thorough rectal examination is necessary to search for referred pain from the prostate, uterus, or spasm in muscles of the pelvic floor. Piriformis muscle spasm can be localized at the end of the examiner's finger at the 2 or 10 o'clock position. Because this is associated with sciatic nerve entrapment, compression of this muscle reproduces painful symptoms.

TREATMENT

Recognition is the first part of treatment because it allows treatment to be directed toward the pain generator. Once the diagnosis is established, controlling the conditions for mechanical malpositioning can start with pain control and move on to education, modalities, and exercises.

Education

Mechanical descriptions of pelvic anatomy and rotations of the pelvic brim help the patient to understand what forces are continuing to stress the SI joint and cause pain. Proper ergonomic training for bending, lifting, and stretching prevents repeated injury from undermining the treatment program and increases the patient's interest and participation.

Modalities

Deep heat is tolerated better than ice and is more likely to reach affected areas. Hot packs feel good and may relax or "soften" muscles before stretching or massage. Ultrasound along the SI joint line is palliative. The addition of 10% steroid gel, which can replace electrode gel required for ultrasonography, can add some benefit by reducing inflammation.

Electricity can be curative by relaxing muscle spasm (electrogalvanic stimulation, functional electrical stimulation, electrical acupuncture) or palliative by blocking the pain signal (transcutaneous electrical nerve stimulation). The pain practitioner can choose from office-based units such as the Matrix, which offers 88 different electrical program choices for treatment, or portable transcutaneous nerve stimulator units such as PGS-3000 or RM-4, which are single-output units for directed treatment.

Traction for the pelvis has not been helpful for SI dysfunction but has proven helpful for some spine lesions. Bracing is a form of traction that applies direct pressure and stabilization over a movable area, which can be helpful in SI joint dysfunction. The SI belt should have a sacral pad directly over the sacrum and covering both SI joints. The belt should cross the pelvic brims, fasten in front, and fit tightly enough to resist AP motion. Ground reaction forces are very strong, however, and eventually will overcome most bracing attempts. Some argue that the real value of bracing is to remind the wearer to use proper body mechanics and limit rotational forces. Whatever the source of benefit, there seems to be some value in using bracing initially, especially if hypermobility exists.

Mobilization is helpful for restoring SI alignment and sacral position. There are many osteopathic, chiropractic, and physiotherapy techniques for restoring alignment. The reader is directed to other texts for full mechanical descriptions. Simple office manipulations are safe, effective, and immediately palliative for SI dysfunction but may be frustrated by muscle spasm along the pelvic floor or spinal attachments. One simple procedure that can be done in the office or by a helper at home is leg lengthening to correct anterior rotation shortening. The patient lies supine on the examining table with the examiner standing at the foot of the table and the examiner's thumbs placed over the medial malleoli to evaluate for leg length discrepancy. The patient is asked to sit up, and leg length is observed. If one leg appears to shorten, it can be grasped with the examiner's hands at the ankle and pulled gently toward the foot of the table. Leg length is checked again after this manipulation.

Self-mobilization is the key to giving the patient tools to correct recurrent malpositioning secondary to ligament laxity. Even proper seating can help to maintain a self-bracing system for the SI joint. A small cushion beneath the proximal thighs distributes weight directly on the ischium, and a second in the lumbar lordotic curve straightens the spine and allows even distribution of reaction forces.

Injections may be the best option for quickly reducing inflammation along the joint line.[16] Typical injections contain both analgesic and corticosteroid and are placed in the lower third of the joint (the true synovial portion). These injections may be performed "blind" or under computed tomographic or fluoroscopic guidance. Other "blind" injections with similar drugs to the upper two thirds of the joint line can also be very effective at reducing pain by reducing ligament irritation. We have substituted ketorolac for corticosteroids on repeated injections, with beneficial results.

The following procedure has been used successfully to inject the SI joint. The goals of this injection technique are first explained to the patient, who is placed in the supine position. The skin overlying the affected SI joint space is prepared with antiseptic solution. A sterile syringe containing the 4.0 mL of 0.25% preservative-free bupivacaine and 40 mg of methylprednisolone is attached to a 3-inch, 25-gauge needle using strict aseptic technique. The PSIS is identified. At this point, the needle is then carefully advanced through the skin and subcutaneous tissues at a 45-degree angle toward the affected SI joint (Fig. 88–5). If bone is encountered, the needle is withdrawn into the subcutaneous tissues and redirected superiorly and slightly more lateral. When the needle is correctly positioned in the joint space, the contents of the syringe is gently injected. There should be little resistance to injection. If resistance is encountered, the needle is probably in a ligament and should be advanced slightly into the joint space until the injection can proceed without significant

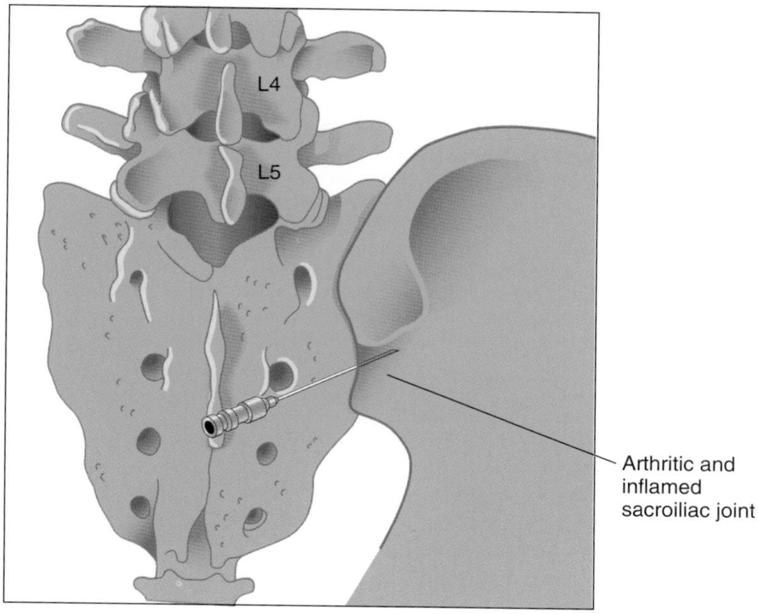

FIGURE 88–5 ■ Sacroiliac joint injection. (From Waldman SD: Atlas of Interventional Pain Management, 2nd ed. Philadelphia, Saunders, 2004, p 432, Figure 94–3.)

resistance. The needle is then removed, and a sterile pressure dressing and ice pack are placed on the injection site.[17]

Proliferant injections instill an irritant (often dextrose) along the joint line, the desired result being thickening of ligaments or muscle attachments to stabilize a hypermobile joint. The operator should be familiar with technique and complications before attempting the procedure.[18]

Surgery should be considered only when pain is intractable and disabling and the patient has failed to respond to conservative treatments. Screw fixation of the ilium to the sacrum has been described.[19]

Exercises

The goals of an exercise program are to provide stretch and strength to connecting muscles, enhance posture, and a means of self manipulation for the patient. These can be done alone or with a helper.

Strengthening Exercises

We suggest a "six pack" of repetitions of these isometric strengthening maneuvers: six sets of six, 6 seconds on, 6 seconds off, six times a day.

Abdominal Crunches

The patient lies supine with hip and knee flexed and feet flat on the floor. A partial sit-up is performed and held as for the aforementioned six-pack regimen.

Hip Abduction, Adduction, and Extension

The patient may be standing, sitting, or lying down. Isometric exercises are performed by resisting the direction of motion, using furniture or hands.

Pelvic Tilt, Anterior and Posterior

The patient stands with hands on hips. The pelvis is tilted up (anterior) then back (posterior); held as for the six-pack regimen.

Isometric Hip Extension

The patient may be sitting, lying down, or standing. The elevated foot must be braced on a pedestal in a vertical position. The hip and knee are flexed maximally against the trunk, held in the flexed position with both hands. Isometric extension is then resisted by the arms, as for the six- pack regimen. Men especially seem to prefer a variation of this maneuver that involves standing against the inside of a door frame with one foot against the opposite side. Resisted extension of hip and knee from pressure against the sole of the foot produces a similar effect.

Posture Enhancement

Correct trunk posture enhances force distribution by maintaining correct spinal alignment. Holding the abdomen "in" (contracting the abdominal and rectus muscles) creates an internal brace against the lower back and helps to maintain adequate pelvic tilt and lumbar lordosis. Holding shoulders and head in proper alignment also enhances spinal positioning and distribution of forces.

References

1. Fortin JD, Aprill CN, Ponthieux B, Pier J: Sacroiliac joint: Pain referral maps upon applying a new injection/arthrography technique. Part I. Spine 19:1475, 1994.
2. Willard FH: The anatomy of the lumbosacral connection. Spine 9:333, 1995.
3. Snijders CJ, et al: Transfer of lumbosacral load to iliac bones and legs. Part I: Biomechanics of self-bracing of the sacroiliac joints and its significance for treatment and exercise. Part II: Loading of the sacroiliac joints when lifting in a stooped posture. Clin Biomech 8:285, 1993.
4. Solonen KA: The sacroiliac joint in the light of anatomical, roentgenological and clinical studies. Acta Orthop Scand 27 (Suppl):27, 1957.
5. Simonian P, Routt ML Jr, Harrington RM, et al: Biomechanical simulation of the anteroposterior compression injury of the pelvis. Clin Orthop 309:245, 1994.
6. Vrahas M, Hem TC, Diangelo D, et al: Ligamentous contributions to pelvic stability. Orthopedics 18:271, 1995.
7. Vleeming A, Pool-Goudzwaard AL, Stoeckert R, et al: The posterior layer of the thoracolumbar fascia. Spine 20:753, 1995.

8. Vrahas M, Hem TC, Diangelo D, et al: Ligamentous contributions to pelvic stability. Orthopedics 18:271, 1995.
9. DonTigny RL: Mechanics and treatment of the sacroiliac joint. J Manual Manip Ther 1:3, 1993.
10. Thorstensson A, Nielsen J, Carlson H, Zomlefer MR: Trunk movements in human locomotion. Acta Physiol Scand 121:9, 1984.
11. Lavignolle B, Vital JM, Senegas J, et al: An approach to the functional anatomy of the sacroiliac joints in vivo. Anatomia Clinica 5:169, 1983.
12. Vlemming A, et al: Towards a better understanding of the etiology of low back pain. Part I. Spine 19:545, 1994.
13. Pierrynowski MR, et al: Three dimensional sacroiliac motion during locomotion in asymptomatic male and female subjects. Presented at the 5th Canadian Society of Biomechanics, Ottawa, Canada. August 1988.
14. Fortin JD, et al: Sacroiliac joint: Pain referral maps upon applying a new injection/arthrography technique, Part II: Clinical evaluation. Spine 19:1483, 1994.
15. Maigne JY, Boulahdour H, Chattellier G: Value of quantitative radionuclide bone scanning in the diagnosis of sacroiliac joint syndrome in 32 patients with low back pain. Eur Spine J 7:328, 1998.
16. Maugars Y, Mathis C, Berthelot JM, et al: Assessment of the efficacy of sacroiliac corticosteroid injections in the spondyloarthropathies: A double-blind study. Br J Rheumatol 35:767, 1996.
17. Waldman SD: Sacroiliac Joint Injection. In Waldman SD: Atlas of Interventional Pain Management, 2nd ed. Philadelphia, Saunders, 2003, p 431.
18. Reeves KD: Technique of prolotherapy. In Lennard TA (ed): Physiatric Procedures in Clinical Practice. Philadelphia, Hanley & Belfus, 1995, p 57.
19. Matta JM, Saucedo T: Internal fixation of pelvic ring fractures. Clin Orthop 242:93, 1989.

chapter 89

Failed Back Surgery Syndrome

J. Antonio Aldrete

In the past 2 decades, a relatively recent entity labeled "failed back surgery syndrome (FBSS)" has been assigned to more and more patients. The rationale for this nomenclature is not clear, but it seems to be related to patients who, after having had one or more operations in the spine, have had their initial complaints appear to have been made worse rather than improve. However, at plain view, this vague diagnosis implies that the patient's back failed to get better, avoiding to list the specific diagnosis derived from the attempts to alleviate the initial symptomatology of the patient. It is not clear whether the terminology was formulated to identify a new category of disease entity (including spinal surgery) or to avoid having to specifically mention some of the diagnoses that may reveal the failure of the treatment given (including spinal surgery). It seems that for lack of a better global term that would list each and every one of these diagnoses, or as some would call it "by default," FBSS has been incorporated into the medical jargon.[1] In a way, this attribute is not fair to the patients because as a negative term they do not understand it. It casts a stigma that assumes that there is nothing else positive that can be done to help them and what is worse they may be considered abusers of the healthcare system and prejudiced as drug seekers. Somehow it seems that most of them, in their journey of sorrow, end up in pain facilities because they no longer fit into any of the conventional specialty clinics because their condition has failed to progress as expected.

Each case varies, but they all have some common denominators; after one or more laminectomies, these factors may include:

- Recurrent disk herniation
- Peridural scarring
- Nerve root compressed by scarring
- Deformity of the dural sac
- Herniation of adjacent disk
- Spinal instability
- Facetectomy
- Pseudomeningocele
- Arachnoid cysts
- Arachnoiditis
- Foraminal re-stenosis

Not uncommonly after one or two laminectomies, the spine becomes "destabilized" as portions of disks are removed and laminectomies are extended laterally, rendering the facet joints dysfunctional and painful. The sequence follows with a spinal fusion to stabilize that portion of the spine. Although spinal fusions are supposed to convert two or more vertebrae into one bony (with or without hardware) union, they may result in one or more of the following:

- Pseudarthrosis
- Malposition of screws
- Protrusion of screws through the vertebral body
- Protrusion of screws into the vertebral canal
- Fracture of screws
- Displacement of hardware (cages)
- Intrathecal scarring
- Intrathecal calcification
- Impingement of nerve roots
- Pedicular pain
- Paravertebral muscle dysfunction and atrophy

HISTORICAL PERSPECTIVE

To best understand this syndrome, a brief historical description of the events that brought about the circumstances, now in play, is in order. Invasive entry into the neuraxis was initiated by Quincke,[2] in 1885, when he performed the first lumbar puncture to sample the CSF. Attempts to visualize the contents of the dural sac were led by Dandy,[3] in 1919, who injected air into the subarachnoid space, which resulted in the advent of pneumomyelography producing only a borderline radiographic visualization of the spinal cord and nerve roots. Myelography was introduced in 1922 by Sicard and Forrestier[4] by injecting Lipiodol (iodized poppy seed oil) intrathecally and taking plain radiographs that allowed them to have a fair visualization of the spinal contents; however, because of its high viscosity and low miscibility with the CSF, it was discarded. Eventually, dyes with lower density, but almost as toxic, such as Abrodil, thorium oxide, and Kontrast[5] were tried, but all showed poor definition of images and frequent complications.[6] Meanwhile, Mixter and Barr,[7] in 1934, defined lumbar herniated disks as the main cause of sciatica; it was then that diskectomy, through a laminectomy, initiated the trend for elective surgical operations of the spine. This was facilitated by the introduction of Pantopaque (ethyl iodophenyl undecylate), first administered to patients in 1944, that provided a good definition and contrast of images, establishing myelography as the standard test to identify spinal pathology.[8] Because it was the contrast medium of choice, Pantopaque was used extensively in spite of multiple reports of arachnoiditis.[9-11] After laminectomies, spinal fusions were proposed for correction of scoliosis and traumatic injuries. Initially they were done with bone graft and later with hardware. These procedures have given the impression that extensive interventions in the spine were feasible and uneventful.

RATIONALIZATION FOR LAMINECTOMY

The removal of a compressive lesion from a tubular osseous structure containing delicate neural elements such as the spinal cord, nerve roots, dural sac, and CSF more often than not eliminates the pain and dramatically improves the affected function(s); however, surgical access into the spine does not occur without risks and consequences.

Zeidman and Long[12] defined this syndrome as "the condition resulting from one or more surgical interventions, with disastrous results with persistence of back pain and exacerbation of the preexisting complaints, characterized by a constellation of symptoms, including referred pain to the lower extremities, sphincter dysfunction and psychological alterations associated to the disease of the spine." What has not been clarified is the fact that patients seek medical attention, requesting help for pain in their backs; whatever procedure performed for this purpose that does not relieve the back pain should be considered a failure. This fact is pertinent to laminectomies and especially to spinal fusions even when a solid arthrodesis is achieved; however, if the patient's pain continues, in reality, the operations have not succeeded. In accordance with Deyo and colleagues[13] from this premise, the objectives of spinal operations need to be redefined directing their aims to only utilize therapeutic modalities that have proven to effectively relieve the specific pain experienced by that specific patient, as demonstrated in a review of the literature.[14]

EPIDEMIOLOGY

Considering that low back pain is one of the most prevalent diseases of middle and older age, the iatrogenic component of this entity adds a threatening aspect to it. More that 300,000 spinal fusions are performed annually in the United States[15]; and, incredibly, from 10% to 40% of these cases end up as a FBSS.[1] Because there is a life time incidence of back pain in about 80% in the general population, these numbers are substantial, because by the time the diagnosis of FBSS is reached, it is estimated that more than $250,000 has already been spent on the care of those patients. At that point their predicament is that they contemplate disability, rejection, and persistent pain and suffering for the remainder of their life.

The frequency of surgical operations of the spine for comparative populations in industrialized countries has been estimated to be 10 times more in the United States than in the Scandinavian countries, 8 times more than in the United Kingdom, and 7 times more than in Germany.[16] The reasons for these disparities are numerous, but the most relevant are as follows:

- Labor protection is given to workers in other countries, where lifting, pulling, and carrying are done mechanically rather than by humans. Lifting in industry, offices, hospitals, and so on is done by pulleys that have been placed strategically to avoid back injuries.
- Back-saving education is a subject taught in schools and is taken seriously by both supervisors and workers.
- The financial incentive is undoubtedly an uncontrollable factor that influences excessive surgical intervention in the private practice of medicine versus conservative therapy in institutional medicine.
- Specific clinical guidelines are lacking as to when and what operations are indicated for each specific condition that produces low back pain.
- Inadequate control is exercised by governmental agencies over new surgical procedures and the implantation of medical devices.
- There is lack of implementation of evidence-based medicine as a necessary proof that new treatments truly benefit patients. The treatments are approved only after comparative, impartial, double-blind control studies have been performed.[14,15]

Most cases start with back pain. After a variable degree of conservative therapy the patients are offered a laminectomy to remove the herniated portion of a disk supposedly because the corresponding nerve root is compressed by such herniation. The usual manifestations include symptoms and signs of radiculopathy. The most common access into the spinal canal is through the posterior approach and usually requires a laminectomy or a laminotomy. Even then, access to the degenerated disk is narrow and frequently complicated by swelling of the affected nerve root that has been compressed.[1] This may improve soon thereafter, but in some cases the distal end of the root can actually become more swollen,[17] depending on the radicular vascular response to the surgical manipulation.

The consequences from spinal surgery have to be considered individually, accepting that the main objective is the relief of the low back pain that motivated the patient to seek help. It is apparent that the outcomes in patients younger than age 30 years having one single degenerated intervertebral disk are more favorable than those in middle-aged individuals with two or three affected disks and some degree of spondylosis, especially smokers.[18] The outcomes are less hopeful in elderly patients who have multiple levels and degrees of disk disease, facet joint arthritis, osteoporosis, and spinal stenosis. However, because of work-related injuries, motor vehicle accidents, and possibly other factors, the middle-aged group, proportionally, undergoes spinal surgery more often.[15,19]

In his classic treatise, Wilkinson[1] admitted that "the conclusion that in America many failed back syndromes result from excessive surgical intervention seems difficult to avoid." He went on to define three culprits:

- *Incorrect diagnosis,* which may include misdiagnosed neoplasms, the so-called flabby back syndrome common in affluent societies where obesity is prevalent, rheumatoid arthritis, osteoarthritis, ankylosing spondylitis, and so on.
- *Unnecessary surgery,* such as operating on a bulging disk without radiculopathy symptoms; slight sensory loss does not necessarily mandate operation. To perform fusions in grade I spondylolisthesis is still under debate.[13]

- *Improper or inadequate surgery,* such as disk excision performed at the wrong level, the wrong side, leaving a loose fragment of disk, or selection of the wrong hardware to execute a fusion.[19]

To these, at least three more predisposing factors may be added:

- Short pedicles, lumbarization of S1, sacralization of L5, and arachnoid cysts may be present.
- Inadequate imaging or inconclusive interpretation may offer misleading diagnosis or fail to recognize associated pathology, such as vertebral hemangiomas and scoliosis. The value of diagnostic invasive tests such as differential blocks, epidurography, diskography, and so on is still in doubt, because most pathology can be identified by MRI. For example, in diskography 1.0 mL of dye produces little pain in normal and ruptured disks alike but 2 mL of dye produces pain in every disk injected, casting doubt on this procedure.
- Cigarette smoking has been found to decrease the threshold of pain,[20] increase perioperative narcotic requirements,[21] affect wound healing,[22] increase postoperative pulmonary morbidity,[20] and add to a patient's stress response[23]; furthermore, it increases dural sac pressure during bouts of coughing, facilitating CSF leaks.[20,24] Nevertheless, this factor is seldom considered a contraindication to proceed with surgery in patients who refuse to stop smoking.

WHAT MAY FAIL IN THE "FAILED BACK" SYNDROME?

The reasons are multiple and at any one time one or more may cause the reappearance of pain and neurologic symptoms after these operations. The following causes are not listed in order of frequency or seriousness of their occurrence:

Incidental Durotomy

Perhaps one of the most underrated complications, incidental durotomy may occur in 6% to 8% of first-time laminectomies, 12% to 20% of repeat laminectomies, and 14% to 30% of spinal fusions.[25,26] Recognition of these tears allows them to be repaired on site. Unrecognized tears not only would result in CSF leak but also would allow for blood accumulated at the bottom of the wound (in patients in the prone position) to therefore enter the subarachnoid space.[27] This usually unexpected development may have serious consequences because blood is an active irritant of nerve tissue and may initiate an arachnoiditic inflammatory response. Depending on the amount of CSF lost, postural headache and even meningismus may occur with a bulging mass under the incision. Occasionally, serosanguineous fluid may leak through the incision, which can be tested for sugar content with a glucose strip. Ultimate confirmation can be obtained by MRI of the lumbar spine. If CSF is contained in the retrospinal tissues, eventually a soft, thin pseudomembrane is formed that contains it. If not initially repaired it may give rise to a pseudomeningocele (see Fig. 89–11).[28] Puncture is not recommended because CSF may leak persistently.[29]

Loose Disk Fragments

With an incidence from 2% to 7%, loose disk fragments of nucleus pulposus may be "dragged out" of the anulus fibrosus cavity by the rongeurs employed to remove the loose portions of the nucleus.[30] Less commonly, loose fragments can also come out of the disk cavity later on, when the patient is mobilized. Pain is sharp, severe, and localized to the dermatome corresponding to the compressed nerve root that is being pressured by the 0.5- to 1.4-cm fibrocartilaginous mass. Confirmation is again done with MRI, requiring immediate surgical re-intervention because the patients are in severe constant pain and may also have bladder dysfunction.[31,32]

Intrathecal and/or Peridural Hematoma

Both intrathecal and peridural hematomas are serious events. A substantial amount of blood in the subarachnoid space is manifested by severe, burning low back pain with or without radicular symptoms appearing immediately on the patient's awakening from the anesthetic.[33] It usually requires considerable dosages of opiates to control it. More common are extradural hematomas (Fig. 89–1), which initially present as light to moderate back pain but with moderate to severe paravertebral muscle spasm. Depending on the size of the hematoma and its proximity to the dural sac, back pain and neurologic symptoms may appear 2 or 3 weeks after surgery. This may result from the degradation of blood elements and products and the subsequent liberation of leukotrienes and cytokines that are able to cross the dural barrier.[34] After 10 days, hemosiderin may be recognized on MRI.

Nerve Root Cysts

Leg pain with minimal back pain may be caused by postoperative cystic outpouchings when dural tears occur in the dural cuff that accompany the emerging nerve roots (Fig. 89–2) during their intraspinal canal passage. They should be differentiated from the congenital or Tarlov arachnoid cysts

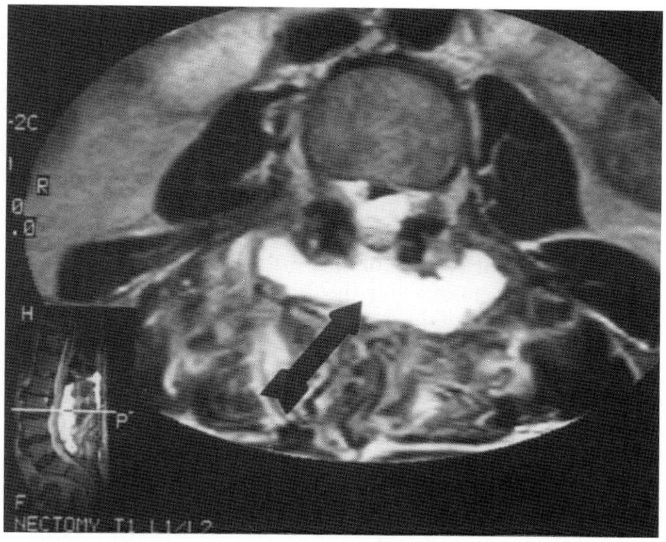

FIGURE 89–1 ■ Axial MR image of the lumbar spine showing an accumulation of blood intrathecally and extradurally *(arrow)*. A bilateral laminotomy had been performed at the L3 level.

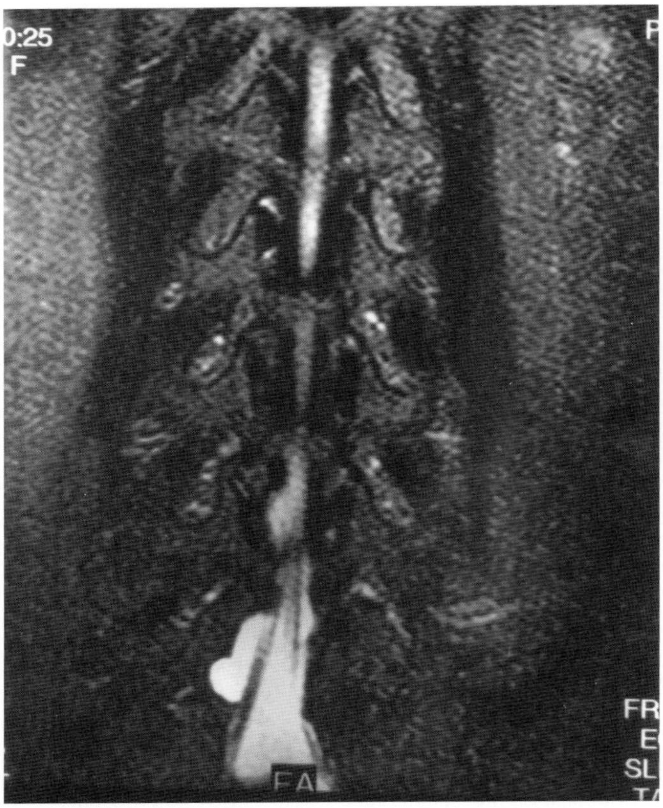

FIGURE 89–2 ■ Coronal MR image of the lumbar spine demonstrating a dural sheath cyst on the right L5 nerve root, 4 months post laminectomy.

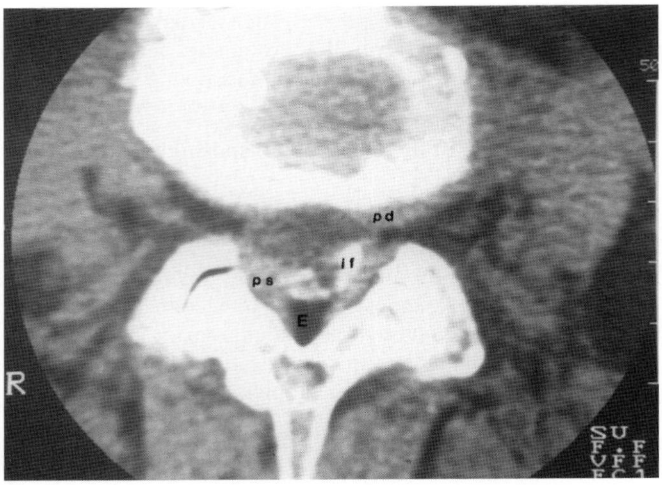

FIGURE 89–3 ■ CT scan of the lumbar spine depicting intrathecal fibrosis (if) on the left inside wall of the dural sac. There is abundant peridural scarring and fibrosis (ps) adhering to the right lamina. The epidural space (E) is preserved. There is a broad protruding disk, mostly to the left, narrowing the lateral foramen and bilateral facet joint hypertrophy.

that occur at the same location. At myelography, they fill immediately. Postoperative arachnoidal cysts are formed at the time of surgery when a small dural tear occurs in this same sheath location; if not corrected, the arachnoid that herniates through this dural tear forms the primary cyst and is usually reinforced by an outer wall of fibrous tissue.[35] They may be identified by fluid pulsations. In any case, at surgery the ostium or opening communicating with the subarachnoid space is very small and difficult to find.[1]

Epidural Fibrosis

Epidural fibrosis is perhaps the most dreadful of complications from spinal surgery and the most frequent cause of FBSS.[36] Most laminectomies are usually followed by a short period (3 to 6 months) of improvement because the excision of the herniated portion of the disk and the removal of a portion of the lamina and the ligamentum flavum provide relief from the stenotic compression with a satisfactory result as the patient's symptoms subside or are markedly improved.[37] All along, as the wound heals, an inflammatory response is occurring around the dural sac and the paravertebral muscles (Fig. 89–3). Eventually, the cellular infiltrate gives way to collagen deposition that proliferates for months and the incision heals, as all tissues in every organ do, with scar tissue. The operated intervertebral space heals with collagen and fibrous tissue, leading to scarring in the peridural space and fibrous adhesions to dura, nerve roots, bone, muscles, and fascia where surgery took place.[38] In some cases, this proliferation of fibrotic tissue and adhesions is exaggerated, and eventually it may indent or compress the dural sac and even encircle a nerve root.[39] If foreign bodies (e.g., Surgicel, Gelfoam, cotton pads),[40] glues (e.g., ADPL),[41] or natural materials[42] are left in the wound or there has been a difficult, traumatic access or a large extradural hematoma, this reaction may be accelerated. Fatal anaphylaxis has occurred after fibrin glue application.[43] Symptoms of radiculopathy may appear according to the nerve root affected. However, not uncommonly, all these materials may provoke more inflammation, resulting in greater fibrosis and scarring.[44] It is here where meticulous surgical technique makes a difference.[45]

The gradual surrounding of a nerve root by scar tissue produces radicular pain and sensory disturbances as it elicits traction and a compressive effect on the root.[46] It is difficult to make the differential diagnosis if a recurrent herniated disk is suspected. In this case, the nerve root is displaced.[17,47] Because electrodiagnostic studies may be inconclusive, MRI with gadolinium is necessary to enhance the scar tissue by the transfer of the dye from the intravascular to the interstitial tissue compartments as it would occur from inflammation or scarring,[28,32,47] whereas disks usually do not enhance. Caution on the interpretation is advised because high doses of contrast agent (0.3 mmol/kg) have been demonstrated to increase the conspicuity of the disk.[48] Repeated attempts to prevent peridural scarring have not been successful.[42,46,49]

Insufficient Decompression

Insufficient decompression may be lateral when it occurs after a decompressive attempt within the lateral foramina that might have compressed the nerve root by an osteophyte within the lumen, soft tissue, or even bone residues from bony spurs. Within the spinal canal, central stenosis may be due to a hypertrophic ligamentum flavum, short pedicles, a loose disk fragment, or a herniated disk, in which case wider

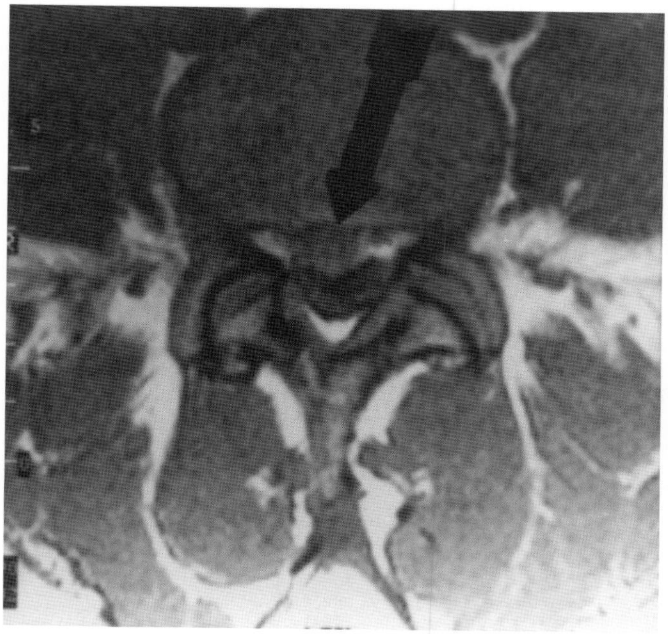

FIGURE 89–4 ■ Axial MR image of the lumbar spine (L3-L4 level) demonstrating a centrally located herniated nucleus pulposus *(arrow)* compressing the dural sac (darker semilunar structure). The posterior epidural space is shown accessible.

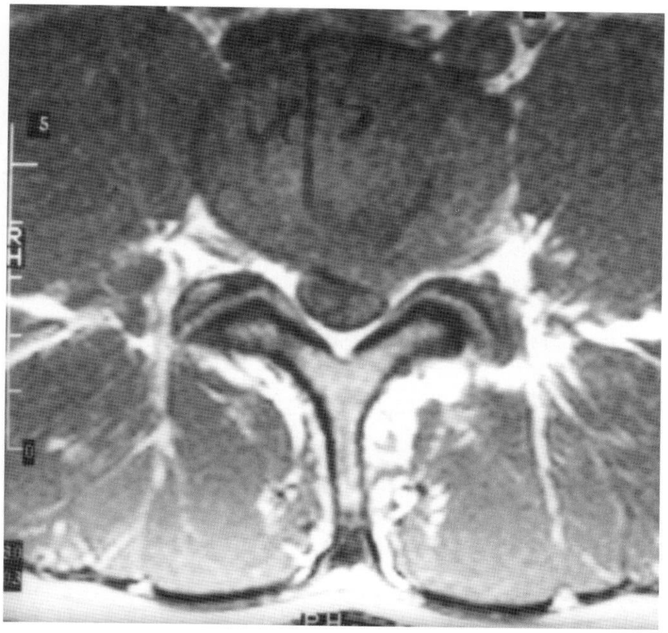

FIGURE 89–5 ■ Axial MR image of the lumbar spine showing a paracentral L4-5 herniated disk, toward the left, narrowing the lateral foramen. There is impingement of the dural sac with reduction in size of the posterior epidural space.

decompression, such as obtained from a bilateral laminotomy or lateral foraminectomy, may be necessary to gain ample access to the lesion generating the pain.[45,47,50]

Residual, Recurrent, or Adjacent Herniated Nucleus Pulposus

An incompletely removed herniation may be extruded again because the anulus fibrosus is usually left open, liberating a free fragment in the vertebral canal.[36,37] A single herniated nucleus pulposus is more frequent in young patients (Fig. 89–4) whereas in middle-aged and elderly patients several lumbar disks may have various degrees of degeneration; thus when a herniated portion of the most degenerated disk is removed, the protruding[30,32,37,51] or slightly herniated disks may not be able to tolerate the new undue pressures applied while in the erect position or during flexion, so adjacent disks continue to degenerate in an accelerated process and soon another disk is fully ruptured, producing radiculopathy.[53] Depending on its extent (>4 mm) or if its location is lateral (Fig. 89–5) or broad when the nerve root is compressed, the apparent need for another laminectomy becomes apparent in sort of a domino effect.[52,54]

Mechanical Instability

There are number of preexisting abnormalities that predispose to lumbosacral spine instability. Among them are sacralization of L5 or lumbarization of S1 and scoliosis from 5 to 15 degrees. Usually these congenital variances can be recognized in MR images.[55] Prior facetectomies, extensive bilateral laminotomies, and severe unilateral spondylosis destabilize the adjacent segments of the spine. Malalignment of adjacent vertebrae may occur after extensive diskectomy, leading to spondylolisthesis. Alteration of the usually even axial surface of each vertebra, by either scoliosis, a degenerated disk, an osteophyte, or one-sided spondylosis may change the individual support given by each segment. In addition, an unstable spinal segment(s) prevents the normal dissipation of the load sharing, thus changing the distribution of stress forces throughout the axial topography of each vertebra.[30,52]

Depending on which lesion predominates, spinal stenosis, spondylolisthesis, or ligament stretching may result, reducing and morphologically changing the transverse diameter of the vertebral canal and/or the neuroforamen. During the aging process, these changes occur gradually; in severe trauma, some of them may appear suddenly. Diskectomies, as helpful as they may be in reducing the compression of neural elements under certain circumstances, may affect the stability of the spine, precipitating the need for a stabilizing fusion.[56]

Pseudarthrosis

After spinal fusions, it is essential to monitor the stability of the fused unit; however, the usual plain films on flexion and extension show only extreme causes of instability.[53,55] To define if bone growth is taking place between vertebrae, either CT or MRI[57] would be required to determine if there are any vacuum phenomena or spaces (Fig. 89–6) in between where new bone growth should be.[56,58] In all fairness, a maximum of 2 years is suggested as a waiting period for a fusion to be successful. If no bone pockets persist, most likely the pseudarthrosis is permanent. If hardware was applied, then as long as the screws and plates are in place and not causing side

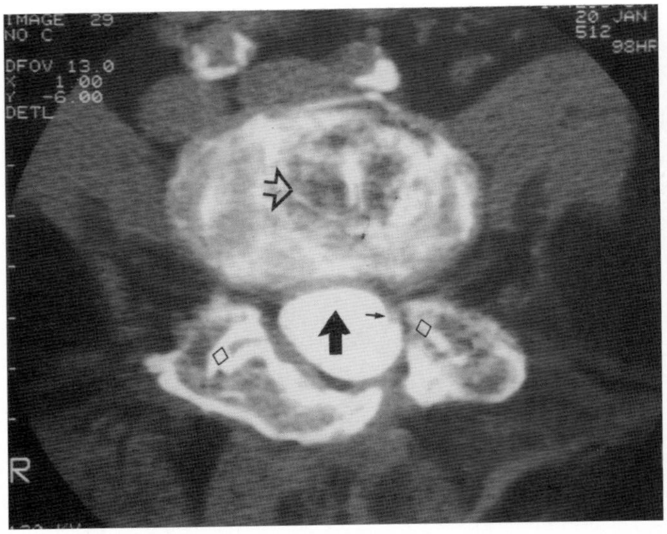

FIGURE 89–6 ■ Lumbar spine CT scan at the L4-L5 level showing areas of nonsolidification implying pseudarthrosis *(open arrow).* In addition there is a pseudomeningocele with a cluster of nerve roots adhering to the left wall of the dural sac *(black arrow),* indicative of arachnoiditis. There is bilateral spondylosis *(open diamonds),* as well as evidence of a left laminectomy.

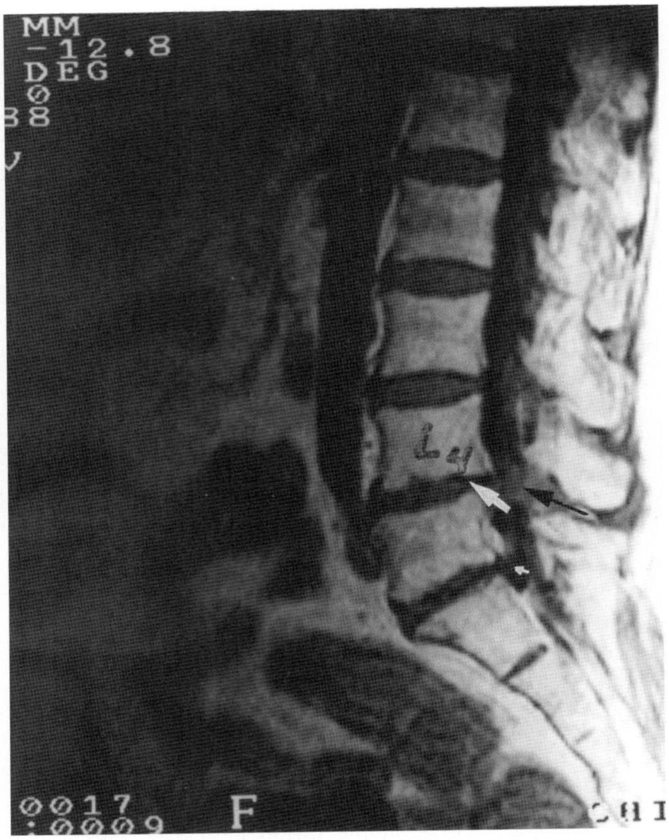

FIGURE 89–7 ■ Sagittal MR image of the lumbosacral spine, post laminectomy, showing posterior peridural scaring at the L4-L5 *(black arrow)* with spondylolisthesis of L4 on L5 *(large white arrow).* There is also a extruded disk fragment located posterior to L5 *(small white arrow).*There is a primitive intervertebral disk between S1 and S2.

effects they can be left in. However, if pain persists and the screw head sites are tender or there is bending or screw fracture, the screws may have to be removed, leaving an unstable spine that is sometimes worse than it was before, because the disks usually had been removed.[52,59] Occasionally when bone fragments are placed in between the vertebral bodies, close to the posterior edge, growing graft bone eventually may protrude into the vertebral canal acting as osteophytes and impinging on the dural sac.[60] Repeat fusions are usually less likely to succeed than the first attempt.[56,57,59]

Spondylolisthesis

The overriding of a vertebra over the posterior plate of the one below results in undue compression of the posterior end of the intervertebral disk, narrowing of the lateral foramen, and possible impingement of the corresponding nerve root, producing moderate constant pain that is exacerbated by standing and walking.[52,58] According to the degree of disparity of the alignment of the two vertebrae involved, it is given one of four grades (I to IV) (Fig. 89–7).[54] Grade I is one that may be treated with conservative measures; higher level of deviation usually requires surgical stability (Fig. 89–8). It is desirable not only to fix the two adjacent vertebrae but to attempt to correct the misalignment and relieve the pain.[55,60]

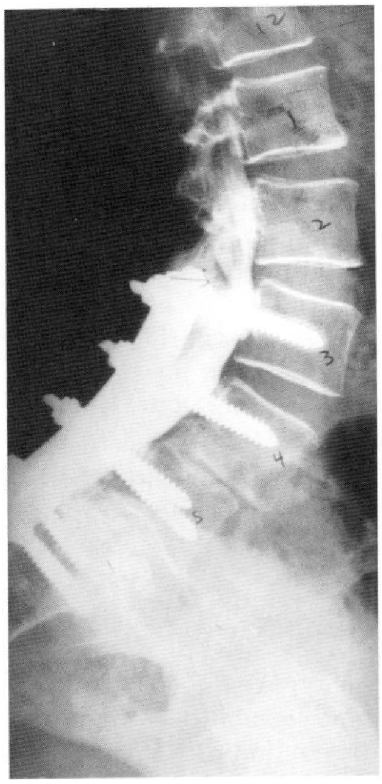

FIGURE 89–8 ■ Lateral view of a myelogram of the lumbar spine 6 months after a spinal fusion with hardware for instability of the spine and spondylolisthesis of L4 on L5 that was not corrected by the fusion. The tip of one of the lowest screws protrudes through the anterior sacral wall.

Infections

Infections can occur in the soft tissue as cellulitis, fasciitis, epidural abscess (Fig. 89–9), or meningitis with delayed clinical manifestations for up to 1 month.[61] Diskitis may also be present and produce localized pain, low-grade fever, and malaise for months.[62] Ultrasound and/or radiologic imaging[63,64] usually identifies the type and location of the infections. Most of them can be treated conservatively,[65] but

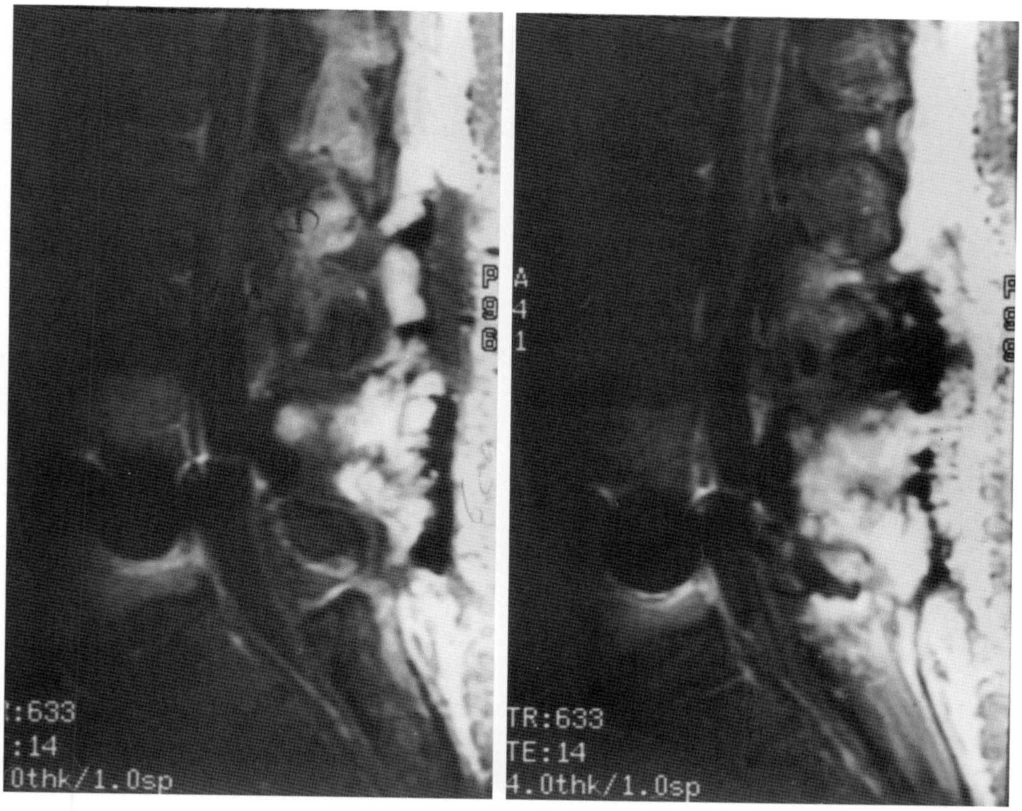

FIGURE 89–9 ■ Sagittal MR images of the lumbosacral spine, 14 days post laminectomy and fusion with hardware at the L3-L4, L4-L5, and L5-S1 levels. An epidural abscess has formed extending to the dural sac anteriorly and the lumbar fascia posteriorly.

if a neurologic deficit persists, surgical drainage and evacuation may be necessary.[61]

Spinal Stenosis

Repeated operations may produce both axial and radicular pain that may be caused by a herniated disk, hypertrophy of the facet joints (Fig. 89–10), progression or overgrowth of a previous spinal fusion, or hypertropic osteophyte, which may coexist with peridural scarring significantly compressing the dural elements.[66] Although bony and ligamentum compression may be mechanically reduced, pain relief may be minimal.

Pseudomeningocele

A pseudomeningocele may occur after laminectomies[28] or fusions usually from unsealed dural tears followed by postural sequelae with or without CSF seeping through the incision.[27] If superficial layers are tightly closed, CSF accumulates in the peridural region encircled by a pseudomeningocele (Fig. 89–11).[29] Palpating the area causes much pain. Repair is difficult, and there is a high incidence of recurrence.[25,30]

Surgery at the Wrong Level

Indeed, the surgeon's nightmare can occur because sometimes the S1-S2 space is mobile or the L5-S1 space is immobile, misleading the surgical team.[34] The only way to avoid operating in the wrong space is by confirming the precise location of the intervertebral space to be operated on by placing a metal object (hemostat) in the intended space and then taking a radiograph or by using two views of fluoroscopy.[66] This may be more likely to occur when microdiskectomies are done when exposure is marginal, and fluoroscopy guidance depends on the interpretation of the operator.[1]

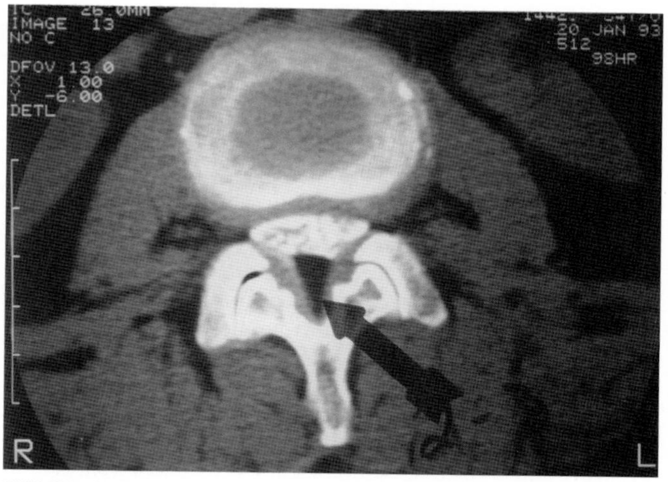

FIGURE 89–10 ■ CT scan of the lumbar spine depicting spinal canal stenosis as result of a broad disk herniation and bilateral facet joint hypertrophy. The epidural space has not been altered.

Arachnoiditis

Arachnoiditis is now recognized as one of the most common and serious complications of spinal operations. Its existence

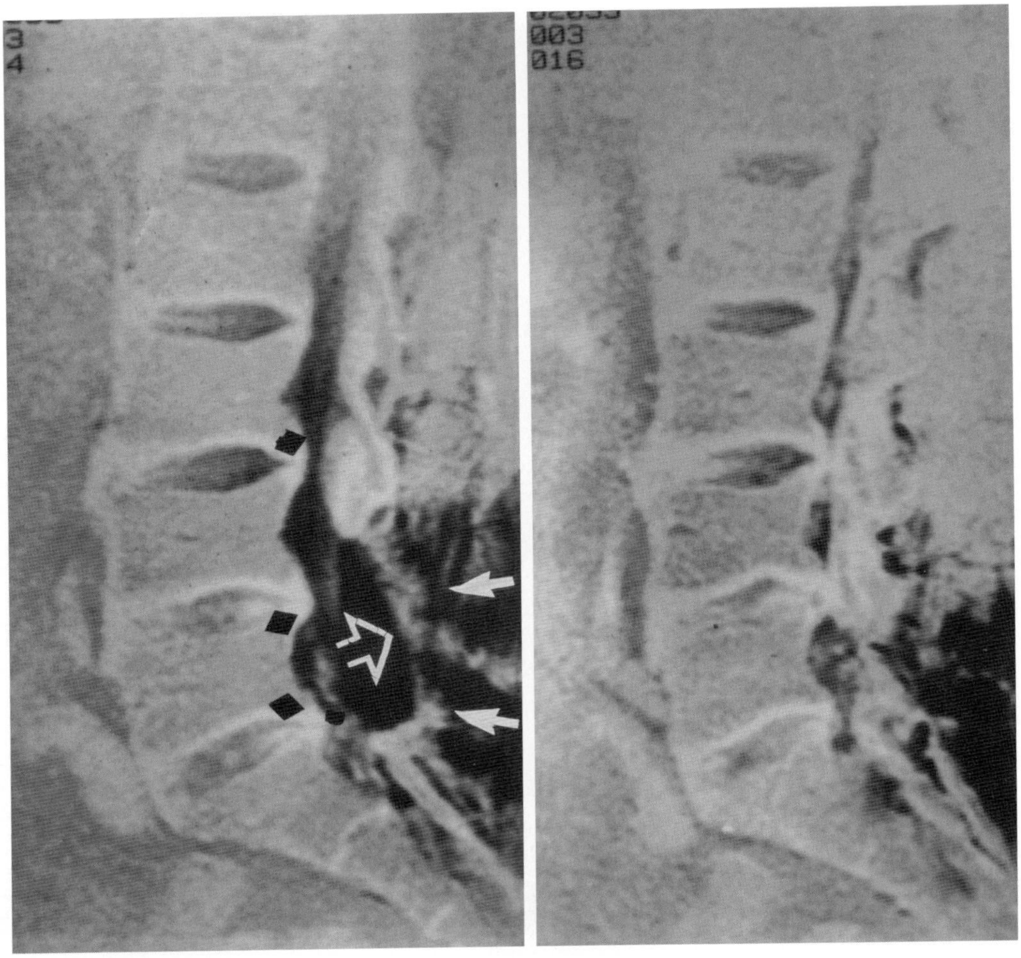

FIGURE 89–11 ■ Sagittal MR image of the lumbosacral spine depicting a post-laminectomy pseudomeningocele from L4 to S1 *(open arrow)*. Recurrent protruding disks at L3-L4, L4-L5 and L5-S1 *(diamonds)*, causing spinal stenosis at the uppermost space (which appears also to have spondylosis). Scar tissue is present anterior and posterior to the pseudosac *(white arrows)*.

has evolved from being questioned, ignored, and overlooked to being recognized as one of the most common complications that has disastrous consequences on patients and enormous expense to the healthcare system because it is not curable. A definite incidence has not been determined, but isolated series have indicated that it occurs from 3% to 16% of the patients having lumbar laminectomies and in 6% to 21% of the patients who undergo spinal fusions.[19,27,61] One of the most revealing studies was conducted by Matsui and colleagues,[67] who performed lumbar spine MRI on the 3rd, 7th, 21st, and 42nd days in 10 patients (7 with herniated nucleus pulposus and 3 with spinal stenosis) who underwent spinal surgery via a posterior approach. In axial views, intrathecal adhesions to the cauda equina were prevalent at the "laminectomized" levels in all patients. Partial adhesions were found at nine levels, 6 weeks after surgery. Most of these resolved by the 42nd day, but in 5 of 14 spaces exposed, partial nerve root adhesions were still present. An initial shrinking of the dural sac returned to near-normal levels at the end of the observation period. This study showed that some of these changes are transitory; however, intradural lesions (clumped nerve roots) are evident even when only extradural surgery had been performed (Figs. 89–12 and 89–13). The possible mechanisms for these events have been described in the section on intrathecal and extradural hematoma (see Fig. 89–1).[33,34]

Nakano and coworkers[68] reported that laminectomy in rats consistently induced an increase in vascular permeability in the cauda equina, as well as an increase in the vesicular transport of the endothelial cells with opening of the "tight junction," which suggests a breakdown of the blood-nerve barrier, facilitating the formation of adhesions. Furthermore, the same group[69] was able to show that the administration of the antiinflammatory agents indomethacin and methylprednisolone, 24 hours after laminectomy, suppressed the formation of such adhesions and the leakage from the nutrient vessels. This phenomenon was only reduced when the drugs were given 3 or 6 weeks after laminectomy.

The importance of conducting serial neurologic examinations and of obtaining imaging studies (preferably an MRI with contrast) of the operated region[70] is crucial in patients who develop severe pain and neurologic deficits after laminectomy. This premise also applies to cases of arachnoiditis in patients who had a fusion with bone or titanium hardware. If the devices are made of other metals, a myelogram, followed by CT would be necessary to visualize the intrathecal structures. Early manifestations would be swollen, enhanced nerve roots that may be located in their normal position or in the anterior half of the sac (Fig. 89–14).[71] Depending on the extent and intensity of the inflammatory reaction, clumping of nerve roots is not seen clearly until 2 or 3 months after the adverse event (Fig. 89–15; see also Fig. 89–13).

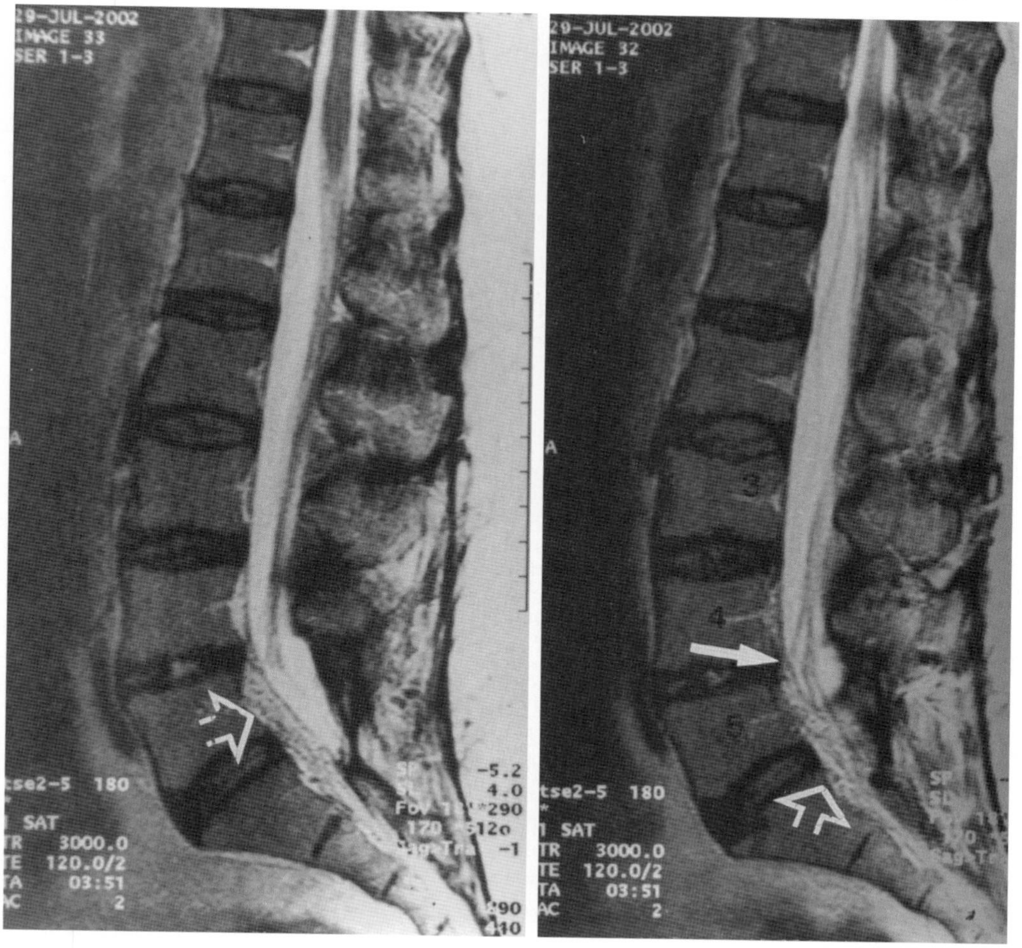

FIGURE 89–12 ■ Sagittal MR image of the lumbosacral spine with extensive scarring on the anterior epidural space, post laminectomy, at L4-L5 and L5-S1 *(open arrow).* Thickened nerve roots are noted displaced anteriorly in the dural sac *(white arrow),* suggestive of arachnoiditis.

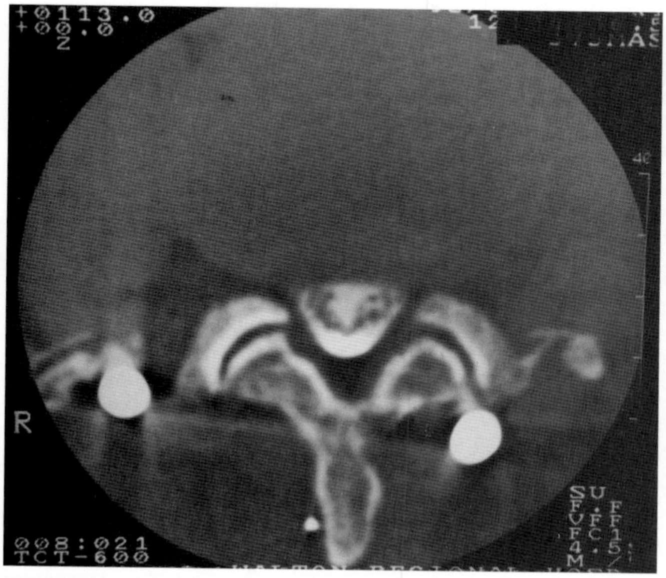

FIGURE 89–13 ■ Post-myelogram CT scan of the lumbar spine illustrating clumped nerve roots noted after spinal fusion with hardware and left laminectomy at L4-L5 typical of arachnoiditis in the permanent proliferative phase.

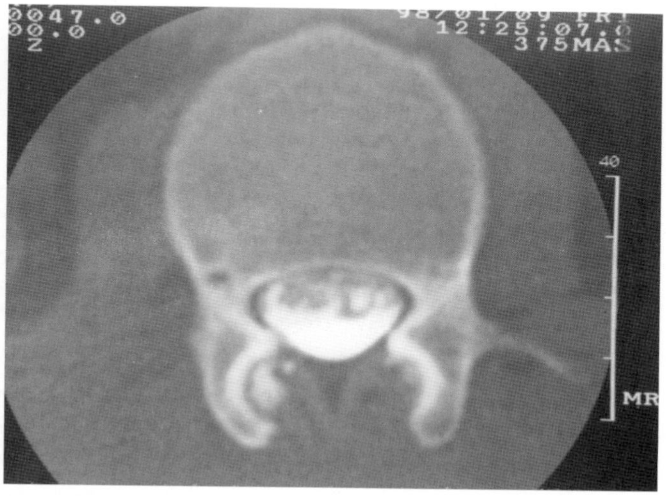

FIGURE 89–14 ■ Post-myelogram CT scan of the lumbar spine showing thickened and swollen nerve roots located in the anterior half of the dural sac, at the level of the L3 vertebra, suggesting arachnoiditis in the early inflammatory phase.

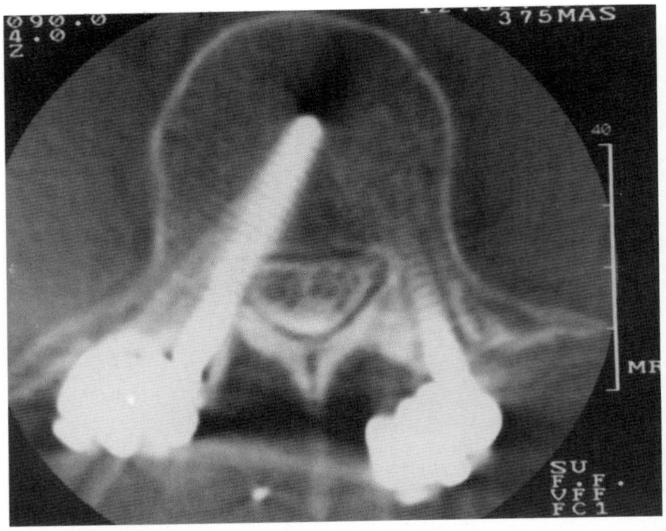

FIGURE 89–15 ■ Post-myelogram CT scan at the L4 vertebra with pedicular screws, bilaterally. The right screw is misplaced, invading the vertebral canal, impinging on the dural sac. The nerve roots are mostly clustered in two clumps, indicative of arachnoiditis in the chronic proliferative phase.

Thereafter, the swelling gradually subsides and the nerve roots remain adhered to each other in clumps or to the interior wall of the dural sac.[72,73] This is a permanent condition. Although arachnoiditis is not present in every case of FBSS, nevertheless it complicates the clinical features of FBSS, making the differential diagnosis difficult, especially if metal hardware has been implanted.

Distal Dural Sac Ectasia

More often than not, the peridural fibrosis that follows any intervention on the spine produces a certain degree of stenosis, impeding the normal circulatory return of the CSF and converting the usual tapering of the dural sac into a ectasia of its caudal end, expanding sometimes into a major dilatation (Fig. 89–16). This complication has not been recognized as a pain generator but manifests as a severe pressure sensation that exacerbates the low back pain.[74] Further operations including fusions will probably worsen this complication because the scarring most likely will be increased.

Other Complications

Other less common complications may be part of FBSS, but because of their rarity they are not mentioned here. Readers are referred to references 19, 36, 37, and 66 for more detailed discussions.

DIAGNOSIS

Practitioners need to have a precise understanding of this disease, because it usually includes a number of diagnoses that have been globalized in the "failed back surgery syndrome." Because adequate noninvasive procedures are available, to further subject these patients to invasive tests such as differential spinal or epidural blocks, diskograms, and

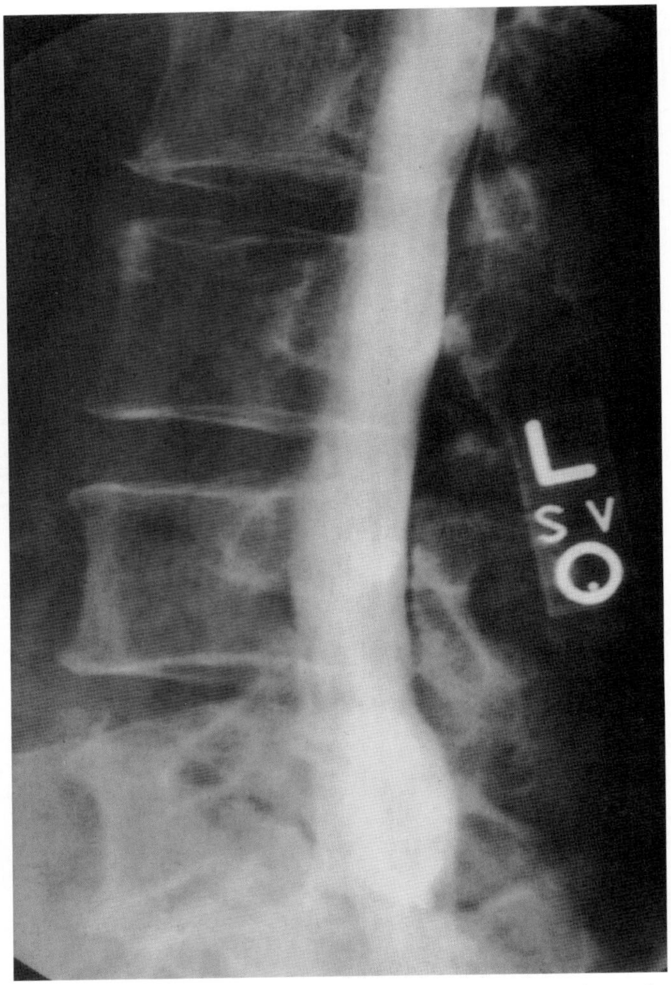

FIGURE 89–16 ■ Lumbar spine myelogram showing narrowing at the L4-L5 level post laminectomy. The distal dural sac, instead of tapering, appears dilated from L5 down.

neuroplasty would be not only futile and wasteful but also hazardous.[75-78]

A complete, detailed history, including diagnostic tests, adverse events, and attempted therapeutic modalities, needs to be listed and described chronologically. Minor injuries and work accidents, as trivial as they may appear, may give clues that explain the patient's actual complaints. The monitoring of spinal evoked potentials in the perioperative period may prevent permanent injury.[79] Specific tracking of the time of appearance of symptoms in relation to one of the operations performed may not only be a determinant of the cause of the FBSS but also assist in including or eliminating certain therapeutic modalities that have not been of benefit in the past (Fig. 89–17). Repeated operations may produce both axial and radicular pain that may be caused by progression or overgrowth of a previous spinal fusion or hypertrophic osteophyte that may coexist with peridural scarring, significantly compressing the dural contents.[59,60] Although bony and ligamentum compression may be mechanically reduced, pain relief would likely be minimal.

Symptoms may be classified as:

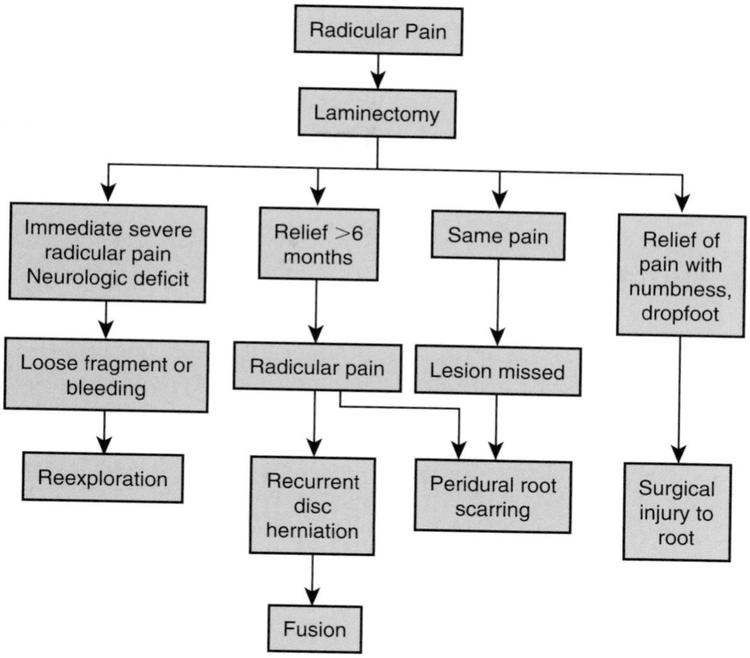

FIGURE 89–17 ■ Algorithm for the diagnosis of postlaminectomy complications.

- *Mechanical,* noted as increased back pain when standing, walking, or sitting
- *Related,* includes referred pain, muscle spasms, pain on the hips or sacroiliac joints, and bone friction as in pseudarthrosis
- *Neurologic,* including headaches, electrical shock–like pain, burning, lacerating pain from stretching of the dural sac or the nerve roots, numbness, and weakness not following a dermatome path.
- *Functional,* implying dysfunction of bladder, bowel, sexual activities, and autonomic dysfunction (e.g., excessive sweating, heat intolerance, hypertension)
- *Aggregated,* caused by other related illnesses such as diabetic neuropathy, rheumatoid arthritis, lupus erythematosus, and so on
- *Psychogenic,* such as fears, depression, anxiety, hopelessness, insomnia, suicidal ideation, and others
- *Radicular,* including pain and sensory alteration (e.g., numbness, tingling, formication) and weakness along a specific dermatome, usually due to extradural compression of a nerve root

Patients usually have several of these clinical manifestations requiring early consultation, understanding, and guidance. A detrimental trend has been the globalization of the radiologic findings referred to by radiologists as "surgical changes" or "peridural enhancement." These statements are difficult to understand and to interpret by nonradiologists. It is imperative to have a detailed and precise description of all the abnormal findings, level by level, in the narrative and a complete listing of the various diagnoses with opinions regarding their possible occurrence. In a retrospective review of the medical records of 684 patients diagnosed with FBSS,[74] after obtaining a history and performing a physical examination followed by imaging studies, the number and percentages of the possible pain generators were identified, correlating them with location, extent, and side of the clinical symptoms. Multiple pain generators were revealed in these patients (Table 89–1).

Table 89–1

Clinical Manifestations of Failed Back Syndrome

	No. Patients	***%***
Epidural scarring	578	84.5
Recurrent herniated nucleus pulposus	316	46.1
Dural sac ectasia	297	43.4
Deformity of dural sac	219	32.0
Herniation at adjacent disk	194	28.3
Arachnoiditis	166	24.2
Spinal instability	104	15.2
Facetectomy	78	11.4
Fusion with hardware	64	9.3
Bony fusion	32	4.6
Pseudomeningocele	21	3.0
Loose disk fragment	6	0.87

All patients had more than two pain generators.

There was no intent to establish incidence of postlaminectomy complications because the surgical interventions were performed by different surgeons. Because some of these pain generators are not surgically correctable, patients with FBSS need to be informed that the presenting symptom, *pain,* will likely continue after any subsequent operation. A list of specific diagnoses is preferable, avoiding the generalized and imprecise diagnosis of FBSS.

Having now objective radiologic findings as evidence, the "Waddell signs evaluation" may be discarded because it was based on nonorganic, attitudinal, and preconceived notions.[80] Waddell and Richardson[76] have already cast certain doubts regarding the reliability of this evaluation,[76] which have been reinforced by the report of Polatin and colleagues,[77] who conducted a prospective study in patients with low back pain, noting the lack of consistency by the evaluating physician.

PROGNOSIS

This prediction relates only to patients who have already been assigned the diagnosis of FBSS. Unfortunately, the prognosis is not hopeful because in itself, by definition, the label implies a hopeless condition, essentially condemning these patients to severe chronic pain, dysfunction, and disability.

Attempts to identify the factors that more affect the eventual symptomatology seen in herniated nucleus pulposus resection have shown that men usually have greater canal compromise than women[21,83] and a more positive sciatic nerve tension,[84-86] both of which correlated with larger disk herniations. In nonoperated groups, shorter duration of sciatica symptoms predicted good outcomes.[87] Moreover, younger patients with symptoms that lasted less than 6 months and had no litigation also had better outcomes. In contrast, larger disks in relation to the vertebral canal diameter, cigarette smoking, involvement in litigation, and age were bad predictors. For the operated groups, larger anteroposterior diameter and smaller central and paracentral herniations indicated better outcomes whereas concurrent and preexistent diseases, cigarette smoking, spondylosis, workers' compensation claims, and middle age and female gender led to poorer outcomes.[18,88] These findings confirm that morphometric features of disk herniation as they relate to the dimensions of the spinal canal, as seen in MRI, appear to be the most reliable predictors.[13,83,89]

The volume of complex operations performed by one specific surgeon in one specific hospital has been shown to impact the outcomes of most operations.[13-15] It is now evident that patients with obesity, who smoke tobacco products, have osteoporosis, or have certain congenital anatomic variances, such as short vertebral pedicles, spondylosis, the presence of a rudimentary disk between L5-S1, lateral recess stenosis, or mild scoliosis of the lumbar region, have greater predisposition to post-laminectomy complications ending in FBSS.[19,62,90]

TREATMENT

Prevention is the best treatment, although a constellation of therapeutic modalities have been attempted in efforts to relieve pain, which is the most significant manifestation of this disease. Most of them have, however, proven not only to be palliative but also to have been inadequately evaluated as the determination of evidence-based effectiveness.[13] In most cases therapeutic approaches have been less than satisfactory, including intrathecal[91] or epidural infusions of opiates,[92] spinal cord stimulation,[93,94] sympathetic blocks,[95] epidural injections of corticosteroids,[96] and antiinflammatory drugs.[97] Other forms of therapy using neurolytic substances[77,98] have a high risk of injury with a low benefit ratio.[78,99-101] Further surgical interventions are only indicated when precisely necessary, such as in the case of a loose disk fragment compressing a nerve root, sudden sensory or motor deficit, or severe infections. When fusions include implanted hardware, a screw may be pressing on a nerve root. If the screw is malpositioned or if there is a screw fracture, screw removal may also be indicated. Because fusions have not been proven to be cost-effective and have a high incidence of complications and of failure to relieve the patient's chief complaint of pain, Deyo and associates[13,93] have emphasized that research should address who should undergo fusion rather than how to perform another fusion.[102] Destructive or neuroablative procedures are not recommended because they may result in added morbidity and neural deficit.[94] For further information, the readers are directed to Chapters 203 and 208 through 210 for in-depth details on these therapeutic modalities.

The selection of patient candidates for spinal surgery is crucial in avoiding further increasing the population of patients with FBSS; the aims of the operation should be reevaluated, focusing on the elimination of pain rather than on the technical success of the operation.[102] Implantation of hardware and spinal interventionism have to prove that they are at least beneficial for 2 years in 400 patients before their application can be generalized to a larger population.

References

1. Wilkinson HA: The Failed Back Syndrome. New York, Springer-Verlag, 1983, pp 2-15.
2. Quinke H: Ueber Lumbalpunction. Berlin Klin Wochenschr 28:889, 1891.
3. Dandy WE: Roentgenography of the brain after the injection of air into the spinal canal. Ann Surg 70:397, 1919.
4. Sicard JA, Forestier J: Méthode general d'éxploration radiologique par-l'huide iodée (Lipiodol). Bull Med Soc Hôp Paris 46:463, 1992.
5. Dale AJ, Love JG: Thorium dioxide myelopathy. JAMA 199:606, 1967.
6. Aldrete JA: Myelography. In Aldrete JA (ed): Arachnoiditis: The Silent Epidemic. Denver, Futuremed, 2000, pp 41-63.
7. Mixter WJ, Barr JS: Rupture of the intervertebral disc with involvement of the spinal canal. N Eng J Med 211:210, 1934.
8. Ramsey GH, French JD, Strain WH: Iodinated organic compounds as contrast media for radiographic diagnosis: IV. Pantopaque myelography. Radiology 43:236, 1944.
9. Luce JC, Leith W, Burrage WS: Pantopaque meningitis due to hypersensitivity. Radiology 57:879, 1951.
10. Imielinski L, Chmielewski JM: Arachnoidite adhesive intraarachidienne à la suite de myelographies a l'ethiodane (Pantopaque). J Radiol Electrol Med Nucl 52:31, 1971.
11. Quiles M, Marchisello PJ, Tsairis P: Lumbar adhesive arachnoiditis: Etiologic and pathologic aspects. Spine 3:45, 1978.
12. Zeidman SM, Long DM: Failed back surgery syndrome. In Menezes AHJ, Sonntag VKH (eds): Principles of Spinal Surgery. New York, McGraw-Hill, 1996, pp 657-680.
13. Deyo RA, Nachefson A, Mirza SK: Spinal fusion surgery—the case for restraint. N Engl J Med 350:722, 2004.
14. Kleuver M, Oner FC, Jacobs WC: Total disc replacement for low back pain: Background and a systematic review of the literature. Eur Spine J 12:108, 2003.
15. Deyo RA, Ciol MA, Cherkin DC, et al: Lumbar spinal fusion: A cohort study of complications, re-operation and resource use in the Medicare population. Spine 18:1463, 1993.
16. Volinn E: The epidemiology of low back pain in the rest of the world. Spine 22:1747, 1997.
17. Matsui H, Kanamori M, Kawaguchi Y, et al: Clinical and electrophysiologic characteristics of compressed lumbar nerve roots. Spine 22:2100, 1997.
18. Jamner ID, Girdler SS, Shapiro D, Jarvik MI: Pain inhibition, nicotine and gender. Exp Clin Psychopharmacol 6:96, 1998.

19. Wilkinson HA: The role of improper surgery in the etiology of the failed back syndrome. In Wilkinson HA (ed): The Failed Back Syndrome, 2nd ed. New York, Springer-Verlag, 1992, pp 4-12.
20. Pauli P, Rau H, Zhuang P, et al: Effect of smoking on thermal pain in deprived and minimally deprived in habitual smokers. Psychopharmacology 111:472, 1993.
21. Woodside J Jr: Females smokers have increase perioperative narcotic requirement. J Addict Dis 19:1, 2000.
22. Silvertein P: Smoking and wound healing. Am J Med 93:225, 1992.
23. Warner DO, Patten CA, Ames SC, et al: Smoking behaviour and perceived stress in cigarette smokers undergoing elective surgery. Anesthesiology 100:1125, 2004.
24. Kwaiatkowski TC, Hanley EN: Cigarette smoking and its orthopedic consequences. Am J Orthop 25:590, 1996.
25. Goodkin R, Laska LL: Unintended "incidental" durotomy during surgery of the lumbar spine: Medicolegal implications. Surg Neurol 43:4, 1994.
26. Eismont FJ, Wiesel SW, Rothman RH: Treatment of dural tears associated with spinal surgery. J Bone Joint Surg Am 63:1132, 1981.
27. Jones AM, Stambough JL, Balderstyon RA, et al: Long-term results of lumbar spine surgery complicated by incidental durotomy. Spine 14:443, 1989.
28. Aldrete JA, Ghaly RF: Post-laminectomy pseudomeningocele: An unsuspected cause of low back pain. Reg Anesth 20:75, 1995.
29. Waisman M, Schweppe Y: Postoperative cerebrospinal fluid leakage after lumbar spine operations: Conservative treatment. Spine 16:52, 1991.
30. Long D: Failed back surgery syndrome. Neurosurg Clin North Am 2:899, 1991.
31. Schellinger D, Manz HJ, Vidic B, et al: Disc fragment migration. Radiology 175:831, 1990.
32. Carrage EJ, Kim DH: A prospective analysis of MRI findings in patients with sciatica and lumbar disc herniation: Correlation of outcomes with disc fragment and canal morphology. Spine 22:1650, 1997.
33. LaRocca H, McNab I: The laminectomy membrane: Studies on its evolution, characteristics, effects and prophylaxis in dogs. J Bone Joint Surg Br 56:545, 1974.
34. DeLeo JA, Colburn RW: The role of cytokines in nociception and chronic pain. In Weinstein JN, Gordon SL (eds): Low Back Pain: A Scientific and Clinical Overview. Philadelphia, American Academy of Orthopedic Surgeons, 1996, pp 163-185.
35. Borgeson SE, Vang PS: Extradural pseudocysts. Acta Orthop Scand 44:12, 1973.
36. North RB, Campbell JN, Javers CS, et al: Failed back surgery syndrome: A 5-year follow-up in 102 patients undergoing repeated operations. Neurosurgery 28:685, 1991.
37. Burton CV: Causes of failure of surgery of the lumbar spine: Ten-year follow-up. Mount Sinai J Med 58:183, 1991.
38. Liu S, Boutrand JP, Bittoun J, Tadie M: A collage-based sealant to prevent in vivo reformation of epidural scar adhesions in an adult rat laminectomy model. J Neurosurg 97:69, 2002.
39. Hogland J, Freemont AJ, Denton J, et al: Retained surgical swab debris in post laminectomy arachnoiditis and peridural fibrosis. J Bone Joint Surg Br 70:659, 1988.
40. Friedman J, Whitecloud TS III: Lumbar cauda equina syndrome associated with the use of Gelfoam: Case report. Spine 26:485, 2001.
41. Gawande AA, Studdert DM, Orav EJ, et al: Risk factors for retained instruments and sponges after surgery. N Engl J Med 348:229, 2003.
42. Brotchi JC, Pirotte B, DeWitt O, et al: Prevention of epidural fibrosis in prospective series of 100 primary lumbosacral discectomy patients: Follow-up and assessment at reoperation. Neurol Res 21:47, 1999.
43. Oswald AM, Joly LM, Gurry C, et al: Fatal intraoperative anaphylaxis related to aprotinin after local application of fibrin glue. Anesthesiology 99:521, 2003.
44. Yamagami T, Matsui H, Tsuji J, et al: Effects of laminectomy and retained extradural foreign body on cauda equina adhesion. Spine 18:1774, 1993.
45. Ghaly RF, Aldrete JA: Surgical treatment. In Aldrete JA (ed): Arachnoiditis: The Silent Epidemic. Denver, Futuremed, 2000, pp 305-322.
46. Matsui H, Kanamori M, Kawaguchi Y, et al: Clinical and electrophysiologic characteristics of compressed lumbar nerve roots. Spine 22:2100, 1997.
47. Hardy RW: Extradural cauda equina and nerve root compression from benign lesions of the lumbar spine. In Youmans JR (ed): Neurological Surgery, 4th ed. Philadelphia, WB Saunders, 1996, pp 2368-2372.
48. Wilmink JT, Hofman PA: MRI of the postoperative lumbar spine: Triple dose gadodiamide and fat suppression. Neuroradiology 39:589, 1997.
49. Kemaloglu S, Ozkan U, Yilmaz F, et al: Prevention of spinal epidural fibrosis by recombinant tissue plasminogen activator in rats. Spinal Cord 41:430, 2003.
50. Horng S, Miller FG: Is placebo surgery unethical? N Engl J Med 347:137, 2002.
51. Simeone F: Lumbar disc disease. In Wilkins RH, Rengachary SS (eds): Neurosurgery, 2nd ed. New York, McGraw-Hill, 1996, vol III, pp 3805-3814.
52. Fujiwara A, Lim T, An HS, et al: The effect of disc degeneration and facet joint osteoarthritis on the segmental flexibility of the lumbar spine. Spine 23:3036, 2000.
53. Panjabi MM, Oxland T, Yamamoto I, Crisco JJ: Mechanical behavior or the human lumbar spine and lumbosacral spine as shown by three-dimensional load displacement curves. J Bone Joint Surg Am 76:413, 1994.
54. Roberts N, Gratin C, Whitehouse GH, et al: MRI analysis of lumbar intervertebral disc height in young and older populations. J Magn Reson Imaging 7:880, 1997.
55. Hutton DC, Ganey TM, Elmer WA, et al: Does long-term compressive loading on the intervertebral disc cause degeneration. Spine 25:2993, 2000.
56. Fritzell P, Hagg O, Nordwall A: Complications in lumbar fusion surgery for chronic low back pain: Comparison of three surgical techniques used in a prospective randomized study. Eur Spine J 12:178, 2003.
57. Ross JS, Masaryk TJ, Schrader M, et al: MR imaging of the postoperative lumbar spine: Assessment with gadopentetate dimeglumine. AJNR Am J Neuroradiol 11:771, 1990.
58. Bennett GJ, Serhan HA, Sorini PM, Willis BH: An experimental study of lumbar destabilization: Restabilization and bone density. Spine 22:1448, 1997.
59. Whiteland TS, Butler JC, Cohen JL, et al: Complications with the variable spinal plating system. Spine 14:472, 1989.
60. Kestler OC: Overgrowth (hypertrophy) of lumbosacral grafts causing a complete spinal block. Bull Hosp Joint Dis 27:51, 1966.
61. Martin RJ, Yuan HA: Neurosurgical care of spinal epidural, subdural and intramedullary abscesses and arachnoiditis. Orthop Clin North Am 27:125, 1993.
62. Carrol SE, Wiesel SW: Neurological complications and lumbar laminectomies. Clin Orthop 25:14, 1992.
63. Linholm TS, Pylkkanen P: Discitis following removal of intervertebral disc. Spine 7:617, 1982.
64. Maiuri F, Iaconetta G, Gallichio B, et al: Spondylodiscitis: Clinical and MRI diagnosis. Spine 22:1741, 1997.
65. Aldrete JA, Williams SK: Infections from extended epidural catheterization in ambulatory patients. Reg Anesth Pain Med 23:491, 1998.
66. Wilkinson HA: Diagnostic errors and inadequate surgery. In Wilkinson HA (ed): The Failed Back Syndrome, 2nd ed. New York, Springer-Verlag, 1992, pp 26-31.
67. Matsui H, Tsuji H, Kanamori M, et al: Laminectomy induced arachnoradiculitis: A postoperative serial MRI study. Neuroradiology 37:660, 1995.
68. Nakano M, Matsui H, Miaki K, et al: Postlaminectomy adhesion of the cauda equina: Changes of postoperative vascular permeability of the cauda equina in rats. Spine 15:22:1005, 1997.
69. Nakano M, Matsui H, Miaki K, Tsuji H: Postlaminectomy adhesion of the cauda equina: Inhibitory effects of anti-inflammatory drugs on cauda equina adhesions in rats. Spine 23:298, 1998.
70. Avidan A, Gomori M, Davison E: Nerve root inflammation demonstrated by MRI in a patient with transient neurologic symptoms after intrathecal injection of lidocaine. Anesthesiology 97:257, 2002.
71. Aldrete JA: Nerve root "irritation" or inflammation diagnosed by MRI. Anesthesiology 98:1294, 2003.
72. Ross JS, Masaryk TJ, Schrader M, et al: MR imaging of the postoperative lumbar spine. Assessment with gadopentate dimeglumine. AJR Am J Roentgenol 167:867, 1996.
73. Ross JS, Masaryk TJ, Modic MT, et al: MR imaging of lumbar arachnoiditis. AJR Am J Roentgenol 149:1025, 1987.
74. Aldrete JA, Aldrete VT: Pain generators in patients with failed back syndrome. XIII Congress WFSA, Paris, France, April 22-27, 2004.

75. Heggeness MH, Watters WC, Gray PM: Discography of lumbar discs after surgical treatment for disc herniation. Spine 22:1606, 1997.
76. Carragge EJ, Chen Y, Tanner CM, et al: Provocative discography in patients after limited lumbar discectomy: A controlled randomized study of pain response in symptomatic and asymptomatic subjects. Spine 25:3065, 2000.
77. Heavner J, Racz GB, Singleton W, et al: Percutaneous epidural neuroplasty. Reg Anesth Pain Med 24:201, 1999.
78. Devulder J, Bogaet L, Castille F, et al: Relevance of epidurography and epidural adhesiolysis in chronic failed back surgery patients. Clin J Pain 11:147, 1995.
79. Straham C, Min K, Boos N, et al: Reliability of perioperative SSEP recordings in spine surgery. Spinal Cord 41:483, 2003.
80. Waddell G, McCulloch J, Kummel E, Venner R: Non-organic physical signs in low back pain. Spine 5:117, 1980.
81. Waddell G, Richardson J: Observation of overt pain behavior by physicians during routine clinical examination of patients with low back pain. J Psychosom Res 36:77, 1992.
82. Polatin PB, Cox, B, Gatchel RJ, Mayer TG: A prospective study of Waddell signs in patients with chronic low back pain. Spine 22:1618, 1997.
83. Junge A, Dvorak J, Ahrens S: Predictors of bad and good outcomes of lumbar disc surgery. Spine 20:460, 1995.
84. Vromen PCA, de Krom CTFM, Wilmink JT: Pathoanatomy of clinical findings in patients with sciatica: A MRI study. J Neurosurg 92:135, 2000.
85. Spencer DL, Irwin GS, Miller JA: Anatomy and significance of fixation of lumbosacral nerve roots in sciatica. Spine 8:672, 1983.
86. Porter R, Bewley B: A ten-year prospective study of vertebral canal size as a predictor of back pain. Spine 19:173, 1994.
87. Van Tulder MW, Boes BW, Bouter LM: Conservative treatment of acute and chronic nonspecific low back pain: A systematic review of randomized control trials of the most common interventions. Spine 22:2128, 1997.
88. Ivar Brox J, Sorenson R, Fris A, et al: Randomized clinical trial of lumbar instrumented fusion and cognitive intervention and exercises in patients with chronic low back pain and disc degeneration. Spine 28:1913, 2003.
89. Ohnmeiss DD, Vanharata H, Ekholm J: Degree of disc disruption and lower extremity pain. Spine 22:1600, 1997.
90. Glassman SD, Anagnost SC, Parker A, et al: The effect of cigarette smoking and smoking cessation on spinal fusion. Spine 25:2608, 2000.
91. Krames ES, Lanning RM: Intrathecal infusion of analgesics for non-malignant pain: Analgesic efficacy. J Pain Symptom Manage 8:539, 1996.
92. Aldrete JA: Temporary epidural infusions in ambulatory patients with severe lumbalgia. Pain Rev 3:1, 1996.
93. Carter ML: Spinal cord stimulation in chronic pain: A review of the evidence. Anaesth Intensiv Care 32:11, 2004.
94. Cameron T: Safety and efficacy of spinal cord stimulation for the treatment of chronic pain: A 20-year literature review. J Neurosurg 100(3 Suppl Spine):254, 2004.
95. Fredman B, Zophar E, Nun MB, et al: The effect of repeated epidural sympathetic nerve block on "failed back surgery syndrome" associated with chronic low back pain. J Clin Anesth 11:46, 1999.
96. Fredman B, Nun MB, Zohar E, et al: Epidural steroids for treating "failed back surgery syndrome": Is fluoroscopy really necessary? Anesth Analg 89:1330, 1999.
97. Aldrete JA: Epidural injections of indomethacin for postlaminectomy syndrome: A preliminary report. Anesth Analg 96:463, 2003.
98. Racz GB, Heavner JE, Haynsworth R: Repeat epidural phenol injection in chronic pain and spasticity. In Racz GB (ed): Techniques of Neurolysis. Amsterdam, Kluwer Academic, 1989, pp 193-212.
99. Kim R, Porter RW, Choi BH, et al: Myelopathy after intrathecal administration of hypertonic saline. Neurosurgery 22:942, 1998.
100. Fibuch EE: Percutaneous epidural neuroplasty: Cutting edge or potentially harmful pain management. Reg Anesth Pain Med 24:198, 1999.
101. Aldrete JA, Zapata JC, Ghaly RF: Arachnoiditis following epidural adhesiolysis with hypertonic saline: Report of two cases. Pain Digest 6:368-370, 1996.
102. Aldrete JA (ed): The failed back surgery syndrome. Buenos Aires, Corpus, 2006, pp 9-20.

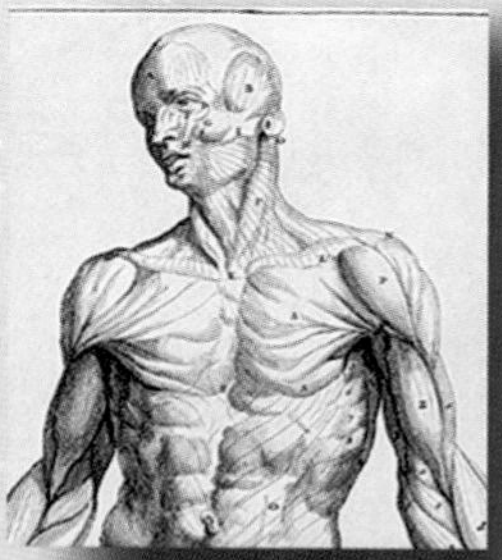

Part I

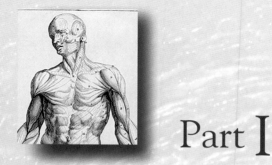

Pain Syndromes of the Pelvis and Genitalia

chapter 90

Osteitis Pubis

Steven D. Waldman

A common cause of anterior pelvic pain, osteitis pubis is relatively straightforward to diagnosis if the clinician thinks of it. A disease of the 2nd through 4th decades, osteitis pubis affects females more frequently than males. Osteitis pubis is a constellation of symptoms consisting of a localized tenderness over the symphysis pubis, pain radiating into the inner thigh and a waddling gait.[1] Characteristic radiographic changes consisting of erosion, sclerosis, and widening of the symphysis pubis are pathognomonic for osteitis pubis (Fig. 90–1). Osteitis pubis occurs most commonly following bladder, inguinal, or prostate surgery and is thought to be due to hematogenous spread of infection to the relatively avascular symphysis pubis.[2] Osteitis pubis can appear without obvious inciting factor or infection.[3]

■ SIGNS AND SYMPTOMS

On physical examination, the patient will exhibit point tenderness over the symphysis pubis. The patient may be tender over the anterior pelvis and note that the pain radiates into the inner thigh with palpation of the symphysis pubis. Patients may adopt a waddling gait to avoid movement of the symphysis pubis. This dysfunctional gait may result in lower extremity bursitis and tendinitis, which may confuse the clinical picture and further increase the patient's pain and disability.

■ TESTING

Plain radiographs are indicated in all patients who present with pain thought to be emanating from the symphysis pubis to rule out occult bony pathology and tumor. Based on the patient's clinical presentation, additional testing including complete blood count, prostate specific antigen, sedimentation rate, serum protein electrophoresis and antinuclear antibody testing may be indicated. MRI scan of the pelvis is indicated if occult mass or tumor is suspected. Radionucleotide bone scanning may be useful to rule out stress fractures not seen on plain radiographs. The injection technique described subsequently will serve as a diagnostic and therapeutic maneuver.

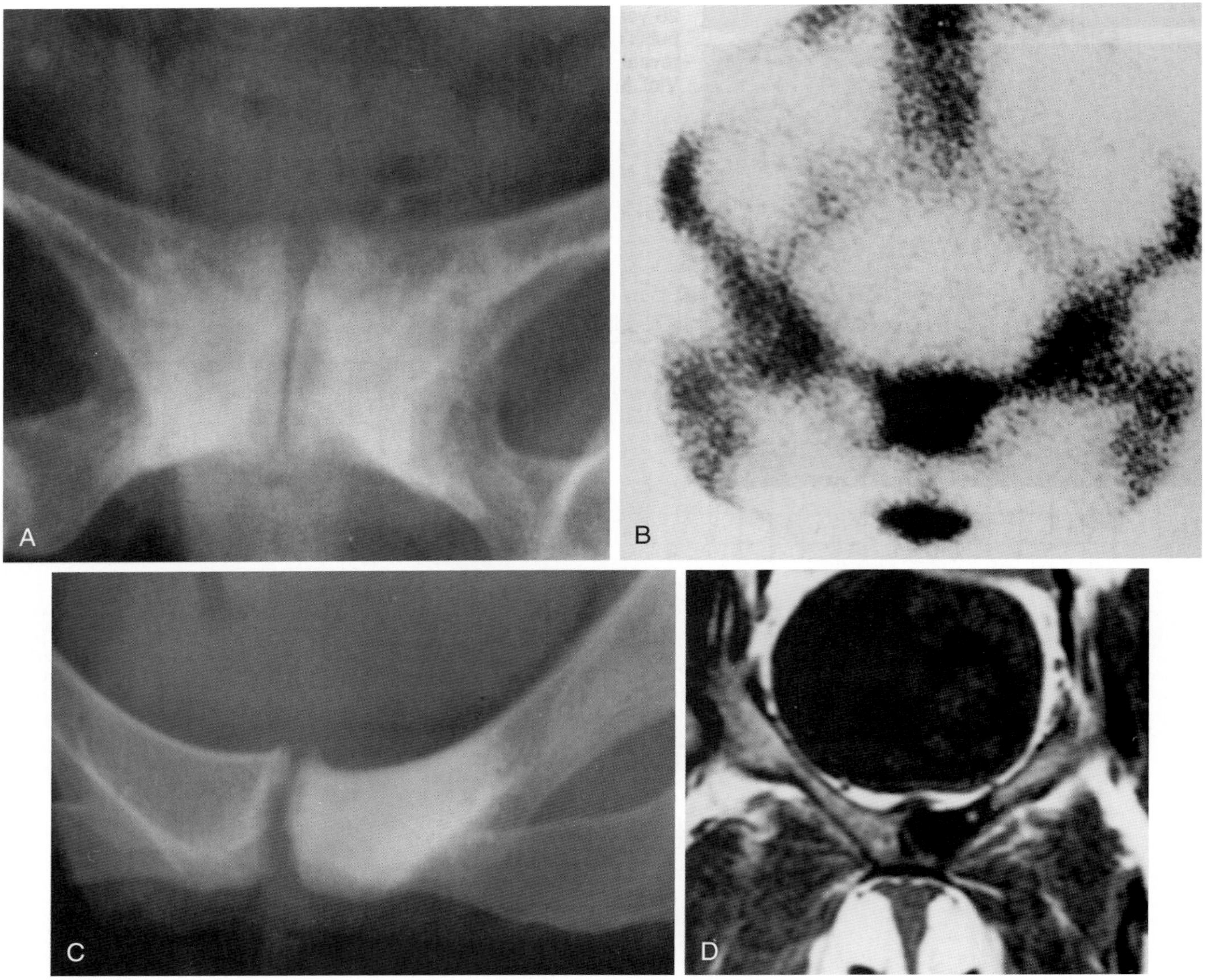

FIGURE 90–1 ■ In this 61-year-old woman, local pain and tenderness about the symphysis pubis were the major clinical abnormalities. The radiograph (**A**) reveals considerable bone sclerosis on both sides of the symphysis with narrowing of the joint space. Marked increased accumulation of the bone-seeking radiopharmaceutical agent (**B**) is observed. In this 34-year-old woman, a routine radiograph (**C**) shows unilateral osteitis pubis. A coronal T1-weighted (TR/TE, 633/17) spin echo MR image (**D**) shows low signal intensity in the involved bone. (**A** and **B**, courtesy of M. Austin, MD, Newport Beach, Calif; **C** and **D**, Courtesy of S. Eilenberg, MD, San Diego, Calif.) (From Resnick D [ed]: Diagnosis of Bone and Joint Disorders, 4th ed. Philadelphia, Saunders, 2002, p 2132.)

DIFFERENTIAL DIAGNOSIS

A pain syndrome clinically similar to osteitis pubis can be seen in patients suffering from rheumatoid arthritis and ankylosing spondylitis, but without the characteristic radiographic changes of osteitis pubis. Multiple myeloma and metastatic tumors may also mimic the pain and radiographic changes of osteitis pubis. Insufficiency fractures of the pubic rami should also be considered if generalized osteoporosis is present.

TREATMENT

Initial treatment of the pain and functional disability associated with osteitis pubis should include a combination of the nonsteroidal antiinflammatory agents or COX-2 inhibitors and physical therapy. The local application of heat and cold may also be beneficial. For patients who do not respond to these treatment modalities, the following injection technique with local anesthetic and steroid may be a reasonable next step.

Injection for osteitis pubis is carried out by placing the patient in the supine position. The midpoint of pubic bones and the symphysis pubis is identified by palpation. Proper preparation with antiseptic solution of the skin overlying this point is then carried out. A syringe containing the 2.0 mL of 0.25% preservative-free bupivacaine and 40 mg of methylprednisolone is attached to a 3 ½-inch, 25-gauge needle.

The needle is then carefully advanced through the previously identified point at a right angle to the skin directly toward the center of the pubic symphysis. The needle is

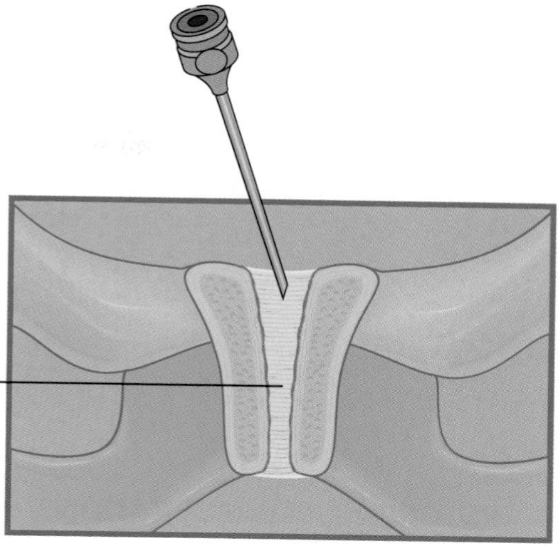

FIGURE 90–2 ■ Injection technique for osteitis pubis. (From Waldman SD: Atlas of Pain Management Injection Techniques. Philadelphia, Saunders, 2000, p 229.)

advanced very slowly until the needle impinges on the fibroelastic cartilage of the joint (Fig. 90–2). The needle is then withdrawn slightly back out of the joint and, after careful aspiration for blood and if no paresthesia is present, the contents of the syringe is then gently injected. There should be minimal resistance to injection.

The proximity to the pelvic contents makes it imperative that this procedure be carried out only by those well versed in the regional anatomy and experienced in performing injection techniques. Many patients will also complain of a transient increase in pain following the aforementioned injection technique. Reactivation of latent infection, although rare, can occur and careful attention to sterile technique is mandatory.

CONCLUSION

Osteitis pubis should be suspected in patients presenting with pain over the pubic symphysis in the absence of trauma. The above injection technique is extremely effective in the treatment of osteitis pubis. This technique is a safe procedure if careful attention is paid to the clinically relevant anatomy in the areas to be injected. Care must be taken to use sterile technique to avoid infection as well as the use of universal precautions to avoid risk to the operator. Most side effects of this injection technique are related to needle-induced trauma to the injection site and underlying tissues. The incidence of ecchymosis and hematoma formation can be decreased if pressure is placed on the injection site immediately following injection.

The use of physical modalities including local heat as well as gentle stretching exercises should be introduced several days after the patient undergoes this injection technique. Vigorous exercises should be avoided as they will exacerbate the patients symptomatology. Simple analgesics, nonsteroidal antiinflammatory agents, and antimyotonic agents such as tizanidine may be used concurrently with this injection technique.

References

1. Waldman SD: Osteitis pubis. In Waldman SD: Atlas of Common Pain Syndromes. Philadelphia, Saunders, 2002, p 266.
2. Michiels E, Knockaert DC, Vanneste SB: Infectious osteitis pubis. Neth J Med 36:297, 1990.
3. Fricker PA, Taunton JE, Ammann W: Osteitis pubis in athletes. Sports Med 12:266, 1991.

chapter 91

Piriformis Syndrome

Lowell W. Reynolds and Thomas F. Schrattenholzer

HISTORICAL CONSIDERATIONS

Initially described in 1928, piriformis syndrome is thought to be responsible for as much as 6% of sciatica.[1,2] Piriformis syndrome may be even more common, because it is often underdiagnosed and undertreated.[3-5] This is frequently because it can resemble more common pain syndromes such as lumbar radiculopathy, sacroiliac joint dysfunction, and greater trochanteric bursitis.[4,5] It is usually caused by compression and/or irritation of the proximal sciatic nerve by the piriformis muscle.[6]

CLINICALLY RELEVANT ANATOMY

The piriformis is a flat and pyramid-shaped muscle. It originates anterior to the S2-S4 vertebrae, near the sacroiliac capsule and the upper margin of the greater sciatic foramen. This muscle passes through the greater sciatic notch and inserts on the superior surface of the greater trochanter of the femur. As the piriformis courses through the sciatic notch, it comes in close proximity to the sciatic nerve (Fig. 91–1). With the hip extended, the piriformis muscle is primarily an external rotator. But when the hip is flexed, it helps to abduct the hip. The muscle is innervated by branches of the L5, S1, and S2 nerve roots. A lower lumbar radiculopathy can also cause secondary irritation of the piriformis muscle.[7,8]

There are many developmental variations between the sciatic nerve and the piriformis muscle. In approximately 20% of the population, the muscle belly is split by the sciatic nerve. In 10% of the population, the tibial/peroneal divisions are not enclosed in a common sheath. The peroneal portion splits the piriformis muscle belly, whereas the tibial division rarely splits the muscle belly.[9,10]

ETIOLOGY

Approximately 50% of patients with piriformis syndrome have a history of direct trauma to the buttock, hip, or lower back.[2] Blunt injury causes hematoma formation and subsequent scarring between the sciatic nerve and piriformis muscle. Sciatic nerve injury can also occur with prolonged pressure on the nerve. Other causes of spontaneous piriformis syndrome are the following[11,12]:

- Pseudoaneurysms of the inferior gluteal artery adjacent to the piriformis muscle
- Bilateral piriformis syndrome due to prolonged sitting during an extended neurosurgical procedure
- Cerebral palsy
- Total hip arthroplasty
- Myositis ossificans
- Vigorous physical activity

DIFFERENTIAL DIAGNOSIS

The differential diagnosis includes the following:

- Lumbosacral radiculopathy
- Lumbar degenerative disk disease
- Lumbar facet arthropathy
- Lumbar spondylolysis and spondylolisthesis
- Myofascial pain
- Trochanteric bursitis
- Ischial tuberosity bursitis

CLINICAL PRESENTATION

When the piriformis muscle spasms or becomes inflamed it may mimic sacroiliac joint dysfunction, greater trochanteric bursitis, and/or lumbar radiculopathy. Generally, the patient complains of low back, buttock, and hip pain that radiates down the ipsilateral leg.[4] Physical examination shows tenderness over the sacroiliac joint region and the superior aspect of the greater trochanter of the femur.[6] It is difficult to palpate the muscle belly because of the overlying gluteal muscles. A more reliable way of palpating the piriformis muscle is during a rectal examination. A sausage-shaped mass may be felt laterally that can reproduce the patient's pain.[13]

Other findings on examination may include the following:

- The Pace test reproduces pain with weakness to resisted abduction/external rotation.[2]
- The Freiberg test elicits pain on forced internal rotation of the extended thigh.[14]
- Shortening of the involved lower extremity may be observed.[15]

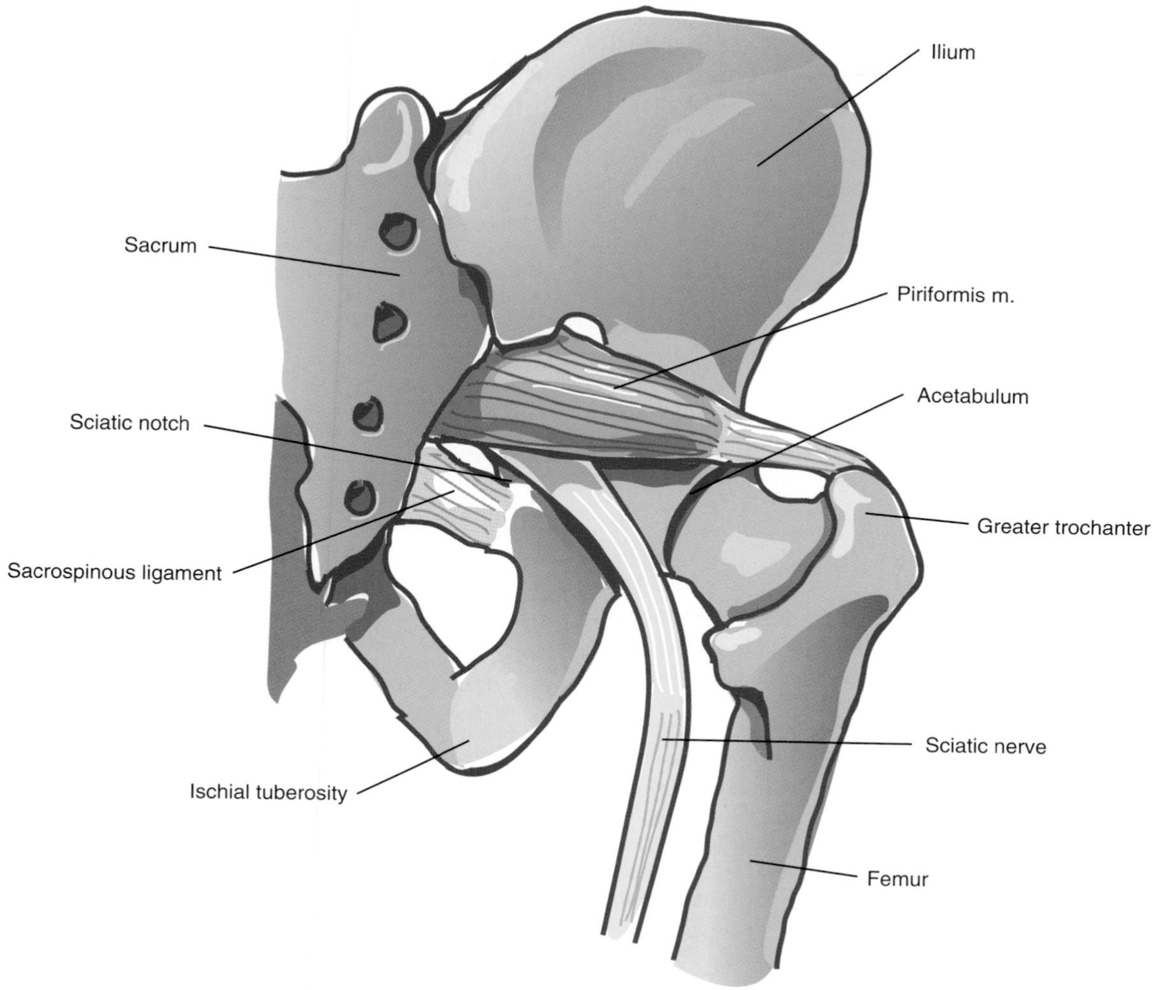

FIGURE 91–1 ■ Clinically relevant anatomy for piriformis syndrome.

TREATMENT

A trial of nonsteroidal antiinflammatory and muscle relaxant medications should be given to reduce inflammation and spasm of the piriformis muscle. Patients should be educated to the possible causes of piriformis syndrome and how to prevent further injury. This may include avoiding or reducing aggravating physical activity until the current flare-up has subsided. Applying heat, massage, and stretching to the muscle in spasm may also significantly reduce the patient's discomfort.

Physical Therapy

Patients with piriformis syndrome often respond to a trial of physical therapy. Stretching exercises are intended to lengthen the contracted piriformis muscle. The most common stretching exercise is to have the patient lie supine with the affected knee bent and pulled into the chest and toward midline. This position should be held for 30 seconds and should be repeated several times a day. A similar stretch can be performed in the standing position.[5] Care should be taken not to pull the affected knee toward the contralateral chest, because this may cause stretching at the sacroiliac joint. Ultrasound, electric stimulation, and the use of vapor-coolant spray over the area in combination with stretching have produced good results.

Acupuncture

Acupuncture has been used for centuries to reduce muscle spasm and promote healing. There are a variety of techniques that can be used such as needling, cupping, and electrical stimulation of inserted needles. Improving blood flow to the affected region seems to be an important component.

Injections

A variety of injection techniques and injectates may be used for treating piriformis syndrome. Traditionally, this has been done using a blind technique. With the patient in a lateral decubitus position with the affected side up, the ipsilateral leg is flexed until the knee rests on the treatment table. A line is then drawn from the greater trochanter to the posterior superior iliac crest. The injection site is then located approximately 5 cm below the midpoint of this line. A 22-gauge spinal needle is then inserted slowly until paresthesias are identified. After negative aspiration, methylprednisolone, 40 mg, and 10 mL 0.25% bupivacaine may be injected. Care must be taken not to inject into the sciatic nerve.[16]

Alternative techniques such as utilizing EMG-assisted fluoroscopy or MRI guidance may be used. This may improve the reliability of proper needle placement and allow for definitive diagnosis and treatment. Botulinum (Botox) is an alternative to the local anesthetic and corticosteroid injectate therapy just described. Botox can prolong the relaxation of the piriformis muscle and reduce the associated radicular symptoms.[17]

Dry needling, synonymous with acupuncture, may also have a role in the treatment of piriformis syndrome. However, unlike trigger points, its efficacy has not been adequately studied.

Surgery

If more conservative treatments prove ineffective, persistent piriformis syndrome may be treated by surgical intervention. Patients who have objective pathologic changes or dysfunction tend to be more responsive to surgical intervention. The procedure involves dissecting out the piriformis muscle and the sciatic nerve. The section of the piriformis muscle overlying the sciatic nerve is often removed. Most patients ambulate 1 day after surgery and progress to weight bearing within a week. Although there are often persistent paresthesias in the distribution of the sciatic nerve for several weeks after surgery, many patients report immediate relief of their sciatic pain.[18,19]

CONCLUSION

Piriformis syndrome often masquerades as lumbar radiculopathy, sacroiliac joint dysfunction, or greater trochanteric bursitis. Performing a careful history and physical examination is imperative in differentiating this from other common ailments. This will then significantly improve the patient's chances of responding to appropriate therapies.

References

1. Yoeman W: The relation of arthritis of the sacro-iliac joint to sciatica, with an analysis of 100 cases. Lancet 2:1119, 1928.
2. Pace JB, Nagle D: Piriformis syndrome. West J Med 124:435, 1976.
3. Durrani Z, Winnie AP: Piriformis muscle syndrome: An underdiagnosed cause of sciatica. J Pain Symptom Manage 6:374, 1991.
4. Parziale JR, Hudgins TH, Fishman LM: The piriformis syndrome. Am J Orthop 25:819, 1996.
5. Barton PM: Piriformis syndrome: A rational approach to management. Pain 47:345, 1991.
6. Fishman LM, Zybert PA: Electrophysiologic evidence of piriformis syndrome. Arch Phys Med Rehabil 73:359, 1991.
7. O'Rahilly R: The gluteal region. In Gardner-Gray-O'Rahilly Anatomy, A Regional Study of Human Structure, 5th ed. Philadelphia, WB Saunders 1986, pp 197-199.
8. Moore KR, Tsuruda JS, Dailey AT: The value of MR neurography for evaluating extraspinal neuropathic leg pain: A pictorial essay. Am J Neuroradiol 22:786, 2001.
9. Hallin RP: Sciatic pain and the piriformis muscle. Postgrad Med 74:69, 1983.
10. Chen WS, Wan YL: Sciatica caused by piriformis muscle syndrome: Report of two cases. J Formos Med Assoc 91:647, 1992.
11. Steiner C, Staubs C, Ganon M: Piriformis syndrome: Pathogenesis, diagnosis, and treatment. J Am Osteopath Assoc 87:318, 1987.
12. Uchio Y, Nishikawa U, Ochi M: Bilateral piriformis syndrome after total hip arthroplasty. Arch Orthop Trauma Surg 117:177, 1988.
13. Jankiewicz JJ, Hennrikus WL, Houkom JA: The appearance of the piriformis muscle syndrome in computed tomography and magnetic resonance imaging. A case report and review of the literature. Clin Orthop 262:205, 1991.
14. Freidberg AH: Sciatic pain and its relief by operation on muscle and fascia. Arch Surg 34:337, 1937.
15. Pecina M: Contribution to the etiological explanation of the piriformis syndrome. Acta Anat (Basel) 105:181, 1979.
16. Waldman S: Piriformis syndrome. In Waldman S (ed): Atlas of Pain Management Injection Techniques. Philadelphia, WB Saunders, 2000, pp 231-233.
17. Fishman LM, Anderson C, Rosner B: BOTOX and the physical therapy in the treatment of piriformis syndrome. Am J Phys Med Rehabil 81:936, 2002.
18. Hughes SS, Goldstein MN, Hicks DG, Pellegrini VD Jr: Extrapelvic compression of the sciatic nerve: An unusual cause of pain about the hip: Report of five cases. J Bone Joint Surg Am 74:1553, 1992.
19. Vandertop WP, Bosma WJ: The piriformis syndrome: A case report. J Bone Joint Surg Am 73:1095, 1991.

chapter 92

Orchialgia

Lowell W. Reynolds and Shawn M. Sills

HISTORICAL CONSIDERATIONS

One of the most frustrating clinical situations for the physician and for the patient is the management of orchialgia, or testicular pain. Also known as orchidynia or orchidalgia, this syndrome frequently has no obvious identifiable, causative factors.[1] In addition, the male psyche, strongly influenced by the genitalia, brings a strong psychological dimension to the management of this problem.[2]

Orchialgia can be classified in a variety of ways. These include time course (acute/chronic), age at onset (pediatric/adult), anatomic site (referred/nonreferred), pathology (mechanical/infectious), severity (severe/mild), treatment (surgical/supportive), mechanism (traumatic/nontraumatic), whether it is medication induced, whether it is physical versus psychiatric (pain disorder due to general medical condition/pain disorder associated with psychological factors), or whether it is reality based (malingering/real).[3]

Chronic orchialgia is defined as intermittent or constant, unilateral or bilateral testicular pain of 3 months or longer in duration that significantly interferes with the daily activities of a patient so as to prompt him to seek medical intervention.[4] In this chapter we explain the nerve supply and innervation of the testis, develop a differential diagnosis for orchialgia, highlight the key components of the history and physical examination, and discuss the common therapeutic approach.

PATHOPHYSIOLOGY (Fig. 92–1)

The innervation of the testis is poorly understood.[5] However, the autonomic supply to the testes and epididymis is mostly sympathetic and originates from the T10-L1 segments.[6] About 10% of the autonomic supply is parasympathetic and originates from the S2-S4 segments.[7] The *spermatic plexus* describes the group of autonomic fibers that accompany the internal spermatic vessels (the testicular artery and vein) and vas deferens to the epididymis and the testis.[6] Three nerve groups contribute to this plexus: (1) the superior spermatic nerves; (2) the middle spermatic nerves; and (3) the inferior spermatic nerves.[8,9] The superior spermatic nerves, composed of fibers from the intermesenteric and renal plexuses, run toward the testicular artery and follow its course to the testis. This association between the intestinal and testicular nerves may account for the visceral symptoms of a "sick stomach" associated with testicular trauma. The middle spermatic nerves arise from fibers of the *superior hypogastric plexus.* The middle spermatic nerves pass to the mid ureter, then travel inferiorly and then laterally along the vas deferens to the internal abdominal ring, where they join the spermatic cord and plexus.[10] The inferior spermatic nerves originate from the *pelvic plexus,* or *inferior hypogastric plexus,* and may provide the predominant sympathetic input to the testis.[7] Hypogastric nerves entering the plexus from the superior hypogastric plexus are joined from pelvic and sacral splanchnic nerves at the prostatovesical junction anterior to the rectum. The inferior spermatic nerves then join the vas deferens to exit the internal abdominal ring. Interestingly, some afferent and efferent fibers cross over to the contralateral pelvic plexus.[11] This neural cross-communication may explain how pathologic processes in one testis affect the function in the contralateral testis.

The somatic supply to the testes and scrotum originates from the L1 and L2 nerve roots via the iliohypogastric, ilioinguinal, and genitofemoral nerves.[12] The iliohypogastric nerve is a branch of the L1 nerve root with a contribution from T12 in some patients.[13] It follows a curvilinear course along the ilium, until it perforates the transversus abdominis muscle to lie between it and the external oblique muscle. The anterior branch goes on to provide cutaneous sensory innervation to the abdominal skin above the pubis. The nerve may interconnect with the ilioinguinal nerve along its course, resulting in the variable sensory distribution of these nerves. The ilioinguinal nerve is a branch of the L1 nerve root with a contribution from T12 in some patients.[14] It follows a curvilinear course along the ilium, until it perforates the transversus abdominis muscle at the level of the anterior superior iliac spine. In general, this nerve supplies sensory innervation to the upper portion of the skin of the inner thigh, the root of the penis, and the upper scrotum. The genitofemoral nerve arises from fibers of the L1 and L2 nerve roots.[15] This nerve passes through the psoas muscle where it divides into a genital and a femoral branch. The femoral branch passes beneath the inguinal ligament along with the femoral artery and provides sensory innervation to a small area of skin on the inside of the thigh. The genital branch passes through the inguinal canal and passes with the spermatic cord to provide innervation to the cremaster muscle, as well as the parietal and visceral tunica vaginalis. The S2 to S4 nerve roots provide

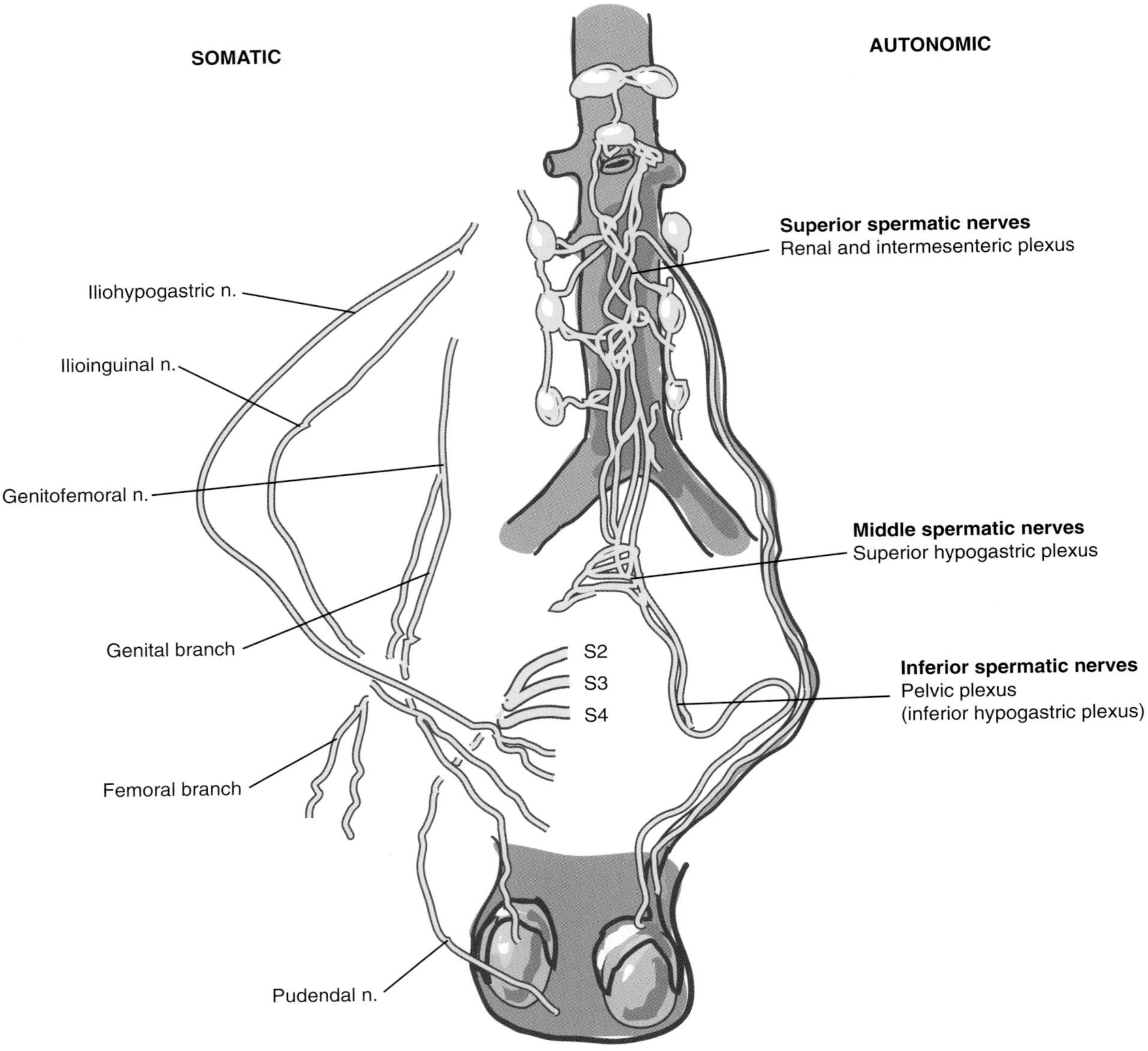

FIGURE 92–1 ■ Innervation of the testis.

innervation to the posterior and inferior scrotum via the pudendal nerve.[16]

Damage to the testes or epididymis or to the nerve supply of these structures will result in orchialgia. Also, lesions affecting somatic structures in the same segmental nerve supply as the testes, namely, L1 and L2, may refer pain to this area. As with other neuropathic pain syndromes, sympathetically maintained and mediated pain may occur after injury to these structures. Thus, patients who do not respond to inguinal denervation or subcutaneous blockade may respond to application of local anesthetics to the pelvic plexus.[17]

■ DIFFERENTIAL DIAGNOSIS

(Table 92–1)

Orchialgia may be due to a host of processes that have nothing to do with intrascrotal pathology.[3] Somatic structures in the same segmental nerve supply as the testis (L1, L2) may refer pain to this area. Radiculitis is the most likely cause of referred orchialgia.[18] Degenerative lesions of the lower thoracic and upper lumbar spine refer an "aching" pain to the groin and testis.[19] Nephrolithiasis masquerades as orchialgia when a midureteric stone is present. This occurs by two mechanisms. First, the ureteric autonomic afferents arising from the same somatic segment at L1 and L2 cross over to the testis afferents in the autonomic ganglia. Second, the genitofemoral nerve lying in contact with the ureter at the L4 vertebral level can become irritated and refer pain along its distribution.[20] Ilioinguinal and genitofemoral neuralgia not uncommonly follow inguinal herniorrhaphy.[21] This is usually caused by the entrapment of neural tissue by suture placement, surgical clips, fibrous adhesions, or a cicatricial neuroma.[22] A small indirect inguinal hernia may irritate the genital branch of the genitofemoral nerve.[19] Tendonitis at the insertion of the inguinal ligament into the pubic tubercle may cause testicu-

Table 92–1

Differential Diagnosis of Orchialgia

Referred Pain
Radiculitis
Nephrolithiasis
Ilioinguinal, genitofemoral neuralgia
Inguinal hernia
Tendinitis of the inguinal ligament
Abdominal aortic aneurysm
Appendicitis
Epilepsy

Causative Factors
Testicular torsion
Torsion of the testicular appendage
Infection: scrotitis, epididymitis
Trauma
Surgery (herniorrhaphy, vasectomy)
Inguinal hernia
Tumor
Vasculitis, Henoch-Schönlein purpura
Idiopathic scrotal edema
"Blue balls" (sexual frustration)
Self-palpation orchitis
Hydrocele
Varicocele
Spermatocele

lar pain.[4] Interestingly, even acute abdominal aortic aneurysm rupture or leakage may produce testicular pain,[23] as can aneurysm of the common iliac artery.[24]

Causative factors for orchialgia include torsion, ischemia, infection, trauma, tumor, inguinal hernia, hydrocele, spermatocele, varicocele, vasculitis, edema, and previous surgery (e.g., herniorrhaphy, vasectomy, or other scrotal procedures).[25,26]

In the acute setting, and especially with the pediatric population, acute testicular pain should be considered testicular torsion until proven otherwise.[27] The prognosis of torsion is poor, with up to 55% of affected boys losing a testis, even with immediate surgical exploration.[28] Typically, this is due to the slow response of the patient to present to a physician. Torsion of the testicular appendage may also occur and is sometimes associated with the "blue dot" sign.[29] Intermittent torsion may present with recurrent severe pain. These patients usually have a "bell-clapper" deformity that puts them at risk for torsion.[30] Any man with a history of recurrent pain and a horizontal testicular lie, even in the absence of pain at the time of physical examination, should have exploration and bilateral testicular fixation.[31] Autoimmune testicular vasculitis, with involvement of medium-sized arteries, may present in the absence of any systemic symptoms.[32]

Acute scrotitis, which is usually bacterial, may also be the cause of acute orchialgia and should especially be considered in the diabetic or otherwise immunocompromised patient. When bacterial infection becomes fulminant, gangrene can set in (Fournier's gangrene).[26] Epididymitis or orchitis often occurs secondary to chlamydial or *Ureaplasma* infection.[25]

Table 92–2

Work-Up for Orchialgia

History and Physical Examination
Past medical history: nephrolithiasis, low back pain, hernia
Past surgical history: herniorrhaphy, scrotal surgery

Laboratory Tests
Complete blood cell count with differential
Urinalysis with culture and sensitivity

Other Tests
Testicular ultrasonography
Color flow Doppler imaging
Radionuclide scans
MRI of testes or low back
Electromyography

Trauma is a leading cause of acute testicular pain and may lead to hematocele, ruptured testes, or sperm granuloma.[33] Self-palpation orchitis, caused by frequent squeezing of the testis by a neurotic man overly concerned about developing testis cancer, may present as orchialgia.[34] Malignancy may present as persistent scrotal pain. If malignancy is suspected, this should be investigated with MRI or scrotal ultrasonography.[35]

Hydrocele, spermatocele, and varicocele are amenable to surgical management, which may be highly effective.[36] However, these lesions may be incidental findings, with surgery exacerbating the pain.[37] Indeed, surgery is often the cause of orchialgia.[4] During herniorrhaphy, if the vascular supply is compromised, acute ischemic orchitis and testicular atrophy may follow.[38] Vasectomy with distention of the epididymis is commonly associated with orchialgia.[39] However, the cause of orchialgia may never be identified. Up to 25% of patients with chronic orchialgia have no obvious cause for the pain.[4] A strong clinical depressive abnormality is often present on psychological tests.[40]

DIAGNOSIS (Table 92–2)

A complete history and physical examination performed with careful attention to the scrotal region is the cornerstone of proper evaluation.[41] The history should include the typical questions regarding onset, duration, exacerbating and alleviating factors, associated symptoms, and so on, but should also include a sexual history with questions about sexual dysfunction, sexually transmitted disease risk factors, and history of sexual abuse.[3] The past medical history is vital and often suggests a potential cause, such as a history of nephrolithiasis, lumbar disk disease, or hernia. The past surgical history may reveal prior inguinal surgery, such as herniorrhaphy, or other urologic procedures. The complaint is usually of a squeezing, deep ache in the testis, often bilateral or alternating from one side to the other, that is intermittent and commonly associated with low back pain.[40] Sometimes the patient reports that it feels as if the testis is pinched in the underwear but that trouser readjustment does not help. The onset of pain is commonly related to particular activities (e.g., long automobile journeys or unsupported seating posture).[40]

Occasionally, a physical examination may reveal an obvious source of pain, but usually the patient has no abnormality on physical examination. A thorough physical examination should be done to help rule out causes of radicular pain. Palpation of the testes while the patient is standing should be done as part of the routine examination. Palpation may reveal a varicocele that classically presents as a "bag of worms." These patients may benefit from semen analysis, because as high as 40% of patients seen in infertility clinics have an associated varicocele.[3] A hydrocele may be diagnosed by transillumination of the testes.

Simple laboratory tests include a complete blood cell count with differential, urinalysis, and cultures. If pyuria or hematuria is detected, these conditions are worked up the same way as they would be in the absence of pain. If these laboratory studies are normal, a good next step is scrotal ultrasound. An obvious abnormality would prompt surgical consultation and intervention. If a tumor is suspected, tumor markers, such α-fetoprotein, β-human chorionic gonadotropin, and lactate dehydrogenase, should be obtained. Other potentially useful tests are color flow Doppler imaging, radionuclide (^{99m}Tc pertechnetate) scans, MRI, and needle aspiration.[42-45] Electromyography may be useful to distinguish ilioinguinal nerve entrapment from lumbar plexopathy, lumbar radiculopathy, and diabetic polyneuropathy.[46] MRI of the thoracic and lumbar spines should be considered if radiculitis is suspected.

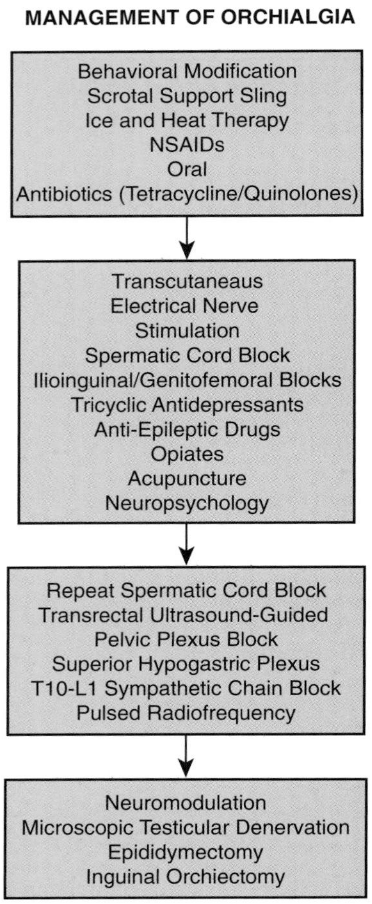

FIGURE 92–2 ■ Algorithm for the management of orchialgia.

CONSERVATIVE MANAGEMENT (Fig. 92–2)

Initial relief may be obtained by modifying exertional and postural habits, the use of a scrotal suspension sling or jock strap, heat and cold therapy, and a trial of anti-inflammatory agents and oral antibiotics. A minimum 1-month trial of at least two NSAIDs is recommended.[4] Even in the presence of normal laboratory findings, a course of oral antibiotics (either from the tetracycline and/or quinolone group) is indicated to cover possible chlamydial or *Ureaplasma* infection.[25]

If this management fails, a multidisciplinary approach, as with other chronic pain syndromes, is best.[37] This may include the addition of a low-dose antidepressant, such as doxepin or amitriptyline of the tricyclic antidepressant class. It is important to start with a low dose at bedtime and titrate the dose to the patient's response. This approach helps to decrease the side effects of sedation and disorientation, factors that cause many patients to stop medication before achieving any therapeutic effect. Chronic opiate therapy may also be indicated. Antiepileptic drugs, such as gabapentin, may be beneficial.[47] Transcutaneous electrical nerve stimulation (TENS) has been useful in many patients with chronic scrotal pain. A trial of TENS for 1 to 3 months is safe and may be beneficial.[37] Biofeedback, acupuncture, and psychotherapy are other adjunctive therapies that can be employed.

Should pain continue, consultation should be sought with an interventional pain specialist for a selective nerve block. Access to a pain management clinic is a strong asset. A spermatic cord block can be tried using a mixture of epinephrine free local anesthetic and corticosteroid. Patients with temporary relief may be considered for repeated cord blocks.[4] Patients with ilioinguinal or genitofemoral neuralgia may be treated with similar blocks to these nerves. Pulsed radiofrequency has been used successfully for chronic groin pain or orchialgia originating from these nerves.[48]

For patients unresponsive to spermatic cord blockade, local anesthetic and corticosteroid applied to the pelvic plexus may be beneficial.[17,49] The pelvic plexus lies anterior to the rectum at the prostatovesical junction. These periprostatic nerves are localized under transrectal ultrasound guidance. The location of these nerves may explain the association of testicular pain with prostatic inflammation or after surgery. As shown by the success of this block, the pelvic plexus may provide the predominant sympathetic and parasympathetic efferent input to the testis. Alternatively, the superior hypogastric plexus may be blocked. In the case of testicular cancer, neurolysis of this plexus using 8 to 10 mL of 10% aqueous phenol or 50% alcohol may produce long-lasting pain relief.[50] A lumbar sympathetic chain block at the T10-L1 level is a third approach.

Occasionally, tendinitis caused by insertion of the inguinal ligament into the pubic tubercle may masquerade as testicular pain. This condition usually responds well to injection of the tubercle and ligament with a mixture of local anesthetics and corticosteroid.[1]

SURGICAL TREATMENT

Surgical treatment may ultimately be necessary if medical management proves unsuccessful. Orchidectomy, with the inguinal approach favored over the scrotal approach, is usually a last resort. The response to this procedure is unpredictable, and the impact on the male psyche may be profound. Consequently, other testis-sparing procedures have been advocated. Neuromodulation, such as spinal cord stimulation, has proven effective in treating groin and testicular pain. This may be indicated in select patients. Many urologists prefer epididymectomy as the initial surgical treatment, especially when the pain seems to be localized to the epididymis.[4] Alternatively, microscopic testicular denervation or laparoscopic testicular denervation may offer patients a significant reduction in pain that is minimally invasive and with minimal morbidity.[51-54] In these procedures, the spermatic plexus and adventitia are stripped away from the vas deferens and vessels and divided or the vessels with nerves themselves are simply divided. Spermatic cord block should be performed before these procedures and is a prognostic indicator of surgical success.

CONCLUSION

Chronic orchialgia is a difficult problem to manage. The clinician should be aware of the unique relationship of the genitalia and the male psyche. Behavioral and psychological issues should be addressed concurrently with medical therapy. Despite the often unclear cause of orchialgia, the possibility of testicular malignancy remains ever present and should be carefully sought in all patients suffering from orchialgia. The ultimate goal of therapy is the patient's return to gainful activity, with minimal loss of function and sparing of the testes. Improved interventional techniques, such as transrectal ultrasound–guided pelvic plexus blockade and microsurgical denervation of the spermatic cord, are helping in achieving this goal.

References

1. Masarani M, Cox R: The aetiology, pathophysiology and management of chronic orchialgia. BJU Int 91:435, 2003.
2. American Psychiatric Association: Diagnostic and Statistical Manual of Mental Disorders, 4th ed. Washington, DC, American Psychiatric Association, 1994.
3. Reynolds LW, Schultz DE, Waldman SD: Testicular pain (orchialgia). Pain Digest 8:177, 1998.
4. Davis B, Noble MJ, Weigel JD, Mebust WK: Analysis and management of chronic testicular pain. J Urol 143:936, 1990.
5. Kim F, Pinto P, Su LM, et al: Ipsilateral orchialgia after laparoscopic donor nephrectomy. J Endourol 17:405, 2003.
6. Gee WF, Arnell JS, Bonica JJ: Pelvic and perineal pain of urologic origin. In Bonica JJ, Malvern N (eds): The Management of Pain. Philadelphia, Lea & Febiger, 1990, pp 1368-1372.
7. Zorn BH, Watson LR, Steers WD: Nerves from pelvic plexus contribute to chronic orchialgia. Lancet 1994;343:1161
8. Colby F: Embryology, anatomy and physiology of the testis and epididymis. In Essential Urology, 2nd ed. Baltimore, Williams & Wilkins, 1953, pp 101-103.
9. Redman JF: Anatomy of the genitourinary system. In Gillenwater JY, Grayhack JT, Howards SS, Duckett JW (eds): Adult and Pediatric Urology, 3rd ed. St. Louis, CV Mosby, 1996, pp 3-44.
10. Peterson DF, Brown AM: Functional afferent innervation of testis. J Neurophysiol 36:425, 1973.
11. Brooks JD: Anatomy of the lower urinary tract and male genitalia. In Walsh PC, Retik AB, Vaughn ED Jr, Wein AJ (eds): Campbell's Urology, 7th ed. Philadelphia, WB Saunders, 1998, pp 89-128.
12. Brown DL: Lower extremity anatomy. In Brown DL: Atlas of Regional Anesthesia, 2nd ed. Philadelphia, WB Saunders, 1999, pp 77-84.
13. Reynolds L, Kedlaya D: Ilioinguinal-iliohypogastric and genitofemoral nerve blocks. In Waldman SD (ed): Interventional Pain Management, 2nd ed. Philadelphia, WB Saunders, 2001, pp 508-511.
14. Waldman SD: Ilioinguinal nerve block. In Waldman SD: Atlas of Interventional Pain Management. Philadelphia, WB Saunders, 1998, pp 281-285.
15. Waldman SD: Genitofemoral nerve block. In Waldman SD: Atlas of Interventional Pain Management. Philadelphia, WB Saunders, 1998, pp 361-365.
16. Waldman SD: Pudendal nerve block. In Waldman SD: Atlas of Interventional Pain Management. Philadelphia, WB Saunders, 1998, pp 378-385.
17. Zorn B, Rauchenwald M, Steers WD: Periprostatic injection of local anesthesia for relief of chronic orchialgia. J Urol 151:411, 1994.
18. Holland JM, Feldman JL, Gilbert HC: Phantom orchialgia. J Urol 152:2291, 1994.
19. Yeats WK: Pain in the scrotum. Br J Hosp Med 33:101, 1985.
20. Brown FR: Testicular pain; its significance and localization. Lancet 1:994, 1994.
21. Starling JR, Harms BA: Diagnosis and treatment of genitofemoral and ilioinguinal neuralgia. World J Surg 13:586, 1989.
22. Holland JM, Feldman JL, Gilbert HC: Phantom orchialgia. J Urol 152:2291, 1994.
23. Crausman RS, Bravo K: Re: Ruptured abdominal aortic aneurysm masquerading as testicular pain [Letter to the Editor]. Am J Emerg Med 15:445, 1997.
24. Ali MS: Testicular pain in a patient with aneurysm of the common iliac artery. Br J Urol 55:447, 1983.
25. Baum N, Defidio L: Chronic testicular pain: A work-up and treatment guide for the primary care physician. Postgrad Med 98:151, 1995.
26. O'Brien WM, Lynch JH: The acute scrotum. Am Fam Physician 37:239, 1988.
27. Lindsey D: Boys with acute testicular pain should be presumed to have torsion until proven otherwise. J Emerg Med 12:531, 1994.
28. Bennett S, Nicholson MS, Little TM: Torsion of the testis: Why is the prognosis so poor? Br Med J 294:824, 1987.
29. Bourne HH, Lee RE: Torsion of spermatic cord and testicular appendage. Urology 5:73, 1975.
30. Stillwell TJ, Kramer SA: Intermittent testicular torsion. Pediatrics 77:908, 1986.
31. Schulsinger D, Glassberg K, Strashum A: Intermittent torsion: Association with the horizontal lie of the testicle [Letter]. J Urol 145:1053, 1991.
32. Raj GV, Ellington KS, Polascik TJ: Autoimmune testicular vasculitis. Urology 61:1035x, 2003.
33. Witherington R: The acute scrotum: Lesions that require immediate attention. Postgrad Med 82:207, 1987.
34. Schneiderman H: Self-palpation orchitis. Gen Intern Med 3:79, 1988.
35. Comiter CV, Benson CJ, Capellouto CC, et al: Nonpalpable intratesticular masses detected sonographically. J Urol 154:1367, 1995.
36. Gray CL, Powell CR, Amling CL: Outcomes for surgical management of orchialgia in patients with identifiable intrascrotal lesions. Eur Urol 39:455, 2001.
37. Costabile RA, Hahn M, McLeod DG: Chronic orchialgia in the pain prone patient: The clinical perspective. J Urol 146:1571, 1991.
38. Wantz GE: Complications of inguinal hernial repair. Surg Clin North Am 64:287, 1984.
39. McCormack M, Lapointe S: Physiologic consequences and complications of vasectomy. Can Med Assoc J 138:223, 1988.
40. Magni G, de Bertalini C: Chronic pain as a depressive equivalent. Postgrad Med 73:79, 1983.
41. Hayden LJ: Chronic testicular pain. Aust Fam Physician 22:1357, 1993.
42. Dewire DM, Begun FP, Lawson RK et al: Color Doppler ultrasonography in the evaluation of the acute scrotum. J Urol 147:89, 1992.
43. Rosenfield AT, Hammers LW: Imaging of the testicle: The painful scrotum and nonpalpable masses. Urol Radiol 14:229, 1992.
44. May DC, Lesh P, Lewis S: Evaluation of acute scrotum pain with testicular scanning. Ann Emerg Med 14:696, 1985.
45. Trambert MA, Mattrey RF, Levine D, et al: Subacute scrotal pain: Evaluation of torsion versus epididymitis with MR imaging. Radiology 175:53, 1990.

46. Waldman SD: Orchialgia. In Waldman SD: Atlas of Uncommon Pain Syndromes. Philadelphia, WB Saunders, 2003, pp 173-175.
47. Sasaki K, Smith CP, et al: Oral gabapentin (Neurontin) treatment of refractory genitourinary tract pain. Tech Urol 7:47, 2001.
48. Cohen SP, Foster A: Pulsed radiofrequency as a treatment for groin pain and orchialgia. Urology 61:645xxi, 2003.
49. Yamamoto M, Hibi H, Katsuno S, Miyake K: Management of chronic orchialgia of unknown etiology. Int J Urol 2:47, 1995.
50. Brown DL: Superior hypogastric plexus block. In Brown DL: Atlas of Regional Anesthesia, 2nd ed. Philadelphia, WB Saunders, 1999, pp 293-302.
51. Choaa RG, Swami KS: Testicular denervation: A new surgical procedure for intractable testicular pain. Br J Urol 70:417, 1992.
52. Chadeddu JA, Bishoff JT, Chan DY, et al: Laparoscopic testicular denervation for chronic orchialgia. J Urol 162:733, 1999.
53. Levine LA, Matkov TG, Lubenow TR: Microsurgical denervation of the spermatic cord: A surgical alternative treatment for chronic orchialgia. J Urol 155:1005, 1996.
54. Levine LA, Matkov TG: Microsurgical denervation of the spermatic cord as primary surgical treatment of chronic orchialgia. J Urol 165:1927, 2001.

chapter 93

Vulvodynia

Lowell W. Reynolds and Brett T. Quave

HISTORICAL CONSIDERATIONS

Vulvodynia is a complex syndrome of vulvar pain, sexual dysfunction, and psychological distress. There have been multiple attempts to categorize varying types of vulvodynia. Some of these classifications include primary vulvodynia, secondary vulvodynia, vulvar pain syndrome, essential vulvodynia, vulval vestibulitis, dysesthetic vulvodynia, and cyclic vulvitis.

CLINICALLY RELEVANT ANATOMY

When addressing a patient with vulvodynia, one must remember to educate the patient. This includes using the appropriate anatomic vocabulary with the patient and even giving her an illustration of the anatomy to take home and study (Fig. 93–1). Not only does this improve the physician's ability to outline a treatment plan with the patient, but it also allows the patient to communicate more comfortably with the physician. Having said this, the vulva consists of the mons pubis, the labia majora, the labia minora, the vestibule of the vagina, the clitoris, the bulb of the vestibule, and the greater vestibular glands.[1] The ilioinguinal and genitofemoral nerves supply the mons pubis, labia majora, and labia minora.[1,2] Any of these structures may be involved in a chronic pain condition. However, the vestibule, glands, and labia are frequently involved in vulvodynia.

CLINICAL PRESENTATION

As noted earlier, this painful condition has many differing terms. Vulvodynia can be divided into primary or essential vulvodynia, which are idiopathic. Secondary vulvodynia is due to an infection or other known cause. Regardless of the primary or secondary classification, vulvodynia typically is described as a burning or aching sensation that is painful to the touch.[3] Patients will frequently scratch and wash the affected area, leading to excoriations and extensive drying.

Vulvar vestibulitis is a painful condition that occurs when something is inserted into the opening of the vagina. This may occur with insertion of a tampon or during sexual activity. Dysesthetic vulvodynia is a painful condition that persists even in the absence of touch or pressure. These burning and aching sensations can be constant, or they can be caused by light normally nonpainful touch. These findings are similar to complex regional pain syndrome, which is known for such things as allodynia and hyperalgesia.[4] Pain that occurs with contact seems to lessen with age, but the overall prevalence of vulvodynia remains fairly consistent at approximately 16% of the female population regardless of age. Hispanic females tend to have an 80% higher likelihood of having chronic vulvar pain than do African American or white women.[5]

Some women experience worsening symptoms before menses or after intercourse, which is referred to as cyclic vulvitis. This may be due to an infectious etiology or simply an increased sensitivity to hormone replacement therapy. They may be completely pain free at other times of the month.

Depression frequently is found in conjunction with vulvodynia but is rarely the cause. The opposite in fact is true. Usually it is the chronic pain of vulvodynia that then leads to depression. This may present as depressed mood and loss of interest in work, recreation, and sexual activity. Sleep disturbances are also common with depression, which leads to further reduced function and worsening pain.

DIAGNOSIS

A thorough history and physical examination are essential in making a diagnosis of vulvodynia (Table 93–1). Various sensory and pain testing modalities can be utilized to make the diagnosis and to assess for severity.[7] Biopsy results consistently reveal a low-grade chronic inflammatory process that is not pathognomonic.[12] Histologic studies may illustrate a neural hyperplasia.[15] Infection should be excluded as the cause of vulvodynia. This can frequently be difficult to do, especially if a fungus is the infective agent. Two of the more common causes of secondary vulvodynia are *Candida albicans* and group B *Streptococcus.* Cultures can be done to help make this diagnosis. Once these have been ruled out or treated, then neuropathic vulvodynia can be addressed.[4]

TREATMENT

Education

Educating the patient about her condition is imperative. This may involve discussing the condition with the patient, giving her handouts, and referring her to support groups. Avoiding

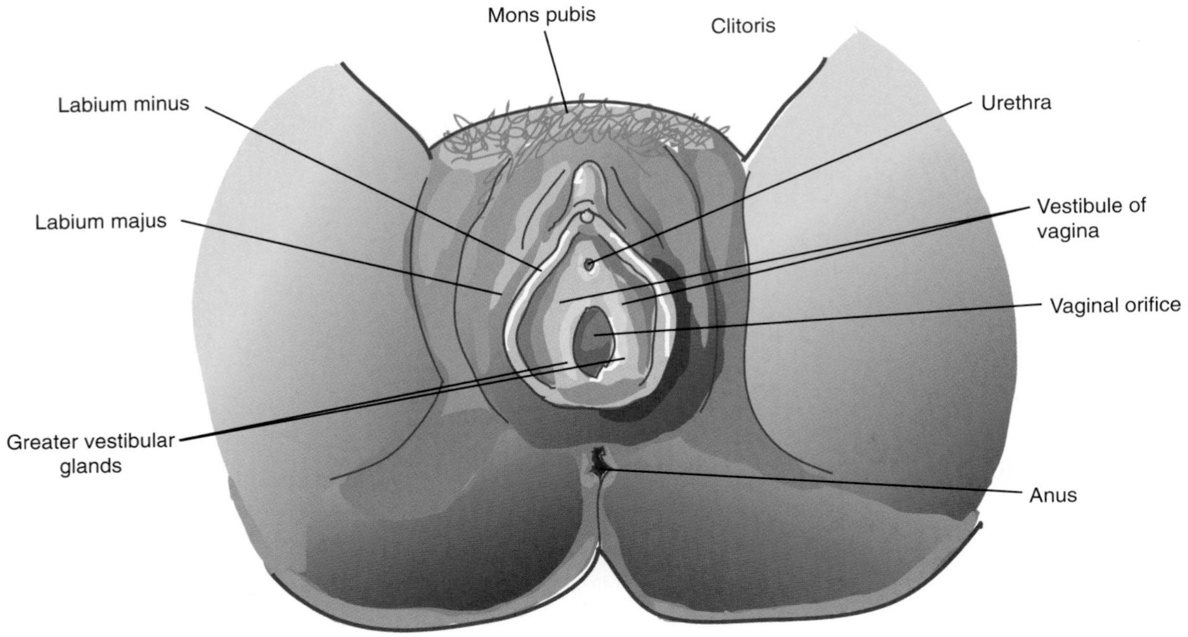

FIGURE 93–1 ■ Female external genitalia.

Table 93–1

Diagnosis of Vulvodynia

- History: illnesses, hygiene, pain, depression
- Physical examination: vulva, vagina, pelvis
- Biopsy lesions
- Microscopic examination
- Culture

harmful habits such as scratching and overcleansing the vulva should be stressed. Most importantly, ways to maintain a normal sex life, exercise regimen, and work routine should also be discussed.

Pharmacology

Agents to fight *C. albicans* or other types of infections should be administered if vulvodynia secondary to an infection is suspected. The avoidance of estrogen and progesterone used in hormone replacement therapies should be considered, because these agents have been implicated in causing vulvodynia. Other irritants should also be avoided, such as certain cleansers and lubricants.[9,14] If these agents are thought to be the cause, they should be removed from the patient's daily regimen. Lidocaine cream may be applied 20 minutes before sexual activity to reduce the pain during and after intercourse.

Amitriptyline and other antidepressants should be used as first-line therapy in treating primary vulvodynia.[8,10] Typically, this involves slowly escalating the dose until the patient achieves pain relief or has to stop secondary to side effects of the medication. The dose of amitriptyline may be as high as 300 mg at bedtime. Night-time dosing is preferred because amitriptyline can be very sedating. Thus it not only serves as a simple analgesic but also may improve the sleep pattern of the patient. This improvement in the sleep-wake cycle may be one reason vulvodynia sufferers, like other chronic pain patients, respond well to tricyclic antidepressants. Other tricyclic antidepressants have also been used successfully to treat vulvodynia, but selective serotonin reuptake inhibitors generally do not seem to offer the same analgesic qualities. However, all antidepressants may reduce the depressive component of the patient's suffering.

Antiepileptic medications have been used for years to treat a variety of neuropathic pain syndromes. For instance, medications such as phenytoin, carbamazepine, and valproic acid have all been used with varying success and side effects. Some newer medications arguably work equally well with fewer side effects. Gabapentin has been used successfully in treating postherpetic neuralgia, complex regional pain syndrome, and vulvodynia.[11] Like most antiseizure medications, gabapentin is slowly titrated upward to find a balance of the lowest effective dose for the patient and the fewest side effects. Frequently, the dose of gabapentin may be as high as 1200 mg three times a day. Common side effects include dizziness, nausea, and sedation. Newer antiepileptic medications such as topiramate, tiagabine, zonisamide, and levetiracetam may also prove effective in cases of vulvodynia caused by a neuropathic process; however, they have not been studied extensively for this purpose.

Injections

The ilioinguinal and genitofemoral nerves supply the external genitalia. In the setting of vulvodynia, blocking these nerves may prove diagnostic or even therapeutic. For pain of the mons pubis or labium majora, the ilioinguinal nerve can be blocked with the patient lying supine. A mark is made on the skin 2 cm medial and 2 cm cephalad to the anterior superior iliac spine. After the skin is sterilely prepped, a 1.5-inch 25-gauge needle connected to a syringe is advanced perpendicular to the skin. When the tip of the needle reaches the fascia of the external oblique muscle, 2.5 mL of 0.25% bupivacaine and 20 to 40 mg of methylprednisolone is injected. An equal amount of solution is then injected in a fanlike manner in the surrounding area[2] (Figs. 93–2 and 93–3).

Blocking the genital branch of the genitofemoral nerve may reduce pain of the labia majora and labia minora. This is done by placing the patient in a supine position. The pubic tubercle is then palpated. After sterile prep, a 1.5-inch, 25-gauge needle is advanced perpendicular to the skin, just lateral to the pubic tubercle below the inguinal ligament. Infiltration of 5 mL of 0.25% bupivacaine and 20 to 40 mg of methylprednisolone is used for the nerve block[2] (Fig. 93–4).

Other procedures may prove effective and should be considered in treating vulvodynia. Two of these include hypogastric plexus blockade and spinal cord stimulation.[6] A discussion of these procedures is beyond the scope of this chapter.

Psychology

Depression and anxiety are very common in patients suffering from vulvodynia. These patients should have their psychologic issues addressed while they are receiving ongoing treatment for the primary physiologic disease.[13] A referral to a psychologist or psychiatrist should be made early in the diagnosis and treatment phase. These referrals should not be made only when an organic cause for a patient's illness is ruled out. This "either/or" mentality should be avoided so as not to give the patient the impression that she is being written off as a "mental case." Patients should be informed about the power of a cognitive behavioral approach to chronic pain. Through biofeedback, visual imagery, and other powerful psychologic tools, the patient can be expected to improve her pain management and coping skills. Medications prescribed by the psychiatrist may not only lessen the depression and anxiety but, as mentioned earlier, directly reduce the pain as an adjuvant analgesic.

Surgery

Various surgical approaches have been employed after nonoperative treatments have failed. Pudendal nerve decompression has been shown to be very effective in cases in which pudendal canal syndrome was suspected and supported by temporary pain relief after pudendal nerve block.[16] Procedures involving resection of the hymen and vestibule with mobilization of the lower vagina to cover the resulting defect have been helpful in cases of intractable vulvar vestibulitis.[17]

■ CONCLUSION

The goal of understanding and treating vulvodynia is not only a reduction of the patient's pain. A return to a normal active lifestyle with a reduction in depression and anxiety should also be addressed. This can be done most easily by using a stepwise approach to diagnosis, treatment, and adjunctive psychologic therapy.

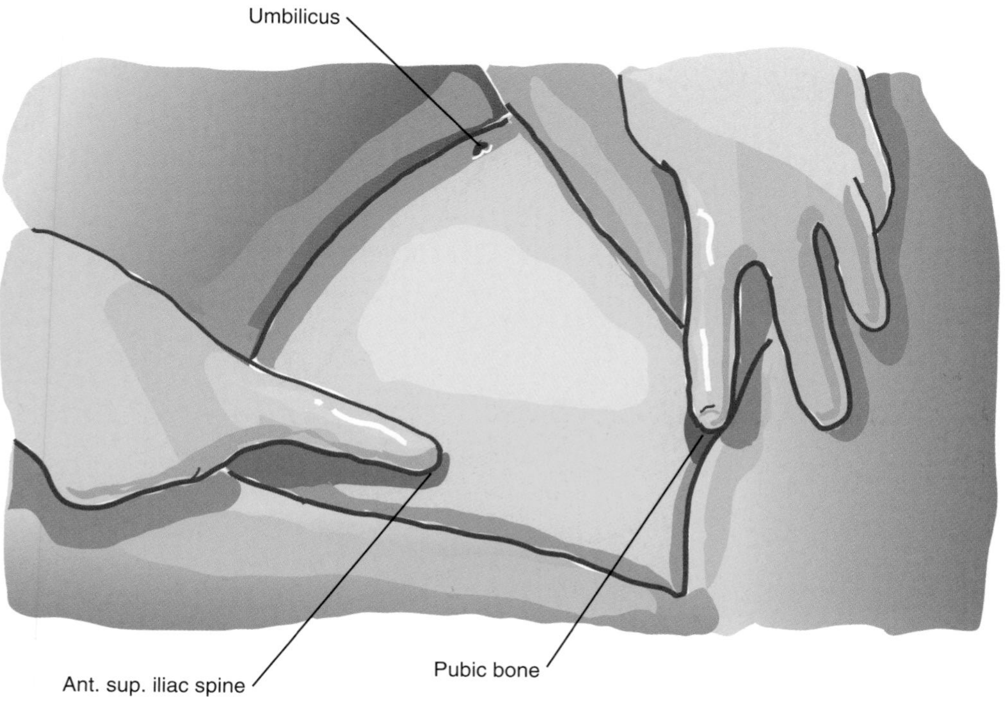

FIGURE 93–2 ■ Anterior view shows important anatomic landmarks for ilioinguinal-iliohypogastric-genitofemoral nerve blocks. ASIS, anterior superior iliac spine.

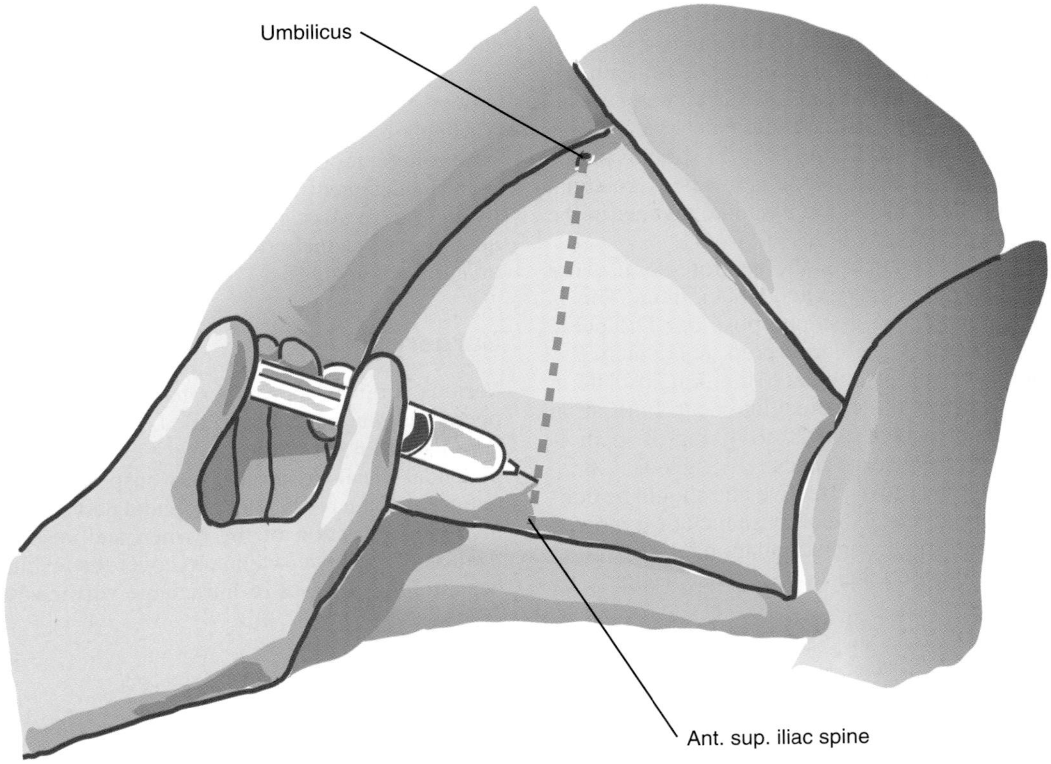

FIGURE 93–3 ■ Technique of ilioinguinal-iliohypogastric nerve block.

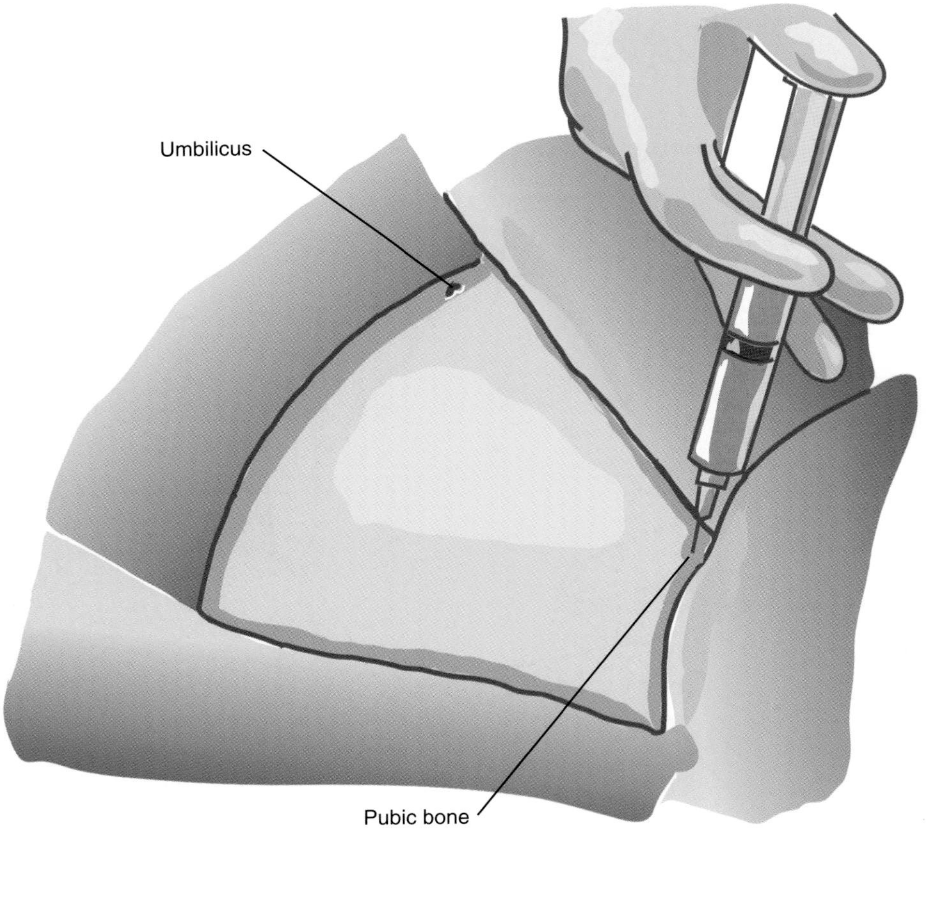

FIGURE 93–4 ■ Technique of genitofemoral nerve block (genital branch).

References

1. O'Rahilly R: The perineal region and external genitalia. In O'Rahilly R: Gardner-Gray-O'Rahilly Anatomy: A Regional Study of Human Structure, 5th ed. Philadelphia, WB Saunders, 1986, pp 502-512.
2. Reynolds L, Kedlaya D: Ilioinguinal-iliohypogastric and genitofemoral nerve blocks. In Waldman SD: Interventional Pain Management, 2nd ed. Philadelphia, WB Saunders, 2001, pp 508-511.
3. Tympanidis P, Terenghi G, Dowd P: Increased innervation of the vulvar vestibule in patients with vulvodynia. Br J Dermatol 148:1021, 2003.
4. Edwards L: New concepts in vulvodynia. Am J Obstet Gynecol 189(3 Suppl):S24, 2003.
5. Harlow BL, Stewart EG: A population-based assessment of chronic unexplained vulvar pain: Have we underestimated the prevalence of vulvodynia? J Am Med Womens Assoc 58(2):82, 2003.
6. Whiteside JL, Walters MD, Mekhail N: Spinal cord stimulation for intractable vulvar pain: A case report. J Reprod Med 48:821, 2003.
7. Lowenstein L: Vulvar vestibulitis severity—assessment by sensory and pain testing modalities. Pain 107:47, 2004.
8. McKay M: Dysesthetic (essential) vulvodynia: Treatment with amitriptyline. J Reprod Med 38:9, 1993.
9. O'Hare PM: Vulvodynia: A dermatologist's perspective with emphasis on an irritant contact dermatitis component. J Womens Health Gend Based Med 9:565, 2000.
10. Munday PE: Response to treatment in dysaesthetic vulvodynia. J Obstet Gynaecol 6:610, 2001.
11. Ben-David B, Friedman M: Gabapentin therapy for vulvodynia. Anesth Analg 89:1459, 1999.
12. Lamont J, Randazzo J, Farad M, et al: Psychosexual and social profiles of women with vulvodynia. J Sex Marital Ther 27:551, 2001.
13. Slowinski J: Multimodal sex therapy for the treatment of vulvodynia: A clinician's view. J Sex Marital Ther 27:607, 2001.
14. Welsh B, Berzins K, Cook K, Fairley C: Management of common vulval conditions. Med J Aust 178:391, 2003.
15. Tympanidis P, Terenghi G, Dowd P: Increased innervation of the vulval vestibule in patients with vulvodynia. Br J Dermatol 148:1021, 2003.
16. Shafik A: Pudendal canal syndrome as a cause of vulvodynia and its treatment by pudendal nerve decompression. Eur J Obstet Gynecol 80:215, 1998.
17. McCormack W, Spence M: Evaluation of the surgical treatment of vulvar vestibulitis. Eur J Obstet Gynecol 86:135, 1999.

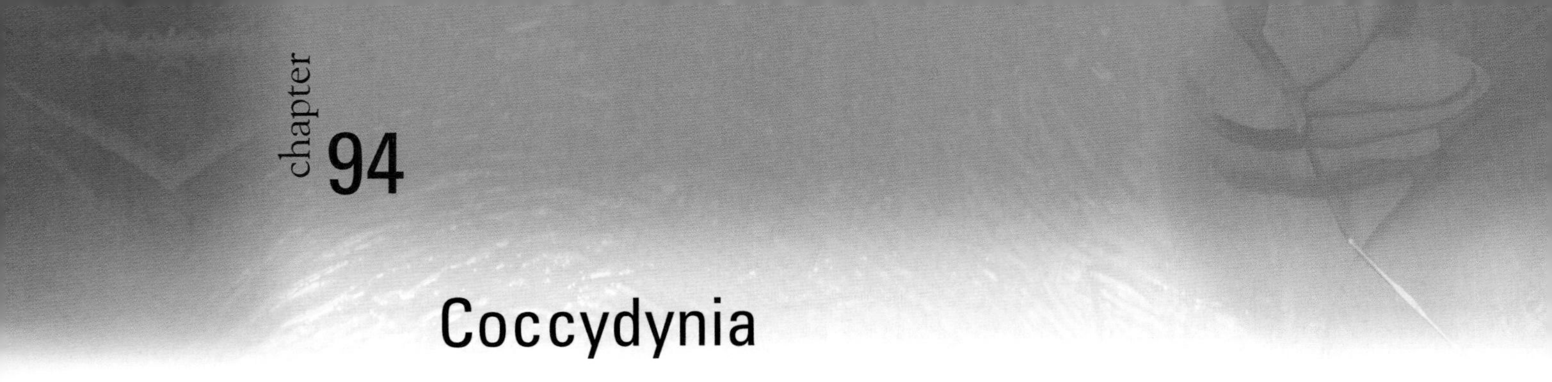

chapter 94

Coccydynia

Steven D. Waldman

Coccydynia is a common pain syndrome that is characterized by pain localized to the tailbone that radiates into the lower sacrum and perineum.[1] It affects females more frequently than males. Coccydynia occurs most commonly after direct trauma to the coccyx from a kick or a fall directly onto the coccyx. It can also occur after difficult vaginal delivery. The pain of coccydynia is thought to be the result of strain of the sacrococcygeal ligament or occasionally due to fracture of the coccyx.[2] Less commonly, arthritis of the sacrococcygeal joint can result in coccydynia, as can tumors affecting the coccyx and adjacent soft tissue.

CLINICAL PRESENTATION

On physical examination, the patient will exhibit point tenderness over the coccyx with the pain being increased with movement of the coccyx. Movement of the coccyx may also cause sharp paresthesias into the rectum, which can be quite distressing to the patient. On rectal examination, the levator ani, piriformis, and coccygeus muscles may feel indurated and palpation of these muscles may induce severe spasm.[2] Sitting may exacerbate the pain of coccydynia, and the patient may attempt to sit on one buttock to avoid pressure on the coccyx (Fig. 94–1).

DIAGNOSIS

Plain radiographs are indicated in all patients who present with pain thought to be emanating from the coccyx to rule out occult bony pathology and tumor. Based on the patient's clinical presentation, additional testing including complete blood cell count, prostate-specific antigen, sedimentation rate, and antinuclear antibody testing may be indicated. MRI of the pelvis is indicated if an occult mass or tumor is suggested (Fig. 94–2). Radionuclide bone scanning may be useful to rule out stress fractures not seen on plain radiographs. The injection technique presented later serves as both a diagnostic and a therapeutic maneuver.

DIFFERENTIAL DIAGNOSIS

Primary pathology of the rectum and anus may occasionally be confused with the pain of coccydynia. Primary tumors or metastatic lesions of the sacrum and/or coccyx may also present as coccydynia.[3] Proctalgia fugax may also mimic the pain of coccydynia but can be distinguished because movement of the coccyx will not reproduce the pain.[4] Insufficiency fractures of the pelvis and sacrum may, on occasion, also mimic coccydynia, as can pathology of the sacroiliac joints.

TREATMENT

A short course of conservative therapy consisting of simple analgesics, nonsteroidal antiinflammatory agents or cyclooxygenase-2 inhibitors, and use of a foam donut to prevent further irritation to the sacrococcygeal ligament is a reasonable first step in the treatment of patients suffering from coccydynia. If the patient does not experience rapid improvement, the following injection technique is a reasonable next step.[5]

To treat the pain of coccydynia, the patient is placed in the prone position. The legs and heels are abducted to prevent tightening of the gluteal muscles, which can make identification of the sacrococcygeal joint more difficult. Preparation of a wide area of skin with antiseptic solution is then carried out so that all of the landmarks can be palpated aseptically. A fenestrated sterile drape is placed to avoid contamination of the palpating finger. The middle finger of the nondominant hand is placed over the sterile drape into the natal cleft with the fingertip palpating the sacrococcygeal joint at the base of the sacrum. After locating the sacrococcygeal joint, a 1.5-inch, 25-gauge needle is inserted through the skin at a 45-degree angle into the region of the sacrococcygeal joint and ligament (Fig. 94–3).

If the sacrococcygeal ligament is penetrated, a "pop" will be felt and the needle should be withdrawn back through the ligament. If contact with the bony wall of the sacrum occurs, the needle should be withdrawn slightly. This will disengage the needle tip from the periosteum. When the needle is satisfactorily positioned, a syringe containing 5 mL of 1.0% preservative-free lidocaine and 40 mg of methylprednisolone is attached to the needle.

Gentle aspiration is carried out to identify CSF or blood. If the aspiration test is negative, the contents of the syringe is slowly injected. There should be little resistance to injection. Any significant pain or sudden increase in resistance during injection suggests incorrect needle placement, and the clinician should stop injecting immediately and reassess the position of the needle. The needle is then

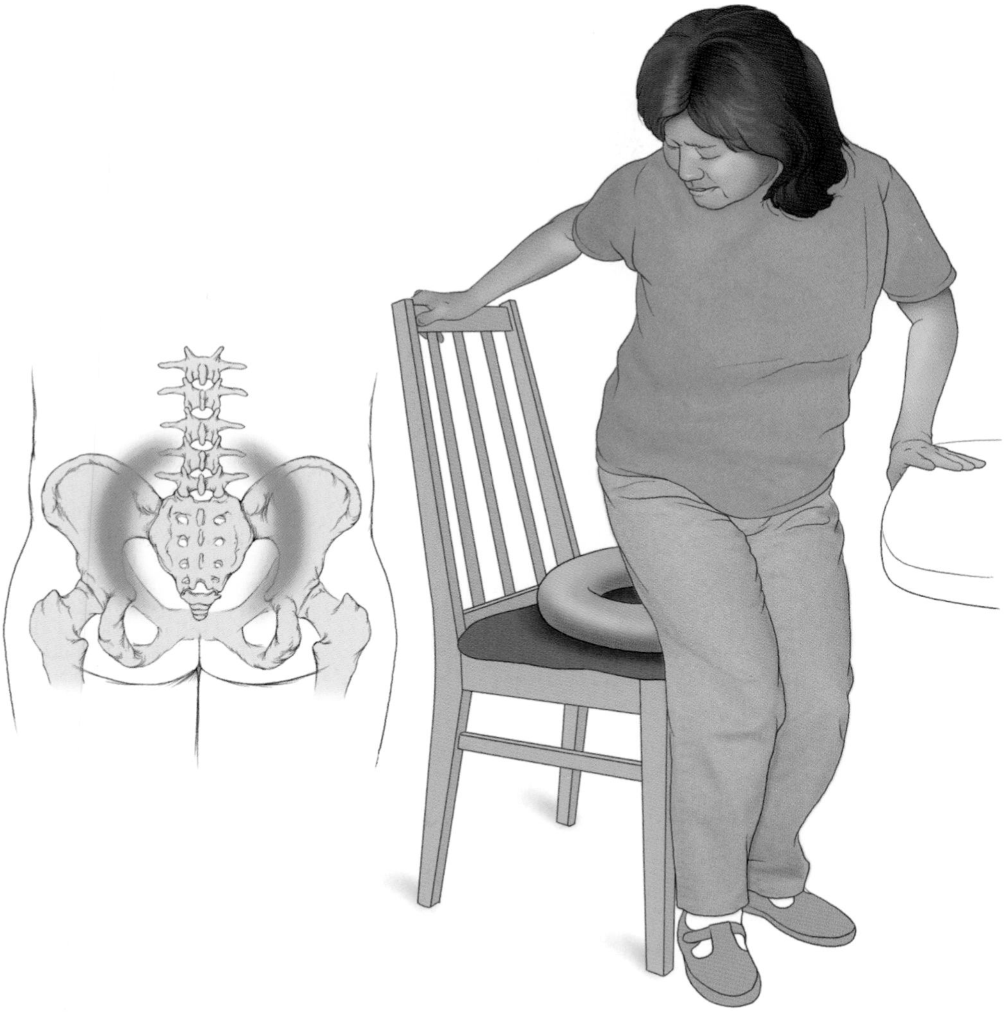

FIGURE 94–1 ■ The pain of coccydynia is localized to the coccyx and is made worse by sitting. (From Waldman SD: Atlas of Common Pain Syndromes. Philadelphia, WB Saunders, 2002, p 227.)

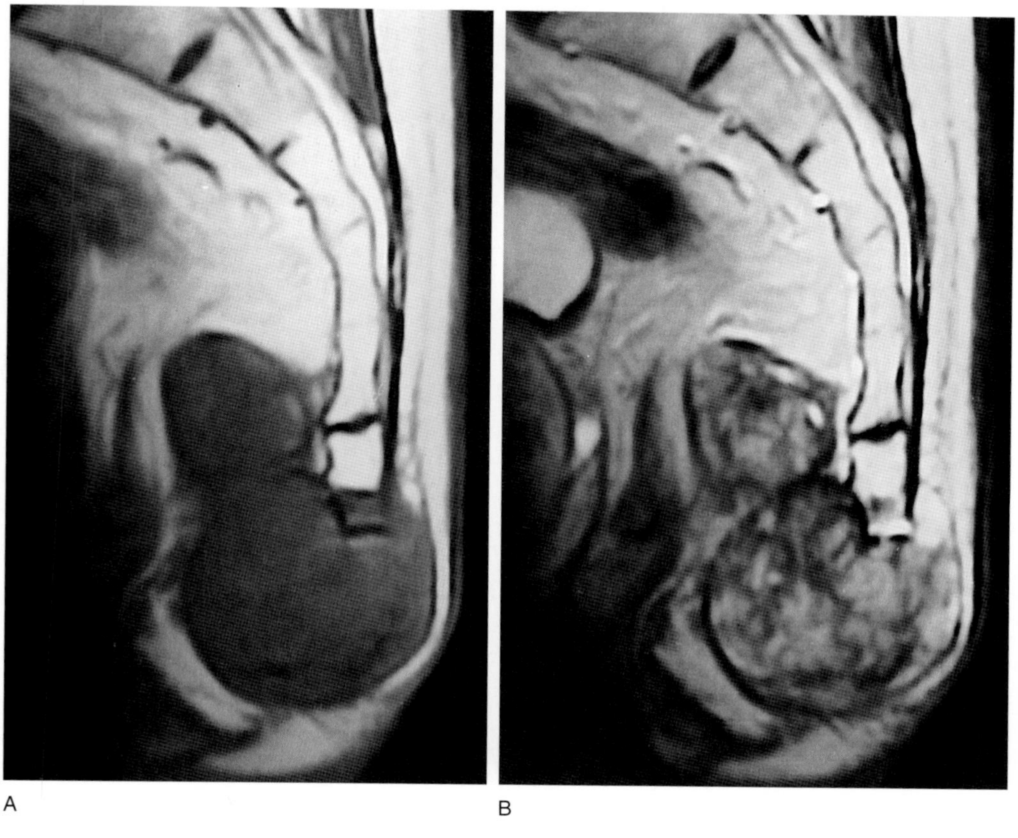

FIGURE 94–2 ■ Chordoma: MRI abnormalities. Sacrococcygeal tumor. Sagittal T1-weighted (TR/TE, 470/10) spin-echo (**A**) and T2-weighted (TR/TE, 5000/136) fast spin-echo (**B**) MR images document a coccygeal tumor with a large soft tissue mass. (Courtesy of Y. Kakitsubata, MD, Miyazaki, Japan; from Resnick D [ed]: Diagnosis of Bone and Joint Disorders, 4th ed. Philadelphia, WB Saunders, 2002, p 4017.)

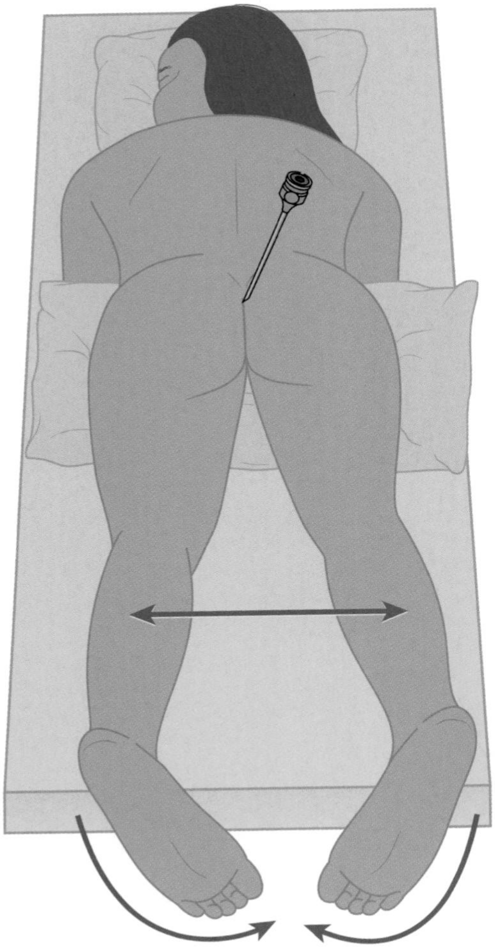

FIGURE 94–3 ■ Injection technique for relieving pain from coccydynia. (From Waldman SD: Atlas of Pain Management Injection Techniques. Philadelphia, WB Saunders, 2000, p 244.)

removed, and a sterile pressure dressing and ice pack is placed at the injection site.

CONCLUSION

Coccydynia should be considered a diagnosis of exclusion in the absence of trauma to the coccyx and its ligaments. Failure to diagnose an underlying tumor can have disastrous consequences. As with all pelvic pain syndromes, a careful evaluation of behavioral abnormalities that may be contributing to the patient's pain and functional disability should be considered.

References

1. Wray CC, Easom S, Hoskinson J: Coccydynia: Aetiology and treatment. J Bone Joint Surg Br 73:335, 1991.
2. Waldman SD: Coccydynia. In Waldman SD: Atlas of Common Pain Syndromes. Philadelphia, WB Saunders, 2002, pp 226-228.
3. Resnick D: Tumors and tumor like lesions of bone: Imaging and pathology of specific lesions. In Resnick D (ed): Diagnosis of Bone and Joint Disorders, 4th ed. Philadelphia, WB Saunders, 2002, pp 4015-4017.
4. Waldman SD: Proctalgia fugax. In Waldman SD: Atlas of Uncommon Pain Syndromes. Philadelphia, WB Saunders, 2003, pp 176-178.
5. Waldman SD: Coccydynia syndrome. In Waldman SD: Atlas of Pain Management Injection Techniques. Philadelphia, WB Saunders, 2000, pp 243-244.

chapter 95

Proctalgia Fugax

Steven D. Waldman

Proctalgia fugax is a disease of unknown etiology that is characterized by paroxysms of rectal pain with pain-free periods in between attacks.[1] The pain-free periods between attacks can last seconds to minutes. Like cluster headache, spontaneous remissions of the disease occur and may last from weeks to years. Proctalgia fugax is more common in females and occurs with greater frequency in those patients suffering from irritable bowel syndrome.

The pain of proctalgia fugax is sharp or gripping in nature and is severe in intensity. Like other urogenital focal pain syndromes such as vulvodynia and prostadynia, the causes remain obscure.[2] Increased stress will often increase the frequency and intensity of attacks of proctalgia fugax, as will sitting for prolonged periods. Patients will often feel an urge to defecate with the onset of the paroxysms of pain (Fig. 95–1). Depression often accompanies the pain of proctalgia fugax but is not thought to be the primary cause. The symptoms of proctalgia fugax can be so severe as to limit the patient's ability to carry out activities of daily living.

CLINICAL PRESENTATION

The physical examination of the patient suffering from proctalgia fugax is usually normal. The patient may be depressed or appear anxious. Rectal examination is normal, although deep palpation of the surrounding musculature may trigger paroxysms of pain. Interestingly, the patient suffering from proctalgia fugax will often report that he or she can abort the attack of pain by placing a finger in the rectum. Rectal suppositories may also interrupt the attacks.

DIAGNOSIS

As with the physical examination, testing in patients suffering from proctalgia fugax is usually within normal limits. Because of the risk of overlooking rectal malignancy that may be responsible for pain that may be attributed to a benign etiology, by necessity proctalgia fugax must be a diagnosis of exclusion.[3] Rectal examination is mandatory in all patients thought to be suffering from proctalgia fugax. Sigmoidoscopy or colonoscopy is also strongly recommended in such patients. Testing of the stool for occult blood is also indicated. Screening laboratory tests consisting of a complete blood cell count, automated blood chemistries, and erythrocyte sedimentation rate should also be performed. MRI or CT of the pelvis should also be considered if the diagnosis is in doubt. If psychological problems are suspected, or if there is a history of sexual abuse, psychiatric evaluation is indicated concurrently with laboratory and radiographic testing.

DIFFERENTIAL DIAGNOSIS

As mentioned earlier, because of the risk of overlooking serious pathology of the anus and rectum, proctalgia fugax must be a diagnosis of exclusion. First and foremost, the clinician must rule out rectal malignancy to avoid disaster. Proctitis can mimic the pain of proctalgia fugax and can be diagnosed on sigmoidoscopy or colonoscopy. Hemorrhoids will usually present as bleeding associated with pain and can be distinguished from proctalgia fugax on physical examination. Prostadynia may sometimes be confused with proctalgia fugax, but the pain is more constant and duller and aching in character.

TREATMENT

Initial treatment of proctalgia fugax should include a combination of simple analgesics and the nonsteroidal anti-inflammatory agents or the cyclooxygenase-2 inhibitors. If these medications do not adequately control the patient's symptoms, a tricyclic antidepressant or gabapentin should be added.

Traditionally, the tricyclic antidepressants have been a mainstay in the palliation of pain secondary to proctalgia fugax. Controlled studies have demonstrated the efficacy of amitriptyline for this indication. Other tricyclic antidepressants including nortriptyline and desipramine have also shown to be clinically useful. Unfortunately, this class of drugs is associated with significant anticholinergic side effects, including dry mouth, constipation, sedation, and urinary retention. These drugs should be used with caution in those suffering from glaucoma, cardiac arrhythmia, and prostatism. To minimize side effects and encourage compliance, the primary care physician should start amitriptyline or nortriptyline at a 10-mg dose at bedtime. The dose can be then titrated upward to 25 mg at bedtime as side effects allow. Upward titration of dosage in 25-mg increments can be carried out each week as side effects allow. Even at lower doses, patients will generally report a rapid improvement in sleep disturbance and will begin to experience some pain relief in 10 to 14 days. If the patient does not experience any

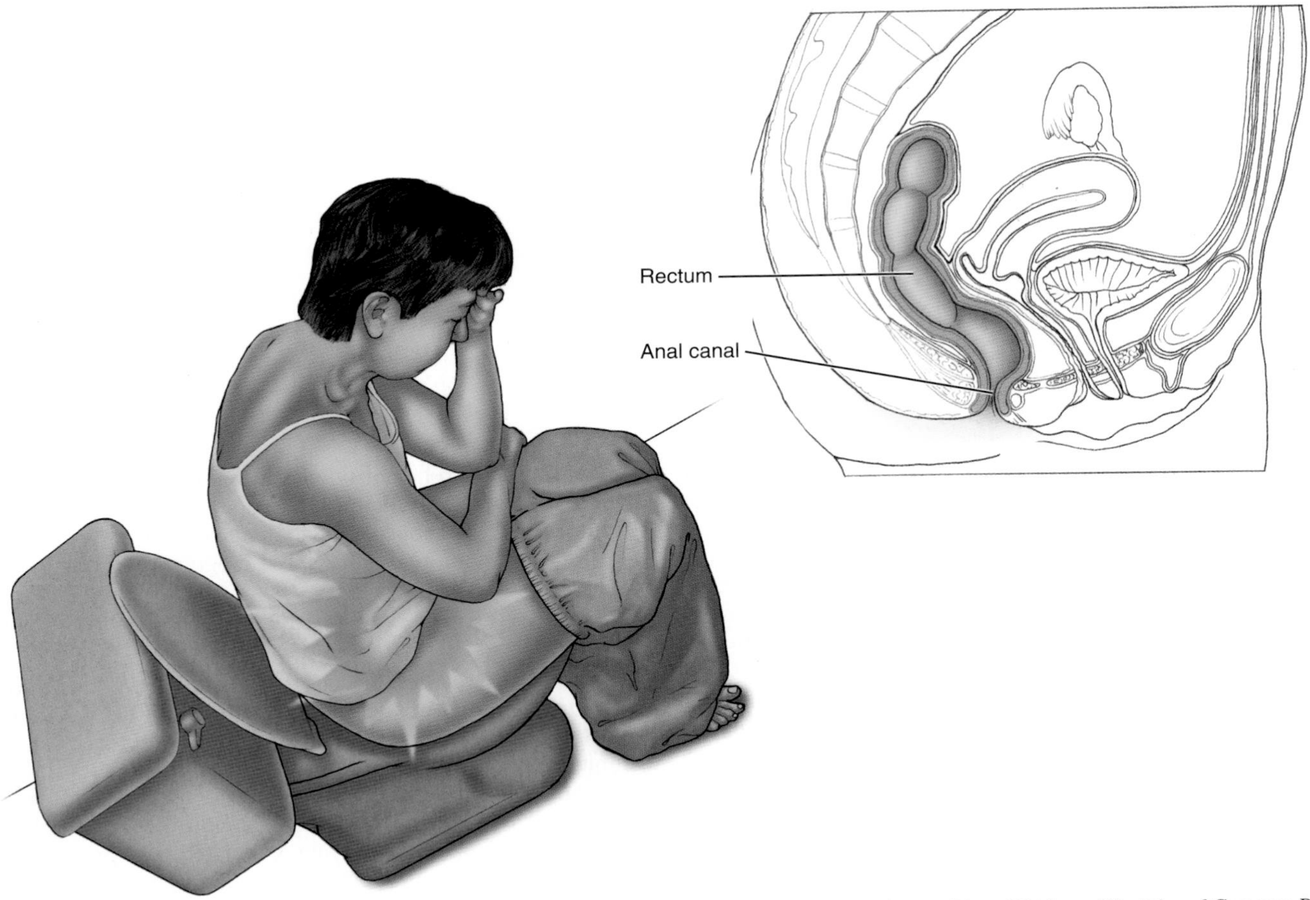

FIGURE 95–1 ■ The onset of pain of proctalgia fugax often causes the patient to feel an urge to defecate. (From Waldman SD: Atlas of Common Pain Syndromes. Philadelphia, WB Saunders, 2002, p 177.)

improvement in pain as the dose is being titrated upward, the addition of gabapentin alone or in combination with nerve blocks of the pudendal nerves with local anesthetics and/or corticosteroid is recommended. The selective serotonin reuptake inhibitors such as fluoxetine have also been utilized to treat the pain of diabetic neuropathy; and although better tolerated than the tricyclic antidepressants, they appear to be less efficacious.

If the antidepressant compounds are ineffective or contraindicated, gabapentin represents a reasonable alternative. Gabapentin should be started with a 300-mg dose at bedtime for two nights. The patient should be cautioned about potential side effects, including dizziness, sedation, confusion, and rash. The drug is then increased in 300-mg increments, given in equally divided doses over 2 days, as side effects allow, until pain relief is obtained or a total dose of 2400 mg daily is reached. At this point, if the patient has experienced partial relief of pain, blood values are measured and the drug is carefully titrated upward using 100-mg tablets. Rarely will more than 3600 mg daily be required.

The local application of heat and cold may also be beneficial to provide symptomatic relief of the pain of proctalgia fugax. The use of bland rectal suppositories may also help provide symptomatic relief. For patients who do not respond to these treatment modalities, injection of the peroneal nerves or caudal epidural nerve block using local anesthetic and corticosteroid may be a reasonable next step.[4] The clinician should be aware that there are anecdotal reports that the calcium channel blockers, topical nitroglycerin, and inhalation of albuterol will provide symptomatic relief of the pain of proctalgia fugax.

The major problem in the care of patients thought to suffer from proctalgia fugax is the failure to identify potentially serious pathology of the anus or rectum due to primary tumor or invasion of these structures by pelvic tumor.[3] Although uncommon, occult rectal infection remains a possibility, especially in the immunocompromised cancer patient. Early detection of infection is crucial to avoid potentially life-threatening sequelae. Given the psychological implications of pain involving the genitalia and rectum, the clinician should not overlook the possibility of psychological abnormality in patients with pain in the rectum.

References

1. Vincent C: Anorectal pain and irritation: Anal fissure, levator syndrome proctalgia fugax, and pruritus ani. Prim Care 26:53, 1999.
2. Mazza L, Formento F, Fonda G: Anorectal and perineal pain: New pathological hypothesis. Tech Coloproctol 8:77, 2004.
3. Wald A: Functional anorectal and pelvic pain. Gastroenterol Clin North Am 30:243, 2001.
4. Waldman SD: Proctalgia fugax. In Waldman SD: Uncommon Pain Syndromes. Philadelphia, WB Saunders, 2003, pp 176-178.

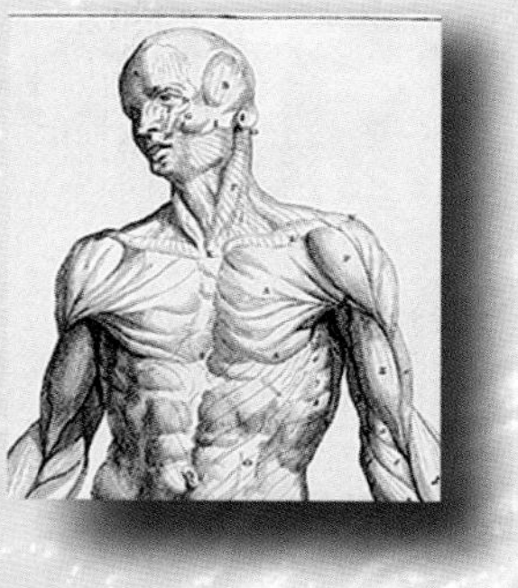

Part J

Pain Syndromes of the Hip and Proximal Lower Extremity

chapter 96

Gluteal and Ischiogluteal Bursitis

Steven D. Waldman

Gluteal and ischiogluteal bursitis are among the myriad causes of buttock pain that are frequently misdiagnosed as primary hip pathology. Frequently coexisting with tendonitis and sacroiliac joint pain, these painful conditions require not only treatment of the acute symptomatology of pain and decreased range of motion but also correction of the functional abnormalities that perpetuate the patient's symptoms.

■ GLUTEAL BURSITIS

The patient suffering from gluteal bursitis will frequently complain of pain at the upper outer quadrant of the buttock and with resisted abduction and extension of the lower extremity. The pain of gluteal bursitis, also known as weaver's bottom, is localized to the area over the upper outer quadrant of the buttock with referred pain noted into the sciatic notch.[1] Often, the patient will be unable to sleep on the affected hip and may complain of a sharp, catching sensation when extending and abducting the hip, especially on first awakening.

The gluteal bursae lie between the gluteus maximus and medius and minimus muscles as well as between these muscles and the underlying bone (Fig. 96–1). These bursae may exist as a single bursal sac or in some patients as a multisegmented series of sacs that may be loculated. The gluteal bursae are vulnerable to injury from both acute trauma and repeated microtrauma. The action of the gluteus maximus muscle includes the flexion of trunk on thigh when maintaining a sitting position when riding a horse (Fig. 96–2). This action can irritate the gluteal bursae and result in pain and inflammation. Acute injuries frequently take the form of direct trauma to the bursa from falls directly onto the buttocks or repeated intramuscular injections as well as from overuse such as running for long distances, especially on soft or uneven surfaces. If the inflammation of the gluteal bursae becomes chronic, calcification of the bursae may occur.

Clinical Presentation

Physical examination of patients suffering from gluteal bursitis may reveal point tenderness in the upper outer quadrant

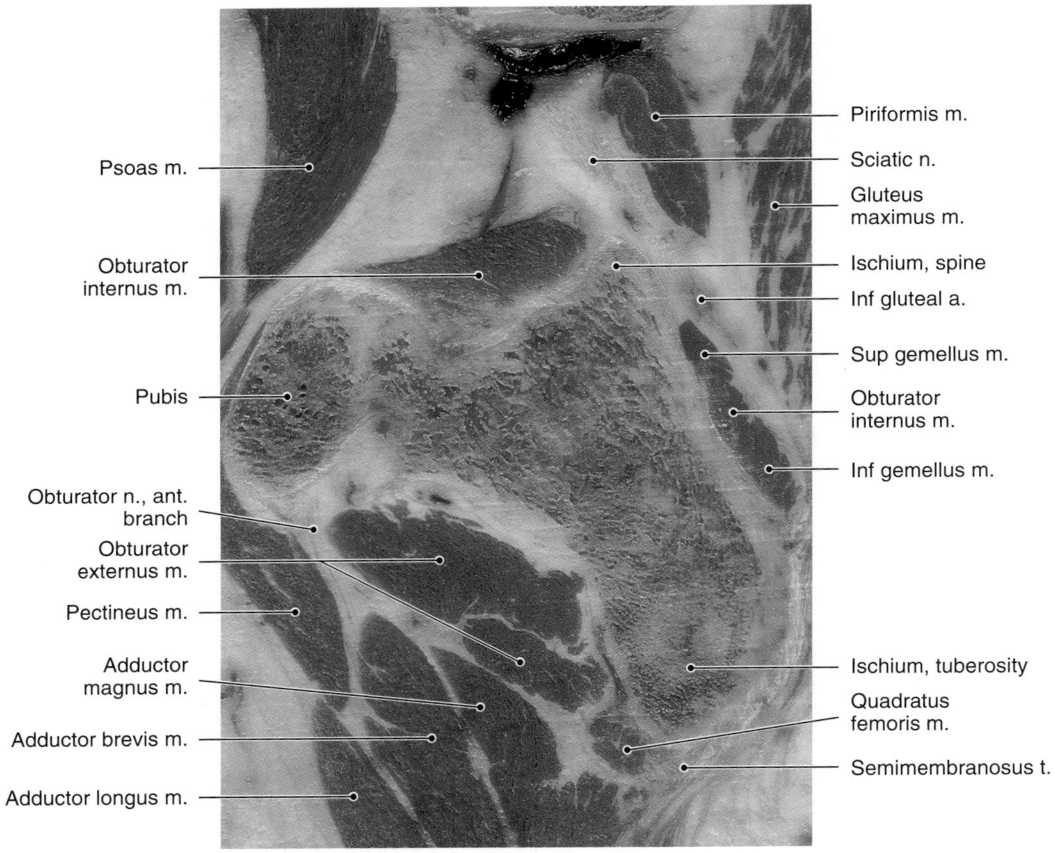

FIGURE 96–1 ■ Anatomy of gluteal bursae. (From Kang HS, Ahn JM, Resnick D (eds): MRI of the Extremities, 2nd ed. Philadelphia, WB Saunders, 2002.)

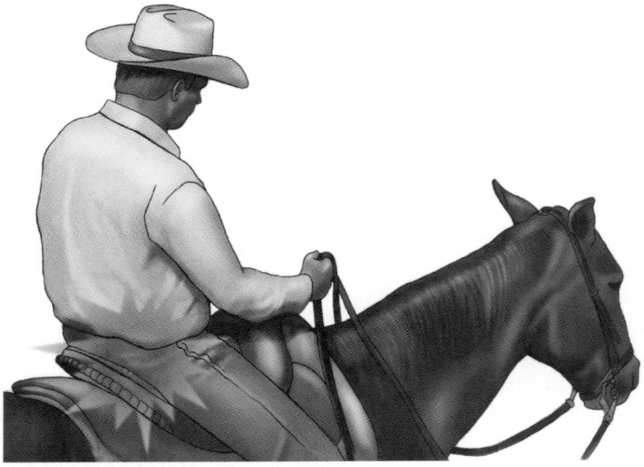

FIGURE 92-2 ■ The action of the gluteus maximus muscle includes the flexion of trunk on thigh when maintaining a sitting position, such as riding a horse. This action can irritate the gluteal bursae and result in pain and inflammation. (From Waldman SD: Atlas of Uncommon Pain Syndromes. Philadelphia, WB Saunders, 2003, p 186.)

of the buttocks. Passive flexion and adduction as well as active resisted extension and abduction of the affected lower extremity will reproduce the pain. Sudden release of resistance during this maneuver will markedly increase the pain.

Examination of the hip will be within normal limits as will examination of the sacroiliac joint. Careful neurologic examination of the affected lower extremity should reveal no neurologic deficits. If neurologic deficits are present, evaluation for plexopathy, radiculopathy, or entrapment neuropathy should be undertaken.[2] It should be remembered that these neurologic symptoms can coexist with gluteal bursitis, confusing the clinical diagnosis.

Differential Diagnosis

Gluteal bursitis is often misdiagnosed as sciatica or attributed to primary hip pathology. Radiographs of the hip and electromyography will help distinguish gluteal bursitis from radiculopathy emanating from the hip. Most patients suffering from a lumbar radiculopathy will have back pain associated with reflex, motor, and sensory changes associated with back pain, whereas patients with gluteal bursitis will have only secondary back pain and no neurologic changes. Piriformis syndrome may sometimes be confused with gluteal bursitis but can be distinguished by the presence of motor and sensory changes involving the sciatic nerve.[3] These motor and sensory changes will be limited to the distribution of the sciatic nerve below the sciatic notch. Lumbar radiculopathy and sciatic nerve entrapment may coexist as the so-called "double crush" syndrome. The pain of gluteal bursitis may cause alteration of gait, which may result in secondary back and radicular symptomatology and which may coexist with this entrapment neuropathy.

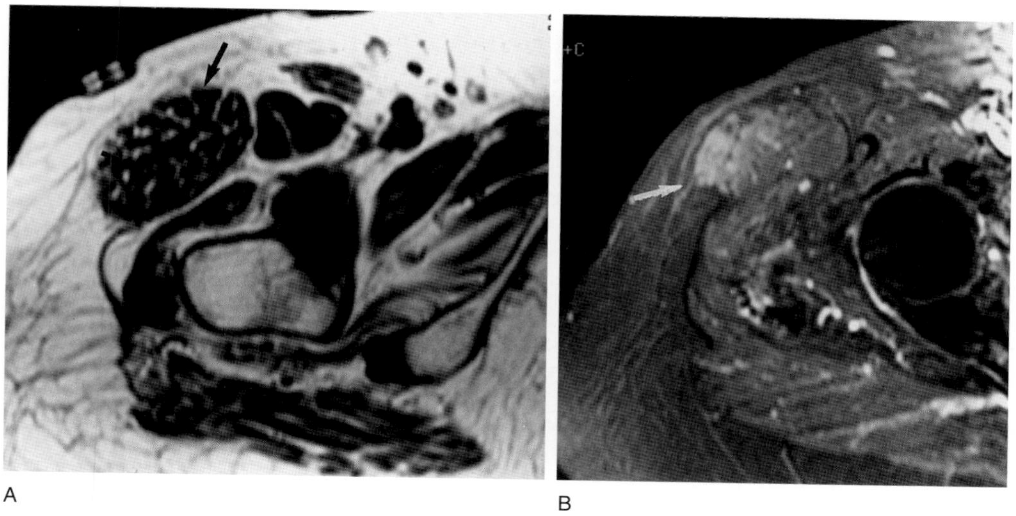

FIGURE 96–3 ■ Possible entrapment of the superior gluteal nerve. Note the denervation hypertrophy of the tensor fasciae latae muscle *(arrow)*, as shown on a transverse T1-weighted (TR/TE, 416/14) spin-echo MR image (**A**), and similar hypertrophy of and high signal intensity in this muscle *(arrow)* on a transverse fat-suppressed T1-weighted (TR/TE 500/14) spin-echo MR image obtained after intravenous administration of gadolinium (**B**). (From Resnick D [ed]: Diagnosis of Bone and Joint Disorders, 4th ed. Philadelphia, WB Saunders, 2002, p 3351.)

Diagnosis

Plain radiographs of the hip may reveal calcification of the bursa and associated structures consistent with chronic inflammation. MRI is indicated if occult mass or tumor of the hip is suspected. Electromyography should be performed if neurologic findings are present to rule out plexopathy, radiculopathy, and/or nerve entrapment syndromes of the gluteal nerve or of the nerves of the lower extremity (Fig. 96–3). Based on the patient's clinical presentation, additional testing including complete blood cell count, HLA-B27 testing, automated serum chemistries including uric acid, sedimentation rate, and antinuclear antibody testing may be indicated. The injection technique described later will serve as both a diagnostic and therapeutic maneuver for patients suffering from gluteal bursitis.[4]

Treatment

Initial treatment of the pain and functional disability associated with gluteal bursitis should include a combination of the nonsteroidal antiinflammatory agents or cyclooxygenase-2 inhibitors and physical therapy. The local application of heat and cold may also be beneficial. Avoidance of the repetitive movements that incite the syndrome should be avoided. For patients who do not respond to these treatment modalities, injection of the gluteal bursa with local anesthetic and corticosteroid may be a reasonable next step.

To inject the gluteal bursae, the patient is placed in the lateral position with the affected side up and the affected leg flexed at the knee. Proper preparation with antiseptic solution of the skin overlying the upper outer quadrant of the buttocks is then carried out. A syringe containing 4.0 mL of 0.25% preservative-free bupivacaine and 40 mg of methylprednisolone is attached to a 1.5-inch, 25-gauge needle. The point of maximal tenderness within the upper outer quadrant of the buttocks is then identified with a sterilely gloved finger. Before needle placement, the patient should be advised to say "there" immediately if he or she feels a paresthesia into the lower extremity, indicating that the needle has impinged on the sciatic nerve. Should a paresthesia occur, the needle should be immediately withdrawn and repositioned more medially. The needle is then carefully advanced perpendicular to the skin at the previously identified point until it impinges on the wing of the ilium (Fig. 96–4). Care must be taken to keep the needle medial and not to advance it laterally or it could impinge on the sciatic nerve. After careful aspiration and if no paresthesia is present, the contents of the syringe are then gently injected into the bursa. There should be minimal resistance to injection.

■ ISCHIOGLUTEAL BURSITIS

The ischial bursa lies between the gluteus maximus muscle and the bone of the ischial tuberosity. If may exist as a single bursal sac or in some patients may exist as a multi-segmented series of sacs that may be loculated. The ischial bursa is vulnerable to injury from both acute trauma and repeated microtrauma. Acute injuries frequently take the form of direct trauma to the bursa from direct falls onto the buttocks and from overuse such as prolonged riding of horses or bicycles. Running on uneven or soft surfaces such as sand may also cause ischial bursitis (Fig. 96–5). If the inflammation of the ischial bursa becomes chronic, calcification of the bursa may occur.

Clinical Presentation

The patient suffering from ischial bursitis will frequently complain of pain at the base of the buttock during resisted extension off the lower extremity. The pain is localized to the area over the ischial tuberosity, with referred pain noted into the hamstring muscle, which may also develop coexistent tendinitis.[5] Often, the patient will be unable to sleep on the affected hip and may complain of a sharp, catching sensation when extending and flexing the hip, especially on first awakening. Physical examination may reveal point tenderness over the ischial tuberosity. Passive straight-leg raising and active resisted extension of the affected lower extremity will reproduce the pain. Sudden release of resistance during this maneuver will markedly increase the pain.

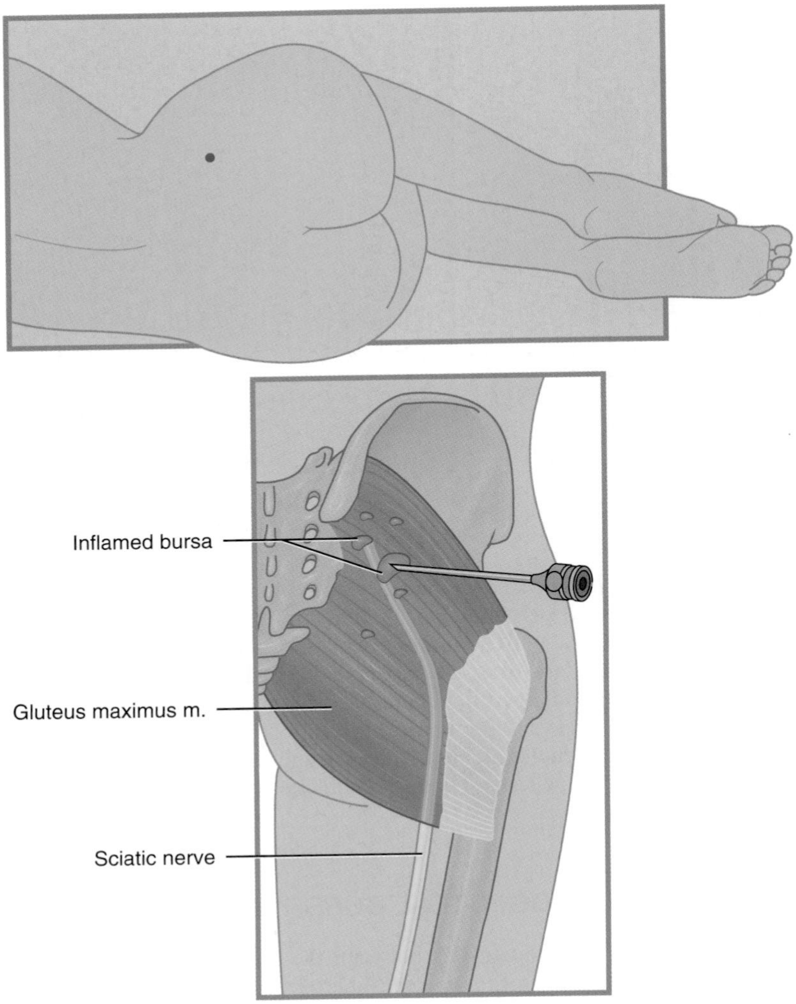

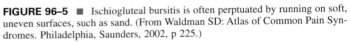

FIGURE 96–4 ■ Injection technique for relieving the pain due to gluteal bursitis. (From Waldman SD: Atlas of Pain Management Injection Techniques. Philadelphia, WB Saunders, 2000, p 211.)

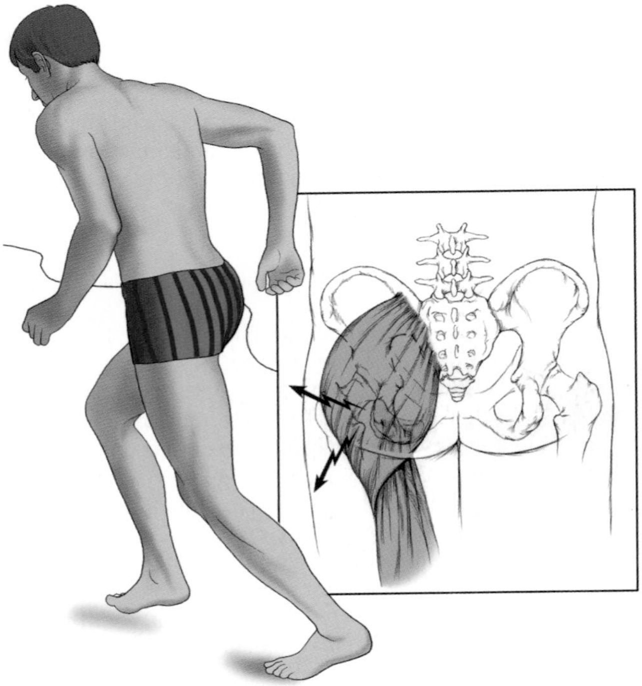

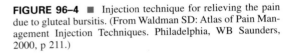

FIGURE 96–5 ■ Ischiogluteal bursitis is often perptuated by running on soft, uneven surfaces, such as sand. (From Waldman SD: Atlas of Common Pain Syndromes. Philadelphia, Saunders, 2002, p 225.)

Diagnosis

Plain radiographs of the hip may reveal calcification of the bursa and associated structures consistent with chronic inflammation. MRI is indicated if disruption of the hamstring musculotendinous unit is suspected. The injection technique described later will serve as both a diagnostic and therapeutic maneuver and will also treat hamstring tendinitis. Screening laboratory tests consisting of a complete blood cell count, erythrocyte sedimentation rate, and antinuclear antibody level are indicated if collagen vascular disease is suspected. Plain radiographs and radionuclide bone scanning are indicated in the presence of trauma or if tumor is a possibility.

Differential Diagnosis

Although the diagnosis of ischiogluteal bursitis is usually straightforward, this painful condition can occasionally be confused with sciatica, primary pathology of the hip, insufficiency fractures of the pelvis, and tendinitis of the hamstrings. Tumors of the hip and pelvis may be overlooked and should be considered in the differential diagnosis of ischiogluteal bursitis.

Treatment

Initial treatment of the pain and functional disability associated with ischiogluteal bursitis should include a combination of the nonsteroidal antiinflammatory agents or cyclooxygenase-2 inhibitors and physical therapy. The local application of heat and cold may also be beneficial. Avoidance of any repetitive activity that may exacerbate the patient's symptomatology should be avoided. For patients who do not respond to these treatment modalities, the following injection technique may be a reasonable next step.[6]

To inject the ischiogluteal bursa, the patient is placed in the lateral position with the affected side up and the affected leg flexed at the knee. Proper preparation with antiseptic solution of the skin overlying the ischial tuberosity is then carried out. A syringe containing 4.0 mL of 0.25% preservative-free bupivacaine and 40 mg of methylprednisolone is attached to a 1.5-inch 25-gauge needle. The ischial tuberosity is then identified with a sterile gloved finger. Before needle placement, the patient should be advised to say "there" immediately if he or she feels a paresthesia into the lower extremity, indicating that the needle has impinged on the sciatic nerve. Should a paresthesia occur, the needle should be

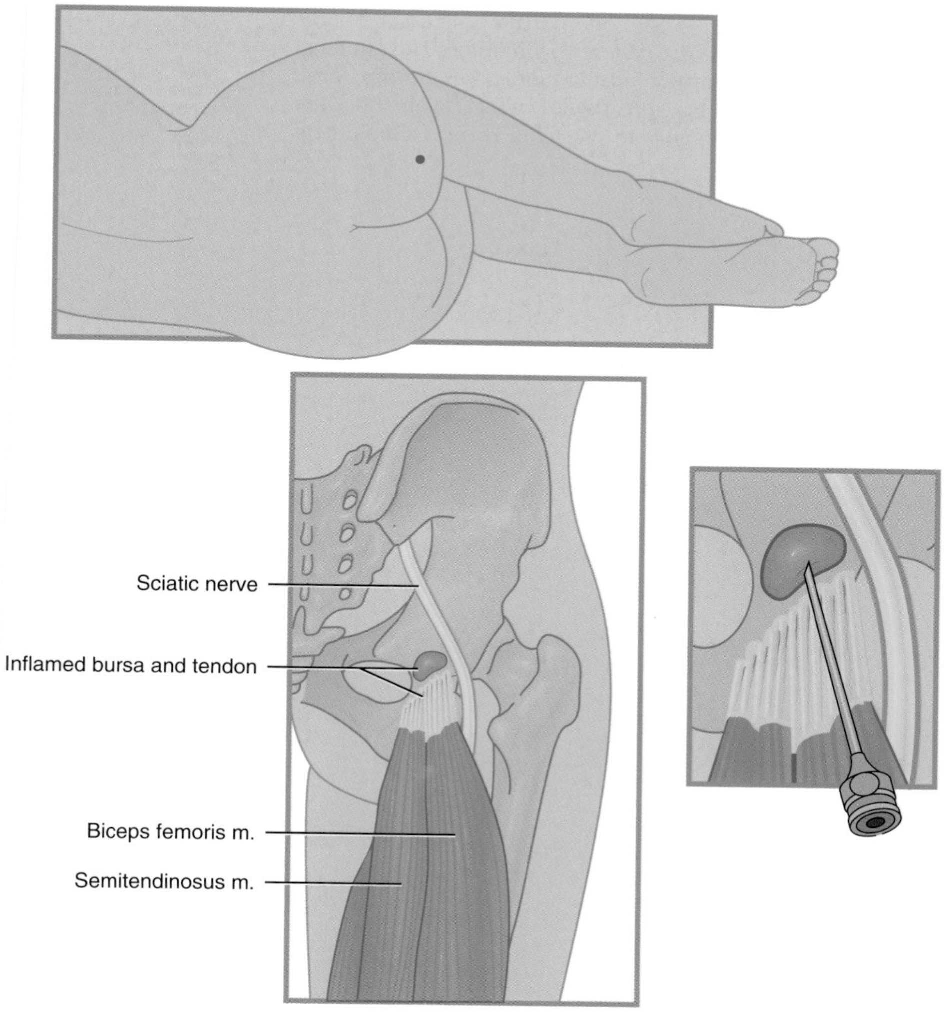

FIGURE 96–6 ■ Injection technique for relieving the pain due to ischial bursitis. (From Waldman SD: Atlas of Pain Management Injection Techniques. Philadelphia, WB Saunders, 2000, p 209.)

immediately withdrawn and repositioned more medially. The needle is then carefully advanced at that point through the skin, subcutaneous tissues, muscle, and tendon until it impinges on the bone of the ischial tuberosity (Fig. 96–6). Care must be taken to keep the needle in the midline and not to advance it laterally or it could impinge on the sciatic nerve. After careful aspiration and if no paresthesia is present, the contents of the syringe is then gently injected into the bursa.

If the patient continues the repetitive activities responsible for the evolution of his or her ischiogluteal bursitis, improvement will be limited and the patient should be warned of such. The proximity to the sciatic nerve makes it imperative that this procedure be carried out only by those well versed in the regional anatomy and experienced in performing injection techniques. Many patients will also complain of a transient increase in pain after injection of the bursa and tendons.

CONCLUSION

Gluteal and ischiogluteal bursitis are among the myriad causes of buttock pain that are encountered in clinical practice. Frequently coexisting with tendinitis and sacroiliac joint pain, these painful conditions require not only treatment of the acute symptomatology of pain and decreased range of motion but also correction of the functional abnormalities that perpetuate the patient's symptoms. The clinician should be sure to consider occult tumors of the hip joint, pelvis, and surrounding soft tissues when evaluating the patient with pain thought to be gluteal or ischiogluteal bursitis.

Although the treatment is the same, ischial bursitis can be distinguished from hamstring tendinitis by the fact that ischial bursitis will present with point tenderness over the ischial bursa and the tenderness of hamstring bursitis is more diffuse over the upper muscle and tendons of the hamstring. The above injection technique is extremely effective in the treatment of ischial bursitis and hamstring tendinitis. This technique is a safe procedure if careful attention is paid to the clinically relevant anatomy in the areas to be injected.

The use of physical modalities including local heat as well as gentle stretching exercises should be introduced several days after the patient undergoes this injection technique. Vigorous exercises should be avoided because they will exacerbate the patient's symptoms. Simple analgesics, nonsteroidal antiinflammatory agents, and antimyotonic agents such as tizanidine may be used concurrently with this injection technique.

References

1. Waldman SD: Gluteal bursitis. In Waldman SD: Atlas of Uncommon Pain Syndromes. Philadelphia, Saunders, 2003, pp 185-187.
2. Resnick D: Neuromuscular disorders. In Resnick D (ed): Diagnosis of Bone and Joint Disorders, 4th ed. Philadelphia, Saunders, 2002, pp 3349-3351.
3. Waldman SD: Piriformis syndrome. In Waldman SD: Atlas of Common Pain Syndromes. Philadelphia, WB Saunders, 2002, pp 220-222.
4. Waldman SD: Gluteal bursitis pain. In Waldman SD: Atlas of Pain Management Injection Techniques. Philadelphia, Saunders, 2000, pp 210-212.
5. Waldman SD: Ischiogluteal bursitis. In Waldman SD: Atlas of Common Pain Syndromes. Philadelphia, Saunders, 2002, pp 223-225.
6. Waldman SD: Ischial bursitis pain. In Waldman SD: Atlas of Pain Management Injection Techniques. Philadelphia, Saunders, 2000, pp 207-208.

chapter 97

Trochanteric Bursitis

Martin Childers

HISTORICAL CONSIDERATIONS

Calcifications of the gluteal tendons associated with the trochanteric bursae were reported as early as 1930 by Nilsonne[1] and were generally considered to be caused by tuberculosis.[2] The condition was also thought to be acute rather than chronic until 1952 when Spear and Lipscomb[3] published a case series of 64 patients. In the late 1950s, a number of journal articles appeared[2,4-7] that challenged the traditional notion that trochanteric bursitis was an acute, rare condition[8] but instead existed as a discrete, and often chronic, clinical entity. However, as Anderson pointed out in 1957, trochanteric bursitis is a complex diagnosis usually associated with other disorders.[2]

CLINICAL PRESENTATION

Patients with trochanteric bursitis generally present with chronic intermittent aching pain over the lateral aspect of the affected hip.[2,4,9] Pain is worsened by sitting in a deep chair or car seat[10] or by climbing stairs.[11] In contrast, in patients with hip osteoarthritis (pain due to pathology of the underlying articular cartilage and bone) pain is usually relieved with sitting.[12] Clinical criteria for trochanteric bursitis have been proposed[2,13,14] to include the first and second and at least one of the remaining findings: (1) history of lateral aching hip pain; (2) localized tenderness over the greater trochanter; (3) radiation of pain over the lateral thigh; (4) pain of resisted hip abduction; and (5) pain at extreme ends of rotation, particularly a positive Patrick (Fabere) test.

Because evidence of bursitis is frequently lacking,[15] the descriptive term *greater trochanteric pain syndrome* (GTPS) is preferred to the term *trochanteric bursitis*. The incidence of GTPS peaks between the fourth and sixth decades of life with a female-to-male ratio of 4:1.[16] The prevalence of patients with GTPS referred to an orthopedic spine clinic was reported to be 20.2% with a mean age of 54 years.[9] In the same study, 20% of patients referred for low back pain were found to have GTPS with higher incidences reported elsewhere.[16,17] Thus, GTPS appears to be a relatively common condition among middle-aged or elderly women evaluated by specialists for the treatment of hip or low back pain. The condition also occurs as a result of a running injury, most commonly in female athletes with a wide pelvis[19] or a cavus foot.[20]

Historically, the general assumption regarding the etiology of GTPS involves one or more of three relatively constant bursae associated with the greater trochanter: two major bursae (subgluteus maximus and subgluteus medius) and one minor bursa (gluteus minimus) (Fig. 97–1).[16,21] It is not entirely clear if pathology of one or more trochanteric bursae directly results in GTPS. During hip replacement surgery in a patient with hip pain and osteoarthritis, the trochanteric bursa was reported to be enlarged and contained calcium pyrophosphate dihydrate (CPPD) crystals.[22] However, recent prospective data from MRI and physical findings of patients with chronic lateral hip pain indicate that fluid distention of the trochanteric bursae (as assessed by MRI) is uncommon[11] whereas gluteus medius tendon pathology appears to be much more common. Yet, tendon pathology and bursae distention are not mutually exclusive because it has been demonstrated in a recent report[23] that tendinopathy and partial tears of the gluteus medius could occur in the presence of bursae fluid distention. In a series of 250 MRI studies of the hip, Kingzett-Taylor and coworkers[15] reported that 14 of 35 patients with gluteal tendon pathology also had discrete fluid collections within the trochanteric bursae. Indeed, in 1961, Gordon proposed that the primary lesion in trochanteric bursitis was injury to the gluteal tendons at their insertion onto the greater trochanter and that the adjacent bursae were damaged as a consequence.[5] Thus, it seems likely that GTPS is caused by gluteal tendinitis in a manner analogous to that of shoulder joint bursitis and rotator cuff tendinitis. Accordingly, some authors[23] urge prompt review of the tendon insertions for signs of tendinopathy and tears when MRI findings demonstrate gluteus medius and minimus atrophy and fatty replacement in patients with chronic lateral hip pain.

The primary presenting symptom of GTPS is chronic, intermittent, aching pain over the lateral aspect of the hip with exacerbation of pain while lying on the affected side.[24] Occasionally, pain may extend from the hip to include the lateral thigh[5] and may radiate down the leg to the level of the insertion of the iliotibial tract on the proximal tibia[23] with associated paresthesia.[17] In fact, Ege and Fano include "pseudoradiculopathy" as one aspect of inclusion criteria for trochanteric bursitis.[13] Groin pain was reported in 10% of GTPS patients presenting to a Dutch rheumatology clinic.[18] Indeed, the fact that patients complain of pain in areas of the body at sites rather far removed from the hip is one of the more fascinating aspects of GTPS.

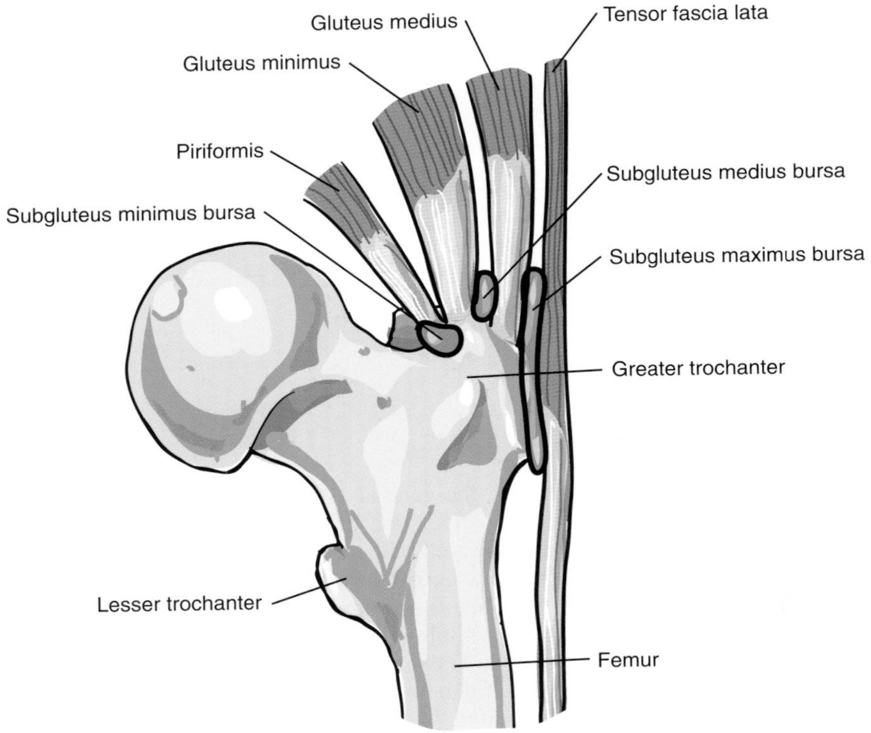

FIGURE 97–1 ■ The bursae associated with the greater trochanter.

DIAGNOSIS

Physical Examination

The examiner should try to localize the patient's usual hip pain by performing a careful palpatory examination of the hip area followed by active and passive range-of-motion testing. GTPS is one cause of hip pain that Roberts and associates[25] categorize into one of three areas: (1) anterior groin pain, (2) posterior buttock pain, or (3) lateral trochanteric pain. Anterior groin pain should alert the clinician of the likelihood of an intra-articular etiology, such as a septic joint or fracture. The most consistent physical finding in patients with GTPS is localized tenderness over the greater trochanter, usually on the posterosuperior aspect over the tendinous insertion of the gluteus medius.[2,4] With the patient in the lateral recumbent position and the painful hip facing the examiner, the clinician should palpate the hip in a caudal to cephalad direction, beginning below the greater trochanteric eminence until the area of maximal tenderness is identified with one fingertip.[16] While the patient is still in the lateral recumbent position, the examiner can typically reproduce the patient's usual lateral hip pain with resistive active hip abduction and external rotation. The examiner should also check for hip pain upon active resisted hip extension and flexion, because this should not elicit pain in patients with GTPS but rather indicate intra-articular hip disease.[14,16]

On observation of gait, a "gluteal limp" is frequently present.[7] Pathology (tears or inflammation) of the gluteus medius tendon results in a positive Trendelenburg sign (upward movement of the pelvis on the weight-bearing side while the pelvis moves downward on the non–weight-bearing side during gait) and is a more accurate predictor of tendon pathology (assessed by MRI) as compared with two other physical signs (pain elicited by resisted hip abduction or internal rotation).[11] Leg-length inequality may be assessed by visual inspection of the height of the iliac crests or by comparing the side-to-side difference between distance from the anterior superior iliac spine to the medial malleolus. However, standing plain radiographs of the pelvis to determine differences in leg length are considered to be more accurate than clinical measurements.[25]

Testing

The diagnosis of GTPS is based upon clinical evidence and no radiographic findings are necessarily diagnostic, although imaging studies may help distinguish GTPS from an intraarticular etiology of hip pain. Gordon[5] reported calcifications of the tendons associated with the greater trochanter in 40% of patients with GTPS, but these data may have reflected tuberculous involvement of the bursa, a diagnosis rarely seen today.[27] Such calcifications may be identified in radiographic images of the hip as linear or small rounded masses of varying size.[16] After hip arthroplasty, some patients may develop bursitis within communicating cavities or "psuedobursae."[28] For these patients, arthrography may be useful to distinguish pain from causes other than loosening and infection.

Plain radiographs may help distinguish rare causes of GTPS. For example, a small percentage (1% to 3%) of patients with tuberculosis have skeletal involvement.[29] Moreover, patients with tuberculosis rarely present with GTPS. Nonetheless, tuberculous involvement of the greater trochanter bursa or its associated tendons may be identified based on imaging features, with a pattern of tendon tethering suggestive of tuberculosis. For instance, in a case series of patients with tuberculous tenosynovitis and bursitis,

Jaovisidha and colleagues found soft tissue swelling on plain radiographs with calcification in three of nine cases.[29] When the tendon sheath was replaced by vascular tuberculous granulation tissue, high signal intensity was observed in T2-weighted MR images. In 6 of 12 cases of tuberculous tenosynovitis, pulmonary tuberculosis was evident on plain chest radiographs.

More advanced imaging methods, such as MRI or bone scans, have characteristic features of GTPS. MRI may demonstrate fluid distention of the trochanteric bursae and associated gluteus medius tendon pathology[23] represented by high signal intensity on short-echo time-inversion recovery sequences in the greater trochanteric region.[16] MRI may also demonstrate gluteus medius and minimus atrophy with fatty replacement. Radioisotope bone scanning may demonstrate a characteristic linear uptake[27] in the lateral aspect of the greater trochanter generally seen in the early blood-pooling phase and on delayed images.[16]

DIFFERENTIAL DIAGNOSIS

Tendinopathy of the gluteal tendons is thought to be responsible for GTPS, but the pathogenesis of GTPS is unclear and is probably multifactorial. A number of common musculoskeletal conditions have been reported in association with GTPS, including leg-length discrepancy, cavus foot,[20] mechanical low back pain, hip osteoarthritis,[30] gluteal tendinitis, and lumbar radiculopathy,[31] but a cause-and-effect relationship between any of these conditions and GTPS has not been definitively established. Infection of the bursae can occur,[32] but reports in the literature are infrequent. In a series of 100 patients with rheumatoid arthritis, 15 patients were found to have GTPS, suggesting a casual association.[31] Biomechanical alteration in gait and associated forces might predispose some patients to GTPS.[15] Gordon[5] postulated that a strain of the hip results in a slight tear in the relatively avascular tendon of the gluteus medius or minimus muscle with subsequent hemorrhage, local necrosis, and organization of scar tissue and tendon calcification. The cause of injury to the gluteal tendons may originate from iliotibial band friction on the tendons and their respective bursae.[15]

A differential diagnosis for GTPS is listed in Table 93–1. Common conditions associated with GTPS include degenerative processes of the hip and spine; thus, patients may initially present with low back pain. Symptoms of GTPS may be confused with a lumbosacral strain, osteoarthritis of the hip, or a herniated lumbar disk.[5] Because of the overlap of the iliotibial tract and the lumbar dermatomes, back and associated lower limb pain can mimic lumbar radiculopathy.[9,33] Collee and colleagues diagnosed GTPS in 35 of 100 consecutive patients presenting to a rheumatology clinic with a primary complaint of low back pain.[17,18] Distinguishing GTPS from lumbar radiculopathy requires a careful history and physical examination, with pain and tenderness most often elicited in the hip rather than in the back.

TREATMENT

Reported benefits of treatment for GTPS are myriad, but few treatment protocols have been rigorously tested using scientific methods. A series of "deep x-ray therapy" was recommended in the 1950s[34] but is no longer suggested. In 1959, Krout and Anderson described short-wave diathermy applied to the trochanteric and low back region as effective in 41 of 50 cases.[6] Today, treatment (Table 93–2) generally consists of rest, ice or heat, nonsteroidal antiinflammatory drugs (NSAIDs), and local injection of a corticosteroid[10] such as methylprednisolone (40 to 80 mg) or triamcinolone hexacetonide (20 to 40 mg), or mixtures of betamethasone sodium phosphate/betamethasone acetate suspension with 1% lidocaine.[13,14] Ultrasound guidance may increase the precision of needle placement.[8] Clinical evidence supports the use of corticosteroids in GTPS. A favorable dose-response relationship with betamethasone was reported in a series of 75 patients with GTPS.[14] As early as 1958, Leonard[7] reported that local injection of hydrocortisone acetate resulted in "complete relief of symptoms in all instances." Gordon's 1961 description[5] outlined the process of local injection for GTPS: "The most successful method of treatment was local infiltration and needling of the bursa, selecting the point of maximum tenderness behind or above the greater trochanter as the point of entry. . . . The tip of the needle was directed against the posterosuperior point of the greater trochanter, and then the solution infiltrated in fanlike fashion adjacent to and above the trochanter."

Conservative treatment that decreases forces placed on the painful hip is generally thought to be helpful in GTPS. Use of a cane in the hand on the side opposite the painful hip reduces forces placed on the affected side equivalent to one half of the body weight.[35] Correction of a leg-length discrepancy with a shoe lift may similarly work to relieve pain.[10] In support of this idea, Swezey and associates[33] noted

Table 97–1

Differential Diagnosis of Trochanteric Bursitis
Lumbosacral strain
Osteoarthritis of the hip
Lumbar radiculopathy
Septic joint
Hip fracture
Avascular necrosis
Synovitis
Lumbar facet syndrome
Iliohypogastric nerve entrapment
Tuberculosis with skeletal involvement

Table 97–2

Treatment of Trochanteric Bursitis
Rest
Ice or heat
Nonsteroidal antiinflammatory drugs
Bisphosphonates
Local corticosteroid injection
Surgery
Release of iliotibial band
Removal of trochanteric osteophytes
Débridement of gluteus maximus bursae

an association between hip disease and/or leg-length discrepancies in a group of elderly patients with GTPS. The authors speculated that gait alterations due to back pain or prolonged bed rest might predispose patients to GTPS. Alternatively, active exercise is considered to be the cornerstone of treatment for friction-induced bursitis in athletes. Increased flexibility and symmetrical strengthening of the muscle involved in adjacent joint motion are thought to improve faulty joint mechanics that may induce excessive tension over the greater trochanter.[36] Exercises that stretch the external rotators of the hip and the iliotibial band were suggested to prevent recurrences of GTPS in young adults.[33] Alternative therapies proposed for GTPS include identification and injections of fibrofatty nodules with corticosteroid/lidocaine.[37]

NSAIDs and acetaminophen have also been reported effective for GTPS. Monteforte and colleagues compared pain relief from use of paracetamol (known as acetaminophen in the United States) (500-mg oral dose twice daily for 15 days, followed by 500 mg daily for 15 days) to that from the bisphosphonate disodium clodronate (100-mg daily intramuscular injection for 30 days) in an open-label comparison trial of 10 patients with GTPS previously unresponsive to conservative treatment.[38] Patients treated with the bisphosphonate demonstrated better pain relief compared with those in the paracetamol-treated group, suggesting that an increase in bone turnover may be implicated in the pathogenesis of GTPS.

In refractory cases, surgical release of tight fascia may be indicated.[5,10,39] In seven athletes with chronic disabling hip pain caused by a snapping iliotibial band and secondary trochanteric bursitis, partial excision of the iliotibial band with excision of the trochanteric bursa resulted in long-term pain relief and return to athletic acitivity.[38]

COMPLICATIONS AND PITFALLS

Fatal necrotizing fasciitis in a non–insulin-dependent diabetic man was reported as a complication of a single corticosteroid injection of the greater trochanteric bursa.[40] Accordingly, the clinician should be wary of performing similar procedures in patients with diabetes or any other condition that might predispose the patient to infection from a corticosteroid injection. Because other syndromes including entrapment neuropathies, radiculopathies, and lumbar facet syndromes can mimic GTPS, the astute clinician should carefully consider the differential diagnoses. Entrapment neuropathy of the iliohypogastric nerve can mimic lateral thigh pain that is commonly observed in GTPS. Perineural injection with local anesthetic over the superior margin of the ilium where the terminal branches of the iliohypogastric nerve cross the iliac crest should confirm the diagnosis.[41] For patients with a presumptive diagnosis of GTPS but who do not respond to local peritrochanteric injection of corticosteroid and local anesthetic, selective neural blockade may help distinguish the underlying cause. Electromyography and/or transforaminal nerve root blocks may identify a lumbar radiculopathy. Lumbar facet blockade may elucidate a lumbar facet syndrome as a cause of lateral hip pain.

CONCLUSION

Trochanteric bursitis, also known as GTPS, is a common cause of lateral hip pain in elderly women, is readily diagnosed by finding localized tenderness over the greater trochanter with radiation of pain over the lateral thigh and increased pain with resistive hip abduction and external rotation. The differential diagnosis includes tendinopathy of the gluteal muscles, degenerative processes of the hip and spine, lumbosacral strain, herniated lumbar disk, or rarely tuberculosis or infection. Treatment of this condition usually consists of rest, ice, heat, and local corticosteroid injection into the most tender area around the greater trochanter, although double-blind placebo-controlled trials have yet to demonstrate efficacy of a particular treatment paradigm.

References

1. Nilsonne H: Ein operierter Fall non Tendinitis calcificans trochanterica. Acta Orthop Scand 1: 231, 1930.
2. Anderson TP: Trochanteric bursitis: Diagnostic criteria and clinical significance. Arch Phys Med Rehabil 39:617, 1958.
3. Spear IM, Lipscomb PR: Noninfectious trochanteric bursitis and peritendinitis. Surg Clin North Am 95:1217, 1952.
4. Barker CS: Treatment of trochanteric bursitis by steroid injections. Can Med Assoc J 78:613, 1958.
6. Krout RM, Anderson TP: Trochanteric bursitis: Management. Arch Phys Med Rehabil 40:8, 1959.
5. Gordon EJ: Trochanteric bursitis and tendinitis. Clin Orthop 20:193, 1961.
7. Leonard MH: Trochanteric syndrome: Calcareous and noncalcareous tendonitis and bursitis about the trochanter major. JAMA 168:175, 1958.
8. Howard CB, Vinzberg A, Nyska M, Zirkin H: Aspiration of acute calcareous trochanteric bursitis using ultrasound guidance. J Clin Ultrasound 21:45, 1993.
9. Tortolani PJ, Carbone JJ, Quartararo LG: Greater trochanteric pain syndrome in patients referred to orthopedic spine specialists. Spine J 2:251, 2002.
10. Reveille JD: Soft-tissue rheumatism: Diagnosis and treatment. Am J Med 102:23S, 1997.
11. Bird PA, Oakley SP, Shnier R, Kirkham BW: Prospective evaluation of magnetic resonance imaging and physical examination findings in patients with greater trochanteric pain syndrome. Arthritis Rheum 44:2138, 2001.
12. Altman RD: Criteria for the classification of osteoarthritis of the knee and hip. Scand J Rheumatol Suppl 65:31, 1987.
13. Ege RK, Fano N: Trochanteric bursitis: Treatment by corticosteroid injection. Scand J Rheumatol 14:417, 1985.
14. Shbeeb MI, O'Duffy JD, Michet CJ, et al: Evaluation of glucocorticosteroid injection for the treatment of trochanteric bursitis. J Rheumatol 23:2104, 1996.
15. Kingzett-Taylor A, Tirman PF, Feller J, et al: Tendinosis and tears of gluteus medius and minimus muscles as a cause of hip pain: MR imaging findings. Am J Roentgenol 173:1123, 1999.
16. Shbeeb MI, Matteson EL: Trochanteric bursitis (greater trochanter pain syndrome). Mayo Clin Proc 71:565, 1996.
17. Collee G, Dijkmans BA, Vandenbroucke JP, Cats A: Greater trochanteric pain syndrome (trochanteric bursitis) in low back pain. Scand J Rheumatol 20:262, 1991.
18. Collee G, Dijkmans BA, Vandenbroucke JP, et al: A clinical epidemiological study in low back pain: Description of two clinical syndromes. Br J Rheumatol 29:354, 1990.
19. Scoggin JF: Common sports injuries seen by the primary care physician: II: Lower extremity. Hawaii Med J 57:502, 1998.
20. McKenzie DC, Clement DB, Taunton JE: Running shoes, orthotics, and injuries. Sports Med 2:334, 1985.
21. Bywaters EG: The bursae of the body. Ann Rheum Dis 24:215, 1965.
22. Lagier R, Vasey H: Calcium pyrophosphate dihydrate (CPPD) crystal deposition in the trochanteric bursa of a patient with hip osteoarthritis. J Rheumatol 13:473, 1986.
23. Walsh G, Archibald CG: MRI in greater trochanter pain syndrome. Australas Radiol 47:85, 2003.
24. Little H: Trochanteric bursitis: A common cause of pelvic girdle pain. Can Med Assoc J 120:456, 1979.
25. Roberts WN, Williams RB: Hip pain. Prim Care 15:783, 1988.

26. Rothenberg RJ: Rheumatic disease aspects of leg length inequality. Semin Arthritis Rheum 17:196, 1988.
27. Allwright SJ, Cooper RA, Nash P: Trochanteric bursitis: Bone scan appearance. Clin Nucl Med 13:561, 1988.
28. Berquist TH, Bender CE, Maus TP, et al: Pseudobursae: A useful finding in patients with painful hip arthroplasty. AJR Am J Roentgenol 148:103, 1987.
28. Jaovisidha S, Chen C, Ryu KN, et al: Tuberculous tenosynovitis and bursitis: Imaging findings in 21 cases. Radiology 201:507, 1996.
30. Roos NP, Lyttle D: Hip arthroplasty surgery in Manitoba: 1973-1978. Clin Orthop (199):248, 1985.
31. Raman D, Haslock I: Trochanteric bursitis—a frequent cause of "hip" pain in rheumatoid arthritis. Ann Rheum Dis 41:602, 1982.
32. Lefebvre C, Lambert M, Bastien P, et al: Septic trochanteric bursitis caused by *Fusobacterium gonidiaformans.* J Rheumatol 12:391, 1985.
33. Swezey RL: Pseudo-radiculopathy in subacute trochanteric bursitis of the subgluteus maximus bursa. Arch Phys Med Rehabil 57:387, 1976.
34. Cloyd WL: Bursitis of the hip. Miss Valley Med J 76:219, 1954.
35. Brady LP: Hip pain: Don't throw away the cane. Postgrad Med 83:89, 1988.
36. Butcher JD, Salzman KL, Lillegard WA: Lower extremity bursitis. Am Fam Physician 53:2317, 1996.
37. Curtis P, Gibbons G, Price J: Fibro-fatty nodules and low back pain: The back mouse masquerade. J Fam Pract 49:345, 2000.
38. Monteforte P, Molfetta L, Grillo G, et al: Disodium clodronate in painful nonresponsive periarthropathy of the hip. Int J Tissue React 22:111, 2000.
39. Zoltan DJ, Clancy WJG, Keene JS: A new operative approach to snapping hip and refractory trochanteric bursitis in athletes. Am J Sports Med 14:201, 1986.
40. Hofmeister E, Engelhardt S: Necrotizing fasciitis as complication of injection into greater trochanteric bursa. Am J Orthop 30:426, 2001.
41. Traycoff RB: "Pseudotrochanteric bursitis": The differential diagnosis of lateral hip pain. J Rheumatol 18:1810, 1991.

chapter 98

Iliopsoas Bursitis

Robert Trout

HISTORICAL CONSIDERATIONS

Although it is often overlooked in the standard evaluation of hip pain, the iliopsoas bursa, is the largest in the body, measuring up to 7 cm in length (Fig. 98–1).[1] Also known as the iliopectineal or iliofemoral bursa, it has been studied as a source of hip pain since 1834 when Fricke described a painful bursitis in a case report.[2] Later a distended bursa was identified with arthrography in 1917 by Kummer and De Senarclens,[3] and for many years arthrography remained the only helpful imaging study for diagnosis until the advent of CT and MRI scanning.

In 1967, Melamad and colleagues described a clinical triad of iliopsoas bursitis as a mass in the inguinal region, effects of pressure on other structures nearby, and osteoarthritis of the hip visualized on radiographs.[4] This triad has become less relevant in recent years because patients with only the most significant symptoms will present with such findings. Along with better imaging techniques, there has been a greater emphasis on earlier conservative treatment that can help to prevent these symptoms from occurring.

SIGNS AND SYMPTOMS

There are two types of patients who will present with iliopsoas bursitis. It most commonly occurs in older individuals who have some type of underlying hip pathology—such as degenerative or rheumatoid arthritis. It is theorized that increased intra-articular pressure leads to the bursa acting as a reservoir for fluid that leaks through the anterior joint capsule, similar to the formation of a Baker's cyst in the knee.[5,6] Eventually, the bursa becomes distended and inflamed. Because these patients will likely exhibit physical signs and radiographic findings of other types of articular problems, a thorough hip examination is essential to differentiate between pain from bursitis versus arthritis or other bony pathology.

The other type of patient is younger and will exhibit completely normal radiographs. These are often athletes who perform repetitive or forceful flexion and extension of the hip. They are at risk for developing bursitis due to the friction of the iliopsoas tendon that overlies it because the purpose of this bursa is to reduce the friction between the tendon and the hip capsule. Thus, for someone who presents with persistent hip pain and normal hip films, iliopsoas bursitis should remain near the top of a differential diagnosis.

Patients will present with pain in the inguinal or hip regions, the pain often radiates to the anterior thigh. Aggravating activities include walking up stairs, putting on shoes and socks, and moving from a sitting to a standing position. Some patients may also describe abdominal pain. Although not as common, edema in the lower extremity or numbness may occur if the bursa is large enough to compress the femoral vein or nerve.

Gait should be observed because a common initial finding will be a shortened stride length when the patient attempts to minimize flexion and extension of the hip. A mass in the area of the inguinal ligament may be palpable and is sometimes mistaken for a hernia, lymph node, or even an aneurysm. It is possible that the mass will be pulsatile due to its proximity to the femoral artery.[7] Pain can be reproduced by placing the hip in flexion, abduction, and external rotation, and then moving it into extension (Fig. 98–2).[8] A palpable or audible snap may occur as the bursa passes underneath the tendon, thus it is sometimes called *snapping hip syndrome* or *iliotibial band syndrome*.

The Thomas test is helpful to evaluate for tight hip flexors. The patient lies supine and fully flexes one knee and hip. If the contralateral hip raises off the examination table, then a contracture is present.

TESTING

Initial testing with plain radiographs of the hip will often demonstrate intra-articular pathology such as degenerative changes, effusion, or calcifications. The diagnostic yield for this specific disorder is limited, however, as it will not identify an inflamed bursa.

For many years, arthrography was the only available means to diagnose a distended iliopsoas bursa, which would fill with contrast if there were a communication with the hip joint. However, because of its invasiveness and its inability to visualize other nearby structures—such as the femoral vessels—it has become essentially obsolete for this purpose.

Ultrasound is fast, noninvasive, and has the advantage of ruling out other possible etiologies for a palpable inguinal mass, including hernia and aneurysm. With bursitis, ultrasound will show a well-defined mass between the anterior hip capsule and the iliopsoas muscle (Fig. 98–3A), although it has

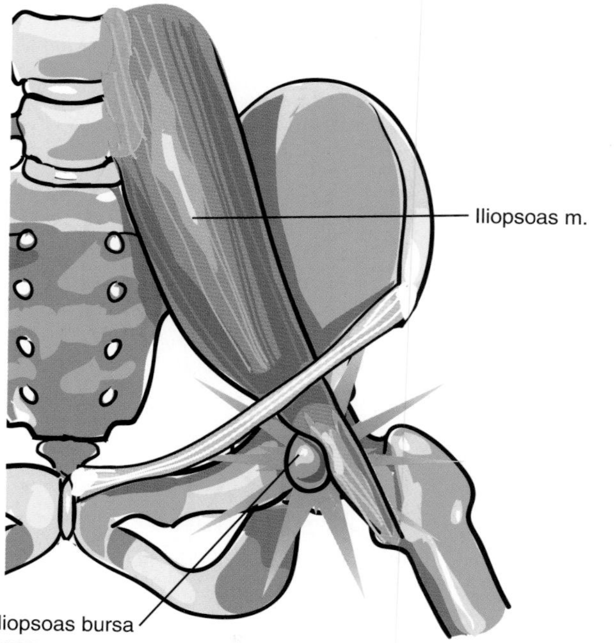

FIGURE 98–1 ■ Iliopsoas bursa, also known as the iliopectineal or iliofemoral bursa.

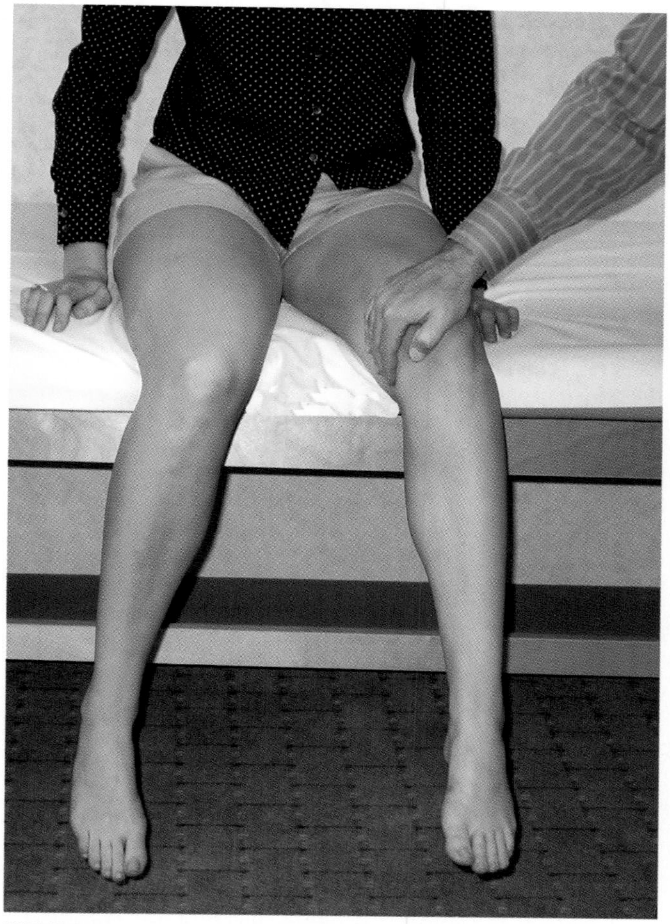

FIGURE 98–2 ■ Resisted hip adduction test for iliopsoas bursitis. (From Waldman SD: Physical Diagnosis in Pain: An Atlas of Signs and Symptoms. Philadelphia, Saunders, 2005, p 313.)

been found to often underestimate the size of the mass. CT scan will also demonstrate an encapsulated mass that has a water density and, if present, a communication with the hip joint. Surrounding structures are well visualized and displacement of the femoral vessels may be observed. MRI is the most sensitive and accurate test in evaluating the characteristics of the bursa—such as its size and shape and its relation to the adjacent soft tissues and structures (see Fig. 98–3B).[8] MRI is also valuable in ruling out other potential

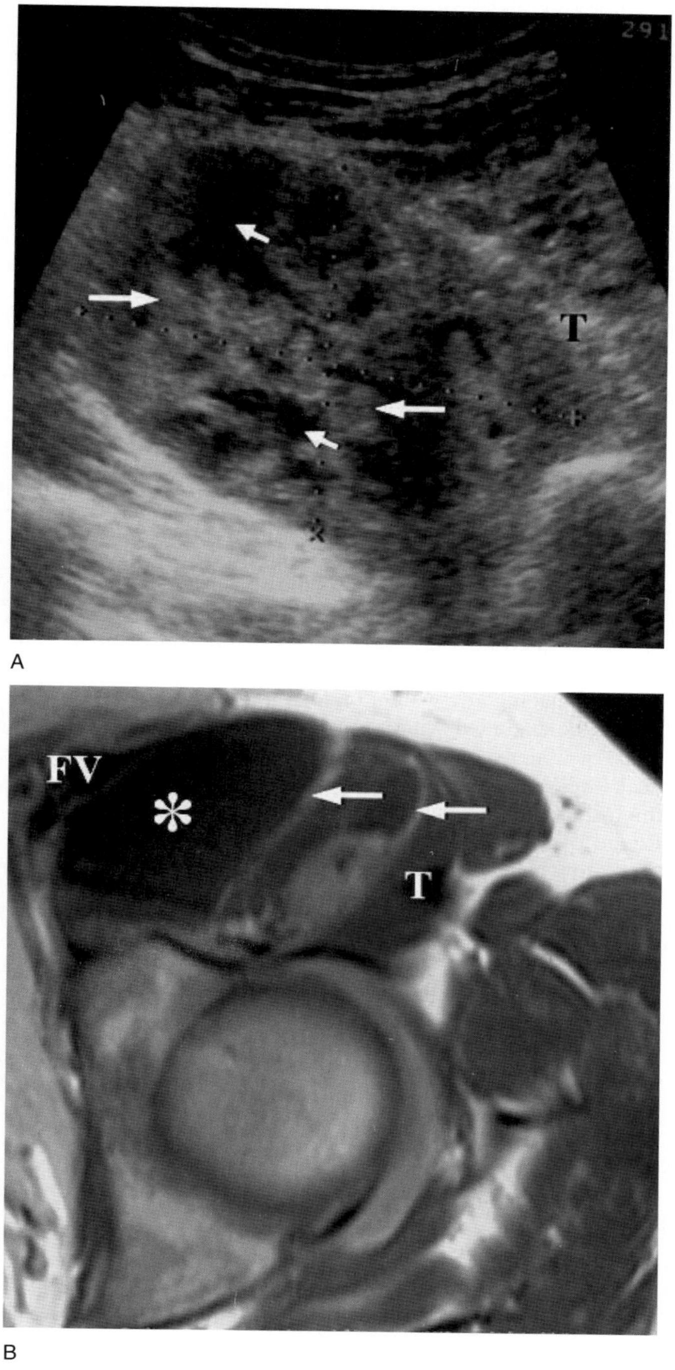

FIGURE 98–3 ■ Imaging studies for iliopsoas bursitis. **A,** Ultrasound. **B,** MRI. (In **B,** *asterisk*, fluid-filled bursa; T, inguinal ligament; *large arrows*, loculations; in **A,** *small arrows*, fluid-filled bursa.

Table 98–1

Differential Diagnosis of Iliopsoas Bursitis
Osteoarthritis
Rheumatoid arthritis
Avascular necrosis
Femoral stress fracture
Osteitis pubis
Pelvic abscess/hematoma
Lymphadenopathy/aneurysm
Metastatic disease
Radiculopathy

causes of hip pain such as avascular necrosis or stress fracture.

DIFFERENTIAL DIAGNOSIS

The differential includes both intra-articular and extra-articular causes of pain around the hip joint (Table 98–1). It may be difficult to differentiate bursitis from osteoarthritis of the hip because many patients will exhibit arthritic hip changes on plain films. The pain of osteoarthritis typically occurs with standing and weight bearing, and these patients will more often demonstrate a Trendelenburg gait in which they will lean toward the affected side during stance phase. On examination, range of motion will be reduced with pain when internally or externally rotating the hip. Avascular necrosis should also remain in the differential for patients with significant hip or groin pain, particularly if they have a history of steroid use. They will also report worsened pain with weight bearing and will have a significantly antalgic gait to avoid placing any weight on the hip joint. Avascular necrosis can be excluded with a bone scan or MRI.

For athletes, primarily long-distance runners, a femoral neck stress fracture will cause an aching pain in the groin or thigh that is exacerbated by activity and improved with rest. Range of motion will be reduced and painful. Radiographs may show callus formation or an actual fracture line, but may be negative early-on. If suspected clinically, a bone scan should be performed because it is sensitive within 2 to 8 days.

Osteitis pubis, or inflammation of the pubic bone, is another condition that is seen in athletes who perform repetitive side-to-side motions as in hockey or soccer. It is also common in pregnant women owing to the instability of the pubic symphysis. These patients will report pain in the groin or thigh areas, but will be most tender at the pubic symphysis. Radiographs will show resorption or sclerosis of the pubic bones, but may be negative initially. A bone scan may also be needed for an early diagnosis.

Radicular pain may manifest with similar symptoms to bursitis with pain extending into the anterior thigh. It is possible for the mass effect of an enlarged bursa on the femoral nerve to cause numbness or paresthesias. Usually the clinician can distinguish between the two with adequate hip and lumbar physical examinations; however, electrodiagnostic studies may be helpful if the diagnosis is unclear.

For the patient who presents with a palpable inguinal mass, the other possibilities include hernia, aneurysm, and lymphadenopathy. Although these other diagnoses may also produce pain, it is usually not clearly related specifically to hip flexion and extension, and the patient should otherwise exhibit a normal hip examination. Ultrasound is a good first line test in this situation when one of these other etiologies is suspected.

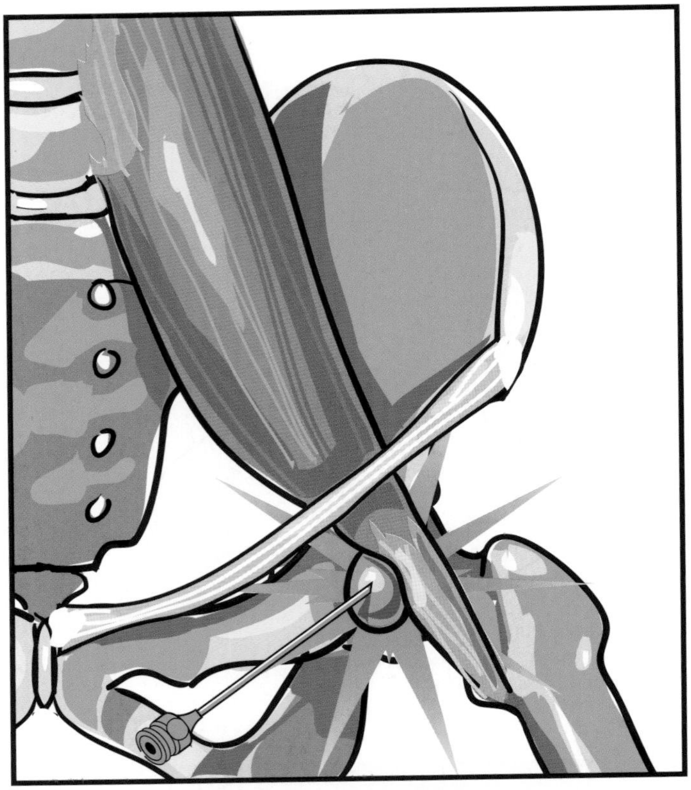

FIGURE 98–4 ■ Injection technique for iliopsoas bursitis.

TREATMENT

Initial treatment for most cases is conservative with relative rest and avoidance of aggravating activities, antiinflammatory medications, and physical therapy for localized hip flexor stretching. Johnston and Wiley also advocated a hip rotation strengthening program with good results to correct subtle muscle imbalances that may lead to the problem over time.[9]

Corticosteroid injection to the bursa is often quite helpful for rapid relief of pain symptoms. A solution of 40 mg methylprednisolone is diluted in 0.25% bupivacaine or similar equivalent in a syringe attached to a 3.5-inch, 25-gauge needle. The patient is place in the supine position and the femoral artery pulse is palpated. The needle is placed at a point 2.5 inches below and 3.5 inches lateral to the femoral pulse. It is then advanced superiorly at a 45-degree angle (Fig. 98–4). The patient should be advised to tell the clinician if he or she feels a paresthesia into the thigh on advancement of the needle, which is a sign that the needle has impinged on the femoral nerve. If no paresthesia occurs, the needle is advanced slowly until it hits bone and then is withdrawn slightly. After initial aspiration, the medication is injected into the bursa with very little resistance.[10] For patients with a significantly distended bursa or if infection is suspected, an empty syringe may be used first to aspirate the excess synovial fluid from the sac. Obviously, if the fluid appears cloudy or infected, the corticosteroid is not injected. If there is difficulty in aspirating a palpable bursa, a CT scan or ultrasound-guided procedure may be performed.

Although the majority of patients respond very well to a regimen of medications, injections, and therapy, recalcitrant cases may still require surgery. This usually consists of a bursectomy with possible release of the iliopsoas tendon, and it has a good outcome rate.

COMPLICATIONS AND PITFALLS

The most common pitfall of this process is a delay in making the proper diagnosis. Often, the problem is mistaken to be osteoarthritis or radicular pain. Iliopsoas bursitis should always be considered in patients with persistent hip pain with negative radiographs and an unremarkable lumbar examination.

Patients will commonly experience soreness or increased pain for 1 to 2 days after an injection to the bursa, but major complications are rare with proper technique. The most serious complication would be abscess or hematoma formation and would manifest with progressively worsening hip or flank pain with guarding of hip movements and possibly fever. Weakness would occur if there is compression on the lumbosacral plexus. If these symptoms occur post-injection, a pelvic CT scan should be obtained immediately. To reduce this risk, patients should be asked about clotting disorders, immune dysfunction, or use of anticoagulants prior to any injection.

SUMMARY

Iliopsoas bursitis is an often overlooked cause of hip pain that will occur in older patients with other underlying hip disease and in young athletes. The diagnosis is usually made clinically with point tenderness in the iliopsoas tendon and reproduction of pain with flexion and extension of the hip. When further information is needed, a CT scan, ultrasound, or MRI may demonstrate the presence of a distended bursa and rule out other potential causes of hip pain. Patients typically respond well to conservative treatment and a well-placed injection, although surgery is a possible option for severe or persistent cases.

References

1. Johnston CA, Wiley JP, Lindsay DM, Wiseman DA: Iliopsoas bursitis and tendinitis: A review. Sports Med 25:271, 1998.
2. Fricke JI: Uber die bursa mucosa iliaca und deren communikation mit dem hueftgelenke. J Chir Augenheilkunde 21:223, 1834.
3. Kummer E, DeSenarclans P: Un cas d' hygroma chronique de la buorse du psoas-ilique ou iliopectinee. Rev Med Suisse Romande 37:574, 1917.
4. Melamad A, Bauer C, Johnson H: Iliopsoas bursal extension of arthritic disease of the hip. Radiology 89:54, 1967.
5. Armstrong P, Saxton H: Iliopsoas bursa. Br J Radiol 45:493, 1972.
6. Carrera GF, Papudakes M, Imray TJ: Retropsoas extension of ruptured hip capsule: Arthrographic demonstration. AJR Am J Roentgenol 135:1293, 1980.
7. Underwood PL, McLeod RA, Ginsburg WW: The varied clinical manifestations of iliopsoas bursitis. J Rheumatol 15:1683, 1988.
8. Mccormack JJ, Demos TC, Lomasney LM: Iliopsoas bursitis: Radiologic case study. Orthopedics 26:1171, 2003.
9. Johnston CAM, Lindsay DM, Wiley MPE: Treatment of iliopsoas syndrome with a hip rotation strengthening program: A retrospective case series. J Orthop Sports Phys Ther 29:218, 1999.
10. Waldman SD: Iliopectineal bursitis. In Waldman SD: Atlas of Pain Management Injection Techniques. Philadelphia, Saunders, 2000, p 216.

chapter 99

Meralgia Paresthetica

Steven D. Waldman

Meralgia paresthetica is caused by compression of the lateral femoral cutaneous nerve by the inguinal ligament as it passes through or under the inguinal ligament.[1] This entrapment neuropathy presents as pain, numbness, and dysesthesias in the distribution of the lateral femoral cutaneous nerve.[2] These symptoms often begin as a burning pain in the lateral thigh with associated cutaneous sensitivity. Patients suffering from meralgia paresthetica note that sitting, squatting, or wearing wide belts that compress the lateral femoral cutaneous nerve will cause their symptoms to worsen (Fig. 99–1).[3] Although traumatic lesions to the lateral femoral cutaneous nerve have been implicated in the onset of meralgia paresthetica, in most patients, no obvious antecedent trauma can be identified.[4]

■ CLINICAL PRESENTATION

Physical findings include tenderness over the lateral femoral cutaneous nerve at the origin of the inguinal ligament at the anterior superior iliac spine.[2] A positive Tinel sign over the lateral femoral cutaneous nerve as it passes beneath the inguinal ligament may be present (Fig. 99–2). Careful sensory examination of the lateral thigh will reveal a sensory deficit in the distribution of the lateral femoral cutaneous nerve. No motor deficit should be present. Sitting or the wearing of tight waistbands or wide belts that compress the lateral femoral cutaneous nerve may exacerbate the symptoms of meralgia paresthetica.

■ DIAGNOSIS

Electromyography will help distinguish lumbar radiculopathy and diabetic femoral neuropathy from meralgia paresthetica. Plain radiographs of the back, hip, and pelvis are indicated in all patients who present with meralgia paresthetica to rule out occult bony pathology. Based on the patient's clinical presentation, additional testing including complete blood cell count, uric acid, sedimentation rate, and antinuclear antibody testing may be indicated. MRI of the back is indicated if herniated disk, spinal stenosis, or a space-occupying lesion is suspected. The injection technique described later serves as both a diagnostic and a therapeutic maneuver.

■ DIFFERENTIAL DIAGNOSIS

Meralgia paresthetica is often misdiagnosed as lumbar radiculopathy or trochanteric bursitis or is attributed to primary hip pathology.[5] Radiographs of the hip and electromyography will help distinguish meralgia paresthetica from radiculopathy or pain emanating from the hip. Most patients suffering from a lumbar radiculopathy will have back pain associated with reflex, motor, and sensory changes accompanied by neck pain, whereas patients with meralgia paresthetica will have no back pain and no motor or reflex changes. The sensory changes of meralgia paresthetica will be limited to the distribution of the lateral femoral cutaneous nerve and should not extend below the knee (see Fig. 99–2). It should be remembered that lumbar radiculopathy and lateral femoral cutaneous nerve entrapment may coexist as the so-called double-crush syndrome. Occasionally, diabetic femoral neuropathy may produce anterior thigh pain, which may confuse the diagnosis.

■ TREATMENT

The patient suffering from meralgia paresthetica should be instructed in avoidance techniques to help reduce the unpleasant symptoms and pain associated with this entrapment neuropathy. A short course of conservative therapy consisting of simple analgesics, nonsteroidal antiinflammatory agents, or cyclooxygenase-2 inhibitors is a reasonable first step in the treatment of patients suffering from meralgia paresthetica. If the patient does not experience rapid improvement, the following injection technique is a reasonable next step.[6]

To treat the pain of meralgia paresthetica, the patient is placed in the supine position with a pillow under the knees if lying with the legs extended increases the patient's pain due to traction on the nerve. The anterior superior iliac spine is identified by palpation. A point 1 inch medial to the anterior superior iliac spine and just inferior to the inguinal ligament is then identified and prepped with antiseptic solution (Fig. 99–3). A 1.5-inch 25-gauge needle is then advanced perpendicular to the skin slowly until the needle is felt to pop through the fascia. A paresthesia is often elicited. After careful aspiration, 5 to 7 mL of 1.0% preservative-free lidocaine and 40 mg of methylprednisolone is injected in a fanlike manner as the needle pierces the fascia of the external oblique muscle. Care must be taken not to place the needle too deep to avoid entering the peritoneal cavity and perforating the abdominal

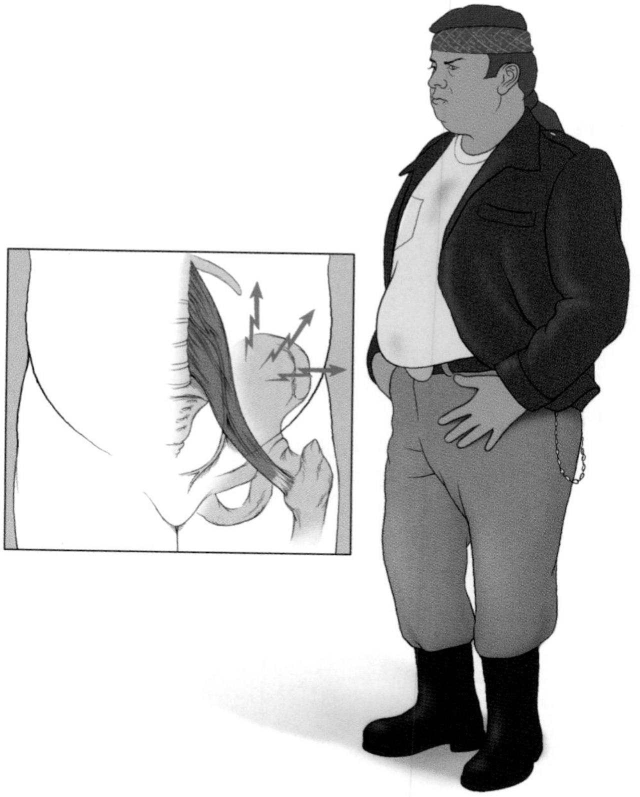

FIGURE 99–1 ■ Obesity and wearing of wide belts may cause compression of the lateral femoral cutaneous nerve and result in meralgia paresthetica. (From Waldman SD: Atlas of Common Pain Syndromes. Philadelphia, WB Saunders, 2002, p 235.)

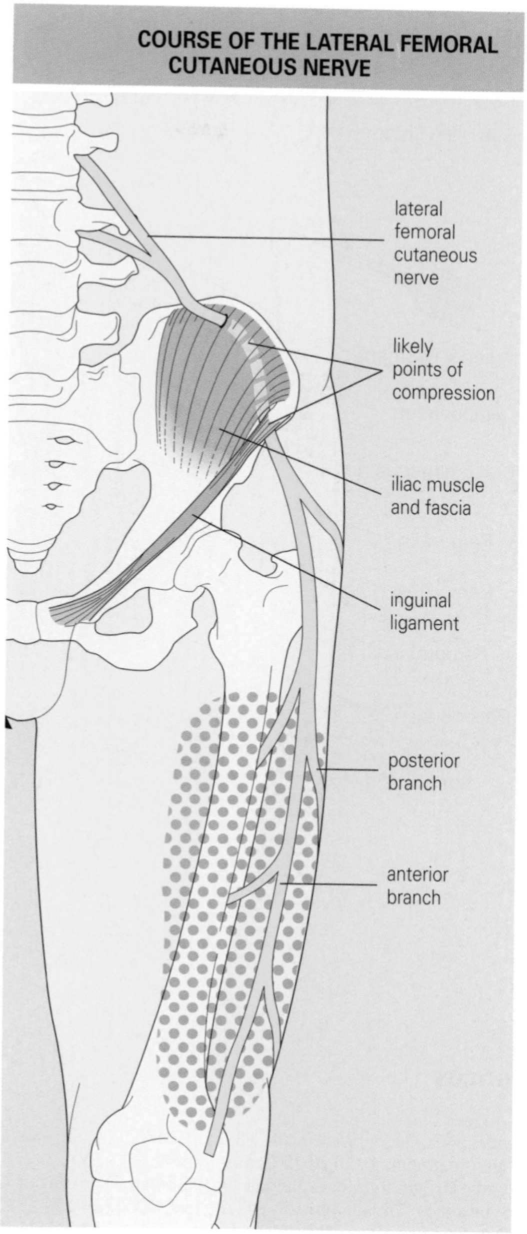

FIGURE 99–2 ■ Course of the lateral femoral cutaneous nerve. The potential for entrapment of the lateral femoral cutaneous nerve can be seen by its course just under the inguinal ligament and medial to the anterior superior iliac spine. (From Klippel JH, Dieppe PA [eds]: Rheumatology, 2nd ed. London, CV Mosby, 1998.)

viscera. After injection of the solution, pressure is applied to the injection site to decrease the incidence of post-block ecchymosis and hematoma formation, which can be quite dramatic, especially in the anticoagulated patient.

Care must be taken to rule out other conditions that may mimic the pain of meralgia paresthetica. The main side effect of the just-described nerve block is post-block ecchymosis and hematoma. If needle placement is too deep and enters the peritoneal cavity, perforation of the colon may result in the formation of intraabdominal abscess and fistula. Early detection of infection is crucial to avoid potentially life-threatening sequelae. If the needle is placed too medial, blockade of the femoral nerve may occur and make ambulation difficult.

CONCLUSION

Meralgia paresthetica is a common pain complaint encountered in clinical practice. It is often misdiagnosed as lumbar radiculopathy. If a patient presents with pain suggestive of lateral femoral cutaneous neuralgia and does not respond to lateral femoral cutaneous nerve blocks, a diagnosis of lesions more proximal in the lumbar plexus or an L2-L3 radiculopathy should be considered. Such patients will often respond to epidural steroid blocks. Electromyography and MRI of the lumbar plexus are indicated in this patient population to help rule out other causes of lateral femoral cutaneous pain, including malignancy invading the lumbar plexus or epidural or vertebral metastatic disease at L2-L3.

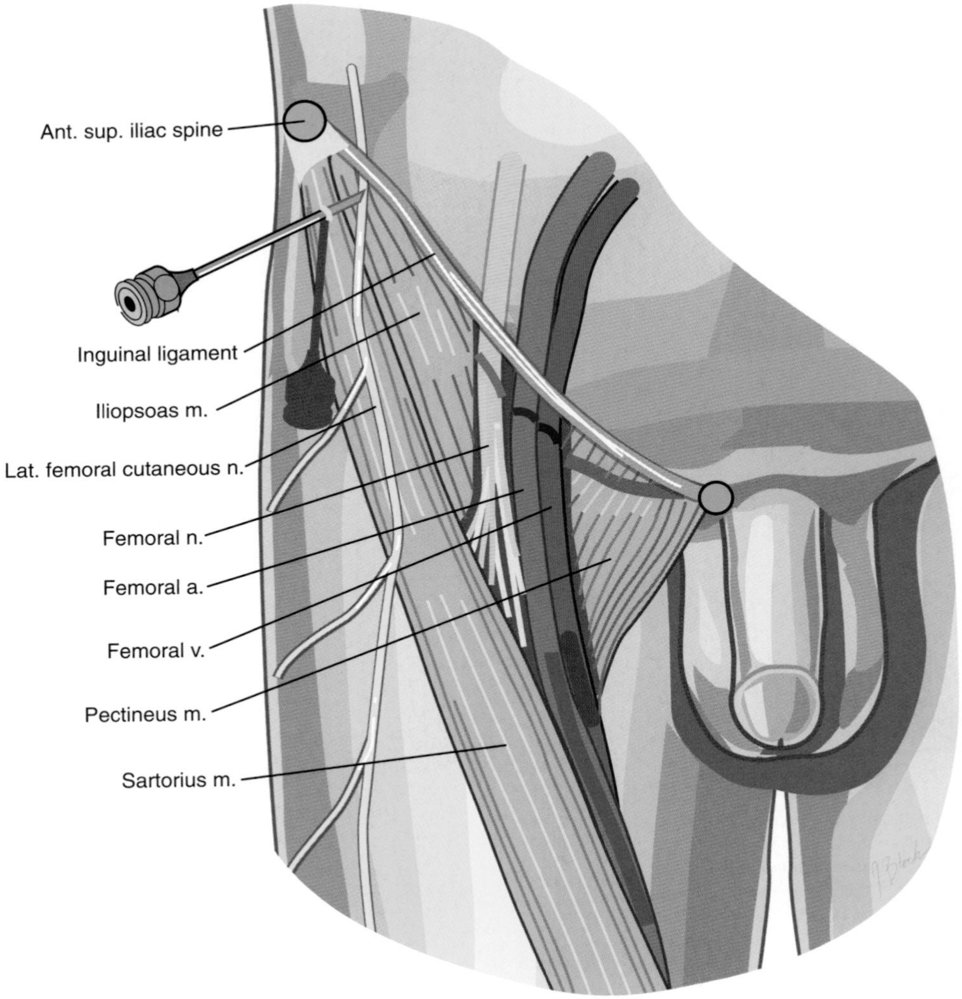

FIGURE 99–3 ■ Injection technique for relieving pain of meralgia paresthetica. (From Waldman SD: Atlas of Interventional Pain Management, 2nd ed. Philadelphia, WB Saunders, 2003, p 457.)

References

1. Grossman MG, Ducey SA, Nadler SS, et al: Meralgia paresthetica: Diagnosis and treatment. J Am Acad Orthop Surg 9:336, 2001.
2. Waldman SD: Meralgia paresthetica. In Waldman SD: Atlas of Common Pain Syndromes. Philadelphia, WB Saunders, 2002, pp 234-237.
3. Dombrowski MA, Hasan IM, Klaas J, et al: Ties that bind: Understanding meralgia paresthestica. Adv Nurse Pract 8:61, 2000.
4. Ahsan MR, Curtin J: Meralgia paresthetica following total hip replacement. Ir J Med Sci 170:149, 2001.
5. Erbay H: Meralgia paresthetica in the differential diagnosis of low-back pain. Clin J Pain 18:132, 2002.
6. Waldman SD: Lateral femoral cutaneous nerve block. In Waldman SD: Atlas of Interventional Pain Management, 2nd ed. Philadelphia, WB Saunders, 2004, pp 454-457.

chapter 100

Femoral and Saphenous Neuropathies

Bernard M. Abrams

Femoral and saphenous neuropathies are uncommon pain-producing conditions. Femoral neuropathy can produce pain into the anterior thigh and midcalf and is associated with weakness of the quadriceps muscle. It can be caused by myriad factors.[1] The saphenous nerve, a pure sensory nerve and anatomic extension of the femoral nerve, can produce medial calf pain which may be confused with medial calf claudication.[2]

HISTORICAL CONSIDERATIONS

Kopell and Thompson described entrapment of the saphenous nerve in 1960[3] but undoubtedly saphenous nerve dysfunction and injury have been known for many years owing to experience with trauma and surgery in the region of the medial thigh. Descriptions of diabetic neuropathy as early as 1890 recognized cases in which there was asymmetrical lower extremity pain and weakness[4] and this concept dates to 1798 when John Rollo mentioned neurologic disorders in his book *Cases of Diabetes Mellitus* and persisted through the 18th, 19th, and 20th centuries until, at least, 1976.[5] Then it became recognized that what had previously been termed *femoral neuropathy* was much more frequently a lumbar plexopathy. Asbury clarified the issue advocating the term *proximal diabetic neuropathy* in view of the ambiguities associated with the earlier term *diabetic amyotrophy*.[8] Unfortunately, the association of the relatively uncommon femoral neuropathy with diabetes mellitus has persisted when, in fact, diabetes is much more commonly associated with a lumbar plexopathy. The long history of this erroneous association terminated only with the advent of modern meticulous electrodiagnostic methods and should serve as a cautionary note not to neglect the multiple possible causes of true femoral neuropathy.[9]

FEMORAL NEUROPATHY

Anatomy

The femoral nerve arises from the lumbar plexus within the psoas major muscle. It is formed form the posterior divisions of the ventral rami of the L2-L4 spinal nerve roots (Fig. 100–1). After emerging from the lateral border of the psoas muscle, it lies in a groove between the psoas and iliacus muscles. As it approaches the external iliac artery (which is anteromedial to it), the nerve and artery descend toward the pelvis. In its descent, the nerve gives off some twigs to innervate the iliacus and psoas muscles.[9] The psoas is also innervated by branches of the L2 and L3 spinal nerve roots. Authorities differ on whether clinically significant innervation of the iliacus and psoas muscles comes from the beginning of the femoral nerve or from fibers of the lumbar plexus proximal to the origin of the femoral nerve. Therefore, weakness of hip flexion due to involvement of the psoas and iliacus may or may not be included in the femoral nerve syndrome depending on which viewpoint is espoused.

The femoral nerve, the psoas muscle, the iliacus muscle, and the iliolumbar vessels, roofed over by the iliacus fascia, form a tight "iliacus compartment," which accounts for femoral nerve lesions due to space-occupying processes in this area.

The femoral nerve then passes beneath the inguinal ligament giving off a branch to the pectineus muscle and then enters the femoral triangle lateral to the femoral artery and separated from the artery by some psoas fibers. About 4 cm distal to the inguinal ligament the artery bifurcates into an anterior and a posterior division. The anterior division innervates the sartorius muscle and forms the medial and intermediate femoral cutaneous nerves that give sensory innervation to the skin of the medial and anterior surfaces of the knee, the medial surface of the lower leg, medial malleolus, and part of the arch of the foot and great toe. It also gives motor branches to the quadriceps muscles composed of the rectus femoris, vastus lateralis, vastus intermedius, and vastus medialis muscles. It continues as the saphenous nerve (see later).

Clinical Presentation

Patients with femoral neuropathies usually complain that their lower extremity buckles at the knee and they cannot maintain their stance, especially when trying to descend stairs.[6] They may have pain, numbness, and paresthesias in the entire femoral nerve and saphenous nerve distribution or sensory abnormalities may be mild or even absent entirely. When pain is felt, it may be in the inguinal region or felt in the iliac fossa. When flank pain is severe with other symptoms and signs of femoral neuropathy, hemorrhage in the iliacus compartment

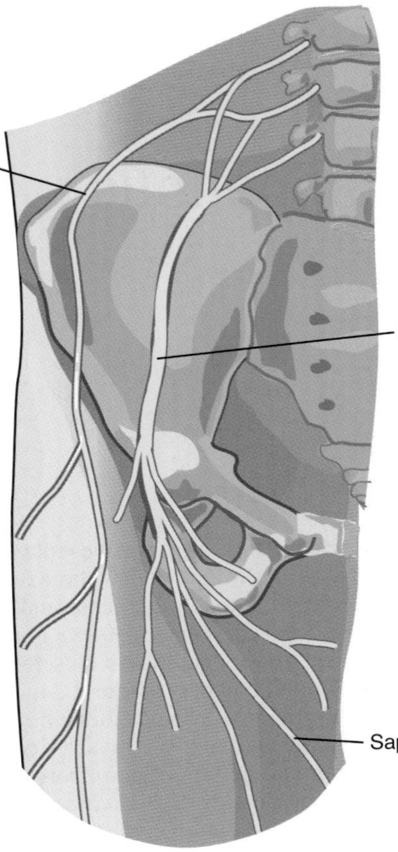

FIGURE 100–1 ■ Anatomy of the femoral nerve.

should be strongly suspected, especially in circumstances conducive to hemorrhage—such as anticoagulation. Severe femoral nerve lesions produce weakness and eventually wasting of the quadriceps group of muscles, loss of the knee reflex (although this may also be seen in high lumbar radiculopathies [L3-L4]), and sensory abnormalities over the anterior aspect of the thigh and the medial part of the lower leg. In the case of the proximal diabetic neuropathy[6,7] (actually a lumbar plexopathy in the vast majority of cases) there is characteristically severe pain radiating from the groin into the anterior thigh, usually worse at night and at rest (in contrast to a lumbar radiculopathy), which subsides over several days to weeks to be followed by severe painless weakness of the quadriceps group of muscles. This pain may be of such severity as to require narcotics for pain relief.

In examination of a patient with suspected femoral neuropathy, the iliopsoas muscle and hip adductor strength must be evaluated to differentiate among femoral neuropathy, combined obturator and femoral neuropathy, and upper lumbar plexopathy or L2, L3 radiculopathy.[10]

Etiology

Numerous etiologies, many of them iatrogenic, can cause femoral neuropathies. The most common causes are listed in Table 100–1.

Iliac Hemorrhage

A hemorrhage in the tight iliacus compartment can compress the femoral nerve. Causes range from the common hemorrhage due to anticoagulation to hemophilia and other coagulopathies. The characteristic clinical picture is femoral nerve dysfunction and severe pain and swelling. The pain is generally in the iliac fossa and groin associated with a flexed posture of the leg at the hip. Ecchymoses may be present in the upper thigh.[9] Hematomas within the psoas muscle characteristically cause widespread lumbar plexopathy but occasionally there is only femoral dysfunction. False aneurysms may form within the psoas muscle.[10-30] Traumatic avulsion of the iliacus muscle may occur in otherwise healthy people, occasionally with only minor trauma.[31,32,34]

Iliac Abscess

Iliac abscess may develop independently or be a result of infection of a hematoma. With the addition of signs of infection, the signs are the same as for a hemorrhage.[33]

Abdominal Aortic Aneurysms

Sometimes abdominal aortic aneurysms rupture into the psoas muscle producing false aneurysms compressing the femoral nerve. Other arteries including the profunda femoral artery and the iliac artery may have aneurysms or false aneurysms that compress the femoral nerve.[35-42]

Trauma, Stretch, or Compression

Direct injury by bullet wounds, stab wounds, blunt injuries, and hip and pelvic fractures can compromise the femoral nerve. Gymnasts and dancers have been reported to have femoral nerve injuries during hyperextension of the hip. Damage during coma and drunken stupors has also been

Table 100–1

Causes of Femoral Neuropathy

Retroperitoneal and iliacus compartment hemorrhage
Spontaneous
Associated with anticoagulants (e.g., heparin, warfarin [Coumadin])
Traumatic iliacus muscle avulsion
Hemophilia and other coagulopathies
Traumatic pseudoaneurysm and iliacus hematoma
Iliacus abscess
Abdominal aortic aneurysm and pseudoaneurysm
Trauma, stretch or compression
Idiopathic
Tumors, enlarged lymph nodes, complications of radiation, chemotherapeutic injection
Diabetes mellitus (usually as part of a lumbar plexopathy)
Pregnancy and labor
Iatrogenic
Hip arthroplasty
Neural blockade and tourniquet use
Abdominal hysterectomy including retractor injury
Renal transplants and other urologic and pelvic surgery
Lithotomy position for delivery and surgery, including vaginal hysterectomy
Inguinal and femoral herniorrhaphies

reported, although alcoholism itself has been reported as a cause.[43-49]

Idiopathic Etiology

One report in 1970[50] found 18 of 50 patients to have no demonstrable cause for their neuropathy. Given that the majority were males older than 50 years of age with eventual resolution over months, some may have had occult diabetic plexopathy.

Tumors, Complications of Cancer Therapy, and other Space-Occupying Lesions

Tumors may arise primarily from the nerve sheath, arise from the iliopsoas muscle or the ilium itself, or rarely be primary malignancies or metastases and cause femoral neuropathy.[50-60] Infusions of chemotherapeutic agents into the femoral artery may also cause femoral neuropathy.[5]

Diabetes Mellitus

Although the older literature described diabetes as the most common cause of femoral neuropathy, modern electrodiagnosis has clearly identified the lumbosacral plexus as the primary pathologic site of the lesion. The femoral nerve is often the most affected portion of the structures involved, although other portions of the lumbosacral plexus can clearly be shown to be involved.[9] An association with renal failure has been noted.[61]

Pregnancy and Delivery

Femoral neuropathy has been reported as a result of pregnancy and delivery, even in uncomplicated situations.[62-68] During pregnancy and before delivery, pressure on the femoral nerve in the pelvis is presumably implicated.[64]

Iatrogenic Causes

Unfortunately iatrogenic femoral neuropathy is all too frequent. It has been associated with a wide variety of surgical procedures in the abdomen, pelvic inguinal and hip areas.[69] It has most frequently been associated with abdominal hysterectomy and self-retaining retractors compressing the femoral nerve directly or within the iliopsoas muscle and the lateral wall of the pelvis. Not using these retractors significantly lowered the incidence. Hip replacement and repair have also been reported frequently as causing femoral neuropathy although not as frequently as sciatic neuropathy.

Other circumstances in which femoral neuropathy may occur are renal transplantation, inguinal or femoral herniorrhaphy, lymph node resection in the groin, femoral artery surgery, cardiac catheterization, and angioplasty. Suturing of the femoral nerve may occur during surgery as well as extrusion of cement, tourniquet use, and untoward effects of neural anesthetic blockage.

Hip Arthroplasty

Femoral neuropathy occurs much less frequently than sciatic neuropathy (0.1% to 2.3%) following hip arthroplasty. When it occurs, it is usually due to retractor compression, heat from bone cement, or nerve encasement in cement, laceration and complicating iliac hematoma. There may be a delay in the onset due to scar formation. Iliacus hemorrhage following prophylactic anticoagulation postoperatively has also been reported.[70-80]

Neural Blockade and Tourniquet Use

Both neural blockade in the psoas compartment and ilioinguinal block for hernia repair have been associated with transient or permanent femoral nerve damage. Use of a tourniquet has produced both femoral and saphenous nerve damage.[81-83]

Abdominal Hysterectomy and Tuboplasty

Abdominal hysterectomy has been the operation most associated with intraoperative femoral nerve palsies. Two studies in the 1980s gave statistical incidences of 11.6% and 7.5%, respectively.[84,85]

The lateral blade of self-retaining retractors was ascribed to be the likely cause of femoral neuropathy based on cadaver anatomic studies and clinical experience. The abandonment of this instrument led to a reduction in femoral neuropathies from 7.5% to 0.7%.[86] Other possible scenarios for femoral neuropathy include suturing the nerve and attempts at tubal ligation and reanastomosis.[87-100]

Laparoscopy

Laparoscopy and suprapubic interventions have been implicated in the development of femoral neuropathy.

Renal Transplantation

Femoral neuropathy has been reported with some frequency in renal transplants that involve retroperitoneal placement of the donated kidney. Again, self-retaining retractors have been implicated but even without their use, delayed femoral neuropathy due to compression of the nerve by hematoma has been seen and confirmed at autopsy. In addition, surgery for genitourinary malignancies and other pelvic urologic surgeries have been attended by femoral neuropathies.[101-116]

Lithotomy Positions

Prolonged and rarely even brief intervals in the lithotomy position have produced femoral neuropathies. This may be due to kinking and compression of the nerve below the inguinal ligament. Prolonged lithotomy position for delivery and for surgeries such as laparoscopy may produce femoral neuropathy.[117-119]

Inguinal and Femoral Herniorrhaphies

Inguinal or femoral herniorrhaphies may cause femoral neuropathy by cutting or placing suture material around the nerve. Delayed involvement may result from later development of scar tissue.[120,121,123]

Diagnosis and Testing

The etiology of a femoral neuropathy may be obvious because of the setting in which it arose—such as immediately postoperatively following a surgery well known to be associated with femoral neuropathy. Renal transplants, abdominal hysterectomy, and prolonged lithotomy positions head this category. Injections, catheterizations, and hernia surgery in the groin provide clear causality on many occasions. Confusion may arise in cases of delayed onset due to scarring or hemorrhage, although hemorrhage is generally connected with severe pain in the iliacus fossa. Again, circumstances may clearly give the etiology in hemorrhagic lesions (e.g., in patients who undergo anticoagulation or in those who have hemophilia or another coagulopathy).

One of the maneuvers necessary in more occult etiologies is to strictly delineate the anatomic boundaries of the patient's deficits. Often, what appears to be a pure femoral neuropathy clinically may actually be part of a radiculoplexopathy. This not only moves the anatomic site of the lesion more proximally, it introduces diagnostic possibilities of diabetes mellitus and other processes such as malignancy in the pelvis. Electromyography is well suited for this task, and should include sufficient interrogation of the quadriceps muscle group, paraspinal, iliopsoas and hip adductor muscles to differentiate femoral neuropathy from more extensive lesions. Motor nerve conduction tests of the femoral nerve(stimulation point above the inguinal ligament and recording from the quadriceps muscle) may be performed but is generally less informative than needle electromyography[122] and may need to be followed up with laboratory tests for diabetes mellitus and imaging of the pelvis by CT scan and, more recently, MRI scan.[124-128]

CT scan has long been shown to image the femoral nerve, as have MRI and ultrasound. CT scan is indicated for suspected iliacus hemorrhages and other masses affecting the femoral nerve. Ultrasound and MRI are also effective in diagnosing iliacus hemorrhage and other masses.[129-137]

Treatment

Obvious inciting lesions should be treated with such curative measures as are available. Exploration of the femoral nerve should be undertaken if complete disruption of the nerve, unintentional suturing or stapling of the nerve is suspected. Management of retroperitoneal or iliopsoas hemorrhage may constitute a surgical emergency.[138-140] Percutaneous relief of hemorrhage has been reported.[140] In acute hemorrhage, anticoagulation, when present, must be reversed. Fluid and blood replacement may be necessary. Persistent pain requires pharmacologic treatment such as gabapentin, pregabalin, other membrane stabilizers (newer anticonvulsants), tricyclic antidepressants, or other medications useful in neuropathic pain. Nerve blocks of the femoral nerve may be helpful for pain. Physical therapy, bracing, and assistive devices may be necessary. Mobility and range of motion should be maintained.

Prognosis

In iatrogenic femoral neuropathy, recovery is the usual outcome. The prognosis is better in incidents induced by the lithotomy position than in hip or inguinal surgical untoward events. The only significant prognostic factor is the percentage of axon loss in the vastus lateralis derived by comparison of vastus lateralis compound muscle action potential on the affected and unaffected sides.[141]

SAPHENOUS NEUROPATHY

Saphenous neuropathies can occur in the thigh due to lacerations, arterial surgery, compression by fibrous bands, entrapment at the subsartorial canal exit[3]; at the knee due to surgery including arthroscopy or external compression; in the lower leg due to surgery; and the infrapatellar branch can be injured by direct compression or knee surgery—including arthroscopy and possibly entrapment in the sartorius muscle tendon.

Anatomy

The saphenous nerve is the distal sensory continuation of the femoral nerve. It descends in the thigh through the quadriceps muscle in the subsartorial canal of Hunter lateral to the femoral artery and gives off an infrapatellar branch supplying sensation to the anterior skin of the patella before entering a fascial layer between the sartorius and gracilis muscles (Fig. 100–2). It emerges from the canal and becomes subcutaneous about 10 cm proximal to the knee.[10]

The nerve crosses the pes anserine bursa at the upper medial portion of the tibia and then goes distally along the medial aspect of the tibia. The saphenous vein is closely apposed to the nerve along most of its descent in the calf, especially in the distal third of the leg. At the lower third of the leg, there is division of the saphenous nerve into two main branches. One continues along the medial border of the tibia, reaching and terminating at the ankle. The other passes anteriorly with the vein to cross the medial surface of the tibia and in front of the medial malleolus to reach the foot; it then continues along the medial surface to the ball of the great toe. The saphenous innervates the medial and anterior sensory portions of the knee and the medial surface of the lower leg, medial malleolus, and a minor part of the medial arch of the foot and great toe.[10]

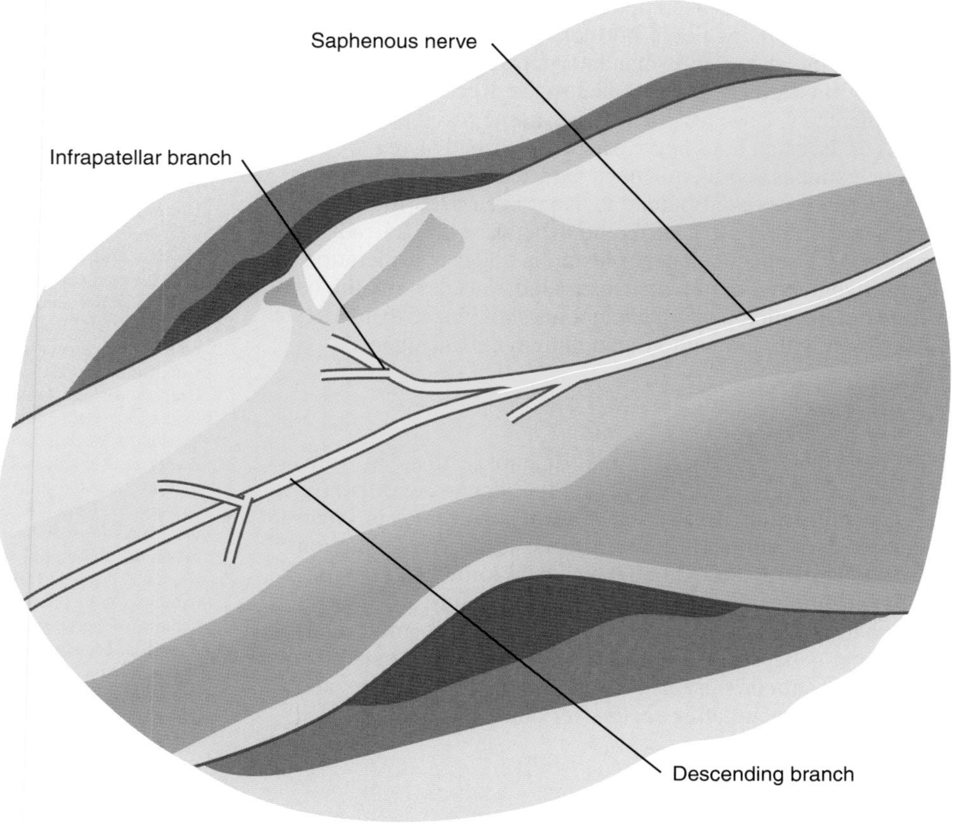

FIGURE 100–2 ■ Anatomy of the saphenous nerve.

Etiology

Causes of saphenous neuropathy are outlined in Table 100–2. The differential diagnosis of saphenous neuropathy depends on the anatomic location. In the thigh, due to its proximity to the femoral artery in the subsartorial canal, it can be damaged by arterial surgery, lacerations, compression by fibrous bands, schwannoma, or nerve entrapment where the nerve pierces a fascial layer to leave the subsartorial canal.[3] At the knee, arthroscopic surgery, medial meniscectomy, external compression from knee-supporting stirrups, and in surfers who habitually grasp the board between their knees. In the lower leg, surgical damage or saphenous nerve cannulation can produce a neuropathy. Spontaneous paresthesias of the infrapatellar branch has been termed *gonyalgia paresthetica*.[146,148] The infrapatellar branch can be injured by direct compression, knee surgery (arthroscopy), and questionably by entrapment in the sartorius tendon.

Clinical Presentation

In saphenous neuropathy, there may be trivial numbness but severe neuropathic pain may occur. The course of the nerve should be palpated for tenderness, a neuroma or Tinel sign. The pain may be at the medial aspect of the knee and may radiate downward to the medial side of the foot. The patient will often state that negotiating stairs causes significant aggravation of the pain.[3] The sensory abnormality in the medial calf that may extend to the medial foot and the great toe may take the form of numbness or paresthesia.

Table 100–2

Causes of Saphenous Neuropathy

Thigh
- Lacerations
- Arterial surgery (femoral artery)
- Compression
- Schwannoma
- Subsartorial canal entrapment

Knee
- Surgery: arthroscopy; medial meniscectomy
- External compression (stirrups)

Lower leg
- Surgical injury (varicose vein operations, vein harvest for arterial surgery)
- Cannulation of saphenous vein

Infrapatellar branch
- Compression and other direct injuries
- Arthroscopy

Possible entrapment in the sartorius tendon

Diagnosis and Testing

Electromyography provides an anatomic method of differentiating plexopathy from radiculopathy or combined lesions. Saphenous nerve conduction studies are technically challenging but may be useful for confirming damage to sensory fibers of the saphenous nerve.[142-144]

Somatosensory evoked potential may document dysfunction of the saphenous nerve but not localize the lesion.[145-147] CT scan of the abdomen is mandatory in suspected lesions in the psoas muscle or retroperitoneal space. Recently, MRI has supplemented CT because of superior tissue resolution. Focal lesions of the saphenous nerve can be confirmed by nerve conduction studies, which may be technically difficult. Somatosensory evoked potentials have been used for saphenous nerve studies. If a differential between an L4 radiculopathy and a saphenous nerve lesion is under consideration, electromyography of the L4-innervated muscles should be carried out. Suspicion of a schwannoma should lead to an MRI of the thigh with and without gadolinium enhancement.[9]

Treatment

Treatment depends on accurate diagnosis that, in turn, depends on setting up and resolving the diagnostic dilemma. Surgical correction of any lesion, when possible, is ideal. When residual pain and disability persist, then rehabilitation efforts must be made. Although medical knowledge is constantly changing, neuropathic pain at this juncture is best dealt with pharmacologic treatment such as NSAIDs, mild analgesics, and gabapentin, pregabalin, other membrane stabilizers (newer anticonvulsants), tricyclic antidepressants, and avoidance of precipitating factors for pain.

References

1. Waldman SD: Femoral neuropathy. In Waldman SD: Atlas of Uncommon Pain Syndromes. Philadelphia, Saunders, 2003, p 194.
2. Waldman, SD: Saphenous neuralgia. In Waldman SD: Atlas of Uncommon Pain Syndromes. Philadelphia, Saunders, 2003, p 200.
3. Kopell HP, Thompson WAL: Knee pain due to saphenous nerve entrapment. N Engl J Med 263:351, 1960.
4. Said G, Thomas PK: Proximal diabetic neuropathy. In Dyck PJ, Thomas PK: Diabetic Neuropathy, 2nd ed. Philadelphia, Saunders, 1999, p 474.
5. Giannini C, Dyck PJ: Pathologic alterations in human diabetic neuropathy. In Dyck PJ, Thomas PK: Diabetic Neuropathy 2nd ed. Philadelphia, Saunders, 1999, p 279.
6. Calverly JR, Mulder DW: Femoral neuropathy. Neurology 10:963, 1960.
7. Goodman JI: Femoral neuropathy in relation to diabetes mellitus: Report of 17 cases. Diabetes 3:266, 1954.
8. Asbury AK: Proximal diabetic neuropathy. Ann Neurol 2:179, 1977.
9. Stewart, John D: The femoral and saphenous nerves. In Focal Peripheral Neuropathies, 2nd ed. New York, Raven, 1993, p 387.
10. Busis NA: Femoral and obturator neuropathies. In Logigian EL: Entrapment and Other Focal Neuropathies. Neurol Clin North Am, Saunders, Philadelphia, 1999, p 633.
11. Wada Y, Yanagihara C, Nishimura Y: Bilateral iliopsoas hematomas complicating anticoagulant therapy. Intern Med 44:641, 2005.
12. Rochman AS, Vitarbo E, Levi AD: Femoral nerve palsy secondary to traumatic pseudoaneurysm and iliacus hematoma. J Neurosurg 102:382, 2005.
13. Forcano M, Garcia-Arilla E: Femoral neuropathy as presentation of psoas iliacus hematoma. Ann Med Interna 20:594, 2003. [Spanish]
14. Tokarz VA, McGrory JE, Stewart JD, Croslin AR: Femoral neuropathy and iliopsoas hematoma as a result of postpartum factor VIII inhibitor syndrome. A case report. J Bone Joint Surg Am 85-A:1812, 2003.
15. Ho KJ, Gawley SD, Young MR: Psoas haematoma and femoral neuropathy associated with enoxaparin therapy. Int J Clin Pract 57(6):553, 2003.
16. Seijo-Martinez M, Castro del Rio M, Fontoira E, Fontoira M: Acute femoral neuropathy secondary to an iliacus muscle hematoma. J Neurol Sci 209:119, 2003.
17. Sipos P, Zubek L, Sperlagh M, Ondrejka P: Femoral neuropathy caused by retroperitoneal hematoma. Magy Seb 55:36, 2002. [Hungarian]
18. Marquardt G, Barduzal Angles S, Leheta F, Seifert V: Spontaneous haematoma of the iliac psoas muscle: A case report and review of the literature. Arch Orthop Trauma Surg 122(2):109, 2000.
19. Nakao A, Sakagami K, Mitsuoka S, et al: Retroperitoneal hematoma associated with femoral neuropathy: A complication under antiplatelet therapy. Acta Med Okayama 55:363, 2001.
20. Andrews FJ: Retroperitoneal haematoma after paracetamol increased anticoagulation. Emerg Med J 19:84, 2002.
21. Pirouzmand F, Midha R: Subacute femoral compressive neuropathy from iliacus compartment hematoma. Can J Neurol Sci. 28:155, 2001.
22. Ha YC, Ahn IO, Jeong ST, et al: Iliacus hematoma and femoral nerve palsy after revision hip arthroplasty: A case report. Clin Orthop Relat Res (385):100, 2001.
23. Robinson DE, Ball KE, Webb PJ: Iliopsoas hematoma with femoral neuropathy presenting a diagnostic dilemma after spinal decompression. Spine 26: E135, 2001.
24. Fealy S, Paletta GA, Jr. Femoral nerve palsy secondary to traumatic iliacus muscle hematoma: Course after nonoperative management. J Trauma 47:1150, 1999.
25. Ahuja R, Venkatesh P: Femoral neuropathy following anticoagulant therapy: A case report and discussion. Conn Med 63:69, 1999.
26. Crosby ET, Reid DR, DiPrimio G, Grahovac S: Lumbosacral plexopathy from iliopsoas haematoma after combined general-epidural anaesthesia for abdominal aneurysmectomy. Can J Anaesth 45:46, 1998.
27. Sasson Z, Mangat I, Peckham KA: Spontaneous iliopsoas hematoma in patients with unstable coronary syndromes receiving intravenous heparin in therapeutic doses. Can J Cardiol 12 490, 1996.
28. Kent KC, Moscucci M, Mansour KA, et al: Retroperitoneal hematoma after cardiac catheterization: Prevalence, risk factors, and optimal management. J Vasc Surg 20:905, 1994.
29. Casoni P, Dalla Valle R: Femoral neuropathy due to a spontaneous hematoma of the iliopsoas muscle during therapy with heparin-calcium. Acta Biomed Ateneo Parmense 65:289, 1994. [Italian]
30. Chevalier X, Larget-Piet B: Femoral neuropathy due to psoas hematoma revisited. Report of three cases with serious outcomes. Spine 17:724, 1992.
31. Green JP: Proximal avulsion of the iliacus with paralysis of the femoral nerve: Report of a case. J Bone Joint Surg Br 54B:154, 1972.
32. Gertzbein SD, Evan DC: Femoral nerve neuropathy complicating iliopsoas haemorrhage without haemophilia. J Bone Joint Surg Br 54B:149, 1972.
33. Aichroth P, Rowe-Jones DC: Iliacus compartment compression syndrome Br J Surg 58:833, 1971.
34. Mukherjee SK: Iliacus hematoma. J Bone Joint Surg Br 53B:149, 1971.
35. Razzuk MA, Linton RR, Darling RC: Femoral neuropathy secondary to ruptured aortic aneurysms with false aneurysms. JAMA 201:817, 1967.
36. Dorrucci V, Dusi R, Rombola G, Cordiano C: Contained rupture of an abdominal aortic aneurysm presenting as obstructive jaundice: Report of a case. Surg Today 31:331, 2001.
37. Crosby ET, Reid DR, DiPrimio G, Grahovac S: Lumbosacral plexopathy from iliopsoas haematoma after combined general-epidural anaesthesia for abdominal aneurysmectomy. Can J Anaesth 45:46, 1998.
38. Jacobs MJ, Gregoric ID, Reul GJ: Profunda femoral artery pseudoaneurysm after percutaneous transluminal procedures manifested by neuropathy. J Cardiovasc Surg (Torino). 33:729, 1992.
39. Mark MD, Kwasnik EM, Wright SC: Combined femoral neuropathy and psoas sign: An unusual presentation of an iliac artery aneurysm. Am J Med 88:435, 1990.
40. Sterpetti AV, Blair EA, Schultz RD, et al: Sealed rupture of abdominal aortic aneurysms. J Vasc Surg 11:430, 1990.
41. Lainez JM, Yaya R, Lluch V, et al: Lumbosacral plexopathy caused by aneurysms of the abdominal aorta. Med Clin (Barc) 92:462, 1989. [Spanish]
42. Boontje AH, Haaxma R: Femoral neuropathy as a complication of aortic surgery. J Cardiovasc Surg (Torino. 28:286, 1987.
43. Shin CS, Davis BA: Femoral neuropathy due to patellar dislocation in a theatrical and jazz dancer: A case report. Arch Phys Med Rehabil 86:1258, 2005.
44. Muellner T, Ganko A, Bugge W, Engebretsen L: Isolated femoral mononeuropathy in the athlete. Anatomic considerations and report of two cases. Am J Sports Med 29(6):814, 2001.

45. Groah SL, Cifu DX: The rehabilitative management of the traumatic brain injury patient with associated femoral neuropathy. Arch Phys Med Rehabil 76:480, 1995.
46. Gorczyca JT, Powell JN, Tile M: Lateral extension of the ilioinguinal incision in the operative treatment of acetabulum fractures. Injury 26:207, 1995.
47. Uterga JM, Martin R, Sadaba F, Eguiluz JI: Acute alcohol proximal (femoral neuropathy). Rev Neurol 23(120):454, 1995. [Spanish]
48. Guha SC, Poole MD: Stress fracture of the iliac bone with subfascial femoral neuropathy: Unusual complications at a bone graft donor site: Case report. Br J Plast Surg 36:305, 1983.
49. Biemond A: Femoral neuropathy. In Vinken PJ, Bruyn GW (eds): Handbook of Clinical Neurology. New York, Elsevier, 1970, p 303.
50. Shamberger JD, LaQuaglia MP: Resection of a tumor of the psoas muscle. J Pediatr Surg 24:933, 1989.
51. Tajima Y, Sudoh K, Matsumoto A, et al: Femoral neuropathy induced by a low-grade myofibroblastic sarcoma of the groin. J Neurol 252 (11):1416-17, 2005.
52. D'Silva KJ, Dwivedi AJ, Barnwell JM: Schwannoma of the psoas major presenting with abdominal and back pain. Dig Dis Sci 48:1619, 2003.
53. Brundel KH: Extensive multinodular schwannoma of femoral nerve. Med Klin (Munich) 97:687, 2002.
54. Schwarz J, Belzberg AJ: Malignant peripheral nerve sheath tumors in the setting of segmental neurofibromatosis. Case report. J Neurosurg 92:342, 2000.
55. Geiger D, Mpinga E, Steves MA, Sugarbaker PH: Femoral neuropathy: Unusual presentation for recurrent large-bowel cancer. Dis Colon Rectum 41:910, 1998.
56. Castellanos AM, Glass JP, Yung WKA: Regional nerve injury after intra-arterial chemotherapy. Neurology 37:834, 1987.
57. Mendes DG, Nawalker RR, Eldar S: Post-irradiation femoral neuropathy. A case report. J Bone Joint Surg Am 73:137, 1991.
58. Lavyne MH, Voorhies RM, Coll RH: Femoral neuropathy caused by an iliopsoas cyst. Case report. J Neurosurg 56:584, 1982.
59. Khella L: Femoral nerve palsy: Compression by lymph glands in the inguinal region. Arch Phys Med Rehabil 60:325, 1979.
60. Yoon TR, Song EK, Chung JY, Park CH: Femoral neuropathy caused by enlarged iliopsoas bursa associated with osteonecrosis of femoral head—a case report. Acta Orthop Scand 71:322, 2000.
61. Brouns R, De Deyn PP: Neurological complications in renal failure: A review. Clin Neurol Neurosurg 107:1, 2004.
62. Pildner von Steinburg S, Kuhler A, Herrmann N, et al: Pregnancy-associated femoral nerve affection.. Zentralbl Gynakol 126:328, 2004.
63. Cohen S, Zada Y: Postpartum femoral neuropathy. Anaesthesia. 56:500, 2001.
64. Dar AQ, Robinson A, Lyons G: Postpartum femoral neuropathy: More common than you think. Anaesthesia 54:512, 1999.
65. Kofler M, Kronenberg MF: Bilateral femoral neuropathy during pregnancy. Muscle Nerve. 21(8):1106, 1998.
66. Gherman RB, Ouzounian JG, Incerpi MH, Goodwin TM: Symphyseal separation and transient femoral neuropathy associated with the McRoberts' maneuver. Am J Obstet Gynecol 178:609, 1998.
67. Pham LH, Bulich LA, Datta S: Bilateral postpartum femoral neuropathy. Anesth Analg 80(5):1036, 1995.
68. Vargo MM, Robinson LR, Nicholas JJ, Rulin MC: Postpartum femoral neuropathy: Relic of an earlier era? Arch Phys Med Rehabil 71:591, 1990.
69. Walsh C, Walsh A: Postoperative femoral neuropathy. Surg Gynecol Obstet 174:255, 1992.
70. Schuh A, Werber S, Zeiler G, Craiovan B: Femoral nerve palsy due to excessive granuloma in aseptic cup loosening in cementless total hip arthroplasty. Zentralbl Chir 129:421, 2004.
71. Schuh A, Durr V, Weier H, et al: Delayed paresis of the femoral nerve after total hip arthroplasty associated with hereditary neuropathy with liability to pressure palsies (HNPP). Orthopade 33:836, 2004.
72. Leinung S, Schonfelder M, Wurl P: Inflammatory pseudotumor of the ileopsoas muscle with femoral paralysis caused by massive metal abrasion of a hip endoprosthesis. Chirurg 73:725, 2002.
73. Tani Y, Miyawaki H: Femoral neuropathy caused by reinforcement ring malposition and extruded bone-cement after revision total hip arthroplasty. J Arthroplasty 17:516, 2002.
74. Mihalko WM, Phillips MJ, Krackow KA: Acute sciatic and femoral neuritis following total hip arthroplasty: A case report. J Bone Joint Surg Am 83A:589, 2001.
75. Ha YC, Ahn IO, Jeong ST, et al: Iliacus hematoma and femoral nerve palsy after revision hip arthroplasty: A case report. Clin Orthop Relat Res 385:100, 2001.
76. Eggli S, Hankemayer S, Muller ME: Nerve palsy after leg lengthening in total replacement arthroplasty for developmental dysplasia of the hip. J Bone Joint Surg Br 81:843, 1999.
77. Simmons C, Jr, Izant TH, Rothman RH, et al: Femoral neuropathy following total hip arthroplasty. Anatomic study, case reports, and literature review. J Arthroplasty 6 (Suppl):S57, 1991.
78. Pess GM, Lusskin R, Waugh TR, Battista AE: Femoral neuropathy secondary to pressurized cement in total hip replacement: Treatment by decompression and neurolysis. Report of a case. J Bone Joint Surg Am 69:623, 1987.
79. Weber EW, Daube JR, Coventry MB: Peripheral neuropathies associated with total hip arthroplasty. J Bone Joint Surg Am 58A:66, 1976.
80. Schmalzried TP, Amshutz HC, Dorey FJ: Nerve palsy associated with total hip replacement: Risk factors and prognosis. J Bone Joint Surg Am 73A:1074, 1991.
81. Al-Nasser B, Palacios JL: Femoral nerve injury complicating continuous psoas compartment block. Reg Anesth Pain Med 29:361, 2004.
82. Ghani KR, McMillan R, Paterson-Brown S: Transient femoral nerve palsy following ilio-inguinal nerve blockade for day case inguinal hernia repair. J R Coll Surg Edinb 47:626, 2002.
83. Kornbluth ID, Freedman MK, Sher L, Frederick RW: Femoral, saphenous nerve palsy after tourniquet use: A case report. Arch Phys Med Rehab 84:909, 2003.
84. Goldman JA, Feldberg D, Dicker D, Samuel N, Dekel A: Femoral neuropathy subsequent to abdominal hysterectomy. A comparative study. Eur J Obstet Gynecol Reprod Biol 20:385, 1985.
85. Kvist-Poulsen H, Borel J: Iatrogenic femoral neuropathy subsequent to abdominal hysterectomy: Incidence and prevention. Obstet Gynecol 60:516, 1982.
86. Dillavou ED, Anderson LR, Bernert RA, et al: Lower extremity iatrogenic nerve injury due to compression during intraabdominal surgery. Am J Surg 173:505, 1997.
87. Corbu C, Campodonico F, Traverso P, Carmignani G: Femoral nerve palsy caused by a self-retaining polyretractor during major pelvic surgery. Urol Int 68:66, 2002.
88. Hsieh LF, Liaw ES, Cheng HY, Hong CZ: Bilateral femoral neuropathy after vaginal hysterectomy. Arch Phys Med Rehabil 79:1018, 1998.
89. Dillavou ED, Anderson LR, Bernert RA, et al: Lower extremity iatrogenic nerve injury due to compression during intraabdominal surgery. Am J Surg 173:504, 1997.
90. Schottland JR: Femoral neuropathy from inadvertent suturing of the femoral nerve. Neurology 47:844, 1996.
91. Balz JB: Retractor-induced femoral neuropathy. Dis Colon Rectum 39 591, 1996.
92. Brasch RC, Bufo AJ, Kreienberg PF, Johnson GP: Femoral neuropathy secondary to the use of a self-retaining retractor. Report of three cases and review of the literature. Dis Colon Rectum 38:1115, 1995.
93. Dalmau Obrador J, Aguilar Babera M, Marco Igual M: Bilateral femoral neuropathy after abdominal hysterectomy. Neurologia 1:266, 1986.
94. [No authors listed.] Femoral neuropathy following tubal microsurgery. Fertil Steril 46:742, 1986.
95. Hassan AA, Reiff RH, Fayez JA: Femoral neuropathy following microsurgical tuboplasty. Fertil Steril 45:889, 1986.
96. Weiss S, Toaff MA, Toaff R: Femoral neuropathy following the use of intra-abdominal retractor. Harefuah 94:226, 1978. [Hebrew]
97. Berger GS: Prevention of femoral neuropathy following abdominal hysterectomy. Am J Obstet Gynecol 125:571, 1976.
98. Georgy FM: Femoral neuropathy following abdominal hysterectomy. Am J Obstet Gynecol 123:819, 1975.
99. Hopper CL, Baker JB: Bilateral femoral neuropathy complicating vaginal hysterectomy. Analysis of contributing factors in 3 patients. Obstet Gynecol 32:543, 1968.
100. Noldus J, Graefen M, Huland H: Major postoperative complications secondary to use of the Bookwalter self-retaining retractor. Urology 60:964, 2002.
101. Sharma KR, Cross J, Santiago F, et al: Incidence of acute femoral neuropathy following renal transplantation. Arch Neurol 59:541, 2002.
102. Dhillon SS, Sarac E: Lumbosacral plexopathy after dual kidney transplantation. Am J Kidney Dis 36:1045, 2000.
103. Chen SS, Lin AT, Chen KK, Chang LS: Femoral neuropathy after pelvic surgery. Urology 46:575, 1995.

104. Kabalin JN: Femoral neuropathy following abdominal operations for genitourinary malignancies. Urology 45:1089, 1995.
105. Monga M, Castaneda-Zuniga WR, Thomas R: Femoral neuropathy following percutaneous nephrolithotomy of a pelvic kidney. Urology 45:1059, 1995.
106. Hall MC, Koch MO, Smith JA, Jr: Femoral neuropathy complicating urologic abdominopelvic procedures. Urology 45:146, 1995.
107. Jog MS, Turley JE, Berry H: Femoral neuropathy in renal transplantation. Can J Neurol Sci 21:38, 1994.
108. Junaid I, Kwan JT, Lord RH: Femoral neuropathy in renal transplantation. Transplantation 56:240, 1993.
109. Arango Toro O, Gelabert Mas A: Femoral neuropathy complicating urologic surgery. Urology 38:394, 1991.
110. Kumar A, Dalela D, Bhandari M, et al: Femoral neuropathy—an unusual complication of renal transplantation. Transplantation 51:1305, 1991.
111. Meech PR: Femoral neuropathy following renal transplantation. Aust N Z J Surg 60:117, 1990.
112. Arango OJ, Gelabert A, Rosales A, et al: Femoral neuropathy after transurethral endoscopic surgery. A rare complication. Actas Urol Esp 11:489, 1987. [Spanish]
113. Vogels M, Buskens F, de Vries J, et al: Femoral neuropathy after renal transplantation. Int J Pediatr Nephrol 8:55, 1987.
114. Yazbeck S, Larbrisseau A, O'Regan S: Femoral neuropathy after renal transplantation. J Urol 134:720, 1985.
115. Probst A, Harder F, Hofer H, Thiel G: Femoral nerve lesion subsequent to renal transplantation. Eur Urol 8:314, 1982.
116. Vaziri ND, Barton CH, Ravikumar GR, et al: Femoral neuropathy: A complication of renal transplantation. Nephron 28:30, 1981.
117. Gombar KK, Gombar S, Singh B, et al: Femoral neuropathy: A complication of the lithotomy position. Reg Anesth 17:306, 1992.
118. Tondare AS, Nadkarni AV, Sathe CH, Dave VB: Femoral neuropathy: A complication of lithotomy position under spinal anaesthesia. Report of three cases. Can Anaesth Soc J 30:84, 1983.
119. Roblee MA: Femoral neuropathy from the lithotomy position: Case report and new leg holder for prevention. Am J Obstet Gynecol 97:871, 1967.
120. Van Hoff J, Shaywitz BA, Seashore JH: Femoral nerve injury following inguinal hernia repair. Pediatr Neurol 1:195, 1985.
121. Pozzati E, Poppi M, Glassi E: Femoral nerve lesion secondary to inguinal herniorrhaphy. Int Surg 67:85, 1982.
122. Gassel MM: A study of femoral nerve conduction time. Arch Neurol 9:607, 1963.
123. Chopra JS, Hurwitz LJ: Femoral nerve conduction in diabetes and chronic occlusive vascular disease. J Neurol Neurosurg Psychiatry 31:28, 1986.
124. Katirji B: Electrodiagnostic approach to the patient with suspected mononeuropathy of the lower extremity. Neurol Clin 20:479, 2002.
125. Lee HJ, Bach JR, DeLisa JA: Medial femoral cutaneous nerve conduction. Am J Phys Med Rehabil 74:305, 1995.
126. Choi IS: Conduction studies of the saphenous nerve in normal subjects and patients with femoral neuropathy. Yonsei Med J 22:49, 1981.
127. Lee HJ, Bach JR, DeLisa JA: Medial femoral cutaneous nerve conduction. Am J Phys Med Rehabil 74:305, 1995.
128. Kuntzer T, van Melle G, Regli F: Clinical and prognostic features in femoral neuropathies Muscle Nerve 20:205, 1997.
129. Gruber H, Peer S, Kovacs P, et al: The ultrasonographic appearance of the femoral nerve and cases of iatrogenic impairment. J Ultrasound Med 22:163, 2003.
130. Dillavou ED, Anderson LR, Bernert RA, et al: Lower extremity iatrogenic nerve injury due to compression during intraabdominal surgery. Am J Surg 173:504, 1997.
131. Eustace S, McCarthy C, O'Byrne J, et al: Computed tomography of the retroperitoneum in patients with femoral neuropathy. Can Assoc Radiol J 45:277, 1994.
132. Giuliani G, Poppi M, Acciarri N, Forti A: CT scan and surgical treatment of traumatic iliacus hematoma with femoral neuropathy: Case report. J Trauma 30:229, 1990.
133. Apter S, Hertz M, Rubinstein ZJ, Morag B: Femoral neuropathy: The role of computed tomography in diagnosis and management in 27 patients. Clin Radiol 40:30, 1989.
134. Woolfitt RA, Brantly PN, Neal RK: CT demonstration of a neurofibrosarcoma causing femoral neuropathy. J Comput Assist Tomogr 6:1013, 1982.
135. Graif M, Olchovsky D, Frankl O, Itzchak Y: Ultrasonic demonstration of iliopsoas hematoma causing femoral neuropathy. Isr J Med Sci 18:967, 1982.
136. Heilbronn YD, Williams VL, Kranzler LI, et al: CT scan of retroperitoneal hematoma with neuropathy. Surg Neurol 12:251, 1979.
137. Simeone JF, Robinson F, Rothman SL, Jaffe CC: Computerized tomographic demonstration of a retroperitoneal hematoma causing femoral neuropathy. Report of two cases. J Neurosurg 47:946, 1977.
138. Brantigan JW, Owens ML, Moody FG: Femoral neuropathy complicating anticoagulant therapy. Am J Surg 132:108, 1976.
139. Chin WS: The syndrome of retroperitoneal hemorrhage and lumbar plexus neuropathy during anticoagulant therapy. South Med J 69:595, 1976.
140. Merrick HW, Zeiss J, Woldenberg LS: Percutaneous decompression for femoral neuropathy secondary to heparin-induced retroperitoneal hematoma: Case report and review of the literature. Am Surg 57:706, 1991.
141. Busis NA: Femoral and obturator neuropathies. Neurol Clin 17:633, 1991.
142. Ertekin C: Saphenous nerve conduction in man. J Neurol Neurosurg Psychiatry 32:530, 1969.
143. Stohr M, Schumm F, Ballier R: Normal sensory conduction in the saphenous nerve in man. Electroencephalogr Clin Neurophysiol 44:172, 1978.
144. Wainapel SF, Kim DJ, Ebel A: Conduction studies of the saphenous nerve in healthy subjects. Arch Phys Med Rehabil 59:316, 1978.
145. Synek,VM, Cowan JC: Saphenous nerve evoked potential and the assessment of intraabdominal lesions of the femoral nerve. Muscle Nerve 6:453, 1983.
146. Tranier S, Durey A, Chevallier B, et al: Value of somatosensory evoked potentials in saphenous entrapment neuropathy. J Neurol Neurosurg Psychiatry 55:461, 1992.
147. Vogel P, Vogel H: Somatosensory cortical potentials evoked by stimulation of leg nerves: Analysis of normal values and variability; diagnostic significance. J Neurol 228:97, 1982.
148. Wartenberg R: Digitalia paresthetica and gonyalgia paresthetica. Neurology 4:106, 1954.

chapter 101

Obturator Neuropathy

Bernard M. Abrams

Obturator neuropathy is an uncommon affliction that can cause medial thigh pain.[1] Although its description as an entrapment neuropathy is historically interesting,[2] the most frequent etiologic agent by far is trauma; and, unfortunately, iatrogenic trauma is the most common cause.

ANATOMY

Anatomically, the obturator nerve is formed within the psoas muscle by the ventral divisions of the ventral primary rami of the L2, L3, and L4 nerve roots (Fig. 101–1). It shares fibers from the same nerve roots as the femoral nerve. After descending through the psoas muscle, it emerges from the medial border of the psoas at the pelvic brim immediately anterior to the sacroiliac joint. In the female, it is separated from the ovary by a thin layer of peritoneum. The nerve then curves downward and forward around the pelvic cavity wall to emerge through the obturator foramen, where it is in company with the obturator vessels. The obturator canal is an osseofibrous canal formed by a hiatus in the obturator membrane up against the pubic bone. Of the anatomic structures in the canal, the nerve is the closest to the bone, leading to its purported involvement in osteitis pubis (Fig. 101–2).[3] In the canal, it divides into anterior and posterior branches.[4] The anterior branch innervates the adductor longus, adductor brevis, and gracilis muscles. The supply to the pectineus muscles is variable. The posterior branch supplies the obturator externus and adductor magnus muscles. The adductor brevis muscle may be supplied by either branch. Articular branches are given off to the hip joint.[4] There is sensory innervation of a limited area of the upper medial thigh. Because of its position the nerve is seldom directly traumatized.

CLINICAL PRESENTATION

Although seldom damaged alone in extensive trauma, the hallmarks of obturator neuropathy are pain and weakness of the adductor musculature. The patient cannot stabilize the hip joint, and leg weakness is usually the predominant complaint, but paresthesias, often painful, may be the main complaint. Maneuvers that stretch the nerve such as extension or lateral leg movement may increase the pain. In an obturator hernia, if still mobile, an increase in abdominal pressure as in coughing, sneezing, or straining will increase the pain.[5]

Careful examination of the strength of the hip adductors and quadriceps muscle, the patella reflexes, as well as the sensory deficit (Fig. 101–3) may serve to differentiate obturator neuropathy from femoral neuropathy, but the two nerves are often damaged together because of their shared nerve root and lumbar plexus origin and course in pelvic trauma or hip surgery. Lumbar radiculopathy of L3 and/or L4 may also account for the weakness and shifts the focus to the lumbar spine for pathology.

ETIOLOGY

Broad categories of etiology are pelvic fractures, complications of hip replacements, malignant pelvic mass or endometriosis (note its proximity to the ovary in the female), obturator hernia, complications of labor, lithotomy position, entrapment, and as a complication in the newborn (Table 101–1).

As stated earlier, isolated obturator nerve injuries are relatively rare and pelvic fractures and penetrating injuries such as gunshot wounds much more frequently injure multiple nerves and/or other neural structures, such as nerve roots or the lumbar plexus.[6-9] The obturator nerve can be injured during hip or pelvic surgery as a result of stretch, retractor compression, injury due to cement (encasement or thermal injury), or electrocautery.[10-14] Massive pelvic hemorrhage, either spontaneously or during gynecologic surgery, can cause obturator neuropathy.[15,16] Obturator hernias can cause pain down the medial thigh, especially with Valsalva maneuvers.[17,18] The lithotomy position has been implicated in obturator neuropathies both in urologic and gynecologic surgeries.[19-23] It also has been reported during pregnancy and delivery, but here multiple factors are at play, including the fetal head, forceps application, hematoma, or other trauma occasioned by cesarean section or improper lithotomy position.[24,25] Malignant tumors can compress or invade the obturator nerve, as can endometriosis and laparoscopic pelvic lymphadenectomy, making visualization of the nerve mandatory during electrocautery.[26,27] Aneurysm of the hypogastric artery can also produce compression of the obturator nerve.[6,28,29]

Obturator neuropathy caused by cardiac catheterization is a special case of retroperitoneal hematoma formation compressing the nerve.[30,31] Bradshaw and associates[32] reported on 32 athletes who had entrapment of the obturator nerve by

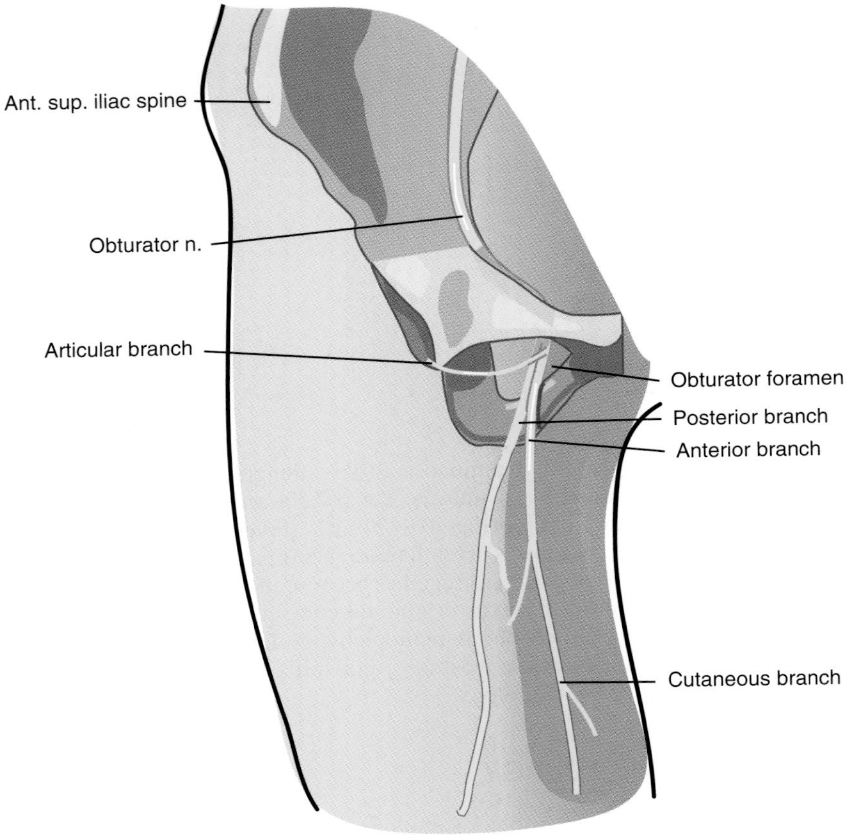

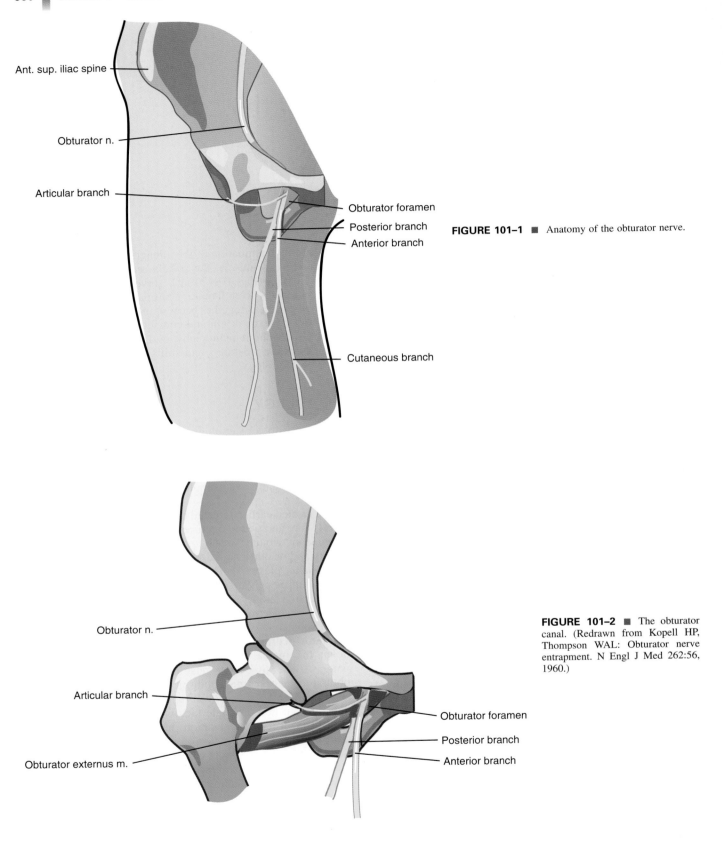

FIGURE 101–1 ■ Anatomy of the obturator nerve.

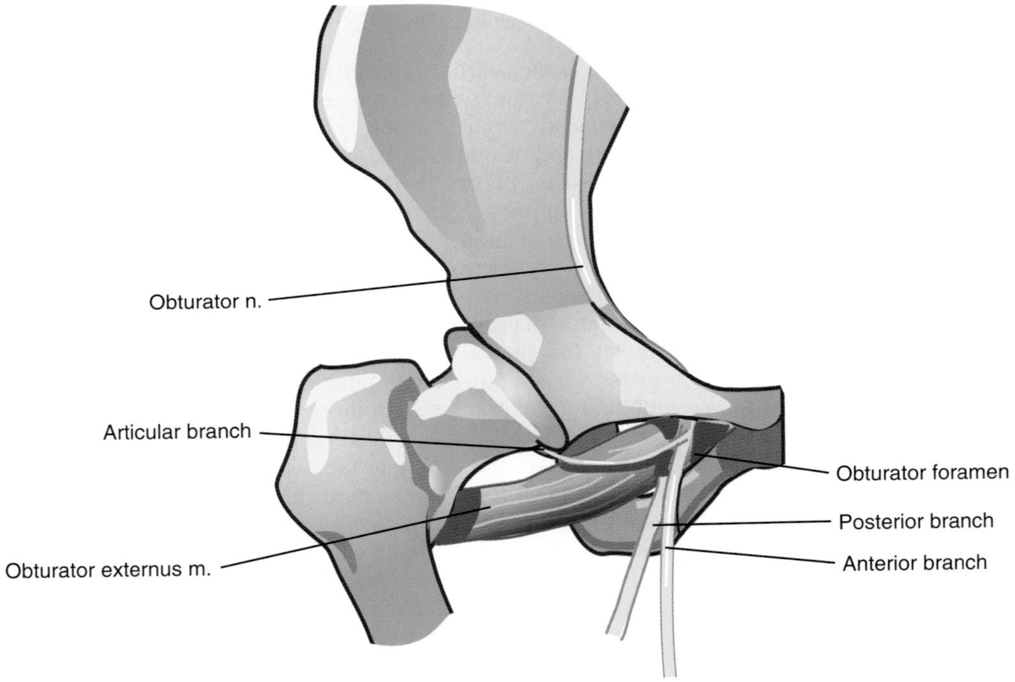

FIGURE 101–2 ■ The obturator canal. (Redrawn from Kopell HP, Thompson WAL: Obturator nerve entrapment. N Engl J Med 262:56, 1960.)

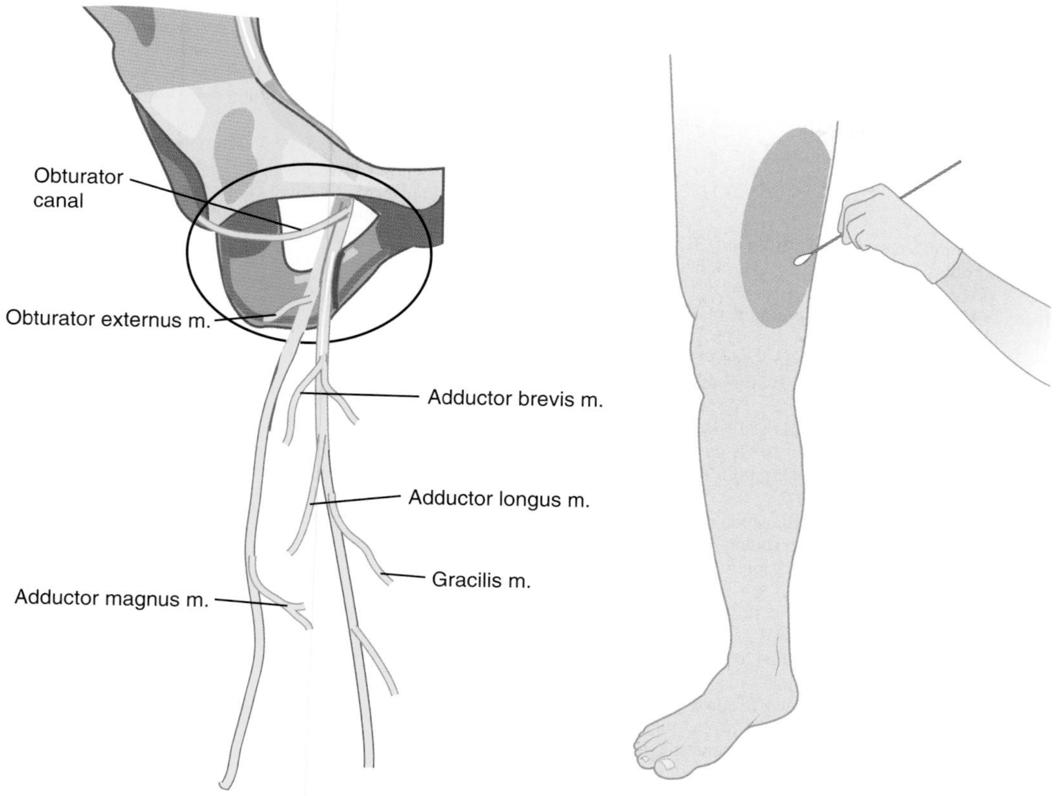

FIGURE 101–3 ■ Sensory testing of the obturator nerve.

Table 101–1

Causes of Obturator Neuropathy

- Pelvic fractures
- Direct penetrating injuries
- Pelvis malignancies
- Endometriosis
- Complications of hip arthroplasty including encasement by cement
- Obturator hernia
- Obturator nerve entrapment
- Lithotomy position
- Pregnancy and labor (multiple mechanisms)
- Pelvic hemorrhage (including as a complication of procedures such as cardiac catheterization)
- Obturator palsy of the newborn

fascial entrapment of the nerve entering the thigh with distal pain radiating along the medial thigh induced by exercise with surgical relief by excising the thickened fascia over the short adductor muscle. All of the afflicted athletes participated in sports with a "leg predominance" such as soccer and rugby. Idiopathic obturator neuropathy has also been described.[33] Finally, infants are not immune to obturator neuropathy, and one case possibly related to prolonged abnormal intrauterine leg position has been reported.[34]

DIAGNOSIS

The clinical examination and the setting in which the neuropathy arose generally suggest its cause. Electromyography is essential for confirmation of anatomic location, and the differential diagnosis includes much more common multiple neuropathies, lumbar plexopathies, and L3-4 nerve root lesions. For possible retroperitoneal hemorrhage or tumor, CT, MRI, and ultrasonography are helpful.[35,36] Angiography may be necessary in the patient suspected of having a hypogastric artery aneurysm.

The question of the possible relationship to diabetes mellitus arises in the same context as that for femoral neuropathy. Muscles innervated by the obturator nerve are almost invariably affected by so-called diabetic amyotrophy. Two reports in the literature[37,38] invoke diabetes as a cause of obturator neuropathy, but this, as in the case of femoral neuropathy, remains problematical. The reader is referred to a recent retrospective study that analyzed causes and outcomes.[39]

TREATMENT

Obvious inciting lesions should be treated with such curative measures as are available, that is, surgery for management of tumors, hemorrhage, or entrapment as indicated. In particular, when hip arthroplasty has been carried out, after a period of observation, re-exploration may be indicated because of the possibility of the nerve's being encased in cement. Persistent pain requires pharmacologic treatment such as with gabapentin, pregabalin, other membrane stabilizers (newer anticonvulsants), tricyclic antidepressants, or other medications useful in neuropathic pain. One report in the literature seems to indicate some promise in the treatment of intractable pain, but further evaluation is warranted.[40]

References

1. Waldman SD: The obturator nerve. In Waldman SD: Atlas of Uncommon Pain Syndromes. Philadelphia, WB Saunders, 2003, pp 197-199.
2. Kopell HP, Thompson WAL: Obturator nerve entrapment. N Engl J Med 262:56, 1960.
3. Kopell HP, Thompson WAL: Obturator nerve. In Kopell HP, Thompson WAL: Peripheral Entrapment Neuropathies. Baltimore, Williams & Wilkins, 1963, pp 610-663.
4. Stewart JD: The obturator nerve. In Stewart JD (ed): Focal Peripheral Neuropathies, 2nd ed. New York, Raven Press, 1993, pp 407-410.
5. Mondelli M, Gianni F, Guazzi G, Corbelli P: Obturator neuropathy due to obturator hernia. Muscle Nerve 26:291, 2002.
6. Dawson DM, Hallett M, Wilbourn AJ: Miscellaneous uncommon syndromes of the lower extremity. In Dawson DM, Hallett M, Wilbourn AJ: Entrapment Neuropathies, 3rd ed. Philadelphia, Lippincott-Raven, 1998, pp 369-379.
7. Patterson FP, Morton KS: Neurological complications of fractures and dislocations of the pelvis. J Trauma 12:1013, 1972.
8. Stoehr M: Traumatic and postoperative lesions of the lumbosacral plexus. Arch Neurol 35:757, 1978.
9. Busis NA: Femoral and obturator neuropathies. Neurol Clin 17:633, 1999.
10. Grant P, Roise O, Ovre S: Obturator neuropathy due to intrapelvic extrusion of cement during total hip replacement—report of patients. Acta Orthop Scand 72:537, 2001.
11. Siliski JM, Scott RD: Obturator-nerve palsy resulting from intrapelvic extrusion of cement during hip replacement: Report of four cases. J Bone Joint Surg Am 67:1225, 1985.
12. Melamed NB, Satya-Murti S: Obturator neuropathy after total hip replacement. Ann Neurol 13:578, 1983.
13. Bischoff C, Schonle PW: Obturator nerve injuries during intra-abdominal surgery. Clin Neurol Neurosurg 93:73, 1991.
14. Schmalzreid TP, Amstutz HC, Dorey FJ: Nerve palsy associated with total hip replacement: Risk factors and prognosis. J Bone Joint Surg Am 73:1074, 1991.
15. Cardosi RJ, Cox CS, Hoffman MS: Postoperative neuropathies after major pelvic surgery. Obstet Gynecol 100:240, 2002.
16. Finan MA, Fiorica JV, Hoffman MS, et al: Massive pelvic hemorrhage during gynecologic cancer surgery: "Pack and go back." Gynecol Oncol 62:390, 1996.
17. Mondelli M, Gianni F, Guazzi G, Corbelli P: Obturator neuropathy due to obturator hernia. Muscle Nerve 26:291, 2002.
18. Mumenthaler M: Some clinical aspects of peripheral nerve lesions. Eur Neurol 2:257, 1969.
19. Litwiller JP, Wells RE Jr, Halliwill JR, et al: Effect of lithotomy position on strain of the obturator and lateral femoral cutaneous nerves. Clin Anat 17:45, 2004.
20. Warner MA, Warner DO, Harper CM, et al: Lower extremity neuropathies associated with lithotomy positions. Anesthesiology 93:938, 2000.
21. Crews DA, Dohlman LE: Obturator neuropathy after multiple genitourinary procedures. Urology 29:504, 1987.
22. Dimachkie MM, Ohanian S, Groves MD, Vriesendorp FJ: Peripheral nerve injury after brief lithotomy for transurethral collagen injection. Urology 56:669, 2000.
23. Pellegrino MJ, Johson EW: Bilateral obturator nerve injuries during urologic surgery. Arch Phys Med Rehabil 69:46, 1988.
24. Lindner A, Schulte-Mattler W, Zierz S: Postpartum obturator nerve syndrome: Case report and review of the nerve compression syndrome during pregnancy and delivery. Zentralbl Gynäkol 119:93, 1997.
25. Warfield CA: Obturator neuropathy after forceps delivery. Obstet Gynecol 64:47S, 1984.
26. Redwine DB, Sharpe DR: Endometriosis of the obturator nerve: A case report. J Reprod Med 35:434, 1990.
27. Fishman JR, Moran ME, Carey RW: Obturator neuropathy after laparoscopic pelvic lymphadenectomy. Urology 42:198, 1993.
28. Kleiner JB, Thorne RP: Obturator neuropathy caused by an aneurysm of the hypogastric artery. J Bone Joint Surg Am 71:1408, 1989.
29. Krupski WC, Bass A, Rosenberg GD, et al: The elusive isolated hypogastric artery aneurysm: Novel presentations. J Vasc Surg 10:557, 1989.
30. Kent KC, Moscucci M, DiMattia ST, Skillman JJ: Neuropathy after cardiac catheterization: Incidence, clinical patterns and outcome. J Vasc Surg 19:1008, 1994.
31. Dingeman RD, Mutz SB: Hemorrhagic neuropathy of the sciatic, femoral and obturator nerves: Case report and review of the literature. Clin Orthop 27:133, 1977.
32. Bradshaw C, McCrory P Bell S, Brukner P: Obturator nerve entrapment: A cause of groin pain in athletes. Am J Sports Med 25:402, 1997.
33. Saurenmann P, Brand S: Obturator neuralgia (Howship-Romberg phenomenon). Schweiz Med Wochenschir 114:1462, 1984.
34. Craig WS, Clark JMP: Obturator palsy in the newborn. Arch Dis Child 37:661, 1962.
35. Rivaasseau T, Vandermarcq P, Boissonnot L, et al: Hematoma of the psoas: Comparative diagnostic contributions of ultrasound and x-ray computed tomography. J Radiol 66:731, 1985.
36. Lazaro RP, Brinker RA, Weiss JJ, Olejniczak S: Femoral and obturator neuropathy secondary to retroperitoneal hemorrhage: Value of the CT scan. Comput Tomogr 5:221, 1981.
37. Hogenhuis LAH, Rose FC: The classification of diabetic neuropathy. Neuroepidemiology 3:169, 1984.
38. Spritz N: Nerve disease in diabetes mellitus. Med Clin North Am 62:787, 1978.
39. Sorenson EJ, Chen JJ, Daube JR: Obturator neuropathy: Causes and outcomes. Muscle Nerve 25:605, 2002.
40. Mukubo Y, Sato K, Kawamata M: Effective radiofrequency lesioning for obturator neuropathy. Masui 52:990, 2003.

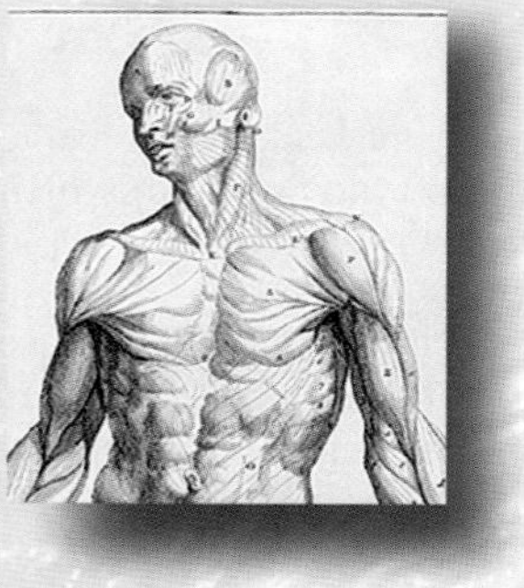

Part K

Pain Syndromes of the Knee and Distal Lower Extremity

chapter 102

Painful Conditions of the Knee

Steven D. Waldman

Knee pain is one of the most common reasons that patients seek medical attention from their primary care physicians, orthopedists, rheumatologists, and pain management specialists. Knee pain can arise from the joint or the periarticular tissues (e.g., the bursae and tendons) or may be referred from the hip joint, femur, and/or proximal tibia and fibula. The largest joint in the body, the knee is subject to an amazing array of forces and injuries.[1] In this chapter an overview is presented of some of the more common knee pain syndromes encountered in clinical practice.

FUNCTIONAL ANATOMY OF THE KNEE

To accurately diagnose and treat knee pain, the clinician must have a clear understanding of the functional anatomy of the knee. The knee is not just a simple hinge joint that flexes and extends. The largest joint in the body in terms of articular surface and joint volume, the knee is capable of amazingly complex movements that encompass highly coordinated flexion and extension. The knee joint is best thought of as a cam capable of locking in a stable position. Even the simplest movements of the knee involve an elegantly coordinated rolling and gliding movement of the femur on the tibia. Because of the complex nature of these movements, the knee is extremely susceptible to functional abnormalities with relatively minor alterations in the anatomy from arthritis or damage to the cartilage or ligaments.

While both clinicians and laypersons think of the knee joint as a single joint, from the viewpoint of understanding its functional anatomy it is more helpful to think of the knee as two separate but interrelated joints: the femoral-tibial and the femoral-patellar joints (Fig. 102–1). Both joints share a common synovial cavity, and dysfunction of one joint can easily affect the function of the other.

The femoral-tibial joint is made up of the articulation of the femur and the tibia. Interposed between the two bones are two fibrocartilaginous structures known as the medial and lateral menisci (Fig. 102–2). The menisci serve to help transmit the forces placed on the femur across the joint onto the tibia. They possess the property of plasticity in that they are able to change their shape in response to the variable forces placed on the joint through its complex range of motion. The

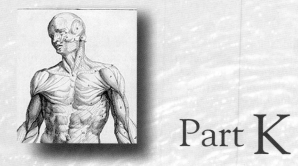

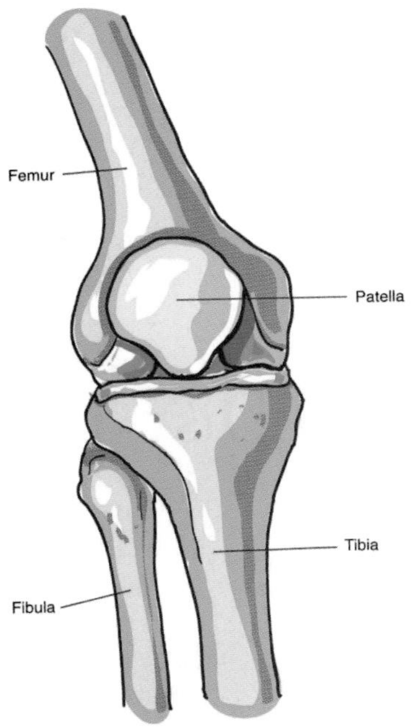

FIGURE 102–1 ■ Functional anatomy of the knee is easier to understand if it is viewed as two separate but interrelated joints—the femoral-tibial and the femoral-patellar joints. (From Waldman SD: Physical Diagnosis of Pain: An Atlas of Signs and Symptoms. Philadelphia, WB Saunders, 2006, p 322.)

medial and lateral menisci are relatively avascular and receive the bulk of their nourishment from the synovial fluid, which means that there is little potential for healing when these important structures are traumatized.

The femoral-patellar joint's primary function is to use the patella, which is a large sesamoid bone embedded in the quadriceps tendon, to improve the mechanical advantage of the quadriceps muscle. The medial and lateral articular surfaces of the sesamoid interface with the articular groove of the femur (Fig. 102–3). In extension, only the superior pole of the patella is in contact with the articular surface of the femur. As the knee flexes, the patella is drawn superiorly into the trochlear groove of the femur.

The majority of the knee joint's stability comes from the ligaments and muscles surrounding it with little contribution from the bony elements. The main ligaments of the knee are the anterior and posterior cruciate ligaments, which provide much of the anteroposterior stability of the knee, and the medial and lateral collateral ligaments, which provide much of the valgus and varus stability (Fig. 102–4). All of these ligaments also help prevent excessive rotation of the tibia in either direction. There are also a number of secondary ligaments that add further stability to this inherently unstable joint.

The main extensor of the knee is the quadriceps muscle, which attaches to the patella via the quadriceps tendon.

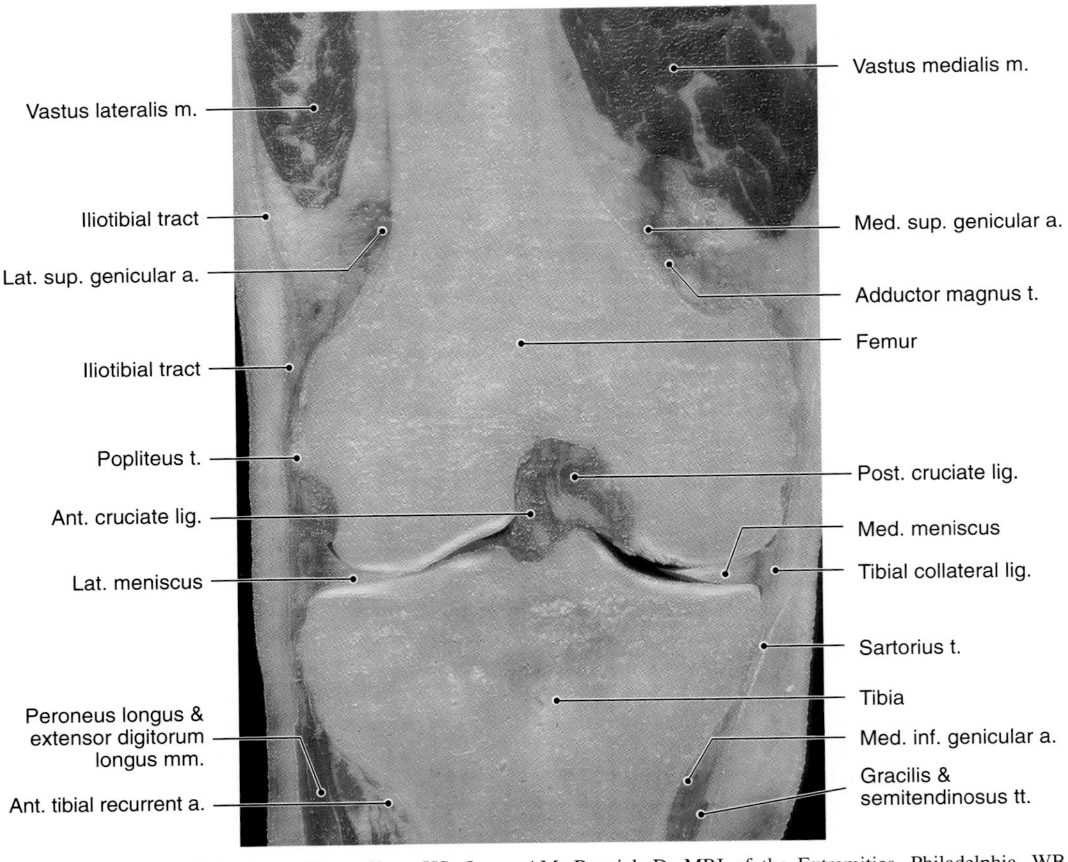

FIGURE 102–2 ■ Coronal view of the knee. (From Kang HS, Joong AM, Resnick D: MRI of the Extremities. Philadelphia, WB Saunders, 2002, p 301.)

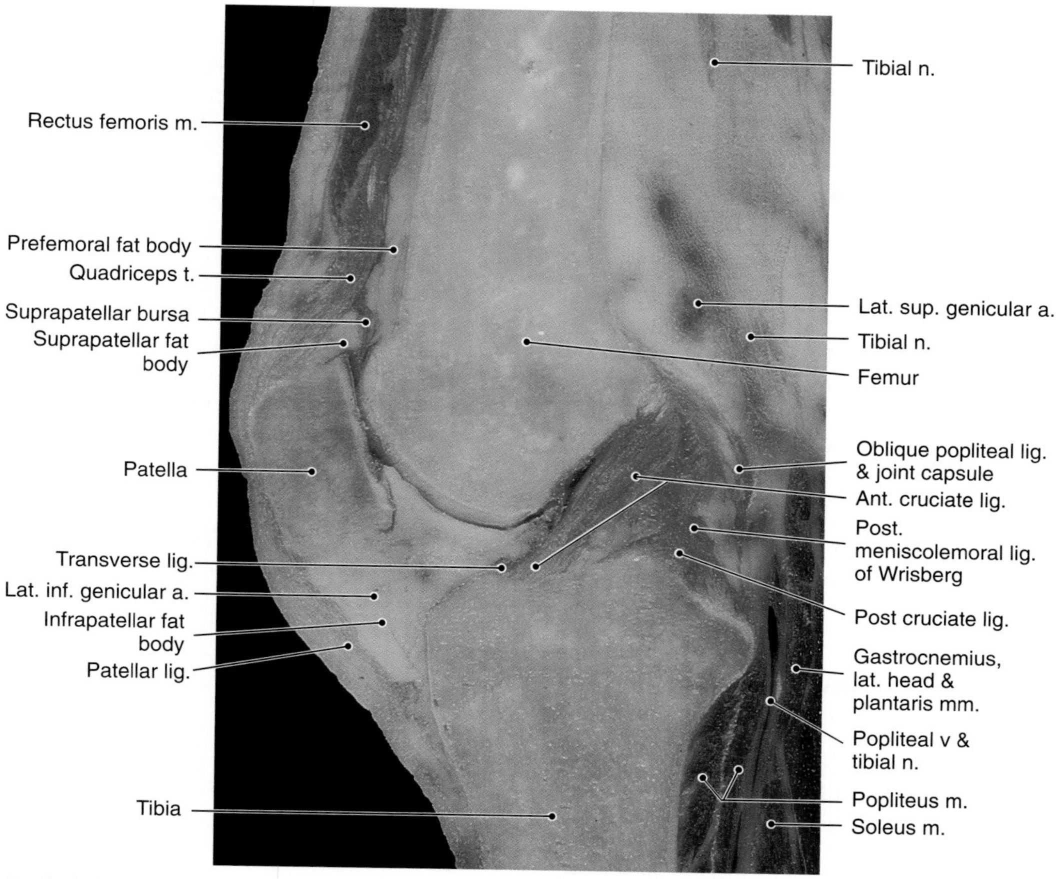

FIGURE 102–3 ■ Sagittal view of the knee. (From Kang HS, Joong AM, Resnick D: MRI of the Extremities. Philadelphia, WB Saunders, 2002, p 341.)

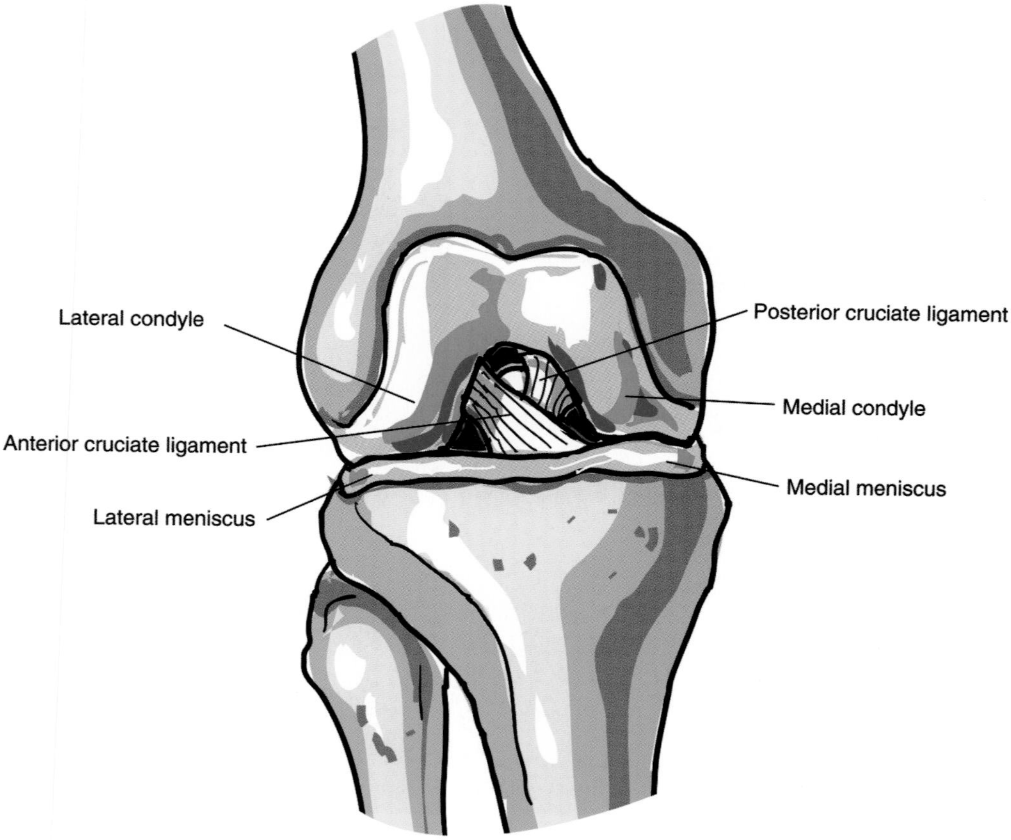

FIGURE 102–4 ■ The main ligaments of the knee. (From Waldman SD: Physical Diagnosis of Pain: An Atlas of Signs and Symptoms. Philadelphia, WB Saunders, 2006, p 325.)

Fibrotendinous expansions of the vastus medialis and vastus lateralis insert into the sides of the patella and are subject to strain and sprain. The hamstrings are the main flexors of the hip, along with help from the gastrocnemius, sartorius, and gracilis muscles. Medial rotation of the flexed knee is via the medial hamstring muscle, and lateral rotation of the knee is controlled by the biceps femoris muscle.

The knee is well endowed with a variety of bursa to facilitate movement. Bursae are formed from synovial sacs whose purpose it is to allow easy sliding of muscles and tendons across one another at areas of repeated movement. These synovial sacs are lined with a synovial membrane that is invested with a network of blood vessels that secrete synovial fluid. Inflammation of the bursa results in an increase in the production of synovial fluid with swelling of the bursal sac. With overuse or misuse, these bursae may become inflamed, enlarged, and, on rare occasions, infected (Fig. 102–5). Given that the knee shares a common synovial cavity, inflammation of one bursa can cause significant dysfunction and pain of the entire knee.

COMMON PAINFUL CONDITIONS OF THE KNEE

It is the initial general physical examination of the knee that guides the clinician in narrowing his or her differential diagnosis and helps suggest which specialized physical examination maneuvers and laboratory and radiographic testing will aid in confirming the cause of the patient's knee pain and dysfunction.[2] For the clinician to make best use of the initial information gleaned from the general physical examination of the knee, a grouping of the common causes of knee pain and dysfunction is exceedingly helpful. Although no classification of knee pain and dysfunction can be all inclusive or all exclusive owing to the frequently overlapping and multifactoral nature of knee pathology, Table 102–1 should help improve the diagnostic accuracy of the clinician confronted with the patient complaining of knee pain and dysfunction and help the clinician avoid overlooking less common diagnoses.

The list of disease processes in Table 102–1 is by no means comprehensive, but it does aid the clinician in organizing the potential sources of pathology presenting as knee pain and dysfunction. It should be noted that the most commonly missed categories of knee pain and the categories that most often result in misadventures in diagnosis and treatment are the last three categories. The knowledge of this potential pitfall should help the clinician keep these sometimes overlooked causes of knee pain and dysfunction in the differential diagnosis.

A RATIONAL APPROACH TO KNEE PAIN

The Targeted History

The starting point for the clinician faced with the patient with knee pain is to obtain a targeted history and perform a targeted physical examination of the affected knee or knees based on that history. Salient features of the targeted history are summarized in Table 102–2. The relevance of each is discussed briefly.

Acute or Chronic?

The onset of acute knee pain in the absence of trauma is a cause for concern in that many of the diseases associated with acute knee pain can cause significant damage to the joint if not promptly diagnosed and treated.[3] The connective tissue diseases, septic arthritis, the crystal arthropathies, and

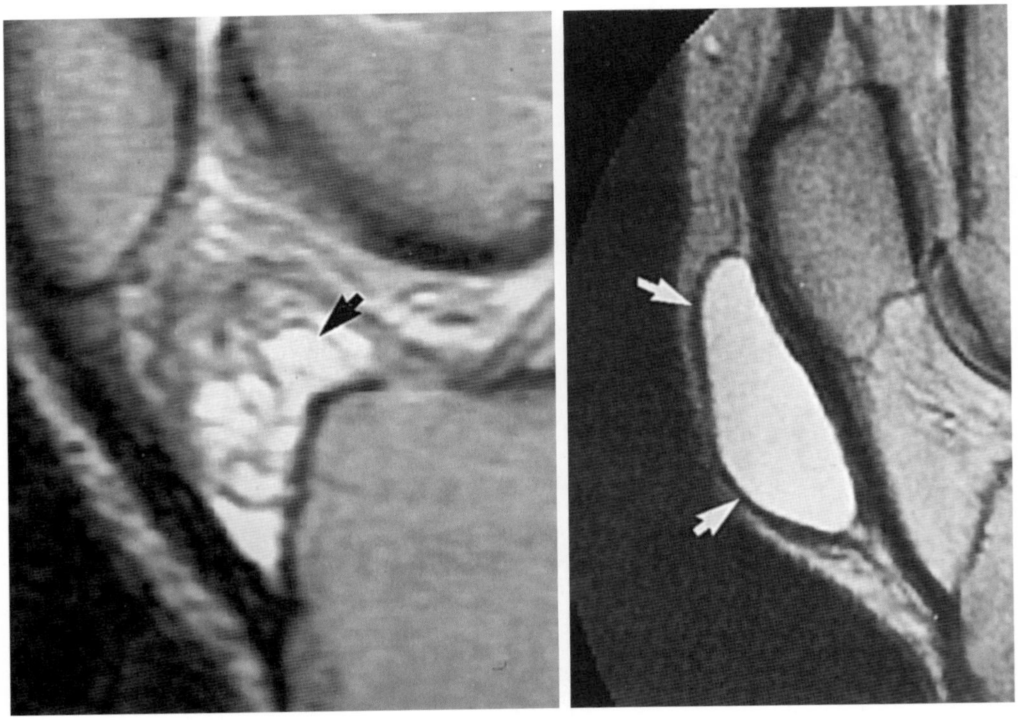

FIGURE 102–5 ■ **A,** Deep infrapatellar bursitis. A sagittal T2-weighted (TR/TE, 2300/70) spin-echo MR image shows fluid of high signal intensity *(arrow)* in the deep infrapatellar bursa. **B,** Prepatellar bursitis. A sagittal T2-weighted (TR/TE, 2000/80) spin-echo MR image shows fluid of high signal intensity *(arrows)* in the prepatellar bursa. (**A,** Courtesy of M Zlatkin, MD, Hollywood, FL; **B,** courtesy of E. M. Bellon, MD, Cleveland, OH; from Resnick D [ed]: Diagnosis of Bone and Joint Disorders, 4th ed. Philadelphia, WB Saunders, 2002, p 3285.)

Table 102–1

Classification of Painful Conditions Affecting the Knee

Knee Pain Resulting from Localized Bony or Joint Space Pathology
Fracture
Primary bone tumor
Primary synovial tissue tumor
Joint instability
Localized arthritis
Osteophyte formation
Joint space infection
Hemarthrosis
Villonodular synovitis
Intra-articular foreign body
Osgood-Schlatter disease
Chronic dislocation of the patella
Patellofemoral pain syndrome
Patella alta
Knee Pain Resulting from Periarticular Pathology
Bursitis
Tendinitis
Adhesive capsulitis
Joint instability
Muscle strain
Muscle sprain
Periarticular infection not involving joint space
Knee Pain Resulting from Systemic Disease
Rheumatoid arthritis
Collagen vascular disease
Reiter syndrome
Gout
Other crystal arthropathies
Charcot's neuropathic arthritis
Knee Pain Resulting from Sympathetically Mediated Pain
Causalgia
Reflex sympathetic dystrophy
Knee Pain Referred from Other Body Areas
Lumbar plexopathy
Lumbar radiculopathy
Lumbar spondylosis
Fibromyalgia
Myofascial pain syndromes
Inguinal hernia
Entrapment neuropathies
Intrapelvic tumors
Retroperitoneal tumors

hemarthrosis in the anticoagulated patient are just a few of the diseases that can permanently damage a knee. Any acute knee pain associated with fever or constitutional symptoms or occurring in an anticoagulated patient should be taken seriously and not automatically attributed to "arthritis."

Age of the Patient

The age of the patient can provide significant direction to the clinician's search for a diagnosis. Table 102–3 provides a grouping of the most common causes of knee pain in different age groups. The presence of knee pain in childhood and early adolescence in the absence of trauma is a cause for concern and should not be attributed to "growing pains."

Table 102–2

Targeted History for Knee Pain

Acute or chronic
Age of patient
History of trauma
Fever
Pain in other joints
Rash
Muscle weakness
Other constitutional symptoms (e.g., malaise, anorexia)
Recent weight gain or loss
Addition of any new medications
Use of anticoagulants
Recent administration of corticosteroids
Recent tapering of corticosteroids
Recent tick bite

Presence of Trauma

Traumatic knee pain is common. Many knee pain syndromes after trauma can be managed conservatively. However, the clinician should remember that many cannot. Early use of MRI of the traumatic knee serves two purposes: (1) It allows the clinician to aggressively rehabilitate those knees in which no internal derangement has be identified, and (2) it allows rapid surgical treatment of those patients suffering from significant ligamentous and cartilaginous injuries before they do more damage to an already compromised joint.[3-5]

Fever

Acute knee pain and fever should be considered a dangerous combination.[6] Although some acute febrile illness such as streptococcal pharyngitis may have large joint arthralgias as part of their constellation of symptoms, the clinician must rule out the septic knee joint, the collagen vascular diseases, and Lyme disease before assuming that the fever and joint pain are unrelated. In younger patients, rheumatic fever must always be considered in the differential diagnosis of knee pain in the presence of fever.

Polyarthralgias

The patient presenting with knee pain who also complains of pain in other joints is a cause for concern. Although in the older, otherwise healthy patient, osteoarthritis is the most common reason for this clinical presentation, the clinician should be careful to avoid jumping to this conclusion without careful consideration.[7] The connective tissue diseases including polymyalgia rheumatica are a common cause of polyarthralgias in older patients.[8] Polyarthralgias in the younger patient should point the clinician toward the diagnosis of juvenile rheumatoid arthritis, among others.

Rash

The presence of rash and knee pain should suggest a number of potentially problematic diseases, such as Lyme disease and

Table 102–3

Common Causes of Knee Pain in Different Age Groups

	Cause		
Age group	***Intra-articular***	***Periarticular***	***Referred***
Childhood (2–10 years)	Juvenile chronic arthritis Osteochondritis dissecans Septic arthritis Torn discoid lateral meniscus	Osteomyelitis	Perthe's disease Transient synovitis of the hip
Adolescence (10–18 years)	Osteochondritis dissecans Torn meniscus Anterior knee pain syndrome Patellar malalignment	Osgood-Schlatter's disease Sinding-Larsen-Johansson Syndrome Osteomyelitis Tumors	Slipped upper femoral epiphysis
Early adulthood (18–30 years)	Torn meniscus Instability Anteroir knee pain syndrome Inflammatory conditions	Overuse syndromes Bursitis	Rare
Adulthood (30–50 years)	Degenerate meniscal tears Early degeneration following injury or meniscectomy Inflammatory arthropathies	Bursitis Tendinitis	Degenerative hip disease secondary to hip dysplasia or injury
Older age (>50 years)	Osteoarthritis Inflammatory arthropathies	Bursitis Tendinitis	Osteoarthritis of the hip

the connective tissue diseases, especially systemic lupus erythematosus and dermatomyositis.[9] In younger patients, it is often the rash that is a harbinger of the onset of a collagen vascular disease or rheumatic fever. Gonococcal arthritis may also present with rash as its first symptom.

Muscle Weakness

The complain of muscle weakness should clue the physician to strongly consider the connective tissue diseases, especially polymyalgia rheumatica and polymyositis.[8] The paraneoplastic syndromes associated with malignancy can also present as large joint pain and muscle weakness. Dermatomyositis in the younger age group is another diagnostic consideration in the setting of knee pain and muscle weakness. It should be remembered that approximately 20% of patients suffering from dermatomyositis will have an occult malignancy, which could include primary or metastatic tumors involving the knee and its related structures.[10]

Constitutional Symptoms

As will all other areas of medicine, the presence of constitutional symptoms should alert the clinician to the potential that a serious systemic illness is present. The association of constitutional symptoms and knee pain should suggest the possibility of primary tumor or metastatic disease, the connective tissue diseases, especially polymyalgia rheumatica, and hypothyroidism.

Recent Weight Gain or Loss

Recent unexplained weight loss in the presence of knee pain has the same implications as the presence of constitutional symptoms as discussed earlier. Recent weight gain may place new forces on the knee joint and exacerbate preexisting problems, such as degenerative arthritis or a torn meniscus.

Addition of New Medications

Many medications can cause joint pain as a side effect unrelated to their intended therapeutic action. In most instance this is an idiosyncratic reaction and will abate with discontinuation of the offending drug. In some, such as procainamide and hydralazine, the drug may cause a syndrome indistinguishable from systemic lupus erythematosus.[11]

Use of Anticoagulants

Anticoagulants and knee pain spell trouble for two reasons: (1) Seemingly minor trauma can cause a hemarthrosis of the knee that if untreated can result in permanent knee damage, and (2) the presence of anticoagulants precludes rapid surgical treatment of otherwise treatable causes of knee pain.[12]

Corticosteroids

Knee pain after treatment with the corticosteroids can be the result of the return of the inflammatory condition originally responsible for the pain or the result of pseudorheumatism.[13] The pain of pseudorheumatism can be quite severe and can also occur with the tapering of corticosteroids used to treat unrelated acute conditions such as poison ivy or in the chronic setting as in the treatment of chronic obstructive pulmonary disease.

Tick Bites

Although uncommon, Lyme disease after a tick bite can cause significant knee pain.[14] Usually associated with a specific rash know as erythema migrans that is the result of an infection

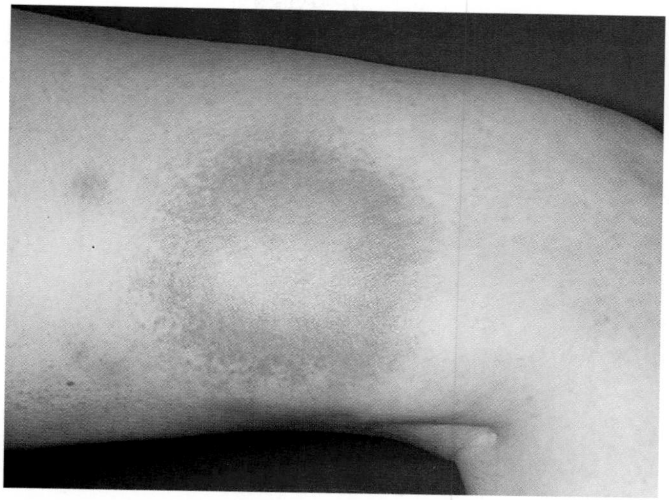

FIGURE 102–6 ■ Erythema migrans. This annular, erythematous lesion developed over a period of 3 weeks around the site of a tick bite. (Reproduced with permission from McKee PH: Pathology of the Skin, 2nd ed. London, CV Mosby, 1996; from Klippel JH, Dieppe PA: Rheumatology, 2nd ed. London, CV Mosby, 1998.)

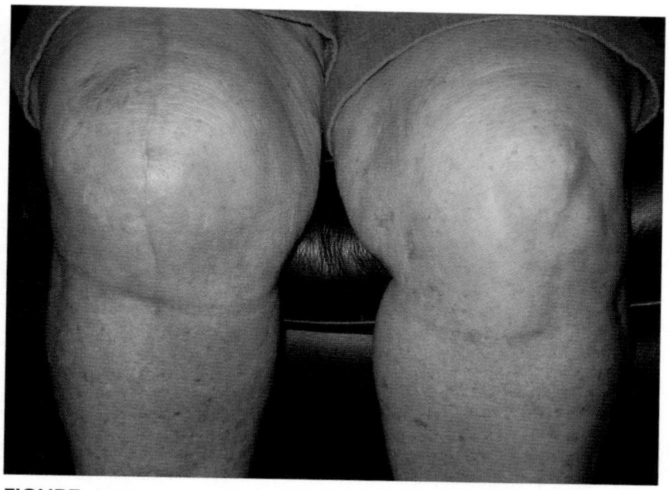

FIGURE 102–7 ■ Visual inspection of the knee. (From Waldman SD: Physical Diagnosis of Pain: An Atlas of Signs and Symptoms. Philadelphia, WB Saunders, 2006, p 326.)

with *Borrelia burgdorferi,* failure to accurately diagnose and treat this uncommon cause of knee pain can result in permanent knee damage (Fig. 102–6).

Targeted Physical Examination

The targeted physical examination when combined with the targeted history will allow the clinician to correctly diagnose the cause of the painful knee in most instances or at least direct further radiographic and laboratory investigations. Because of the lack of soft tissue overlying the knee joint, visual inspection can provide the clinician with important clues to the cause of knee pain and dysfunction. The starting point to visual inspection of the knee is an observation of the patient both standing and walking. The degree of valgus or varus of the knee with weight bearing should be noted as should any other obvious bony deformity (Fig. 102–7). The clinician should then look for evidence of quadriceps wasting, which if identified can be quantified with careful measurement at a point 12 cm above the upper margin of the patella with the knee fully extended. The presence of rubor suggestive of infection and/or swelling above, below, and along side of the patella suggestive of an inflammatory process including bursitis and tendonitis is also noted. The posterior knee is then inspected for presence of a popliteal fossa mass suggestive of Baker's cyst.

Palpation of the Knee

Careful palpation of the knee will often provide the examiner valuable clues to the cause of the patient's knee pain and dysfunction. The examiner palpates the temperature of both knees because localized increase in temperature may indicate inflammation and/or infection. The presence of swelling in the suprapatellar, prepatellar, or infrapatellar regions suggestive of suprapatellar, prepatellar, or infrapatellar bursitis is then identified. Generalized joint effusion may be identified by performing the ballottement test (Fig. 102–8). The bony ele-

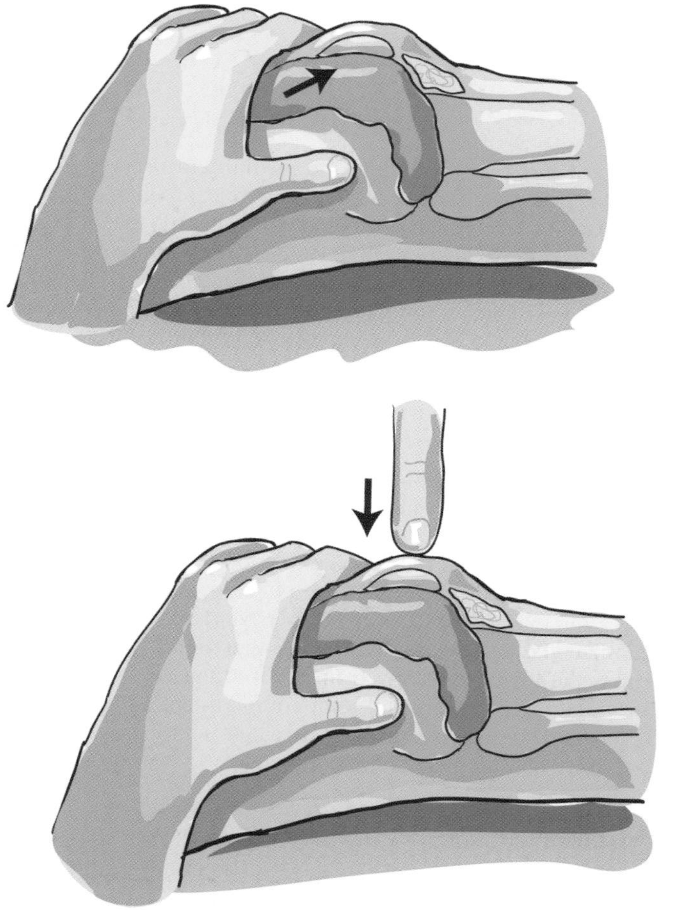

FIGURE 102–8 ■ The ballottement test for large joint effusions. (From Waldman SD: Physical Diagnosis of Pain: An Atlas of Signs and Symptoms. Philadelphia, WB Saunders, 2006, p 332.)

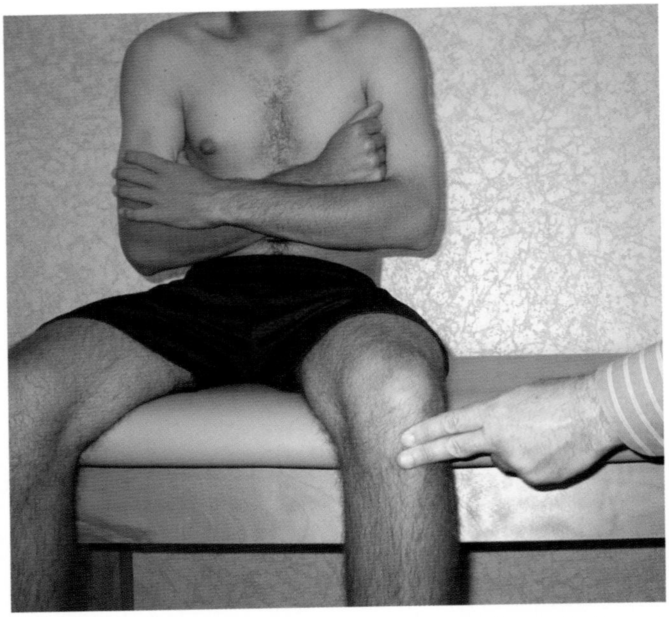

FIGURE 102–9 ■ Palpation of the knee. (From Waldman SD: Physical Diagnosis of Pain: An Atlas of Signs and Symptoms. Philadelphia, WB Saunders, 2006, p 327.)

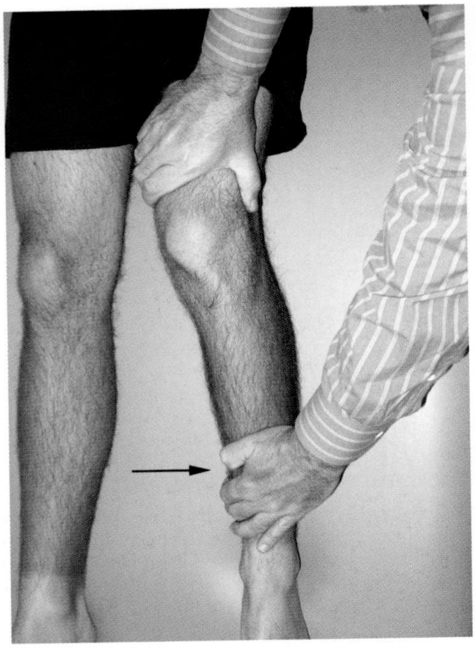

FIGURE 102–10 ■ Valgus stress test for medial collateral ligament integrity. (From Waldman SD: Physical Diagnosis of Pain: An Atlas of Signs and Symptoms. Philadelphia, WB Saunders, 2006, p 334.)

ments of the knee, including the medial and lateral femoral condyles, the patella, and the tibial tubercle, are then palpated. The patellar tendon is then palpated to identify patellar tendonitis or jumper's knee (Fig. 102–9). The popliteal fossa is then palpated for evidence of a mass or Baker's cyst. The knee joint is then ranged through flexion, extension, and medial and lateral rotation to identify crepitus or limitation of range of motion

Valgus Stress Test for Medial Collateral Ligament Integrity

The valgus stress test provides the clinician with useful information regarding the integrity of the medial collateral ligaments. To perform the valgus stress test, the patient is placed in a supine position on the examination table with the knee flexed 35 degrees and the entire affected extremity relaxed. The examiner then places his or her hand above the knee to stabilize the upper leg. With the other hand the examiner forces the lower leg away from the midline while observing for widening of the medial joint compartment and pain (Fig. 102–10). The maneuver is then repeated with the other lower extremity and the results are compared.

Varus Stress Test for Lateral Collateral Ligament Integrity

The varus stress test provides the clinician with useful information regarding the integrity of the lateral collateral ligaments. To perform the varus stress test, the patient is placed in a supine position on the examination table with the knee flexed 35 degrees and the entire affected extremity relaxed. The examiner then places his or her hand above the knee to stabilize the upper leg. With the other hand the examiner forces the lower leg toward from the midline while observing for widening of the medial joint compartment and pain (Fig. 102–11). The maneuver is then repeated with the other lower extremity and the results are compared.

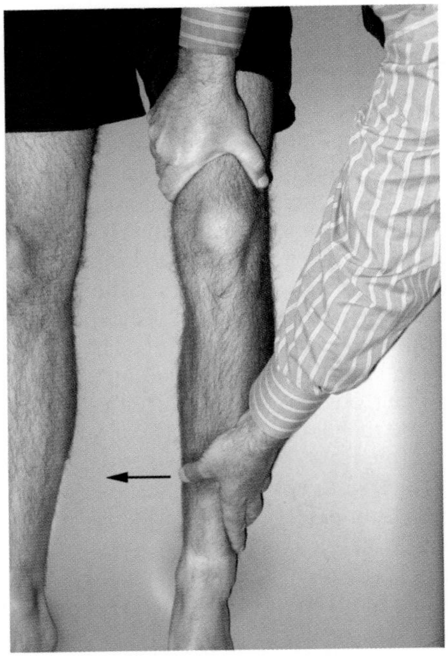

FIGURE 102–11 ■ Varus stress test for lateral collateral ligament integrity. (From Waldman SD: Physical Diagnosis of Pain: An Atlas of Signs and Symptoms. Philadelphia, WB Saunders, 2006, p 335.)

Anterior Drawer Test for Anterior Cruciate Ligament Integrity

The anterior drawer test is useful in helping the clinician assess the integrity of the anterior cruciate ligament. To

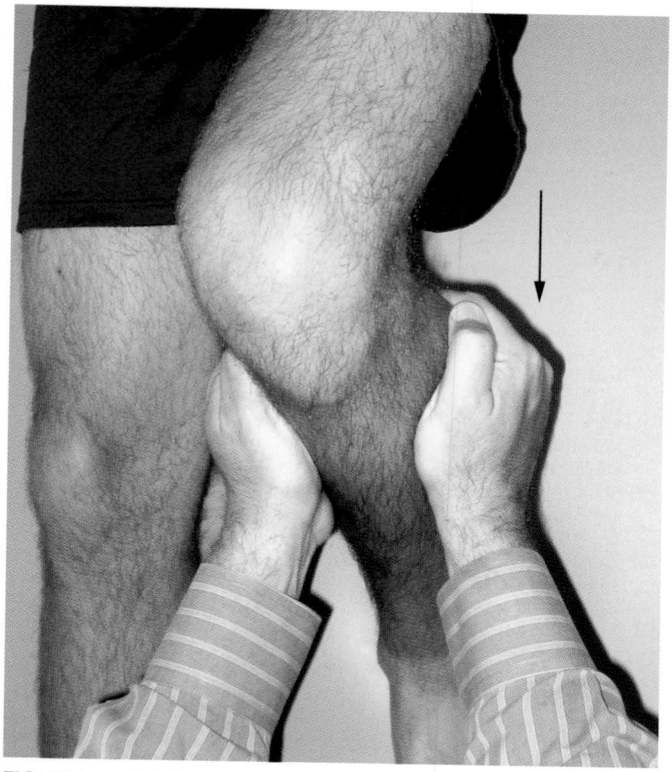

FIGURE 102–12 ■ Anterior drawer test for anterior cruciate ligament integrity. (From Waldman SD: Physical Diagnosis of Pain: An Atlas of Signs and Symptoms. Philadelphia, WB Saunders, 2006, p 336.)

perform the anterior drawer test, the patient is placed in the supine position on the examination table with the patient's head on a pillow to help relax the hamstring muscles. The patient's hip is then flexed to 45 degrees with the patient's foot placed flat on the table. The examiner then grasps the affected leg below the knee with both hands and pulls the lower leg forward while stabilizing the foot (Fig. 102–12). The test is considered positive if there is more than 5 mm of anterior motion.

Posterior Drawer Test for Posterior Cruciate Ligament Integrity

The posterior drawer test is useful in helping the clinician assess the integrity of the posterior cruciate ligament. To perform the posterior drawer test, the patient is placed in the supine position on the examination table with the patient's head on a pillow to help relax the hamstring muscles. The patient's hip is then flexed to 45 degrees with the patient's foot placed flat on the table. The examiner then grasps the affected leg below the knee with both hands and pushes the lower leg backward while stabilizing the foot (Fig. 102–13). The test is considered positive if there is more than 5 mm of posterior motion.

McMurray Test for Torn Meniscus

The McMurray test for torn meniscus can provide the clinician with useful information as to the whether a torn medial or lateral meniscus is responsible for the patient's knee pain. To perform the McMurray test for torn meniscus the examiner has the patient assume the supine position on the examination table with the knee maximally flexed. With the affected extremity relaxed the examiner grasps the ankle and palpates the knee while simultaneously rotating the lower leg internally and externally and extending the knee (Fig. 102–14). The test is considered positive for a torn meniscus

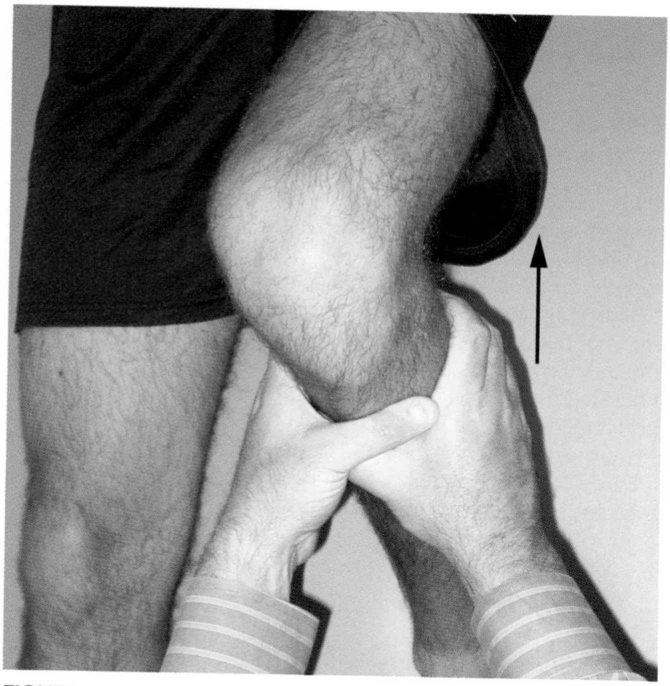

FIGURE 102–13 ■ Posterior drawer test for posterior cruciate ligament integrity. (From Waldman SD: Physical Diagnosis of Pain: An Atlas of Signs and Symptoms. Philadelphia, WB Saunders, 2006, p 337.)

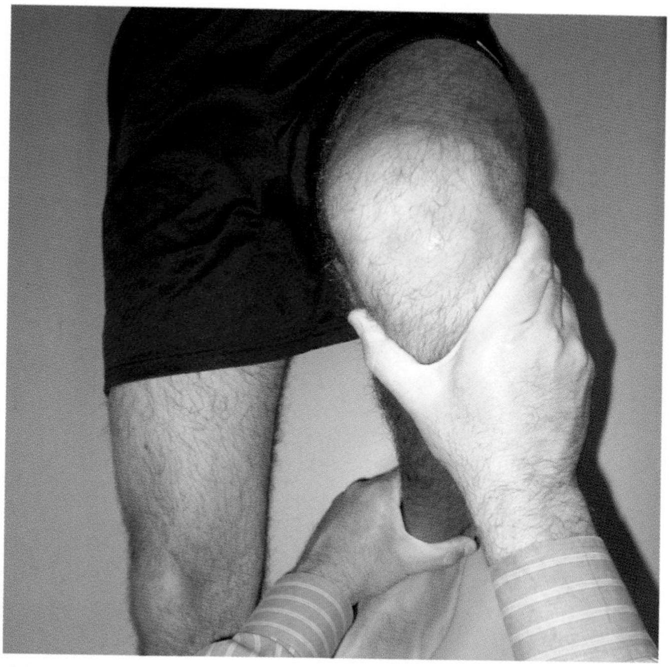

FIGURE 102–14 ■ McMurray test for torn meniscus. (From Waldman SD: Physical Diagnosis of Pain: An Atlas of Signs and Symptoms. Philadelphia, WB Saunders, 2006, p 342.)

if the examiner appreciates a palpable or auditory click while rotating and extending the knee.

Use of Testing Modalities for Evaluation of the Painful Knee

Plain radiographs are indicated in all patients who present with knee pain. Based on the patient's clinical presentation, additional testing including complete blood cell count, sedimentation rate, and antinuclear antibody testing may be indicated. Magnetic resonance imaging of the knee is indicated if internal derangement is suspected. Radionuclide bone scan is indicated if metastatic disease or primary tumor involving the knee is being considered. Synovial fluid analysis should be performed in all patients suspected of having a septic joint or suffering from a crystal arthropathy. Titers for Lyme disease are indicated in patients with rash suggestive of erythema migrans or in patients with a history of tick bite who also complain of knee pain.[14]

CONCLUSION

The diagnosis of knee pain should be a relatively straightforward clinical endeavor as long as the clinician performs a careful targeted history and physical examination. The clinician faced with the patient with knee pain should have a relatively low threshold for the ordering of MRI especially in the presence of trauma. A failure to heed the warning signs just discussed can result in much unneeded pain and functional disability and permanent damage to the knee.

References

1. Shrive NG, O'Connor JJ, Goodfellow JW: Load-bearing in the knee joint. Clin Orthop (131):279, 1978.
2. Magee DJ: Examination of the knee. In Orthopedic Physical Assessment, 3rd ed, Philadelphia, WB Saunders, 1997, pp 519-577.
3. Ricklin P, Ruttimann A, Del Buono MS: Meniscus Lesions: Diagnosis, Differential Diagnosis and Therapy, 2nd ed. Stuttgart, Thieme Medical, 1983, p 16.
4. Lobst CA, Stanitski CL: Acute knee injuries. Clin Sports Med 19:621, 2000.
5. Reicher MA, Hartzman S, Duckwiler GR: Meniscal injuries: Detection using MR imaging. Radiology 159:753, 1986.
6. Weil EK: Pain and pyrexia. In Resident's Prescribing Reference, Reston, VA, American Society of Health System Pharmacists, 1996, vol 5, pp 164-168.
7. Goldstein J, Zuckerman JD: Selected orthopedic problems in the elderly. Rheum Dis Clin North Am 26:593, 2000.
8. Miller D, Allen SE, Walker SE: A primary care physician's guide to polymyalgia rheumatica. Primary Care Rep 4:91, 1998.
9. Malawista SE: Lyme disease. In Wyngarden JB, Smith LH (eds): Cecil Textbook of Medicine, 21st ed. Philadelphia, WB Saunders, 2000, pp 1757-1761.
10. Banker BQ, Engel AG: The polymyositis and dermatomyositis syndromes. In Engel AG, Banker BQ (eds): Myology. New York, McGraw-Hill, 1986, vol 2, pp 1385-1422.
11. Rich MW: Drug-induced lupus: The list of culprits grows. Postgrad Med 100:299, 1996.
12. Stanitski CL, Harvell JC, Fu F: Observations on acute knee hemarthrosis in children and adolescents. J Pediatr Orthop 13:506, 1993.
13. Rotstein J: Steroid pseudorheumatism. Postgrad Med 31:459, 1962.
14. Callister SM, Schell RF: Laboratory serodiagnosis of Lyme borreliosis. J Spirochetal Tick-Borne Dis 5:7, 1998.

chapter 103

Bursitis Syndromes of the Knee

Steven D. Waldman

Bursitis of the knee is one of the most common causes of knee pain encountered in clinical practice. The bursae of the knee are vulnerable to injury from both acute trauma and repeated microtrauma. The bursae of the knee may exist as single bursal sacs or in some patients as a multi-segmented series of sacs that may be loculated. Acute injuries to the bursae of the knee frequently take the form of direct trauma to the bursa from falls or blows directly to the knee or of patellar, tibial plateau, and proximal fibular fractures, as well as of overuse injuries, including running on soft or uneven surfaces or from jobs requiring crawling on the knees such as laying carpet. If the inflammation of the bursae of the knees becomes chronic, calcification of the bursa may occur.

SUPRAPATELLAR BURSITIS

The suprapatellar bursa extends superiorly from beneath the patella under the quadriceps femoris muscle (Fig. 103–1). The patient suffering from suprapatellar bursitis will frequently complain of pain in the anterior knee above the patella, which can radiate superiorly into the distal anterior thigh.[1] Often, the patient will be unable to kneel or walk down stairs (Fig. 103–2). The patient may also complain of a sharp, catching sensation with range of motion of the knee, especially on first arising. Suprapatellar bursitis often coexists with arthritis and tendinitis of the knee joint, and these other pathologic processes may confuse the clinical picture.[2]

Clinical Presentation

Physical examination may reveal point tenderness in the anterior knee just above the patella. Passive flexion as well as active resisted extension of the knee will reproduce the pain. Sudden release of resistance during this maneuver will markedly increase the pain.[1] There may be swelling in the suprapatellar region with a boggy feeling to palpation. Occasionally, the suprapatellar bursa may become infected as evidenced by systemic symptoms including fever and malaise as well as local signs of rubor, color, and dolor.

Diagnosis

Plain radiographs of the knee may reveal calcification of the bursa and associated structures including the quadriceps tendon consistent with chronic inflammation. MRI is indicated if internal derangement, occult mass, or tumor of the knee is suspected. Electromyography will help distinguish suprapatellar bursitis from femoral neuropathy, lumbar radiculopathy, and plexopathy. The injection technique described later serves as a diagnostic and therapeutic maneuver. A complete blood cell count and an automated chemistry profile including determinations of uric acid, the erythrocyte sedimentation rate, and the antinuclear antibody value are indicated if collagen vascular disease is suspected. If infection is considered, aspiration, Gram stain, and culture of bursal fluid are indicated on an emergent basis.

Differential Diagnosis

Because of the unique anatomy of the region, not only the suprapatellar bursa but also the associated tendons and other bursae of the knee can become inflamed and confuse the diagnosis. The suprapatellar bursa extends superiorly from beneath the patella under the quadriceps femoris muscle and its tendon. The bursa is held in place by a small portion of the vastus intermedius muscle called the articularis genus muscle. Both the quadriceps tendon as well as the suprapatellar bursa are subject to the development of inflammation after overuse, misuse, or direct trauma. The quadriceps tendon is made up of fibers from the four muscles that comprise the quadriceps muscle: the vastus lateralis, the vastus intermedius, the vastus medialis, and the rectus femoris. These muscles are the primary extensors of the lower extremity at the knee. The tendons of these muscles converge and unite to form a single exceedingly strong tendon. The patella functions as a sesamoid bone within the quadriceps tendon with fibers of the tendon expanding around the patella forming the medial and lateral patella retinacula that help strengthen the knee joint. These fibers are called expansions and are subject to strain, and the tendon proper is subject to the development of tendinitis. The suprapatellar, infrapatellar, and prepatellar bursae may also concurrently become inflamed with dysfunction of the quadriceps tendon. It should be remembered that anything that alters the normal biomechanics of the knee can result in inflammation of the suprapatellar bursa.

Treatment

A short course of conservative therapy consisting of simple analgesics, nonsteroidal antiinflammatory agents, or

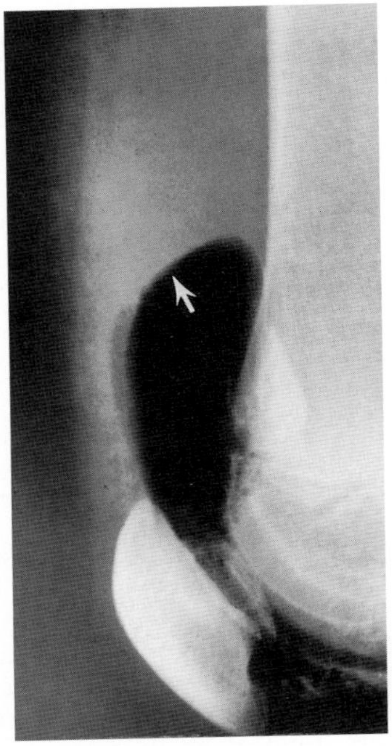

FIGURE 103–1 ■ Noncommunicating suprapatellar pouch cyst. A lateral view from a double-contrast knee arthrogram demonstrates minimal extrinsic impression on the suprapatellar pouch *(arrow)* by an adjacent fluid-filled mass. (From Resnick D [ed]: Diagnosis of Bone and Joint Disorders, 4th ed. Philadelphia, WB Saunders, 2002, p 284.)

cyclooxygenase-2 inhibitors and a knee brace to prevent further trauma is a reasonable first step in the treatment of patients suffering from suprapatellar bursitis. If the patient does not experience rapid improvement, the following injection technique is a reasonable next step.[3] The goals of this injection technique are explained to the patient. The patient is placed supine with a rolled blanket underneath the knee to gently flex the joint. The skin overlying the medial aspect of the knee joint is prepped with antiseptic solution. A sterile syringe containing the 2.0 mL of 0.25% preservative-free bupivacaine and 40 mg of methylprednisolone is attached to a 1.5-inch 25-gauge needle using strict aseptic technique. The superior margin of the medial patella is identified. Just above this point, the needle is inserted horizontally to slide just beneath the quadriceps tendon (Fig. 103–3). If the needle strikes the femur, it is then withdrawn slightly and redirected in a more anterior trajectory. When the needle is in position just below the quadriceps tendon, the contents of the syringe are then gently injected. There should be little resistance to injection. If resistance is encountered, the needle is probably in a ligament or tendon and should be advanced or withdrawn slightly until the injection proceeds without significant resistance. The needle is then removed and a sterile pressure dressing and ice pack are placed at the injection site. Physical therapy to restore function is a reasonable next step after the acute pain and swelling has subsided after injection with local anesthetic and corticosteroid.

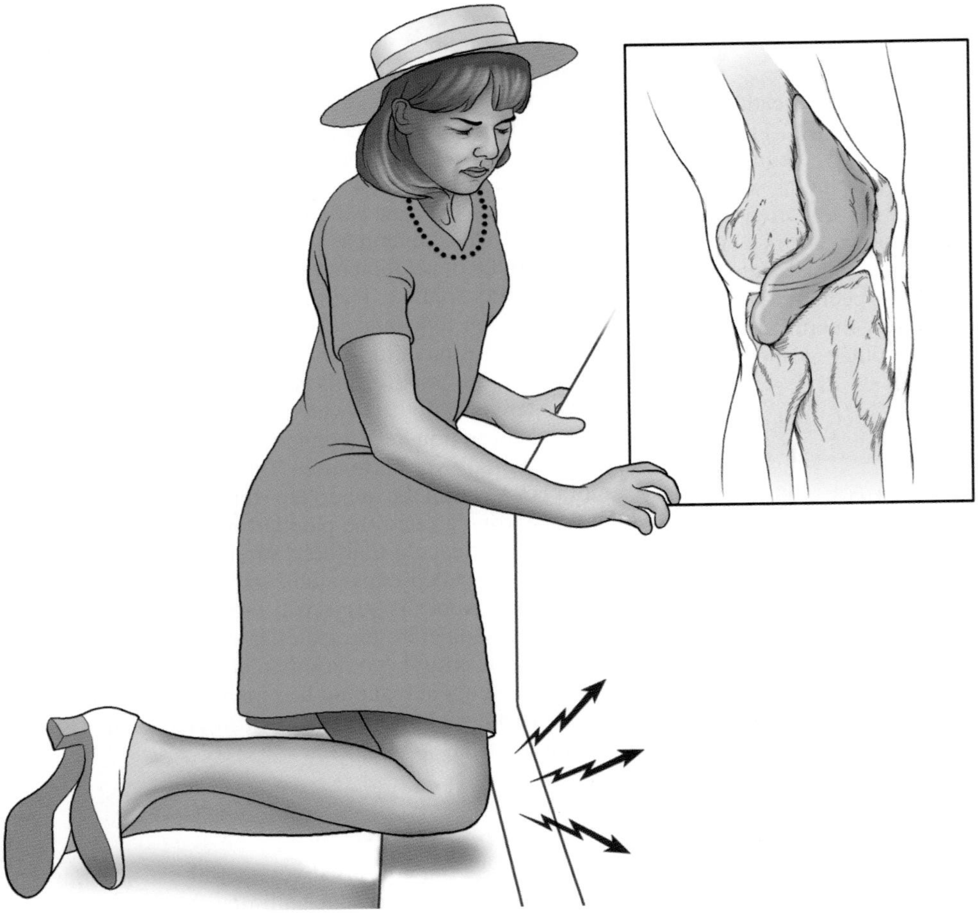

FIGURE 103–2 ■ Suprapatellar bursitis is usually the result of direct trauma to the suprapatellar bursa from either acute injury or repeated microtrauma. (From Waldman SD: Atlas of Common Pain Syndromes. Philadelphia, WB Saunders, 2002, p 255.)

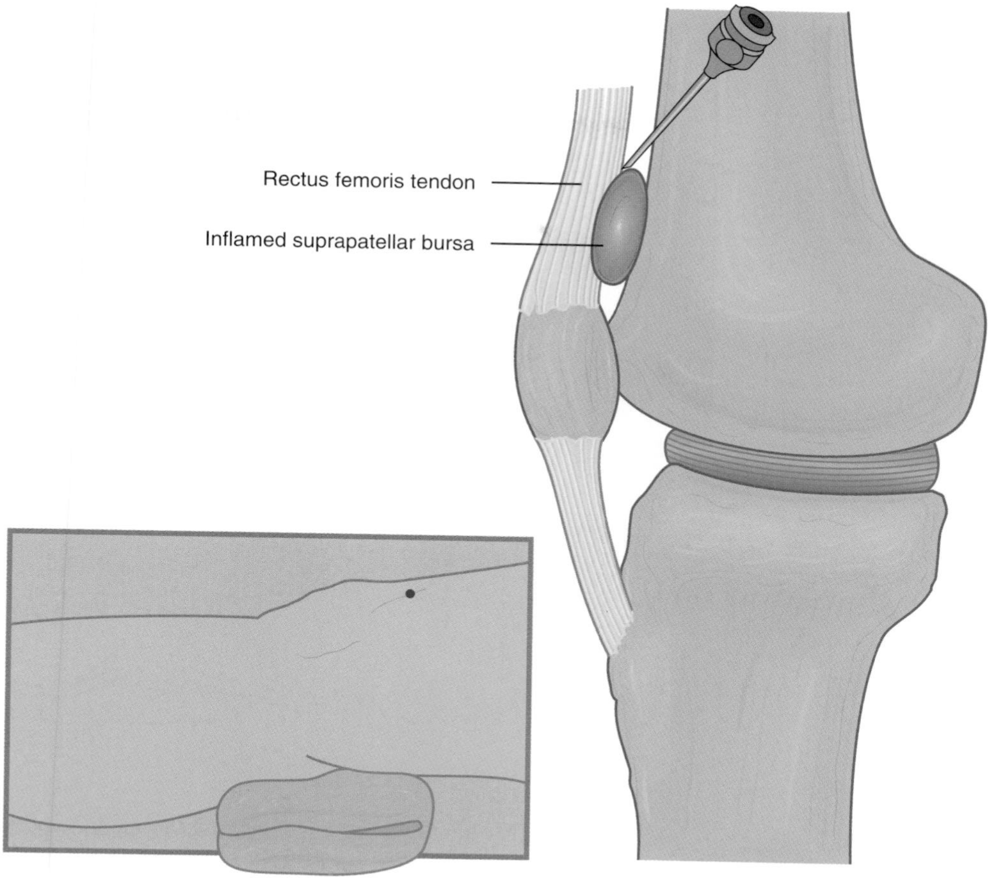

FIGURE 103–3 ■ Injection technique for relieving the pain due to suprapatellar bursitis. (From Waldman SD: Atlas of Pain Management Injection Techniques. Philadelphia, WB Saunders, 2000, p 269.)

■ PREPATELLAR BURSITIS

The prepatellar bursa is vulnerable to injury from both acute trauma and repeated microtrauma. The prepatellar bursa lies between the subcutaneous tissues and the patella (Fig. 103–4). This bursa may exist as a single bursal sac or in some patients as a multi-segmented series of sacs that may be loculated. Acute injuries frequently take the form of direct trauma to the bursa from falls directly onto the knee or from patellar fractures as well as from overuse injuries, including running on soft or uneven surfaces. Prepatellar bursitis may also result from jobs requiring crawling on the knees such as laying carpet or scrubbing floors; hence the other name for prepatellar bursitis is housemaid's knee (Fig. 103–5). If the inflammation of the prepatellar bursa becomes chronic, calcification of the bursa may occur.

Clinical Presentation

The patient suffering from prepatellar bursitis will frequently complain of pain and swelling in the anterior knee over the patella that can radiate superiorly and inferiorly into the area surrounding the knee.[4] Often, the patient will be unable to kneel or walk down stairs. The patient may also complain of a sharp, catching sensation with range of motion of the knee, especially on first arising. Prepatellar bursitis often coexists with arthritis and tendinitis of the knee joint, and these other pathologic processes may confuse the clinical picture.

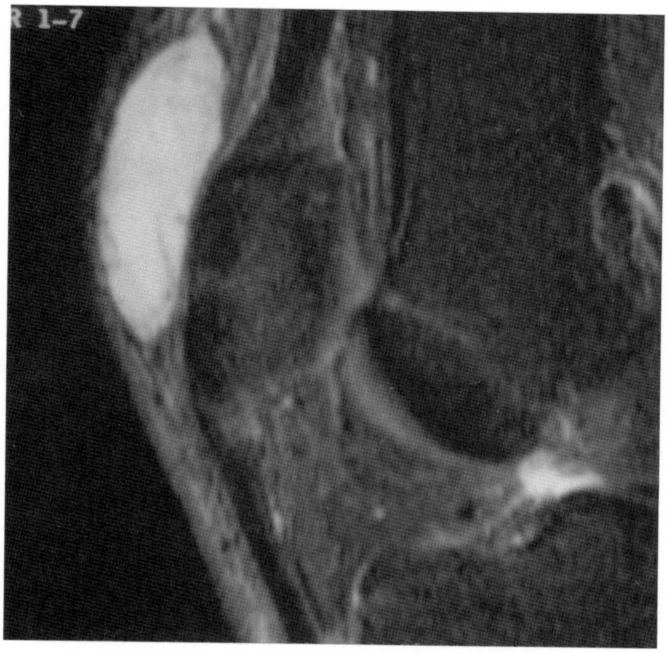

FIGURE 103–4 ■ Prepatellar bursitis. A sagittal STIR (TR/TE, 5300/30; inversion time, 150 ms) MR image shows fluid and synovial tissue in the prepatellar bursa. (From Resnick D [ed]: Diagnosis of Bone and Joint Disorders, 4th ed. Philadelphia, WB Saunders, 2002, p 4257.)

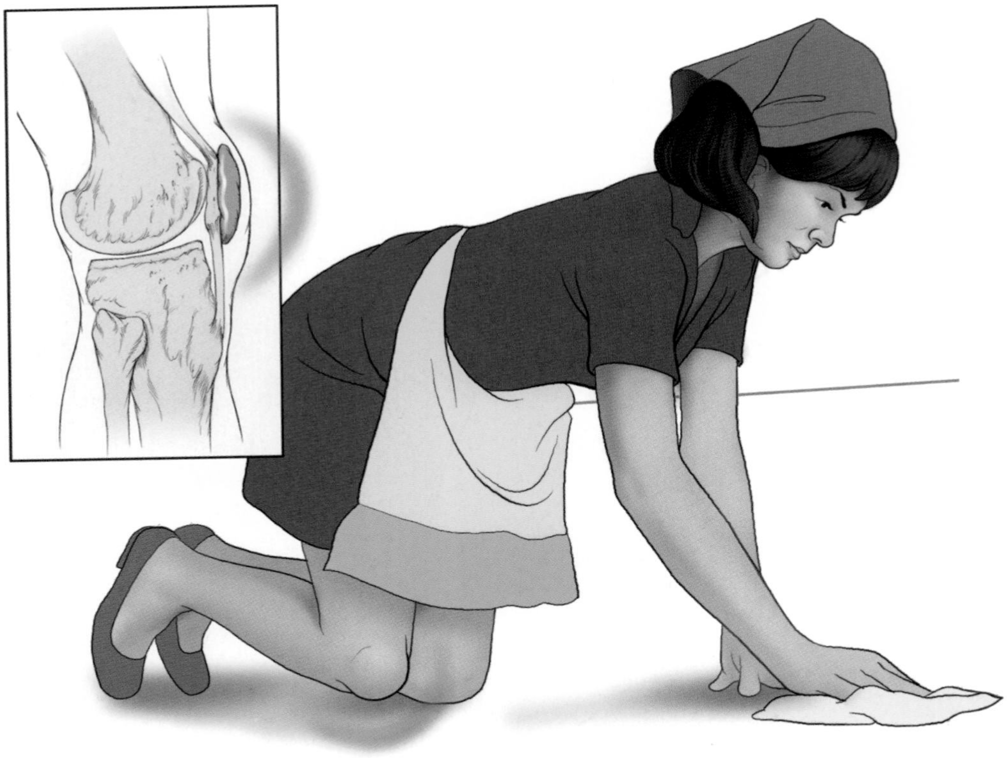

FIGURE 103–5 ■ Prepatellar bursitis is also known as housemaid's knee because of its prevalence in people whose work requires prolonged crawling or kneeling. (From Waldman SD: Atlas of Common Pain Syndromes. Philadelphia, WB Saunders, 2002, p 259.)

Diagnosis

Plain radiographs of the knee may reveal calcification of the bursa and associated structures including the quadriceps tendon consistent with chronic inflammation. MRI is indicated if internal derangement, occult mass, or tumor of the knee is suspected. Electromyography will help distinguish prepatellar bursitis from femoral neuropathy, lumbar radiculopathy, and plexopathy. The injection technique described in the section on treatment serves as a diagnostic and therapeutic maneuver. Testing for antinuclear antibody is indicated if collagen vascular disease is suspected. If infection is considered, aspiration, Gram stain, and culture of bursal fluid is indicated on an emergent basis

Differential Diagnosis

Because of the unique anatomy of the region, not only the prepatellar bursa but also the associated tendons and other bursae of the knee can become inflamed and confuse the diagnosis. The prepatellar bursa lies between the subcutaneous tissues and the patella. The bursa is held in place by the ligamentum patellae. Both the quadriceps tendon as well as the prepatellar bursa are subject to the development of inflammation after overuse, misuse, or direct trauma. The quadriceps tendon is made up of fibers from the four muscles that comprise the quadriceps muscle: the vastus lateralis, the vastus intermedius, the vastus medialis, and the rectus femoris. These muscles are the primary extensors of the lower extremity at the knee. The tendons of these muscles converge and unite to form a single, exceedingly strong tendon. The patella functions as a sesamoid bone within the quadriceps tendon with fibers of the tendon extending around the patella forming the medial and lateral patella retinacula, which help strengthen the knee joint. These fibers are called expansions and are subject to strain, and the tendon proper is subject to the development of tendinitis. The suprapatellar, infrapatellar, and prepatellar bursae may also concurrently become inflamed with dysfunction of the quadriceps tendon. It should be remembered that anything that alters the normal biomechanics of the knee can result in inflammation of the prepatellar bursa.

Treatment

A short course of conservative therapy consisting of simple analgesics, nonsteroidal antiinflammatory agents, or cyclooxygenase-2 inhibitors and use of a knee brace to prevent further trauma is a reasonable first step in the treatment of patients suffering from prepatellar bursitis. If the patient does not experience rapid improvement, the following injection technique is a reasonable next step.[5] The patient is placed supine with a rolled blanket underneath the knee to gently flex the joint. The skin overlying the patella is prepped with antiseptic solution. A sterile syringe containing the 2.0 mL of 0.25% preservative-free bupivacaine and 40 mg of methylprednisolone is attached to a 1.5-inch 25-gauge needle using strict aseptic technique. With strict aseptic technique, the center of the medial patella is identified (Fig. 103–6). Just above this point, the needle is inserted horizontally to slide subcutaneously into the prepatellar bursa. If the needle strikes the patella, it is then withdrawn slightly and redirected in a more anterior trajectory. When the needle is in position in proximity to the prepatellar bursa, the contents of the syringe are then gently injected. There should be little resistance to injection. If resistance is encountered, the needle is probably

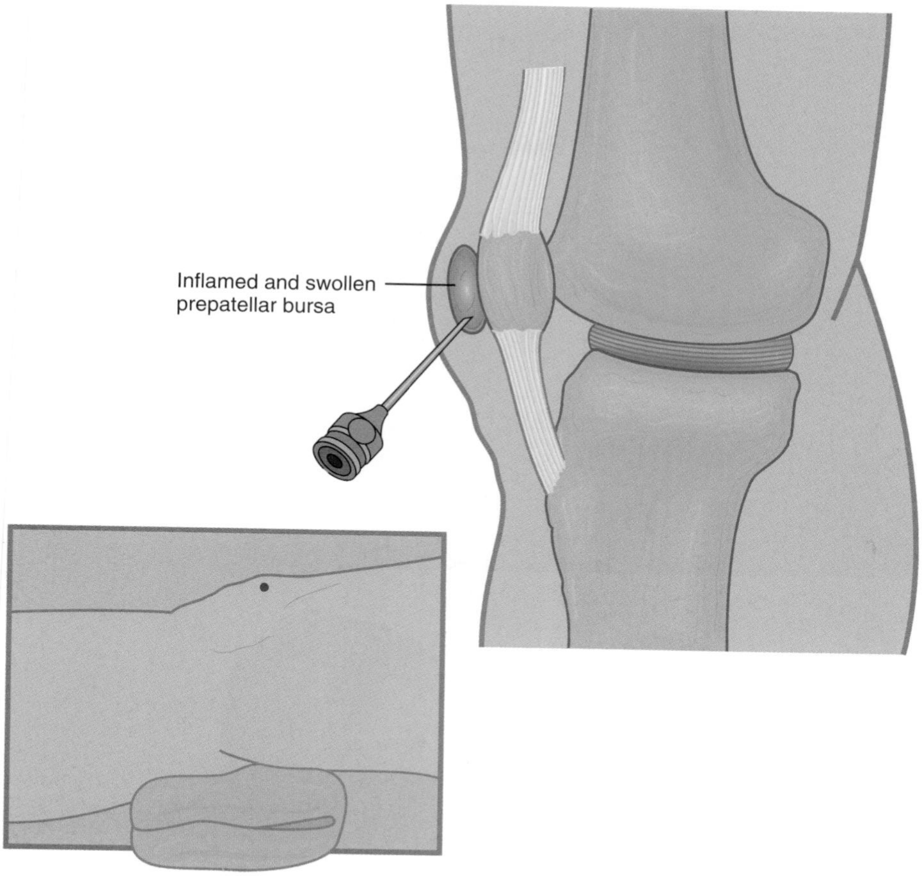

FIGURE 103–6 ■ Injection technique for relieving the pain due to prepatellar bursitis. (From Waldman SD: Atlas of Pain Management Injection Techniques. Philadelphia, WB Saunders, 2000, p 272.)

in a ligament or tendon and should be advanced or withdrawn slightly until the injection proceeds without significant resistance. The needle is then removed, and a sterile pressure dressing and ice pack are placed at the injection site.

Complications and Pitfalls

Failure to identify primary or metastatic distal femur or joint disease that is responsible for the patient's pain may yield disastrous results. The major complication of this injection technique is infection. This complication should be exceedingly rare if strict aseptic technique is adhered to. Approximately 25% of patients will complain of a transient increase in pain after injection of the suprapatellar bursa of the knee and should be warned of such. The use of physical modalities including local heat as well as gentle range-of-motion exercises should be introduced several days after the patient undergoes this injection technique for prepatellar bursitis pain. Vigorous exercises should be avoided because they will exacerbate the patient's symptoms.

■ SUPERFICIAL INFRAPATELLAR BURSITIS

The superficial infrapatellar bursa is vulnerable to injury from both acute trauma and repeated microtrauma. The superficial infrapatellar bursa lies between the subcutaneous tissues and the upper part of the ligamentum patellae (Fig. 103–7). The deep infrapatellar bursa lies between the ligamentum patellae and the tibia. These bursae may exist as single bursal sacs or in some patients as a multi-segmented series of sacs that may be loculated. Acute injuries frequently take the form of direct trauma to the bursa from falls directly onto the knee or from patellar fractures as well as from overuse injuries, including running on soft or uneven surfaces. Superficial infrapatellar bursitis may also result from jobs requiring crawling on the knees such as laying carpet or scrubbing floors (Fig. 103–8). If the inflammation of the superficial infrapatellar bursa becomes chronic, calcification of the bursa may occur.

Clinical Presentation

The patient suffering from superficial infrapatellar bursitis will frequently complain of pain and swelling in the anterior knee over the patella that can radiate superiorly and inferiorly into the area surrounding the knee.[6] Often, the patient will be unable to kneel or walk down stairs. The patient may also complain of a sharp, catching sensation with range of motion of the knee, especially on first arising. Superficial infrapatellar bursitis often coexists with arthritis and tendinitis of the knee joint, and these other pathologic processes may confuse the clinical picture.

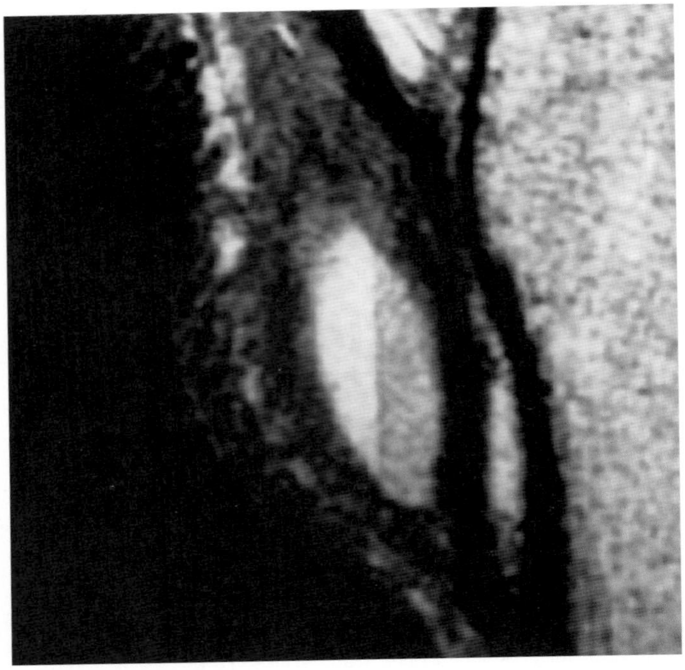

FIGURE 103–7 ■ Superficial infrapatellar bursitis. A fluid level within the bursa is evident on a sagittal fast spin-echo (TR/TE, 2600/22) MR image. (From Resnick D [ed]: Diagnosis of Bone and Joint Disorders, 4th ed. Philadelphia, WB Saunders, 2002, p 4257.)

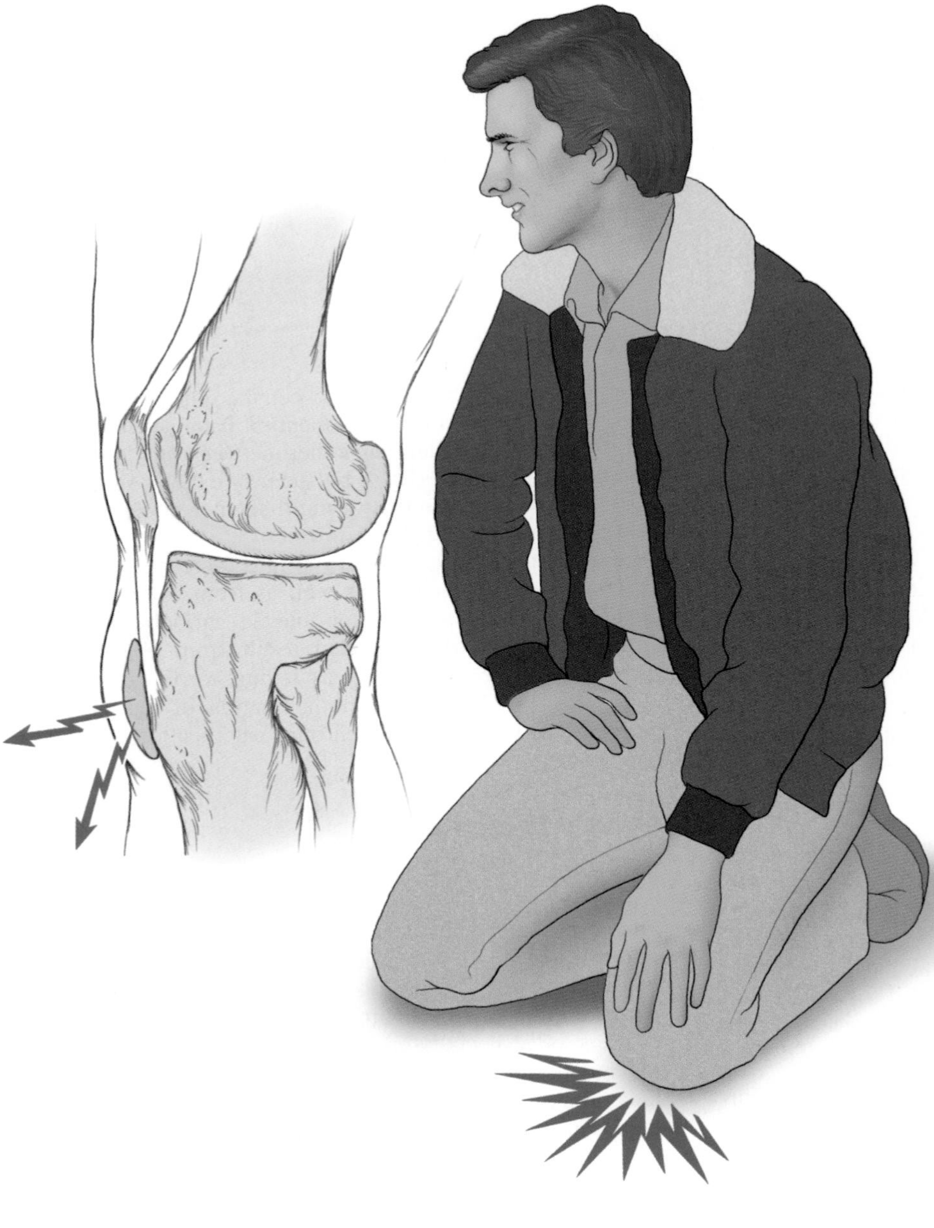

FIGURE 103–8 ■ Infrapatellar bursitis is a common cause of inferior knee pain. (From Waldman SD: Atlas of Common Pain Syndromes. Philadelphia, WB Saunders, 2002, p 261.)

Diagnosis

Plain radiographs of the knee may reveal calcification of the bursa and associated structures including the quadriceps tendon consistent with chronic inflammation. MRI is indicated if internal derangement, occult mass, or tumor of the knee is suspected. Electromyography will help distinguish superficial infrapatellar bursitis from femoral neuropathy, lumbar radiculopathy, and plexopathy. The injection technique described in the section on treatment will serve as a diagnostic and therapeutic maneuver. Testing for antinuclear antibody is indicated if collagen vascular disease is suspected. If infection is considered, aspiration, Gram stain, and culture of bursal fluid is indicated on an emergent basis.

Differential Diagnosis

Because of the unique anatomy of the region, not only the superficial infrapatellar bursa but also the associated tendons and other bursae of the knee can become inflamed and confuse the diagnosis. Both the quadriceps tendon as well as the superficial infrapatellar bursa are subject to the development of inflammation after overuse, misuse, or direct trauma. The quadriceps tendon is made up of fibers from the four muscles that comprise the quadriceps muscle: the vastus lateralis, the vastus intermedius, the vastus medialis, and the rectus femoris. These muscles are the primary extensors of the lower extremity at the knee. The tendons of these muscles converge and unite to form a single, exceedingly strong tendon. The patella functions as a sesamoid bone within the quadriceps tendon, with fibers of the tendon extending around the patella forming the medial and lateral patella retinacula, which help strengthen the knee joint. These fibers are called expansions and are subject to strain, and the tendon proper is subject to the development of tendinitis. The suprapatellar, infrapatellar, and superficial infrapatellar bursae may also concurrently become inflamed with dysfunction of the quadriceps tendon. It should be remembered that anything that alters the normal biomechanics of the knee can result in inflammation of the superficial infrapatellar bursa.

Treatment

A short course of conservative therapy consisting of simple analgesics, nonsteroidal antiinflammatory agents, or cyclooxygenase-2 inhibitors and use of a knee brace to prevent further trauma is a reasonable first step in the treatment of patients suffering from superficial infrapatellar bursitis. If the patient does not experience rapid improvement, the following injection technique is a reasonable next step.[7]

To inject the superficial infrapatellar bursa, the patient is placed in the supine position with a rolled blanket underneath the knee to gently flex the joint. The skin overlying the patella is prepped with antiseptic solution. A sterile syringe containing 2.0 mL of 0.25% preservative-free bupivacaine and 40 mg of methylprednisolone is attached to a 1.5-inch 25-gauge needle using strict aseptic technique. The center of the lower pole of the patella is identified. Just below this point, the needle is inserted at a 45-degree angle to slide subcutaneously into the superficial infrapatellar bursa (Fig. 103–9). If the needle strikes the patella, it is then withdrawn slightly and

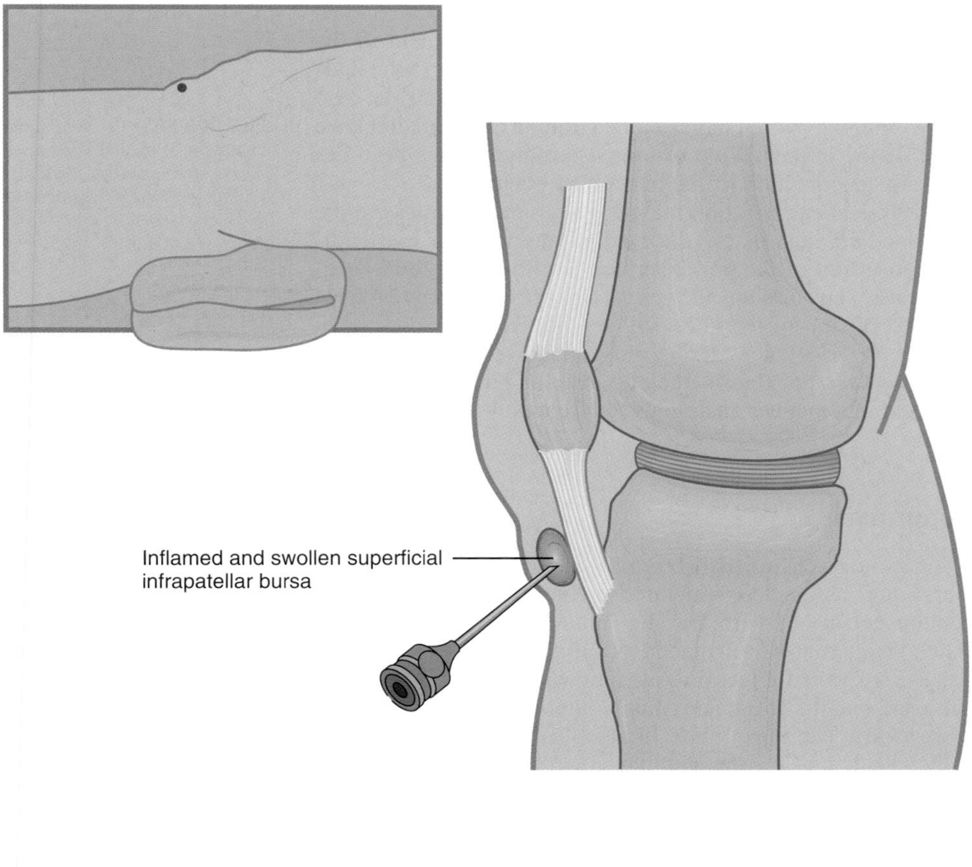

FIGURE 103–9 ■ Injection technique for relieving the pain due to infrapatellar bursitis. (From Waldman SD: Atlas of Pain Management Injection Techniques. Philadelphia, WB Saunders, 2000, p 275.)

redirected in a more inferior trajectory. When the needle is in position in proximity to the superficial infrapatellar bursa, the contents of the syringe is then gently injected. There should be little resistance to injection. If resistance is encountered, the needle is probably in a ligament or tendon and should be advanced or withdrawn slightly until the injection proceeds without significant resistance. The needle is then removed, and a sterile pressure dressing and ice pack are placed at the injection site. The use of physical modalities including local heat as well as gentle range of motion exercises should be introduced several days after the patient undergoes this injection technique for prepatellar bursitis pain. Vigorous exercises should be avoided because they will exacerbate the patient's symptoms.

PES ANSERINE BURSITIS

The pes anserine bursa lies beneath the pes anserine tendon, which is the insertional tendon of the sartorius, gracilis, and semitendinous muscles to the medial side of the tibia (Fig. 103–10). This bursa may exist as a single bursal sac or in some patients may exist as a multi-segmented series of sacs that may be loculated. Patients with pes anserine bursitis will present with pain over the medial knee joint and increased pain on passive valgus and external rotation of the knee.[8] Activity, especially involving flexion and external rotation of the knee will make the pain worse, with rest and heat providing some relief. Often, the patient will be unable to kneel or walk down stairs.

Clinical Presentation

The pain of pes anserine bursitis is constant and characterized as aching. The pain may interfere with sleep. Coexistent bursitis, tendinitis, arthritis, and/or internal derangement of the knee may confuse the clinical picture after trauma to the knee joint. Frequently, the medial collateral ligament is also involved if the patient has sustained trauma to the medial knee joint. If the inflammation of the pes anserine bursa becomes chronic, calcification of the bursa may occur.

Physical examination may reveal point tenderness in the anterior knee just below the medial knee joint at the tendinous insertion of the pes anserine.[8] Swelling and fluid accumulation surrounding the bursa is often present. Active resisted flexion of the knee will reproduce the pain. Sudden release of resistance during this maneuver will markedly increase the pain. Rarely, the pes anserine bursa will become infected in a manner analogous to infection of the prepatellar bursa.

Diagnosis

Plain radiographs of the knee may reveal calcification of the bursa and associated structures including the pes anserine tendon consistent with chronic inflammation. MRI is indicated if internal derangement, occult mass, or tumor of the knee is suspected. Electromyography will help distinguish pes anserine bursitis from neuropathy, lumbar radiculopathy, and plexopathy. The injection technique described later serves as a diagnostic and therapeutic maneuver.

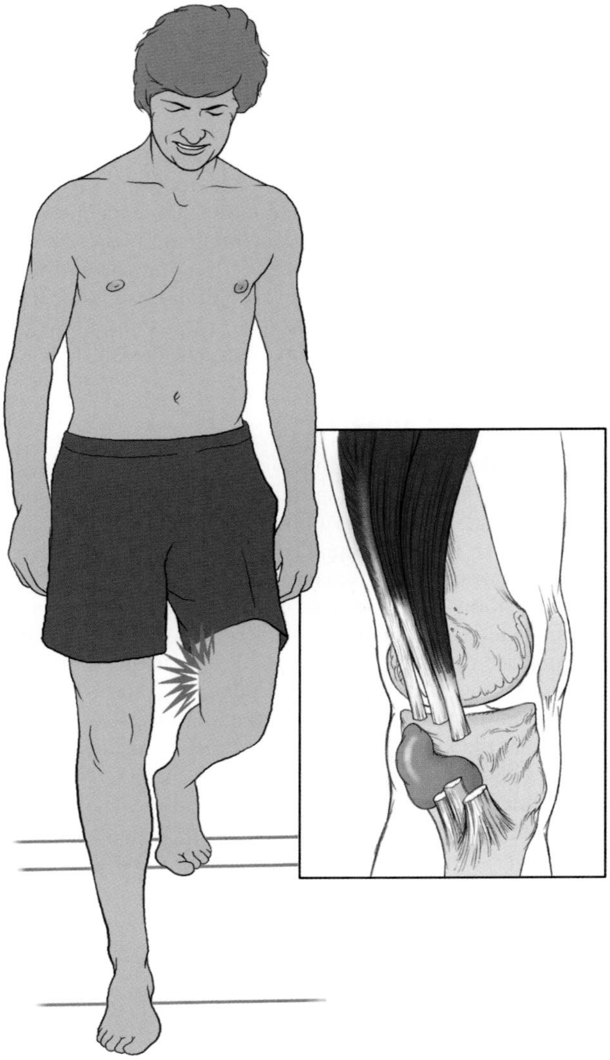

FIGURE 103–10 ■ Patients with pes anserine bursitis will frequently complain of medial knee pain that is made worse with kneeling or walking down stairs. (From Waldman SD: Atlas of Common Pain Syndromes. Philadelphia, WB Saunders, 2002, p 271.)

Differential Diagnosis

The pes anserine bursa is prone to the development of inflammation after overuse, misuse, or direct trauma. The medial collateral ligament also often is involved if the medial knee has been subjected to trauma. The medial collateral ligament is a broad, flat bandlike ligament that runs from the medial condyle of the femur to the medial aspect of the shaft of the tibia where it attaches just above the groove of the semimembranosus muscle attaches. It also attaches to the edge of the medial semilunar cartilage. The medial collateral ligament is crossed at its lower part by the tendons of the sartorius, gracilis, and semitendinosus muscles. Because of the unique anatomic relationships of the medial knee, it is often difficult on clinical grounds to accurately determine which anatomic structure is responsible for the patient's pain. MRI will help sort things out and rule out lesions such as tears of the medial meniscus that may require surgical intervention. It should be remembered that anything that alters the normal biomechanics of the knee can result in inflammation of the pes anserine bursa.

Treatment

A short course of conservative therapy consisting of simple analgesics, nonsteroidal antiinflammatory agents, or cyclooxygenase-2 inhibitors and a knee brace to prevent further trauma is a reasonable first step in the treatment of patients suffering from pes anserine bursitis. If the patient does not experience rapid improvement, the following injection technique is a reasonable next step.[9]

To inject the pes anserine bursa, the patient is placed in the supine position with a rolled blanket underneath the knee to gently flex the joint. The skin just below the medial knee joint is prepped with antiseptic solution. A sterile syringe containing 2.0 mL of 0.25% preservative-free bupivacaine and 40 mg of methylprednisolone is attached to a 1.5-inch, 25-gauge needle using strict aseptic technique. With strict aseptic technique, the pes anserine tendon is identified by having the patient strongly flex his or her leg against resistance. The point distal to the medial joint space at which the pes anserine tendon attaches to the tibia is the location of the pes anserine bursa. The bursa will usually be identified by point tenderness at that spot. At this point, the needle is inserted at a 45-degree angle to the tibia to pass through the skin, subcutaneous tissues, and into the pes anserine bursa (Fig. 103–11). If the needle strikes the tibia, it is then withdrawn slightly into the substance of the bursa. When the needle is in position in proximity to the pes anserine bursa, the contents of the syringe is then gently injected. There should be little resistance to injection. If resistance is encountered, the needle is probably in a ligament or tendon and should be advanced or withdrawn slightly until the injection proceeds without significant resistance. The needle is then removed, and a sterile pressure dressing and ice pack are placed at the injection site. The use of physical modalities including local heat as well as gentle range-of-motion exercises should be introduced several days after the patient undergoes this injection technique for prepatellar bursitis pain. Vigorous exercises should be avoided because they will exacerbate the patient's symptoms.

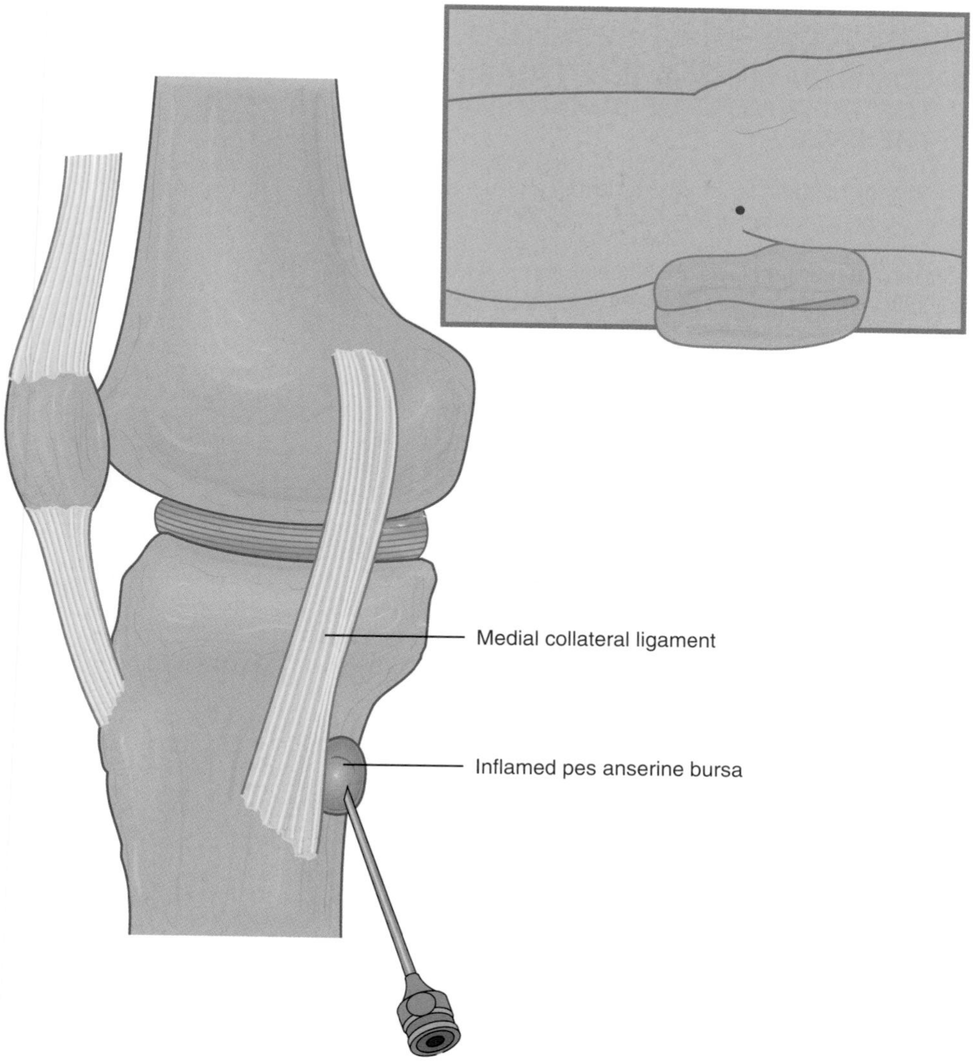

FIGURE 103–11 ■ Injection technique for relieving the pain due to pes anserine bursitis. (From Waldman SD: Atlas of Pain Management Injection Techniques. Philadelphia, WB Saunders, 2000, p 280.)

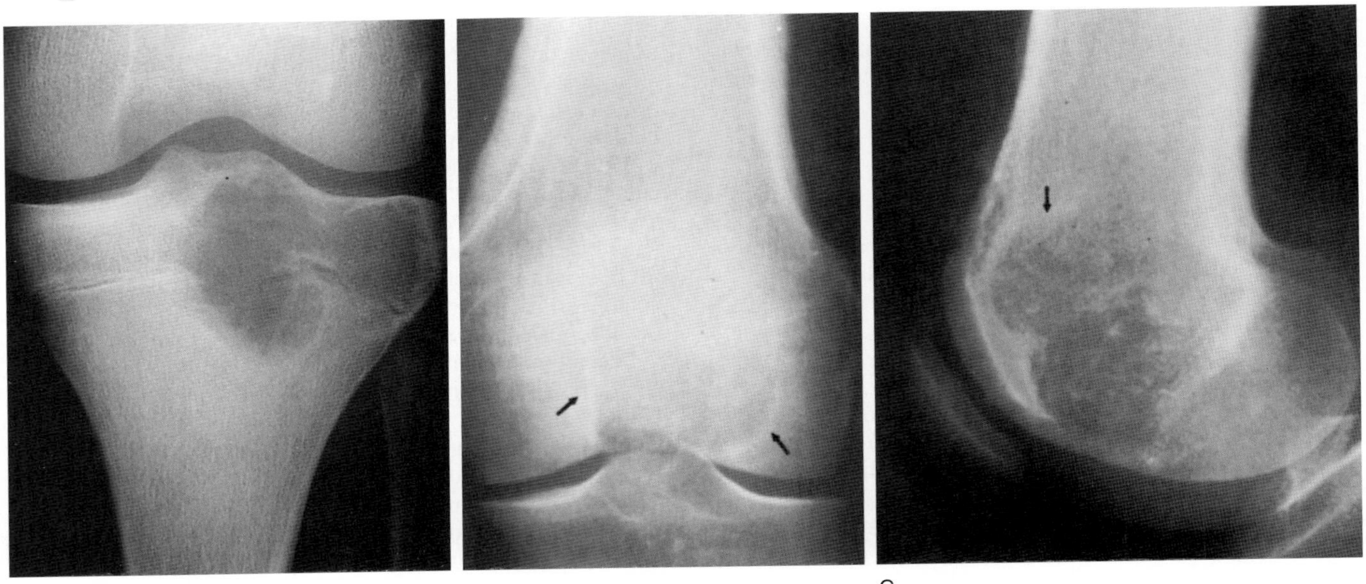

FIGURE 103–12 ■ Chondroblastoma: Radiographic abnormalities of long tubular bones. **A**, Tibia. Note the radiolucent lesion involving the metaphysis and epiphysis of the proximal portion of the tibia. **B** and **C,** Frontal and lateral radiographs of the femur in a 22-year-old man show a large epiphyseal and metaphyseal lesion *(arrows)* that contains foci of calcification. An unusual degree of periostitis is apparent in the metaphysis and diaphysis. (From Resnick D [ed]: Diagnosis of Bone and Joint Disorders, 4th ed. Philadelphia, WB Saunders, 2002, p 3856.)

COMPLICATIONS AND PITFALLS IN THE TREATMENT OF BURSITIS OF THE KNEE

Coexistent bursitis, tendinitis, arthritis, and internal derangement of the knee may also contribute to the patient's pain and may require additional treatment. The simple analgesics and nonsteroidal antiinflammatory agents are a reasonable starting place in the treatment of bursitis of the knee. If these agents are ineffective, the injection of the inflamed bursa with a local anesthetic and corticosteroid is a reasonable next step. The previously described injection techniques are generally safe procedures if careful attention is paid to the clinically relevant anatomy in the areas to be injected. The use of physical modalities including local heat as well as gentle range-of-motion exercises should be introduced several days after the patient undergoes the injection techniques. Vigorous exercises should be avoided because they will exacerbate the patient's symptoms. The clinician should remember that failure to identify infection or primary or metastatic tumors of the distal femur, joint, or proximal tibia and fibula that may be responsible for the patient's pain may yield disastrous results (Fig. 103–12).

References

1. Waldman SD: Suprapatellar bursitis. In Waldman SD: Atlas of Common Pain Syndromes. Philadelphia, WB Saunders, 2002, pp 254-256.
2. Yamamoto T, Akisue T, Marui T: Isolated suprapatellar bursitis: Computed tomographic and arthroscopic findings. Arthroscopy 19:E10, 2003.
3. Waldman SD: Suprapatellar bursitis. In Waldman SD: Atlas of Pain Management Injection Techniques. Philadelphia, WB Saunders, 2000, pp 267-269.
4. Waldman SD: Prepatellar bursitis. In Waldman SD: Atlas of Common Pain Syndromes. Philadelphia, WB Saunders, 2002, pp 257-259.
5. Waldman SD: Prepatellar bursitis. In Waldman SD: Atlas of Pain Management Injection Techniques. Philadelphia, WB Saunders, 2000, pp 270-272.
6. Waldman SD: Superficial infrapatellar bursitis. In Waldman SD: Atlas of Common Pain Syndromes. Philadelphia, WB Saunders, 2002, pp 257-259.
7. Waldman SD: Superficial infrapatellar bursitis. In Waldman SD: Atlas of Pain Management Injection Techniques. Philadelphia, WB Saunders, 2000, pp 273-275.
8. Waldman SD: Pes anserine bursitis. In Waldman SD: Atlas of Common Pain Syndromes. Philadelphia, WB Saunders, 2002, pp 269-271.
9. Waldman SD: Pes anserine bursitis. In Waldman SD: Atlas of Pain Management Injection Techniques. Philadelphia, WB Saunders, 2000, pp 279-281.

chapter 104

Baker's Cyst of the Knee

Steven D. Waldman

A common cause of knee pain, Baker's cyst is the result of an abnormal accumulation of synovial fluid in the medial aspect of the popliteal fossa.[1] Overproduction of synovial fluid from the knee joint results in the formation of a cystic sac. This sac often communicates with the knee joint with a one-way valve effect, causing a gradual expansion of the cyst.[2] Often a tear of the medial meniscus or a tendinitis of the medial hamstring tendon is the inciting factor responsible for the development of Baker's cyst.[3] Patients suffering from rheumatoid arthritis are especially susceptible to the development of Baker's cysts.

CLINICAL PRESENTATION

Patients with Baker's cysts will complain a feeling of fullness behind the knee. Often, they will notice a lump behind the knee that becomes more apparent when they flex the affected knee (Fig. 104–1). The cyst may continue to enlarge and may dissect inferiorly into the calf. Patients suffering from rheumatoid arthritis are prone to this phenomenon, and the pain associated with dissection into the calf may be confused with thrombophlebitis and inappropriately treated with anticoagulants.[4]

On physical examination, the patient suffering from Baker's cyst will have a cystic swelling in the medial aspect of the popliteal fossa. Baker's cysts can become quite large, especially in patients suffering from rheumatoid arthritis. Activity including squatting or walking makes the pain of Baker's cyst worse, with rest and heat providing some relief. The pain is constant and characterized as aching and may interfere with sleep. Baker's cyst may spontaneously rupture, and there may be rubor and color in the calf that may mimic thrombophlebitis.[5] Homan's sign will be negative, and no cords will be palpable.

DIAGNOSIS

Plain radiographs are indicated in all patients who present with Baker's cyst. Based on the patient's clinical presentation, additional testing including complete blood cell count, erythrocyte sedimentation rate, and antinuclear antibody testing may be indicated. MRI of the knee is indicated if internal derangement or occult mass or tumor is suspected and is also useful in confirming the presence of Baker's cyst (Fig. 104–2).

DIFFERENTIAL DIAGNOSIS

As mentioned earlier, Baker's cyst may rupture spontaneously and may be misdiagnosed as thrombophlebitis. Occasionally, tendinitis of the medial hamstring tendon may be confused with Baker's cyst, as may injury to the medial meniscus. Primary or metastatic tumors in the region, although rare, must be considered in the differential diagnosis.

TREATMENT

Although surgery is often required to successfully treat Baker's cyst, conservative therapy consisting of an elastic bandage combined with a short trial of nonsteroidal antiinflammatory drugs or cyclooxygenase-2 inhibitors is warranted. If these conservative treatments fail, the following injection technique represents a reasonable next step.[6]

To inject a Baker's cyst, the patient is placed in the prone position with the anterior ankle resting on a folded towel to slightly flex the knee. The middle of the popliteal fossa is identified and at a point two fingerbreaths medial and two fingerbreaths below the popliteal crease the skin is prepped with antiseptic solution. A syringe containing 2.0 mL of 0.25% preservative-free bupivacaine and 40 mg of methylprednisolone is attached to a 2-inch, 22-gauge needle.

The needle is then carefully advanced through the previously identified point at a 45-degree angle from the medial border of the popliteal fossa directly toward the Baker's cyst (Fig. 104–3). While continuously aspirating, the needle is advanced very slowly to avoid trauma to the tibial nerve or popliteal artery or vein. On entering the cyst, synovial fluid will suddenly be aspirated into the syringe. At this point, if there is no paresthesia in the distribution of the common peroneal or tibial nerve, the contents of the syringe is then gently injected. There should be minimal resistance to injection. A pressure dressing is then placed over the cyst to prevent reaccumulation of fluid.

Failure to diagnose primary knee pathology (e.g., tears of the medial meniscus) may lead to further pain and disability. MRI should help identify internal derangement of the knee. The proximity to the common peroneal and tibial nerves as

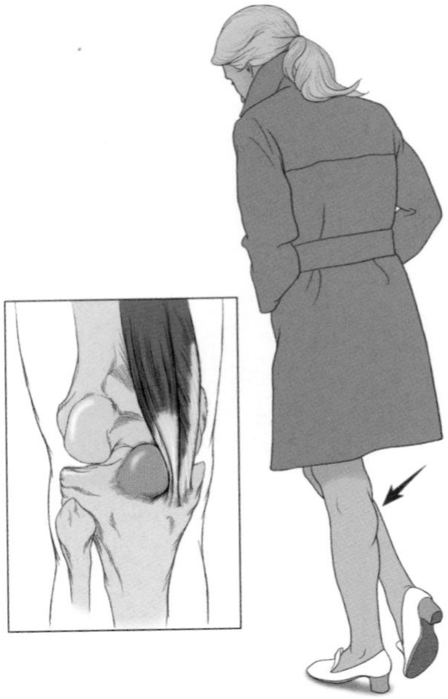

FIGURE 104–1 ■ The patient suffering from Baker's cyst will often complain of a sensation of fullness or a lump behind the knee. (From Waldman SD: Atlas of Common Pain Syndromes. Philadelphia, WB Saunders, 2002, p 267.)

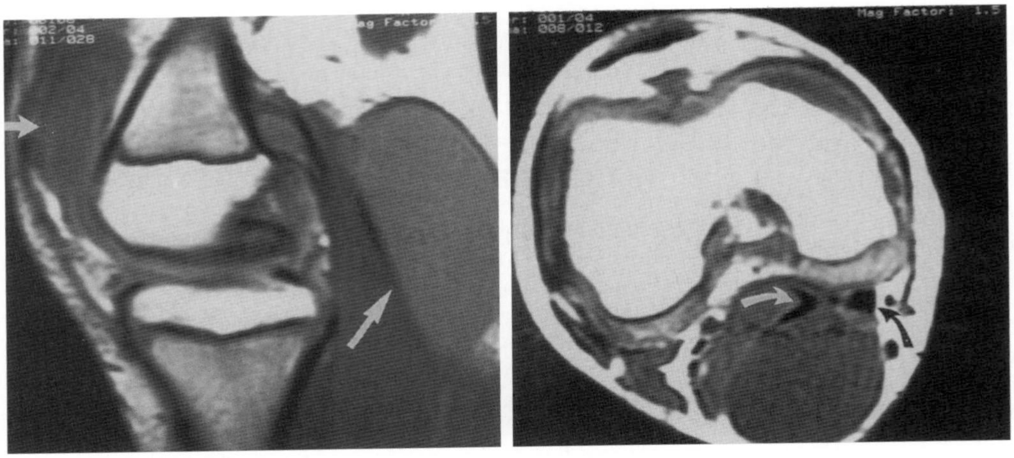

FIGURE 104–2 ■ MRI of the knee is useful in confirming the presence of Baker's cyst. (From Haaga JR, Lanzieri CF, Gilkeson RC: CT and MR Imaging of the Whole Body, 4th ed. Philadelphia, CV Mosby, 2003, p 1808.)

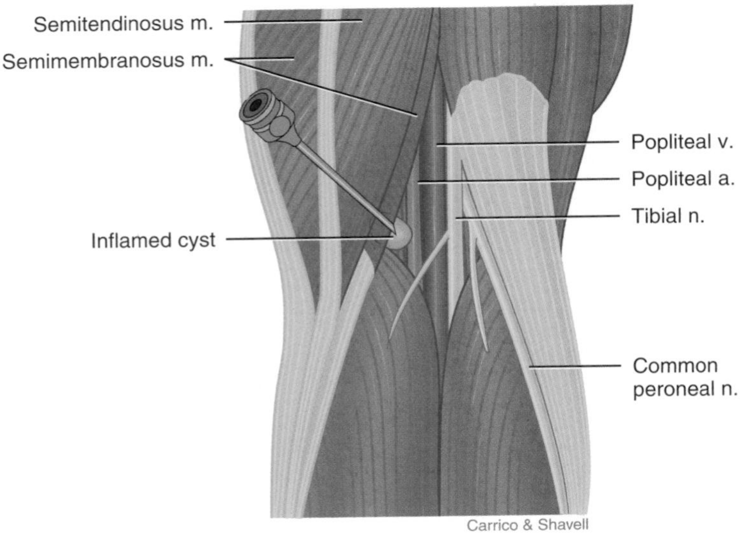

FIGURE 104–3 ■ Technique for injecting Baker's cyst. (From Waldman SD: Atlas of Pain Management Injection Techniques. Philadelphia, WB Saunders, 2000, p 289.)

well as the popliteal artery and vein makes it imperative that this procedure be carried out only by those well versed in the regional anatomy and experienced in performing injection techniques. Many patients will also complain of a transient increase in pain after this injection technique. Although rare, infection may occur if careful attention to sterile technique is not followed.

CONCLUSION

When bursae become inflamed, they may overproduce synovial fluid, which can become trapped in saclike cysts due to a one-way valve phenomenon. This occurs commonly in the medial aspect of the popliteal fossa and is called Baker's cyst. The injection technique described is extremely effective in the treatment of pain and swelling secondary to this disorder. Coexistent semimembranosus bursitis, medial hamstring tendinitis, or internal derangement of the knee may also contribute to knee pain and may require additional treatment with more localized injection of local anesthetic and depot corticosteroid.

References

1. Waldman SD: Baker's cyst. In Waldman SD: Common Pain Syndromes. Philadelphia, WB Saunders, 2002, p 266-268.
2. Rauschning W, Lingren PG: The clinical significance of the valve mechanism in communicating popliteal cysts. Arch Orthop Trauma Surg 95:251, 1979.
3. Stone KR, Stoller D, DeCarli A: The frequency of Baker's cysts associated with meniscal tears Am J Sports Med 24:670, 1996.
4. Scott WN, Jacobs B, Lockshin MD: Posterior compartment syndrome resulting from a dissecting popliteal cyst. Clin Orthop Relat Res 122:189, 1977.
5. Langsfeld M, Matteson B, Johnson W: Baker's cysts mimicking the symptoms of deep venous thrombosis: Diagnosis with venous duplex scanning. J Vasc Surg 25:658, 1997.
6. Waldman SD: Baker's cyst of the knee. In Waldman SD: Atlas of Pain Management Injection Techniques. Philadelphia, WB Saunders, 2000, pp 288-290.

chapter 105

Quadriceps Expansion Syndrome

Steven D. Waldman

The quadriceps expansion syndrome is an uncommon cause of anterior knee pain encountered in clinical practice. This painful condition is characterized by pain at the superior pole of the patella.[1] It is usually the result of overuse or misuse of the knee joint such as running marathons or direct trauma to the quadriceps tendon from kicks or head butts during football. The quadriceps tendon is also subject to acute calcific tendinitis, which may coexist with acute strain injuries. Calcific tendinitis of the quadriceps tendon will have a characteristic radiographic appearance of whiskers on the anterosuperior patella.

The quadriceps tendon is made up of fibers from the four muscles that comprise the quadriceps muscle: the vastus lateralis, the vastus intermedius, the vastus medialis, and the rectus femoris (Fig. 105–1). Fibers of the quadriceps tendon expanding around the patella form the medial and lateral patella retinacula, which help strengthen the knee joint. These fibers are called expansions and are subject to strain, and the tendon proper is subject to the development of tendinitis.

Patients with quadriceps expansion syndrome will present with pain over the superior pole of the sesamoid, more commonly on the medial side. The patient will note increased pain on walking down slopes or down stairs (Fig. 105–2). Activity of the knee will make the pain worse, with rest and heat providing some relief. The pain is constant and characterized as aching and may interfere with sleep.

CLINICAL PRESENTATION

On physical examination, patients suffering from quadriceps expansion syndrome will have tenderness under the superior edge of the patella occurring more commonly on the medial side.[2] Active resisted extension of the knee will reproduce the pain. Coexistent suprapatellar and infrapatellar bursitis, tendinitis, arthritis, and/or internal derangement of the knee may confuse the clinical picture after trauma to the knee joint.[3]

DIAGNOSIS

Plain radiographs of the knee are indicated in all patients who present with quadriceps expansion syndrome pain. Based on the patient's clinical presentation, additional testing including complete blood cell count, erythrocyte sedimentation rate, and antinuclear antibody testing may be indicated. MRI of the knee is indicated if tendinosis, internal derangement, or occult mass or tumor is suspected (Fig. 105–3). Bone scan may be useful to identify occult stress fractures involving the joint, especially if trauma has occurred.

DIFFERENTIAL DIAGNOSIS

The most common cause of anterior knee pain is arthritis of the knee. This should be readily identifiable on plain radiographs of the knee and may coexist with quadriceps expansion syndrome. Another common cause of anterior knee pain that may mimic or coexist with quadriceps expansion syndrome is suprapatellar or prepatellar bursitis.[3] Internal derangement of the knee and a torn medial meniscus may also confuse the clinical diagnosis but should be readily identifiable on MRI of the knee.

TREATMENT

Initial treatment of the pain and functional disability associated with quadriceps insertion syndrome should include a combination of the nonsteroidal antiinflammatory agents or cyclooxygenase-2 inhibitors and physical therapy. Local application of heat and cold may also be beneficial. For patients who do not respond to these treatment modalities, injection of the quadriceps expansion, as described next, with a local anesthetic and a corticosteroid may be a reasonable next step.[4]

To inject the quadriceps expansion, the patient is placed supine with a rolled blanket underneath the knee to gently flex the joint. The skin overlying the medial aspect of the knee joint is prepped with antiseptic solution. A sterile syringe containing the 2.0 mL of 0.25% preservative-free bupivacaine and 40 mg of methylprednisolone is attached to a 1.5-inch 25-gauge needle using strict aseptic technique. The medial edge of the superior patella is identified (Fig. 105–4). At this point, the needle is inserted horizontally toward the medial edge of the patella. The needle is then carefully advanced through the skin and subcutaneous tissues until it impinges on the medial edge of the patella. The needle is withdrawn slightly out of the periosteum of the patella, and the contents of the syringe is then gently injected. There should be little resistance to injection. If resistance is encountered, the needle is probably in a ligament or tendon and should be advanced or withdrawn

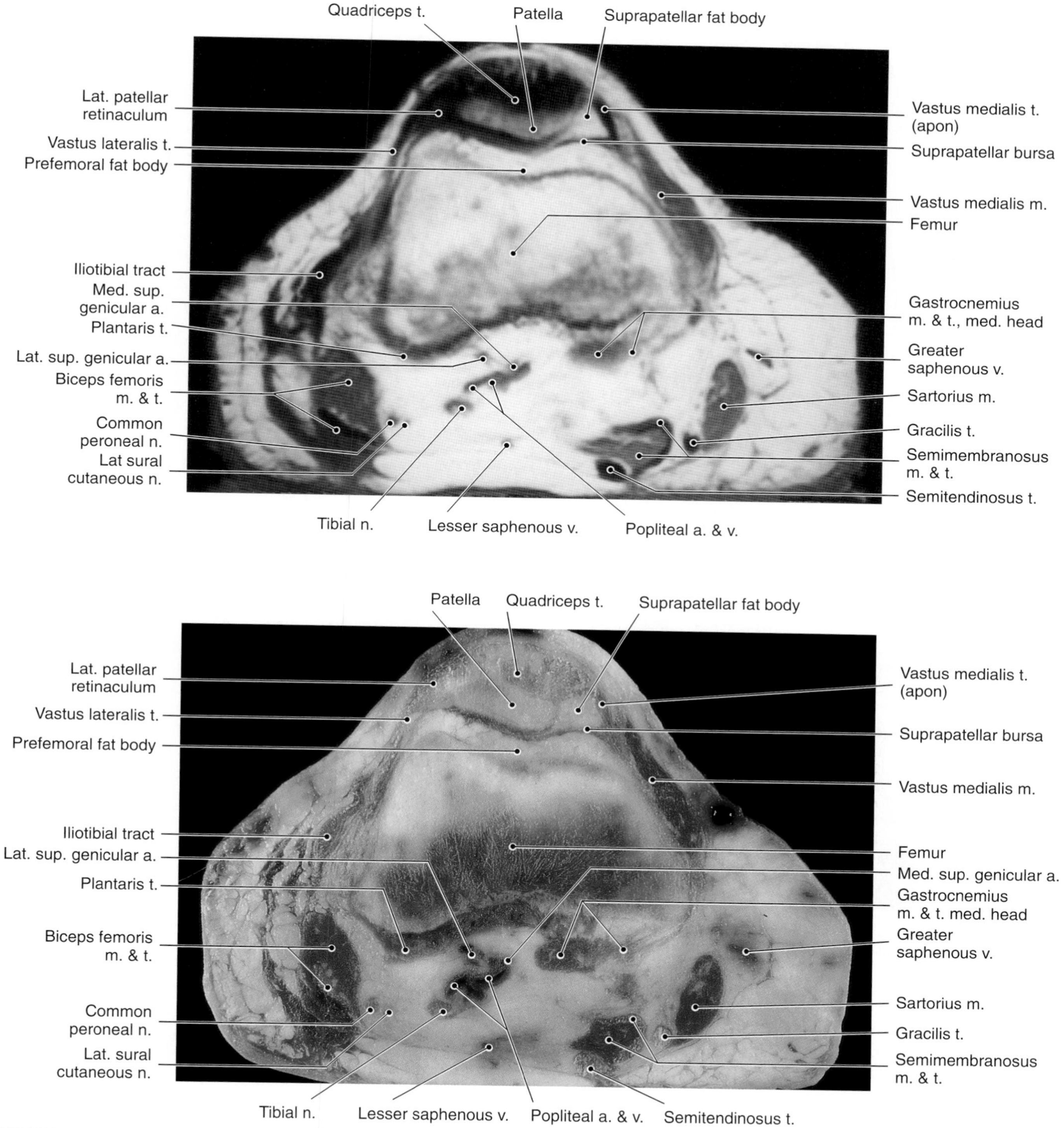

FIGURE 105–1 ■ The quadriceps tendon is made up of fibers from the four muscles that comprise the quadriceps muscle: the vastus lateralis, the vastus intermedius, the vastus medialis, and the rectus femoris. (From Kang HS, Ahn JM, Resnick D et al [eds]: MRI of the Extremities, 2nd ed. Philadelphia, WB Saunders, 2002, p 315.)

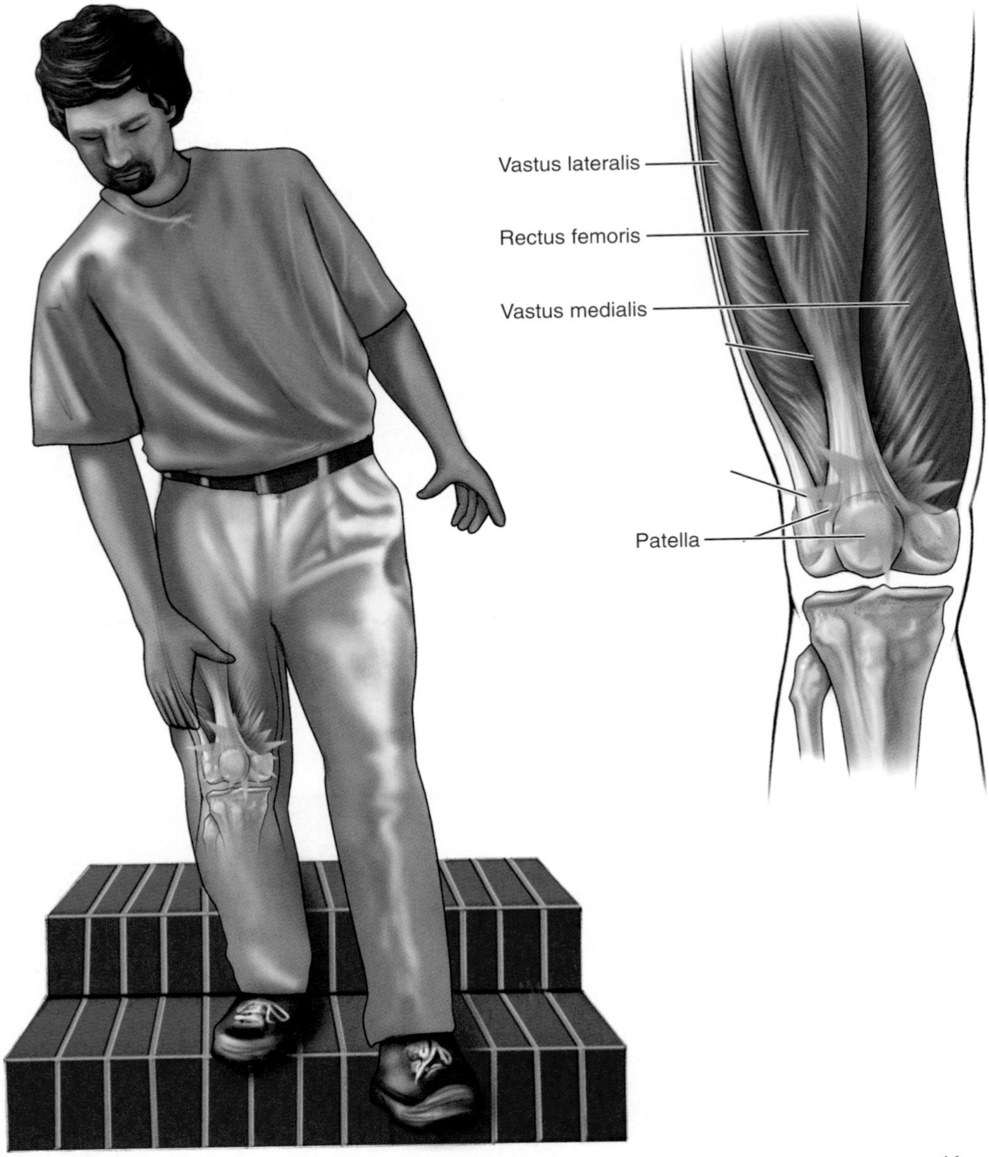

FIGURE 105–2 ■ Patients with quadriceps expansion syndrome will present with pain over the superior pole of the sesamoid, more commonly on the medial side. (From Waldman SD: Atlas of Uncommon Pain Syndromes. Philadelphia, WB Saunders, 2003, p 216.)

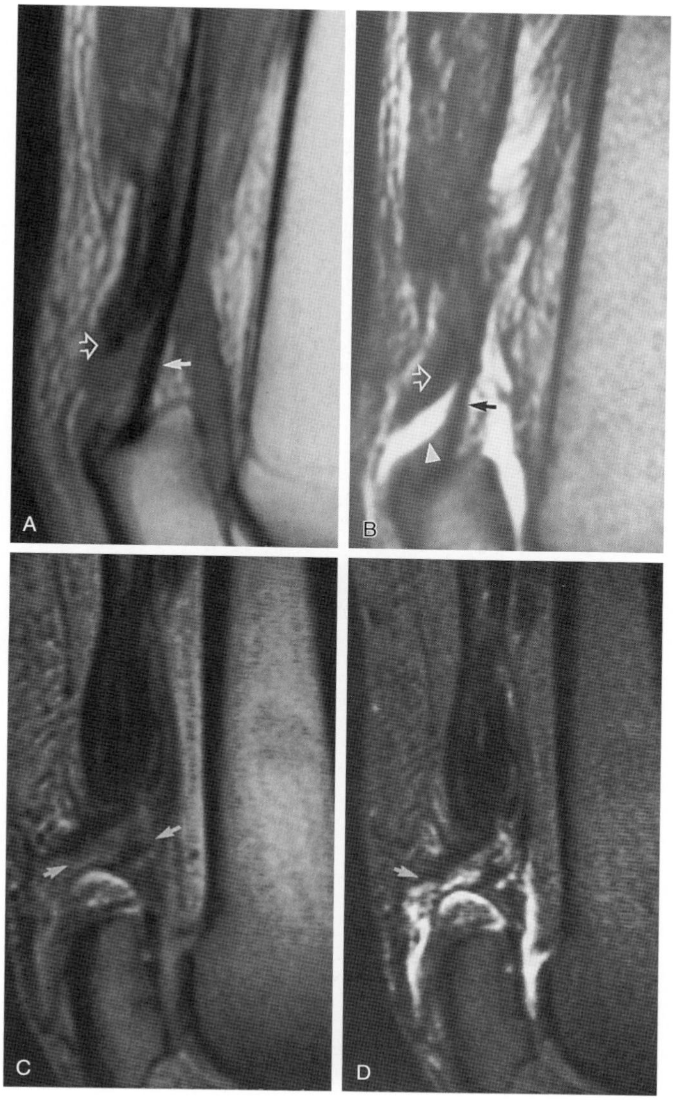

FIGURE 105–3 ■ Partial and complete tears of the quadriceps tendon: **A** and **B,** Partial tear. Sagittal intermediate-weighted (TR/TE, 2500/20) (**A**) and T2-weighted (TR/TE, 2500/80) (**B**) spin-echo MR images show disruption of the normal trilaminar appearance of the quadriceps tendon. The tendon *(solid arrows)* of the vastus intermedius muscle appears intact. The other tendons have retracted *(open arrows)*. Note the high signal intensity at the site of the tear *(arrowhead)* and in the soft tissues and muscles in **B**. **C** and **D,** Complete tear. Sagittal intermediate-weighted (TR/TE, 2500/30) (**C**) and T2-weighted (TR/TE, 2500/80) (**D**) spin-echo MR images show a complete tear *(arrows)* of the quadriceps tendon at the tendo-osseous junction. Note the high signal intensity at the site of the tear in **D**. The patella is displaced inferiorly. (From Resnick D [ed]: Diagnosis of Bone and Joint Disorders, 4th ed. Philadelphia, WB Saunders, 2002, p 3229.)

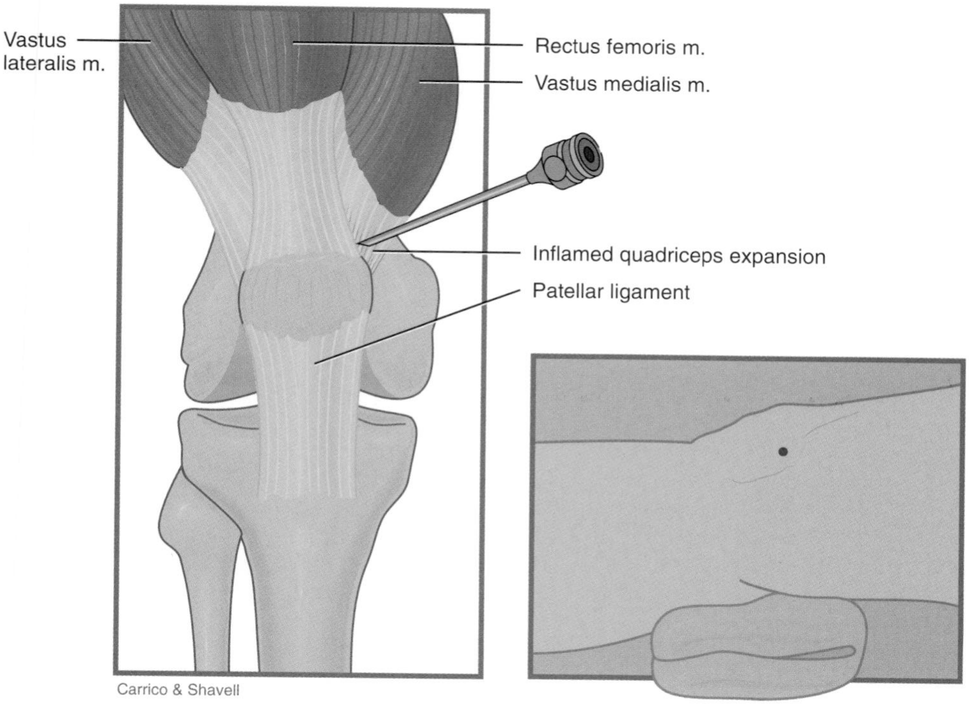

FIGURE 105–4 ■ Injection technique for relieving the pain due to quadriceps expansion syndrome. (From Waldman SD: Atlas of Pain Management Injection Techniques. Philadelphia, WB Saunders, 2000, p 266.)

slightly until the injection proceeds without significant resistance. The needle is then removed and a sterile pressure dressing and ice pack are placed at the injection site.

The major complication of this injection technique is infection. This complication should be exceedingly rare if strict aseptic technique is adhered to. Approximately 25% of patients will complain of a transient increase in pain after injection of the quadriceps tendon of the knee and should be warned of such. The clinician should also identify coexisting internal derangement of the knee, primary and metastatic tumors, and infection, which if undiagnosed may yield disastrous results.

References

1. Kirkendall DT, Garrett WE: Injuries to the muscle-tendon unit. In Fitzgerald RH, Kaufer H, Malkani AL (eds): Orthopaedics. St. Louis, CV Mosby, 2002, pp 555-556.
2. Waldman SD: Quadriceps expansion syndrome. In Waldman SD: Atlas of Uncommon Pain Syndromes. Philadelphia, WB Saunders, 2003, pp 215-217.
3. Waldman SD: Suprapatellar bursitis. In Waldman SD: Atlas of Common Pain Syndromes. Philadelphia, WB Saunders, 2002, pp 254-256.
4. Waldman SD: Quadriceps expansion syndrome. In Waldman SD: Atlas of Pain Management Injection Techniques. Philadelphia, WB Saunders, 2000, pp 264-266.

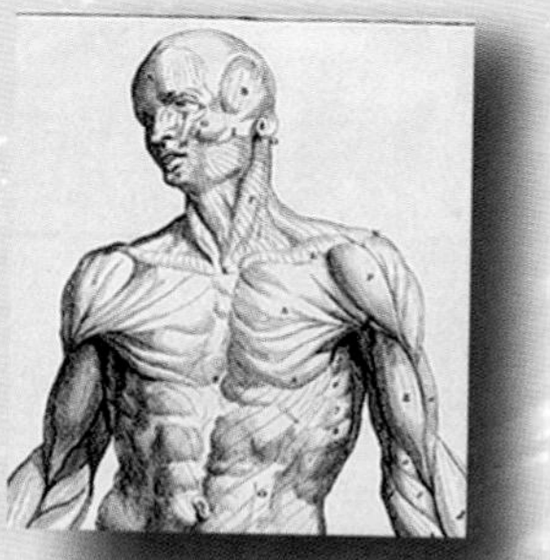

Part L

Pain Syndromes of the Ankle and Foot

chapter 106

Arthritis of the Ankle and Foot

Adel G. Fam

Painful disorders of the ankle and foot are a common presentation in general, rheumatologic, orthopedic, and physiatric practices. The pain may arise from the bones and joints of the ankle and foot, periarticular structures (tendon sheaths, tendon insertions, or bursae), plantar fascia, nerve roots and peripheral nerves, or vascular system or be referred from the lumbar spine or knee joint.[1,2] A classification of painful disorders of the ankle and foot, based on the site of origin and predominant location of the pain, is outlined in Table 106–1. Static disorders due to inappropriate footwear, foot deformities, and/or weak intrinsic muscles account for most painful foot conditions. Precise diagnosis depends on knowledge of anatomy, a detailed history, and an assessment of the joints, periarticular soft tissue structures, nerve and blood supply, and lumbar spine. Diagnostic studies include routine laboratory tests, synovial fluid analysis (when available), plain radiographs, nerve conduction studies, vascular (Doppler) studies, bone scintiscan, sonography, CT, and MRI.[3] Special radiographic views, arthrography, arteriography, gait analysis, and footprint studies are occasionally required.[1,2]

The *ankle or talocrural joint* is a hinge joint between the distal ends of the tibia and fibula and the trochlea of the talus. The synovial cavity does not normally communicate with other joints, adjacent tendon sheaths, or bursae. Tendons crossing the ankle region are invested for part of their course in tenosynovial sheaths (Figs. 106–1 and 106–2). Posteriorly, the common tendon of the gastrocnemius and soleus (Achilles tendon or tendocalcaneus) is inserted into the posterior surface of the calcaneus.[1-4] The tendon does not have a synovial sheath but is surrounded by a loose connective tissue, paratenon, or peritenon.

The retrocalcaneal bursa is located between the Achilles tendon insertion and the posterior surface of the calcaneus. It is surrounded anteriorly by Kager's fat pad. The bursa serves to protect the distal Achilles tendon from frictional wear against the posterior calcaneus. The retroachilleal bursa lies between the skin and the Achilles tendon and protects the tendon from external pressure. The subcalcaneal bursa is located beneath the skin over the plantar aspect of the calcaneus. Two bursae, the medial and lateral subcutaneous malleolar or "last" bursae, are located near the medial and lateral malleoli, respectively (see Figs 106–1 and 106–2).[1,4]

Table 106–1

Painful Disorders of the Ankle and the Foot

Type	*Example*
Articular	
Arthritis	Rheumatoid arthritis, osteoarthritis, psoriatic arthritis, gout
Toe disorders	Hallux valgus, hallux rigidus, hammertoe
Arch disorders	Pes planus, pes cavus
Periarticular	
Cutaneous	Corn, callosity
Subcutaneous	Rheumatoid arthritis nodules, tophi
	Ingrowing toenail
Plantar fascia	Plantar fasciitis
	Plantar nodular fibromatosis
Tendons	Achilles tendonitis
	Achilles tendon rupture
	Tibialis posterior tenosynovitis
	Peroneal tenosynovitis
Bursae	Bunion, bunionette
	Retrocalcaneal and retroachilleal bursitis
	Medial and lateral malleolar bursitis
Acute calcific periarthritis	Hydroxyapatite pseudopodagra (first metatarsophalangeal joint)
Osseous	Fracture (traumatic and stress)
	Sesamoiditis
	Neoplasm
	Infection
	Epiphysitis (osteochondritis)
	Second metatarsal head (Frieberg disease)
	Navicular (Kohler disease)
	Calcaneus (Sever disease)
	Painful accessory ossicles
	Accessory navicular
	Os trigonum (near talus)
	Os intermetatarseum (first to second)
Neurologic	Tarsal tunnel syndrome
	Interdigital (Morton) neuroma
	Peripheral neuropathy
	Radiculopathy (lumbar disc)
Vascular	Ischemic (atherosclerosis, Buerger disease)
	Vasospastic disorder (Raynaud phenomenon)
	Cholesterol emboli with "purple toes"
Referred	Lumbosacral spine
	Knee
	Reflex sympathetic dystrophy syndrome

ETIOLOGY AND CLINICAL PRESENTATION

The main causes of arthritis of the ankle and subtalar and other joints of the foot include rheumatoid arthritis, psoriatic arthritis, systemic lupus erythematosus, gout, trauma, and osteoarthritis.

Ankle arthritis is characterized by a diffuse swelling, joint line tenderness, restricted movements, and synovial thickening anteriorly with obliteration of the two small depressions that are normally present in front of the malleoli. A large ankle effusion may bulge both medial and lateral to the extensor tendons and produce fluctuance; pressure with one hand on one side of the joint produces a fluid wave transmitted to the second hand placed on the opposite side of the ankle. A traumatic tear of the talofibular ligament allows forward movement of the tibia and fibula on the talus (positive anterior draw sign).[1] Ankle tenosynovitis, by contrast, presents as a linear, superficial, tender, swelling localized to the distribution of the tendon sheath and extending beyond the joint margins. Movements of the involved tendon often produce pain.[1]

The *subtalar (talocalcaneal) joint* lies between the talus and the calcaneus. It permits about 30 degrees of foot inversion (sole of the foot turned inward), and 10 to 20 degrees of eversion (sole turned outward).[1,4] Subtalar arthritis is associated with painful restriction of inversion and eversion, diffuse swelling, and tenderness in the subtalar region, but direct palpation of the joint is difficult.

The *midtarsal (transverse tarsal) joint* comprises the combined talonavicular and calcaneocuboid joints.[1,4] The cuboid and navicular are usually joined by fibrous tissue, but

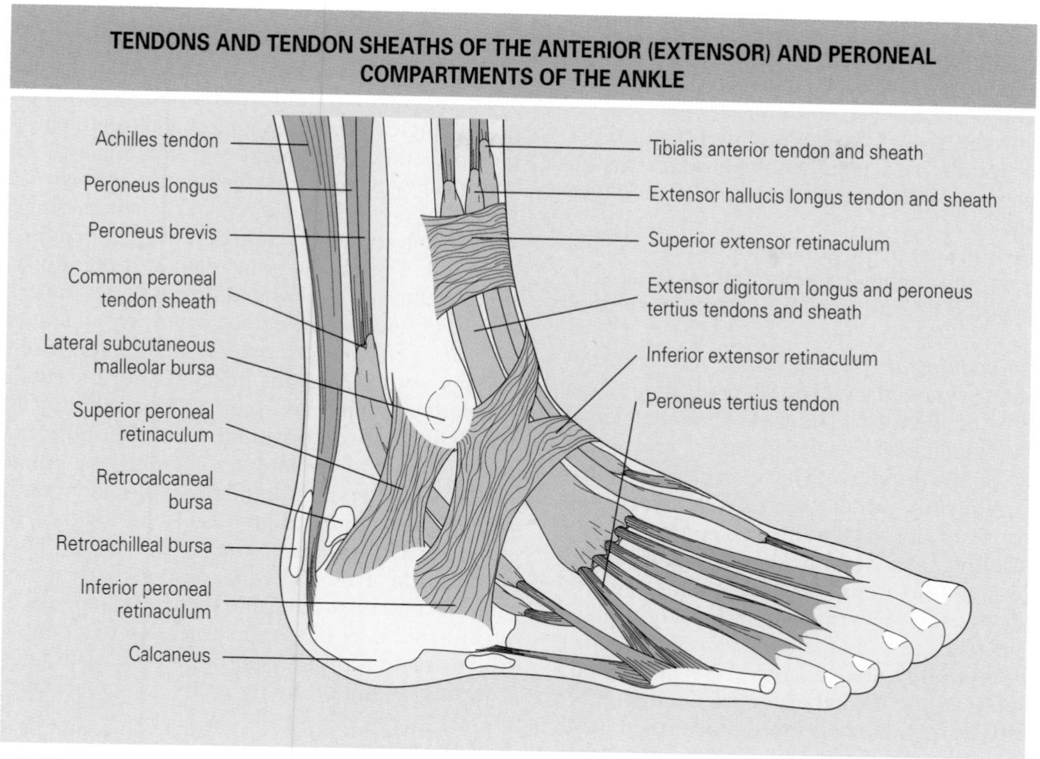

FIGURE 106–1 ■ Bursae, tendons, and tendon sheaths of the anterior tibial (extensor) and peroneal compartments of the ankle.

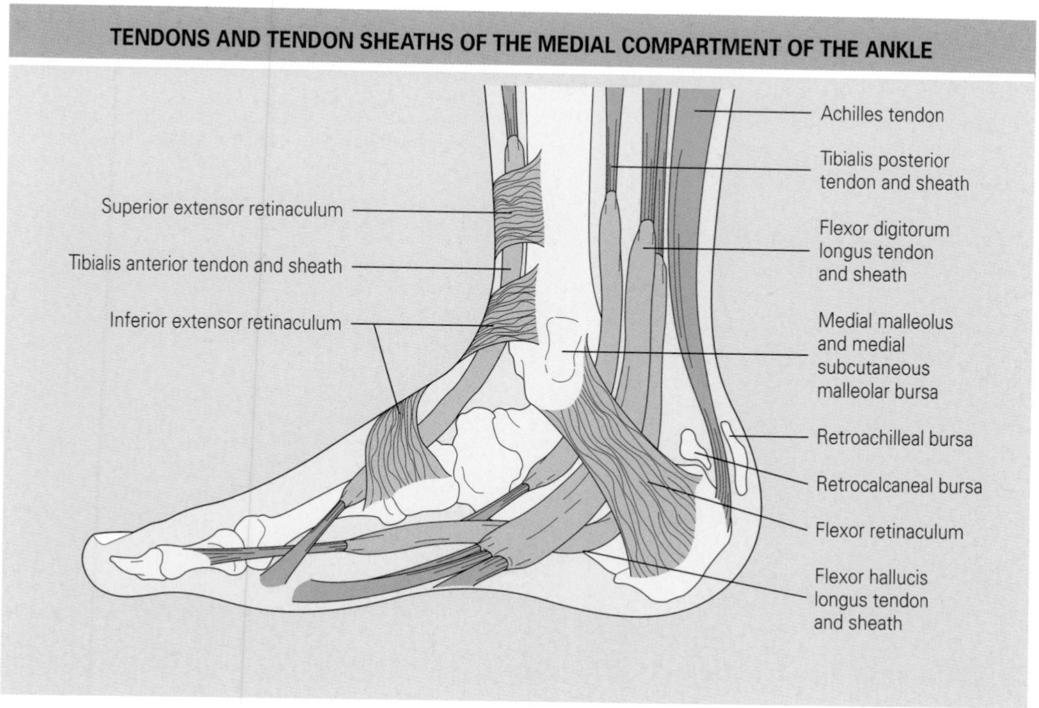

FIGURE 106–2 ■ Bursae, tendons, and tendon sheaths of the medial (flexor) compartment of the ankle.

a synovial cavity may exist between them. The midtarsal joint contributes to inversion (supination) and eversion (pronation) movements at the subtalar joint. It also allows 20 degrees of adduction (foot turned toward the midline) and 10 degrees of abduction (foot turned away from the midline). Arthritis of the transverse tarsal joint is associated with painful restriction of inversion and eversion, diffuse tenderness, and swelling of the midtarsal region.

The *intertarsal joints* are plane gliding joints between the navicular, cuneiforms, and cuboid that intercommunicate with one another and with the intermetatarsal and tarsometatarsal joints.

The *metatarsophalangeal (MTP) joints* are ellipsoid joints lined by separate synovial cavities. They lie about 2 cm proximal to the webs of the toes.[1] The transverse metatarsal ligament binds the metatarsal heads together preventing excessive splaying of the forefoot. The intermetatarsophalangeal bursae are frequently present between the metatarsal heads. Chronic arthritis of the MTP joints is characterized by local tenderness, swelling, synovial thickening, and a painful "metatarsal compression test" (pain on gentle compression of the metatarsal heads together with one hand). Forefoot splaying or spread, from weakness of the transverse metatarsal ligaments, and toe deformities are frequent. A bursa (bunion) is commonly located over the medial aspect of the first MTP joint. Less frequently, a small bursa is present over the lateral aspect of the fifth metatarsal head (bunionette or tailor's bursa).

The proximal and distal interphalangeal (PIP and DIP) joints are hinge joints.[1] The digital flexor tendon sheaths enclose the long and short flexor tendons extending proximally along the length of the toes to the distal third of the sole.

Arthritis of the PIP and DIP joints is associated with tender swelling, synovial thickening, restriction of movements, and often toe deformities.

TREATMENT

Management of arthritis of the ankle, subtalar, midtarsal, MTP, PIP, and DIP joints of the toes depends primarily on the underlying cause. For symptomatic treatment, rest, local heat therapy, and nonsteroidal antiinflammatory drugs are often helpful. For persistent inflammatory synovitis, corticosteroid injections are often beneficial.[5] The ankle joint can be injected via an anteromedial approach with the joint slightly plantarflexed. The needle is inserted at a point just medial to the tibialis anterior tendon and distal to the lower margin of the tibia. The needle is directed posteriorly and laterally to a depth of 1 to 2 cm, and 20 mg of methylprednisolone acetate or another corticosteroid is injected.[5] For the subtalar joint, with the patient supine and the leg-foot-ankle at 90 degrees, the needle is inserted horizontally into the subtalar joint just inferior to the tip of the lateral malleolus at a point just proximal to the sinus tarsi.[5] The midtarsal, other intertarsal, and tarsometatarsal joints cannot easily be injected without fluoroscopic or CT guidance. The MTP, PIP, and DIP joints can be entered via a dorsomedial or dorsolateral route. The joint space is first identified, and then a 28-gauge needle is inserted on either side of the extensor tendon to a depth of 2 to 4 mm. Slight traction on the appropriate toe facilitates entry before injecting 10 mg of methylprednisolone acetate.[5]

References

1. Fam AG: The ankle and foot. In Hochberg H, Silman A, Smolen J, et al (eds): Rheumatology, 3rd ed. London, Mosby, 2003, pp 681-692.
2. Pyasta RT, Panush RS: Common painful foot syndromes. Bull Rheum Dis 48:1, 1999.
3. Schweitzer ME, Karasick D: MR imaging of disorders of the Achilles tendon. AJR Am J Roentgenol 175:613, 2000.
4. Perry J: Anatomy and biomechanics of the hindfoot. Clin Orthop 177:9, 1983.
5. Fam AG: The ankle and foot. In Klippel JH, Dieppe PA (eds): Rheumatology. St. Louis, CV Mosby, 1993, pp 13.1-13.12.

chapter 107

Achilles Tendinitis and Bursitis and Other Painful Conditions of the Ankle

Adel G. Fam

ACHILLES TENDINITIS

Etiology

Achilles tendinitis is usually caused by repetitive trauma and microscopic tears due to excessive use of the calf muscles as in ballet dancing, distance running (about 10% of runners), track and field, jumping, and other athletic activities or from wearing faulty footwear with a rigid shoe counter.[1-7] Tendon microtears are often associated with both focal mucoid degeneration and neovascularization.[8] Insertional Achilles tendinitis, often associated with enthesopathy and retrocalcaneal bursitis, occurs frequently in patients with spondyloarthropathies, such as ankylosing spondylitis or psoriatic arthritis. The tendon is also a common site for gouty tophi, rheumatoid nodules, and xanthomas.[1]

Clinical Presentation

Tendinitis of the Achilles tendon is characterized by activity-related pain, swelling, tenderness, and sometimes crepitus over the tendon 2 to 6 cm from its insertion.[1-7] Thickening and irregularity of the tissues surrounding the tendon and sometimes a palpable nodule may be present. Passive dorsiflexion of the ankle intensifies the pain. The "painful arc sign" (movements of the tender swollen area within the tendon with active dorsiflexion and plantarflexion of the ankle) and the "Royal London Hospital test" (tenderness on re-palpating a tender swollen area within the tendon with the ankle in maximum active dorsiflexion and plantarflexion) are often positive.[7]

Diagnosis

Abnormalities of the tendon and peritendinous tissues can be demonstrated by both ultrasonography[9] and MRI.[3] By ultrasound, Achilles tendinitis is characterized by swelling and a hypoechogenic area within the substance of the tendon with loss of the normal, well-organized, ribbon-like intratendinous echostructure.[9] The ultrasound demonstration of a spindle-shaped thickening of the Achilles tendon in asymptomatic athletes may also predict those at risk of subsequently developing symptoms.[9]

Treatment

Treatment consists of a period of rest, weight reduction in obese patients, avoidance of the provocative occupational or athletic activity, shoe modification, a heel raise to reduce stretching of the tendon during walking, nonsteroidal antiinflammatory drugs, and physiotherapy, including local ice or heat application, gentle stretching exercises, and sometimes a temporary splint with slight ankle plantarflexion.[1-3] Avoidance of hills and uneven running surfaces and diligent stretching before sport activities are often beneficial. Symptoms may persist for several months. The Achilles tendon is vulnerable to rupture, particularly in elderly individuals. Corticosteroid injections in or near the tendon are of questionable value. These can predispose to tendon rupture and are, therefore, strongly discouraged.[1-7,10] Color Doppler ultrasound-guided injection of a sclerosing solution into new vessels within the tendon is a promising but unproven new treatment.[8] Surgical treatment, including open tenotomy with excision of the inflamed peritendinous tissue, open tenotomy with paratenon stripping, or percutaneous longitudinal tenotomy, is rarely required in those not responding to more than 6 months of nonoperative management.[1-7,11]

ACHILLES TENDON RUPTURE

Etiology

The area of the Achilles tendon, located 2 to 6 cm proximal to its calcaneal insertion, has the poorest blood supply, predisposing this region to tendinopathy and possible rupture.[6] Achilles tendon rupture occurs most commonly in active men between 30 and 50 years old, typically during a burst of unaccustomed physical activity involving forced ankle dorsiflexion. It may also result from a sharp blow, from a fall, or from intense athletic activities, particularly football, basketball, baseball, and tennis.[1-7,12,13] It may occur spontaneously or after minor trauma in elderly patients with preexisting Achilles tendinitis or retrocalcaneal bursitis, patients with systemic lupus erythematosus or rheumatoid arthritis receiving corticosteroids, in those on long-term hemodialysis, after local corticosteroid injections in the vicinity of the tendon, and in patients treated with fluoroquinolone antibiotics.[14]

Clinical Presentation

The onset is often sudden, with pain in the region of the tendon, sometimes with a faint "pop" sound and difficulty walking or standing on the toes.[1-7,12,13] Swelling, ecchymosis, tenderness, and sometimes a palpable gap are present at the site of the tear. In partial tendon rupture, active plantarflexion of the ankle may be preserved but painful. In those with complete rupture it is still possible to actively plantarflex the ankle with the adjacent intact flexor tendons. However, gentle squeezing of the calf muscles with the patient prone, sitting, or kneeling on a chair produces little or no passive ankle plantarflexion (positive Thompson calf squeeze test).[1-7,12,13] If the Thompson test is equivocal, a sphygmomanometer cuff is inflated to 100 mm Hg around the calf with the patient lying prone and knee flexed 90 degrees.[13] If the tendon is intact, the pressure rises to about 140 mm Hg with passive dorsiflexion of the ankle, but it changes very little if the tendon is ruptured.[13] Rupture is typically associated with inability to perform single-leg toe raise on the affected side.

Diagnosis

It is estimated that 20% to 30% of Achilles tendon ruptures are not diagnosed on initial assessment.[6,13] The tendon defect can be disguised by hematoma, and the patient may retain some plantarflexion power because of the actions of the flexor digitorum, flexor hallucis longus, tibialis posterior, and peronei. The Thompson test should, therefore, be performed in all patients with suspected Achilles tendon injury. If the diagnosis is still in doubt, the extent and orientation of the rupture can be confirmed and accurately assessed by either ultrasonography[15] or MRI.[1,3]

Treatment

Open operative or percutaneous repair of the ruptured Achilles tendon is indicated in the majority of patients, particularly in young athletes.[1-7,13,16] Surgery is followed by 6 weeks of immobilization, including 2 weeks of non–weight bearing using crutches. Nonoperative treatment, with cast immobilization for 8 to 12 weeks with 4 weeks of non–weight bearing, is sometimes advocated in older, less active persons.[4-7,12] However, immobilization is associated with a higher rerupture rate, a more prolonged recovery time, and a less favorable functional outcome.[1-7,12,16]

RETROCALCANEAL, SUB-ACHILLES, OR SUBTENDINOUS BURSITIS

Etiology

Retrocalcaneal bursitis usually occurs in middle-aged and elderly individuals. Known causes include rheumatoid arthritis, psoriatic arthritis, and ankylosing spondylitis.[1,2,6,17] It may also occur in association with both Haglund's deformity (abnormal prominence of the posterosuperior surface of the calcaneus causing chronic irritation of Achilles tendon and bursa)[18] and Achilles tendinitis resulting from overactivity. Haglund's deformity is often associated with a varus hindfoot. When viewed from behind, it presents as a round bony swelling just lateral to the distal part of the Achilles tendon.[18]

Clinical Presentation

Retrocalcaneal bursitis is associated with posterior heel pain that is aggravated by passive dorsiflexion of the ankle.[1,2,6,17] It is often worse in the beginning of an activity, such as walking and running, and diminishes as the activity continues. Symptoms seem to improve on weekends and during vacations. Patients may develop a limp, and wearing shoes can become painful. On examination, the bursitis is associated with tenderness and sometimes erythema on the posterior aspect of the heel at the tendon insertion. Bursal distention produces a tender swelling behind the ankle with bulging on both sides of the tendon.[1,2,6,17] The diagnosis can be confirmed by radiography (showing obliteration of the retrocalcaneal recess, a Haglund deformity, and sometimes calcified distal Achilles tendon), ultrasonography,[19] or MRI.[17]

Treatment

Rest, activity modification, heat application, a slight heel elevation using a felt heel pad or cup, and NSAIDs constitute sufficient therapy for most patients.[1,2,6] A walking cast and/or a cautious ultrasound-guided corticosteroid injection into the bursa are sometimes required. Surgical bursectomy and resection of the superior prominence of the calcaneal tuberosity are rarely indicated.[1,2,6,18]

RETROACHILLEAL OR SUBCUTANEOUS CALCANEAL BURSITIS

Retroachilleal bursitis, also known as "pump bumps," produces a painful tender subcutaneous swelling overlying the Achilles tendon, usually at the level of the shoe counter.[1-4] The overlying skin may be hyperkeratotic or reddened. It occurs predominantly in women and is frequently caused and aggravated by improperly fitting shoes or pumps with a stiff, closely contoured heel counter. It may also occur in patients with Haglund's deformity and varus hindfoot.[1,2,4,6,18]

Treatment

Treatment consists of rest, heat application, NSAIDs, padding, and relief from shoe pressure by wearing a soft, nonrestrictive shoe without a counter. Local corticosteroid injections should be avoided. Surgical excision is rarely indicated.[1,2,6]

References

1. Fam AG: The ankle and foot. In Hochberg H, Silman A, et al (eds): Rheumatology, 3rd ed. London, Mosby, 2003, pp 681-692.
2. Pyasta RT, Panush RS: Common painful foot syndromes. Bull Rheum Dis 48:1-4, 1999.
3. Schweitzer ME, Karasick D: MR imaging of disorders of the Achilles tendon. AJR Am J Roentgenol 175:613, 2000.
4. Plattner PF: Tendon problems of the foot and ankle. Postgrad Med 86:155, 1989.
5. Scioli MW: Achilles tendinitis. Orthop Clin North Am 25:177, 1994.
6. Mazzone MF, McCue T: Common conditions of the Achilles tendon. Am Fam Physician 65:1805, 2002.
7. Maffuli N, Kenward MG, Testa V, et al: Clinical diagnosis of Achilles tendinopathy with tendinosis. Clin J Sport Med 13:11, 2003.

8. Ohberg L, Alfredson H: Ultrasound guided sclerosis of neovessels in painful Achilles tendinosis: Pilot study of a new treatment. Br J Sports Med 36:173, 2002.
9. Fredberg U, Bolvig L: Significance of ultrasonographically detected asymptomatic tendinosis in the patellar and Achilles tendons of elite soccer players: A longitudinal study. Am J Sports Med 30:488, 2002.
10. Shrier I, Matheson GO, Kohl HW III: Achilles tendonitis: Are corticosteroid injections useful or harmful? Clin J Sports Med 6:245, 1996.
11. Tallon C, Coleman BD, Khan K, Maffulli N: Outcome of surgery for chronic Achilles tendinopathy: A critical review. Am J Sports Med 29:315, 2001.
12. Maffulli N: Rupture of the Achilles tendon. J Bone Joint Surg Am 81:1019, 1999.
13. Copeland SA: Rupture of the Achilles tendon: A new clinical test. Ann R Coll Surg Engl 72:270, 1990.
14. Harrell RM: Fluoroquinolone-induced tendinopathy: What do we know? South Med J 92:622, 1999.
15. Kainberger FM, Engel A, Barton P, et al: Injury of the Achilles tendon: Diagnosis with sonography. AJR Am J Roentgenol 155:1031, 1990.
16. Webb JM, Bannister GC: Percutaneous repair of the ruptured tendo Achillis. J Bone Joint Surg Br 81:877, 1999.
17. Olivieri I, Barozzi L, Padula A, et al: Retrocalcaneal bursitis in spondyloarthropathy: Assessment by ultrasonography and magnetic imaging resonance. J Rheumatol 25:1352, 1998.
18. Stephens MM: Haglund's deformity and retrocalcaneal bursitis. Orthop Clin North Am 25:41, 1994.
19. Bottger BA, Schweitzer ME, El-Noueam K, Desai M: MR imaging of the normal and abnormal retrocalcaneal bursae. AJR 170:1239, 1998.

chapter 108

Morton Interdigital Neuroma and Other Causes of Metatarsalgia

Adel G. Fam

ETIOLOGY

Metatarsalgia, or pain and tenderness in and about the metatarsal heads or metatarsophalangeal (MTP) joints, is a common symptom of diverse causes (Table 108–1).[1-6] The condition often follows years of disuse and weakness of the intrinsic muscles owing to chronic foot strain from improper footwear with the toes cramped into tight or pointed shoes.

CLINICAL PRESENTATION

Metatarsalgia may either be limited to a single joint or generalized across the ball of the foot. Pain in the forefoot on standing and walking and tenderness on palpation of the metatarsal heads and sometimes the MTP joints are the main clinical findings.[1,3-6] Prominent, dropped central metatarsal heads, plantar calluses, and clawed toes are frequently present.

MORTON INTERDIGITAL NEUROMA

Historical Aspects

Detailed description of interdigital neuroma was first reported by T. G. Morton in 1876.[7]

Etiology

Morton neuroma is commonly unilateral and occurs most often in middle-aged women. It often results from chronic foot strain and repetitive trauma caused by inappropriately fitting shoes or from mechanical foot problems such as pronated flatfoot and pes cavus.[1-8] It represents an entrapment neuropathy (rather than a true neuroma) of an interdigital nerve, typically between the third and fourth, or the second and third, metatarsal heads but rarely in the first or fourth. The nerve is entrapped under the transverse metatarsal ligament, causing endoneural edema, demyelination, axonal injury, and perineurial fibrosis. An intermetatarsophalangeal bursa or synovial cyst may also cause compression of the nerve.

Clinical Features

Although Morton neuroma can be clinically silent, typical symptoms include paroxysms of lancinating, burning, or neuralgic pain in the affected interdigital cleft and occasionally paresthesia or anesthesia of contiguous borders of adjacent toes.[1-9] Relief of pain when the shoe is removed and the foot is massaged is characteristic. Walking on hard surfaces or wearing tight or high-heeled shoes increases the discomfort. The metatarsal arch is often depressed and tenderness is present over the entrapped nerve between the third and fourth metatarsal heads.[1-9] The pain is made worse by compression of the metatarsal heads together with one hand while squeezing the affected web space between the thumb and index finger of the opposite hand (web space compression test). Injection of 1% lidocaine into the symptomatic interspace often temporarily relieves the pain.[1,7] Altered sensation may be found on the lateral aspect of the third toe and the medial aspect of the fourth toe. A soft tissue mass (neuroma) may be palpable between the metatarsal heads. Movements of the adjacent toes may produce a clicking sensation produced by extrusion of the neuroma from between the metatarsal heads as it moves beneath the transverse metatarsal ligament (Mulder's sign).[1,2,3-8] The affected nerve may show slow sensory conduction velocity on electrophysiologic testing. The exact location and extent of the lesion can be determined by both sonography[10] and MRI.[11] MRI is more sensitive and often shows a well-demarcated mass on the plantar side of the transverse metatarsal ligament. The lesion is hypointense relative to fat on T2-weighted fast spin-echo sequences.[11]

Treatment

Symptomatic management of metatarsalgia includes a metatarsal pad placed proximal to the metatarsal heads, weight reduction in obese patients, strengthening of the intrinsic muscles by toe flexion exercises, and shoe modification, including a wide toe box and, in patients with a pronated foot, an arch support.[1-9] If these measures fail, metatarsal osteotomy and/or metatarsal head resection are indicated. In Morton neuroma, nonoperative measures, including proper footwear, metatarsal pad, and local corticosteroid injections

Table 108–1

Causes of Metatarsalgia

- Chronic foot strain and weakness of intrinsic muscles from improper footwear with the toes crammed into tight or pointed shoes
- Altered foot biomechanics due to flat, cavus, or splay foot
- Interdigital (Morton) neuroma
- Attrition of the plantar fat pad in elderly patients
- Painful plantar callosities, including "intractable plantar keratosis" (discrete or diffuse painful callus beneath one or more of the lateral metatarsals)
- Plantar plate rupture with secondary metatarsophalangeal joint instability (usually the second)
- Hallux valgus, hallux rigidus, hammertoes, and mallet toes
- Arthritis of the metatarsophalangeal joints: osteoarthritis, rheumatoid arthritis, psoriatic arthritis, gout, trauma
- Overlapping and underlapping toes
- Bunion, bunionette and intermetatarsophalangeal bursitis
- Osteochondritis of the second metatarsal head (Freiberg disease)
- Metatarsal stress (march) fracture
- Sesamoiditis, sesamoid fracture, or osteonecrosis
- Failed forefoot surgery
- Tarsal tunnel syndrome, neuropathy
- Ischemic forefoot pain: peripheral vascular disease, vasospastic disorder, vasculitis

delivered from the dorsal aspect into the intermetatarsal space are often helpful. Surgical excision of the neuroma (interdigital neurectomy), epineurolysis, or simple division of the transverse metatarsal ligament are required in patients whose condition is refractory to conservative treatment.[1-9] After neurectomy, regeneration of the proximal cut end of the interdigital nerve, blocked by scar tissue, can result in a painful, recurrent, interdigital neuroma. This can be managed by implanting the proximal cut end of the nerve into an intrinsic arch muscle.[12]

References

1. Fam AG: The ankle and foot. In Hochberg H, Silman A, et al (eds): Rheumatology, 3rd ed. London, Mosby, 2003, pp 681-692.
2. Pyasta RT, Panush RS: Common painful foot syndromes. Bull Rheum Dis 48:1, 1999.
3. Mann RA: Metatarsalgia. Postgrad Med 75:150, 1984.
4. Gould JS: Metatarsalgia. Orthop Clin North Am 20:553, 1989.
5. Wu KK: Morton neuroma and metatarsalgia. Curr Opin Rheumatol 12:131, 2000.
6. Coughlin MJ: Common causes of pain in the forefoot in adults. J Bone Joint Surg Br 82:781, 2000.
7. Coughlin MJ, Pinsonneault T: Operative treatment of interdigital neuroma: A long-term follow-up study. J Bone Joint Surg Am 83:1321, 2001.
8. Morris MA: Morton's metatarsalgia. Clin Orthop 127:203, 1977.
9. Bencardino J, Rosenerg ZS, Beltran J, et al: Morton's neuroma: Is it always symptomatic? AJR Am J Roentgenol 175:649, 2000.
10. Quinn TJ, Jacobson JA, Craig JG, van Holsbeeck MT: Sonography of Morton's neuromas. AJR Am J Roentgenol 174:1723, 2000.
11. Weishaupt D, Treiber K, Kundert H-P, et al: Morton neuroma: MR imaging in prone, supine, and upright weight-bearing body positions. Radiology 226:849, 2003.
12. Wolfort SF, Dellon AL: Treatment of recurrent neuroma of the interdigital nerve by implantation of the proximal nerve into muscle in the arch of the foot. J Foot Ankle Surg 40:404, 2001.

chapter 109

Hallux Valgus, Bunion, Bunionette, and Other Painful Conditions of the Toe

Adel G. Fam

HALLUX VALGUS

Etiology

Hallux valgus refers to lateral deviation of the first (great) toe on the first metatarsal more than 10 to 15 degrees. It is more common in women and may be caused by a genetic predisposition aggravated by wearing short, narrow, high-heeled or pointed shoes.[1-5] Other causes include congenital splay foot deformity, metatarsus primus varus with or without metatarsus adductus of the adjacent second and third metatarsals,[6] and arthritis of the first metatarsophalangeal (MTP) joint due to rheumatoid arthritis or osteoarthritis.[1-5]

Clinical Presentation

There is medial deviation and splaying of the first metatarsal (metatarsus primus varus) with an increased intermetatarsal angle of more than 9 degrees. The condition is often asymptomatic, but pain may arise from wearing of improper footwear, bursitis over the medial aspect of the first MTP joint (bunion), or secondary osteoarthritis.[1-5] As the first metatarsal moves into varus at its joint with the first cuneiform, its head also moves dorsally, resulting in a transfer of weight to the second metatarsal head. This is known as "transfer lesion." Altered weight bearing results in a callosity under the second metatarsal head with a hammertoe deformity and a flattened transverse metatarsal arch. If the deformity is marked, the great toe may overlie or underlie the second toe and the sesamoids are displaced laterally.[1-5] The severity of the deformity and its progression over time can be assessed radiographically by measuring the hallux valgus angle between the first metatarsal and first proximal phalanx.[7] Structural abnormalities of metatarsal head and sesamoids and the presence of bunion bursitis can be clearly delineated by MRI.[8]

Treatment

Treatment of hallux valgus consists of shoe correction to accommodate the bunion, a bunion pad, and, in the presence of a transfer lesion, a metatarsal pad.[1-5] Surgical correction (osteotomy of the first metatarsal base, resection of metatarsal head, and/or base of proximal phalanx [Keller procedure], with or without distal soft tissue lateral release, and realignment of the sesamoids) is indicated in patients with severe deformity and intractable pain.[1-5,9] Corrective osteotomies for the adduction deformities of the second and third metatarsals are often required to correct the metatarsus primus varus deformity in those with hallux valgus associated with metatarsus adductus.[6] Patients with symptomatic, recurrent hallux valgus, following failed prior surgery, may benefit from a modified Lapidus procedure (reduction of the first to second intermetatarsal angle and arthrodesis of both the first tarsometatarsal and first to second intermetatarsal joints).[10]

HALLUX RIGIDUS

Hallux limitus refers to painful limitation of dorsiflexion of the first MTP joint. In hallux rigidus, there is marked limitation of movement or immobility of the first MTP joint, usually due to advanced osteoarthritis.[1-3,8,11] Intermittent aching pain, joint tenderness, crepitus, osteophytic lipping, and painful limitation of movement, particularly toe dorsiflexion, are common. It usually occurs in elderly patients with osteoarthritis. A primary type is seen in younger persons, and the condition may follow repetitive trauma as in ballet dancing. The "toe-off" is accomplished by the outer four toes and the distal phalanx of the great toe, thereby bypassing and protecting the first MTP joint from painful dorsiflexion. Calluses often develop beneath the second, third, and fourth metatarsal heads. In advanced stages, the first MTP joint becomes completely rigid in slight plantarflexion.[1-3,8,11]

Treatment

Treatment consists of a stiff-soled shoe with a wide toebox and a bar across the metatarsal heads to allow walking with little movement at the first MTP joint.[1-3,8,11] Intraarticular corticosteroid injections may produce temporary relief. In patients with severe pain and disability, cheilectomy (excision of irregular osteophytic lipping that interferes with MTP movements), arthrodesis, or arthroplasty of the first MTP joint is indicated.[1-3,,8,11]

BUNIONETTE

A bunionette (tailor's bunion) is a painful callus and/or an adventitious bursa overlying a prominent, laterally deviated fifth metatarsal head (metatarsus quintus valgus) and a medially deviated fifth toe.[1-3,12-15] It often occurs in conjunction with hallux valgus or splay foot deformity due to an incompletely developed transverse metatarsal ligament. The mean fourth to fifth intermetatarsal angle varies between 3 and 11 degrees with a mean of 6.5 to 8.0 degrees. The angle is often more than 10 degrees in patients with symptomatic bunionette deformity. The fifth metatarsophalangeal angle is normally less than 14 degrees and is more than16 degrees in those with bunionette.[12,13] Enlargement of the fifth metatarsal head due to exostosis is commonly present. Bunionette deformity is common in athletes, especially downhill skiers. It is often asymptomatic, but patients may present with pain, tenderness, and swelling over the head of the fifth metatarsal. The pain is made worse by both activity and wearing constricting shoes. There is callosity with hyperkeratosis of the skin over the fifth metatarsal head, and an adventitious bursa, skin ulceration, or infection may develop.[1-3,12]

Treatment

Shoe modification with a wide toe box, shaving of the callus, a bunion pad, nonsteroidal antiinflammatory drugs, and intrabursal corticosteroid injections may reduce symptoms, particularly in those with inflamed bunionette bursitis.[1-3,12] Distal osteotomy of the fifth metatarsal,[12,14] proximal dome-shaped osteotomy of the fifth metatarsal,[15] or resection of the lateral one third of the fifth metatarsal prominence (head)[12] may be necessary in those conditions that are refractory to nonoperative treatment.

References

1. Fam AG: The ankle and foot. In Hochbert H, Silman A, et al (eds): Rheumatology, 3rd ed. London, Mosby, 2003, pp 681-692.
2. Pyasta RT, Panush RS: Common painful foot syndromes. Bull Rheum Dis 48:1, 1999.
3. Coughlin MJ: Common causes of pain in the forefoot in adults. J Bone Joint Surg Br 82:781, 2000.
4. Inman VT: Hallux valgus: A review of etiologic factors. Orthop Clin North Am 5:59-66,1974.
5. Coughlin MJ: Hallux valgus: Causes, evaluation and treatment. Postgrad Med 75:174-187.1984.
6. Okuda R, Kinoshita M, Morikawa J, et al: Adult hallux valgus with metatarsus adductus: A case report. Clin Orthop 396:179, 2002.
7. Budiman-Mak E, Roach KE, Stuck R, et al: Radiographic measurement of hallux valgus in the rheumatoid arthritic foot. J Rheumatol 21:623, 1994.
8. Schweitzer ME, Maheshwari S, Shabshin N: Hallux valgus and hallux rigidus: MRI findings. Clin Imag 23:397, 1999.
9. Sammarco GJ, Idusuyi OB: Complications after surgery of the hallux. Clin Orthop 391:59, 2001.
10. Coetzee JC, Resig SG, Kuskowski M, Saleh KJ: The Lapidus procedure as salvage after failed surgical treatment of hallux valgus. J Bone Joint Surg Am 85:60, 2003.
11. Shereff MJ, Baumhauer JF: Hallux rigidus and osteoarthrosis of the first metatarsophalangeal joint. J Bone Joint Surg Am 80A:898, 1998.
12. Koti M, Maffulli N: Bunionette. J Bone Joint Surg Am 83:1076, 2001.
13. Karasick D: Preoperative assessment of symptomatic bunionette deformity: Radiologic findings. AJR Am J Roentgenol 164:147, 1995.
14. London BP, Stern SF, Quist MA, et al: Long oblique distal osteotomy of the fifth metatarsal for correction of tailor's bunion: A retrospective review. J Foot Ankle Surg 42:36, 2003.
15. Okuda R, Kinoshita M, Morikawa J, et al: Proximal dome-shaped osteotomy for symptomatic bunionette. Clin Orthop 396:173, 2002.

chapter 110

Heel Spur Pain, Plantar Fasciitis, and Related Disorders

Daneshvari R. Solanki

Plantar fasciitis is one of the most common conditions treated by orthopedists. It is an orthopedic syndrome that can occur in athletes and nonathletes, yet little is known about its pathophysiology. It is presumed to be synonymous with the inflammation of the plantar fascia. But is it really an inflammatory disorder?

The diagnosis of plantar fasciitis is made on the basis of the patient's history and presence of tenderness on the medial aspect of the heel. Clinical and histologic signs of inflammation are typically absent. Histologic studies show marked thickening and fibrosis as well as degenerative changes of the fascia. Microtears in the plantar fascia and perifascial edema are seen on MRI. All of this evidence indicates that plantar fasciitis is not an inflammatory but a degenerative disease. Thus the correct term to describe this condition would be *plantar fasciosis.*[1]

ANATOMY OF THE PLANTAR FASCIA

The plantar fascia is a longitudinal fibrous tissue with its origin at the medial tubercle of the calcaneus. It traverses the sole of the foot, dividing into five bands at mid foot. It is thickest at its center, and each band attaches distally to the proximal phalanx of the toes (Fig. 110–1).[2] It is a static support for the longitudinal arch and acts as a bowstring on the plantar surface of the foot (Fig. 110–2). A normal plantar fascia has a dorsoplanar thickness of 3 mm. In plantar fasciitis it can increase to 15 mm.[3]

CLINICAL PRESENTATION

Plantar fasciitis has been reported in patients aged 7 to 85 years. The skin at the heel is thicker than in other areas and is designed to deal with constant friction. The fat pad at the heel absorbs the shock. Thickness of this fat pad decreases after the age of 40, so plantar fasciitis is more common after this age. Additionally, the syndrome is more common in women. Normally it is unilateral, but in 15% of the cases it can be bilateral.

Some of the risk factors for developing plantar fasciitis include the following:

- Obesity or sudden increase in weight
- Poorly fitting shoes
- Increase in running intensity or distance
- Change in running or walking surfaces
- Occupations involving prolonged standing (e.g., policeman)

Other causes of heel pain include heel spur, stress fracture of the calcaneum, tarsal tunnel syndrome, and injury to the first branch of the lateral plantar nerve. Heel pain could also occur in patients with systemic diseases such as gout and rheumatoid arthritis. Bilateral heel pain in a young person could be secondary to Reiter syndrome.

DIAGNOSIS

The diagnosis of plantar fasciitis is based on history and physical examination. There is no history of trauma. The patient provides a history of pain of gradual onset that progressively gets worse. It is worse on awakening in the morning and the patient often limps to the bathroom because weight bearing increases the pain. This pain eases after taking a few steps, decreases through the day, and gets worse toward the end of the day. Rest in the evening produces pain relief. Pain of the calcaneal stress fracture worsens on walking. If the pain persists during sleep, other causes such as infection, tumors, and neuropathic pain must be sought. Investigations should be done to rule out other pathologic processes that could cause the heel pain.

The most cardinal finding is localized tenderness on palpation of the anteromedial aspect of the heel. It is often necessary to apply firm pressure to determine the maximum point of tenderness. There is tightness of the Achilles tendon. This limits the dorsiflexion of the foot in about 78% of the patients. There are no other clinical findings in the foot or the ankle.

Tenderness in the posterior part of the heel may be indicative of subcalcaneal bursitis. Mediolateral tenderness on the heel is due to calcaneal stress fracture. A positive Tinel sign on the medial aspect of the heel may be due to tarsal tunnel syndrome or to entrapment of the nerve to the abductor digiti quinti.

Plain radiographs of the heel are obtained to rule out causes such as stress fracture, bony erosion due to bursitis, or bony heel spurs, which could cause heel pain. Isotope

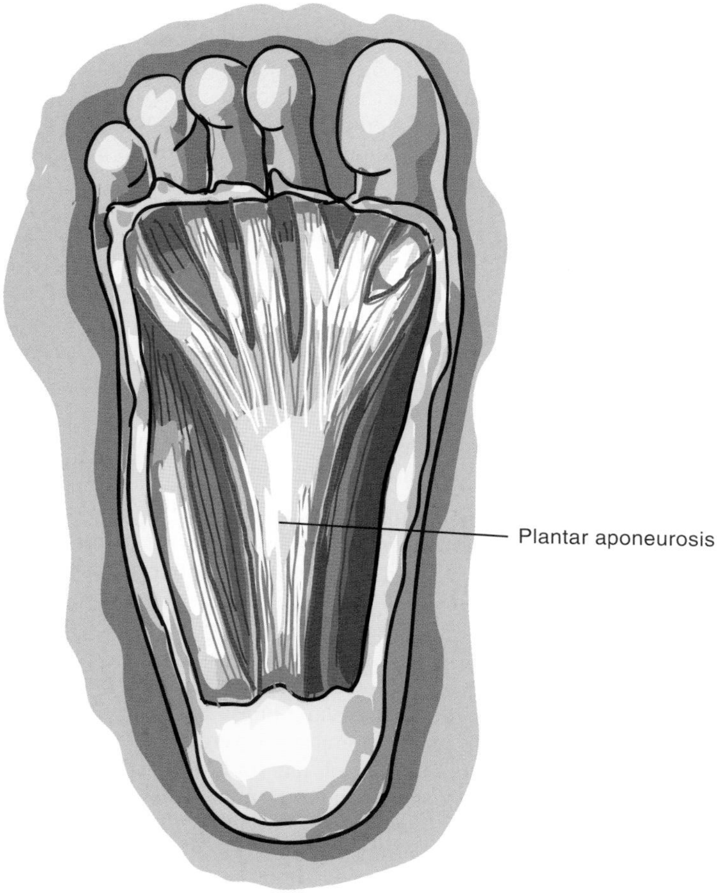

FIGURE 110–1 ■ Anatomy of the plantar fascia.

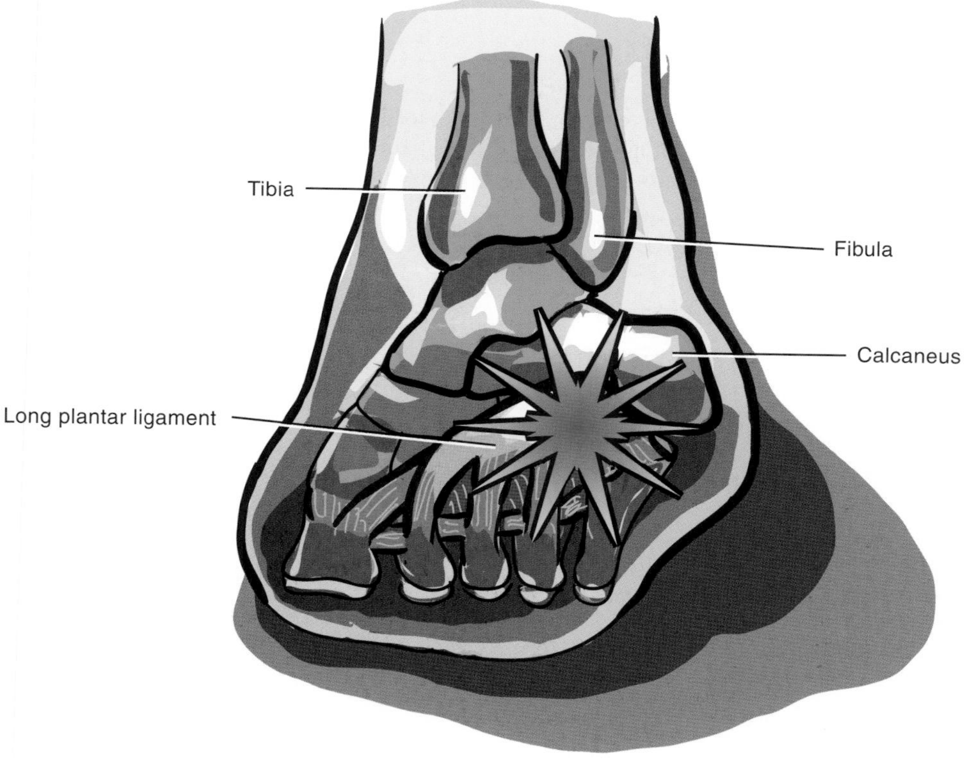

FIGURE 110–2 ■ Increased dorso-planar thickness of the fascia in plantar fasciitis.

scanning should be considered only when the plain radiographs are normal and calcaneal fracture is suspected.[4] MRI is rarely indicative, but it can define the thickness of the plantar fascia. Ultrasound of the fascia also can provide information on the thickness of the fascia. A complete blood cell count and erythrocyte sedimentation rate should be done in patients presenting with bilateral heel pain or atypical symptoms.[5]

TREATMENT

Conservative Treatment

Plantar fasciitis is a self-limiting condition. The conservative treatment, if started within 6 weeks of the onset of the symptoms, hastens the recovery process.[6] Such conservative means should be tried for 12 months before surgical intervention is contemplated. Such conservative treatments are as follows:

1. The patient should not walk barefoot.
2. Footwear must have heel pads and arch support. It must be emphasized that a laced shoe provides better support than a sandal.
3. The shoes should be changed at regular intervals because the loss of the cushion can aggravate the pain.
4. Patients should be treated with oral nonsteroidal anti-inflammatory drugs during the acute phase only.
5. Patients must be taught stretching exercises for the Achilles tendon. Dorsiflexion of the foot with the knee extended stretches the gastrocnemius muscle. The same movement with the knee flexed stretches the soleus muscle. These gentle stretches with 8 to 10 repetitions must be done three to five times a day.
6. Night splints can help because they can help to keep the Achilles tendon in a stretched position.
7. Patients with severe pain can benefit from a below-the-knee cast for 4 weeks.

Invasive Treatment

Injection of a corticosteroid in combination with a local anesthetic on the medial aspect of the heel can provide pain relief. However, corticosteroids are implicated in increasing the microtears in the fascia and in iatrogenic rupture of the plantar fascia,[7] which can aggravate the pain.

Surgery

Surgery should be considered only when the patient has not responded to the previously described treatments for 12 months.[8] The surgical procedures that are considered for treatment of plantar fasciitis are release of plantar fascia, calcaneal spur excision, Steindler stripping, neurolysis, and endoscopic procedures.[9] Surgery provides relief in 50% to 60% of the patients, but there could be significant complications as well.

CONCLUSION

Plantar fasciitis is the most common cause for the heel pain. Review of the literature provides ample evidence that conservative management is the treatment of choice. Surgical intervention should only be considered when the pain and disability persist despite adequate trial with nonsurgical therapies.

References

1. Lemont H, Ammirati KM, Usen N: Plantar fasciitis: A degenerative process (fasciosis) without inflammation. J Am Podiatr Med Assoc 93:234-237, 2003.
2. Schepsis AA, Leach RE, Gorzyca J: Plantar fasciitis. Etiology, treatment, surgical results, and review of the literature. Clin Orthop 266:185-196, 1991.
3. Kier R: Magnetic resonance imaging of plantar fasciitis and other causes of heel pain. Magn Reson Imaging Clin North Am 2:97-107, 1994.
4. Tudor GR, Finlay D, Allen MJ, Belton I: The role of bone scintigraphy and plain radiography in intractable plantar fasciitis. Nucl Med Commun 18:853-856, 1997.
5. DeMaio M, Paine R, Mangine RE, Drez D Jr: Plantar fasciitis. Orthopedics 16:1153-1163, 1993.
6. Singh D, Angel J, Bentley G, Trevino SG: Fortnightly review. Plantar fasciitis. BMJ 315:172-175, 1997.
7. Sellman JR: Plantar fascia rupture associated with corticosteroid injection. Foot Ankle Int 15:376-381, 1994.
8. Pfeffer GB: Plantar heel pain. In Baxter DE (ed): The Foot and Ankle in Sports. St. Louis, Mosby, 1995, pp 195-206.
9. Anderson RB, Foster MD: Operative treatment of subcalcaneal pain. Foot Ankle 9:317-323, 1989.

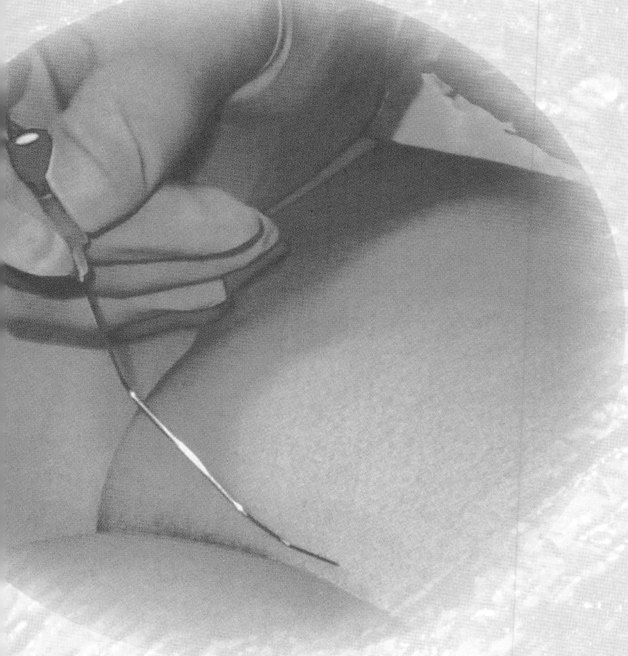

section 5

Specific Treatment Modalities for Pain and Symptom Management

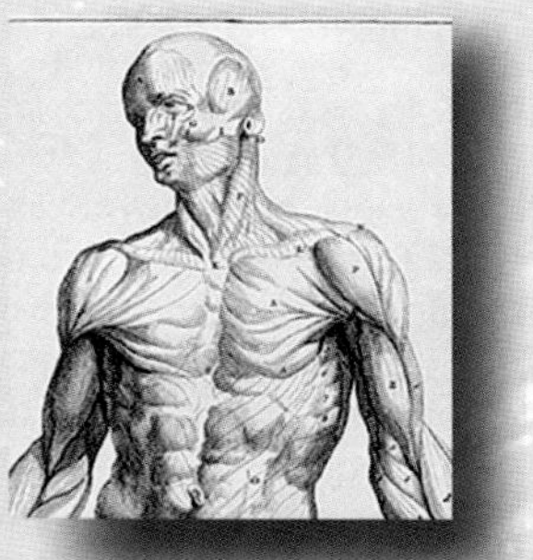

Part A

Pharmacologic Management of Pain

chapter 111

Simple Analgesics

Robert B. Supernaw

For most pain phenomena, pharmacotherapy represents an indispensable therapeutic tool. However, pharmacotherapy—even over-the-counter (OTC) pharmacotherapy—has the dual feature of combating the principal condition while potentially provoking undesired adverse effects. Therefore, even in cases of mild, uncomplicated pain, the best therapeutic approach is to combat the pain with physical methods (e.g., ice packs, heat, massage) if the condition is amenable to such treatment. However, the option of not employing pharmacotherapy in managing many painful conditions is not realistic. If the clinician has determined that the symptom of pain cannot be effectively treated with physical intervention, drug therapy is indicated. To determine the best pharmacotherapeutic response to pain, the nature and severity of the pain must be assessed and considered. If the pain is uncomplicated and nonpsychogenic and the pain intensity is mild or moderate, simple analgesics, including OTC agents, represent first-line treatment options.

Even in cases of mild or moderate pain, treatment plans are formulated on the basis of the specific nature of the complaint. For example, moderate headache pain may be treated differently than moderate pain of a sprained ankle. In one case, it may be important to consider the pain of inflammation while in another case inflammation may not be at the root of the pain. And, unlike the basic therapeutic approach to other commonly encountered problems (e.g., hypertension, hyperlipidemia) where drug therapy is initiated in relatively small doses and slowly increased until the therapeutic threshold or desired outcome is achieved, the therapeutic approach to pain is predicated on the basis of matching the complete pain presentation to the appropriate agent and a reasoned dose of the agent chosen.

In many instances, there is no need to begin drug therapy for the pain complaint with a less potent, OTC analgesic before attempting more potent drug therapy. The severe pain of a cluster headache will not respond to aspirin or acetaminophen therapy; therefore, there is little to be gained in trying. This treatment principle underscores the need for an accurate categorization of the pain complaint. When, in the judgment of the clinician, the nature (i.e., relatively uncomplicated pain) and intensity (i.e., mild or moderate pain) of the pain complaint is deemed appropriate, first-line pharmacotherapy (i.e., simple OTC analgesics) may be initiated. These conditions include uncomplicated headache, facial pain, muscle ache, toothache, joint pain, foot pain, and uncomplicated back pain, to name a few of the more commonly encountered pain problems.

The OTC simple analgesics are the most widely used drugs for mild-to-moderate nociceptive pain, and sales of these agents (i.e., aspirin, acetaminophen, ibuprofen, naproxen sodium, and ketoprofen) totaled more than $2.18 billion in the United States in 2004.

NONPRESCRIPTION SIMPLE ANALGESICS

Mild *acute* pain is limited in its duration; therefore it need not be aggressively treated if it does not affect an individual's quality of life, and the patient has not indicated significant or distracting discomfort. In some instances, it need not be treated at all. Mild *chronic* pain may prove to be more problematic in its negative impact on an individual's quality of life, family relations, and ability to work. It will usually require active treatment. If a decision is made to treat mild acute or chronic pain, first consideration should be given to simple analgesics. These agents are available without a prescription on an OTC basis. The principal OTC simple analgesics include members of two major families of drugs—the nonsteroidal antiinflammatory drugs (NSAIDs) and acetaminophen. A useful categorization of the OTC NSAIDs includes two principal groupings—the salicylates and the nonsalicylates. And finally, the salicylates can be further divided into two families of drugs, the acetylated and the nonacetylated salicylates. A helpful representation of the categorization of the simple analgesics is depicted in Figure 111–1.

When a decision is made to treat mild to moderate nociceptive pain, consideration should be given to the nature of the pain and the patient. If the patient is not allergic to aspirin and tolerates aspirin well, then aspirin is a good first-line choice and is the most widely prescribed analgesic.[1] Acetaminophen should be considered if the patient is aspirin sensitive, aspirin intolerant, or is allergic to aspirin. However, as is the case with most choices in pharmacotherapy, the rules are not quite that simple. There are many other considerations to be taken into account before the choice of a simple analgesic can be made. These considerations are detailed in the following sections of this chapter.

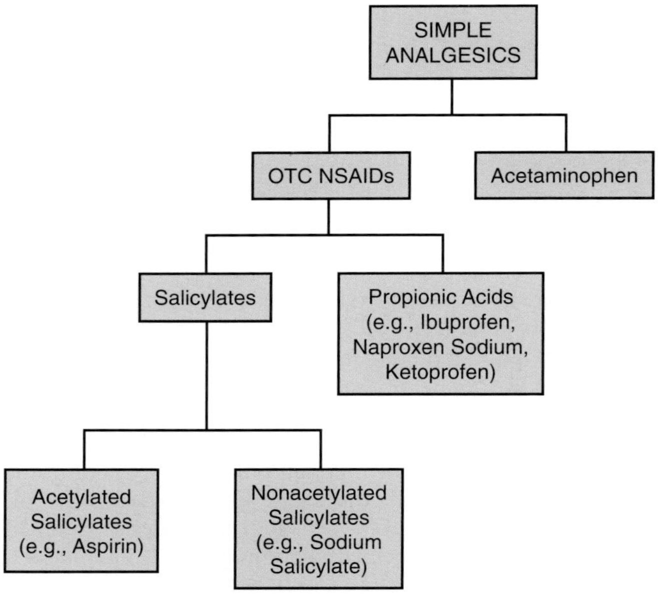

FIGURE 111–1 ■ Classification and relationships of simple analgesics.

OVER-THE-COUNTER NONSTEROIDAL ANTIINFLAMMATORY DRUGS

Over-the-counter nonsteroidal antiinflammatory drugs (OTC NSAIDs) are the most commonly employed of the simple analgesics. This category of drugs includes the salicylates and the propionic acids (see Figure 111–1). The salicylates are further divided into the acetylated and the nonacetylated compounds.

The salicylates

There are two forms of salicylates in the OTC analgesic armamentarium. The most commonly used member of the acetylated salicylate family is aspirin and the combination products enteric-coated aspirin and buffered aspirin. The OTC nonacetylated salicylate family includes sodium salicylate.

Aspirin

Acetylsalicylic acid, more commonly known as aspirin, is the most commonly used simple analgesic and has been for many years. According to the Aspirin Foundation, approximately 100-billion aspirin tablets are produced annually. Aspirin represents a reasonable first choice for common mild to moderate pain, if the pain is nociceptive in nature. The forerunner of aspirin, sodium salicylic acid, was widely used as an analgesic and antipyretic from the 1700s on. A much improved acetyl derivative of sodium salicylic acid—acetylsalicylic acid or aspirin—was introduced into the U.S. market in 1899. By definition, it is a nonsteroidal antiinflammatory drug (NSAID) that predates all other modern NSAIDs. Aspirin is the prototypical salicylate, and, as such, aspirin has a long history of safe and effective use. However, as is the case with almost all drugs, whether OTC or prescription, aspirin is not without its risks.

The benefits of aspirin therapy are well known. It is cheap, readily available, has a very long track record, is effective in the relief of mild to moderate nociceptive pain, improves function, and reduces inflammation especially at higher doses. Additional benefits include its ability to reduce fever and its anti-platelet adhesion properties. Given as a 650-mg dose (two regular-strength tablets) every 4 hours, aspirin may be considered first-line drug therapy in various mild to moderate pain-related problems including chronic joint pain, minor arthritis flare-ups, common and tension-type headaches, dysmenorrhea, minor postoperative pain and inflammation, and chronic minor low back pain.

Action

Aspirin and the acetylated salicylates have analgesic, antiinflammatory, antiplatelet, and antipyretic activity. They are most effective in general pain, common headache pain, and especially pain of a musculoskeletal origin, including arthritis and muscle pain. When peripheral tissue is insulted in trauma or when a pain-triggering event occurs, prostaglandins enhance the transmission of pain impulses and the sensitivity of the pain receptors, and an inflammatory response may ensue. Aspirin's principal mechanism of action is inhibition of prostaglandin (eicosanoid) synthesis in peripheral tissue.[2] Therefore, pain relief is not instantaneous, as eicosanoid levels dissipate. Aspirin appears to acetylate the active site of the enzyme cyclooxygenase (COX), also known as PGH synthase, which is the specific enzyme necessary for the conversion of arachidonic acid to eicosanoids. This acetylation permanently (irreversibly) deactivates the COX enzyme, thereby effectively inhibiting prostaglandin production.[3] This irreversibility is an important distinction between aspirin, an acetylated salicylate, and the other nonsteroidal antiinflammatory agents. It is likely that aspirin also mitigates pain through central mechanisms. It is hypothesized that the acetate components of aspirin pass into the brain and spinal cord and exert their activity on prostaglandins within in the central nervous system that are involved in the perception and transmission of pain.

Dosing

Aspirin is available in 325-mg and 500-mg tablet, caplet, and effervescent tablet strengths. It is also available as an 81-mg chewable tablet and 81-mg enteric coated tablet. It is available in a controlled release 800-mg oral dosage form, and embedded in chewing gum in the 228-mg strength. For rectal use, it is available in 125- and 300-mg suppositories.

For administration in adult patients, for general musculoskeletal and common headache pain, aspirin is most often given orally in doses ranging from 325 mg to 650 mg every 3 to 4 hours as needed, not to exceed 4 gm in a 24-hour period. If the condition warrants the more potent dosage form (i.e., extra strength 500 mg), it is suggested that it be dosed at 500 mg every 3 to 4 hours or 1000 mg every 6 to 8 hours. For significant inflammatory processes, including arthritis, it can be given in divided doses equivalent to 3.2 to 6.0 gm daily, provided every 3 to 4 hours. For severe headache pain, aspirin has been demonstrated to show added analgesic activity when doses are pushed to 1000 mg.[4] For the pain and discomfort of niacin induced flushing, 325 mg aspirin should be given before the administration of the niacin dose. Because the potential for gastrointestinal irritation is related to a local effect as well as a pharmacologic effect, aspirin should always be taken with a full glass of water. Studies have also shown that doses should be slightly increased in obese patients because peak levels do not match those seen in nonobese individuals.[5]

For administration in pediatric patients over the age of 2 years, 10 to 15 mg/kg/dose every 4 hours, up to 60 to 80 mg/kg/day is appropriate for general pain, discomfort, or fever. For infants and children into their teens, aspirin is contraindicated—should not be given—in cases of viral infections, including flu and chicken pox because it has been implicated in Reye syndrome. For infants and children suffering from juvenile rheumatoid arthritis, an initial dose of 90 to 130 mg/kg/day, in divided doses every 4 to 6 hours, is appropriate for oral administration. This dose may be increased as needed to maximize antiinflammatory efficacy to achieve a plasma salicylate level objective of 150 to 300 mg/mL.

An alternative dosing guideline for pediatric patients is based on age and weight. For children ages 2 to 11, a total of 64 mg/kg/day in 4 to 6 doses is appropriate. Another guideline[6,7] is as follows, if the child's weight is within normal limits:

- Children >11 years (weight greater than 43.2), 650 mg every 4 hours, not to exceed 4 g/day
- Children age 11 (weight 32.4 kg to 43.2 kg), 480 mg every 4 hours
- Children age 9 to 10 (weight 26.9 kg to 32.3 kg), 400 mg every 4 hours
- Children age 6 to 8 (weight 21.5 kg to 26.8 kg), 325 mg every 4 hours
- Children age 4 to 5 (weight 16.0 kg to 21.4 kg), 240 mg every 4 hours
- Children age 2 to 3 (weight 10.6 kg to 15.9 kg) 160 mg every 4 hours
- For children younger than 2 years (up to 23 months and up to 10.5 kg in weight), aspirin is not recommended.

Pharmacokinetics

Oral aspirin is absorbed very rapidly in the stomach and upper small intestine by passive diffusion.[8] There are moderate differences in absorption between buffered and nonbuffered varieties; buffered tablets are absorbed in 30 to 45 minutes and nonbuffered are absorbed within 60 minutes[9]; however, significant levels are detectable in plasma in less than 30 minutes after a single dose of aspirin.[1] In buffered aspirin, minute quantities of antacid are added to aid in the dissolution of the tablet. In theory, this would enhance absorption, but studies have not demonstrated significant differences in total absorption. Although enteric coating does delay aspirin's absorption, it does not affect total absorption or the resultant salicylate levels.[10] Taking aspirin with food or with meals does not affect its absorption.[11] Peak levels of oral aspirin occur at about 1 hour post-administration. Unlike salicylic acid, aspirin is not effectively absorbed through the skin. Percutaneous absorption is significantly less than 10% of oral absorption.[12] Rectal absorption from aspirin administered in a suppository dosage form is incomplete and variable; therefore, it is not advisable unless other routes are not feasible.[13]

The distribution of the salicylates is throughout most body tissues and is patient and drug concentration dependent. Approximately 68% (± 3%) of the aspirin dose is available (at the initial stages post-administration) as the unchanged drug, but this may be significantly different in the elderly and in those individuals with compromised liver function.[14] Of course, aspirin (acetylsalicylic acid) is hydrolyzed to salicylic acid, which is not accounted for in this 68% figure. At usual or higher concentrations of salicylates, albumin binding will vary but may approach 80%.[13] At lower concentrations, inactive binding to albumin may approach 90%. On average, at therapeutic concentrations, approximately 80% of the aspirin dosed is inactively bound.[1,13] Because of this significant albumin binding, caution is warranted when aspirin is given to a patient who is taking an oral anticoagulant (OAC) in that the OAC is approximately 97% albumin bound. The aspirin binding will displace some of the OAC, causing an increase in the active dose (drug level) of the OAC and significantly increasing bleeding time. If as little as 3% of the OAC is displaced by the aspirin, the effective dose of the OAC will be doubled. The process of inactive albumin binding can saturate the system; therefore, high doses of aspirin (e.g., single doses above 650 mg) will saturate the binding system and lead to very high blood levels. That is, increasing the dose of aspirin above 650 mg will increase the blood levels of aspirin in a disproportionate manner and significantly increase the half-life of the drug. The volume of distribution of aspirin is 0.15 L/kg (±0.03 L/kg).[1] Aspirin crosses the placental barrier and is not advised in the third trimester of pregnancy (Pregnancy Category C/D).

Aspirin is hydrolyzed in circulation and in the liver to form salicylate and acetic acid. Within 30 minutes, only 27% of the orally administered dose remains as acetylsalicylic acid, the active remainder as salicylate.[1] As with all salicylates, aspirin is metabolized in the liver by esterases. The major metabolite of salicylates is salicyluric acid.

Salicylates are excreted in the urine; and alkalinization of the urine increases the rate of excretion.[13] Aspirin exhibits a two-compartment half-life. It has a half-life of 15 minutes as aspirin (acetylsalicylic acid) and 3 to 5 hours as its salicylate metabolite. So, although normally the half-life of pure aspirin is 15 minutes, and 3 to 5 hours for salicylate, when the inactive albumin binding system is saturated, the half-life may increase up to threefold normal (e.g., 3 to 5 hours for dosing at 600 mg daily versus 12 to 16 hours for dosing at 3.6 gm daily for significant antiinflamatory effects).[13] Only about 10% of aspirin is excreted as free salicylic acid; 75% is excreted as salicyluric acid.[1] Aspirin is excreted in breast milk making it unsafe to use in breastfeeding mothers.

Indications in Pain

As a nonselective COX-1 and COX-2 inhibitor, aspirin is indicated for the treatment of general complaints of pain associated with inflammatory processes, menstruation (e.g., dysmenorrhea), dental pain, headache, joint pain, muscle pain, and integumentary pain. It is less effective in treating visceral pain. In synovial fluid, aspirin reaches approximately 78% of plasma concentrations,[15,16] making it a good option in treating arthritis pain and, at higher doses, inflammation.

Cautions

Aspirin should never be given to children or teenagers who exhibit symptoms of influenza or chicken pox. In these cases, aspirin administration has been associated with Reye syndrome, although rare, with mortality rates up to 30% and severe brain damage in those who survive.

Ringing in the ears may indicate toxicity. Any complaints of such a symptom indicate the basis for discontinuation of aspirin. Dizziness may also indicate the onset of toxicity. Because of its irreversible antiplatelet effects, aspirin should be discontinued at least 7 days before surgery to preclude the chances of aspirin-induced postoperative bleeding.

Caution is warranted with the use of aspirin in asthmatics. Bronchospasms occur in up to 19% of these patients. As with all drugs metabolized in the liver, caution is warranted in liver-function compromised patients. Aspirin should not be considered in the third trimester of pregnancy and should not be considered in lactating mothers who are breastfeeding.

Because of local and pharmacologic induced gastrointestinal irritation, aspirin should be used with caution in patients who complain of gastrointestinal burning and in those with ulcers. Rectal bleeding and fecal blood loss should be monitored. When plasma concentration monitoring is possible, the therapeutic range should not exceed 300 mg/mL (30 mg/dL). Acidification of the urine will increase plasma levels, and alkalinizing the urine will decrease levels. Aspirin has also been implicated in blood-related problems including decreased white blood cell and platelet counts and hemolytic anemia.

Clinicians should warn patients to discard aspirin that has an odor of vinegar; this indicates that the aspirin has undergone chemical degradation. Extra caution is indicated if the patient (1) is taking an anticoagulant; (2) is taking an oral antidiabetic agent; (3) has a history of peptic ulcer disease; (4) has systemic lupus erythematosus; (5) is pregnant or contemplating pregnancy; (6) is scheduled for surgery; (7) is receiving a new prescription; or (8) any time the patient experiences a new significant adverse effect.

Analgesic effects result from plasma levels approaching 10 mg/dL. Antiinflammatory effects result from plasma levels from 10 to 40 mg/dL. Ringing in the ears occurs at approximately 50 mg/dL. Toxicity will occur as a function of levels above this; and doses leading to levels above 160 mg/dL are lethal.[17]

Aspirin interacts with several other drugs and chemical entities. Alcohol increases the risk of gastrointestinal irritation. Ascorbic acid acidifies the urine and decrease the excretion of aspirin. Antacids and urinary alkalinizers increase the excretion of aspirin, thereby decreasing the effects of aspirin Oral anticoagulant levels will be increased with concomitant use of aspirin because of inactive binding displacement. Aspirin and other NSAIDs will exhibit additive gastrointestinal irritative effects. Aspirin will decrease the antihypertensive effects of angiotensin converting enzyme agents (ACE inhibitors) and beta-blockers. Aspirin and the salicylates antagonize the action of uricosuric agents, and salicylates should not be given with methotrexate.

Sodium Salicylate

Sodium salicylate is the "other" nonprescription salicylate. Its characteristics are similar to those of aspirin with one major exception: sodium salicylate is not acetylated. As such, it does not have a two-compartment half-life as does aspirin. That is, although aspirin has a "first" half-life as acetylsalicylic acid that is approximately 15 minutes followed by an active metabolite, salicylate, half-life of 3 to 5 hours, sodium salicylate has a single compartment active drug half-life of 3 to 5 hours, but can be prolonged up to 19 hours.[13] The second major difference between aspirin and sodium salicylate is that aspirin acetylates and irreversibly blocks cyclooxgenase. Therefore, platelet aggregation is effectively inhibited for the life of the platelet with aspirin, whereas the antiplatelet adhesion effect is only temporary with the nonacetylated salicylates.

Sodium salicylate is considered somewhat less effective in reducing pain when compared with aspirin. However, some patients who are hypersensitive to aspirin may tolerate sodium salicylate. The dose of sodium salicylate is the same as for aspirin—325 mg to 650 mg every 4 hours, as needed.

Ibuprofen

Ibuprofen is available as an OTC analgesic in modest doses of 200 mg per tablet. For a complete description of the

NSAIDs used in pain management, please see Chapter 149. Although OTC doses of ibuprofen are effective in mild to moderate pain, the drug, at this low dose does not have antiinflammatory effects. It is marketed generically and as Motrin, Nuprin, and Advil. It is relatively safe to give to children. The children's OTC dose is 50 mg every 6 to 8 hours for children weighing 12 to 17 pounds (not more than 4 doses per day); 75 mg every 6 to 8 hours for children weighing 18 to 23 pounds (not more than 4 doses per day); 100 mg every 6 to 8 hours for children weighing 24 to 35 pounds (not more than 4 doses per day); 150 mg every 6 to 8 hours for children weighing 35 to 47 pounds (not more than 4 doses per day); 200 mg every 6 to 8 hours for children weighing 48 to 59 pounds (not more than 4 doses per day); 250 mg every 6 to 8 hours for children weighing 60 to 71 pounds (not more than 4 doses per day); and 300 mg every 6 to 8 hours for children weighing 72 to 95 pounds (not more than 4 doses per day). Children age 12 and older may be dosed at 200 mg every 4 to 6 hours with a maximum 24-hour total dose of 1200 mg. The recommended OTC dose for mild to moderate pain patients older than the age of 16 is 200 to 400 mg every 4 to 6 hours as needed up to a maximum of 1200 mg in a 24-hour period. Absorption is approximately 85%, but it is 90% to 99% albumin bound. The time to peak concentrations is 1 to 2 hours, and its half-life is 2 to 4 hours. In OTC doses (i.e., 200 mg), this medication is safe to use in the elderly, with caution.

Naproxen Sodium

Naproxen sodium is available as an OTC analgesic in modest doses of 220 mg per tablet. For a complete description of NSAIDs used in pain management, please see Chapter 149. Although OTC doses of naproxen sodium are effective in mild-to-moderate pain, the drug at this low dose does not have antiinflammatory effects. It is marketed on an OTC basis as Aleve. It should not be given to children under the age of 12. The recommended OTC dose for mild to moderate pain in adults over the age of 12 is two tablets initially (440 mg), followed by one tablet (220 mg) every 8 to 12 hours. For individuals over the age of 65, the recommended OTC dose is one tablet every 12 hours. It is virtually completely absorbed, but it is highly albumin bound. The time to peak concentrations is 1 to 4 hours, and its duration of action is approximately 12 hours. Therefore, it is an excellent choice when an OTC NSAID is indicated and extended duration of action is desired.

Ketoprofen

Ketoprofen is available as an OTC analgesic in modest doses of 12.5 mg per tablet. For a complete description of the nonsteroidal antiinflammatory agents used in pain management, please see Chapter 149. Although OTC doses of ketoprofen are effective in mild-to-moderate pain, the drug at this low dose does not have antiinflammatory effects. It is marketed for OTC use as Orudis KT. It should not be given to children. The recommended OTC dose for mild to moderate pain in adults over the age of 16 is 12.5 mg every 4 to 6 hours as needed up to a maximum of six tablets in a 24-hour period. It is virtually completely absorbed, but it is highly albumin bound. The time to peak concentrations is 30 minutes up to 2 hours, and its half-life is 2.5 hours. In OTC doses, this medication is safe to use in the elderly.

Acetaminophen

Acetaminophen is *not* an NSAID. It has a different mechanism of action than the NSAIDs, and it has little antiinflammatory and no antiplatelet activity. However, it is a very good OTC analgesic, and it has significantly less potential for gastrointestinal irritation when compared to aspirin and the NSAIDs. On an equivalent-dose basis, acetaminophen is comparable to aspirin in its analgesic abilities.

Acetaminophen is *N*-acetyl-aminophenol. (The last three letters of ace*tyl* and the last four letters of aminoph*enol* have lent themselves to the naming of the most popular tradenamed acetaminophen product, Tylenol. Acetaminophen is an active metabolite of phenacetin. Analogs of acetaminophen were used in the late-1800s. Although these analogs exhibited good analgesic and antipyretic effects, most had significant adverse effects. Acetaminophen was used sparingly from 1893 until 1950. In 1951, research revealed that acetaminophen was as effective as aspirin for temporary pain relief and fever reduction. McNeil Pharmaceuticals then marketed acetaminophen as an aspirin alternative in 1953 and as an elixir for children in 1955.

Today, acetaminophen is available generically and as brand-named products including Tylenol, Acephen, Aspirin Free Anacin, Tempra, Panadol, Genipap, Liquiprin, and Datril to name but a few.

Action

The mechanism of acetaminophen's analgesic action has not been fully determined; however, research indicates that acetaminophen inhibits prostaglandin synthesis in a manner somewhat similar to that of aspirin. Although aspirin clearly nonselectively blocks the COX-1 and COX-2 enzymes to inhibit prostaglandin synthesis, it appears that acetaminophen only partially blocks the COX-1 and, perhaps, COX-2 enzymes. Most likely, acetaminophen inhibits specific prostaglandin synthesis associated with the newly identified COX-3 enzyme as well as a subtype of the COX-1 enzyme.[18] Other researchers have opined that the COX-3 enzyme is a subtype of the COX-2 enzyme.[25] Regardless of the nature of the COX-3 entity, blocking the activity of this newly discovered enzyme provides a reasonable explanation that accounts for acetaminophen's ability to inhibit or diminish pain impulse transmission and perception while having little effect on inflammation and platelet aggregation, and does not diminish the production of the prostaglandin that is protective of the gastrointestinal tract lining.

Dosing

Acetaminophen is available in tablet, capsule, extended-release dosage forms, chewable tablets, rectal suppositories, and in liquid elixirs for oral pediatric use. The recommended OTC dose for adults is similar to that of aspirin—325 mg to 650 mg every 4 hours as needed, up to 1 gm every 6 hours or 1300 mg every 8 hours. At these higher doses, the self-medicating patient should be carefully reviewed by the physician if the condition does not improve within 10 days. It is essential not to exceed 4 gm of acetaminophen per day. The accumulation of the drug will cause hepatotoxicity.[19]

Dosing in children should be guided by the formula, 1.5 gm per day, in divided doses, for each square meter of body surface. Alternatively, a more convenient guideline[20] has been developed by McNeil Laboratories:

- Infants up to 3 months—oral 40 mg every 4 hours as needed
- Infants 4 to 14 months—oral, 80 mg every 4 hours as needed
- Children 1 to 2 years—oral, 120 mg every 4 hours as needed
- Children 2 to 4 years—oral, 160 mg every 4 hours as needed
- Children 4 to 6 years—oral, 240 mg every 4 hours as needed
- Children 6 to 9 years—oral, 320 mg every 4 hours as needed
- Children 9 to 11 years—oral, 320 to 400 mg every 4 hours as needed
- Children 11 to 12 years—oral, 320 to 480 mg every 4 hours as needed

It is recommended that children up to the age of 12 receive no more than five doses in any 24-hour period. For children, liquid dosage forms are preferred; however, instruction to parents and caregivers on the dosage calibration when dosing liquids using teaspoons or droppers must be clear.

Pharmacokinetics

Acetaminophen is rapidly and almost completely absorbed when taken orally.[21,22] Absorption may be decreased if it is taken following a meal high in carbohydrates. Rectal absorption is variable and depends largely on the vehicle base. After oral administration, peak levels are reached in 30 to 60 minutes.[21,22] The plasma half-life is approximately 2 hours, and its duration of action is approximately 4 hours. The drug is widely distributed, and it is approximately 20% to 50% plasma protein bound. Acetaminophen does appear in breast milk, but only reaches levels of 10 to 15 mg per mL approximately 1 to 2 hours after administration of a 650-mg dose. The metabolism of acetaminophen occurs primarily in the liver. One of the metabolites may accumulate when the system is saturated; this metabolite is hepato- and nephrotoxic. With doses up to 650 mg, plasma concentrations will reach levels of from 5 to 20 mg/mL. Elimination is by the renal pathway; approximately 3% of the dose is excreted unchanged.

Indications in Pain

Acetaminophen is an excellent OTC analgesic drug to be considered in place of aspirin in patients who are sensitive to aspirin or aspirin-like medications; in patients who have ulcers; in patients who experience pain without an inflammatory process; in patients who should not receive antiplatelet drug therapy— including those who are receiving anticoagulant therapy; and in patients receiving uricosuric agents. Although acetaminophen has little or no antiinflammatory capabilities and should not be considered in rheumatoid arthritis, it can be used in patients who have mild osteoarthritis (OA). In fact, it is recommended as a first-line agent for the treatment of pain associated with OA of the hip and knee by the American College of Rheumatology, Subcommittee on Osteoarthritis Guidelines.[23] Additionally, acetaminophen is widely used and is effective in treating general complaints of pain associated with menstruation (e.g., dysmenorrhea), dental pain, headache, joint pain, muscle pain, and integumentary pain. It is less effective in treating visceral pain.

Cautions

The metabolites of acetaminophen are toxic and may accumulate when high doses are employed and in liver-impaired individuals. Special concern should be exercised in alcoholic patients, patients with eating disorders, and patients who are fasting.

Acute hepatotoxicity may occur when a single dose of 10 to 15 gm or more is taken (150 to 250 mg/kg).[21,22] Doses of 20 to 25 gm or more can be fatal.[21,22] Chronic daily use of 4 gm or more for extended periods of time may also lead to serious toxicity. Symptoms of chronic toxicity include significant gastrointestinal disturbance.

If an acute toxic dose is caught within 4 hours, gastric lavage is indicated.[21,22] For many poison control centers, *N*-acetylcysteine (Mucomyst) is the treatment of choice if it can be administered less than 36 hours post-ingestion; however, it is most effective if given within 10 hours post-ingestion[24] and consisting of 140 mg/kg orally (loading) followed by 70 mg/kg every 4 hours for 17 doses. In any cases of acetaminophen overdose or suspected toxicity, the caregiver should immediately call a poison control center and emergency services. While awaiting recommendations, activated charcoal may be administered. It is effective in binding acetaminophen in cases of acute toxicity.

The therapeutic effects of acetaminophen may be decreased when dosed concomitantly with barbiturates, carbamazepine, hydantoins, rifampin, and sulfinpyrazone which may decrease the drug's analgesic effects. Cholestyramine may decrease acetaminophen absorption; so it is prudent to separate concomitant dosing of acetaminophen and cholestyramine by at least 1 hour.

Barbiturates, carbamazepine, hydantoins, isoniazid, rifampin, and sulfinpyrazone may have additive effects when dosed concomitantly with acetaminophen, thereby increasing their cumulative hepatotoxic potential when combined with acetaminophen. The effects of warfarin may also be enhanced when employed in a patient taking acetaminophen. Consuming alcohol while taking acetaminophen may increase the risk of hepatotoxicity, as will the concomitant use of NSAIDs and acetaminophen.

References

1. Roberts LJ, Morrow J: Analgesic-Antipyretic and anti-inflammatory agents and drugs employed in the treatment of gout. In Hardman JG, Limbird LE (eds): Goodman and Gilman's The Pharmacological Basis of Therapeutics, 10th ed. New York, McGraw-Hill, 2001, p. 696.
2. Brooks PM, Day RO: Nonsteroidal anti-inflammatory drugs: Differences and similarities. N Engl J Med 324:1716, 1991.
3. Smith WL: Prostanoid biosynthesis and mechanism of action. Am J Physiol 263:F181, 1992.
4. Steiner TJ, Lange R, Voelker M: Aspirin in episodic tension-type headache: Placebo-controlled dose-ranging comparison with paracetamol. Cephalalgia 23(1):59, 2003.
5. Greenblatt DJ, Abernethy DR, Boxenbaum HG, et al: Influence of age, gender, and obesity on salicylate kinetics following single doses of aspirin. Arthritis Rheum 29(8):971, 1986.
6. Benitz WE, Tatro DS: The Pediatric Drug Handbook, 2nd ed. Chicago, Year Book, 1988.
7. Boyd JR (ed): Facts and Comparisons. Philadelphia, JB Lippincott, 1997.

8. Brunton L, Lazo J, Parker K (eds): Goodman and Gilman's The Pharmacological Basis of Therapeutics, 11th ed. New York, McGraw-Hill, 2005.
9. Leonards JR: The influence of solubility on the rate of gastrointestinal absorption of aspirin. Clin Pharmacol Ther 4:476, 1963.
10. Mielants H, Veys EM, Verbruggen G, et al.: Salicylate-induced gastrointestinal bleeding. J Rheumatol 6:210, 1979.
11. Mason WD, Winer N: Influence of food on aspirin absorption from tablets and buffered solutions. J Pharm Sci 72(7):819, 1983.
12. Cryer B, Kliewer D, Hubert S, et al.: Effects of cutaneous aspirin on the human stomach and duodenum. Proc Assoc Am Physicians 111(5):448, 1999.
13. Furst DE, Munster T: Nonsteroidal anti-inflammatory drugs, disease-modifying antirheumatic drugs, nonopioid analgesics, and drugs used in gout. In: Katzung BG (ed): Basic and Clinical Pharmacology 8th ed. New York, Lange, 2001, p 596.
14. Roberts MS, Runble RH, Wanwimolruk S, et al: Pharmacokinetics of aspirin and salicylate in elderly subjects and in patients with alcoholic liver disease. Eur J Clin Pharmacol 25:253, 1983.
15. Sitar DS, Chalmers IM, Hunter T: Plasma and synovial fluid concentrations of salicylic acid and its metabolites in patients with joint effusions. J Rheumatol 12:134, 1985.
16. Soren A: Kinetics of salicylates in blood and joint fluid. Eur J Clin Pharmacol 16:279, 1979.
17. Holander J, McCarty D: Arthritis and allied conditions. Philadelphia, Lea & Febiger, 1972.
18. Chandrasekharan NV, Dai H, Roos KL, et al: COX-3, a cyclooxygenase-1 variant inhibited by acetaminophen and other analgesic/antipyretic drugs: Cloning, structure, and expression. Proc Natl Acad Sci USA. 99(21):13926, 2002.
19. McClain CJ, Prince S, Barve S, et al:. Acetaminophen hepatotoxicity: An update. Curr Gastroenterol Rep 1:42, 1999.
20. PDR Physicians' Desk Reference for Nonprescription Drugs, 14th ed. Montvale, NJ, Medical Economics Data, 1993, p 586.
21. Furst DE, Munster T: Nonsteroidal anti-inflammatory drugs, disease-modifying antirheumatic drugs, nonopioid analgesics, and drugs used in gout. In: Katzung BG, (ed): Basic and Clinical Pharmacology 8th ed. New York, Lange, 2001, p 615.
22. Roberts LJ, Morrow J. Analgesic-antipyretic and anti-inflammatory agents and drugs employed in the treatment of gout. In Hardman JG, Limbird LE (eds): Goodman and Gilman's The Pharmacological Basis of Therapeutics, 10th ed. New York, McGraw-Hill, 2001, p 703.
23. Anon: Recommendations for the medical management of osteoarthritis of the hip and knee. Arthritis and Rheumatism 43(9):1905, 2000.
24. Smilkstein MJ, Knapp GL, Kulig KW, Rumack BH: Efficacy of oral *N*-acetylcysteine in the treatment of acetaminophen overdose. N Engl J Med 319:1557, 1988.
25. Botting RM: Mechanism of action of acetaminophen: Is there a cyclooxygenase 3? Clin Infect Dis 31:S202, 2000.

chapter 112

Nonsteroidal Antiinflammatory Drugs and COX-2 Inhibitors

Steven D. Waldman

The nonsteroidal antiinflammatory drugs are among the most widely used drugs in the world. This heterogeneous group of drugs includes aspirin, the nonacetylated salicylates, and an ever-increasing number of chemically diverse nonsalicylate compounds commonly referred to as the nonsteroidal antiinflammatory drugs (NSAIDs) and a subclass of drugs within this group that are known as the cyclooxygenase-2 (COX-2) inhibitors. These drugs have become an integral part of the routine treatment of a variety of painful conditions.

Although it was initially assumed that the pain-relieving properties of the NSAIDs could be attributed solely to their inhibition of prostaglandins, recent research suggests that at least some of the NSAIDs may exert an antinociceptive effect that is separate and apart from their antiinflammatory properties. This chapter focuses on the pharmacology, mechanisms of action, adverse effects, and clinical use of NSAIDs. It also provides the clinician with a practical framework for the safe and optimal use of this class of drugs.

PROSTAGLANDIN SYNTHESIS AND THE ANALGESIC EFFECTS OF THE NONSTEROIDAL ANTIINFLAMMATORY DRUGS

It was initially believed that the pain-relieving properties of the NSAIDs were primarily the result of these drugs' ability to inhibit the peripheral formation of prostaglandins.[1] Further understanding of how the NSAIDs produce both their beneficial and harmful effects has led to the concept that this class of drugs most likely works by inhibition of the enzyme cyclooxygenase (COX). Currently it is known that at least two forms of the enzyme exist. These have been named COX-1 and COX-2.[2] COX-1 activation leads to the production of prostacyclin, which exhibits antithrombogenic and gastric cytoprotective properties. COX-2 is induced by inflammatory stimuli and cytokines and exhibits an antiinflammatory response. The antiinflammatory actions of the NSAIDs appear to be due to inhibition of COX-2, whereas many of the unwanted side effects, such as gastrointestinal bleeding, are due to inhibition of COX-1. Therefore, in theory, drugs that have the highest COX-2 activity and a more favorable COX-2 to COX-1 activity ratio should have a potent antiinflammatory activity with fewer side effects than drugs with a less favorable COX-2 to COX-1 activity ratio. Although this conclusion is the logical result of years of basic science research and has led to the development of a number of new NSAIDs with this seemingly desirable profile, the recent withdrawal of rofecoxib (Vioxx) and other COX-2 inhibitors from the market owing to unwanted cardiovascular side effects has called this logic into question—or at least has pointed to our incomplete understanding of how the NSAIDs affect the various organ systems.[3]

Although the foregoing discussion provides an explanation for how the NSAIDs can relieve pain mediated via the inflammatory response, it does not fully explain the antinociceptive properties of this group of drugs in the treatment of acute pain from a single noxious stimuli on otherwise healthy tissue. This apparent disparity between the relative antiinflammatory and antinociceptive effects is termed "dissociation".[4] The proposed reasons for dissociation include (1) that NSAIDs produce pain relief in the absence of the physicochemical changes induced by inflammation; (2) that the NSAIDs appear to exert some central modulation of pain via attenuation of the phenomena of "central sensitization" independent of peripheral events including prostaglandin synthesis; and (3) that there is little correlation between the efficacy of a given NSAID to relieve pain and its ability to inhibit prostaglandin synthesis.[4] The clinical importance of these findings is currently the subject of much clinical research.

BODY'S RESPONSE TO INFLAMMATION

Inflammation is the body's response to tissue injury. Many of the major events in the inflammatory process have been identified, but the reasons for these events and the roles of the different chemical mediators in this process remain unclear. Factors such as the severity of tissue injury and the patient's ability to mount an inflammatory response determine the intensity of inflammation in each individual case.[5] Histamine mediates the initial inflammatory response by producing a transient period of vasoconstriction. Subsequently, vasodilation and increased permeability of blood vessels are a process which is sustained by prostaglandins.[5] In addition to these vascular events, cellular events contribute to the production of inflammation. At the site of inflammation, complement activation causes the release of chemotactic peptides called *leukotrienes*. These peptides diffuse into the adjoining capillaries, causing passing phagocytes to adhere to the endothelium. This process is called *pavementing*. The phagocytes insert pseudopods between the endothelial cells and dissolve the basement membrane (diapedesis). The neutrophils then pass out of the blood vessel and move up the concentration gradient of the chemotactic peptides toward the site of inflammation.[4,6] The result of this phagocytic process is the eventual destruction of the neutrophil. When this occurs, intracellular free radicals and lysosomal enzymes are released from the cell into the extracellular space. These substances cause further tissue damage.[6]

As the process continues, other chemical mediators, including complement fragments and interleukin-1, stimulate increased release of leukocytes from the bone marrow.[7] As leukocytes, leukocyte fragments, damaged tissue, and plasma accumulate in the area of injury, an exudate (pus) forms.[6,7] These events characterize acute inflammation. When the precipitating stimulus is removed or destroyed, inflammation resolves. If, however, the precipitating stimulus cannot be eliminated by these body defenses, inflammation will progress from an acute to a chronic state.[5,8,9]

INDIVIDUAL CHARACTERISTICS OF VARIOUS NONSTEROIDAL ANTIINFLAMMATORY DRUGS

Salicylates

Aspirin (acetylsalicylic acid) is the prototype of non-opioid antiinflammatory drugs (Fig 112–1). Aspirin and aspirin-like drugs are most often administered as analgesics, antipyretics, and inhibitors of platelet aggregation.[10] To achieve antiinflammatory activity, doses of aspirin greater than 3.6 g/day are necessary.[10] The serum half-life of salicylates ranges from 2 hours for analgesic doses to more than 20 hours for antiinflammatory doses.[10]

Orally administered salicylates are rapidly absorbed from the small intestine and, to a lesser extent, from the stomach. There is no conclusive evidence that sodium bicarbonate given with aspirin (buffered aspirin) results in a faster onset of action, greater peak intensity, or longer analgesic effect. Aspirin available in buffered effervescent preparations, however, undergoes a more rapid systemic absorption and achieves higher plasma concentrations than the corresponding tablet formulations. These effervescent preparations also cause less gastrointestinal irritation.[11] Food delays the absorption of salicylates.

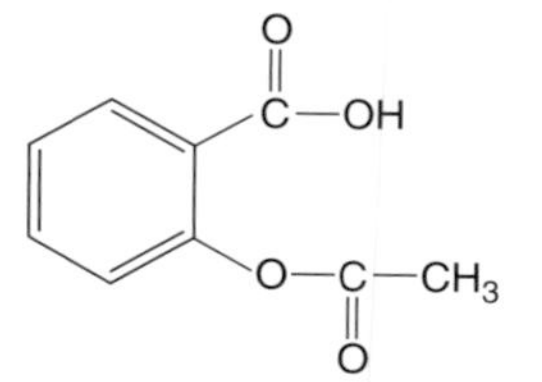

FIGURE 112–1 ■ Chemical structure of aspirin.

Aspirin, by acetylating cyclooxygenase, decreases the formation of both thromboxane (a potent vasoconstrictor and stimulant of platelet aggregation) and prostacyclin (a potent vasodilator and inhibitor of platelet aggregation). Low doses of aspirin, 60 to 100 mg daily, selectively suppress the synthesis of platelet thromboxane without inhibiting the production of endothelial prostacyclin.[9] This selective suppression may explain the favorable effect of low doses of aspirin in preventing coronary artery thrombosis.[12] Aspirin-induced platelet dysfunction seen with higher doses of aspirin lasts for the normal life span of platelets, which is 8 to 11 days.

The decreased platelet aggregation observed with aspirin is not seen with the nonacetylated salicylate products such as choline magnesium trisalicylate (Trilisate) and salsalate (Disalcid).[14,15] These nonacetylated salicylates are a much safer alternative in patients with a bleeding disorder or in those patients scheduled to undergo a surgical procedure.[15] Aspirin should be avoided in patients with severe hepatic dysfunction, vitamin K deficiency, hypoprothrombinemia, or hemophilia because platelet inhibition in such patients can result in hemorrhage.[14] Aspirin should also be avoided in children with chicken pox and flu-like illnesses, because the drug has been implicated as a possible causative or contributory factor in the evolution of Reye syndrome. Patients with asthma and nasal polyposis should also avoid aspirin and aspirin-like drugs because acute allergic reactions may result.

Salicylates may cause gastric irritation and ulceration by a reduction in prostaglandins, which normally inhibit gastric acid secretion and the ability to inhibit COX-1.[15] Alcohol ingestion may exacerbate the problem. To minimize these effects, the salicylates should be taken with food or milk or administered with cytoprotection agents. Being highly bound to albumin (80% to 90%), aspirin and aspirin-like drugs may displace other drugs such as warfarin, oral hypoglycemics, and methotrexate from protein-binding sites.[14]

Diflunisal

Diflunisal (Dolobid) is a difluorophenyl derivative of salicylic acid. This drug has pharmacodynamic and pharmacokinetics profiles similar to the other salicylates. It has been used primarily for musculoskeletal pain. It is less likely to cause the tinnitus associated with higher doses of aspirin. The initial loading dose for diflunisal is 1000 mg followed by 250 to 500 mg every 8 to 12 hours.

Nonacetylated Salicylates

Choline magnesium trisalicylate (Trilisate) and salsalate (Disalcid) are two nonacetylated salicylate derivatives that appear to lack many of the side effects of the other members of the salicylate family. These drugs exert significantly fewer effects on platelets and cause fewer gastrointestinal side effects.[13] These unique qualities are especially useful in the oncology patient who may have chemotherapy-induced clotting abnormalities. Both drugs appear to exert analgesic and antiinflammatory effects similar to the acetylated salicylates.

Choline magnesium trisalicylate is available in a liquid form, making it useful for those patients who are unable to swallow pills.

Other Nonsteroidal Antiinflammatory Drugs

Although technically the salicylates and para-amino-phenol derivatives (acetaminophen) are included in this class of drugs, the term *nonsteroidal antiinflammatory drug* has gained common acceptance for describing the chemically heterogeneous group of drugs that exhibit aspirin-like analgesic and antiinflammatory properties. NSAIDs provide analgesic effects at lower doses and antiinflammatory effects at higher doses. Many NSAIDs from a variety of chemical classes are available. More products are in various phases of clinical testing in Europe and the United States. Although the drugs referred to in common parlance as the COX-2 inhibitors are also technically NSAIDs, here they will be considered separately subsequently.

In general, the NSAIDs are indicated after simple analgesics have failed to relieve pain, toxic effects have developed, or inflammation is present.[14] All NSAIDs appear to be as effective as aspirin in terms of analgesia or antiinflammatory properties and may cause fewer gastrointestinal complaints than aspirin, although this relationship may be dose dependent.[14,15] These characteristics have encouraged many physicians to select NSAIDs before aspirin in spite of the increased cost to the patient.

The pharmacokinetics of all individual NSAIDs are similar.[16] All are well absorbed after oral administration, are highly protein bound (greater than 90%), and have a low volume of distribution (less than 0.21/kg). The NSAIDs readily penetrate synovial fluid in concentrations approximately one half those found in blood. Elimination is dependent on hepatic biotransformation to inactive metabolites (except sulindac which is metabolized to an active form), with renal excretion of less than 5% of the unchanged drug.[16]

DRUG SELECTION

Many NSAIDs are available. Busy clinicians need not be familiar with each drug, but they should have a working knowledge of one or two agents in each class of drugs. For each drug, physicians should be aware of the need for a loading dose, the time from onset of activity to peak effect, routes of administration, cost, and the side-effect profile. Also, efficacy may be enhanced by choosing a drug that can be given by a non-oral route (e.g., rectal administration of indomethacin, intramuscular administration of ketorolac tromethamine). By capitalizing on the unique properties of each drug, physicians can tailor a treatment plan to meet each patient's needs. Practical suggestions for choosing an NSAID are offered in Table 112–1.

Because of the great variation in dosage ranges and dosing frequency of NSAIDs, physicians should carefully review the properties of the agent chosen. In general, dosing should be started at the low end of the recommended range and be titrated upward as therapeutic response and side effects dictate. A loading dose should be used if indicated, especially when treating acute pain syndromes.[16,17] Extreme caution should be exercised whenever the recommended ceiling dose is exceeded.[18]

Table 112–1

Guidelines for Choosing an Optimal NSAID

- Assess patient's renal status and history of peptic ulcer disease before starting drug.
- Determine best route of administration.
- Identify drugs that are appropriate for route of administration desired.
- Select familiar agent among these drugs whose time between onset of activity and peak effect is appropriate for pain syndrome being treated.

Patient response to NSAIDs is typically variable and highly individual.[19,20] Therefore, it is reasonable to try other NSAIDs in a selective manner after an adequate trial (2 to 3 weeks) at an adequate dose (either antiinflammatory or analgesic).[16,21] Patients should always be instructed that a trial with more than one drug may be necessary and compliance with the scheduled regimen is important in evaluating effectiveness. Combination of one NSAID with other NSAIDs or aspirin increases toxic effects while providing no added benefit.[20] If additional analgesic effects are needed, a narcotic analgesic may be used during the acute phase of the pain problem.

SIDE EFFECTS

Considering their diversity in chemical structure, NSAIDs are extremely well tolerated and, when compared with all of the other non-opioid drugs currently used to treat acute pain, they have among the most favorable risk-benefit ratios. However, as with all medications, NSAIDs can cause side effects ranging from minor annoyances (e.g., dyspepsia, diarrhea, constipation) to life-threatening conditions (e.g., gastrointestinal hemorrhage, hepatic dysfunction, renal insufficiency).[22,23] Consequently, physicians need to anticipate the potential for side effects and use this important group of drugs appropriately.

NSAIDs have also been shown to cause a variety of renal complications, including peripheral edemas, transient acute renal insufficiency, tubulointerstitial nephropathy, hyperkalemia, and renal papillary necrosis.[23] Piroxicam, tolmetin, and especially sulindac are considered less likely to have renal side effects. Higher incidences of adverse effects on kidney function have been seen with indomethacin, ibuprofen, fenoprofen, mefenamic acid, naproxen, and diclofenac.[24] Prostaglandin-mediated renal effects are usually reversible on discontinuation of therapy if identified early. Identifying a patient with borderline renal function purely on clinical grounds is often impossible. For this reason, a baseline measurement of the serum creatinine level should be obtained before NSAID therapy is begun. This alerts physicians to preexisting renal problems that may be exacerbated by NSAID use and enables the physician to attribute any changes in renal function that occur during nonsteroidal antiinflammatory therapy in patients who had normal function before therapy.[25]

In general, NSAIDs should be taken with food to minimize gastrointestinal side effects. A past history of dyspepsia and gastrointestinal upset may indicate the need for the concurrent use of gastric cytoprotective agents. A past history of gastric ulceration or hemorrhage requires that NSAIDs be used only after medications that are free of gastrointestinal side effects have failed to adequately control the pain. In this event, histamine-blocking and cytoprotective agents should be given concurrently with NSAIDs and patients should be carefully monitored for occult gastrointestinal blood loss. NSAID therapy should be discontinued at the first sign of gastrointestinal difficulties.[22] The concurrent use of two or more NSAIDs increases the risk of side effects (as may the concurrent use of an NSAID and a simple analgesic, (such as acetaminophen). Thus, patients with acute pain must be carefully questioned about their use of over-the-counter agents.

COX-2 INHIBITORS

With increased understanding of the role the enzyme cyclooxygenase played in the efficacy and side effects of the NSAIDs, it was thought that the majority of side effects associated with this clinically useful class of drugs was the result of their inhibition of cyclooxygenase-1 (COX-1). It was believed that developing drugs with increased affinity for cyclooxygenase-2 (COX-2) would lead to drugs with better clinical efficacy and fewer side effects. This logic was somewhat correct and a new subclass of NSAIDs with fewer gastrointestinal side effects was developed, called the COX-2 inhibitors.[2] The first of these drugs in widespread clinical use was celecoxib (Celebrex). It became an enormous commercial success and encouraged the development and release of similar drugs. With widespread clinical use it became apparent that, although they did produce fewer gastrointestinal side effects, the COX-2 inhibitors appeared to increase the risk of cardiovascular side effects, including an increased risk of myocardial infarction.[26] As a consequence, several COX-2 inhibitors were withdrawn from the U.S. market. The actual risk profile of this class of drugs has yet to be fully elucidated and whether these drugs should remain available to patients suffering from inflammatory arthritides and connective tissue diseases remains to be answered.

Celecoxib (Celebrex)

One of the first COX-2 inhibitors available for clinical use, celecoxib, found widespread acceptance as an analgesic and antiinflammatory drug (Fig. 112–2). The initial promise of decreased gastrointestinal side effects, while not absolute, represented a positive advance for patients and prescribing physicians alike.[27] Supplied as 100-mg, 200-mg, and 400-mg tablets, celecoxib should be started at 100 mg twice a day by mouth or as a single 200-mg dose by mouth. It may be increased carefully while observing for hepatic, renal, gastrointestinal or cardiovascular side effects to a maximum daily dose of 400 mg. Higher doses have been used for the treatment of familial polyposis, but are not generally recommended for pain management indications.

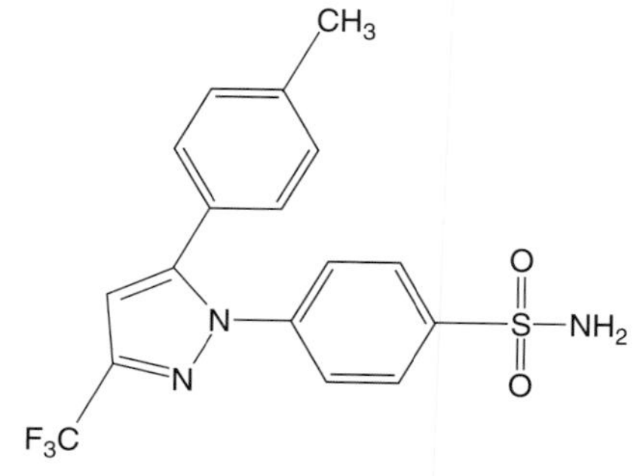

FIGURE 112–2 ■ Chemical structure of celecoxib.

Clinical experience with the drug has been positive, but the increased incidence of stroke and cardiac abnormalities led the United States Food and Drug Administration to mandate a "black box" warning to ensure that the patients and prescribing physicians are aware of these potentially fatal side effects. Whether the risk of these side effects warrants the discontinuation of this drug in patients that have tolerated it is unclear, as well as whether these drugs should be used as first-line analgesic or antiinflammatory therapeutics at all.

SUMMARY

The NSAIDs are a heterogeneous group of compounds that have been shown to be effective in the management of a variety of acute and chronic painful conditions. The clinician must understand the basic pharmacokinetics data of each NSAID that he or she prescribes to optimize pain relief and avoid side effects.

References

1. Olin BR (ed): Drug Facts and Comparisons. Philadelphia, JB Lippincott, 1991, p 2512.
2. Hawkey CJ: Cox-2 inhibitors. Lancet 353:307, 1999.
3. Couzin J: Withdrawal of Vioxx casts a shadow over COX-2 inhibitors. Science 306:384, 2004.
4. McCormack K, Brune K: Dissociation between the antinociceptive and anti-inflammatory effects of the nonsteroidal anti-inflammatory drugs, a survey of their analgesic efficacy. Drugs 41:333, 1991.
5. Graziano FM, Bell CL: The normal immune response and what can go wrong. Med Clin North Am 69:439, 1985.
6. Koch-Wesner J, Simon LS, Mills JA: Drug therapy. Nonsteroidal anti-inflammatory drugs. N Engl J Med 302:1237, 1980.
7. Crowe J, Sister JP: Nonsteroidal anti-inflammatory drugs. Am Drug 202:27, 1990.
8. Schuna AA, Vejraska BD: Rheumatoid arthritis and the seronegative spondyloarthropathies. In DiPiro JT, Talbert RL, Hayes PE, et al (eds): Pharmacotherapy: A Pathophysiologic Approach. Amsterdam, Elsevier, p 881.
9. Benigni A, Gregorini G, Frusca T, et al: Effect of low-dose aspirin on fetal and maternal generation of thromboxane by platelets in women at risk for pregnancy-induced hypertension. N Engl J Med 321:357, 1989.
10. Brunton L, Lazo JS, Parker KL (eds): Goodman & Gilman's The Pharmacological Basis of Therapeutics, 11th ed. New York, McGraw-Hill, 2006, p 644.
11. Stoelting RK, Hillier SC: Physiology and Pharmacology in Anesthetic Practice, 4th ed. Philadelphia, Lippincott, 2006.
12. Hunink MG, Goldman L, Tosteson AN, et al: The recent decline in mortality from coronary heart disease, 1980-1990. The effect of secular trends in risk factors and treatment. JAMA 277:535, 1997.
13. Estes D, Kaplan K: Lack of platelet effect with salsalate. Arthritis Rheum 23:1303, 1980.
14. Marsh CC: A review of selected investigational nonsteroidal anti-inflammatory drugs of the 1980s. Pharmacotherapy 6:10, 1986.
15. Fries JF, Bruce B: Rates of serious GI events from low-dose use of ASA, acetaminophen, and ibuprofen in patients with OA and RA . Rheumatology 30:2226, 2003.

16. Waldman SD: Management of acute pain. Refresher course in Anesthesiology. Am Soc Anesthesiol 205:1, 1990.
17. Ziegler DK, Ellis DJ: Naproxen in prophylaxis of migraine. Arch Neurol 42:582, 1995.
18. Verbeeck RK: Clinical pharmacokinetics of nonsteroidal anti-inflammatory drugs. Clin Pharmacokinet 8:297, 1983.
19. Boh LE: Osteoarthritis Pharmacotherapy: A Pathophysiologic Approach. New York, Elsevier, 1989, p 990.
20. Simon LS, Mills JA: Drug therapy: Nonsteroidal anti-inflammatory drugs. N Engl J Med 302:1179, 1980.
21. Portenoy RK, Waldman SD: Recent advances in the management of cancer pain, part 1. Pain Management 4:10, 1991.
22. Rainsford KD: Profile and mechanisms of gastrointestinal and other side effects of nonsteroidal anti-inflammatory drugs (NSAIDs). Am J Med 107(6A):27S, 1999.
23. Wilson DE, Galati JS: NSAID gastropathy: Prevention and treatment. Musculoskeletal Med 21:55, 1991.
24. Sandier DP, Smith JC, Weinberg CR, et al: Analgesic use and chronic renal disease. N Engl J Med 320:1238, 1980.
25. Clive DM: Medical progress: Renal syndromes associated with nonsteroidal antiinflammatory drugs. N Engl J Med 310:563, 1984.
26. Juni P, Rutjes AW, Dieppe PA: Are selective COX 2 inhibitors superior to traditional nonsteroidal anti-inflammatory drugs? BMJ 324:1287, 2002.
27. Lane NE: Pain management in osteoarthritis: The role of Cox-2 inhibitors. J Rheumatol 49:20, 1997.

chapter 113

Opioid Analgesics

Dhanalakshmi Koyyalagunta

Morphine is the prototypic opioid and is thus the standard against which all opioids are compared. Morphine and its related compounds exert their effects by mimicking naturally occurring substances—endogenous opioid peptides. There is an immense amount of literature available to clinicians concerning the basic biology of this endogenous opioid system and the available opioids, with new information becoming available on what seems like a daily basis. Opioids appear to be the drugs of choice for most pain syndromes, but they are associated with tolerance and abuse. Research is ongoing to discover an efficacious opioid that does not display the potential for abuse.

There is still some confusion about the terminologies used to describe these compounds. On the one hand, opiates refer to any agent derived from opium (alkaloids). On the other hand, opioids are all endogenous and exogenous substances with morphine-like properties.[1] The word opium is derived from the Greek word *opos*, meaning juice. The term narcotic is derived from the Greek word *stupor*. This chapter focuses on the description of the endogenous opioid system, its anatomy and diversity, the mechanism of opioid analgesia, and the pharmacokinetic and pharmacodynamic differences among opioid agonists and antagonists. A brief review of the various routes of administration will be presented. The focus of the chapter is to establish a basis of understanding of the various clinically used opioid medications.

HISTORY

The medicinal use of opium and morphine in different cultures and ancient civilizations is well documented. It is probable that primitive human beings, while experimenting with various plants to ascertain what was edible, discovered the value of some of these in relieving pain. The pharmacologic effects of opium were well documented 5000 years ago when, at the dawn of history, the Sumerians mentioned the poppy in their pharmacopoeia and called it "*HU GIL*," the plant of joy.[2] The Ebers Papyrus, written in 1552 BC, describes early Egyptian formulae, some of which contain opium. The first authentic reference to opium dates back to 3rd century BC in the writings of Theophrastus.[3] Scribonius Largus, in his *Compositiones Medicamentorum* (40 AD), described the method for procuring opium and mentioned that opium was derived from the unripe seed capsule of the poppy plant (Fig. 113–1).[4] Arabic physicians used opium extensively, and even wrote special treatises (Avicenna 980 to 1037) on some of its preparations.[3] Arabs introduced opium to China, where it was used to treat dysenteries. Sertuner isolated the active constituent of opium in 1805. He experimented with it on animals, himself, and his friends. He called his new discovery *Principium Somniferum*; in 1817 he renamed it *morphine* after Morpheus, the Greek god of dreams. The discovery of the other alkaloids soon followed, with codeine being discovered in 1832, papaverine in 1848, and, most recently, the endogenous opioids in the 1970s.

ENDOGENOUS OPIOID PEPTIDES

The observation that electrical stimulation of certain areas in the rat brain elicits profound analgesia and that this analgesia[5] is readily reversible by the opioid antagonist naloxone[6] implies the presence of an endogenous opioid system.[7] In 1975, an endogenous, opiate-like factor was identified and named enkephalin (from the head).[8] Soon after, two more classes of endogenous opioid peptides were isolated—the dynorphins and the endorphins. Each of these peptides is derived from a distinct precursor polypeptide and has a characteristic anatomic distribution. The precursors are preproenkephalin, preprodynorphin and preproopiomelanocortin (Pre-POMC). Each of these precursors undergoes complex cleavages and modifications to yield multiple active peptides. All the opioid peptides have a common amino-terminal sequence of Tyr-Gly-Gly-Phe- (met or leu), which has been called the *opioid motif.'*[9] ß-Endorphin is derived from proopiomelanocortin (POMC), and met-enkephalin and leu-enkephalin are derived from the processing of proenkephalin and dynorphin arises from cleavage of prodynorphin. Pre-POMC is also processed into other nonopioid peptides, such as adrenocorticotropic hormone (ACTH), melanocyte-stimulating hormone (MSH) and ß-lipoprotein (ß-l-LPH). In 1995, a novel peptide was cloned by two groups of investigators and named *orphanin FQ* (OFQ) by one group and *nociceptin (N)* by another group. N/OFQ has behavioral and pain modulatory properties distinct from the classic opioid peptides. The endogenous opioids are degraded by peptidases, and their action is very short-lived. The relative distributions of these endogenous peptides have been established by biochemical and histochemical studies. The production of ß-

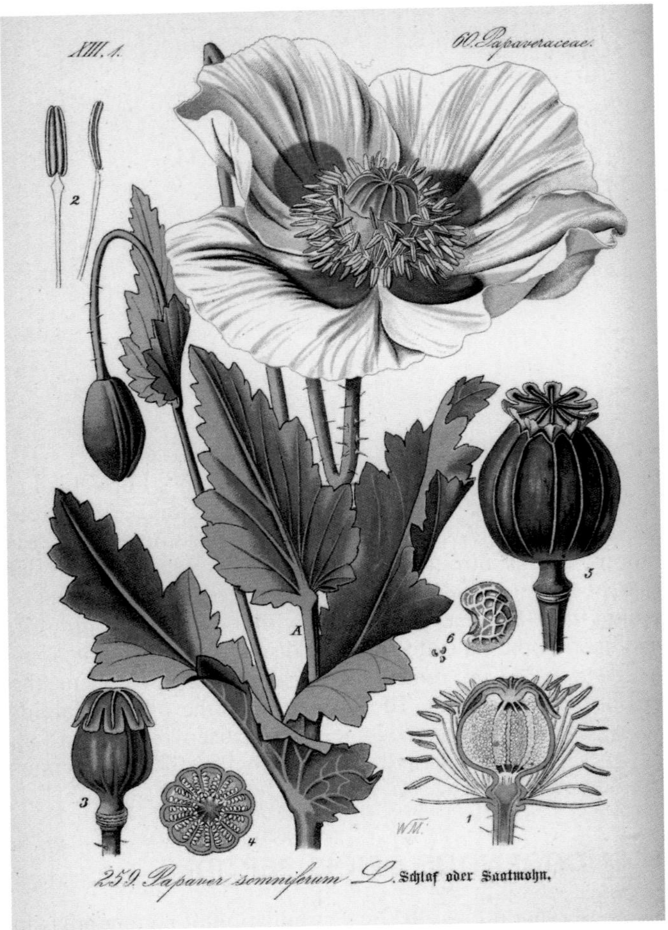

FIGURE 113–1 ■ The poppy plant (*Papaver somniferum*, Papaveraceae). (From Prof. Dr. Otto Wilhelm Thomé: Flora von Deutschland, Österreich, und der Schweiz. Gera, Germany, 1885.)

endorphin is relatively limited to the nervous system and is found in the pituitary, arcuate nucleus, medial basal hypothalamus, nucleus of the solitary tract, and the nucleus commissuralis. The second major neuronal pathway (proenkephalin) is very widespread and also includes endocrine and central nervous system (CNS) distributions. Proenkephalin peptides are present in areas of CNS that are involved in perception of pain (laminae I and II of the spinal cord, spinal trigeminal nucleus, and the periaqueductal gray), modulation of affective behavior (cerebral cortex, amygdala, hippocampus, and locus ceruleus), modulation of motor control (caudate nucleus and globus pallidus), regulation of autonomic nervous system (medulla oblongata) and neuroendocrinologic functions (median eminence).[9] Proenkephalin peptides are also present in the gastrointestinal tract and adrenal medulla. In spite of prodynorphin's having an anatomic distribution similar to proenkephalin, dynorphins are weak analgesics. N/OFQ precursor is distributed in the hippocampus, cortex, and other sensory sites. N/OFQ has a complex pharmacology and is capable of eliciting opposing actions that depend on the dose and paradigm employed.[10] It produces a naloxone-sensitive analgesia and has also been shown to exhibit an anti-opioid effect. Opioid peptides exert their pharmacologic effects through membrane bound G-protein–coupled receptors.

■ OPIOID RECEPTORS

The existence of opiate receptors was first hypothesized in 1954. The first convincing evidence regarding the existence of multiple opioid receptors was proposed by Martin and colleagues, in 1976, based on addiction, cross tolerance, and abstinence syndromes in dogs with chronic spinal transaction.[11] Using receptor-binding studies and subsequent cloning, he showed the existence of three main receptor types and named them based on the drugs used in their studies: μ or morphine receptor, σ or SKF-10047 receptor, and κ or ketocyclazocine receptor. Existence of the δ (deferens) receptor was proposed by Lord and colleagues.[12] The N/OFQ receptor opioid receptor-like-1 (ORL-1) was cloned in 1994. Other subtypes include iota, lambda and zeta. Subtypes of the μ receptor (μ_1 and μ_2), δ receptor (δ_1 and δ_2), and κ receptor (κ_1, κ_2 and κ_3) have been described. There are several other nomenclatures put forth to describe these receptors. Molecular biologists have renamed the δ, κ, μ, and N/OFQ receptors as DOR, KOR, MOR, and NOR, respectively. The International Union of Pharmacology (IUPHAR) has set guidelines that receptors should be named after their endogenous ligands followed by a numerical subscript depicting the chronologic order of the demonstration of the existence of these receptors, OP_1 (δ receptor), OP_2 (κ receptor), and OP_3 (μ-receptor).

Opioid receptors consist of seven transmembrane domains with conserved proline and aromatic residues, a characteristic of G-protein–coupled receptors.[13] Significant structural homology has been observed among the three opioid receptor cDNA clones. The μ receptor is 66% identical to the δ receptor and 68% identical to the κ receptor, whereas the δ and κ receptors have 58% identical amino acid sequences.[12] Charged residues located in the transmembrane domains have been implicated in the high affinity binding of most opioid ligands. The μ receptors bind to endorphins more so than enkephalins, the δ receptors bind to enkephalins, and the κ receptors potently bind to dynorphins. N/OFQ binds to ORL-1, a protein with a structure typical of a G-protein–coupled receptor.[14]

Opioid receptors are distributed within the CNS and periphery. The μ receptors are distributed throughout the neuraxis with the highest density in the caudate nucleus. They are also present in the neocortex, thalamus, nucleus accumbens (NAcc), hippocampus, amygdala, and superficial layers of the dorsal horn of the spinal cord.[15] A majority of the spinal μ-receptor ligand binding sites are located presynaptically on the terminals of primary afferent nociceptors. The μ receptor is most identified with the analgesic and addicting properties of opioid drugs. Morphine has been shown to exhibit a 50-fold higher affinity for μ than for δ receptors.[16] The μ receptor controls various physiologic functions, including nociception, respiration, cardiovascular functions, intestinal transit, feeding, learning and memory, locomotor activity, thermoregulation, hormone secretion, and immune function.[12]

δ Receptors have a more restricted distribution in the CNS. They are located in the olfactory bulb, caudate, putamen, neocortex, NAcc, thalamus, hypothalamus, and brain stem. The δ receptor is involved in analgesia, motor integration, cognitive function, mood driven behavior, gastrointestinal motility, olfaction, and respiration. Activation of the δ receptor produces spinal analgesia without concomitant respiratory depression.

The κ receptor is involved in the regulation of nociception, diuresis, feeding, immune function, neuroendocrine function, and possibly thermoregulation. Diuresis is due to inhibition of release of antidiuretic hormone. κ Agonist application to the spinal cord produces facilitation and inhibition of the C-fiber-evoked nociceptive responses.[17] Activation of κ receptors cause spinal analgesia, dysphoria, and sedation without concomitant respiratory depression.[1] Dynorphins may have a role in modulating the development of central plasticity and hyperalgesia (Table 113–1).

The μ-receptor mRNA is present in medium- and large-diameter DRG cells, whereas the δ-receptor mRNA is found in large-diameter cells and the κ-opioid receptor mRNA is found in small- and medium-diameter cells.[18] This differential localization may be the reason for functional differences in pain modulation.

N/OFQ stimulates food intake, produces anxiolysis, and has a role in memory and information processing. Drugs interacting with the ORL-1 receptor appear to be free of abuse potential.[14]

Table 113–1

Opioid Receptors and Their Clinical Effects

Receptor	*Effect*
Mu (μ)	
μ_1	Supraspinal analgesia
μ_2	Spinal analgesia
	Respiratory depression
	Slowing of gastric transit
	Pruritus, nausea, vomiting
	Most cardiovascular effects
	Physical dependence
	Euphoria
Kappa (κ)	
κ_1	Spinal analgesia
	Diuresis
	Sedation
	Miosis
κ_2	Low potential for abuse
κ_3	Supraspinal analgesia
Delta (δ)	Modulation of μ-receptor activity
	Spinal analgesia
Sigma (Σ)	No analgesia
	Dysphoria
	Hypertonia
	Respiratory and vasomotor stimulation
	Mydriasis

Adapted from Pasternak GW: Pharmacological mechanisms of opioid analgesics. Clin Neuropharmacol16:1, 1993 and Reisine T, Pasternak G: Opioid analgesics and antagonists. In Hardman JG, Limbard LE (eds): Goodman and Gilman's the Pharmacologic Basis of Therapeutics, 9th ed. New York, McGraw-Hill, 1996, p 521.

■ CLASSIFICATION OF OPIOIDS

There are three schemes used to classify opioids. Based on their intrinsic action at the receptor site, opioids can be classified as partial agonists (buprenorphine), agonists (morphine, codeine, methadone, fentanyl, etc.), agonists/antagonists (butorphanol, nalbuphine, pentazocine, and dezocine), and antagonists (naloxone, naltrexone, cholecystokinin) (Table 113–2). Based on their affinity for the opioid receptor, they are considered weak (codeine, propoxyphene) or strong opioids. The other classification is based on how the opioids are derived-naturally occurring (morphine and codeine) or semisynthetic or synthetic compounds. Opium contains two distinct alkaloid types: phenanthrenes and benzylisoquinolones. The phenanthrene derivatives are morphine, codeine, and thebaine. The benzylisoquinolone alkaloids are papaverine (vasodilator, no analgesic property) and noscapine.

Opium still remains the main production source for morphine because laboratory synthesis is not possible. Morphine consists of five condensed ring systems. The morphine molecule has six chiral centers, present on the nitrogen atom and on the carbon atom 5, 6, 8, 9 and 13. The pentacyclic structure conforms to a "T" shape with a piperidine ring forming one cross bar and a hydroxylated aromatic ring lying in the vertical axis (Fig. 113–2).

Modification of functional groups on the skeleton gives rise to semisynthetic opioids, diacetylmorphine, hydromorphone, oxymorphone, hydrocodone, and oxycodone (Fig. 113–3). Synthetic opioids are created by progressive reduction of the number of fused rings on the phenanthrene moiety (Fig. 113–4). Codeine is a methylmorphine, the phenolic hydroxyl group possessing the methyl substitution. Thebaine has very little analgesic property but is a precursor for the strong analgesic compound oxycodone and the antagonist naloxone. Etorphine, a derivative of thebaine is more than 1000 times as potent as morphine.

■ MECHANISM OF ACTION

Opioid receptors, as mentioned earlier, are widespread across the CNS and the periphery. These receptors are bivalent, with one portion (transmembrane regions) mediating signal transduction and the other (extracellular loop) determining receptor selectivity.[14] The recognition site on these receptors is specific and only the levorotatory isomers exhibit analgesic activity.[19] Alkaloids are small enough to fit completely inside or near the mouth of the receptor core, whereas peptides bind

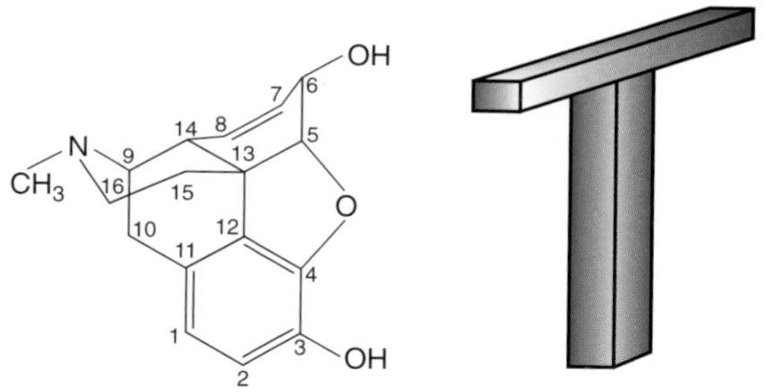

FIGURE 113–2 ■ The T-shaped molecule of morphine.

Table 113–2

Classification of Opioids on the Basis of Intrinsic Activity* and Synthetic Origin

Agonists	*Agonist-Antagonists*	*Antagonists*
Phenanthrene alkaloids	Semisynthetic opioids	Naloxone
Morphine	Buprenorphine	Naltrexone
Codeine	Nalbuphine	
Thebaine	Synthetic opioids	
Semisynthetic opioids	Benzomorphan derivatives pentazocine	
Diacetylmorphine (heroin)	Morphinan derivatives butorphanol dezocine	
Hydrocodone		
Hydromorphone		
Oxycodone		
Oxymorphone		
Synthetic opioids		
Morphinan derivatives levorphanol		
Phenylpiperidine derivatives		
Meperidine		
Fentanyl		
Sufentanil		
Alfentanil		
Propioanilide derivatives		
Methadone		
Propoxyphene		

*Intrinsic activity refers to the intensity of the pharmacologic effect initiated by the drug-receptor complex.

From Ferrante M: Opioids. In Ferrante M, VadeBoncouer T (eds): Postoperative pain management. New York, Churchill Livingstone, 1993, p 145.

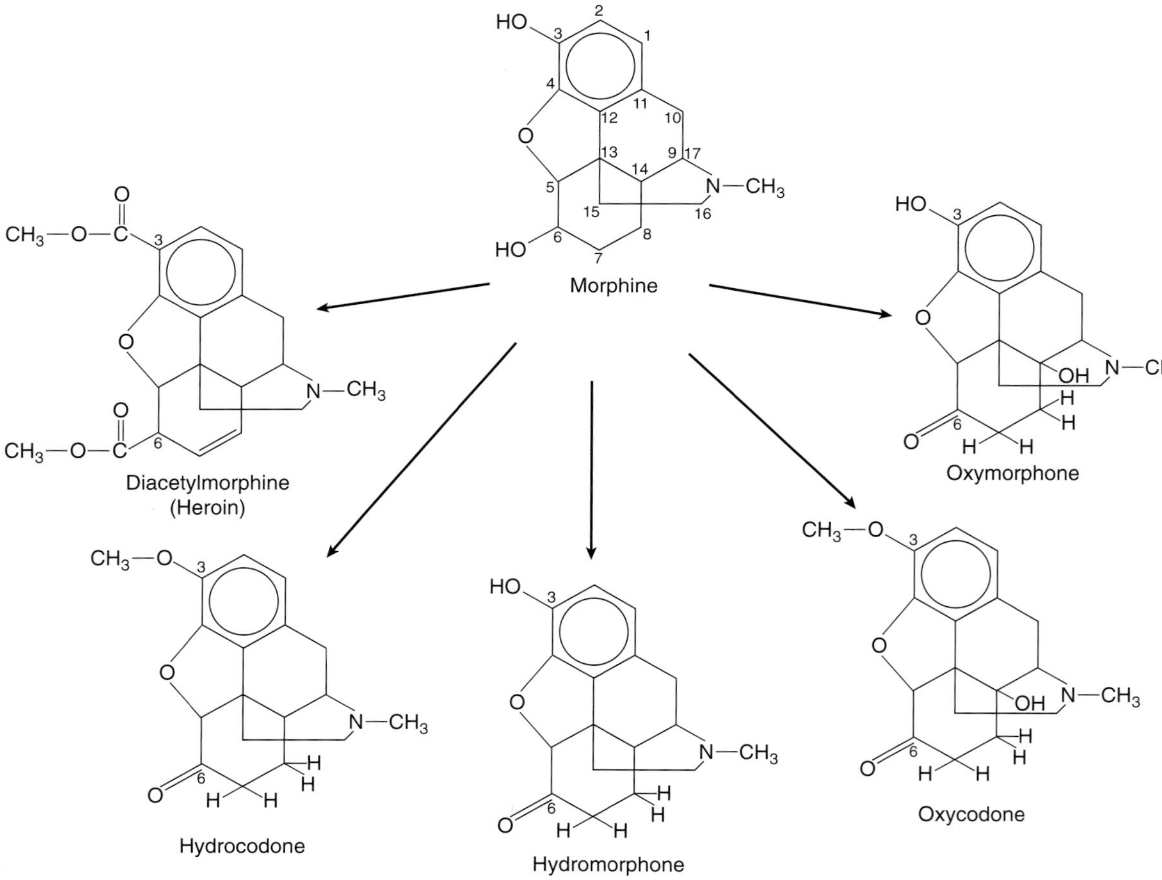

FIGURE 113–3 ■ Chemical structure of semisynthetic opioids diacetylmorphine, hydromorphone, oxymorphone, hydrocodone and oxycodone. (Adapted from Ferrante M: Opioids. In Ferrante M, VadeBoncouer T (eds): Postoperative Pain Management. New York, Churchill Livingstone, 1993, p 145.)

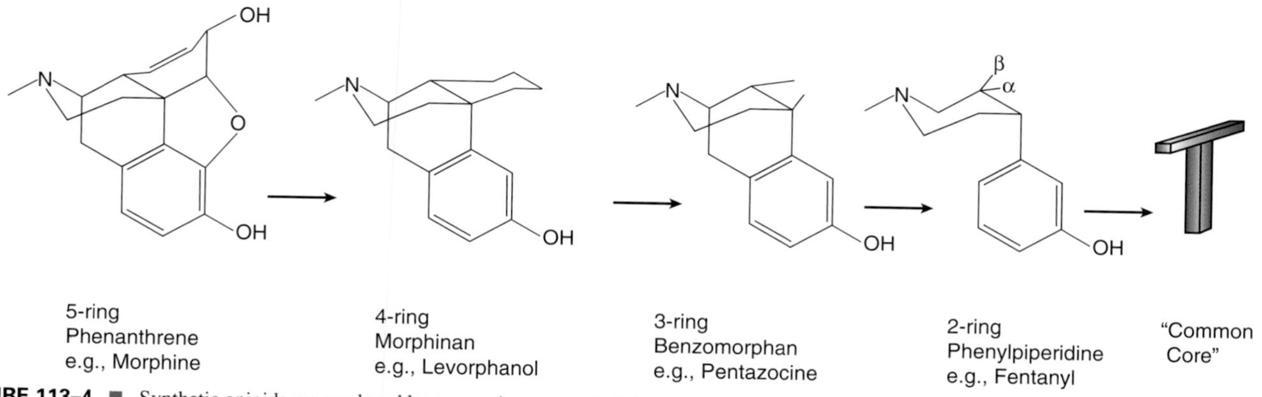

FIGURE 113–4 ■ Synthetic opioids are produced by successive removal of ring structures from the five-ring phenanthrene structure of morphine. However, a common core, resembling a "T" shape, is shared by all opioids. A piperidine ring (which is believed to confer "opioid-like" properties to a compound) forms the cross bar and a hydroxylated phenyl group forms the vertical axis. (Adapted from Ferrante M: Opioids. In Ferrante M, VadeBoncouer T (eds): Postoperative Pain Management. New York, Churchill Livingstone, 1993, p 145.)

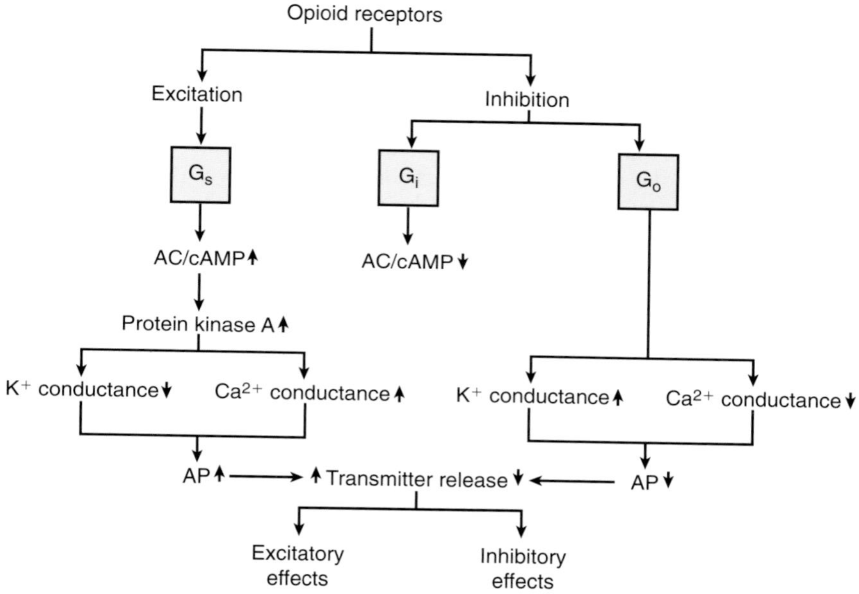

FIGURE 113–5 ■ Opioid agonists in micromolar concentrations are primarily inhibitory, decreasing the activity of adenylyl cyclase (AC), intracellular cAMP, and the action potential (AP), resulting in neuronal hyperpolarization. In contrast, nanomolar concentrations cause the opposite effects, resulting in increased neuronal excitability. (Adapted from Bovill JG: Update on opioid and analgesic pharmacology. Anesth Analg 92(3S):1, 2001.)

to the extracellular loops and simultaneously extend to the receptor core to activate the common binding site. Opioids bind to the receptors with varying affinities. The analgesic potency of an opioid is determined by its affinity to the receptor. Using various bioassay systems, the rank order of the binding affinities has been determined, with sufentanil exhibiting the highest binding affinity.[20]

The spatial orientation of the various amino acids in the transmembrane regions and the extracellular loops determine the formation of the binding pocket of the receptor. The opioid receptor is anionic in nature and an opioid has to be in an ionic state for binding to occur.[21] Activation of the opioid receptors produces effects that are primarily inhibitory in nature. Direct inhibitory effects of opioids are mediated by opioid receptors coupled to pertussis-sensitive G_I/G_O proteins and direct excitatory effects via a cholera toxin-sensitive G_S protein.[22-24] Opioid agonists inhibit adenylyl cyclase and thereby decrease cyclic AMP production. They close N-type voltage-operated calcium channels and open receptor-operated potassium channels. This results in hyperpolarization and a decrease in neuronal excitability. Nanomolar concentrations of opioids can produce excitatory effects by activating excitatory G_S proteins (Fig. 113–5). This antagonism of excitatory activity may explain the observation that co-treatment with extremely low doses of an antagonist can enhance the analgesic efficacy of opioid agonists.[22] Another mode of opioid action is the inhibition of GABAergic transmission in a local circuit (e.g., in the brain stem where GABA acts to inhibit pain-inhibitory neurons). The net effect of this disinhibitory action would be exciting a descending inhibitory circuit. Opioids also decrease the pain-evoked release of tachykinins from primary afferent nociceptors.[25] Opioid agonists have a peripheral analgesic effect. Opioid receptors synthesized in the dorsal root ganglion (DRG) are transported to the peripheral tissues.[26,27] Locally released endogenous opioid compounds are up-regulated during inflammatory pain states.[28] Peripheral opioid analgesia is possibly mediated by G protein coupled inhibition of cAMP in peripheral terminals.[27]

PHARMACODYNAMICS

Pharmacodynamics is the study of the relation of the concentration of the drug at the site of action and the body's biological and physiologic response (what the drug does to the body).

Central Nervous System

Analgesia

Opioids produce analgesia by mimicking the action of endogenous opioids. Opioids act to produce analgesia at several levels of the CNS. Most of the clinically used opioids produce analgesia by binding to the μ receptor and share a common spectrum of pharmacodynamic effects. δ-Receptor agonists are potent analgesics in animals and in some isolated cases in humans, but the clinical use of δ agonists is limited, as they do not cross the blood-brain barrier.[29] κ Agonists produce analgesia mediated primarily at spinal sites. Some opioids (meperidine, methadone, ketobemidone and dextropropoxyphene) have antihyperalgesic and anti-allodynic effect by their *N*-methyl-D-aspartate (NMDA) antagonist properties. Preclinical studies have shown the NMDA receptor antagonists reverse or prevent the development of morphine tolerance.[30] Analgesic effects of opioids arise from their ability to inhibit the ascending transmission of nociceptive information from the spinal cord dorsal horn and to activate the descending inhibitory pathways. Opioids, by their action on the limbic system, alter the emotional response to pain, making it bearable. In addition to central effects, opioid agonists have peripheral analgesic effects. Opioids depress the spontaneous firing of nociceptors of inflamed skin in a naloxone-reversible manner. *Equianalgesia* is the same degree of pain relief obtained by different drugs at specified doses (Table 113–3) and is a way of comparing the analgesic effects of drugs.

Mood Alteration and Rewarding Properties

Opioids produce euphoria, tranquility, and rewarding behavior. Euphoria is mediated by μ receptors. Activation of κ receptors produces dysphoria. The dopaminergic pathways, particularly involving the NAcc, are responsible for drug-induced reward.[9] Opioid agonists with an affinity for μ and δ opioid receptors are rewarding, whereas opioid agonists with affinity for κ receptors are aversive.[31] High concentrations of opioid receptors and noradrenergic neurons present in the locus ceruleus are thought to play a major role in feelings of alarm, panic, fear, and anxiety. Exogenous and endogenous opioid peptides inhibit neural activity in the locus ceruleus. At high doses, opioids produce sleep; there is a replacement of rapid α waves by slower δ waves on the electroencephalogram (EEG).[32]

Antitussive

Opioids have an antitussive effect by depressing the cough center in the medulla. There is no correlation between suppression of coughing and the respiratory depressant effect of opioids. Opioids differ in their capacity to depress the cough reflex (Table 113–4). Suppression of coughing seems to be less sensitive to naloxone reversal.

Nausea

All opioids produce some degree of nausea. Certain opioids cause more nausea than others. This is due to direct stimulation of the chemoreceptor trigger zone for emesis in the area postrema of the medulla. There is also a vestibular component to the nausea caused by opioids because nausea and vomiting are more common in ambulatory patients who have received opioids. Delay in gastric transit may also contribute to the nausea produced by opioids.

Miosis

Miosis is caused by stimulation of the Edinger-Westphal nucleus of the oculomotor nerve. Patients display a delayed tolerance to miosis, which is seen with most μ- and κ-agonist use. Pinpoint pupils are characteristic of opioid poisoning unless there is profound hypercarbia associated with the respiratory depression.

Convulsions

Morphine and related compounds at high doses cause convulsions by stimulating neurons, especially in the hippocampal pyramidal cells. The M3G metabolite may play a part in EEG spiking and epileptiform discharges.[33] Smith and

Table 113–3

Relative Potencies of Opioid Analgesics

Drug	*Relative Potency IM*	*Relative Potency PO*
Morphine	10	30
Hydromorphone	1.5	7.5
Meperidine	75	300
Methadone	10	12.5
Codeine	120	200
Levorphanol	2	4
Nalbuphine	10	
Oxycodone		30
Pentazocine	60	180

IM, intramuscularly; PO, by mouth.
From Katz JA: Opioids and nonsteroidal analgesics. In Raj PP (ed): Pain Medicine: A Comprehensive Review. St Louis, Mosby, 1996, p 126.

Table 113–4

Antitussive Effects of Opioids (Decreasing Order of Potency)

Diacetylmorphine = fentanyl = hydromorphone = hydrocodone
Methadone
Codeine
Morphine
Levorphanol
Meperidine = pentazocine

From Ferrante M: Opioids. In Ferrante M, VadeBoncouer T (eds): Postoperative Pain Management. New York, Churchill Livingstone, 1993, p 145.

colleagues, showed seizure-like activity in humans with no EEG evidence and concluded that what was demonstrated was muscular rigidity. Normeperidine (a metabolite of meperidine) and norpropoxyphene (a metabolite of propoxyphene) are known to cause CNS excitation.

Muscular Rigidity

The exact mechanism for muscular rigidity is not known but it is postulated to be centrally located in the striatum, which is known to be rich in opioid binding sites.[34] High doses and rapid injection of intravenous opioids are notorious for causing muscular rigidity, which is more common in the elderly population (>60 years). The rigidity of the striatal muscles is characterized by an increased muscle tone, which may progress to severe stiffness. In particular, thoracic and abdominal muscles are involved, resulting in so-called "wooden chest," which impedes ventilation.

Respiratory System

All μ-agonists produce a dose-dependent respiratory depression. The agonist-antagonists also depress respiration but have a ceiling effect. Opioids primarily cause respiratory depression by reducing brain stem respiratory center responsiveness to carbon dioxide. They also depress the respiratory centers in the pons and medulla, which are involved in regulating respiratory rhythmicity.[35] There is an increase in the resting CO_2 and a shift of the CO_2 response curve to the right. Equianalgesic doses of μ-agonists produce the same degree of respiratory depression. A decrease in respiratory rate is characteristic of μ-agonist-induced respiratory depression. There is some compensatory increase in the minute volume, which is incomplete, as evidenced by an increase in $PaCO_2$. Patients must rely on hypoxic drive to stimulate ventilation. Pain is an effective antagonist to the respiratory depressant effects of opioids. κ-Agonists produce less respiratory depression, even after administration of large doses. Opioid antagonists antagonize the respiratory depressant effects of opioids. Partial opioid agonists have also been used to antagonize the respiratory depression caused by pure opioid agonists. Physostigmine also has been shown to reverse the respiratory depressant effect while preserving the analgesic effect.[36]

Cardiovascular System

The cardiovascular effects of opioids depend not only on the dosage; they are also linked with the product and the prevailing vegetative basic tone of the patient. Opioids produce a dose-dependent bradycardia by increasing the centrally mediated vagal stimulation. Meperidine produces tachycardia due to its structural similarity to atropine (Fig. 113–6). Morphine and some other opioids (meperidine and codeine) provoke release of histamine, which plays a major role in producing hypotension. Naloxone does not inhibit the histamine release produced by opioids. Morphine also has a direct effect on the vascular smooth muscle. Morphine exerts its well-known therapeutic effect in the treatment of angina pectoris by decreasing preload, inotropy, and chronotropy, thereby decreasing myocardial oxygen consumption.[9] Pentazocine and butorphanol cause an increase in systemic and pulmonary artery pressure, left ventricular filling pressure, systemic vascular resistance, and a decrease in left ventricular ejection fraction. Opioids should be used with caution in patients with decreased blood volume because they can aggravate hypovolemic shock.

Gastrointestinal Tract

μ-Agonists decrease gastric, biliary, pancreatic, and intestinal secretions. Even small doses decrease gastric motility and prolong gastric emptying time. Resting tone in the small and large intestine is increased to the point of spasm, and the propulsive peristaltic waves are decreased. Opioids exert their effect on the submucosal plexus, decrease the secretion by enterocytes, and inhibit the stimulatory effects of acetylcholine, prostaglandin E_2, and vasoactive intestinal peptide. These effects are mediated in large part by the release of norepinephrine and stimulation of α_2 receptors on the enterocytes.[37] The gastrointestinal effects of opioids are primarily mediated by μ- and δ-receptors in the bowel. However, neuraxial application of opioids can also cause these effects as long as the extrinsic innervation of the bowel is intact. Patients usually develop very little tolerance to the constipating effects of opioids. Opioids constrict the sphincter of Oddi and raise the common bile duct pressure. Opioids in patients with biliary disease may cause severe sphincter constriction and pain. Delayed respiratory depression associated with opioids is postulated to be caused by enterosystemic circulation of opioids. Secondary peaks are often seen in plasma concentration-time graphs during pharmacokinetic studies of the more lipid-soluble opioids.[38] This is thought to be caused by absorption of the opioids first sequestered in the acidic gastric juices then absorbed from the small intestine.

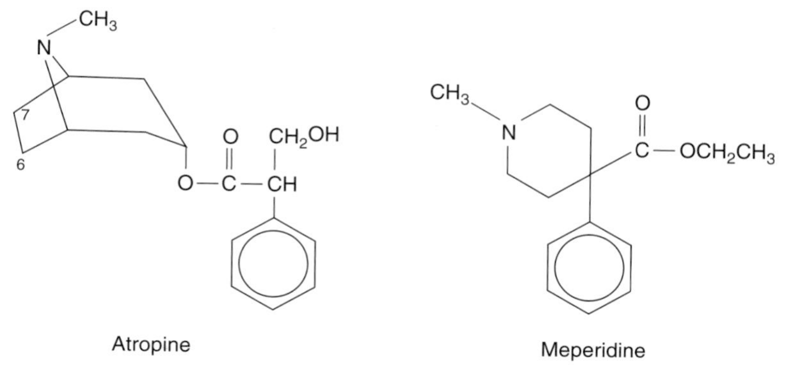

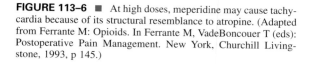

FIGURE 113–6 ■ At high doses, meperidine may cause tachycardia because of its structural resemblance to atropine. (Adapted from Ferrante M: Opioids. In Ferrante M, VadeBoncouer T (eds): Postoperative Pain Management. New York, Churchill Livingstone, 1993, p 145.)

Genitourinary System

Retention of urine is a frequent finding with opioid analgesics, which increase urinary sphincter pressure and decrease the central inhibition of detrusor tone. The hypothesized site of action of opioids is in the thoracic spinal cord, where some preganglionic cell bodies are surrounded by terminals containing enkephalins and substance P.[39]

Neuroendocrine System

μ-Agonists inhibit the release of gonadotropin-releasing hormone and corticotropin-releasing hormone, thereby decreasing the circulating concentrations of luteinizing hormone (LH), follicle-stimulating hormone (FSH), ACTH, and ß-endorphin. As a result of decreased pituitary trophic hormones, there is also a decrease in testosterone and cortisol levels in the plasma. With chronic administration, patients develop a tolerance to these effects. κ-Receptor agonists inhibit the release of antidiuretic hormone and cause diuresis, and μ-receptor agonists tend to produce an antidiuretic effect.

Uterus

Opioids in therapeutic doses prolong labor by decreasing uterine contractions.[40] Parenteral opioids given within 2 to 4 hours of delivery can produce neonatal respiratory depression as they cross the placenta.

Skin

Morphine, in therapeutic doses can cause dilation of cutaneous blood vessels. This is in part caused by histamine release and a decrease in peripheral vascular resistance. The skin of the face, neck, and upper thorax become flushed. Morphine- and meperidine-induced histamine release accounts for the urticaria at the site of injection; this is not reversed by naloxone.[9] Oxymorphone, methadone, fentanyl, and sufentanil are not associated with histamine release. Pruritus is a disabling side effect associated with opioid use. Pruritus is more intense with the intrathecal application of opioids,[41] and the effect appears to be mediated in large part by dorsal horn neurons and reversible by naloxone.[42]

Immune System

Opioids affect host defense mechanisms in a complex manner. Acute, central immunomodulatory effects seem to be mediated by activation of the sympathetic nervous system and the chronic effects may involve modulation of hypothalamic-pituitary-adrenal axis function.[43] Morphine alters a number of mature immunocompetent cells that are involved in cell-mediated and humoral immune responses. Individuals exposed to opioid treatment for pain management or those on methadone maintenance show no effect or a suppressed immune system. Heroin addicts present an altered and impaired immune system and show a higher prevalence of infectious diseases than non-addicts.[44]

TOLERANCE

Tolerance refers to a phenomenon in which exposure to a drug results in the diminution of an effect or the need for a higher dose to maintain an effect. Tolerance can be innate (genetically determined) or acquired. There are three types of acquired tolerance-pharmacokinetic, pharmacodynamic, and learned. Pharmacokinetic tolerance comes from changes in the metabolism and distribution of the drug after repeated administration (i.e., enzyme induction). Pharmacodynamic tolerance comes from adaptive changes (i.e., drug-induced changes in receptor density). Learned tolerance is a result of compensatory mechanisms that are learned.[45] Short-term tolerance probably involves phosphorylation of the μ- and δ-receptors via protein kinase C,[46] whereas long-term tolerance is associated with increases in adenylyl cyclase activity, a counter regulation to the decrease in cyclic AMP levels seen after acute opioid administration.[47] In opioid tolerance, a functional decoupling of opioid receptors from the G-protein-regulated cellular mechanisms occurs in addition to down-regulation of endogenous opioids and/or opioid receptors and behavioral changes.[48]

Tolerances to different opioid side effects develop at different rates; this has been termed selective tolerance. Tolerance to nausea, vomiting, sedation, euphoria, and respiratory depression develop rapidly, whereas tolerance to constipation and miosis is minimal.[49] Repeated doses of a drug in a given category confer tolerance not only to the drug being used but also to other drugs in the same structural and mechanistic category; this effect is known as cross-tolerance. Cross-tolerance has been shown to be incomplete in animal studies and has been reported in humans as well.[50] Incomplete cross-tolerance is frequently attributed to opioids, having differing opioid-receptor subtype affinity.[51] NMDA antagonists have been shown to block the antinociceptive tolerance to morphine.[52]

ADDICTION AND PHYSICAL DEPENDENCE

Addiction has been defined by the World Health Organization as "a state, psychic and sometimes also physical, resulting from the interactions between a living organism and a drug, characterized by a behavioral and other responses that always include a compulsion to take the drug on a continuous or periodic basis in order to experience its psychic effects, and sometimes to avoid the discomfort of its absence. Tolerance may or may not be present." There is increasing evidence to implicate the mesolimbic dopamine system in the rewarding effects of drugs of abuse such as opioids; in addition, endogenous opioids may play a key role in the underlying adaptive mechanisms.[31] Opioid agonists with affinity for μ- and δ-receptors are rewarding, whereas opioid agonists with affinity for κ-receptors are aversive. Experiments with opioid antagonists have demonstrated the presence of an endogenous opioidergic tone in the reward system. The dopaminergic mesolimbic system, originating in the ventral tegmental area (VTA) of the midbrain has been implicated in the rewarding effects seen with opioid use (Fig. 113–7). The D_1 subtype of dopamine (DA) receptors mediates a tonic activation of this pathway. The basal release of DA in the NAcc is under tonic control of both opposing opioid systems: μ-receptor (and possibly

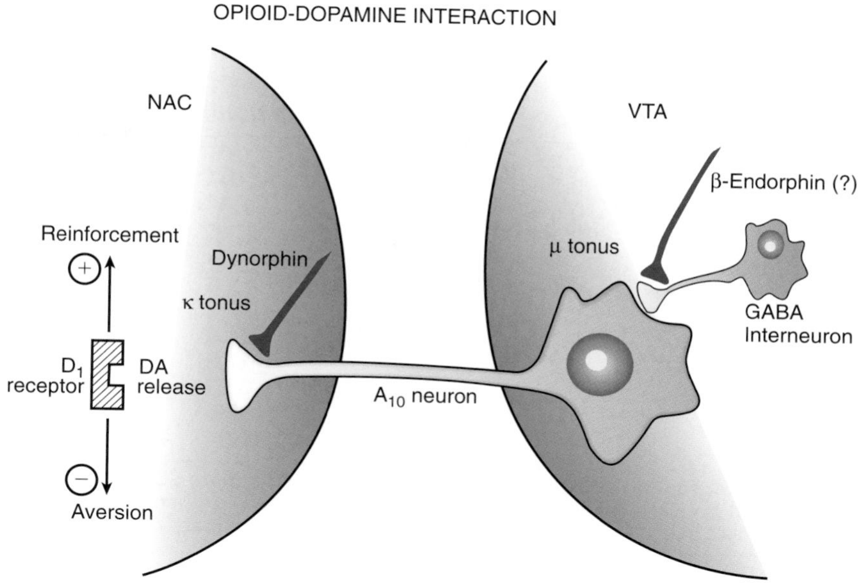

FIGURE 113–7 ■ Model for the modulation of mesolimbic A_{10} neurons by endogenous opioid systems. (Adapted from Spanagel R, Herz A, Shippenberg TS: Opposing tonically active endogenous opioid systems modulate the mesolimbic dopaminergic pathway. Proc Natl Acad Sci U S A 89:2046, 1992.)

Table 113–5

Symptoms and Signs of Opioid Withdrawal

Symptoms	***Signs***
Craving for opioids	Pupillary dilatation
Restlessness	Sweating
Irritability	Piloerection
Increased sensitivity to pain	Tachycardia
Nausea	Vomiting
Abdominal cramps	Diarrhea
Myalgia	Hypertension
Dysphoria	Yawning
Insomnia	Fever
Anxiety	Rhinorrhea

From Collett BJ: Opioid tolerance: The clinical perspective. Br J Anaesth 81:58, 1998.

δ-receptor) activity originating from the VTA increases and κ-receptor activity (originating from the NAcc) decreases basal activity of the mesolimbic reward system.[53] *Pseudo-addiction* has been used to describe the iatrogenic syndrome of behavioral changes similar to addiction that can develop as a result of inadequate pain management. *Opiophobia* is the phenomenon of failure to administer legitimate opioid analgesics because of fear of the power of these drugs to produce addiction.

Physical dependence is defined as the potential for an abstinence syndrome, or withdrawal, after abrupt dose reduction, discontinuation of the drug, or administration of an antagonist or agonist-antagonist drug. This is a physiologic phenomenon and is associated with disabling symptoms (Table 113–5). The lowest dose and shortest duration of treatment that may predispose to a significant abstinence syndrome is not known.[31] Clinically, the dose can be decreased by 10% to 20% every other day and eventually stopped without signs and symptoms of withdrawal.[9]

■ PHARMACOKINETICS

Pharmacokinetics is the study of drug disposition in the body (what the body does to the drug) over time, including absorption, distribution, biotransformation, and elimination. Opioids have similar pharmacodynamic properties but have widely different kinetic properties (Tables 113–6 and 113–7).

Absorption and Routes of Administration

Absorption refers to the rate and extent of removal of the drug from the site of administration. This process is determined by the drug's molecular shape and size, ionization constant, lipid solubility, and physicochemical properties of the membrane it must cross.[54]

Oral Route

This is the preferred route for long-term administration of opioids because it is convenient and cost effective. Most opioids are well absorbed after oral administration. Aqueous solutions are absorbed the best, followed by oily solutions, suspensions, and oral solids. Drugs absorbed from the gut are subject to first-pass metabolism in the liver and some degree of metabolism by enzymes in the intestinal wall. The onset of action is slower and variable in comparison to parenteral administration. Some opioids (e.g., codeine, oxycodone) have a high oral-to-parenteral potency ratio because they are protected from conjugation by substitution on C3 aromatic hydroxyl residue.[55] Oral opioids are available in tablet and liquid form and in immediate-release and controlled-release preparations. Morphine and oxycodone are available in controlled-release forms. The controlled-release form of hydromorphone is not available in the United States.

Subcutaneous

In comparison to the oral route, subcutaneous administration is faster and does not have to rely on gastrointestinal function. The absorption can be variable and erratic. The

Table 113–6

Pharmacokinetic and Physiochemical Variables of Opioid Analgesics

Drug	*Vc (L/kg)*	*Vd (L/kg)*	*Cl (mL/min/kg)*	*T1/2β (min)*	*Partition Coefficient (octanol/water)*
Morphine	0.23	2.8	15.5	134	1
Hydromorphone	0.34	4.1	22.7	15	1
Meperidine	0.6	2.6	12	180	21
Methadone	0.15	3.4	1.6	23 hr	115
Levorphanol		10.0	10.5	11 hr	
Alfentanil	0.12	0.9	7.6	94	130
Fentanyl	0.85	4.6	21	186	820
Sufentanil	0.1	2.5	11.3	149	1750
Buprenorphine	0.2	2.8	17.2	184	10,000
Nalbuphine	0.45	4.8	23.1	222	
Butorphanol		5.0	38.6	159	
Dezocine		12.0	52	156	

Vc, central volume of distribution; Vd, volume of distribution; Cl, clearance; T1/2β, elimination half-life.
Adapted from Hill H, Mather L: Patient-controlled analgesic, pharmacokinetic and therapeutic considerations. Clin Pharmacokinet 24:124, 1993 and O'Brien JJ, Benfield P: Dezocine: A preliminary review of its pharmacodynamic and pharmacokinetic properties and therapeutic efficacy. Drugs 38:226, 1989.

Table 113–7

Plasma Half-Life Values for Opioids and Their Active Metabolites

	Plasma Half-Life (hr)
Short half-life opioids	
Morphine	2-3.5
Morphine-6-glucuronide	2
Hydromorphone	2-3
Oxycodone	2-3
Fentanyl	3.7
Codeine	3
Meperidine	3-4
Pentazocine	2-3
Nalbuphine	5
Butorphanol	2.5-3.5
Buprenorphine	3-5
Long half-life opioids	
Methadone	24
Levorphanol	12-16
Propoxyphene	12
Norpropoxyphene	30-40
Normeperidine	14-21

From Inturrisi CE: Clinical pharmacology of opioids for pain. Clin J Pain 18(Suppl 4):S3, 2002.

subcutaneous route can be used for continuous infusion, patient-controlled analgesia, and intermittent boluses. The drawbacks are that only small volumes can be infused and there could be pain and necrosis at the site of injection.

Intramuscular

The intramuscular route is painful and inconvenient and absorption can show some variability. As compared to the subcutaneous route, larger volumes and oil-based solutions can be used intramuscularly.

Intravenous

The intravenous route provides the most rapid onset of analgesia, but the duration of analgesia after a bolus dose is shorter than with other routes. This route provides a more reliable absorption and drug levels in the plasma. Intravenous drugs must be water soluble or the oil-based solutions need to be diluted and given in larger volumes.

Rectal

The rectal route is an alternative when the upper gastrointestinal tract cannot be used and the parenteral route is not available or acceptable. The rectal route is contraindicated if there are lesions of the anus or rectum. Absorption of medications is similar to the oral route. The bioavailability of drugs is variable; the bioavailability of morphine is 55% to 60%, suggesting that this route partially avoids the first-pass metabolism.

Transnasal

Intranasal administration is particularly familiar to the recreational abuser of opioids. Reliable absorption across the nasal mucosa is determined by the lipid solubility. This route avoids first-pass metabolism. Opioids administered by this route can be used either as a dry powder or dissolved in water. Butorphanol is the only opioid available formulated in a metered-dose spray form. Many opioids dissolved in water or saline have been investigated. Intranasal administration of opioids for acute pain settings is not superior to parenteral administration. It may have a role in patients with difficult intravenous access.

Inhalational

This is a novel route for administration of opioids. Use of this technique has been encouraging due to the suggestion that this method may target opioid receptors in the lung. After inhalation of morphine and diamorphine, morphine has been detected in the plasma after 1 minute with t_{max} in 10 and 6 minutes, respectively.[56,57] Fentanyl administered by this route achieves a t_{max} in 2 minutes.[58] Inhaled opioids have been investigated for several indications; dyspnea at rest, postoperative pain, and provision of pain relief in the general population.

Transdermal

The transdermal route is used in two forms: passive system and active (iontophoresis) system. Fentanyl is the only opioid currently available in a transdermal form. Fentanyl can be used for transdermal delivery due to its physicochemical properties: low molecular weight, adequate water and lipid solubility, and high potency. Transdermal fentanyl uses the passive system. Its two principal components are a fentanyl-containing reservoir and a rate-controlling membrane. Four patch sizes are available and provide delivery of fentanyl at 25, 50, 75, or 100 μg/hour. The transdermal system is not ideal for rapid dose titration. Transdermal fentanyl should be considered when patients have relatively constant pain with infrequent episodes of breakthrough pain. The transdermal therapeutic system (TTS) used to administer fentanyl is designed to release the drug for 72 hours at a controlled rate dictated by the system rather than the skin.[59] Fentanyl is dissolved in ethanol and gelled with hydroxyl cellulose and held in a reservoir between a clear occluding polyester/ethylene backing layer and a rate-controlling membrane (ethylene-vinyl acetate copolymer film) on an adhesive base (Fig. 113–8). The amount of fentanyl administered per hour is proportional to the surface area of the patch. Multiple patches need to be applied if higher doses are needed. The major obstacle to diffusion is the stratum corneum, where diffusion occurs primarily via the intracellular lipid medium.[60] As a depot is established in the dermis, absorption continues even after patch removal. After the first patch application, initial detection of fentanyl in the blood has been reported to be at 1 to 2 hours.[61] The plasma fentanyl concentration increases over 12 to 18 hours until a plateau develops. Under normal physiologic conditions, skin temperature and regional blood flow do not influence fentanyl absorption significantly.[59] Absorption rises by approximately one third with a rise in body temperature to 40°C.[61] The plasma concentration remains constant as long as the patch is changed every 72 hours. After patch removal, the plasma fentanyl concentration will slowly decline, with an apparent half-life of 15 to 21 hours.[60]

Iontophoresis is a method of transdermal delivery of drugs in an ionized state using an electric current. Morphine has been administered using this route for postoperative analgesia.[62] The delivery of fentanyl by iontophoresis is being investigated more extensively than that of other opioids. Iontophoresis has the advantage of achieving a rapid steady state and the ability to vary delivery rate.[63]

Neuraxial

Intrathecal, epidural, and intraventricular administration of opioids has the advantage of producing profound analgesia with relatively small doses. The mechanism of analgesia produced by epidural morphine is bimodal and synergistic. During the first 20 minutes, the vascularly absorbed morphine activates the descending inhibitory system. Then, as the cerebrospinal fluid (CSF) morphine concentration increases, the spinal cord receptors are activated.[2] The short-term use of this route is most commonly advocated for postsurgical pain relief. It is indicated for long-term use when other routes do not control the pain and/or are associated with significant side effects. Opioids injected in the neuraxis should be preservative free. Duramorph (preservative-free morphine) is commercially available. Other opioids like fentanyl, sufentanil, meperidine, methadone and hydromorphone are used intrathecally and epidurally. Remifentanil cannot be given intraspinally; it is prepared with glycine, which can cause temporary motor paralysis. The most common side effects are pruritus, nausea, vomiting, somnolence, urinary retention, and respiratory depression. The most worrisome side effect is delayed respiratory depression, which may occur 12 hours after the intraspinal administration of morphine. Lipophilic drugs such as fentanyl do not spread much after intrathecal administration, but hydrophilic drugs such as morphine can spread rostrally and cause the delayed respiratory depression. This is also seen sporadically after epidural administration.

Intraventricular opioids are a satisfactory analgesic method that should be reserved for patients who have intractable pain and a short life expectancy and who have exhausted other modalities of pain management. Small doses of intraventricular morphine provide satisfactory control of otherwise intractable pain in terminal cancer patients.[64]

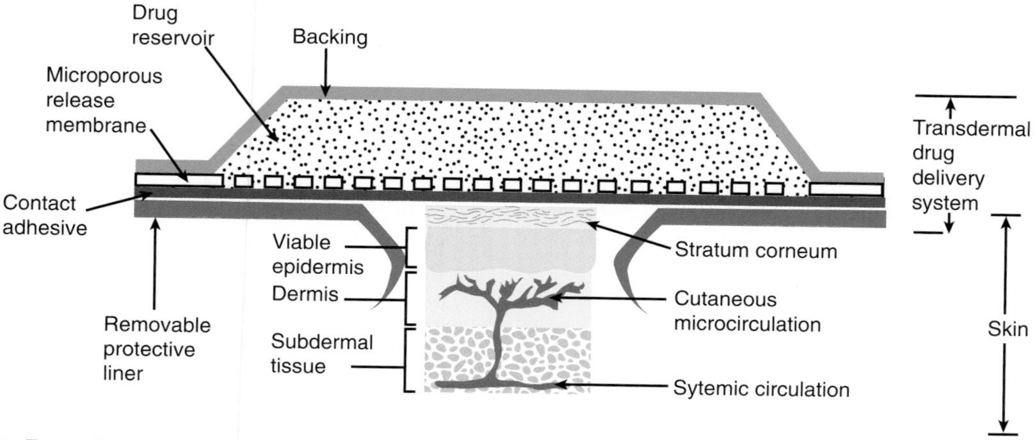

FIGURE 113–8 ■ Fentanyl transdermal therapeutic system. Schematic representation (not to scale) of the delivery system and the pathway of absorption across the skin.

Distribution

After being injected into the circulation or being absorbed, opioids are distributed within the body. This occurs in two phases. In the early phase, the drug is distributed to highly perfused tissues such as the heart, liver, kidney, and brain. This is a function of the cardiac output and regional blood flow. In the second phase, there is a slow diffusion to less-perfused areas such as muscle, fat, viscera, and skin. Volume of distribution is the extent to which a drug is distributed within the body (calculated as the amount of drug in the plasma divided by the plasma concentration).

The differences in distribution determine the onset of activity. A highly diffusible drug that acts on a highly diffusible organ will have a very rapid onset of action. The nonionized and unbound fraction of the drug is diffusible and this fraction leaves the circulation to be distributed. Highly protein-bound drugs are poorly diffusible and have a small volume of distribution. Lipid-insoluble drugs diffuse poorly and also have a small volume of distribution, whereas highly lipid-soluble drugs have a large volume of distribution. The measure of acid strength (pKa) determines the ionized versus the nonionized fraction at a particular pH. The apparent potency of an opioid will depend on the ease with which the unbound, nonionized fraction of a lipid-soluble opioid diffuses across membranes to reach the receptors. This explains the greater potency of fentanyl and sufentanil in comparison to morphine.

The potency or analgesic effect can be corrected clinically by adjusting the ultimate dose. The clinical effects of the highly lipophilic opioids are determined by the apparent volume of distribution (tissue:blood partition coefficient). For a given opioid, the larger the volume of distribution, the lesser the concentration in the plasma. Alfentanil has a small volume of distribution and, therefore, has a rapid onset of action and a short duration.

Metabolism

Opioids containing a hydroxyl group are conjugated in the liver with glucuronic acid to form opioid glucuronides that are then excreted by the kidney. Uridine 5-diphosphate-glucuronyltransferase (UGT) performs an important group of conjugation reactions.[55] UGTs are involved in metabolism of many opioid analgesics. Some natural opioids and semisynthetic opioids are metabolized by the cytochrome P_{450} isoforms. The phenylpiperidine derivatives undergo oxidative metabolism. *N*-demethylation is a minor pathway for metabolism of opioids.

Excretion

The kidneys excrete most polar metabolites and a small amount is excreted unchanged. Glucuronide conjugates are also excreted in bile and may undergo enterohepatic circulation.

PHENANTHRENE ALKALOIDS

Morphine

Morphine is the prototypic μ-agonist and remains the standard against which new analgesics are compared. It is a naturally occurring alkaloid derived from opium, and, to date, chemical synthesis is difficult. The milky juice obtained from the unripe seed capsule of the poppy plant is dried and powdered to make powdered opium, which contains a number of alkaloids: the principal phenanthrenes are morphine (10% of opium), codeine (0.5%), and thebaine (0.2%). The morphine molecule consists of five fused ring systems (see Fig. 113–2).[65] The carbon atoms are numbered 1 to 16. There are five asymmetrical carbon atoms (5, 6, 8, 9, 13), resulting in strong levorotation, the levo isomer being pharmacologically active and the dextro isomer inactive.[66] The pKa for the morphine base is 7.9, and at physiologic pH, it is 76% nonionized. It is relatively water soluble and poorly lipid soluble, because of the hydrophilic OH^- groups present.[67] This poor lipid solubility limits movement of morphine across membranes and is a barrier to accessing the CNS.

Pharmacokinetics

Morphine is absorbed, to some extent, through all mucosa and the spinal dura, so that multiple routes are available for drug administration. Protein binding of morphine in plasma is 45%. Mean elimination half-life ranges from 1.4 to 3.4 hours. After intravenous administration, morphine is rapidly distributed to tissues and organs. Within 10 minutes of administration, 96% to 98% of the drug is cleared from the plasma. Mean volume of distribution is large, ranging from 2.1 to 4.0 L/kg. Intramuscular absorption is rapid, and the peak occurs at 10 to 20 minutes.[68] Peak plasma concentrations after subcutaneous administration occurs at approximately 15 minutes, and plasma levels equivalent to those obtained with the intravenous route can be achieved.[69,70] Morphine is rapidly distributed out of the plasma after intravenous administration. Intramuscular or subcutaneous injection creates a depot, which continues to release morphine into the plasma for distribution.

After oral administration, plasma levels of morphine peak at 30 to 90 minutes. Absorption is mainly from the upper small intestine; morphine is poorly absorbed from the stomach.[67] Bioavailability from the oral route is low owing to extensive first-pass metabolism in the liver. There is a great inter-individual variability for bioavailability (20% to 30% reported in various studies). Low bioavailability of oral morphine is a factor in determining oral to parenteral conversion ratios, 1:3 in chronic pain states.[69,71,72] Peak plasma levels after controlled release morphine occur two to three times later (at 150 minutes) than with immediate-release oral morphine preparations.

Bioavailability of controlled release morphine is 85% to 90% that of immediate release formulations. Rectal absorption appears to be as good as or better than oral route absorbtion. Morphine can be administered intrathecally, epidurally, or intraventricularly. Epidural morphine is rapidly absorbed into the systemic circulation, producing significant plasma levels. Plasma levels after intrathecal administration are too low to be of any clinical significance. Neuraxial administration of morphine produces CSF morphine levels many times greater than systemic routes.

There is a rostral distribution of morphine in the CSF, and this causes a delayed respiratory depression (12 to 18 hours). Morphine is not suited to be administered transdermally or via the nasal route as it is poorly lipid soluble. Morphine has been delivered by iontophoresis for postoperative analgesia after total hip and knee replacement surgery.[62] Absorption after buccal and sublingual administration is similar to oral administration in terms of peak plasma level and time to peak, low bioavailability, and large degree of inter-individual variation.[72] After being absorbed, morphine is rapidly distributed throughout the body to highly perfused tissues, such as the lungs, kidney, liver, and spleen.[68,69]

Morphine and its highly polar metabolites morphine-3-glucuronide (M3G) and M6G, cross the blood-brain barrier to a small extent. CSF morphine levels are 4% to 60% after systemic administration.[73] Mean volume of distribution is large, ranging from 2.1 to 4.0 L/kg. It is affected by the hemodynamic status of the patient, alterations in plasma protein binding, and variations in tissue blood flow. Morphine binds to albumin and gamma-globulin. Morphine is 20% to 40% protein bound.[74,75] Major changes in binding would be required to influence plasma morphine levels because of its normally low extent of binding.

The predominant metabolic fate of morphine in man is glucuronidation, and the liver is the predominant site for this biotransformation. About 90% of injected morphine is converted into metabolites, the major ones being M3G (45% to 55%) and M6G (10% to 15%) (Fig. 113–9). Other metabolites include morphine-3, 6-diglucuronide, morphine-3-ethereal sulfate, normorphine, normorphine-6-glucuronide, normorphine-3-glucoronide[76] and codeine.[77]

M3G is the major metabolite quantitatively. It has a very low affinity for the μ receptor and as a consequence no analgesic potency. M3G has been found to antagonize morphine and M6G-induced analgesia and respiratory depression in the rat and has led to the hypothesis that M3G may influence the development of morphine tolerance.[78] M3G has shown to cause non-opioid mediated hyperalgesia and allodynia after intrathecal administration in rats.

M6G has a higher affinity for μ receptors than for δ- or κ-receptors. M6G is poorly lipid soluble and very little crosses the blood-brain barrier. M6G can accumulate in patients with renal insufficiency and is a likely factor in prolonged opioid effects after morphine administration. Increase in M6G levels in patients with renal failure causes an increase in CSF concentration and is due to the mass effect of the accumulated M6G. Within the CSF, M6G is 45 to 100 times more potent than morphine in its analgesic activity and 10 times more potent in depressing the ventilation. Normorphine is produced in small amounts and is pharmacologically active. Normorphine may be neurotoxic, analogous to normeperidine.[79] Excretion of morphine is predominantly renal, by glomerular filtration of water-soluble conjugates. Up to 85% of a dose of morphine is recovered from the urine as free morphine and metabolites. Some morphine (10% to 20%) is unaccounted for by renal excretion and is presumably excreted in urine as unidentified metabolite or excreted via other routes.[65] Enterohepatic circulation of morphine and its glucuronides accounts for the presence of small amounts of morphine in the feces and in the urine for several days after the last dose.

Pharmacodynamics

Morphine remains the reference against which all other opioids are compared. The clinical effects and side effects are

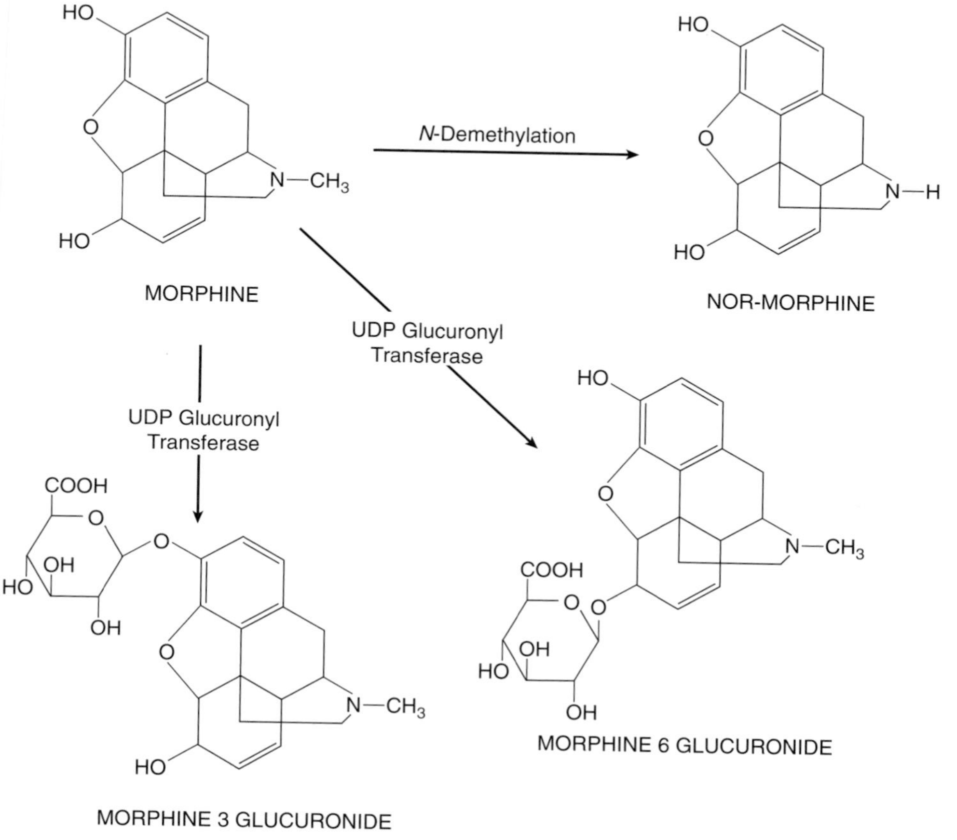

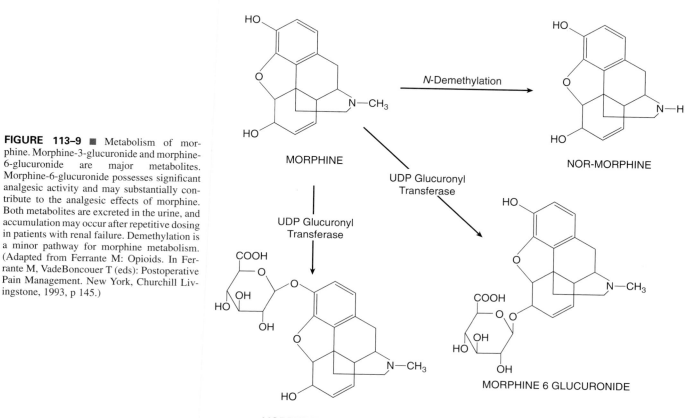

FIGURE 113–9 ■ Metabolism of morphine. Morphine-3-glucuronide and morphine-6-glucuronide are major metabolites. Morphine-6-glucuronide possesses significant analgesic activity and may substantially contribute to the analgesic effects of morphine. Both metabolites are excreted in the urine, and accumulation may occur after repetitive dosing in patients with renal failure. Demethylation is a minor pathway for morphine metabolism. (Adapted from Ferrante M: Opioids. In Ferrante M, VadeBoncouer T (eds): Postoperative Pain Management. New York, Churchill Livingstone, 1993, p 145.)

those that are seen with all μ-agonists. These have been detailed in the previous section of pharmacodynamics of opioids.

Clinical Uses and Preparations

Morphine is available as its sulfate and hydrochloride forms. It is the most commonly used medication for moderate-to-severe pain in the acute and chronic setting. Oral morphine is available as tablets and suspension in immediate-release and sustained-release forms. Immediate-release formulations have the disadvantage of frequent dosing. Various sustained-release forms are available that can be dosed every 8 to 12 hours (MS Contin, Oramorph) or every 24 hours (Kapalon, MXL). The majority of sustained-release formulations adsorb morphine onto a hydrophilic polymer that is embedded in some form of a wax or hydrophobic matrix, granulated and finally compressed into tablets.[80] Following oral administration, the gastric fluid dissolves the tablet surface and hydrates the hydrophilic polymer to produce a gel, the formation of which is controlled by higher aliphatic alcohols. Varying the hydrophilic polymer, the type of hydrophobic matrix, or their ratio, can control the release rate. There is also a suspension formulation, wherein morphine is attached to small beads of an ion exchange resin. Rectal suppositories are available; a specific sustained-release formulation contains morphine, sodium alginate, and a calcium salt in a suitable vehicle that melts in the rectum. Parenteral formulations are available for intravenous, intramuscular, and subcutaneous use. A preservative-free formulation for intrathecal and epidural use is available. Morphine has also been used intra-articularly with varying results.

Codeine

Like morphine, codeine is a naturally occurring alkaloid. Codeine is methylmorphine, the methyl substitution being on the phenolic hydroxyl group. With the exception of aspirin, codeine has perhaps been the most widely used oral analgesic and is generally accepted as the alternative to aspirin as a standard of comparison of drugs in this category[81] (e.g., 60 mg of codeine is comparable to 600 mg of aspirin). Codeine is approximately 60% as effective orally as parenterally, both as an analgesic and as a respiratory depressant. Compared to morphine, codeine has a high oral-to-parenteral potency ratio as a result of less first-pass metabolism in the liver. Codeine is metabolized by the liver to inactive forms (90%), which are excreted in the urine. Free and conjugated forms of morphine are found in urine after codeine administration: 10% of administered codeine is O-demethylated to morphine. The cytochrome P_{450} enzyme CYP2D6 effects the conversion of codeine to morphine. In the white population, 10% have a well-characterized genetic polymorphism in the CYP2D6 enzyme, and they are not able to convert codeine to morphine and thus do not attain an analgesic effect from codeine administration.

Codeine's major disadvantage is its lack of effectiveness in treating severe pain. Codeine has a low affinity for opioid receptors and is a weak analgesic; the analgesic effect is due to its conversion to morphine. It has a limited propensity to produce sedation, nausea, vomiting, constipation and respiratory depression. It also produces a lower incidence and degree of physical dependence than most other opioids. Codeine is used for mild-to-moderate pain conditions. The addiction potential of codeine is low. Codeine has excellent antitussive effect at doses as low as 15 mg; greater cough suppression is seen at higher doses. The antitussive effects are mediated by the active metabolites depressing the cough reflex in the medulla. There may be distinct receptors that bind to codeine itself.[54] Codeine is available in the United States in oral, subcutaneous, intramuscular and intravenous formulations. Oral forms of codeine are formulated with acetaminophen. Parenteral forms of codeine are also available; 130 mg of codeine is equianalgesic to 10 mg of intramuscular morphine. Codeine should not be used intravenously as the histamine-releasing potency of codeine is even greater than that of morphine.[1]

Thebaine

Thebaine is a naturally occurring alkaloid derived from opium. Thebaine has little analgesic action but is a precursor of several important 14-OH such as oxycodone and naloxone. A few derivatives of thebaine are more than 1000 times as potent as morphine (e.g., etorphine).[9]

SEMISYNTHETIC OPIOIDS

Heroin

Diacetylmorphine, or heroin, is derived from acetylation of morphine at the 3 and 6 positions (Fig. 113–10). Heroin is deacetylated to 6-monoacetylmorphine (6-MAM) and subsequently to morphine. The liver has the greatest capacity for the production of morphine from 6-MAM. In serum, the conversion to 6-MAM is mediated by a serum cholinesterase, which is present also in kidney, liver, and brain tissues and could be responsible for conversion in these organs as well.[82] Direct renal clearance of heroin is less than 1% of the administered dose.[83] Both heroin and 6-MAM are more lipid soluble than morphine and cross the blood-brain barrier more readily.

Heroin should be given orally; it is approximately 1.5 times more potent than morphine in controlling chronic pain. Given parenterally, heroin is two to four times more potent than morphine and faster in onset of action. Heroin has a short half-life, but the effects of its active metabolites last longer. Heroin has a high addiction potential and it is not known to have any real advantage over morphine. It is banned from the manufacture and medicinal use in the United States.[1]

Hydrocodone

Hydrocodone is a semisynthetic opioid with multiple actions qualitatively similar to codeine. It has a bioavailibity of 50% and is available as oral formulations in combination with non-opioid analgesics.

Hydrocodone undergoes O-demethylation, *N*-dealkylation, and 6-ketoreduction to the corresponding 6-α and 6-ß hydroxymetabolites. The O-demethylation to dihydromorphine is mediated by polymorphically expressed cytochrome P_{450} CYP2D6 enzyme. Some of the hydrocodone metabolites (dihydromorphine, dihydrocodeine, and hydromorphone) are pharmacologically active and may produce adverse effects if their excretion is impaired.[55]

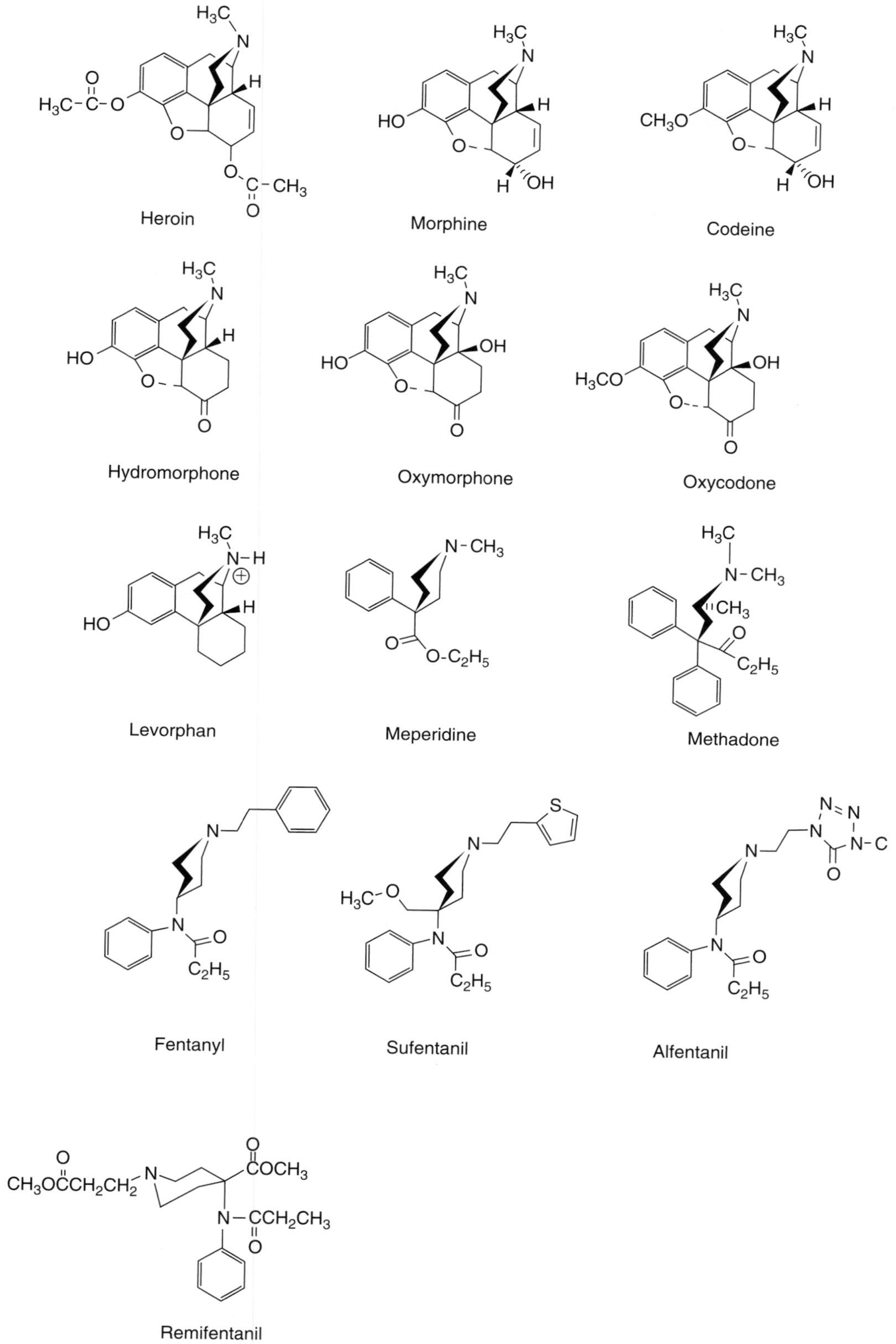

FIGURE 113–10 ■ μ-Opioid receptor agonists.

Hydrocodone is considered a weak analgesic. It has excellent antitussive properties. Like other opioids, hydrocodone can cause respiratory depression, sedation, and impairment of mental and physical performance, constipation and urinary retention. Drug dependence and addiction are seen with long-term use. Hydrocodone is available only for oral use in combination with acetaminophen or acetylsalicylic acid. These combinations provide a synergistic effect and the side effects are reduced.

Hydromorphone (Dilaudid)

Hydromorphone, a direct derivative of morphine, was first synthesized in the 1920s. Like morphine, hydromorphone has a basic amino group as well as a phenolic group but is more lipophilic than morphine because its 6-alcoholic hydroxyl group has been converted to a less hydrophilic ketone group (see Fig. 113–10).[84] The global pharmacokinetics are generally similar to morphine. It is six to eight times as potent as morphine; the most agreed on conversion is that 1.5 mg of hydromorphone is equianalgesic to 10 mg of morphine. It is easily absorbed from the gastrointestinal tract and so is effective after oral and rectal administration. Hydromorphone has a rapid distribution phase; about 90% of a specific dose is lost from the plasma in 10 minutes.[85] Hydromorphone elimination, like morphine, is dependent on tissue uptake with subsequent slow release from tissue to plasma.

Hydromorphone has no active metabolites and, therefore, is a particularly useful drug in treating patients with renal insufficiency. The side effects profile is very similar to other opioids. Despite anecdotal reports of reduced incidence of nausea, vomiting, respiratory depression, urinary retention and constipation, there is little evidence to prove this.[86]

Hydromorphone is available in 1-, 2-, 3- and 4-mg tablets for oral administration and as rectal suppositories. A controlled-release form for administration every 12 hours is available in some countries. Injectable preparations are available, and hydromorphone is particularly useful for subcutaneous use due to its relatively high solubility. Hydromorphone is used intrathecally and epidurally with good effect. Hydromorphone is hydrophilic: when given epidurally, its long half-life resembles that of epidural morphine, and its short latency of analgesia is similar to meperidine.[87]

Oxycodone

Oxycodone (14-hydroxyl-7, 8-dihydrocodeine) is derived from modification of the morphine molecule. It has different pharmacokinetics and opioid-receptor binding characteristics from morphine. Oxycodone is a μ-receptor agonist and also exhibits some κ-mediated antinociceptive effects.[88] It is available in immediate and sustained release forms and also in combination with non-opioid analgesics. The parenteral forms are currently not available in the United States.

The oral bioavailability is superior to morphine; 50% to 80%. Bioavailability and peak plasma concentration are altered by high-fat meals; there is a delayed absorption but improved bioavailability. NR oxycodone absorption is mono-exponential; mean half-life is 3.5 to 5.6 hours. CR oxycodone is absorbed in a bi-exponential fashion. There is a rapid phase with a half-life of 37 minutes and a slow phase with a half-life of 6.2 hours.[89] In uremic patients, the mean half-life of oxycodone is increased by increased volume of distribution and reduced clearance, and plasma concentrations of noroxycodone are higher.[84] Oxycodone is metabolized by the liver to the active metabolite oxymorphone (10%) through O-demethylation by the cytochrome P_{450} enzyme CYP2D6 and to the dominant nonactive metabolite, noroxycodone through *N*-demethylation.[90] Oxymorphone is 14 times as potent as oxycodone. The metabolites are excreted in the urine; noroxycodone in an unchanged form and oxymorphone in the form of a conjugate. Women eliminate oxycodone 25% more slowly than do men.[91] Protein binding is low (i.e., 38% to 45%). Lipid solubility is very similar to morphine.

Oxycodone is a μ-receptor agonist but part of its antinociceptive effect is mediated by κ-opioid receptors.[88] The relative potency of parenteral oxycodone is 70% that of morphine. The wide variability of oral morphine bioavailability, unequal incomplete cross-tolerance depending on the drug sequence and delayed oxycodone clearance in women account for bioequivalent ratios between 1:1 and 2.3:1.[90] There is less cross-tolerance with a switch from morphine to oxycodone than from oxycodone to morphine.[92] The side effects of oxycodone are similar to those normally attributed to opioids. The incidence of constipation is more than with morphine but there is a decreased incidence of nausea. Oxycodone causes drowsiness, lightheadedness, nausea, vomiting, pruritus, constipation, and sweating. Fluoxetine and its metabolite norfluoxetine inhibit CYP2D6 and prevent O-demethylation of oxycodone to oxymorphone, which may lead to higher plasma oxycodone levels.[93] Presumably, sertraline does the same.

Oxymorphone

Oxymorphone is a congener of morphine with a substitution of a ketone group at the C-6 position, conferring a more rapid onset of action, greater potency, and slightly longer duration of action than morphine.[94] Oxymorphone has a short half-life but has a prolonged duration of action owing to slow dissociation from its receptor sites.[54] It has a high affinity for μ-opioid receptors, being approximately 10 times more potent than morphine in the parenteral form. Like heroin, it has a high addiction potential. Oxymorphone and naloxone have significant structural similarities; naloxone is the *N*-allyl ($-CH_2-CH{=}CH_2$)-substituted analog of oxymorphone.[1] The structural similarities between the μ-receptor antagonist naloxone and agonist oxymorphone have been used to study and develop new agonists and antagonists.

Oxymorphone is available in the United States in injectable and rectal forms (Numorphan). The adult subcutaneous or intramuscular dose is 1 to 1.5 mg every 4 to 6 hours, with the starting intravenous dose being 0.5 mg. Rectal administration is approximately one-tenth as potent as intramuscular administration.

SYNTHETIC OPIOIDS

Levorphanol and Congeners

Levorphanol is the only commercially available opioid agonist of the morphinan series. Only the l-isomer has analgesic effect. The d-isomer (dextromethorphan) is relatively devoid of analgesic effect but may have inhibitory effects at NMDA receptors and it also has an antitussive activity. Levorphanol has activity mainly at the μ-opioid receptors and some effect at κ- and δ-receptors. Because of its effect on multiple receptors, levorphanol is used as a second-line agent or in patients who are tolerant to morphine.[95]

The pharmacologic profile of levorphanol closely parallels that of morphine. The analgesic effects are similar to morphine, but it has a lower incidence of nausea and vomiting. Levorphanol is available in forms that can be administered subcutaneously, intramuscularly, intravenously or orally. It is less effective when given orally; the oral-to-parenteral potency ratio is comparable to codeine and oxycodone. Levorphanol is seven times more potent than oral morphine and five times more potent than parenteral morphine.

Levorphanol has a half-life of 12 to 16 hours but its duration of analgesia is similar to morphine (i.e., 4 to 6 hours). The longer half-life may lead to systemic accumulation with repeated dosing. Levorphanol is available for oral administration in 2-mg tablets and as an injectable solution for parenteral administration.

Meperidine and Congeners

Meperidine is a synthetic phenylpiperidine opioid analgesic. The other opioids in the phenylpiperidine series are fentanyl, sufentanil, alfentanil and remifentanil.

Pharmacokinetics

Oral bioavailability is 45% to 75% due to extensive first-pass metabolism. Its absorption is slow and peaks at 2 hours. Meperidine is absorbed by all routes of administration but absorption after intramuscular injection is very erratic.[96] About 60% of meperidine is protein bound. Meperidine is metabolized in the liver; *N*-demethylated to meperidinic acid and normeperidine. Normeperidine has a half-life of 15 to 40 hours. Meperidine has a half-life of 3 hours but in patients with liver disease, the half-life of meperidine and the half-life of normeperidine are prolonged. Patients with renal insufficiency accumulate normeperidine, causing systemic toxicity.

Normeperidine is an active metabolite possessing one half the analgesic potency of meperidine. It has twice the potency of the parent compound as a proconvulsant. Normeperidine has CNS stimulant effects, and toxicity may be manifested as myoclonus and seizures.[97,98] Meperidine is no longer recommended for chronic pain; use for longer than 48 hours or doses greater than 600 mg/24 hours are not advocated (Agency for Health Care Policy and Research, 1992).[9]

Pharmacodynamics

Meperidine is 7 to 10 times less potent than morphine in producing analgesia; 75 to 100 mg of meperidine is equivalent to 10 mg of morphine. The peak analgesic effect is seen 1 to 2 hours after oral administration and in less than an hour after parenteral administration. The analgesic effect lasts 2 to 3 hours, which is shorter than that of morphine. Meperidine also produces sedation; respiratory depression, euphoria, and a few patients experience dysphoria. Like other opioids, it produces nausea and vomiting, pupillary dilation with large doses, and has effects on pituitary hormones. The accumulation of normeperidine can cause CNS excitation, which may present as tremors, myoclonus and seizures. Unlike other opioids, meperidine causes tachycardia and this is due to its structural similarity to atropine. Meperidine can cause hypotension owing to its histamine releasing effect. In large doses, meperidine can cause a decrease in myocardial contractility, stroke volume, and a rise in filling pressures.[99] No deleterious effects were seen with therapeutic doses of meperidine used in patients with acute myocardial infarction.[100] Like other opioids, meperidine is known to cause spasm of smooth muscle but to a lesser degree. It is a preferred agent in patients with pain due to renal colic and biliary spasm. Therapeutic doses of meperidine during active labor, do not delay the birth process. The adverse effects associated with meperidine are qualitatively similar to those produced by morphine. Meperidine is associated with a lower incidence of constipation and urinary retention. Tolerance develops to the actions of meperidine, and there is a high addiction potential. CNS excitation is seen with long-term use of meperidine, especially in patients with compromised renal and liver function owing to the accumulation of normeperidine. Naloxone does not reverse meperidine-induced seizures.

Meperidine administration is relatively contraindicated in patients on monoamine oxidase inhibitors. Two types of interactions are seen—with the most prominent being an excitatory one. It presents as hyperthermia, hyper- or hypotension, muscular rigidity, convulsions, coma, and death.[9] This reaction is probably the result of the ability of meperidine to block neuronal reuptake of serotonin and thereby cause an increase in local serotonin activity.[101] The other type of interaction is seen as a potentiation of opioid effect due to inhibition of hepatic microsomal enzymes in patients taking monoamine oxidase inhibitors.

Therapeutic Uses and Preparations

The major use of meperidine is for acute pain control. It is no longer recommended for chronic use owing to its active metabolite. Meperidine, in single doses is used to treat post-anesthesia shivering. Congeners of meperidine, diphenoxylate and loperamide, are used to treat diarrhea. Meperidine is available for oral administration in the form of tablets and elixir. It is available for parenteral administration in varying concentrations. Intramuscular doses of 50 to 100 mg are used to treat severe pain and need to be repeated every 2 to 4 hours.

Fentanyl

Fentanyl is a synthetic opioid, a meperidine congener of the phenylpiperidine series. It is a pure opioid agonist with a high affinity for the μ receptor. It is about 75 to 100 times more potent than morphine as an analgesic. Fentanyl is very commonly used in anesthetic practice owing to its high potency and quick onset and offset of action.

Pharmacokinetics

Fentanyl is a highly lipid-soluble opioid and crosses the blood-brain barrier rapidly. The plasma level equilibrates with the CSF levels within 5 minutes. It has a rapid onset of action (30 seconds) and a short duration of action owing to redistribution to fat and skeletal muscle. There is a fairly rapid decline in plasma concentration reflecting the redistribution.

But with repeated dosing or continuous infusion, there is saturation of the fat and muscle depots. This leads to a prolonged effect due to systemic accumulation and a slower decline in the plasma concentration. Fentanyl is 50% protein bound. Fentanyl is primarily metabolized in the liver by cytochrome P_{450} 3A4 to phenylacetic acid, norfentanyl, and small amounts of the pharmacologically active compound, *p*-hydroxyl fentanyl[102]; which are excreted in the bile and urine. A small portion (8%) is excreted unchanged in the urine. It is the drug of choice in patients with renal disease because all but a small percentage of the metabolites are inactive. Fentanyl has a large volume of distribution and this is reflected by its long (3 to 4 hours) elimination half-life.[1] Similar to other highly lipid-soluble opioids, the half-life of fentanyl is influenced by duration of administration, which is a function of extent of fat sequestration. The elimination half-life is 7 to 12 hours in steady-state conditions.[102] Liver disease does not prolong the half-life, but a prolonged effect is seen in the elderly.[103]

Pharmacodynamics

Fentanyl has a high affinity for the μ-opioid receptor, is almost 100 times more potent than morphine, and produces the same degree of respiratory depression as morphine in equianalgesic doses. Because it is highly lipid soluble, the risk of delayed respiration due to rostral spread of intrathecally-administered drug to medullary respiratory centers is greatly reduced. When administered intravenously, the peak analgesic effect is seen after 5 minutes and a quick recovery is also seen with single doses. With repeated dosing or prolonged infusions, a prolonged effect is seen. Muscle rigidity is commonly seen with intravenous fentanyl administration. Like other μ agonists, it produces nausea, vomiting, and itching. Respiratory depression is noted, and the onset is much more rapid than with morphine. As with morphine and meperidine, delayed respiratory depression seen after the use of fentanyl is possibly caused by enterohepatic circulation.[9] High doses of fentanyl can cause neuroexcitation and, rarely, seizure-like activity. Fentanyl decreases heart rate and mildly decreases blood pressure. It also causes minimal myocardial depression. Fentanyl does not release histamine and provides a marked degree of cardiovascular stability.

Therapeutic Uses and Preparations

Fentanyl is used very commonly as an anesthetic agent because of its rapid onset and offset of action and relative cardiovascular stability. Because of its short duration of action, it is generally not the drug of choice for single shot parenteral administration for chronic pain. It is one of the drugs of choice for intravenous patient-controlled analgesia in patients with renal disease. It is used frequently via the epidural and intrathecal routes. Its high lipophilicity and small molecular weight make it well suited for use in a transdermal preparation. Fentanyl is not used for oral administration because of extensive first-pass metabolism and poor bioavailability (32%). It is available as a preparation for oral-transmucosal use; bioavailability is 52%. This form is used for breakthrough cancer pain and is not recommended for acute postoperative pain. Transdermal fentanyl has a lower incidence of constipation than oxycodone and morphine.[104]

Alfentanil

Alfentanil and remifentanil were developed in search of analgesics with a more rapid onset of action and predictable termination of effects.[9] Alfentanil is 5 to 10 times less potent than fentanyl and has a shorter duration of effect.

Pharmacokinetics

Alfentanil has a rapid onset (1 to 2 minutes) of analgesic effect after intravenous administration. This is because 90% of the drug is nonionized at physiologic pH owing to a low pKa value. It has a smaller volume of distribution, lower lipid solubility, and slightly greater protein binding compared to fentanyl.[105] Its analgesic effect is terminated rapidly as a result of redistribution. Hepatic metabolism accounts for most of the elimination of alfentanil. A small percentage (1%) is excreted unchanged in urine. The elimination half-life is 70 to 98 minutes.[106] The elimination half-life is significantly increased in patients with cirrhosis. Renal disease does not affect alfentanil clearance.

Therapeutic Uses and Preparations

Alfentanil is used for epidural analgesia and intravenous patient-controlled analgesia. Owing to its short duration of analgesic effect, it is not an ideal choice for patient-controlled analgesia use. It is available for injection in a concentration of 500 μg/mL.

Sufentanil

Sufentanil is a synthetic opioid that is a member of the phenylpiperidine series. Sufentanil is the most potent μ-receptor agonist available for human clinical use.[54] It is 5 to 10 times more potent than fentanyl and 1000 times more potent than morphine. It has an affinity for opioid receptors 30 times greater than fentanyl.[107]

Pharmacokinetics

Sufentanil is highly lipid soluble, more so than fentanyl and alfentanil. It rapidly crosses the blood-brain barrier and equilibrates with the CSF and, therefore, has a rapid onset of action. The analgesic effect is terminated quickly as a result of rapid redistribution to fat and skeletal muscle. Sufentanil has a volume of distribution, distribution half-life, and elimination half-life that falls between those of fentanyl and alfentanil.[108] More than 90% of sufentanil is protein bound. The shorter elimination half-life is due to a small volume of distribution and higher hepatic mobilization. Sufentanil is metabolized in the liver; products of *N*-dealkylation are inactive, and O-demethylation product (methylsufentanil) is active. Sufentanil metabolites are excreted in the urine.

Pharmacologic Effects

The profile of sufentanil is very similar to fentanyl. Like other opioids, it produces bradycardia, respiratory depression, nausea, vomiting, itching, and smooth muscle spasm.

Therapeutic Uses and Formulations

Sufentanil is available only in an injectable form. It is administered parenterally and via epidural and intrathecal routes.

Remifentanil

Remifentanil is an esterase-metabolized opioid of the phenylpiperidine series. Its potency is approximately equal to that of fentanyl.

Pharmacokinetics

Analgesic effect occurs within 1 to 1.5 minutes. Remifentanil undergoes rapid hydrolysis by nonspecific esterases in blood and tissues.[109,110] Clearance is unaffected by cholinesterase inhibition. Renal and liver disease does not alter remifentanil pharmacokinetics. Remifentanil has a distribution half-life of 2 to 4 minutes and an elimination half-life of 10 to 20 minutes.

Therapeutic Uses and Preparations

Remifentanil is available only for parenteral administration. Its short duration of effect does not make it an ideal drug for use in intravenous patient-controlled anesthesia. It is currently formulated with glycine and is, therefore, not recommended for epidural or intrathecal use.

Methadone and Congeners

Methadone, a synthetic drug developed approximately 60 years ago, is an opioid of the structural class of diphenylpropylamines. It was originally synthesized during World War II by the German pharmaceutical industry. It bears no structural resemblance to morphine. Methadone is used clinically as a racemic mixture, the levorotatory (L) form being 8 to 50 times more potent than the dextrorotatory (D) form. Methadone is popular as a maintenance drug for heroin addicts and is a time-honored therapy for cancer pain.[111,112] It has an excellent bioavailability and a long half-life, making it an ideal drug for outpatient use.[113]

Pharmacokinetics

The oral bioavailability of methadone is high (i.e., 81% to 95%).[114] Methadone is rapidly absorbed from the gastrointestinal tract and measurable concentrations in plasma are seen in 30 minutes,[115] but the analgesic effect peaks at 4 hours. After parenteral administration, methadone can be detected in plasma within 10 minutes and CSF levels peak at 1 to 2 hours. Methadone is a basic and lipophilic drug subject to considerable tissue distribution.[116] The sequestration of methadone at extravascular binding sites, followed by slow release into plasma, contributes to the prolonged duration of methadone half-life in plasma. The protein (alpha-1-acid-glycoprotein, AAG) binding of methadone is 60% to 90%, which is double that of morphine. It binds to AAG with a relatively high affinity. Methadone can be displaced from AAG by a number of drugs: propranolol, chlorpromazine, prochlorperazine, thioridazine, and tricyclic antidepressants.[117] Biotransformation, as well as renal and fecal excretions are important determinants for the elimination of methadone. Methadone undergoes extensive metabolism in the liver via *N*-demethylation and cyclization to form the inactive metabolites pyrroline and pyrrolidines. These inactive metabolites are excreted in the urine and bile along with small amounts of unchanged drug. Urinary pH is an important determinant of elimination half-life of methadone, with the half-life increasing with rising pH. The elimination half-life of methadone after a single dose is approximately 15 hours and with chronic administration it is 22 hours. Methadone has a secondary half-life of more than 55 hours (from release of tissue stores).

Pharmacodynamics

Methadone is a μ-receptor agonist with pharmacologic properties qualitatively similar to morphine. While being a potent μ-receptor agonist, methadone also has considerable affinity for δ-opioid receptor.[118] Methadone also has some agonist actions at the κ- and σ-opioid receptors.[119] Methadone binds with low affinity to NMDA receptors and acts as a noncompetitive NMDA receptor antagonist in the brain and spinal cord.[120,121] The analgesic potency is equal to or slightly greater than that of morphine. The duration of analgesia after a single dose of methadone is 4 to 6 hours, which is governed by the rapid initial absorption-distribution phase.[116,122] Methadone and many of its congeners retain a considerable degree of their effectiveness when given orally. Methadone, when given orally, is about 50% as effective as the same dose administered intramuscularly; the oral to parenteral potency ratio is 1:2.[123] With repeated dosing, cumulative effects are seen because of slow release from tissues. Dosage should be tailored accordingly; either decrease the dose or decrease the frequency of doses. The occurrence of side effects with equianalgesic doses was similar for both morphine and methadone.

Therapeutic Uses and Preparations

Methadone is an excellent analgesic with a good bioavailability. Its low cost and long half-life makes it a good choice for outpatient use in chronic pain states. It is also used for treatment of opioid abstinence syndromes and in heroin users. The NMDA blocking property of methadone makes it a choice of opioid for the treatment of neuropathic pain. It is available for oral administration in tablets (5 and 10 mg) and as a solution (10 mg/5 mL). Methadone is also available for parenteral administration and is used for intravenous patient-controlled analgesia. Methadone has also been used epidurally and intrathecally.

Levo-Alpha Acetyl Methadol

An alternative to methadone for individuals who are addicted to opioids, levo-alpha acetyl methadol (LAAM) is a medication that is a derivative of methadone; it was first developed in 1948 by German chemists as a painkiller. In 1993, the Food and Drug Administration approved LAAM for use in medication therapy for opiate addiction.[124]

LAAM itself is not effective; its metabolites, nor-LAAM and dinor-LAAM, are the active agents. LAAM is not effective through intravenous injection and, therefore, is not attractive for illegal use.[125] There is a delay before the effects of LAAM can be detected and it remains in the body much longer than methadone (72 hours for most people at doses of 80 mg or above). LAAM has a pharmacologic cross-tolerance to other opioids and thereby blocks the euphoric effects seen with these drugs—but still controls opiate craving. It is available for oral administration in a suspension form. Dosages range from 10 to 140 mg, three times a week.[54] It requires a

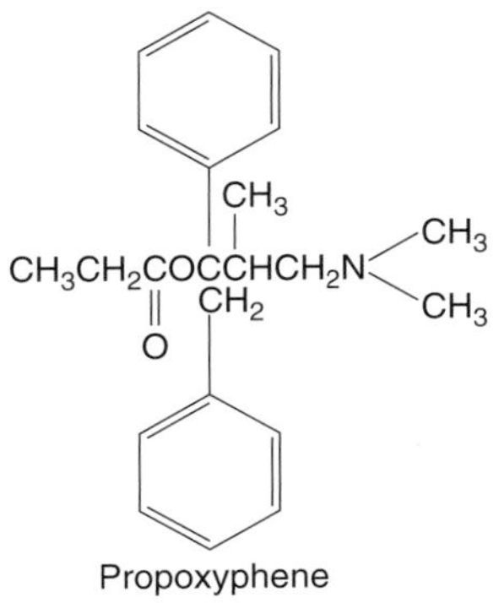

FIGURE 113–11 ■ Chemical structure of propoxyphene.

dosing every 2 to 3 days and can be given at treatment centers by itself with no take-home medications.

Propoxyphene

Propoxyphene is structurally related to methadone (Fig. 113–11) and is a weak analgesic. The analgesic activity of the racemate was found to reside in the dextroisomer, and it is this compound that is currently used as a mild analgesic. The levoisomer, which lacks analgesic activity, has been introduced as an antitussive.[81]

Pharmacokinetics

After oral administration, propoxyphene undergoes first-pass metabolism and has a bioavailability of 30% to 70 %.[1] Plasma concentration peaks at 1 to 2 hours. Propoxyphene undergoes extensive redistribution and tissue binding because its redistribution volume (960 L) is much greater than the other opioid analgesics.[84] Propoxyphene is metabolized in the liver by *N*-demethylation to from norpropoxyphene. Propoxyphene has an average half-life of 6 to 12 hours, which is much longer than that of codeine. Norpropoxyphene has a half-life of about 30 hours, and its accumulation with repeated doses may be responsible for toxicity seen with propoxyphene administration. Norpropoxyphene also undergoes extensive first-pass metabolism and liver disease can enhance accumulation.

Pharmacodynamics

Propoxyphene is a weak analgesic, with a relative potency one half to one third that of codeine. The classic triad of physical dependence, psychological dependence, and tolerance accompanies the use of propoxyphene. Moderately toxic doses produce CNS and respiratory depression, but increasing doses cause CNS excitation, cardiotoxicity, and pulmonary edema. These are attributed to the effects of the active metabolite, norpropoxyphene.

Therapeutic Uses and Preparations

Propoxyphene is recommended for the treatment of mild-to-moderate pain. A dose of 90 to 120 mg of propoxyphene is equianalgesic to 60 mg of codeine or 600 mg of aspirin. Propoxyphene hydrochloride is available in 32- and 65-mg tablets; it is formulated with acetaminophen or aspirin to give a synergistic effect. It is also available as propoxyphene napsylate in a suspension form and in 100-mg tablets.

Tramadol

Tramadol is a synthetic opioid structurally related to morphine and codeine. It is a centrally acting opioid agonist with some selectivity for the μ-receptor and also binds weakly to κ- and δ-receptors. It also acts on the monoamine system by inhibiting the reuptake of noradrenaline (NA) and serotonin (5-hydroxytryptamine, 5-HT).[126]

Pharmacokinetics

Tramadol undergoes some first-pass metabolism after oral administration and has a bioavailability of 68%.[9] It is O-demethylated by the cytochrome P_{450} enzyme CYP2D6 to the therapeutically active O-desmethyltramadol and *N*-demethylated by CYP34A to the inactive *N*-desmethyltramadol. O-desmethyltramadol is two to four times more potent than tramadol itself. A significant amount (10% to 30%) of tramadol is excreted unchanged in the urine. Whereas plasma protein binding is low (20%), its apparent volume of distribution is large (2.7l/kg), indicating considerable tissue uptake.[126] The elimination half-life for tramadol is 6 hours and the active metabolite has a slightly longer half-life of 7.5 hours.

Pharmacodynamics

Tramadol produces analgesia by its opioid-like activity and also by inhibiting the reuptake of noradrenalin and serotonin. It is contraindicated in patients taking monoamine oxidase inhibitors. Tramadol produces nausea, vomiting, sedation, dizziness, dry mouth, hot flashes, and headache. It produces less respiratory depression than morphine in equianalgesic doses. The incidence of seizures in patients receiving tramadol is <1%. Tramadol-induced seizures are not reversed by the μ-opioid antagonist naloxone.

Therapeutic Uses and Preparations

With its dual mode of action (opioid agonist, NA and 5-HT reuptake inhibition), tramadol is a useful drug in nociceptive and neuropathic pain. Unlike other opioids, tramadol produces only a weak and clinically irrelevant respiratory depression at the recommended analgesic doses.[127] Tramadol has a low potential for drug abuse and dependence. It is available as 50-mg tablets, to be dosed every 6 hours. The daily dose should not exceed 400 mg. It is also available formulated in combination with acetaminophen.

Agonist-Antagonists

The agonist-antagonists act to produce opposing action at the μ- and κ-receptors; they are μ-antagonists and κ-agonists. They were initially developed in search of an analgesic with less respiratory depression and addiction potential. These compounds are less efficacious than pure μ-agonists in their analgesic effect and seem to have a lower abuse potential.[54]

Pentazocine

Pentazocine is a synthetic opioid of the benzmorphan (Fig. 113–12) series that is a weak competitive antagonist at the μ-receptor and agonist at the $κ_1$- and possibly $κ_2$-receptors.

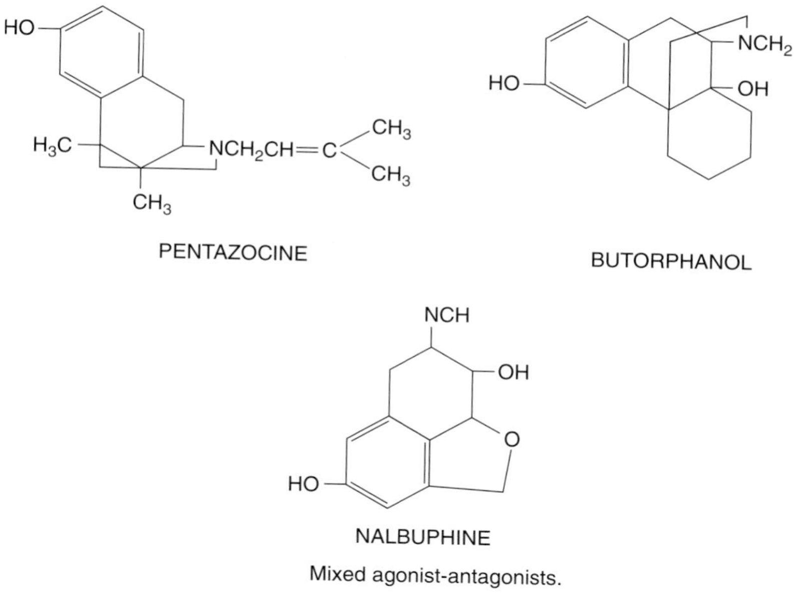

FIGURE 113–12 ■ Chemical structure of pentazocine, butorphanol, and nalbuphine.

Pharmacokinetics

Pentazocine is well absorbed after oral and parenteral administration. It undergoes extensive first-pass metabolism and only 20% of the drug enters the systemic circulation. It has a peak analgesic effect in 15 minutes to 1 hour after intramuscular injection and in 1 to 3 hours after oral administration.[9] Pentazocine has a plasma half-life of 3 to 4 hours. Its action is terminated by hepatic metabolism to inactive glucuronide conjugates and renal excretion. Less than 2% of the given dose is excreted in the bile.

Pharmacodynamics

Pentazocine is an agonist at the κ-receptors and produces analgesia. Higher doses of pentazocine elicit psychotomimetic and dysphoric effects. The exact mechanism for these effects is not known but is thought to be caused by weak σ-receptor agonist activity[1] and activation of supraspinal κ-receptors.[9] Like other agonist-antagonists, pentazocine exhibits a ceiling effect for respiratory depression and analgesic effect. The ceiling effect is seen with 60 to 100 mg of pentazocine.[128] Pentazocine does not reverse the respiratory depression produced by morphine. Pentazocine may, however, precipitate withdrawal if given to patients taking pure μ-agonists. Unlike other opioids, pentazocine does not cause bradycardia. High doses of pentazocine increase heart rate and blood pressure. In patients with acute myocardial infarction, pentazocine produces substantial elevation in cardiac preload and afterload and thereby increases the cardiac workload.[100] In addition, an increase in systemic and pulmonary artery pressure, left ventricular filling pressure, and systemic vascular resistance and a decrease in left ventricular ejection fraction are seen. This may be caused by a rise in the plasma concentration of catecholamine. Pentazocine also produces smooth muscle spasm but appears to cause less of a biliary spasm than morphine.[129] The most common adverse effects are sedation, sweating, dizziness, and nausea. With parenteral doses above 60 mg, psychotomimetic effects are seen. This manifests as anxiety, strange thoughts, nightmares, and hallucinations. With prolonged use, tolerance develops to the analgesic and subjective effects.

Therapeutic Uses and Preparations

Pentazocine is used to treat mild to moderate pain; an oral dose of 50 mg is equianalgesic to 60 mg of codeine orally. Oral forms are available compounded with aspirin and acetaminophen. To reduce the incidence of parenteral injection, tablets for oral use are formulated with naloxone. Naloxone is completely degraded with oral administration, but if injected, the combination would have no effect because of the antagonist effects of naloxone. Abuse patterns seem to be low with the oral forms of pentazocine.

Nalbuphine

Nalbuphine is a semisynthetic mixed agonist-antagonist that is chemically related to naloxone and oxymorphone.

Pharmacokinetics

Bioavailability of oral nalbuphine is <20% as a result of extensive first-pass metabolism. It is lipophilic and has a large volume of distribution. Nalbuphine is metabolized in the liver to inactive glucuronide conjugates. Nalbuphine and its metabolites are excreted to a great extent in the feces. The elimination half-life of nalbuphine is 3 to 6 hours.[130]

Pharmacodynamics

Compared to pentazocine, nalbuphine is a more potent antagonist at the μ-receptor. Intramuscularly administered nalbuphine produces analgesia that is comparable to morphine (potency ratio of 1:1). It exhibits a ceiling effect at approximately 0.45 mg/kg [1] and no further respiratory depression or analgesia is obtained. In contrast to pentazocine and butorphanol, nalbuphine does not increase cardiac index, pulmonary artery pressure, or cardiac work. The systemic blood pressure does not change significantly.[9] The most common adverse effects are sedation, sweating, and headache. Higher doses can produce dysphoria and psychotomimetic effects.

Nalbuphine can precipitate withdrawal symptoms in individuals taking μ-opioid receptor agonists. Nalbuphine also reverses the respiratory depression[131] associated with opioids and can be used to treat pruritus seen with opioid use.[132] Long-term use of nalbuphine can cause physical dependence.

Butorphanol

Butorphanol is a synthetic mixed agonist-antagonist compound of the morphinan series. It has a profile of action similar to pentazocine but with greater analgesic efficacy and fewer side effects.[54]

Pharmacokinetics

Bioavailability after oral administration is low (5% to 17%)[133] as a result of extensive first-pass metabolism. There is no first-pass metabolism with parenteral or transnasal administration and they produce similar plasma levels.[9] Butorphanol is rapidly absorbed after parenteral administration and has a distribution half-life of 5 minutes. Transnasal administration results in rapid absorption with onset of analgesia within 15 minutes. Plasma protein binding is approximately 85%. Butorphanol is converted to the inactive metabolites hydroxybutorphanol and norbutorphanol.[1] The plasma terminal half-life of butorphanol is 3 hours with parenteral administration and 4.5 to 5.5 hours with transnasal administration.

Pharmacodynamics

Butorphanol has agonistic activity at the κ-receptor and antagonistic activity at the μ-receptor. It also exhibits partial agonistic activity at the σ-receptor.[134] A dose of 2 to 3 mg of parenteral butorphanol is equivalent to 10 mg of parenteral morphine. Like other agonist-antagonists, it has a ceiling effect for respiratory depression and analgesia. Common adverse effects of butorphanol are sedation and diaphoresis. It also exhibits dysphoria because of its σ-agonist activity. Like pentazocine, analgesic doses of butorphanol produce an increase in heart rate, systemic blood pressure, and pulmonary artery pressure.[135] Its effects on the biliary tract are milder than morphine. Butorphanol can reverse the analgesia produced by pure μ-agonists but does not reverse the respiratory depression. Physical dependence is noted with long-term use of butorphanol.

Therapeutic Uses and Preparations

Due to its high analgesic potency, butorphanol is indicated for the treatment of moderate to severe pain. The recommended parenteral dose is 1 to 2 mg intramuscularly and 0.5 to 2 mg intravenously every 3 to 4 hours. Butorphanol is also available for intranasal administration in a spray form.

Buprenorphine

Buprenorphine is a semisynthetic, highly lipophilic opioid derived from the naturally occurring alkaloid thebaine (Fig. 113–13). It is 25 to 50 times more potent than morphine[9] and is a partial μ-agonist.

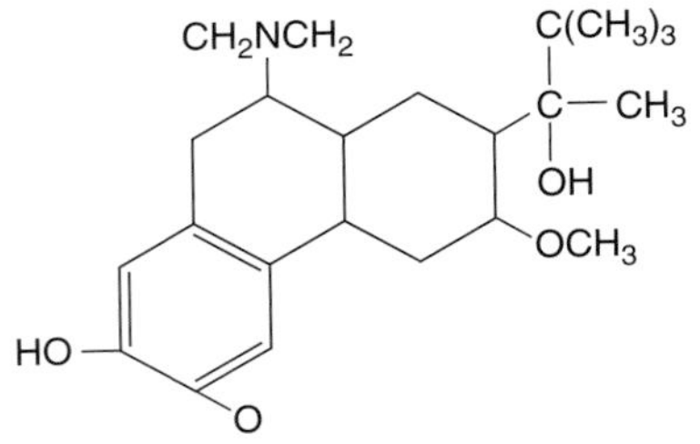

FIGURE 113–13 ■ Chemical structure of buprenorphine.

Pharmacokinetics

Bioavailability after oral administration is 16% due to extensive first-pass metabolism.[136] Buprenorphine displays a bell-shaped dose-response curve, with peak antinociceptive opioid effects at approximately 0.5 mg/kg (subcutaneous), 60 minutes after the dose and a gradual decline of the effects in the dosage range of 0.5 to 10 mg/kg.[137] Buprenorphine is highly lipophilic and is approximately 96% bound to plasma proteins. After parenteral administration, the analgesic response is governed by the kinetics of receptor dissociation.[138] The half-life of dissociation from the μ-receptor is 166 minutes for buprenorphine versus 7 minutes for fentanyl.[139] It has an elimination half-life of 3 to 4 hours but a prolonged duration of effect because of slow dissociation from receptor site.[136] There is limited information concerning the metabolism of buprenorphine. In animal studies, buprenorphine disposition is by hepatic conjugation to glucuronides, which is eliminated in the bile (92%).

Pharmacodynamics

A dose of 0.3 mg of parenteral buprenorphine produces analgesia equivalent to that of 10 mg of parenteral morphine.[140] Buprenorphine acts as a partial agonist at the μ-receptor and as an antagonist at the κ-receptor. Buprenorphine has a less well-defined effect on respiratory function than that usually expected for opioids, with a ceiling effect on respiratory depression with increasing dose. The adverse effects associated with buprenorphine are sedation and nausea. Usual parenteral doses of buprenorphine can reduce adrenocortical response after surgery.[141] Buprenorphine partially reverses the effects of large doses of μ-agonists and can reverse the ventilatory depression seen with these opioids. The cardiovascular hemodynamic responses are similar to morphine.

Therapeutic Uses and Preparations

Buprenorphine is used to treat moderate to severe pain conditions. Parenteral buprenorphine can be given in a dose of 0.3 mg every 6 to 8 hours. It may not be a good choice for intravenous patient-controlled analgesia because of slow onset of action. Few studies have described effective analgesia with minimal respiratory depression associated with buprenorphine via intravenous patient-controlled analgesia. Sublingual buprenorphine 0.4 mg every 8 hours provides analgesia equivalent to 10 mg of morphine intramuscularly every 4 hours. Literature is available describing the use of epidural buprenorphine for cesarean section and postoperative pain.

ANTAGONISTS

Pohl developed the first opioid antagonist in 1915 by minor changes in the codeine molecule (Fig. 113–14). Naloxone

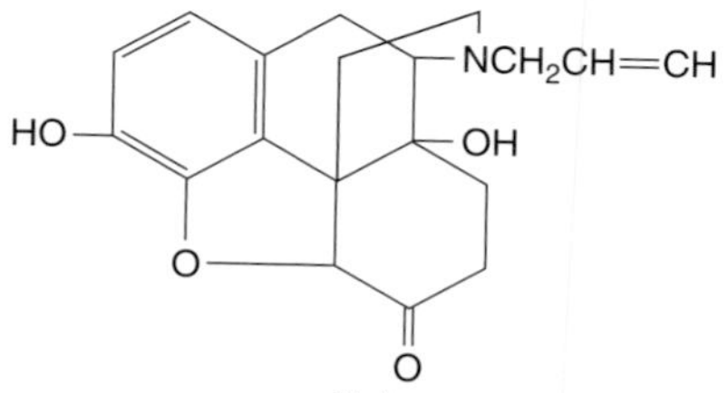

FIGURE 113–14 ■ Chemical structure of naloxone.

and naltrexone are pure antagonists at the μ-, κ-, δ-, and σ-receptors.

Naloxone

Naloxone is the first opioid antagonist to be developed that is devoid of agonist activity. Naloxone is a synthetic *N*-allyl derivative of oxymorphone.

Pharmacokinetics

Naloxone is rapidly absorbed after oral administration, but high pre-systemic metabolism makes this route unreliable. The oral-to-parenteral potency ratio has been estimated as 1:50. Effects are seen 1 to 2 minutes after intravenous dose and 2 to 5 minutes after a subcutaneous dose. Naloxone is highly lipid soluble and is rapidly distributed throughout the body. As a result of this rapid redistribution, naloxone has a very short duration (30 to 45 minutes) of action. Supplementation of the initial dose of naloxone is usually necessary if sustained antagonism is desired. Approximately 50% of the drug is bound to plasma proteins, mainly albumin. The plasma half-life is 1 to 2 hours. Naloxone undergoes extensive biotransformation in the liver to inactive metabolites. The metabolites are, in large part, excreted in the urine.

Pharmacodynamics

The effects produced by naloxone are the result of antagonism of endogenous and exogenous opioids. It has no effects when administered in clinical doses to normal human volunteers. On administration in humans with pain who have not received exogenous opioids, naloxone demonstrates a biphasic response. Low doses produce analgesia and higher doses produce hyperalgesia.[142] Naloxone reverses all the effects of exogenous opioids (i.e., analgesia, respiratory depression, pupillary constriction, delayed gastric transit, sedation). Naloxone also reverses the analgesic effects of placebo medications and acupuncture. Small doses (0.4 to 0.8 mg) of naloxone given parenterally reverse the effects of μ-receptor agonists. Naloxone can be titrated to reverse the respiratory depression produced by opioids while maintaining some analgesic effect. Naloxone infusions of 5 μg/kg/hour have been shown to reverse the respiratory depression with epidural morphine and not affect the quality of analgesia.[143] Rebound release of catecholamines may cause hypertension, tachycardia, and ventricular arrhythmias. Pulmonary edema has also been observed after naloxone administration. Small doses of naloxone can precipitate a withdrawal syndrome in subjects that are opioid-dependent. Long-term administration of naloxone increases the density of opioid receptors and produces a temporary exaggeration of response to subsequently administered opioids.[9]

Therapeutic Uses and Preparations

The treatment of life-threatening consequences of known or suspected opioid overdose is the prime indication for naloxone use. It is also used in small doses to reverse some of the side effects (respiratory depression and pruritus) associated with opioid use. Oral naloxone given in a dose of 8 to 12 mg has been used to ameliorate constipation in patients taking opioids. Naloxone is also used in formulation with oral pentazocine to prevent diversion. To reverse sedation and respiratory depression, an intravenous dose of 10 μg of naloxone (followed by increasing doses) is given. An infusion may be necessary to maintain the antagonism. Naloxone is available for parenteral administration in concentrations of 0.02 mg/mL, 0.4 mg/mL, and 1 mg/mL.

References

1. Ferrante M: Opioids. In Ferrante M, VadeBoncouer T (eds): Post-operative Pain Management. New York, Churchill Livingstone, 1993, p 145.
2. Benedetti C: Intraspinal analgesia: An historical overview. Acta Anaesthesiol Scand Suppl 85:17, 1987.
3. Macht D: The history of opium and some of its preparations and alkaloids. JAMA 46:477, 1915.
4. Tainter M: Pain. Ann NY Acad Sci 51:3, 1948
5. Reynolds DV: Surgery in the rat during electrical analgesia induced by focal brain stimulation. Science 164:444, 1969.
6. Akil H, Mayer DJ, Liebeskind JC: Antagonism of stimulation produced analgesia by naloxone. Science 191:961, 1976.
7. Pasternak G, Goodman R, Snyder SH: An endogenous morphine like factor in mammalian brain. Life Sci 16:1765, 1975.
8. Hughes J, Smith TW, Kosterlitz HW, et al: Identification of two related pentapeptides from the brain with potent opiate agonist activity. Nature 258:577-80, 1975.
9. Gutstein HB, Akil H: Opioid analgesics, In Goodman and Gillman's Pharmacological Basis of Therapeutics, 10th ed. New York, McGraw-Hill, 2001, pp 569-619.
10. King M, Chang A, Pasternak G: Functional blockade of opioid analgesia by orphanin FQ/nociceptin. Biochem Pharmacol 55:1537-1540, 1998.
11. Akil H, Watson SJ, Young E, Lewis ME, et al: Endogenous opioids: Biology and function. Annu Rev Neurosci 7:223-55, 1984.
12. Singh VK, Bajpai K, Biswas S, et al: Molecular biology of opioid receptors: Recent advance. Neuroimmunomodulation 4:285-297, 1997.
13. Probst WC, Synder L, Brosius J, Sealfon SC: Sequence alignment of the G protein coupled receptor super family. DNA Cell Biol 11:1-20, 1992.
14. Bovill JG: Update on opioid and analgesic pharmacology. Anesth Analg 92(3S):1-5, 2001.
15. Besse D, Lombard MC, Zajac JM, et al: Pre and post synaptic distribution of μ, delta and kappa opioid receptors in the superficial layers of the dorsal horn of the rat spinal cord. Brain Res 521:15-22, 1990.
16. Emmerson PJ, Liu MR, Woods JH, Medzihradsky F: Binding affinity and selectivity of opioids at μ, d and ? receptors in monkey brain membranes. J Pharmacol Exp Ther 271:1630-1637, 1994.
17. Knox RJ, Dickenson AH: Effects of selective and nonselective kappa-opioid agonists on cutaneous C fiber evoked responses of rat dorsal horn neurons. Brain Res 415:21-29, 1987.
18. Mansour A, Taylor LP, Fine JL, et al: Key residues defining the μ-opioid receptor binding pocket: A site directed mutagenesis study. J Neurochem 68:344-353, 1997.
19. Beckett AH, Casey AF: Synthetic analgesics, stereochemical considerations. Pharm Pharmacology 6:986, 1954.
20. Kosterlitz HW: Opiate actions in guinea pig ileum and vas deferens. Neurosci Res Program Bull 13:68. 1975.
21. Herz A, Teschemacher HJ: Activities and sites of antinociceptive action of morphine like analgesics and kinetics of distribution following intr-

venous, intracerebral and intraventricular application. Adv Drug Res 6:79, 1971.

22. Crain BM, Shen SM: Opioids can evoke direct receptor mediated excitatory effects on sensory neurons. Trends Pharmacol Sci 11:77-81, 1990.
23. Cox BM: Opioid receptor G protein interactions. In Herz A (ed): Handbook of Experimental Pharmacology: Opioids I. Berlin, Springer-Verlag, 1993, pp 145-188.
24. Johnson PS, Wang JB, Wang WF, Uhl GR: Expressed μ opiate receptor couples to adenylate cyclase and phosphatidyl inositol turnover. Neuro-Report 1:507-509, 1994.
25. Jessell TM, Iversen LL: Opiate analgesics inhibit substance P release from the rat trigeminal nucleus. Nature 268:549-551, 1977.
26. Hassan A, Ableitner A, Stein C, Herz A: Inflammation of the rat paw enhances axonal transport of opioid receptors in the sciatic nerve and increases their density in inflamed tissue. Neuroscience 185-195, 1993.
27. Levine JD, Fields HL, Basbaum AI: Peptides and the primary afferent nociceptor. Neuroscience 13:2273-2286, 1993.
28. Stein C: Peripheral mechanisms of opioid analgesia. Anesth Analg 76:182-191, 1993.
29. Coombs DW, Saunders RL, Lachance D, et al: Intrathecal morphine tolerance: Use of intrathecal clonidine, DADLE, and intraventricular morphine. Anesthesiology 62:358-363, 1985.
30. Elliot K, Kest B, Man A, et al: NMDA receptors, Mu and Kappa opioid tolerance, and perspectives on new analgesic drug development. Neuropsychopharmacology 13:347-356, 1995.
31. Herz A: Opioid reward mechanisms: A key role in drug abuse? Can J Physiol Pharmacol 76:252-258, 1998.
32. Bovill JG, Sebel PS: Electroencephalographic effects of sufentanyl anesthesia in man. Br J Anaesth 54:45, 1982.
33. Labella FS, Pinsky C, Havlecik V: Morphine derivatives with diminished opiate receptor potency show enhanced central excitatory activity. Brain Res 174:263-271, 1979.
34. Freye E: Opioid Agonists, Antagonists and Mixed Narcotic Analgesics: Theoretical Background and Considerations for Practical Use. Berlin, Springer-Verlag, 1987.
35. Martin WR: Pharmacology of opioid. Pharmacol Rev 35:283, 1967.
36. Weinstock M, Davidson JT, Rosin AJ, Shnieden H: Effect of physostigmine on morphine induced postoperative pain and somnolence. Br J Anaesth 54:429, 1982.
37. Manara L, Bianchetti A: The central and peripheral influences of opioids on gastrointestinal propulsion. Ann Rev Pharmacol Toxicol 25:249, 1985.
38. Duthie DJR, Nimmo WS: Adverse effects of opioid analgesic drugs. Br J Anaesth 59:61, 1987.
39. Murray K: Prevention of urinary retention associated phenoxybenzamine during epidural morphine. Br Med J 288:645, 1984.
40. Campbell C, Phillips OC, Frazier TM: Analgesia during labor: A comparison of pentobarbital, meperidine and morphine. Obstet Gynecol 17:714, 1961.
41. Ballantyne JC, Loach AB, Carr DB: Itching after epidural and spinal opiates. Pain 331:149, 1988.
42. Thomass DA, Williams GM, Iwata K, et al: Effects of central administration of opioids on facial scratching in monkeys. Anesth Analg 585:315, 1992.
43. Mellon RD, Bayer BM: Evidence for central opioid receptors in the immunomodulatory effects of morphine: Review of potential mechanisms of action. J Neuroimmunol 83:19, 1998.
44. Alonzo NC, Bayer BM: Opioids immunology and host defenses of intravenous drug abusers. Infect Dis Clin North Am 16:553, 2002.
45. Collett BJ: Opioid tolerance: The clinical perspective. Br J Anaesth 81:58, 1998.
46. Mestek A, Hurley JH, Bye LS, et al: The human mu-opioid receptor; modulation of function desensitization by calcium, calmodulin-dependent protein kinase and protein kinase C. J Neurosci 15:2396, 1995.
47. Sharma S, Nirenberg M: Opioid dependent modulation of adenylate cyclase. Proc Natl Acad Sci USA 74:3365, 1977.
48. Trujillo KA, Akil H: Opiate tolerance and dependence: Recent findings and synthesis. New Biol 3:915, 1991.
49. Taub A: Opioid analgesics in the treatment of chronic intractable pain of non-neoplastic origin. In Kitahata LM, Collins JG (eds): Narcotic Analgesics in Anesthesiology. Baltimore, Williams & Wilkins, 1982, p 199.
50. Foley KM: Clinical tolerance to opioids. In Basbaum AI, Besson JM (eds): Towards a New Pharmacotherapy of Pain. New York, Wiley, 1991, p 181.
51. Moulin DE, Ling GSF, Pasternak G: Unidirectional cross-tolerance between morphine and levorphanol in the rat. Pain 33:233, 1988.
52. Bilsky EJ, Inturissi C, Sadee W, et al: Competitive and non-competitive antagonists block the antinociceptive tolerance to morphine, but not to selective mu or delta opioids in mice. Pain 68:229, 1996.
53. Spanagel R, Herz A, Shippenberg TS: Oppposing tonically active endogenous opioid systems modulate the mesolimbic dopaminergic pathway. Proc Natl Acad Sci USA 89:2040, 1992.
54. Miyoshi HR, Leckband SG: Systemic opioid analgesics. In Loeser JD, Butler SH, Chapman CR, Turk DC (eds): Bonica's Management of Pain, 3rd ed. Philadelphia, Lippincott Williams & Wilkins, 2001, p 1682.
55. Janicki PK, Parris WC: Clinical pharmacology of opioids. In Smith H (ed): Drugs for Pain. Philadelphia, Hanley & Belfus, 2003, p 97.
56. Masood AR, Thomas SHL: Systemic absorption of nebulized morphine compared with oral morphine in healthy subjects. Br J Clin Pharmacol 41:250, 1996.
57. Masters N, Heap G, Wedley J, Moore A: Inhaled nebulized morphine and diamorphine. Useful in general practice. Practitioner 232:910, 1988.
58. Worsley MH, Macleod AD, Brodie MJ, et al: Inhaled fentanyl as a method of analgesia. Anaesthesia 45:449, 1990.
59. Gupta SK, Southam M, Gale R: System functionality and physiochemical model of fentanyl transdermal system. J Pain Symptom Manage (3 Suppl):17S, 1992.
60. Hill HF: Clinical pharmacology of transdermal fentanyl. Eur J Pain 11:81-91, 1990.
61. Southam M: Transdermal fentanyl therapy: System design, pharmacokinetics and efficacy. Anticancer Drugs (Suppl) 3: 29, 1995.
62. Ashburn MA, Stephen RL, Ackerman E, et al: Iontophoretic delivery of morphine for postoperative analgesia. J Pain Symptom Manage 7:27, 1992.
63. Alexander-Williams JM, Rowbotham DJ: Novel routes of opioid administration. Br J Anaesth 81:3, 1998.
64. Lobato RD, Madrid JL, Fatela LV, et al: Intraventricular morphine for intractable cancer pain: Rationale, methods, clinical results. Acta Anaesthesiol Scand (Suppl) 85: 68, 1987.
65. Boerner U, Abbott S, Roe RL: The metabolism of morphine and heroin in man. Drug Metab Rev 4:39, 1975.
66. Mather LE: Opioid pharmacokinetic and pharmacodynamic factors. Clin Anesthesiol 17, 1983.
67. Glare PA, Walsh TD: Clinical pharmacokinetics of morphine. Ther Drug Monitoring 13:1, 1991.
68. Stanski D, Lowenstein E: Kinetics of intravenous and intramuscular morphine. Clin Pharmacol Ther 24:52, 1978.
69. Brunk F, Delle M: Morphine metabolism in man. Clin Pharmacol Ther 16:51, 1974.
70. Waldman CS, Eason JR, Rambohul E: Serum morphine levels. A comparison between continuous subcutaneous and intravenous infusion. Anaesthesia 39:768, 1984.
71. Gourlay GK, Cherry D, Cousins MJ: A comparative study of the efficacy and pharmacokinetics of oral methadone and morphine in the treatment of severe pain in patients with cancer. Pain 25:297, 1986.
72. Hoskin PJ, Hanks GW, Aherne GW, et al: The bioavailibility and pharmacokinetics of morphine after intravenous, oral and buccal administration in healthy volunteers. Br J Anaesth 27:499, 1989.
73. Laitnen L, Kanto J, Vapaavouri M, Vijanen MK: Morphine concentrations in plasma after intramuscular injection. Br J Clin Pharmacol 47:1265, 1975.
74. Spector S, Vessell ES: Disposition of morphine in man. Science 174(4):421, 1971
75. Olsen GD: Morphine binding to human plasma proteins. Clin Pharmacol Ther 17:31, 1975.
76. Yeh SYCW, Krebs HA: Isolation and identification of morphine 3- and 6- glucuoronides, morphine 3,6- glucuronide, morphine 3,6- diglucuronide, morphine 3- ethereal sulphate, nor-morphine and normorphine glucuronide as morphine metabolites in humans. J Pharm Sci 66:1288, 1977.
77. Hoskin PJ, Hanks GW: Morphine: Pharmacokinetics and clinical practice. Br J Cancer 62:705, 1990.
78. Christrup LL: Morphine metabolites. Acta Anaesthesiol Scand 41:116, 1997.

79. Glare PA, Walsh D, Pippenger CE: Normorphine, a neurotoxic metabolite? Lancet 335:725, 1990.
80. Gourlay GK: Sustained relief of chronic pain. Pharmacokinetics of sustained release morphine. Clin Pharmacokinet 35:173, 1998.
81. Beaver WT: Mild analgesics, review of their clinical pharmacology. Am J Med Sci 251:576-599, 1966.
82. Lockridge O, Mottershaw-Jackson N, Eckerson HW: Hydrolysis of diacetylmorphine by human serum cholinesterase. J Pharmacol Exp Ther 215:1, 1980.
83. Sawynok J: The therapeutic use of heroin: A review of pharmacological literature. Can J Physiol Pharmacol 64:1, 1986.
84. Mather L: Clinical pharmacokinetics of analgesic drugs. In Raj PP (ed): Practical Management of Pain, 3rd ed. St Louis, Mosby, 2000, p 462.
85. Hill HF, Coda BA, Schaffer R, Akira T: Multiple dose evaluations of intravenous hydromorphone pharmacokinetics in normal human subjects. Anesth Analg 72:330-336, 1991.
86. Mahler DL, Forrest WH: Relative potencies of morphine and hydromorphone in postoperative pain. Anesthesiology 42:602, 1975.
87. Brose WG, Tanelian DL, Brodsky JB: CSF and blood pharmacokinetics of hydromorphone and morphine following lumbar epidural administration. Pain 45:11, 1991.
88. Ross FB, Wallis SC, Smith MT: Co-administration of sub-antinociceptive synergy with reduced CNS side effects in rats. Pain 84:421, 2000.
89. Mandema JW, Kaiko A, Oshlak B: Characterization and validation of a pharmacokinetic model for controlled-release oxycodone. Br J Clin Pharmacol 42:747, 1996.
90. Davis M, Varga J, Dickerson D, et al: Normal release and controlled release oxycodone: Pharmacokinetics, pharmacodynamics, and controversy. Support Care Cancer 84, 2003.
91. Kaiko RF, Benziger DP, Fitzmartin RD: Pharmacokinetic-pharmacodynamic relationships of controlled release oxycodone. Clin Pharmacol Ther 59:52, 1996.
92. Heiskanen T, Kalso E: Controlled release oxycodone and morphine in cancer elated pain. Pain 73:37, 1997.
93. Otton SV, Wu D, Joffe RT: Inhibition of fluoxetine of cytochrome P450 2D6 activity. Clin Pharmacol Ther 53:401, 1993.
94. Sinatra RS, Hyde NH, Harrison JM: Oxymorphone revisited. Semin Anesth 7:208, 1988.
95. Cherney NI: Opioid analgesics: Comparative features and prescribing guidelines. Drugs 51:713, 1996.
96. Austin KL, Stapleton JV, Mather LE: Multiple intramuscular injections: A major source of variability in analgesic response to meperidine. Pain 8:47, 1980.
97. Armstrong PJ, Bersten A: Normeperidine toxicity. Anesth Analg 65:536, 1986.
98. Kaiko RR, Foley KM, Grabinski PY: Central nervous system excitatory effects of normeperidine in cancer patients. Ann Neurol 13:180, 1983.
99. Freye E: Cardiovascular effects of high doses of fentanyl, meperidine and naloxone in dogs. Anesth Analg 53:40-47, 1974.
100. Garrett L, DeMaria AN, Amsterdam EA, Realyvasquez F: Comparative effects of morphine, meperidine and pentazocine on cardiocirculatory dynamics in patients with acute myocardial infarction. Am J Med Sci 60:949, 1976.
101. Stack CG, Rogers P, Linter SP: Monoamine oxidase inhibitors and anesthesia. Br J Anaesth 60:222, 1988.
102. Jeal W, Benfield P: Transdermal fentanyl. A review of its pharmacological properties and therapeutic efficacy in pain control. Drugs 53:109, 1997.
103. Singleton MA, Rosen JI, Fisher DM: Pharmacokinetics of fentanyl in the elderly. Br J Anaesth 60:619, 1988.
104. Staats PS, Markowitz J, Schein J: Incidence of constipation associated with long-acting opioid therapy: A comparative study. South Med J 97:1, 2004.
105. Bovill JG, Sebel PS, Blackburn CL, Heykants J: The pharmacokinetics of alfentanil: A new opioid analgesic. Anesthesiology 57:439, 1982.
106. Camu F, Gepts E, Rucquoi M, Heykants J: Pharmacokinetics of alfentanil in man. Anesth Analg 61:657, 1982.
107. Celleno D: Spinal sufentanil. Anaesthesia 53:417, 1998.
108. Scholz J, Steinfath M, Schulz M: Clinical pharmacokinetics of alfentanil, fentanyl and sufentanil. Clin Pharmacokinet 31:275, 1996.
109. Rushton AR, Sneyd JR: Opioid analgesics. Br J Hosp Med 57:105, 1997.
110. Egan TD: Remifentanil pharmacokinetics and pharmacodynamics: A preliminary appraisal. Clin Pharmacokinet 29:80, 1995.
111. Ettinger DS, Vitale PJ, Trump DL: Important clinical pharmacological considerations in the use of methadone in cancer patients. Cancer Treat Rep 63:457, 1979.
112. Novick DM, Pascarelli EF, Joseph H, et al: Methadone maintenance patient in general medical practice. JAMA 259(22):3299, 1988.
113. Gorman ES, Warfield CA: The use of opioids in the management of pain. Hosp Pract 48A-48H, 1986.
114. Nilsson MI, Meresar U, Anggard E: Clinical pharmacokinetics of methadone. Acta Anaesthesiol Scand (Suppl) 74:66, 1982.
115. Inturrisi CE, Verebely K: Disposition of methadone in man after a single oral dose. Clin Pharmacol 13:923, 1972.
116. Sawe J: High dose methadone and morphine in cancer patients: Clinical pharmacokinetic consideration of oral treatment. Clin Pharmacol 11:87, 1986.
117. Abramson FP: Methadone plasma protein binding: Alterations in cancer and displacement from alpha 1-acid glycoprotein. Clin Pharmacol Ther 32:652, 1982.
118. Gourlay GK: Different opioids-same actions? Prog Pain Res Manage 14:97, 1999.
119. Dollery C, Boobis A, Rawlins M (eds): Therapeutic Drugs, 2nd ed. London, Churchill Livingstone, 1999.
120. Gorman AL, Elliott KJ, Inturrisi CE: The d and l-isomers of methadone bind to the non-competitive site on the NMDA receptor in rat forebrain and spinal cord. Neurosci Lett 223:5, 1997.
121. Procter MJ, Headley PM: Comparison of NMDA receptor involvement in the anti-nociceptive effects of methadone, morphine and fentanyl in anaesthetised rats. Presented at the Ninth World Congress of the International Association for the Study of Pain, A535, 1999.
122. Inturrisi CE, Colburn WA, Kaiko RF, et al: Pharmacokinetics and pharmacodynamics of methadone in patients with chronic pain. Clin Pharmacol Ther 41:392, 1987.
123. Beaver WT, Wallenstein SL, Houde RW, Rogers AA: A clinical comparison of the analgesic effects of morphine and methadone administered intramuscularly, and of orally and parenterally administered methadone. Clin Pharmacol Ther 8:415, 1967.
124. Finn P, Wilcock K: Levo-alpha acetyl methadol (LAAM). Its advantages and drawbacks. J Subst Abuse Treat 14:559, 1997.
125. Vormfelde SV, Poser W: Death attributed to methadone. Pharmacopsychiatry 34:217, 2001.
126. Klotz U: Tramadol: The impact of its pharmacokinetic and pharmacodynamic properties on the clinical management of pain. Drug Res 53:681, 2003.
127. Gibson TP: Pharmacokinetics, efficacy and a safety of analgesia with a focus on tramadol. Am J Med 101(Suppl 1A):47S, 1996.
128. Bailey PL, Stanley TH: Intravenous opioid anesthetics. In Miller RD (ed): Anesthesia, 4th ed. New York, Churchill Livingstone, 1994, p 291.
129. Radnay PA, Brodman E, Mankikar D, Duncalf D: The effect of equi-analgesic doses of fentanyl, morphine, meperidine and pentazocine on common bile duct pressure. Anaesthesiology 29:26, 1980.
130. Lake CL, DiFazio CA, Duckworth EN: High performance liquid chromatographic analysis of plasma levels of nalbuphine in cardiac surgical patients. J Chromatogr 233:410, 1982.
131. Latasch L, Probst S, Dudziak R: Reversal by nalbuphine of respiratory depression caused by fentanyl. Anesth Analg 63:763, 1984.
132. Davies GG, From R: A blinded study using nalbuphine for prevention of pruritus induced by epidural fentanyl. Anesthesiology 65:216, 1986.
133. Gillis JC, Benfield P, Goa KL: Transnasal butorphanol. A review of its pharmacodynamic and pharmacokinetic properties, and therapeutic potential in acute pain management. Drugs 50:157, 1995.
134. Pallasch TJ, Gill CJ: Butorphanol and nalbuphine: A pharmacologic comparison. Oral Surg Oral Med Oral Pathol 59:15, 1985.
135. Popio KA, Jackson DH, Ross AM: Hemodynamic and respiratory effects of morphine and butorphanol. Clin Pharmacol Ther 23:281, 1978.
136. McQuay HJ, Moore RA, Bullingham RES: Buprenorphine kinetics. In Foley K, Inturissi C (eds): Opioid Analgesics in the Management of Clinical Pain. New York, Raven, 1985.
137. Sadee W, Rosenbaum JS, Herz A: Buprenorphine: Differential interaction with opiate receptor subtypes in vivo. J Pharmacol Exp Ther 223:157, 1982.
138. Mather LE: Opioid pharmacokinetics in relation to their effects. Anaesth Int Care 15:15, 1987.

139. Boas RA, Villiger JW: Clinical actions of fentanyl and buprenorphine. The significance of receptor binding. Br J Anaesth 247:192, 1985.
140. Tigerstedt I, Tammisto T: Double-blind, multiple-dose comparison of buprenorphine and morphine in postoperative pain. Acta Anaesthesiol Scand 24:462, 1980.
141. McQuay HJ, Bullingham RES, Paterson GMC, Moore RA: Clinical effects of buprenorphine during and after operation. Br J Anaesth 52:1018, 1980.
142. Levine JD, Gordon NC, Fields HL: Naloxone dose dependently produces analgesia and hyperalgesia in postoperative pain. Nature 278:740, 1979.
143. Rawal N, Schott U, Dahlstrom B: Effect of naloxone infusion on analgesia and respiratory depression following epidural morphine. Anesthesiology 64:194, 1986.

chapter 114

Role of Antidepressants in the Management of Pain

Steven D. Waldman

The antidepressant compounds have been used in patients suffering from a variety of painful conditions since first released almost 50 years ago; their use in this clinical setting was predicated on the logical notion that most patients with unremitting pain were depressed. It was not until the early 1970s that Merskey and others put forth the notion that this group of drugs might also have analgesic properties separate and apart from their primary mood-altering purpose.[1] This notion has stood the test of time and the results of numerous controlled studies have confirmed it.[2] Given the widespread use of the antidepressant compounds as a first line treatment for pain, one must wonder that if the pharmaceutical companies that first introduced these drugs as antidepressants could turn back the hands of time, they would have introduced them as analgesics. This chapter will review the clinical relevant pharmacology of the various antidepressant compounds that are thought to be useful in the management of pain with an eye to providing the clinician with a practical roadmap on how to implement, manage, and discontinue therapy with this heterogeneous group of drugs.

CLASSIFICATION OF ANTIDEPRESSANTS

For the purposes of this chapter, the antidepressant compounds can be divided into the following six groups: (1) the tricyclic antidepressants (TCAs); (2) the selective serotonin reuptake inhibitors (SSRIs); (3) the serotonin and noradrenergic reuptake inhibitors (SNaRIs); (4) the noradrenergic and specific serotoninergic antidepressants (NaSSAs); (5) the noradrenergic reuptake inhibitors (NaRIs); and (6) the monoamine oxidase inhibitors (MAOIs) (Table 114–1). Although many of the characteristics of the various types of antidepressant compounds are similar to the tricyclic antidepressants, the unique properties of each class of drugs will be discussed individually.

Tricylic (Heterocyclic) Antidepressants

The tricyclic antidepressants are the prototypical antidepressant compounds in clinical use for the treatment of pain and are, by far, the most studied. Their name is derived from their molecular structure which is composed of three rings (Fig. 114–1). It is the modification of the middle ring and the alteration of the amine group on the terminal side chain that has resulted in a variety of clinically useful drugs. More recently, the addition of a fourth ring to the tricyclic antidepressants in drugs such as trazodone and amoxapine has complicated the nomenclature of this class of drugs (Fig. 114–2). In terms of chemical structure, these drugs are now correctly referred to as heterocyclic antidepressants; however, the more familiar term *tricyclic antidepressants* is still used by most clinicians to indicate the amitriptyline-like drugs, regardless of their actual chemical structure and to differentiate them from other classes of antidepressants such as the SSRIs and the MAOIs.

Mechanism of Action

The mechanism of action of tricyclic antidepressants is thought to be via their ability to alter monoamine transmitter activity at the synapse by blocking the reuptake of serotonin and norepinephrine.[3] Although this pharmacologic effect begins with the first dose of the drug, most clinicians believe that clinically demonstrable improvement in the patient's pain complaints requires 2 to 3 weeks of treatment. This lag in onset of clinically demonstrable improvement suggests that there may be more at play than the simple alteration of monoamine transmitter activity.[4] Some investigators have postulated that it is the normalization of a disturbed sleep pattern that is ultimately responsible for the analgesic properties of these drugs rather than their direct action on monoamine transmitter activity per se.

Absorption and Metabolism

The tricyclic antidepressants are well absorbed orally and are bound to serum proteins. This class of drugs undergo rapid first pass hepatic metabolism but have relatively long elimination half-lives of 1 to 4 days owing to their lipophilic nature. Diseases that affect serum proteins or decrease liver function can alter the serum levels of these drugs. These drugs are excreted in the urine and feces.

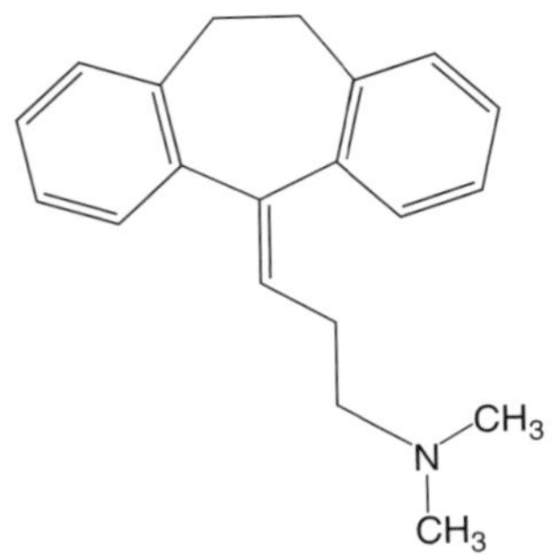

FIGURE 114–1 ■ The chemical structure of amitriptyline, the prototypical tricyclic antidepressant.

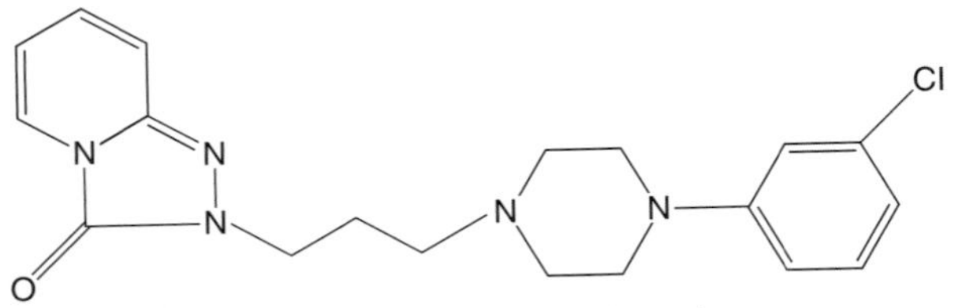

FIGURE 114–2 ■ The chemical structure of trazodone.

Table 114–1

The Classification of Antidepressant Compounds

Tricyclic antidepressants
Selective serotonin reuptake inhibitors
Serotonin and noradrenergic reuptake inhibitors
Noradrenergic and specific serotoninergic antidepressants
Noradrenergic reuptake inhibitors
Monoamine oxidase inhibitors

Side Effects

In addition to blocking the synaptic reuptake of serotonin and norepinephrine, the tricyclic antidepressants also interact with a number of other receptors, which accounts for the wide and varied side effect profile (Table 114–2). Many of the early tricyclic antidepressants as typified by amitriptyline, exert significant anticholinergic side effects via the muscarinic receptors. Such side effects include xerostomia, xerophthalmia, constipation, urinary retention, tachycardia, decreased gastric emptying, and difficulties in visual accommodation.[5]

In addition to the anticholinergic side effects of the tricyclic antidepressants, many of these drugs cause significant blockade of the alpha-adrenergic receptors with resulting orthostatic hypotension. The orthostatic hypotension is most likely the result of venous blood pooling in the lower extremities and viscera. This potentially dangerous side effect can range from a mild annoying sensation of transient lightheadedness when arising to near syncopal episodes with falling and head injury a distinct possibility.

Other side effects include the blocking of the H_2 receptors with resultant decrease in gastric acid production, as well

Table 114–2

Common Side Effects of the Tricyclic Antidepressants

Xerostomia
Xerophthalmia
Urinary retention
Blurred vision
Constipation
Sedation
Cardiac arrhythmias
Sleep disruption
Weight gain
Headache
Nausea
Gastrointestinal disturbance/diarrhea
Abdominal pain
Inability to achieve an erection
Inability to achieve an orgasm (men and women)
Loss of libido
Agitation
Anxiety

as a variety of psychomimetic side effects that can be most upsetting to the patient. These psychomimetic side effects include vivid "Technicolor" dreams, prolonged, intense dreaming, restlessness, and occasionally psychic activation. Some drugs in this class seem to produce increased appetite and weight gain, whereas others seem to suppress appetite. Increased and decreased libido, as well as sexual dysfunction, can occur and should be discussed with patients when assessing the efficacy of therapy with the tricyclic antidepressant compounds. The unique side effect of priapism, which occurs in approximately 1:10,000 men when taking trazodone, should also be discussed when implementing treatment with this drug.

These side effects can usually be managed by proper dosing techniques when implementing therapy with the tricyclic antidepressants as discussed subsequently but may necessitate switching to a drug with a different side effect profile to achieve patient compliance.

Abuse Potential and Side Effects of Withdrawal of the Drug

The tricyclic antidepressants do not appear to interact significantly with the opioid, benzodiazepine, gamma-aminobutyric acid, or beta-adrenergic receptors. There is no clinical evidence of addiction that occurs when these drugs are discontinued, but some drugs in this class have a propensity to cause a variety of symptoms including insomnia, restlessness, lack of energy, and increased cholinergic activity as manifested by excessive salivation and occasional gastrointestinal distress. These side effects can be avoided by slowly tapering the tricyclic antidepressant over 10 to 14 days.

Overdosage

Overdosage of significant amounts of the tricyclic antidepressants is a serious event that, if not aggressively managed, can result in death.[6] In general, the dosages that are required to treat pain are lower than those required to treat severe depression; however, the advent of mail order pharmacies with their 90-day prescription requirements has made overdose a real issue because doses of amitriptyline of greater that 2000 mg can be fatal—well within the amounts prescribed in a 90-day prescription. Sedation progressing to coma, combined cardiac abnormalities including delays in cardiac conduction as manifested by a prolonged QT interval, and bizarre cardiac dysrhythmias can make the management of tricyclic antidepressant overdose most challenging. Further complicating this clinical picture is the potential for grand mal seizures and a hypercholinergic state consisting of mydriasis, urinary retention, dry mouth and eyes, and delirium. Because of the potential for disastrous results with tricyclic antidepressant overdosage, all such events should be taken seriously and all patients suspected of overdosage should be immediately evaluated and treated in an emergency department equipped to managed the attendant life-threatening symptoms.

Some Common Tricyclic and Tetracyclic Antidepressants

Amitriptyline (Elavil)

Amitriptyline is the prototype of all antidepressants (see Figure 114–1). Its efficacy as an analgesic has been studied extensively and there is significant clinical experience in this setting.[7,8] Blocking both norepinephrine as well as serotonin, amitriptyline is an efficacious analgesic, but with significant side effects including sedation, orthostasis, as well as most of the troublesome anticholinergic side effects. It should be used cautiously in patients with cardiac conduction defects owing to its propensity to cause tachycardia and should not be used in patients with narrow-angle glaucoma and significant prostatism. In spite of its side-effect profile, amitriptyline remains a reasonable starting point for implementation of tricyclic antidepressant therapy owing to its proven efficacy, low cost, availability of liquid and parenteral formulations, ability to treat sleep disturbance, dosing flexibility, and universal availability—even for those patients on Medicaid or in managed care plans with restrictive formularies. Because of its sedative properties, amitriptyline should be given as a bedtime dose starting at 10 to 25 mg. The drug can be titrated upward as side effects allow in 10- to 25-mg doses with care being taken to identify the increases in side effects as the dose is raised. In particular, orthostatic hypotension can be insidious in onset as the dosage of the drug is raised and may lead to falls at night when the patient gets up to use the bathroom. If analgesia is not achieved by the time the dose is raised to 150 mg, the patient should be switched to a different antidepressant compound, preferably from another class of drugs, and/or another adjuvant analgesic could be added, such as gabapentin if appropriate. If the patient has partial relief of pain, this drug can be carefully titrated upward to a single bedtime dose of 300 mg.

Desipramine (Norpramin) and Nortriptyline (Pamelor)

Both desipramine and nortriptyline are good choices for initial tricyclic antidepressant therapy if sedation is not desired or the sedative side effects of amitriptyline are too great (Fig. 114–3).[9,10] Given as an AM dose, these drugs are good first choices in those patient suffering from pain who have complained of lack of energy or risk for the orthostatic side effects of amitriptyline (e.g., patients on warfarin (Coumadin). Dosed at 10 to 25 mg every morning and titrated upward to a

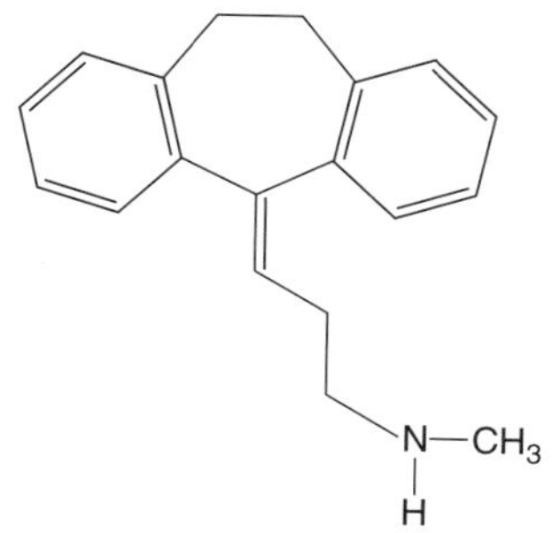

FIGURE 114–3 ■ The chemical structure of nortriptyline.

maximum dose of 150 mg, pain relief will usually be seen at doses of 50 to 75 mg after 2 to 3 weeks of therapy—although improvement in sleep may occur much sooner. These drugs should be used cautiously in patients with cardiac arrhythmia and in those prone to psychic activation or agitation. Such psychic activation or agitation may be exacerbated by the concomitant administration of steroids (e.g., epidural steroid injections).

Trazodone (Deseryl)

Although the unique side effect of priapism may limit the use of this drug in men, trazodone has the sedating characteristic of amitriptyline, which is desirable in those patients suffering from sleep disturbance as part of their pain symptomatology without the cardiac, anticholinergic, and orthostatic side effects (see Fig. 114–2).[11] The drug should be started at 75 mg at bedtime and titrated upward to 300 mg as side effects allow. Pain relief will usually occur at a dosage range of 150 to 200 mg.

Selective Serotonin Reuptake Inhibitors

Although generally less efficacious that the tricyclic (heterocyclic) antidepressants in the treatment of pain, the selective serotonin reuptake inhibitors (SSRIs) have a proven efficacy in this clinical setting. Their lack of side effects relative to the tricyclic antidepressants make the SSRI a good choice for those pain patients who cannot or will not tolerate the side effects of the tricyclic antidepressants, albeit at greater monetary cost.[12]

Mechanism of Action

The SSRIs selectively block the reuptake of serotonin by blocking the sodium/potassium adenosine triphosphate pump resulting in increased levels of serotonin at the synaptic cleft. They also affect other serotonin receptors, most notably in the gut, which probably accounts for their propensity to cause gastrointestinal side effects, especially during initiation of therapy.

Absorption and Metabolism

The SSRIs are well absorbed orally. This class of drugs undergoes rapid first pass hepatic metabolism by hepatic enzymes and may compete with other drugs for these enzymes—resulting in increased blood levels of warfarin (Coumadin) and the benzodiazepines, among others. These drugs have relatively long serum elimination half-lives and given the fact that many of the SSRIs have active metabolites, side effects may persist for a long time after this class of drugs is discontinued. The SSRIs are excreted in the urine and feces.

Side Effects

As mentioned, the SSRI interaction with the serotonin receptors of the gut may result in the side effects of cramping, nausea, and diarrhea—especially during the initial implementation of therapy. These symptoms are usually self-limited and will actually decrease as the gut accommodates to the increased serotoinnergic milieu. In addition to the GI side effects associated with the SSRI, side effects associated with central nervous system activation, including tremors, insomnia, and physic activation can limit the use of these drugs as can the increased incidence of sexual side effects relative to the tricyclic antidepressants. These side effects include alterations in libido, erectile and orgasmic difficulties, ejaculatory delay, and impotence. The allegation that the SSRI fluoxetine may cause increased suicidal ideations has not appeared to be a problem with the use of this drug as an analgesic although its relative lack of efficacy for this purpose when compared with the tricyclic antidepressants has. It should be noted that the SSRI can interact with the monamine oxidase inhibitors to produce a potentially life-threatening constellation of symptoms known as the *central serotonergic syndrome*. The central serotonergic syndrome is characterized by hypertension, fever, myoclonus, and seizures. Tachycardia, and in extreme instances, cardiovascular collapse and death may occur.[13] For this reason, these classes of drugs should never be used together and a long drug-free period of at least 10 half-lives should be implemented when stopping the SSRI and starting the monoamine oxidase inhibitors. This class of drugs also appears to interact with St. John wort, and hypertensive crises have been reported when the drugs were taken together.

Abuse Potential and Side Effects on Withdrawal of the Drug

Like the tricyclic antidepressants, the SSRIs do not appear to interact significantly with the opioid, benzodiazepine, gamma-aminobutyric acid or beta-adrenergic receptors. No clinical evidence of addiction occurs when these drugs are discontinued, but some drugs in this class have a propensity to cause a variety of symptoms including lack of energy and decreased serotoninergic activity as manifested by constipation. These side effects can be avoided by slowly tapering the SSRI over 10 to 14 days.

Overdosage

In general, overdosage with the SSRI is much less serious than overdosage with the tricyclic antidepressants.[14] There have been remarkably few fatal overdoses reported in the literature or to the FDA involving ingestion only of an SSRI. Moderate overdoses of up to 30 times the daily dose are associated with minor or no symptoms, whereas ingestions of greater amounts typically result in drowsiness, tremor, nausea, gastrointestinal disturbances, and vomiting. At very high doses of greater that 75 times the common daily dose, the more serious adverse events, including seizures, electrocardiogram (ECG) changes, and decreased consciousness may occur. SSRI overdoses in combination with alcohol or other drugs are associated with increased toxicity, and almost all fatalities involving SSRIs have involved co-ingestion of other substances.

Some Common Selective Serotonin Reuptake Inhibitors

Fluoxetine (Prozac, Serafem)

Fluoxetine is available in capsule, tablet, and liquid forms, which are usually taken once a day in the morning or twice a day, in the morning and at noon—as well as a fluoxetine delayed-relayed capsule that is usually taken once a week (Fig. 114–4). Because the side-effect profile is minimal, it is usually possible to start this drug at the lower range of the dosages thought to provide analgesia, 20 mg, and titrate upward to 60 mg as side effects allow and efficacy demands. The onset of analgesic action of fluoxetine usually occurs within 2 to 3 weeks.[15]

Paroxetine (Paxil)

Well tolerated by most patients, paroxetine is another reasonable choice for patients who do not tolerate the tricyclic antidepressants. It comes in both an immediate-release and a controlled-release form. It is taken as a once-a-day dose or twice-a-day at morning to noon to minimize the side effects of tremors or irritability. There are anecdotal reports that paroxetine may have a lower incidence of ejaculatory side effects when compared with fluoxetine. Paroxetine should be started at a dose of 20 mg and titrated upward to 40 mg as side effects allow and efficacy dictates.

Sertraline (Zoloft)

Sertraline is available as an immediate-release tablet or capsule as well as an oral liquid concentrate. Generally well tolerated, sertraline is take once a day as an AM dose starting at 50 mg and titrated upward to 200 mg as side effects and efficacy allow.[16] This drug may also have efficacy for those patients suffering from pain and who also exhibit obsessive-compulsive tendencies.

Serotonin and Noradrenergic Reuptake Inhibitors

Venlafaxine (Effexor)

Venlafaxine has been shown to be useful as an analgesic in controlled clinical trials.[17,18] It has a structure that is different from that of any of the other clinically useful antidepressant compounds (Fig. 114–5). With a better side effect profile than the SSRI, this drug is a good starting point for those patients who seem to have side effects with most adjuvant analgesics. Like amitriptyline, venlafaxine affects both serotonin and norepinephrine, which theoretically should make it more efficacious for pain than the SSRIs. It remains to be seen if widespread clinical use will bear this out. A reasonable starting dose for pain is 25 mg of venlafaxine every 12 hours with

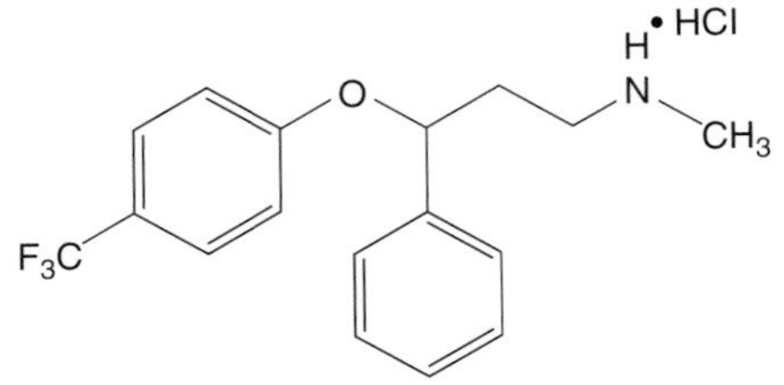

FIGURE 114–4 ■ The chemical structure of fluoxetine.

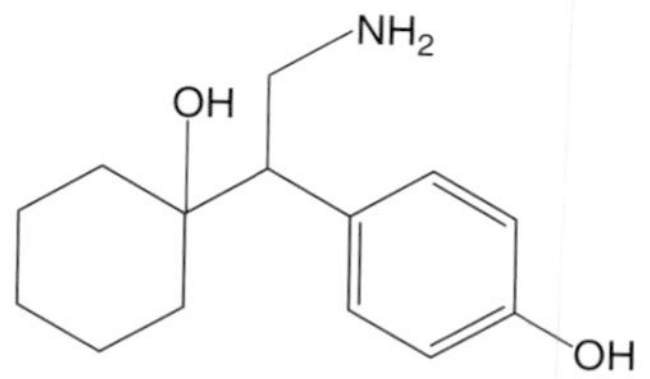

FIGURE 114–5 ■ The chemical structure of venlafaxine.

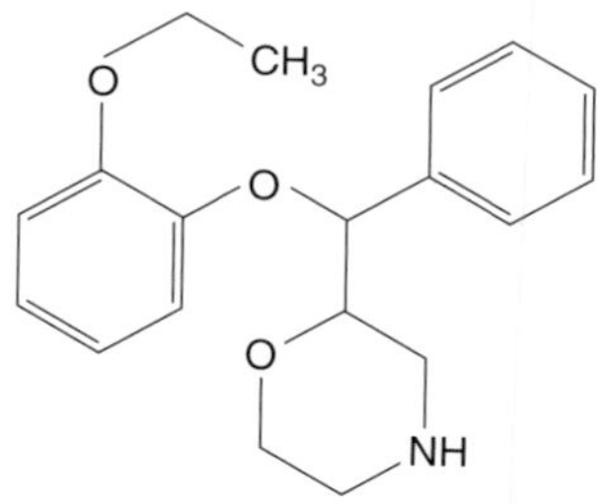

FIGURE 114–6 ■ The chemical structure of reboxetine.

the dose increased by 25 mg every week as side effects allow and efficacy dictates.

Noradrenergic Reuptake Inhibitors

Reboxetine (Edronax)

The newest class of antidepressants, the noradrenergic reuptake inhibitors (NaRIs) are among the least studied of the antidepressant compounds in the role as analgesics.[19,20] Given the fact that reboxetine acts primarily on the noradrenergic system, theoretically it is most useful for those patients with pain who are also suffering from significant anergia and depression and cannot tolerate desipramine or nortriptyline (Fig. 114–6). Not yet unavailable in the United States but available in more than 50 countries, reboxetine is given as a 4-mg twice daily dose titrating upward by 1 mg each week to 10 mg as side effects allow and efficacy dictates. There are anecdotal reports that painful ejaculation can occur at higher dosages of this drug.

Monoamine Oxidase Inhibitors

Isoniazid and its derivative iproniazid were introduced in 1951 as pharmacologic treatments for tuberculosis. It was found that iproniazid inhibited the enzyme monoamine oxidase and that tuberculosis patients treated with this drug experienced an elevation of mood. This discovery, along with the introduction of the phenothiazines, ushered in the modern era of the pharmacologic treatment of psychiatric disorders. Widespread experience with this class of drugs led to an understanding that these drugs were also useful in patients suffering from chronic pain, most notably intractable headache as well as the realization that their side effect profile limited their clinical utility.[21] The introduction of the tricyclic antidepressants in the early 1960s led to the almost complete abandonment of the monoamine (MAO) inhibitors except in the most severely disturbed psychiatric patients and a few recidivist headache patients. Through the almost single-handed efforts of Diamond and his colleagues at the Diamond Headache Clinic in Chicago, the efficacy and the safety of the MAO inhibitors in combination with the tricyclic antidepressants in the treatment of intractable headache have been firmly established.

Table 114–3

Dietary Restrictions When Taking MAO Inhibitors
Aged food or meat
Over-ripe fruit
Fermented food
Chicken liver
Soy sauce
Smoked or pickled meat, poultry, or fish
Cold cuts, including bologna, pepperoni, salami, summer sausage
Alcoholic beverages (especially Chianti, sherry, liqueurs, and beer)
Alcohol-free or reduced-alcohol beer or wine
Anchovies
Caviar
Cheeses (especially strong or aged varieties)
Figs
Raisins, bananas
Meat prepared with tenderizers
Meat extracts

The MAO inhibitors are a heterogeneous group of drugs that work by blocking the oxidative deamination of the biogenic amines at the nerve synapse.[22] This leads to the release of a larger than normal amount of these amines by the synapse when there is an action potential. The MAO inhibitors are well absorbed by mouth and are metabolized in the liver—primarily by acetylation. Some potential for liver damage from this class of drugs exists and appropriate monitoring of liver function tests should be part of the patient's overall treatment plan to avoid permanent liver damage.[23] In spite of their efficacy in the treatment of intractable pain, the unpredictable and sometimes severe side effects of this class of drugs limit their use in pain management to patients who have failed other less problematic treatments and are willing and able to strictly adhere to the dietary and medication restrictions required with these drugs. These restrictions are extremely important as many drugs and foods can potentiate the adrenergic and serotonergic effects of MAO inhibitors (Tables 114–3 and 114–4).[24]

Commonly used MAOIs include phenelzine, isocarboxazid, and tranylcypromine, which are nonselective inhibitors of monoamine oxidase—with phenelzine being the most commonly used in pain management (Fig. 114–7).[25] Phenelzine is started at an initial AM dose of 15 mg. The dose may be increased by 15 mg per week with the second dose being given at noon as side effects allow and as efficacy dictates to a total dose of 60 mg. If there is no relief of pain at this point, amitriptyline at a dose of 10 mg should be added with careful monitoring for side effects. Phenelzine should not be abruptly discontinued and the patient should be cautioned of such, but tapered over a 2 to 3 week period.[26]

PRACTICAL CONSIDERATIONS FOR CLINICAL USE OF ANTIDEPRESSANTS AS ANALGESICS

There are as many ways to use antidepressants to treat pain as there are antidepressant drugs. The following is an

Table 114–4

Drug Interactions and MAO Inhibitors

Allergy medicines (including nose drops or sprays)
Appetite suppressants
Antihistamines (Actifed DM, Benadryl, Benylin, Chlor-Trimeton, Compoz, etc.)
Antipsychotics
Antivert
Asthma drugs
Atrovent
Blood-pressure medicine
Buclazine
BuSpar
Cocaine
Cold medicines
Demerol (deaths have occurred when combining MAOIs and a single dose of meperidine)
Dextromethorphan
Ditropan
Dopar, Larodopa
Flexeril
Insulin (MAOIs may change amount of insulin needed)
Ludiomil
Marezine
Other MAOIs, such as Norflex
Norpace
Phenergan
Pronestyl
Prozac and other SSRIs
Quinidex
Ritalin
Sinus medicine
Symmetrel
Tegretol
Temaril
Tricyclic antidepressants
Tryptophan
Urispas
Wellbutrin

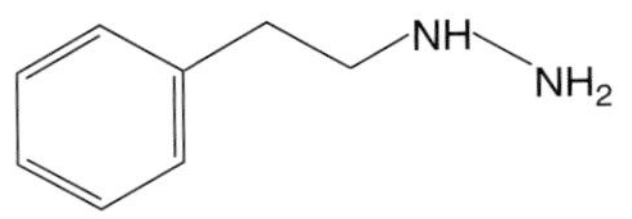

FIGURE 114–7 ■ The chemical structure of phenelzine.

approach that has proved beneficial in the management of patients with a variety of painful conditions in a variety of clinical settings.

The first step in the practical implementation of antidepressant treatment for pain is to explain to the patient that you are treating pain as the primary symptom, not depression. Patients have an unfortunate tendency to attribute motive to the act of prescribing antidepressants and that motive is that the doctor thinks they are crazy enough to need medications or in some patients that the pain is not real and it is "all in their head." Referring to the drugs as tricyclic analgesics and providing patient information sheets that reflect this nomenclature will also help. Beware that the recent efforts by pharmacies to provide written patient information materials with each prescription may undermine the best of intentions. With patients where the motive for prescribing is an issue, a call to the pharmacist to enlist his or her help in patient education is beneficial.

The second step in the practical implementation of antidepressant treatment for pain is to explain to the patient that the medication will not work immediately, but will take a period of weeks for the patient to experience meaningful pain relief. Explain that you are starting at a low dose and for them not to be surprised when you tell them to increase the amount of medication they are taking. This helps alleviate concerns that they are taking "too much medicine." Again, the pharmacist can be of great help in this setting.

The third step is to educate the patient in the role of normal sleep in health and its importance in pain relief. Reinforce the salutary effects of normalization of the patient's sleep cycle as a benefit of most of the drugs discussed earlier. Let the patient know that this drug is not a "sleeping pill" but actually will help treat the sleep disturbance and, most importantly, the pain.

The fourth step is to discuss side effects without setting the stage for medication noncompliance. For the most part, this class of drugs is well tolerated because the chosen drug is started at the lower range of the dosage spectrum and increases in dosage are done slowly. Preempting common early side effects of the tricyclic antidepressants such as xerostomia by having the patient suck on cough drops to stimulate saliva production and to treat xerophthalmia with lubricating eye drops before bedtime will improve patient compliance. Telling the patient that they may feel a little "hung over" for the first few days of treatment but that this bothersome side effect will go away will also help.

The final step is to remain positive regarding the potential for the patient to obtain pain relief. Let the patient know that there will, in all likelihood, be some adjustment of drug dosage and that in some cases switching to another drug will be required to obtain pain relief. Most importantly, the message should be one of hope, not negativity.

References

1. Merskey H, Hester RA: The treatment of pain with psychotropic drugs. Postgrad Med J 48:594, 1972.
2. Frazer A, Conway P: Pharmacologic mechanisms of action of antidepressants. Psychiatr Clin North Am 7:575., 1984.
3. Sternbach RA, Janowsky DS, Huey IY, et al: Effects of altering brain serotonin activity on human chronic pain. In Bonica JJ, Albe Fessard D (eds): Advances in Pain Research and Therapy. New York, Raven, 1976, p 601.
4. Basbaum AI, Fields HL: Endogenous pain control mechanisms: Review and hypothesis. Ann Neurol 4:451, 1978.
5. Kerr GW, McGuffie AC, Wilkie S: Tricyclic antidepressant overdose: A review. Emerg Med J 18:236, 2001.
6. Roose S P, Glassman AH: Antidepressant choice in the patient with cardiac disease: Lessons from the Cardiac Arrhythmia Suppression Trial (CAST) Studies. J Clin Psychiatry (Suppl A):83, 1994.
7. Kalso E, Tasmuth T, Neuvonen PJ: Amitriptyline effectively relieves neuropathic pain following treatment of breast cancer. Pain 64:293, 1995.
8. Stein D, Floman Y, Elizur A, et al: The efficacy of amitriptyline and acetaminophen in the management of acute low back pain. Psychosomatics 37:63, 1996.
9. Watson CPN, Vernich L, Chipman M, et al: Amitriptyline versus nortriptyline in postherpetic neuralgia. Neurology 51:1166, 1998.
10. Atkinson JH, Slater MA, Williams RA, et al: A placebo-controlled randomized clinical trial of nortriptyline for chronic low back pain. Pain 76:287, 1998.

11. Goodkin K, Gullion CM, Agras WS: A randomized double-blind placebo controlled trial of trazodone hydrochloride in chronic low back pain syndrome. J Clin Psychopharmacol 10:269, 1990.
12. Carter GT, Sullivan MD: Antidepressants in pain management. Curr Opin Investig Drugs. 3(3):454, 2002.
13. Sternback H: The serotonin syndrome. Am J Psychiatry 148:705, 1991.
14. Barbey JT, Roose SP: SSRI safety in overdose. J Clin Psychiatry 59 (Suppl 15):42, 1998.
15. Saper JR, Silberstein SD, Lake AE III, et al: Double-blind trial of fluoxetine: Chronic daily headache and migraine. Headache 34:497, 1994.
16. Engel CC Jr, Walker EA, Engel AL, et al: A randomized, double-blind, crossover trial of sertraline in women with chronic pelvic pain. J Psychosom Res 44:203, 1998.
17. Songer DA, Schulte H: Venlafaxine for the treatment of chronic pain. Am J Psychiatry 153:737, 1996.
18. Brita H, Kalso E: Venlafaxine in neuropathic pain following treatment of breast cancer. Eur J Pain 6:17, 2002.
19. Berzewski H, Van Moffaert M, Gagiano CA: Efficacy and tolerability of reboxetine compared with imipramine in a double-blind study in patients suffering from major depressive episodes. Eur Neuropsychopharmacol 7(Suppl 1):S37, 1997.
20. Versiani M, Amin M, Chouinard G: Double-blind, placebo-controlled study with reboxetine in inpatients with severe major depressive disorder. J Clin Psychopharmacol 20:28, 2000.
21. Larsen JK: MAO inhibitors: Pharmacodynamic aspects and clinical implications. Acta Psychiatr Scand (Suppl) 345:74, 1988.
22. Tollefson GD: Monoamine oxidase inhibitors: A review. J Clin Psychiatry 44:280, 1983.
23. Jarrott B, Vajda FJ: The current status of monoamine oxidase and its inhibitors. Med J Aust 146:634, 1987.
24. Lucena MI, Carvajal A, Andrade RJ, Velasco A: Antidepressant-induced hepatotoxicity. Expert Opin Drug Saf 2:249, 2003.
25. Dawson JK, Earnshaw SM, Graham CS: Dangerous monoamine oxidase inhibitor interactions are still occurring in the 1990s. J Accid Emerg Med 12:49, 1995.
26. Dilsaver SC: Monoamine oxidase inhibitor withdrawal phenomena: Symptoms and pathophysiology. Acta Psychiatr Scand 78:1, 1988.

chapter 115

Anticonvulsants

Steven D. Waldman

It is not surprising that with the introduction of each new anticonvulsant into clinical practice, the drug has been tried as a treatment for neuropathic pain, albeit with varying degrees of success. This chapter reviews the anticonvulsant compounds that have proven efficacy in the treatment of a variety of painful conditions and provides the clinician with a practical step-by-step guide for their use.

What is striking about the anticonvulsants that are used to treat pain is their heterogenicity. Unlike the antidepressants that can readily be grouped into classes based on their chemical structure (e.g. the tricyclic antidepressants) or their mechanism of action (e.g., the selective serotonin reuptake inhibitors), the anticonvulsants defy simple classification. However, some generalizations can be made. The anticonvulsants useful in the treatment of pain can be placed into two broad categories (Table 115–1). Category 1 includes those drugs whose primary mechanism of action is to modulate the function of the voltage-dependent sodium channels, whereas category 2 drugs have mechanisms other than modulation of the sodium channel.

CATEGORY 1 ANTICONVULSANTS

Category 1 anticonvulsants modulate the voltage-dependent sodium channels. Although the exact mechanism of neuropathic pain has not been fully explained, some generalizations can be made that may help describe how the anticonvulsants exert their analgesic effect in this clinical setting. If one begins with an assumption that neuropathic pain is the result of abnormal nerve firing, it is reasonable to assume that anything that modulates this abnormal nerve firing downward should decrease the pain—regardless of the drug's exact mechanism of action.

Conceptually, the category 1 anticonvulsant drugs exert their pain-relieving effect by raising the firing threshold required to open the sodium channel and allow the nerve to reach its action potential and fire (Fig. 115–1).[1] Although overly simplistic and ignoring the role of pain modulation at the spinal cord and central levels, the idea that it requires more subthreshold stimuli to elicit an action potential in the presence of category 1 anticonvulsants and that there is a dose-response curve that is roughly linear, fits with our overall clinical observations in this setting—given the diverse nature of pain syndromes we seek to treat with the anticonvulsant drugs. Again, it must be remembered that to attribute a solely peripheral mechanism of action to the anticonvulsants is probably incorrect given the fact that all of the drugs discussed subsequently have the ability to cross the blood-brain barrier and that many of the drugs exert other pharmacologic actions at both the peripheral and higher levels (e.g., the ability of phenytoin to modulate the calcium and potassium channels).

Phenytoin (Dilantin)

The first modern anticonvulsant drug to be use to treat neuropathic pain, phenytoin has seen extensive use as an adjuvant analgesic over the last 60 years with mixed results (Fig. 115–2). Reasonably well absorbed after oral administration, phenytoin is extensively protein bound with only approximately 10% existing in its free state. The drug is metabolized by the liver with only a small amount excreted in the urine. Phenytoin is available in a large array of formulations including immediate-release and sustained-release oral products in a variety of dosages as well as liquid solutions and an injectable preparation. In clinical dosage ranges, it is relatively nonsedating and reasonably well tolerated. Side effects of phenytoin are summarized in Table 115–2 and include nystagmus, behavioral changes, peripheral neuropathy, gingival hyperplasia (Fig. 115–3), gastrointestinal disturbance, osteomalacia, rash, Stevens-Johnson syndrome, liver dysfunction, blood dyscrasias, and a unique side effect of pseudolymphoma which is clinically difficult to distinguish from Hodgkin disease. Because phenytoin is so highly protein bound, any drugs that compete with the binding sites on serum albumin have the potential to increase the free fraction of the drug and can result in toxicity.

To treat neuropathic pain with phenytoin, a dose of 100 mg at bedtime is a reasonable starting point. After 1 week, an additional 100-mg AM dose may be added. If the patient is not experiencing limiting side effects, an additional 100-mg noontime dose may be added. At this point, a complete blood count and liver function tests should be performed. If the patient is tolerating the 300-mg dosing regimen and has experienced partial pain relief, the drug may be titrated upward by 30 mg per week to a maximum dose of 400 mg as side effects allow and efficacy dictates. If at the 300-mg dose the patient is experiencing no diminution of pain, it may be reasonable to switch to another anticonvulsant. Like other

Table 115–1

Classification of Anticonvulsants Based on Their Mechanism of Action
Category 1 anticonvulsants: drugs that modulate voltage-dependent sodium channels
Phenytoin
Carbamazepine
Lamotrigine
Topiramate
Category 2 anticonvulsants: drugs whose primary mechanism of action is unrelated to modulation of the voltage-dependent sodium channel
Gabapentin
Tiagabine
Valproic acid

Table 115–2

Side Effects Associated with Phenytoin
Nystagmus
Behavioral changes
Peripheral neuropathy
Gingival hyperplasia
Gastrointestinal disturbance
Osteomalacia
Rash
Stevens-Johnson syndrome
Liver dysfunction
Blood dyscrasias
Pseudolymphoma

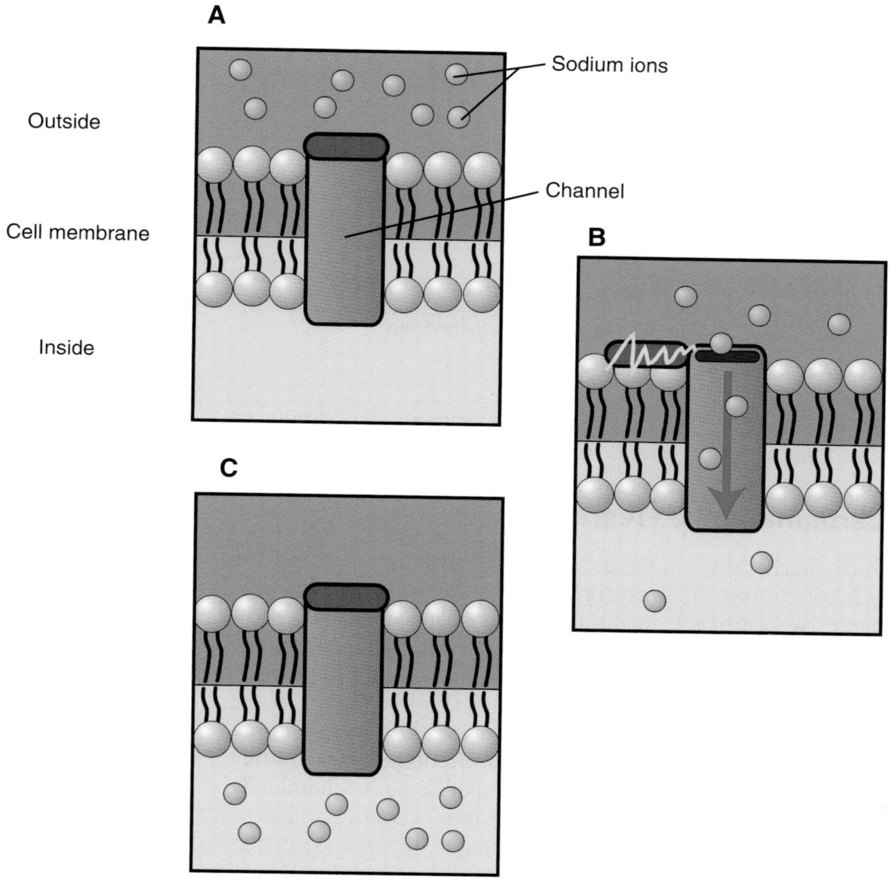

FIGURE 115–1 ■ Modulation of voltage-gated sodium channels by category 1 anticonvulsants. **A,** Voltage-gated sodium channel closed. **B,** Depolarization opens the voltage-gated sodium channel. **C,** Sodium ions inside the cell result in a positive change within the cell and the "gate" closes.

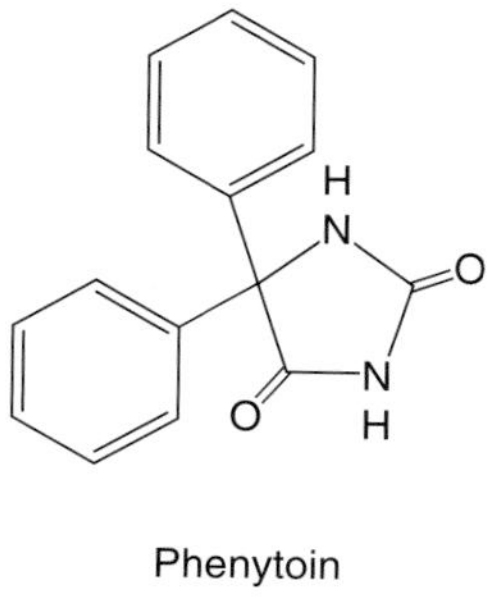

FIGURE 115–2 ■ Chemical structure of phenytoin.

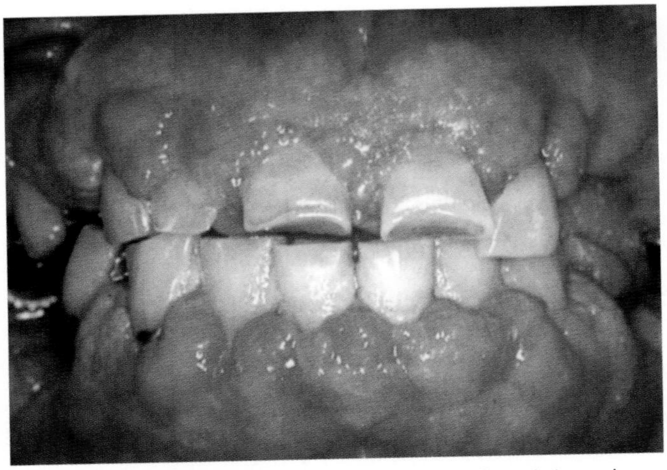

FIGURE 115–3 ■ Gingival hyperplasia as a side effect of phenytoin.

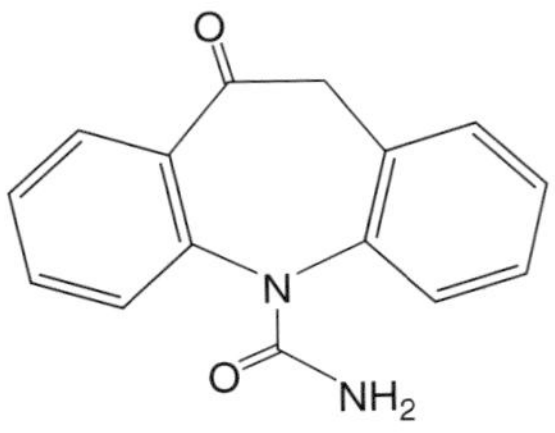

Carbamazepine

FIGURE 115–4 ■ Chemical structure of carbamazepine.

anticonvulsants, this drug should be discontinued slowly to avoid any rebound effect.

Carbamazepine (Tegretol)

Particularly useful in the treatment of lancinating and neuritic pain syndromes such as trigeminal neuralgia, carbamazepine has proven efficacy in the treatment of a variety of neuropathic pain syndromes including diabetic polyneuropathy, trigeminal neuralgia, glossopharyngeal neuralgia, postherpetic neuralgia, and central pain states (Fig. 115–4).[2-4] There are many anecdotal reports supporting the efficacy of carbamazepine in a number of other painful conditions including HIV and chemotherapy-related neuropathic pain. Chemically related to the tricyclic antidepressants, carbamazepine is highly protein bound and is metabolized in the liver. After glucuronidation, it is excreted in the urine. Like phenytoin, interaction with other drugs that are protein bound—such as isoniazid and warfarin (Coumadin) can effect free fraction concentrations and lead to toxicity. In addition to raising the firing threshold of the voltage-dependent sodium channel, carbamazepine suppresses noradrenalin reuptake and, in all likelihood, exerts some of its actions centrally—given it tendency to cause sedation at the higher end of the therapeutic dosage range. In addition to sedation, carbamazepine can cause a variety of central nervous system side effects including vertigo, ataxia, diplopia, dizziness, and blurred vision. Gastrointestinal side effects and rash may occur but the most worrisome side effect of carbamazepine is its potential to cause aplastic anemia. This side effect can generally be avoided if careful and systematic monitoring of hematologic parameters is followed in *all* patients being considered for treatment with this drug. Table 115–3 provides a recommended monitoring protocol for patients who are to receive carbamazepine. A failure to scrupulously monitor the patient on carbamazepine can have fatal consequences. It should be noted that this drug should be used with extreme caution in those patients suffering from neuropathic pain who have previously undergone chemotherapy or radiation therapy for malignancy, even if their hematologic parameters have returned to normal. These patients are extremely sensitive to hematologic side effects from carbamazepine.

Table 115–3

Monitoring Protocol for Carbamazepine Use

1. Obtain baseline complete blood count (CBC), chemistry profile, including creatinine and liver function tests, and urinalysis before first dose of carbamazepine.
2. Repeat CBC and chemistry profile after 1 week of therapy.
3. Repeat CBC and chemistry profile after 2nd week of therapy.
4. Repeat CBC and chemistry profile after 4th week of therapy.
5. Repeat CBC and chemistry profile after 6th week of therapy.
6. Repeat CBC after 8th week of therapy and every 2 months thereafter.
7. Stop carbamazepine immediately at the first sign of hematologic or liver function abnormalities.

Given the reasonably high incidence of CNS side effects associated with carbamazepine therapy, this drug should be started at a low nighttime dose of 100 mg. The drug may then be increased in 100-mg increments given the drug on a four times a day dosing schedule to a maximum dose of 1200 mg as side effects allow and efficacy dictates. With patients with pain emergencies such as intractable trigeminal neuralgia that is limiting the patient's ability to maintain adequate nutrition and hydration, hospitalization is recommended so more rapid upward titration may be safely accomplished. Regardless of the speed at which the drug is titrated upward, the monitoring protocol outlined in Table 115–3 must be followed to avoid disaster. Like all other anticonvulsants, this drug should be discontinued slowly to avoid any rebound effect.

Lamotrigine (Lamictal)

Lamotrigine is another anticonvulsant whose mechanism of action involves modulation of the voltage-dependent sodium channel (Fig. 115–5). Useful in the treatment of a variety of neuropathic pain states including HIV-induced polyneuropathy, trigeminal neuralgia and post-stroke pain, lamotrigine is worth a try in those patients who have lancinating or sharp neuropathic pain that has not responded to carbamazepine or in those patients where carbamazepine is contraindicated.[5-7] Lamotrigine is rapidly and completely absorbed following oral administration, reaching peak plasma concentrations

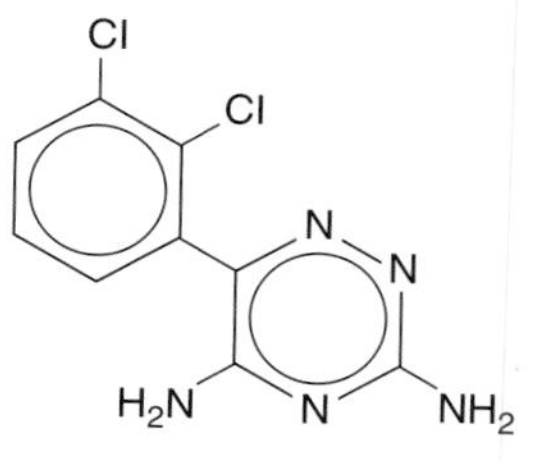

Lamotrigine

FIGURE 115–5 ■ Chemical structure of lamotrigine.

(T_{max}) 1.4 to 4.8 hours post-dosing. When administered with food, the rate of absorption is slightly reduced, but the extent remains unchanged. Lamotrigine is approximately 55% bound to human plasma proteins. Unlike many of the other anticonvulsants, protein binding is unaffected by therapeutic concentrations of phenytoin, phenobarbital, or valproic acid although valproic acid significantly increases the plasma half life of lamotrigine and, therefore, the dose should be decreased with concurrent use of these drugs. Lamotrigine is metabolized predominantly in the liver by glucuronic acid conjugation. The major metabolite is an inactive 2-H-glucuronide conjugate that can be hydrolyzed by beta-glucuronidase. Approximately 70% of an oral lamotrigine dose is recovered in urine as this drug metabolizes. Side effects of lamotrigine include central nervous system side effects similar to carbamazepine, although less severe, as well as occasional gastrointestinal upset and liver function test abnormalities. Although free of the hematologic side effects associated with carbamazepine, lamotrigine has 10% of significant dermatologic side effects ranging from rash to fatal Stevens-Johnson syndrome. Severe dermatologic side effects associated with lamotrigine occur with great enough frequency that they must be carefully looked for and the drug discontinued immediately at the first sign of even the slightest rash or skin irritation. Most dermatologic side effects of lamotrigine occur within the first week of therapy. No monitoring of hematologic parameters is required with this drug.

Lamotrigine is supplied in a chewable and an oral tablet formulation in a variety of dosage strengths making titration of the drug reasonably easy. When treating patients suffering from neuropathic pain with lamotrigine, a reasonable starting dose is 25 mg at bedtime titrating upward in 25-mg increments using a twice daily dosing schedule to a maximum dose of 400 mg as side effects allow and efficacy dictates. Like other anticonvulsants, this drug should be discontinued slowly to avoid any rebound effect.

Topiramate (Topamax)

With demonstrated efficacy in the treatment of the pain associated with diabetic polyneuropathy, topiramate is a reasonable next choice for those patients with neuropathic pain who have not responded to the tricyclic antidepressants—either alone or in combination with other anticonvulsants (Fig. 115–6).[8,9] Topiramate's mechanism of action is thought to be related to its ability to modulate the voltage-dependent sodium channel and, in part, to its ability to inhibit carbonic anhydrase. Topiramate is well absorbed orally with its absorp-

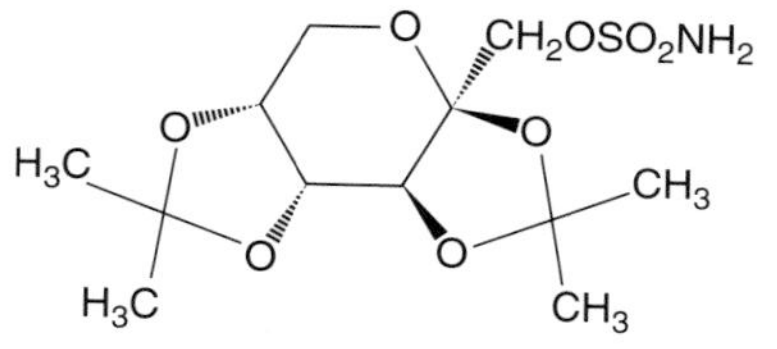

Topiramate

FIGURE 115–6 ■ Chemical structure of topiramate.

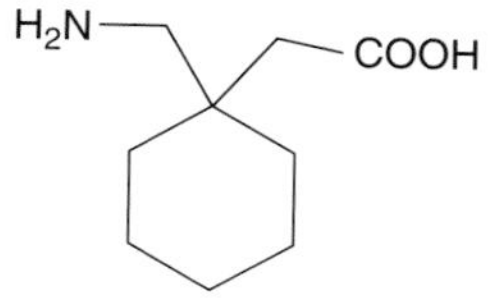

Gabapentin

FIGURE 115–7 ■ Chemical structure of gabapentin.

tion unaffected by food. Topiramate is not extensively metabolized, and approximately 70% is primarily eliminated unchanged in the urine. Available in tablet and sprinkle formulations, topiramate is dispensed in a variety of dosages making titration easy. A reasonable starting dose of topiramate is 25 mg at bedtime. The dosage is then increased in weekly intervals by 25 mg with a twice daily dosing schedule to a maximum dose of 400 mg as side effects allow and efficacy dictates. Central nervous system side effects similar to carbamazepine occur in approximately 15% of patients taking topiramate. Like other anticonvulsants, this drug should be discontinued slowly to avoid any rebound effect.

■ CATEGORY 2 ANTICONVULSANTS

Category 2 anticonvulsants are drugs whose primary mechanism of action is unrelated to modulation of the voltage-dependent sodium channel. They comprise gabapentin, tiagabine, and valproic acid.

Gabapentin (Neurontin)

One of the most extensively used anticonvulsants in the management of neuropathic pain, gabapentin has proven efficacy in the management of diabetic polyneuropathy, postherpetic neuralgia, phantom limb pain, and pain following spinal cord injury (Fig. 115–7).[10-13] An analog of gamma-aminobutyric acid (GABA), gabapentin is thought to exert its analgesic effect by modulating high-voltage calcium channels as well as interacting at the NMDA receptors. Generally well tolerated, gabapentin's oral absorption is not dose dependent in that as the oral dose increases, the proportion that is absorbed decreases. Less than 3% of orally administered gabapentin is protein bound with negligible drug metabolism. The drug is excreted unchanged in the urine. Treatment with gabapentin is begun with a 100-mg bedtime dose and then increased on a weekly basis by 100-mg increments using a four times a day dosing schedule. Gabapentin can be increased to a maximum dose of 3600 mg as side effects allow and efficacy dictates.

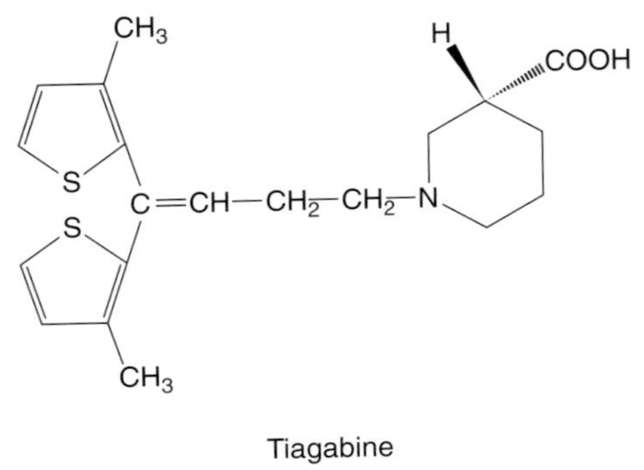

FIGURE 115–8 ■ Chemical structure of tiagabine.

Central nervous system side effects are similar to the other anticonvulsants, but are generally milder. Occasional gastrointestinal side effects including nausea and gastrointestinal upset can occur. Like other anticonvulsants, this drug should be discontinued slowly to avoid any rebound effect.

Tiagabine (Gabitril)

A number of anecdotal reports have suggested that tiagabine may be efficacious in the treatment of neuropathic pain (Fig. 115–8).[14] Tiagabine blocks *GABA uptake* into *presynaptic* neurons, permitting more *GABA* to be available for *receptor* binding on the surfaces of post-synaptic cells. Some investigators have suggested that tiagabine is especially effective in preventing the wind-up phenomenon often seen in many neuropathic pain states. Well absorbed orally, fatty food may decrease absorption and should be avoided when taking the drug. Like phenytoin, tiagabine is highly protein bound and the possibility for drug/drug interactions with other highly protein-bound drugs exists. Tiagabine is partially metabolized in the liver and is excreted in the feces and urine. Therapy with tiagabine should begin with a 4-mg daily dose with the dose being increased in weekly intervals by 4 mg to a maximum dose of 56 mg as side effects allow and efficacy dictates. Side effects of tiagabine include dizziness, sedation, difficulty thinking, and gastrointestinal intolerance. Reports of painful urination and hematuria have also been associated with the use of tiagabine. Like other anticonvulsants, this drug should be discontinued slowly to avoid any rebound effect.

Divalproex Sodium (Depakote)

Divalproex sodium, which is metabolized to valproic acid in the gastrointestinal tract, has been used to treat a variety of neuropathic pain syndromes.[15] Although its mechanism of action has not yet been established, it has been suggested that divalproex sodium's activity is related to its ability to increase levels of gamma-aminobutyric acid (GABA). Valproic acid is well absorbed orally and rapidly distributed throughout the body; more than 90% of the drug is strongly bound to human plasma proteins giving the potential for drug/drug interactions with other drugs that are highly protein bound. Divalproex sodium is metabolized in the liver and excreted in the urine. Central nervous system side effects are similar to those observed with tiagabine. Fatal hepatic side effects have been reported with this drug and patients started on divalproex sodium require careful monitoring of liver function studies throughout therapy. Like other anticonvulsants, this drug should be discontinued slowly to avoid any rebound effect.

■ CONCLUSION

The anticonvulsant compounds have demonstrable efficacy in the treatment of a variety of neuropathic pain syndromes. Much like the antidepressants, the art of using these drugs correctly is paramount if high levels of patient compliance and satisfaction and the avoidance of potentially serious side affects are to be achieved. The admonition to "start low and go slow" is quite apt when contemplating starting a patient on an anticonvulsant drug to treat neuropathic pain. An initial dose of 250 mg bid for a period of 7 to 10 days represents a reasonable starting dose. The dosage may be slowly increased to a maximum of 250 mg qid. Clear and frequent communication with the patient emphasizing the "trial and error" nature of the use of this class of drugs is mandatory to avoid noncompliance. Maintaining a positive and hopeful attitude toward the probability of success will often enhance the therapeutic outcome for the patient in this challenging clinical setting.

References

1. Black JA, Dib-Hajj S, Cummins TR, et al: Sodium channels as therapeutic targets in neuropathic pain. In Hansson PT, Fields HC, Hill RG, Marchettini P (eds): Neuropathic Pain: Pathophysiology and Treatment. Progress in Pain Research and Management, vol 21. Seattle, IASP Press, 2001.
2. Killian JM, Fromm GH: Carbamazepine in the treatment of neuralgia. Use of side effects. Arch Neurol 19:129, 1968.
3. Nicol C: A four-year double-blind randomized study of Tegretol in facial pain. Headache 9:54, 1969.
4. Waldman SD: Glossopharyngeal neuralgia. In Waldman SD: Atlas of Uncommon Pain Syndromes. Philadelphia, Saunders, 2003, p 36.
5. Klamt J, Posner J: Effects of lamotrigine on pain-induced chemo-somatosensory evoked potentials. Anaesthesia 54:774, 1999.
6. McCleane GA: Prospective audit of the use of lamotrigine in 300 chronic pain patients. Pain Clinic 11:97, 1998.
7. Simpson DM, McArthur JC, Olney R, et al: Lamotrigine for HIV-associated painful sensory neuropathies: A placebo-controlled trial. Neurology 60:1508, 2003.
8. Raskin P, Donofrio PD, Rosenthal NR, et al: Topiramate vs. placebo in painful diabetic neuropathy: Analgesic and metabolic effects. Neurology 63:865, 2004.
9. Rosenfield WE: Topiramate: A review of preclinical, pharmacokinetic, and clinical data. Clin Ther 19:1294, 1997.
10. Serpell MG: Gabapentin in neuropathic pain syndromes: A randomized, double-blind, placebo-controlled trial. Pain 99:557, 2002.
11. Backonja M, Beydoun A: Gabapentin for the symptomatic treatment of painful neuropathy in patients with diabetes mellitus: A randomized controlled trial. JAMA 280:1831, 1998.
12. Rice AS, Maton S: Gabapentin in postherpetic neuralgia: A randomized, double-blind, placebo-controlled study. Pain 94:215, 2001.
13. Levendoglu F, Ogun CO, Ozerbil O, et al: Gabapentin is a first-line drug for the treatment of neuropathic pain in spinal cord injury. Spine 29:743, 2004.
14. Laughlin TM, Tram KV, Wilcox GL, Birnbaum AK: Comparison of antiepileptic drugs tiagabine, lamotrigine, and gabapentin in mouse models of acute, prolonged, and chronic nociception. J Pharmacol Exp Ther 302:1168, 2002.
15. Kochar DK, Jain N, Agarwal RP, et al: Sodium valproate in the management of painful neuropathy in type 2 diabetes: A randomized placebo-controlled study. Acta Neurol Scand 106:248, 2002.

chapter 116

Centrally Acting Skeletal Muscle Relaxants and Associated Drugs

Howard J. Waldman, Steven D. Waldman, and Katherine A. Waldman

Numerous painful conditions have associated muscle spasm. These are most frequently musculoskeletal disorders (such as muscle strain) or central nervous system disorders associated with spasticity. Various therapeutic interventions, including pharmacologic agents, have been utilized in an attempt to reduce or obliterate muscle spasm in the belief that this will secondarily alleviate pain and improve function.[1-4]

Although associated with some controversy, centrally acting skeletal muscle relaxants (SMRs) are the most frequently prescribed drugs for this purpose (Table 116–1).[5] Studies have suggested that these drugs are effective, have tolerable side effects, and can be an adjunct in the treatment of painful musculoskeletal conditions with associated muscle spasm.[5-8] Their use is limited by somnolence[9-13] and the potential for abuse and dependency.[14-17] The SMRs should not be confused with peripherally acting skeletal muscle relaxants (such as curare and pancuronium), which block neuromuscular junction function and are generally confined to use in surgical anesthesia.

MECHANISM OF ACTION

The exact mode of action of the SMRs is not known. The SMRs appear to preferentially depress polysynaptic reflexes. At higher dosages, the SMRs may influence monosynaptic reflexes. In animal studies, these drugs appear to produce their muscle-relaxation effects by inhibiting interneuronal activity and blocking polysynaptic neurons in the spinal cord and descending reticular formation in the brain.[5,10,12] In man, the SMRs do not appear to directly relax skeletal muscle. Rather, they may produce their effects through sedation, with resultant depression of neuronal activity at therapeutic doses.[6,9,12,18]

PHARMACOKINETICS

The SMRs are generally well absorbed after oral ingestion. They have a rapid onset of action, generally within 1 hour. Some SMRs may be administered parenterally, and this route yields a more rapid onset of action. The drugs undergo biotransformation in the liver and are excreted primarily in the urine as metabolites. There is significant variability between individual drugs, plasma half-life, and duration of action (Table 116–2).[10-13]

CLINICAL EFFICACY

There have been numerous clinical trials of SMRs. Unfortunately, study design deficiencies have made interpretation of results and comparisons between studies difficult. These deficiencies include ill-defined patient selection criteria, noncomparable musculoskeletal disorders studied, variability of disease severity and duration, and subjective assessment of the patient's response to therapy.[5,18-24] Despite these difficulties, certain conclusions are possible. In almost all studies, SMRs were more effective than placebo in the treatment of acute painful musculoskeletal disorders and muscle spasm. Efficacy was less consistent in the treatment of chronic disorders. When used alone, SMRs were not consistently superior to simple analgesics (for example, aspirin, acetaminophen, and nonsteroidal antiinflammatory medications) in pain relief. However, when SMRs were used in combination with an analgesic, pain relief was superior to that of either drug used alone. Comparative studies of SMR efficacy have failed to document superiority of one drug over another.[25-27]

SIDE EFFECTS

The most commonly reported side effect of the SMRs is drowsiness. Manufacturers of these agents warn against activities that require mental alertness (for example, driving, operation of machinery) while taking these medications. Other central nervous system (CNS) side effects include dizziness, blurred vision, confusion, hallucinations, agitation, and headaches. Gastrointestinal (GI) side effects have also been frequently reported, including anorexia, nausea, vomiting, and epigastric distress. Allergic reactions, including skin rash, pruritus, edema, and anaphylaxis, have also been observed. SMRs are generally not recommended for use in children or in pregnant or lactating women. Because SMRs undergo hepatic metabolism and renal excretion, they must be used cautiously in patients with compromised hepatic or renal

Table 116–1

Commonly Used Centrally Acting Skeletal Muscle Relaxants

Generic Name	*Brand Name*
Carisoprodol	Soma
Chlorphenesin	Maolate
Chlorzoxazone	Paraflex, Parafon Forte DSC
Cyclobenzaprine	Flexeril
Metaxalone	Skelaxin
Methocarbamol	Robaxin
Orphenadrine	Norflex
Tizanidine	Zanaflex

Table 116–2

Skeletal Muscle Relaxant Onset of Action, Duration, and Half-Life

Drug	*Onset*	*Duration (hr)*	*Half-life*
Carisoprodol	30 min	4-6	8 hr
Chlorphenesin	30 min	NR	2.5-5 hr
Chlorzoxazone	1 hr	3-4	1-2 hr
Cyclobenzaprine	1 hr	4-6	2-3 hr
Metaxalone	30 min	NR	1-2 hr
Methocarbamol	1 hr	4-5	14 hr
Orphenadrine	1 hr	12-24	1-3 days

Data are based on oral administration.
NR, duration of action not reported.
From Basmajian JV: Acute back pain and spasm: A controlled multicenter trial of combined analgesic and antispasm agents. Spine14:438, 1989.

function. SMRs should be used cautiously in combination with alcohol and other CNS depressants because their effects may be cumulative.[9-13] Excessive doses of SMRs may result in significant toxicity with CNS depression consisting of stupor, coma, respiratory depression, and even death.[14,17-28] Abrupt cessation of some SMRs may cause withdrawal symptoms similar to barbiturate or alcohol withdrawal.

POTENTIAL FOR ABUSE

It has been recently recognized that SMRs have the potential for abuse and dependence. Although abuse potential of the SMRs is less than that for benzodiazepines or opioids, numerous incidences have been reported in the medical literature.[14,17,29-31]

The SMRs may be the primary drug of abuse, presumably to obtain their sedative or mood-altering effects. More frequently, SMRs are used in combination with other CNS depressants, such as opioids or alcohol. These combinations may be taken to prolong the effect of the opioid or benzodiazepines or achieve the same effect with a lesser amount of the primary drug of abuse. Prescriptions for the SMRs are more readily obtainable than prescriptions for opioids or benzodiazepines and elicit less suspicion when they are frequently refilled.[14,15,17] Because of their potential for abuse, it has been recommended that SMRs be prescribed only for acute conditions and for short periods of time. The SMRs should be used cautiously in known or suspected drug abusers, especially if they are already using other CNS depressants.

INDIVIDUAL SKELETAL MUSCLE RELAXANTS

Carisoprodol (Soma)

Carisoprodol is a precursor of meprobamate (Miltown and Equanil), and meprobamate is one of the three primary metabolites produced by hepatic biotransformation. Meprobamate dependency secondary to carisoprodol usage has been reported with associated drug-seeking behavior and withdrawal symptoms. Withdrawal symptoms are similar to those seen in withdrawal from barbiturates and include restlessness, anxiety, insomnia, anorexia, and vomiting. Severe withdrawal symptoms have included agitation, hallucinations, seizures, and, rarely, death. Because of this potential for physical dependency, carisoprodol should be tapered rather than abruptly discontinued following long-term use. Idiosyncratic adverse effects include weakness, speech disturbances, temporary visual loss, ataxia, and transient paralysis.

The onset of action of carisoprodol is 30 minutes. The plasma half-life is 8 hours and the duration of action is 4 to 6 hours. The drug is supplied as 350-mg tablets and the recommended dose is one tablet taken four times daily. Carisoprodol is also available in combination with aspirin (Soma Compound) or aspirin and codeine (Soma Compound with Codeine).[4,10-13]

Chlorzoxazone (Parafon Forte DSC)

Chlorzoxazone is similar to other SMRs, with the exception of a limited number of reported cases of significant hepatotoxicity in individuals taking this drug.[9,11,32] Chlorzoxazone has an onset of action within 1 hour and a plasma half-life of 1 to 2 hours. The duration of action is 3 to 4 hours. The drug is available in 250- and 500-mg caplets, and the recommended adult dosage is 250 to 750 mg taken three to four times daily. A pediatric dose of 20 mg/kg divided into three or four doses is suggested by the manufacturer.[9,11-13]

Cyclobenzaprine Hydrochloride (Flexeril)

Cyclobenzaprine is related structurally and pharmacologically to the tricyclic antidepressants (TCA). Like other SMRs, cyclobenzaprine produces its effects within the CNS, primarily at the brain stem level. Like the TCAs, cyclobenzaprine has anticholinergic properties and may cause dry mouth, blurred vision, increased intraocular pressure, urinary retention, and constipation. The drug should, therefore, be used with caution in individuals with angle-closure glaucoma or prostatic hypertrophy. As with other TCAs, cyclobenzaprine should not be used in patients with cardiac arrhythmias, conduction disturbances, congestive heart failure, or during the acute phase of recovery from myocardial infarction. Cyclobenzaprine may interact with monoamine oxidase inhibitors and should not be used concurrently or within 14 days of discontinuation of these drugs. Withdrawal symptoms consisting of nausea, headache, and malaise have been reported following abrupt cessation of cyclobenzaprine after prolonged use.[9,11-13,28]

Cyclobenzaprine has an onset of action within 1 hour. The plasma half-life is 1 to 3 days and the duration of action is 12 to 24 hours. Cyclobenzaprine is supplied as 10-mg tablets and has a recommended dose of 10 mg three times per day. Up to 40 mg daily in divided doses may be prescribed.[9,11-13,28]

Metaxalone (Skelaxin)

Metaxalone is comparable in effect to the other SMRs. Adverse effects are also similar, with the exception of drug-associated hemolytic anemia and impaired liver function. Hepatotoxicity associated with metaxalone has not been as severe as that reported with chlorzoxazone. Monitoring of liver function is recommended with long-term usage. Metaxalone has an onset of action of 1 hour, a plasma half-life of 2 to 3 hours, and a duration of action of from 4 to 6 hours. This drug is supplied as 400-mg tablets and has a recommended dose of 800 mg three to four times daily.[9,11-13]

Methocarbamol (Robaxin)

Methocarbamol is available in oral and parenteral form for intravenous (IV) or intramuscular (IM) injection. Subcutaneous injection is not recommended. Taken orally, this drug is similar to the other SMRs. Parenteral use of methocarbamol has been associated with pain, sloughing of skin, and thrombophlebitis at the injection site. Additionally, overly rapid IV injection has been associated with syncope, hypotension, bradycardia, and convulsions. Because of the risk of convulsion, parenteral use of the drug is not recommended for use in patients with epilepsy.

Onset of action is 30 minutes following oral ingestion and is almost immediate following parenteral administration. The plasma half-life of the drug is 1 to 2 hours. The duration of action has not been reported. Methocarbamol is produced in 500- and 750-mg tablets and has a recommended dosage range of 4000 to 4500 mg daily in three to four divided doses. For severe conditions, dosage as high as 6 to 8 g may be given for the first 48 to 72 hours. This drug is available for IV or IM injection in 10-mL single-dose vials containing 10 mg/mL. Methocarbamol tablets are also available in combination with aspirin (Robaxisal).[9,12-15]

Orphenadrine Citrate (Norflex)

Orphenadrine is an analog of the antihistamine diphenhydramine (Benadryl). Orphenadrine shares some of the antihistaminic and anticholinergic effects of diphenhydramine. Unlike the other SMRs, orphenadrine produces some independent analgesic effects that may contribute to its efficacy in relieving painful skeletal muscle spasm. In addition to adverse effects commonly associated with other SMRs, dry mouth, blurred vision, and urinary retention may occur as a result of the drug's anticholinergic activity. Rare instances of aplastic anemia have been reported. Like methocarbamol, orphenadrine is available for IV or IM injection. Anaphylactoid reactions have been reported following parenteral administration.

Orphenadrine has an onset of action of 1 hour following oral administration. Onset of action is approximately 5 minutes after IM injection and is almost immediate with IV administration. The drug's plasma half-life is 14 hours with a duration of action of 4 to 6 hours. Orphenadrine is available in 100-mg tablets with a recommended dose of one tablet twice daily. Orphenadrine is available for parenteral use in 2-mL ampules containing 60 mg of the drug and is also administered once every 12 hours. Orphenadrine tablets are also produced in combination with aspirin and caffeine (Norgesic and Norgesic Forte, respectively).[9-13,31]

Tizanidine Hydrochloride (Zanaflex)

Tizanidine hydrochloride is a centrally acting α_2-adrenergic agonist. Tizanidine is thought to exert its antispasticity properties by increased presynaptic inhibition of motor neurons; this reduces facilitation of spinal motor neuron firing. There does not appear to be any direct effect on the neuromuscular junction or any direct effect on skeletal muscle fibers by tizanidine. The drug is well absorbed after oral administration with a half-life of approximately 2.5 hours. Tizanidine is metabolized by the liver and 95% is excreted in the urine and feces. The drug is available in 2-mg and 4-mg tablets for oral administration.

Because of the drug's short half-life, it must be administered on an every 6 to 8 hour dosing schedule. Because of the common side effects of weakness and sedation, it is best to start the patient on a 2-mg bedtime dose and then titrate upward every 4 to 6 days in 2-mg doses given every 6 to 8 hours. Faster upward titration is best accomplished in an inpatient setting. The maximum daily divided dose should not exceed a total of 36 mg.

ASSOCIATED DRUGS USED IN THE TREATMENT OF MUSCLE SPASM AND SPASTICITY

Two additional drugs with muscle relaxant effects may be useful in the treatment of the pain patient, specifically the benzodiazepine, diazepam, and the antispasmodic agent, baclofen. A third drug, dantrolene sodium, a peripherally acting spasmolytic agent, is limited to controlling chronic spasticity associated with upper motor neuron (UMN) disorders. Finally, the cinchona alkaloid, quinine sulfate, may help to reduce nocturnal leg cramps. A discussion of each drug follows.

Diazepam (Valium)

Diazepam is the most frequently prescribed benzodiazepine utilized in the treatment of muscle spasm and pain.[33] Other available benzodiazepines have not been proven superior to diazepam for this use.[10,33] Diazepam has anxiolytic, hypnotic, and antiepileptic properties in addition to its antispasmodic actions.

The muscle relaxant effects of this drug are thought to result from enhancement of gamma-aminobutyric acid (GABA)-mediated presynaptic inhibition at spinal and supraspinal sites. Numerous studies have been performed comparing diazepam to placebo and to other SMRs in the treatment of painful musculoskeletal disorders. Results have been inconsistent; in general, however, diazepam has been found to be superior to placebo, but not consistently superior to other SMRs in the relief of muscle spasm and pain.[5-21,33-35] Diazepam did appear to offer greater relief of associated anxiety than the other SMRs tested.[5,6,33] Diazepam is superior, however, to other SMRs in the treatment of spasticity associated with CNS disorders such as spinal cord injury and cerebral palsy.[11,12,36,37] Efficacy is similar to baclofen and dantrolene sodium for the latter use. Diazepam's long-term use in these disorders is limited primarily by sedation, abuse potential, and dependence.[36,38]

Diazepam is well absorbed from the GI tract although it may also be administered via IV or IM injection. The drug undergoes biotransformation in the liver and is excreted in the urine. Diazepam is highly lipid soluble and rapidly crosses the blood-brain barrier. Onset of action is rapid following oral and parenteral administration. Diazepam's plasma half-life is 20 to 50 hours and active metabolites of the drug have plasma half-lives ranging from 3 to 200 hours. Duration of action is variable, depending on rate and extent of drug distribution and elimination.

Abuse and dependence have been reported with the use of diazepam and the other benzodiazepines. The incidence of these problems is somewhat controversial. The potential for abuse varies among individuals and also varies with dosages and length of therapy.[33,39-41] Withdrawal symptoms may occur with abrupt cessation of the drug and are similar to symptoms of barbiturate or alcohol withdrawal, including anxiety, dysphoria, insomnia, diaphoresis, vomiting, diarrhea, tremor, and seizures. Diazepam may have an additive effect when taken with other CNS depressants. Diazepam may have reduced plasma clearance and an increased half-life when taken in combination with disulfiram (Antabuse) or cimetidine (Tagamet).

Diazepam's most common adverse effects are related to its CNS-depressant activity: sedation, impairment of psychomotor performance, cognitive dysfunction, confusion, dizziness, and behavioral changes. Paradoxical CNS stimulation has also been reported. Other reported adverse effects include GI complaints, skin rash, blood dyscrasias, and elevation of liver enzymes. Parenteral administration has been associated with pain and thrombophlebitis at the injection site. IV and IM administration have produced more serious side effects especially in seriously ill or geriatric patients; these include cardiopulmonary depression, apnea, hypotension, bradycardia, and cardiac arrest.

Diazepam is available in 2-mg, 5-mg, and 10-mg tablets. The recommended dose for relief of painful musculoskeletal conditions is 2 to 10 mg three to four times daily. An extended-release 15-mg capsule (Valrelease) is produced and has a daily single dose of 1 to 2 capsules. Diazepam is available for parenteral administration in 2-mL ampules or 10-mL vials with 5 mg/mL. The recommended IM or IV dose is 5 to 10 mg every 3 to 4 hours as necessary.[9-13]

Baclofen (Lioresal)

Baclofen is a chemical analog of GABA, which is an inhibitory neurotransmitter. The drug produces its effects primarily by inhibiting monosynaptic and polysynaptic transmission in the spinal cord, although some supraspinal activity may also occur. Baclofen is used chiefly in the management of spasticity associated with CNS disorders such as spinal cord lesions and multiple sclerosis.[9-13] The drug is reported to be equal or superior in efficacy when compared to diazepam and dantrolene sodium. It is less sedating than diazepam and has fewer serious side effects than dantrolene sodium.[12,36,38,42,43] Baclofen may be administered intrathecally to manage severe spasticity in patients who are intolerant to, or who do not respond to, oral therapy.[44-48]

Baclofen has been useful in the treatment of trigeminal neuralgia. Because of a more favorable side-effect profile, some researchers consider baclofen to be the drug of first choice in the treatment of this condition. The coadministration of baclofen and carbamazepine may be more effective than either drug used singly owing to a synergistic effect; however, adverse effects may be cumulative.[33,49-51] L-Baclofen has been reported to be more effective and have fewer side effects than racemic baclofen.[52]

Baclofen is well absorbed from the GI tract and undergoes limited hepatic biotransformation. Most of the drug is excreted unchanged in the urine. Onset of action is highly variable, ranging from hours to weeks. The drug has a plasma half-life of 2.5 to 4 hours. Onset of action following intrathecal injection is 0.5 to 1 hour.

The most frequent side effects associated with the use of baclofen are drowsiness, dizziness, weakness, confusion, nausea, and hypotension. Side effects may be minimized by starting the drug at a low dose and gradually increasing it to the desired level. Abrupt discontinuation of the drug has been associated with hallucinations, psychiatric disturbances, and seizures; therefore, the drug should be gradually withdrawn.[9,10,53] Baclofen is produced in 10- and 20-mg tablets. The recommended starting dose is 5 mg three times daily for 3 days with an incremental increase of 5 mg per dose every 3 days. The therapeutic range is 40 to 80 mg daily.[9-13]

Dantrolene Sodium (Dantrium)

Dantrolene sodium is a peripherally acting skeletal muscle relaxant that produces its effect on skeletal muscle by interfering with the release of calcium ions from the sarcoplasmic reticulum. The primary indication for this drug is reduction of spasticity associated with upper motor neuron disorders, including spinal cord injury, stroke, multiple sclerosis, and cerebral palsy. It is also used in the treatment of malignant hyperthermia by reducing the hypometabolic processes associated with this disorder. Dantrolene sodium is not indicated in the treatment of other painful musculoskeletal disorders.[10-13]

Dantrolene sodium is incompletely absorbed from the GI tract. It is metabolized by the liver and is excreted in the urine primarily as metabolites. Onset of action may require a week or more in the treatment of CNS-associated spasticity. The drug's plasma half-life is 8.7 hours. The most frequent side effects associated with its use are muscle weakness, drowsiness, dizziness, malaise, and diarrhea, which may be severe. Serious idiosyncratic and hypersensitive hepatocellular injury may occur that may be fulminant and fatal. This has occurred most frequently in women older than the age of 35 years. The drug is supplied in 25-mg, 50-mg, and 100-mg tablets. For treatment of spasticity, the recommended starting dose is 25 mg, which is gradually increased to a maximum daily dose of 400 mg.[9-13,18]

Quinine Sulfate (Quinamm)

Quinine sulfate is a cinchona alkaloid best known for its use as an antimalarial. Although controversial, many clinicians believe that the drug is useful in the treatment of nocturnal leg cramps.[54-57] The drug reportedly produces its effect on skeletal muscle via an increased refractory period, reduced excitability of the motor end plate to acetylcholine, and redistribution of calcium within the muscle fiber. After oral ingestion, the drug is well absorbed, metabolized by the liver, and excreted in the urine. Quinine sulfate has a plasma half-life of 4 to 5 hours.

Some individuals are hypersensitive to quinine sulfate and develop thrombocytopenic purpura, which may be life threatening. Visual disturbances, nausea, vomiting, and skin rash have also been reported. The drug may increase plasma levels of digoxin and may potentiate the effects of neuromuscular blocking agents owing to its curariform-like effects. Cinchonism does not usually occur at doses used to treat leg cramps. The drug is supplied as 260-mg tablets and the recommended dose is one or two tablets nightly.[9-12]

SUMMARY

The centrally acting skeletal muscle relaxants are efficacious in the treatment of painful musculoskeletal disorders. They are generally more effective in combination with analgesics and may potentiate the effects of other CNS depressants. Their use may be limited by sedation and other undesirable side effects, as well as by their potential for abuse and dependence. Diazepam may also be useful as a muscle relaxant and an anxiolytic, but it also causes sedation and has potential for abuse. Baclofen is used primarily to treat spasticity due to CNS lesions. It is also useful in the treatment of trigeminal neuralgia and may be the drug of first choice for this condition. Dantrolene sodium is a peripherally acting agent used to treat spasticity. It is not useful in the treatment of other painful musculoskeletal disorders. Quinine sulfate is an antimalarial that may be useful in the treatment of nocturnal leg cramps. Numerous evaluations have failed to demonstrate clear superiority of one skeletal muscle relaxant over another. Practitioners should base their choice of an agent on careful consideration of individual variables in a given clinical situation.

References

1. Basmajian JV: Acute back pain and spasm: A controlled multicenter trial of combined analgesic and antispasm agents. Spine14:438, 1989.
2. Dillin W, Uppal GS: Analysis of medications used in the treatment of cervical disk degeneration. Orthop Clin North Am 23:421, 1992.
3. Butler SH: Pharmacologic treatment of low back pain. Neurosurg Clin North Am 2:891, 1991.
4. DiPalma JR, DiGregorio GJ: Management of low back pain by analgesics and adjuvant drugs. Mt Sinai J Med 58:101, 1991.
5. Elenbaas JK: Centrally acting oral skeletal muscle relaxants. Am J Hosp Pharm 37:1313, 1980.
6. Stanko JR: A review of oral skeletal muscle relaxants for the craniomandibular disorder (CMD) practitioner. J Craniomandib Prac 8:234, 1990.
7. Cullen AP: Carisoprodol (Soma) in acute back conditions: A double-blind, randomized, placebo-controlled study. Curr Ther Res Clin Exp 20: 557, 1976.
8. Roszkowaki AP: A pharmacological comparison of therapeutically useful centrally-acting skeletal muscle relaxants. J Pharmacol Exp Ther 129:75, 1970.
9. Physicians' Desk Reference. Chicago: Montvale, NJ, Thompson, 2006.
10. Drug information for the health care professional. United States Pharmacopeial Convention, Rockville, Md, 1993.
11. McEvoy GK, Litvak K, Welsh OH, Kester LS: AHFS drug information. Bethesda, Md. American Society of Hospital Pharmacists, 1993.
12. American Medical Association. AMA drug evaluations. Chicago, American Medical Association, 1993.
13. Drug Facts and Comparisons. Philadelphia, Wolters Kluwer, 2006.
14. Littrell RA, Hayes LR, Stillner V: Carisoprodol (Soma): A new and cautious perspective on an old agent. South Med J 86:753, 1993.
15. Preston KL, Guarino JJ, Kirk WT, Griffiths RR: Evaluation of the abuse potential of methocarbamol. J Pharmacol Exp Ther 248:1146, 1989.
16. Littrell RA, Safe T, Miller W: Meprobamate dependence secondary to carisoprodol (Soma) use. Am J Drug Alcohol Abuse 19:133, 1993.
17. Elder NC: Abuse of skeletal muscle relaxants. Am Fam Physician 44:122S, 1991.
18. Gilman AG, Rail TW, Nies AS, Taylor P: The Pharmacological Basis of Therapeutics. New York, Pergamon, 1990.
19. Dent W, Ervin DK: Relief of acute musculoskeletal symptoms with intravenous methocarbamol (Robaxin injectable): A placebo-controlled study. Curr Ther Res Clin Exp 20:661, 1976.
20. Hunskaar S, Donnell D: Clinical and pharmacological review of the efficacy of orphenadrine and its combination with paracetamol in painful conditions. J Int Med Res 19:71, 1991.
21. Basmajian JV: Cyclobenzaprine hydrochloride effect on skeletal muscle spasm in the lumbar region and neck: Two double-blind controlled clinical and laboratory studies. Arch Phys Med Rehabil 59:58, 1978.
22. Katz WA, Dube J: Cyclobenzaprine in the treatment of acute muscle spasm: Review of a decade of clinical experience. Clin Ther 10:216, 1988.
23. Swannell PA, Doherty M: Chlormezanone in primary fibromyalgia syndromes: A double-blind placebo controlled study. Br J Rheumatol 32: 55, 1993.
24. Deyo RA: Conservative therapy for low back pain: Distinguishing useful from useless therapy. JAMA 250:1057, 1983.
25. Gready DM: Parafon Forte versus Robaxisal in skeletal muscle disorders: A double-blind study. Curr Ther Res 20:666, 1976.
26. McGuinness BW: A double-blind comparison in general practice of a combination tablet containing orphenadrine citrate and paracetamol (Norgesic) with paracetamol alone. J Int Med Res 11:42, 1983.
27. Scheiner JJ: Evaluation of a combined muscle relaxant-analgesic as an effective therapy for painful skeletal muscle spasm. Curr Ther Res 14:168, 1972.
28. O'Riordan W, Gillette P, Calderon J, Stennes RL: Overdose of cyclobenzaprine, the tricyclic muscle relaxant. Am Emerg Med 15:592, 1986.
29. Grosshandler S: Letter to the editor. Headache Q 3:4, 1992.
30. National Institute on Drug Abuse Statistical Series: Data from the Drug Abuse Warning Network (DAWN). Rockville, Md: Department of Health and Human Services, ser 1, no. 7, 1988.
31. Millar WM: Deaths after overdoses of orphenadrine. Lancet 2:566, 1977.
32. Powers BJ, Cattail EL, Zimmerman HJ: Chlorzoxazone hepatotoxic reactions. Arch Intern Med 146:1183, 1986.
33. Raj PP: Practical management of pain. St Louis, Mosby Year Book, 1992.
34. Brown BR, Womble J: Cyclobenzaprine in intractable pain syndromes with muscle spasm. JAMA 240:1151, 1978.
35. Aiken DW: A comparative study of the effects of cyclobenzaprine, diazepam, and placebo. Postgrad Med J 34, 1978.
36. Rudick RA, Schiffer RB, Herndon RM: Drug treatment of multiple sclerosis. Semin Neurol 7:150, 1987.
37. Davidoff RA: Antispasticity drugs: Mechanisms of action. Ann Neurol 17:107, 1985.
38. Rice GPA: Pharmacothcrapy of spasticity: Some (theoretical and practical) considerations. Can J Neurol Sci 14:510, 1987.

39. Murphy SM, Tyrer P: A double-blind comparison of the effects of gradual withdrawal of lorazepam, diazepam and bromazepam in benzodiazepine dependence. Br J Psychiatry 158:511, 1991.
40. Ayd FJ: Benzodiazepine dependence and withdrawal. JAMA 242:1401, 1979.
41. Ricklcs K, Case WG, Downing RW: Long-term diazepam therapy and clinical outcome. JAMA 250:767, 1983.
42. Smith CR, LaRocca MG, Giesser BS, Schcinberg LC: High-dose oral baclofen: Experience in patients with multiple sclerosis. Neurology 41:1829, 1991.
43. Karzung BG (ed): Basic and Clinical Pharmacology. Norwalk, Conn, Appleton and Lange, 1992.
44. Penn RD: Intrathecal baclofen for spasticity of spinal origin: Seven years of experience. J Neurosurg 77:236, 1992.
45. Hankey GJ, Stewart-Wynne EG, Perlman D: Intrathecal baclofen for severe spasticity. Med J Aust 147:261, 1987.
46. Lazorthes Y, Sallerin-Caute B, VerdieJC: Chronic intrathecal baclofen administration for control of severe spasticity. J Neurosurg 72:393, 1990.
47. Loubser PG, Narayan RK, Sandin KJ: Continuous infusion of intrathecal baclofen: Long-term effects on spasticity in spinal cord injury. Paraplegia 29:48, 1991.
48. Ochs G, Struppler A, Meyerson BA: Intrathecal baclofen for long-term treatment of spasticity: A multicentre study. J Neurol Neurosurg Psychiatry 52:933, 1989.
49. Zakrzewska JM, Patsalos PN: Drugs used in the management of trigeminal neuralgia. Oral Surg Oral Med Oral Pathol 74:439, 1992.
50. Fromm GH: Clinical pharmacology of drugs used to treat head and face pain. Clin Neuropharmacol 8:143, 1990.
51. Fromm GH, Terrance CF, Chattha AS: Baclofen in the treatment of trigeminal neuralgia: Double-blind study and long term follow-up. Am Neurol 15:240, 1984.
52. Fromm GH, Terrance CF: Comparison L-baclofen and racemic baclofen in trigeminal neuralgia. Neurology 37:1725, 1987.
53. Yassa RY, Iskandar IIL: Baclofen-induced psychosis: Two cases and a review. J Clin Psychiatry 49: 318, 1988.
54. Kaji DM: Prevention of muscle cramps in haemodialysis patients by quinine sulphate. Lancet 2:66, 1976.
55. Fung MC, Holbrook JH: Placebo-controlled trial of quinine therapy for nocturnal leg cramps. West J Med 151:42, 1989.
56. Lim SH: Randomised double-blind trial of quinine sulphate for nocturnal leg cramp. Br J Clin Pract 40:462, 1986.
57. Warburton A: A quinine a day keeps the leg cramps away? Br J Clin Pharmacol 23:459, 1987.

chapter 117

Topical and Systemic Local Anesthetics

James E. Heavner

Local anesthetics are widely used to prevent or treat acute pain—to treat cancer, chronic, and inflammatory pain—and for diagnostic and prognostic purposes. Koller is credited with introducing local anesthetics into medical practice when he used cocaine to numb the cornea before performing surgery on the eye.[1] Drugs classified as local anesthetics reversibly block action potential propagation in axons by preventing the sodium entry that produces the potentials.[2] However, other actions of these drugs, such as antiinflammatory by interaction with G-protein receptors,[3] also are thought to be useful to prevent or treat pain. Nociceptive pain, as well as neuropathic pain, is targeted with this group of drugs. Any part of the nervous system, from the periphery to the brain, may be where local anesthetics act to produce a desired anesthetic or analgesic effect. A variety of formulations of local anesthetics, routes of administration, and methods of administration are used. The drugs are formulated commercially or by medical personnel according to intended route of administration and/or to address specific concerns or needs. In this chapter, I will provide a concise review of the pharmacology of local anesthetics. Details regarding some specific indications, e.g., dentistry, will not be considered.

CHEMISTRY

All local anesthetic molecules in clinical use have three parts: lipophilic (aromatic) end, hydrophilic (amine) end, and a link between the ends (Fig. 117–1). The link contains either an aminoester or an aminoamide bond and local anesthetics are designated as belonging to one of two groups, the aminoester-linked local anesthetics or aminoamide-linked local anesthetics. Procaine is the prototypic aminoester-linked local anesthetic and lidocaine is the prototypic aminoamide-linked local anesthetic (Fig. 117–2). Procaine was first synthesized in 1904 and lidocaine was first synthesized in 1943. Fundamental to the development of synthetic local anesthetics was isolation of cocaine from coca beans, and elucidation of its chemical structure. Synthesis of molecules with local anesthetic activity paved the way for "tinkering" with the molecules by systematically modifying chemical structure and testing for a desired result (e.g., reduced toxicity) to develop new local anesthetics. Figure 117–3 presents a chronology of the introduction of local anesthetic into clinical practice. Four aminoester-linked local anesthetics are shown in this figure: cocaine, procaine, tetracaine, and chloroprocaine. The other local anesthetics are aminoamide-linked. What is evident from the figure is that, since 1955, the focus has been on the development of aminoamide—rather than aminoester-linked—local anesthetics. Reasons for this include the allergenic potential of aminoester-linked local anesthetics and the instability of aminoester bonds.

Testing various modifications to the basic procaine and lidocaine structure revealed that increasing the molecular weight of the molecules by adding carbon atoms to either end of the structure or to the link generally increases the lipid solubility, protein binding, duration of action and toxicity, and influences biotransformation of the molecule (Figs. 117–4 and 117–5). There is a positive correlation between intrinsic local anesthetic potency and lipid solubility of local anesthetics.

Most local anesthetics have a tertiary amine on the hydrophilic end. Exceptions include prilocaine, which has a secondary amine and benzocaine, which has a primary amine. Tertiary amines have a positive charge (cation) or are uncharged (base). The ratio of cation to base is determined by the pKa of the local anesthetic and the pH of the solution. The "state" of the amine determines how well local anesthetic molecules move through biological membranes. The unchanged forms of local anesthetics pass readily through cell membranes and, hence, speed of onset of local anesthetic block, at least theoretically, is increased by increasing the concentration of uncharged local anesthetic molecules injected.

Because local anesthetics are weak bases, increasing the pH ("alkalinization") of solution increases the ratio of base to cation. The Henderson-Hasselbach equation can be used to quantitate the ratio.

$$\text{Log}([\text{cation}]/[\text{base}]) = \text{pKa (local anesthetic)} - \text{pH (solution)}$$

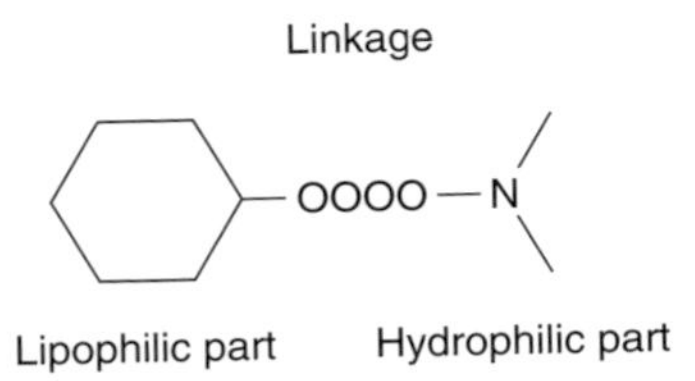

FIGURE 117–1 ■ All local anesthetic molecules in clinical use have three parts: lipophilic (aromatic) end, hydrophilic (amine) end, and a link between the ends.

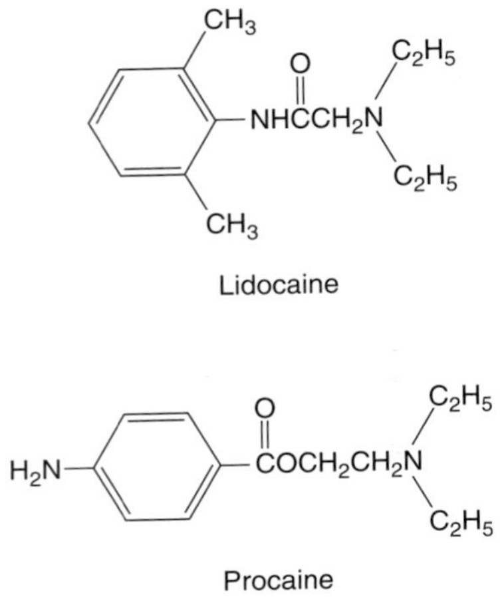

FIGURE 117–2 ■ Chemical structures of the prototypic aminoester-linked local anesthetic (procaine) and the prototypic aminoamide-linked local anesthetic (lidocaine).

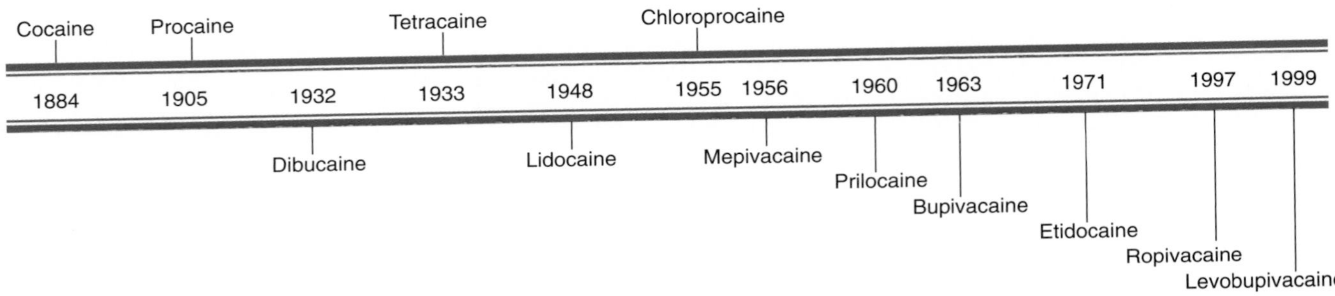

FIGURE 117–3 ■ Chronology of the introduction of different anesthetics into clinical practice. Chloroprocaine (1955) is the last aminoester-linked local anesthetic introduced that is still in clinical use. (Courtesy of David A. Scott, Melbourne, Australia.)

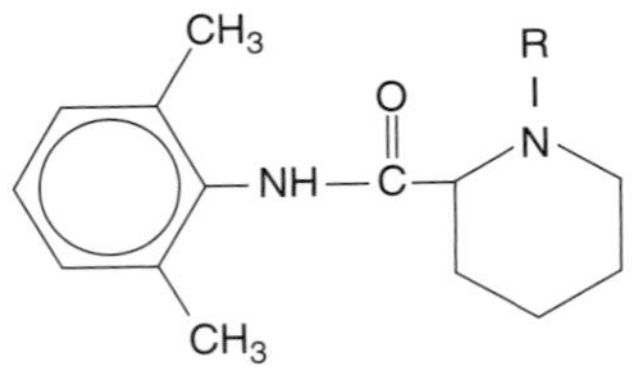

	Mepivacaine	Ropivacaine	Bupivacaine
R=	CH_3	C_3H_6	C_4H_9
Equieffective	1	0.37	0.25
Lipid/H_2O	0.8	2.8	27.5
Protein-bound (%)	77.5	94	95.6

FIGURE 117–4 ■ Results of structure alterations—amide linked. The aminoamide-linked local anesthetics mepivacaine, ropivacaine, and bupivacaine vary only by substitution at R on the basic molecule shown *above*. As the number of carbon atoms increases at R, potency, lipid solubility, and protein binding increase. (Adapted from Heavner JE: Pain mechanisms and local anesthetics: Scientific foundations for clinical practice. In Raj PP [ed]: Textbook of Regional Anesthesia. New York, Churchill Livingstone, 2002, p 105.)

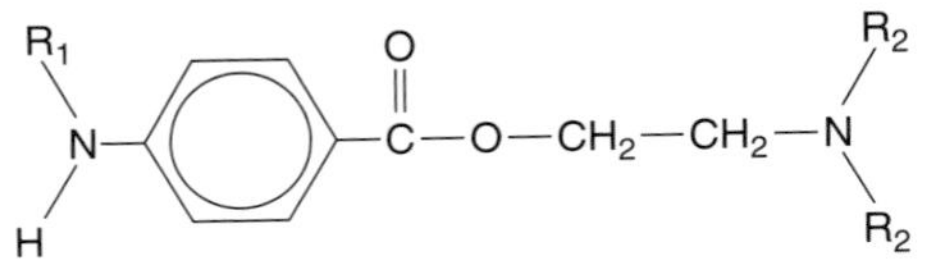

	Procaine	Tetracaine
R_1	H	C_4H_9
R_2	C_2H_5	CH_3
Hydrolysis rate (uM/ml/hr)	1.1	0.25
=potent	2	0.25
Duration (min)	50	175
LD50 (mice)	615	48

FIGURE 117–5 ■ Results of structure alterations—ester linked. The aminoester-linked local anesthetics procaine and tetracaine vary only by substitution at R1 and R2 on the basic molecule shown *above*. (Adapted from Heavner JE: Pain mechanisms and local anesthetics: Scientific foundations for clinical practice. In Raj PP [ed]: Textbook of Regional Anesthesia. New York, Churchill Livingstone, 2002, p 105.)

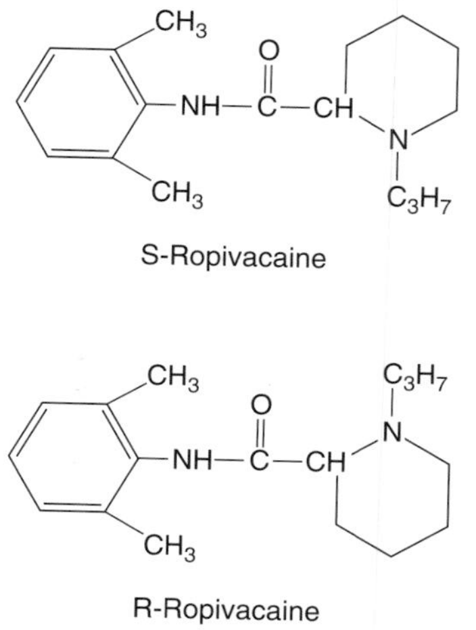

FIGURE 117–6 ■ Chisal forms of ropivacaine. The only difference between the S- and R- isomers is their spatial orientation.

Table 117–1

Anesthetic Duration and Toxicity of Local Anesthetic Isomers

Drug	*Duration*	*Toxicity*
Etidocaine	S = R	S = R
Mepivacaine	S > R	S = R
Bupivacaine	S > R	S < R
Ropivacaine	S > R	S < R

R, R enantiomer; S, S enantiomer.

Sodium bicarbonate is used clinically to increase pH of local anesthetic solutions. Important to note is that commercial solutions of local anesthetics are acidified, so the hydrophilic (cationic) state is favored. Overzealous alkalinization can cause local anesthetic molecules to precipitate from solution.

The newest additions to clinically available local anesthetics, ropivacaine (Fig. 117–6) and levobupivacaine represent (1) the exploitation of technology that permits cost-favorable separation of racemic mixtures of local anesthetics into pure enantiomers; and (2) the search for local anesthetics with greater safety margins. Simply stated, molecules with an asymmetrical carbon atom exist in forms that are mirror images (i.e., exhibit "handedness, chirality"), with images (enantiomer, stereoisomers) distinguished by how they rotate light according to the orientation of the structures in three dimensions. Various terms are used to refer to the different enantiomers; I will use S and R to designate two different enantiomers. A racemic mixture contains equal amounts of the R and S isomers. Commercial formulations of ropivacaine and levobupivacaine contain the S enantiomer. Note that levobupivacaine is the S form of bupivacaine. The motive for marketing pure enantiomers is evidence that the S form is less toxic, more potent, and longer acting than the R form or the racemic mixture (Table 117–1).

■ PHARMACODYNAMICS

Reversible block of voltage-gated sodium channels in axons is generally thought to be how local anesthetic blocks sensory and motor function. Some evidence supporting this is (1) action potentials do not develop in axons exposed to local anesthetic; (2) sodium currents responsible for generation of action potentials are blocked by these drugs; and (3) local anesthetics do not affect the transmembrane potential of axons. The "state" of the sodium channel (resting, open, inactivated) changes during the cycles of polarized, depolarized, and repolarized. The order of affinity of local anesthetics for different channel states is open > inactivated > resting. Many investigators have shown that the block of propagation of action potentials is a function of frequency of depolarization, which supports the conclusion that the open state of the sodium channel is the primary target of local anesthetic molecules. This is referred to as "state-dependent block."

There are a number of sodium channel subtypes that are generally divided into those that are tetrodotoxin sensitive (TTXs) and resistant (TTXr).[4] Most sensory neurons generate TTXs currents. However, TTXr currents are present in a high proportion of smaller dorsal root ganglion neurons associated with nociceptive A-δ and C fibers. Available evidence indicates that channels from both groups are involved in pain states as a result of changes in channel function and expression caused by disease or injury. Arguments have been put forth that local anesthetics might exert their pharmacologic action not only on Na^+ conductance, but also on other ionic conductances (e.g., K^+ and Ca^{++}).[5,6]

Differential block, the block of pain perception without motor block, for example, is observed clinically but the mechanism responsible for this is poorly understood. The clinical manifestations of differential block vary depending on the local anesthetic used.[7] For many years, differential block was ascribed to smaller axons being more sensitive than large ones to local anesthetics[8] but this "size principle" was challenged.[9] Berde and Strichartz[7] cite a number of different factors that might contribute to differential block, including anatomic, and relative sensitivity of different local anesthetics for sodium and potassium channels. Oda and colleagues[10] suggested that preferential block of tetrodotoxin-resistant sodium channels by ropivacaine in small dorsal root ganglia neurons (associated with nociceptive sensation) underlies differential block observed during epidural anesthesia with this drug.

Another pharmacodynamic puzzle is the mechanism whereby systemically administered local anesthetic relieves pain. Analgesia effect has been reported following intravenous lidocaine administration in many acute and chronic conditions.[11-18] Subcutaneously injected bupivacaine reportedly produces analgesia via a systemic effect.[19] Normal or altered sodium channels located in various areas of the brain, spinal cord, dorsal root ganglia, or in peripheral axons are mentioned most frequently as the action sites. Zhang and associates[20] reported that in rats, systemic lidocaine delivered via implanted osmotic pump reduces sympathetic nerve sprouting in dorsal root ganglion that is associated with some neuropathic pain behaviors.

Local anesthetics have effects on a number of other biological processes that are potentially important pharmacodynamic actions of value in treating pain. These include inhibition of G protein-coupled receptor signaling.[3]

Table 117–2

Disposition Kinetics in Adult Males

Local Anesthetic	*V_{dss} (L)*	*Cl (L/min)*	*$T_{1/2}$ (hr)*	*Hepatic Extraction*	*Lipid Solubility*	*Protein Binding*	*Blood/Plasma Partitioning*
Mepivacaine	84	0.78	1.9	0.40	0.8	78%	0.92
Ropivacaine	59	0.73	1.8	0.40	2.8	94%	0.69
Bupivacaine	73	0.58	2.7	0.51	27.5	96%	0.73
Lidocaine	91	0.95	1.6	0.72	2.9	60%	0.84

PHARMACOKINETICS

Usual pharmacokinetic parameters (Table 117–2) for drugs incompletely describe important details regarding distribution of local anesthetics from application sites to target and nontarget structures. It is well established that systemic absorption of local anesthetics correlates positively with the vascularity of the injection site: intravenous > tracheal > intracostal > paracervical > epidural > brachial plexus > sciatic > subcutaneous. The spinal cord meninges influence distribution of local anesthetics from the epidural and subarachnoid spaces. Intact skin is nearly a complete barrier to local anesthetic penetration. In the latter case, special local anesthetic formulations (e.g., EMLA cream, an eutectic mixture of lidocaine and prilocaine) or delivery methods (e.g., electrophoresis) are employed to facilitate transcutaneous transfer. The large number of different injection sites used by pain physicians (e.g., epidural, intrathecal, intrapleural, intraarticular, intramuscular, perineural, topical) and the variety of dosing methods (e.g., single injection, continuous infusion, intermittent infusion) make more than superficial discussion of the distribution kinetics of local anesthetics from injection sites beyond the scope of this chapter.

Aminoester-linked local anesthetics are hydrolyzed by esterases in tissues and blood. Aminoamide-linked local anesthetics are biotransformed primarily in the liver by cytochrome P-450 enzymes. Metabolites may retain local anesthetic activity and toxicity potential, albeit usually at lower potency than the parent compound.

Vasoconstrictors (e.g., epinephrine 1:400,000 [2.5 mg/mL]) are used to reduce absorption of local anesthetics into systemic circulation. The value of doing so depends on the vascularity of injection site and tissue binding of different local anesthetics. The value of the addition of sodium bicarbonate to solutions to enhance speed of onset of local anesthetics also depends on injection site as well as physiochemical properties of different local anesthetics. Addition of sodium bicarbonate increases the pH of solutions, which increases the ratio of uncharged to charged molecules. This increases the number of local anesthetic molecules in the form that most readily pass through biological membranes.

Hyaluronidase (tissue spreading factor) is sometimes added to local anesthetic solutions to facilitate spread of solution at the injection site, thereby affecting speed of onset and extending a block. This seems to be useful only when local anesthetic is injected behind the eyes preparatory to ophthalmologic surgery. Hyaluronidase may be injected with local anesthetic during epidural neurolysis to treat pain with positive benefit. An issue of *Techniques in Regional Anesthesia and Pain Medicine* (volume 8, issue 3, July 2004) discussed in detail additives to local anesthetics. Various attempts have been made to prolong the duration of action of local anesthetics by loading them into liposomes or microcapsules, but no such formulations have been approved by the U.S. Food and Drug Administration for marketing.

Localized or Systemic
Allergic Reactions

Localized
Tissue Toxicity

Systemic
Cardiac/Vascular
Central Nervous System
Methemoglobin

FIGURE 117–7 ■ Categories of local anesthetic toxic reactions.

TOXICITY

The toxic effects of local anesthetics can be categorized as shown in Figure 117–7. True allergic reactions are associated with aminoester-linked local anesthetics, not amino amide linked ones. In a study of anaphylactic and anaphylactoid reactions (n = 789) occurring during anesthesia, Mertes and coworkers[21] found no such reactions to local anesthetics. However, Mackley and colleagues[22] reported that of 183 patients patch tested, four had positive reactions to lidocaine, two of whom had histories of sensitivity to local injections of lidocaine manifested by dermatitis. They concluded that contact type IV sensitivity to lidocaine may occur more frequently than previously thought. It is common, but inappropriate, to refer to all adverse events as "allergic reactions." Tissue toxicity, primary myotoxicity and neurotoxicity can be produced by all local anesthetics if "high" concentrations are used. Signs and symptoms of varying degrees of neuropathy (e.g., transient neurologic symptoms, cauda equina syndrome) have been reported following spinal anesthesia with 2% and 5% lidocaine. A recent systematic review[23] compared the frequency of transcutaneous nerve stimulation (TNS) and neurologic complications after spinal anesthesia with lidocaine with that after other local anesthetics. They found that the risk for developing TNS after spinal anesthesia with lidocaine was higher than with bupivacaine, prilocaine, procaine, or mepivacaine.[24] Symptoms in all patients disappeared spontaneously by the tenth postoperative day. The lithotomy position seems to be a predisposing factor. In 1980, Foster and Carlson reported that of the local anesthetics tested, procaine produces the least and bupivacaine the most severe muscle injury. More recently, Zink and coworkers[25] concluded that the myotoxic

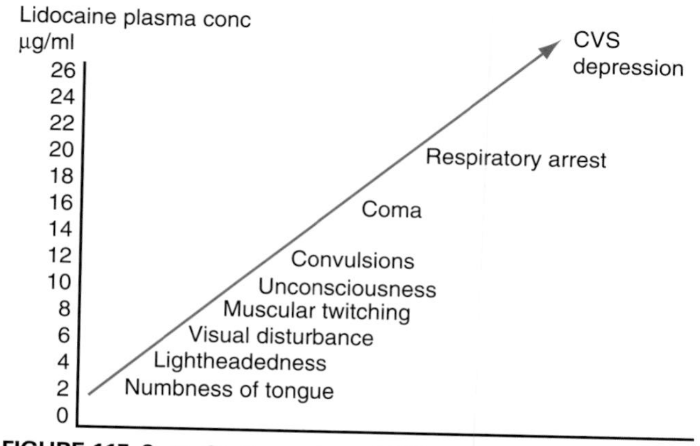

FIGURE 117–8 ■ Cardiovascular and CNS side effects of local anesthetics depending on their concentration in systemic circulation. CVS, cardiovascular system.

potential of ropivacaine is less than the potential of bupivacaine. But both drugs produce morphologically identical patterns of calcified myonecrosis, formation of scar tissue, and a marked rate of muscle fiber regeneration in animals after continuous peripheral nerve blocks.[26]

A variety of local anesthetics reportedly may produce methemoglobulinemia. Prilocaine is the local anesthetic for which there appears to be greatest risk for this to occur. As concentration of local anesthetic in systemic circulation increases, various cardiovascular system (CVS) and central nervous system (CNS) signs and symptoms appear (Fig. 117–8). The relative CVS and CNS toxicity of local anesthetics has been of interest, especially after Albright[27] reported unexpected cardiovascular toxicity of bupivacaine. In animal studies, the ratio of doses of bupivacaine that produced convulsive activity and cardiovascular collapse[7] was lower than for other local anesthetics such as lidocaine. Human volunteer studies of doses required to produce early features of CNS and CVS toxicity by ropivacaine and levo-bupivacaine demonstrated the doses were about equal and higher than for bupivacaine.[28-30]

Brown and colleagues[31] reviewed records of patients who had seizures while undergoing brachial plexus, epidural and caudal regional anesthetics. No adverse cardiovascular, pulmonary or nervous system events were associated with any of the seizures, including 16 patients who received bupivacaine blocks.

Measures to prevent systemic toxic reactions to local anesthetics include following dose recommendations, injecting aliquots over time, avoiding inadvertent intravascular injections, and monitoring vital signs during injection. Blanket recommended doses versus block specific recommended doses were discussed recently.[32,33] Drug administration must be stopped should signs or symptoms of toxicity develop. Seizures induced by local anesthetics are usually self-limiting, require maintenance of respiratory gas exchange, and control of muscle contractions (e.g., intubation, oxygenation, short acting muscle paralysis). Drugs such as propofol, thropental, and diazepam are effective against these seizures.

Cardiovascular toxicity is treated according to American Heart Association guidelines, depending on the nature of the toxicity. Recent evidence suggests that in some instances, lipid emulsion infusion may be beneficial.[34]

Table 117–3

Generic and Trade Names of Local Anesthetics

Generic Name	*Trade Name(s)*
Benoxinate	Dorsacaine; Novesine
Bupivacaine	Marcaine; Sensorcaine
Butacaine	Butyn
Chloroprocaine (2-chlorprocaine)	Nesacaine
Cyclomethycaine	Surfacaine
Dibucaine	Nupercaine; Percaine
Etidocaine	Duranest
Hexylcaine	Cyclaine
Levobupivacaine	Chirocaine
Lidocaine	Xylocaine; Xylotox
Mepivacaine	Carbocaine; Polocaine
Piperocaine	Metycaine
Prilocaine	Citanest
Procaine	Novocain
Proparacaine	Ophthaine
Ropivacaine	Undecided
Tetracaine	Pontocaine; Pantocaine

These local anesthetics are administered chiefly as the chloride or sulfate salts and it would be more accurate to specify procaine hydrochloride rather than just procaine. Because the latter is the active species, it is the commonly used term.

Adapted from de Jong RH: Local Anesthetics. St. Louis, Mosby-Year Book, 1994.

Table 117–4

Topical Local Anesthetics and Their Available Preparations

Benzocaine	**Lidocaine/prilocaine**
Cream	Cream
Ointment	**Lidocaine/tetracaine**
Topical aerosol	Patch
Benzocaine and menthol	**Pramoxine**
Lotion	Cream
Topical aerosol solution	Lotion
Butamben	**Pramoxine and menthol**
Ointment	Gel
Dibucaine	Lotion
Cream	**Tetracaine**
Ointment	Cream
Lidocaine	**Tetracaine and menthol**
Film-forming gel	Ointment
Ointment	
Patch	
Cream	

Adapted from http://www.nlm.nih.gov/medlineplus/druginfo/uspdi/202042.html

LOCAL ANESTHETICS IN CLINICAL USE

Generic and trade names of local anesthetics are listed in Table 117–3. Undoubtedly, lidocaine is most commonly used to prevent procedure-related pain and for diagnostic tests. Immediate- to long-acting local anesthetics such as ropivacaine, levobupivacaine, or bupivacaine are used for therapy. Table 117–4 lists topical anesthetics and their preparations.

Most of the forms are available without prescription. A 5% lidocaine patch (Lidoderm) is approved by the FDA for controlling postherpetic neuralgia.

References

1. de Jong RH: Local Anesthetics. St. Louis, Mosby-Year Book, 1994.
2. Hille B: Ionic Channels of Excitable Membranes, 3rd ed. Sunderland, Sinauer Associates, Inc., 2001.
3. Hollmann MW, Herroeder S, Kurz KS, et al: Time-dependent inhibition of G protein-coupled receptor signaling by local anesthetics. Anesthesiology 100:852, 2004.
4. Baker MD, Wood JN: Involvement of Na+ channels in pain pathways. Trends in Pharmacol Sci 22:1, 2001.
5. Kindler CH, Yost CS: Two-pore domain potassium channels: New sites of local anesthetic action and toxicity. Reg Anesth Pain Med 30:260, 2005.
6. Xu F, Garavito-Aguilar Z, Pecio-Pinto E, et al: Local anesthetics modulate neuronal calcium signaling through multiple sites of action. Anesthesiology 98:1139, 2003.
7. Berde CB, Strichartz GR: Local anesthetics. In Miller RD (ed): Anesthesia, 5th ed. Philadelphia, Churchill Livingstone, 2000, p 491.
8. Gisson AJ, Covino BG, Gregus J: Differential sensitivities of mammalian nerve fibers to local anesthetic agents. Anesthesiology 53:467, 1980.
9. Fink BR, Cairns A: Lack of size-related differential sensitivity to equilibrium conduction block among mammalian myelinated axons exposed to lidocaine. Anesth Analg 66:948, 1987.
10. Oda A, Ohashi H, Komori S, et al: Characteristics of ropivacaine block of Na+ channels in rat dorsal root ganglion neurons. Anesth Analg 91:1213, 2000.
11. Atkinson RL: Intravenous lidocaine for the treatment of intractable pain of adiposis dolorosa. Int J Obesity 56:351, 1982.
12. Cassuto J, Wallin G, Hagstrom S, et al: Inhibition of postoperative pain by continuous low-dose intravenous infusion of lidocaine. Anesth Analg 64:971, 1985.
13. Kastrup J, Petersen P, Dejgard A, et al: Intravenous lidocaine infusion: A new treatment of chronic painful diabetic neuropathy? Pain 25:69, 1987.
14. Glazer SAB, Portenoy K: Systemic local anesthetics in pain control. J Pain Symptom Manage 6:30, 1991.
15. Williams DR, Stark RJ: Intravenous lignocaine (lidocaine) infusion for the treatment of chronic daily headache with substantial medication overuse. Cephalalgia 23:963, 2003.
16. Finnerup NB, Biering-Sorensen F, Johannesen IL, et al: Intravenous lidocaine relieves spinal cord injury pain: A randomized controlled trial. Anesthesiology 102:1023, 2005.
17. Koppert W, Weigand M, Neumann F, et al: Perioperative intravenous lidocaine has preventive effects on postoperative pain and morphine consumption after major abdominal surgery. Anesth Analg 98:1050, 2004.
18. Attal N, Rouaud J, Brasseur L, et al: Systemic lidocaine in pain due to peripheral nerve injury and predictors of response. Neurology 62:218, 2004.
19. Duarte AM, Pospisilova E, Reilly E, et al: Reduction of postincisional allodynia by subcutaneous bupivacaine. Anesthesiology 103:113, 2005.
20. Zhang JM, Li H, Munir MA: Decreasing sympathetic sprouting in pathologic sensory ganglia: A new mechanism for treating neuropathic pain using lidocaine. Pain 109:143, 2004.
21. Mertes PM, Laxenaire MC, Alla F: Anaphylactic and anaphylactoid reactions occurring during anesthesia in France in 1999-2000. Anesthesiology 99:536, 2003.
22. Mackley CL, Marks JG, Anderson BE: Delayed-type hypersensitivity to lidocaine. Arch Dermatol 139:343, 2003.
23. Zaric D, Christiansen C, Pace NL, et al: Transient neurologic symptoms after spinal anesthesia with lidocaine versus other local anesthetics: A systematic review of randomized, controlled trials. Anesth Analg 100:1811, 2005.
24. Foster AH, Carlson BM: Myotoxicity of local anesthetics and regeneration of the damaged muscle fibers. Anesth Analg 59: 727, 1980.
25. Zink W, Seig FC, Bohl JRE, et al: The acute myotoxic effects of bupivacaine and ropivacaine after continuous peripheral nerve blockades. Anesth Analg 97:1173, 2003.
26. Zink W, Bohl JRE, Hacke N, et al: The long term myotoxic effects of bupivacaine and ropivacaine after continuous peripheral nerve blocks. Anesthesia and analgesia 101:548, 2005.
27. Albright GA: Cardiac arrest following regional anesthesia with etidocaine or bupivacaine. Anesthesiology 51:285, 1979.
28. Stewart J, Kellett N, Castro D: The central nervous system and cardiovascular effects of levobupivacaine and ropivacaine in healthy volunteers. Anesth Analg 97:412, 2003.
29. Knudsen K, Beckman-Suurkula M, Blomberg S, et al: Central nervous and cardiovascular effects of IV infusions of ropivacaine, bupivacaine and placebo in volunteers. Br J Anaesth 78:507, 1997.
30. Scott DB, Lee A, Fagan D, et al: Acute toxicity of ropivacaine compared with that of bupivacaine. Anesth Analg 69:563, 1989.
31. Brown DL, Ransom DM, Hall JA, et al: Regional anesthesia and local anesthetic-induced systemic toxicity: Seizure frequency and accompanying cardiovascular changes. Anesth Analg 81:321, 1995.
32. Heavner JE: Let's abandon blanket maximum recommended doses of local anesthetics. Reg Anesth Pain Med 29:524, 2004.
33. Rosenbert H, Veering BT, Urmey WF: Maximum recommended doses of local anesthetics: A multifactorial concept. Reg Anesth Pain Med 29:564, 2004.
34. Weinberg G, Ripper R, Feinstein DL, et al: Lipid emulsion infusion rescues dogs from bupivacaine-induced cardiac toxicity. Reg Anes Pain Med 28:198, 2003.

chapter 118

Alternative Pain Medicine

Winston C.V. Parris and Salahadin Abdi

Pain and illness continue to be the scourge of mankind even with the tremendous strides that have been made in the cure and relief of several diseases. Over the past 10 to 20 years, great progress has been made in the management of pain derived from disease, trauma, or idiopathic origin. However, pain continues to be a major problem in the very young, the very old, cancer patients, diabetic patients, post-stroke patients, and almost all patients whose disorder produces unrelenting pain. Pain in the injured worker is a major problem because of the occupational, legal, emotional, economic, political, psychosocial, and societal factors that influence or modify the patient's ultimate perception of pain.

Since the advent of the pain medicine specialty, significant developments have contributed to modest success in resolving chronic pain,[1] although much remains to be done in optimizing pain control. While we await these advances, patients become disappointed, disenchanted, and at times disgusted with the inadequacy of their pain management. This disillusionment has led many people to seek nontraditional, unconventional, and at times dangerous remedies to control pain. Unfortunately, a few unscrupulous "practitioners" take advantage of this situation, but it is heartening to note that a number of these nontraditional remedies are effective in controlling, if not eliminating, chronic pain syndromes in selected patients. This whole arena is known as alternative or complementary medicine.[2] This chapter explores the role of alternative medicine in chronic pain management and examines how these methods can contribute to traditional or conventional pain medicine.

Some traditional physicians scoff at any remedy that is not well described in standard medical textbooks or is not thoroughly investigated in peer-reviewed journals and supported by placebo-controlled, randomized, scientifically conducted studies. These methods reflect the standard approach by which medical information is disseminated and passed on from teacher to student or from colleague to colleague. If a given alternative medicine practitioner proposed that snake oil is effective for migraine headaches, most traditional physicians would laugh. This reaction would be based on the fact that no Pharmacopoeia or Physicians' Desk Reference (PDR) or medical journal describes snake oil as a pharmacologic agent or as having any therapeutic value. Yet, if snake oil were analyzed and one of its active principles were absorbed transdermally and had a specific effect on cerebral vasculature, ultimately relieving migraine headaches, this originally preposterous idea would become a multimillion-dollar scientific breakthrough. Although this hypothetical scenario is unlikely, it is possible. The major challenge is to determine how to evaluate those "preposterous ideas" that, after all, may not have any deleterious effect on a patient and may, in fact, be beneficial.

The existing scientific, medical, and academic structure does not leave much room for this kind of investigation. Except for a few cases (e.g., The University of New Mexico in Albuquerque), most medical school administrators adhere rigidly, and in many situations blindly, to the curricula handed down by tradition. Change takes place, but most changes are insignificant and do not reflect the realities of medicine today and the needs of today's patient. Thus, while recent medical school graduates may be highly skilled in many new and sophisticated techniques of medicine, they may be relatively uninformed about the principles and practice of pain medicine. A needlessly defensive posture may be adopted when new and unconventional techniques are proposed. It takes approximately 1 to 2 decades of physician experience to allow for exploration or, at least, intelligent examination of nontraditional information.

PREVALENCE OF ALTERNATIVE MEDICINE

The prevalence of alternative medicine in the United States was studied by Eisenberg and coworkers[3] and their results were published in the *New England Journal of Medicine* in 1993. They found that one in three Americans used unconventional or alternative medicine for various illnesses, most of which were associated with pain. This study also highlighted the cost of alternative medicine and the fact that most of the modalities used in alternative medicine are not subject to governmental scrutiny, regulation, or supervision. Nevertheless, a number of patients use alternative medicine as their main therapeutic option, and a majority of patients use alternative medicine along with conventional medicine, occasionally with the assent of a traditional physician. There is some regional bias, in that alternative medicine, including herbal medicine,[4] is used more commonly in the western United States and, to a lesser extent, in the southern than in the northern and eastern regions of the United States.

To address the burgeoning business of alternative medicine and its impact on citizens, the government, through the Department of Health and Human Services, created the Office of Alternative Medicine via congressional mandate under the 1992 National Institutes of Health (NIH) appropriations bill. The creation of this office was motivated by the ground swell from citizens who demanded that government look into the efficacy of nontraditional medicine and its modalities.[5]

Toward the end of the 1980s there was great interest in the Mexican herbal medicine called laetrile. Thousands of United States citizens crossed the Mexican border in search of that elusive cancer cure. Most were not successful in that search. These events, and many others like it, politicized the issue and led to the formation of the Office of Alternative Medicine. The major objective of the Office of Alternative Medicine[6] was to facilitate evaluation of alternative medical treatment modalities to determine their effectiveness in treating disease. Its congressional mandate provided for a public information clearing-house to gather and appropriately categorize information and to fund and organize research training programs for alternative medicine.

DEFINITION

In this chapter, alternative medicine may be defined as unconventional or unorthodox medical interventions not routinely taught at American medical schools or not generally available in American hospitals.[7] Some alternative therapies are benign; others are invasive. Some have been used for a long period of time; others are more recent. Some alternative therapies are well known; others are mysterious and, on occasion, dangerous. Although some alternative therapies have sound scientific principles to recommend their use in clinical practice, they may not have been subjected to the scientifically conducted placebo-controlled randomized studies that most conventional medical therapies undergo and they may not have been exposed to the peer review process necessary before any therapy is accepted as clinically useful. Thus, the claims of many alternative therapies are usually anecdotal, and, at times, inappropriate or inconsistent assumptions have been made regarding their clinical efficacy.

Alternative medicine covers a wide scope of healing philosophies, methodologic approaches, and clinical therapies. In addition to the fact that they are not taught in medical schools, most alternative medical practices are not reimbursed by medical insurance companies. This situation is changing slowly; for example, acupuncture services now not only are recognized as effective but also are reimbursed by several medical insurers.

Alternative medicine has been labeled "holistic medicine," and although there are some common areas, the comparison is not an accurate one. The term *holistic* generally implies that the health care practitioner considers the whole person, including physical, mental, emotional, and spiritual aspects. In today's health-conscious society, many therapies are labeled as "preventive," implying that the practitioner is involved primarily in educating the patient about the disease, its symptoms, its complications, and its treatment—but, even more important, is committed to instructing the patient regarding the techniques and methods of preventing the disease. Using the principle that prevention is better than cure, many preventive practitioners lay heavy emphasis on cessation of smoking, promotion of exercise, a healthy diet, and similar measures to prevent heart disease, metabolic disorders (e.g., diabetes), morbid obesity, and some forms of cancer.

Whereas some forms of alternative medicine are consistent with the fundamental physiologic principles involving the circulation and the central nervous system as understood by Western medicine, other approaches are based on different and unfamiliar healing systems. Gradually, some "non-Western" systems are being absorbed into the mainstream of Western medicine.

CLASSIFICATION

To a large extent, alternative medicine has not been evaluated or scrutinized according to accepted scientific principles or methods. Consequently, the architects of individual alternative modalities have been more concerned with acceptance and positive results rather than an open and unconditional evaluation of their efficacy. As a result, no consistent organization existed before the creation of the Office of Alternative Medicine,[6] and there were no attempts at classifying modalities used for alternative medicine. Under the aegis of the NIH, a task force was created to address classification issues. The result is seven categories of complementary or alternative medical practices, including

1. Alternative systems of practice
2. Bioelectromagnetic applications
3. Diet, nutrition, and lifestyle changes
4. Herbal medicine
5. Manual healing methods
6. Mind-body interventions
7. Pharmacologic and biological treatments

The task force also reported on corresponding issues, such as research methodology, research and training needs, the peer review process, and information dissemination activities.[7]

The classification of alternative medicine practices was designed primarily to facilitate the review process for grant allocation. It was not designed as an arbitrary or definitive classification of alternative medicine. A summary of the classification is listed in Table 118–1.

OFFICE OF ALTERNATIVE MEDICINE

Since its inception, the Office of Alternative Medicine has served a number of important functions that have helped to legitimize some modalities of alternative medicine. Most notably, it has served as an institution that compiles data and serves as a granting agency for sponsoring some of those research projects.

Other functions can be outlined as follows[8]:

1. To provide and evaluate a research data base. The research data base program provides a framework for identifying and organizing scientific literature on alternative medical practices. This literature has grown to more than 100,000 specific citations on complementary and alternative

Table 118–1

Classification of Alternative Medicine Practices

Alternative Systems of Medical Practice	
Acupuncture	***Manual Healing***
Anthroposophically extended medicine	Acupressure
Ayurveda	Alexander technique
Community-based health care practices	Aromatherapy
Environmental medicine	Biofield therapeutics
Homeopathic medicine	Chiropractic medicine
Latin American rural practices	Feldenkrais method
Native American practices	Massage therapy
Natural products	Osteopathy
Naturopathic medicine	Reflexology
Past life therapy	Rolfing
Shamanism	Therapeutic touch
Tibetan medicine	Trager method
Traditional Asian (Oriental) medicine	Zone therapy
Biolectromagnetic Applications	***Mind/Body Control***
Blue light treatment and artificial lighting	Art therapy
Electroacupuncture	Biofeedback
Electromagnetic fields	Counseling
Electrostimulation and neuromagnetic stimulation devices	Dance therapy
Low-level laser	Guided imagery
Magnetic resonance spectroscopy	Humor therapy
Diet, Nutrition, Lifestyle Changes	Hypnotherapy
Changes in lifestyle	Meditation
Diet	Music therapy
Macrobiotics	Prayer therapies
Megavitamins	Psychotherapy
Nutritional supplements	Relaxation techniques
Herbal Medicine	Support groups
Echinacea (purple coneflower)	Virtual reality
Ginger rhizome	Yoga
Ginkgo biloba extract	***Pharmacologic and Biological Treatments***
Ginseng root	Antioxidizing agents
Wild chrysanthemum flower	Cell treatment
Witch hazel	Chelation therapy
Yellow wood	Metabolic therapy
	Oxidizing agents (ozone, hydrogen peroxide)

medical topics. Currently, the program is involved in implementing a process of developing systematic reviews and meta-analyses of the alternative medicine scientific literature.

2. To serve as a clearing house of alternative medicine data. The agency disseminates information to the public, the media, and health care professionals to promote awareness and to provide education about alternative medical research.
3. To optimize media relations. The media relations section provides accurate coverage and subsequent follow-up of relevant stories on alternative medicine to the news media and provides information about the Office of Alternative Medicine and its activities for mass media audiences.
4. To facilitate sponsored research. Shortly after its inception, the agency provided 30 grants to fund research applications to study different aspects of complementary and alternative medicine.
5. To create and fund alternative medicine specialty research centers. The agency has funded 10 specialty research centers designed to study complementary and alternative medicine treatments for specific health conditions.
6. To facilitate an international and professional liaison program that participates in and promotes cooperative efforts in research and education.
7. To organize intramural research training. This program allows scientists to conduct basic and clinical research in alternative medicine and supports postdoctoral training for appropriate candidates. The agency also evaluates specific alternative medical modalities by other institutes and centers within the NIH structure. Furthermore, several other governmental agencies interact with the Office of Alternative Medicine, including the Health Care Finance Agency, the Food and Drug Administration, the Agency for Health Care Policy and Research, and the Centers for Disease Control and Prevention.

SCOPE

In an attempt to determine prevalence, costs, and patterns of use of alternative medicine in the United States, Eisenberg and colleagues[3] demonstrated that alternative modalities are used not only for chronic pain but also for cancer, arthritis, acquired immunodeficiency syndrome (AIDS), gastrointestinal problems, chronic renal failure, and eating disorders. Among the commonly used therapies were

- Relaxation techniques
- Chiropractic manipulation
- Massage
- Imagery
- Spiritual healing
- Promotional weight loss programs
- Lifestyle diets (e.g., macrobiotics, herbal medicine, megavitamin therapy)
- Self-help groups
- Energy healing
- Biofeedback
- Hypnosis
- Magnetic therapy
- Low-power laser therapy
- Homeopathy
- Acupuncture
- Folk remedies
- Exercise
- Prayer

More than 60% of the patients who used unconventional therapy did so without medical supervision and without active consultation with a provider of either conventional or unconventional therapy. The medical conditions for which most patients sought alternative therapy included back pain, allergies, arthritis, insomnia, sprains, strains, headaches, high blood pressure, digestive problems, anxiety, and depression. Most of the medical conditions listed above are associated with some form of chronic pain.

Another criterion for considering the efficacy of alternative therapeutic modalities is based on reimbursement by either patients or third-party payers. Reimbursement for alternative therapy in 1990 was approximately $11.7 billion. It is important to keep in perspective that this criterion is not a scientific index of efficacy; however, the magnitude of this sum of money does highlight the importance that patients placed on these modalities. Thus, unconventional or alternative medicine has a major presence in the American healthcare system. The magnitude of this presence may be underestimated by conventional or traditional healthcare providers, but in 1990, approximately 22 million Americans used alternative therapy modalities as a means of treating their health problems. Occasionally, these methods are used simultaneously with traditional medicine.

A satisfying observation is that most of the users of alternative therapy do not replace conventional therapy but use those alternative therapy modalities as adjuncts to conventional therapy. For example, few patients use alternative therapy modalities for the treatment of high blood pressure or digestive problems, which suggests that patients have been satisfied with the validity and efficacy of traditional therapy for these ailments. Yet many patients do use alternative medicine for the treatment of chronic back pain, headaches, arthritis, strains, or sprains.

As a part of the medical evaluation of chronic pain patients, an attempt should be made to determine whether the patient is receiving alternative therapy and the frequency, amount (units), or intensity with which that particular modality is used. Currently, medical students are being taught very little about unconventional alternative therapy.[9] Perhaps including some information about the subject in the medical school curriculum might not only broaden physicians' outlook on what patients are seeking but might also provide the sensitivity necessary to evaluate these modalities scientifically.

ALTERNATIVE THERAPY MODALITIES

Many unorthodox modalities may be effective in patient care. The laws of consumerism may be influential in dictating not only the popularity but also the longevity of various medical modalities directly related to their therapeutic efficacy. Thus, patients seldom seek an alternative modality for a fractured bone because the conventional orthopedic maneuvers for treating a fractured bone are associated with satisfactory results. Many conditions do not respond to conventional therapy and in frustration, patients are prompted to seek alternative therapy even if the therapeutic efficacy of the alternative modality is not established. Some cancer pain patients who receive satisfactory results and for whom death is imminent may seek not only unconventional treatments but also risky ones out of desperation. Many of the alternative and unconventional therapies do not fit the Western medical paradigm. More research is needed to evaluate the most widely used modalities. Although it is impossible to describe all of the modalities used in alternative medicine, a few have been arbitrarily selected and are discussed here.

Music Therapy

Schorr[10] demonstrated in a study of 30 women with chronic pain secondary to rheumatoid arthritis that chronic pain may be effectively controlled using music as a unitary-transformative intervention. Pain measurements used in the study were obtained from the Pain Rating Index rank (PRI-R) of the McGill Pain Questionnaire. Hanser[11] also described the effective use of music as a distraction during lumbar punctures. Unfortunately, this study was a series of anecdotal reports and not a scientifically conducted investigation. Nevertheless, it is reasonable to propose that for some patients with well-defined pathology, music therapy may not be effective by itself but can be a useful adjunct to conventional modalities for pain management.

Intercessionary Prayer and Spiritual Healing

Several claims have been made regarding the effectiveness of intercessionary prayer, spiritual healing, divine intercessions, and meditation in controlling chronic pain.[12] Certainly, it is not good medical practice for providers to be arbitrary about patients' respective spiritual or religious persuasions.

In fact, those persuasions may be passively supported as long as they do not interfere with the delivery of medical care necessary for treatment. Many anecdotal reports regarding the efficacy of those modalities have been made, but few scientifically controlled studies have been done to determine efficacy.

Sundblom and associates[13] in a well-conducted clinical trial, demonstrated that spiritual healing was not only harmless but was subjectively helpful in managing patients with idiopathic chronic pain syndrome. In this study, 24 patients with idiopathic chronic pain were randomly assigned to one of two groups; one group received spiritual healing, and the other received no active treatment. All patients had passed a pretreatment psychological interview. The main outcome measures used included Visual Analogue Scale, International Association for the Study of Pain (IASP) data base outline, and various psychological measures. Patients were evaluated at baseline and 2 weeks after treatment and were studied over 1½ years. A final assessment was performed at 1 year after treatment using a modified IASP data base outline, and it revealed a minor decrease in analgesic drug intake and an improvement in the sleep pattern in patients treated by the spiritual healer. The group exposed to spiritual healing also experienced a decrease in the feeling of hopelessness and an increased acceptance of psychological factors as reasons for pain. One half of the treated patients felt that spiritual healing gave them satisfactory pain relief. Although this therapeutic approach is not effective for everyone, for selected patients, particularly those with terminal illness, spiritual healing may be used as an adjunct to their conventional treatment if the patient or the family requests it.

Relaxation Therapy

Relaxation therapy is a well-established psychogenic modality for managing chronic pain. Several variations of relaxation strategies have been used. Jacobson's progressive muscle relaxation techniques[14] have been widely used to manage chronic pain syndromes, particularly myofascial pain syndromes, including low back pain.

The use of relaxation to promote comfort and pain relief in patients suffering from advanced cancer pain has been demonstrated to be effective by Sloman and coauthors.[15] Relaxation strategies, including deep breathing, muscle relaxation, and imagery, were tested as a nursing intervention for the promotion of comfort and pain relief in a group of hospitalized cancer patients. This intervention was implemented in accordance with Oren's self-care approach to nursing practice. Sixty-seven cancer patients were randomly assigned to one of three groups to receive relaxation training by audiotapes, live relaxation training by nurses, or no relaxation training at all. The relaxation training was administered twice a week over a 3-week period. All patients were tested before and after the study using the McGill Pain Questionnaire and the Visual Analogue Scale for pain. Furthermore, analgesic medication administered to the patients who received relaxation training led to significant reduction in subjective pain ratings, and there was also a significant decrease in the non-opioid, as-needed (p.r.n.) analgesic intake, which probably suggested a reduced incidence of breakthrough pain. The study suggests that relaxation techniques can be effective in chronic cancer pain management, especially when used concurrently with conventional modalities.

Hypnosis

Until recently, various modalities were considered "unconventional." With their widespread acceptance not only by the patient population but also by the medical establishment, these formerly unconventional modalities have now become conventional. Unfortunately, at times they have not undergone the clinical trials necessary to be considered truly conventional. Hypnosis and acupuncture may fall into this category.

It should be noted that some well-established medical interventions, including surgical procedures, would not be used in clinical practice today if rigorous clinical trials had been instituted. A good example is the use of epidural steroids for chronic diskogenic back pain. The use of epidural steroids has rapidly become widespread, although few well-conducted scientific studies have been carried out to evaluate their efficacy.[16] Hypnosis has been used with sufficient frequency to warrant investigation. Unfortunately, some providers of hypnotic therapy are not necessarily competent in the method's principles, applications, and nuances.[17] This is precisely the danger of using a modality that has not been rigorously subjected to peer review evaluations. Hypnotherapy or hypnotic relaxation has been used as a sedative for some medical procedures (e.g., colonoscopy). Although this procedure is not exquisitely painful, it is associated with significant emotional and physical discomfort.

Cadranel and colleagues[18] investigated the usefulness of hypnotic relaxation in 24 patients scheduled for colonoscopy in whom other forms of anesthesia were not available. Using hypnotic relaxation before the procedure resulted in moderate to deep sedation in 12 of the 24 patients. In the patients for whom hypnosis was successful, the pain and discomfort from the colonoscopy were less intense than in the patients for whom hypnosis was unsuccessful. All patients who received successful hypnotherapy were able to undergo colonoscopy uneventfully, whereas only 50% of the patients who did not receive hypnotic relaxation were able to undergo the procedure. All the patients in the successful group agreed to another examination under the same conditions using hypnotic relaxation, whereas only 2% of the patients in the unsuccessful group agreed to have hypnotic relaxation as the primary means of sedation after their experience. This study suggests that in a subgroup of hypnotizable patients, hypnotic relaxation may be a safe alternative to drug sedation for colonoscopy and related procedures.

Chiropractic Therapy

The use of chiropractic therapy is widespread in the United States and is legal. No doubt it has a place in the management of musculoskeletal dysfunction and various myofascial pain syndromes. This modality has continued to develop, and, properly conducted, it can be effective. Although research into chiropractic is not very widespread, the method is said to be much more effective than other conservative approaches, including bed rest, medication, physical therapy, and massage therapy.

Unfortunately, chiropractic practitioners and medical practitioners have not been able to work together for the good of the patient with chronic musculoskeletal dysfunction. Indeed, inappropriately applied and incompetently administered, chiropractic can be dangerous in some patients and may lead to a worsening of the patient's general condition. A classic case in point would be the application of chiropractic measures for the management of back pain in a patient not recognized as having multiple myeloma or metastatic prostate cancer. By the time the misdiagnosis is recognized, major and irreversible harm may be done. In an ideal situation, chiropractic therapy would be administered to a patient in conjunction with and concurrent with conventional medical treatment.

Comfort Measures

In addition to its being a science, medicine is also an art. In today's busy practice, physicians may appear to be uncaring, arrogant, and inattentive to a patient's real needs. The application of comfort measures goes a long way toward making patients feel comfortable and optimizing their immunosuppressant mechanisms to promote rapid healing and recuperation.[19]

Buchko and associates[20] have demonstrated that comfort measures in breast-feeding primiparous women have been very effective in treating postpartum nipple pain. This same principle may be applied to a number of relatively minor but uncomfortable procedures patients undergo, such as bone marrow biopsy, burn dressing changes, acquisition of vascular access, and cataract surgery. When properly applied, these comfort measures may obviate the need for pharmacologic intervention and may help to introduce a soft touch into a medical experience that may appear cold and uncaring.

Transcutaneous Electrical Nerve Stimulation

Initially, transcutaneous electrical nerve stimulation (TENS)[21] was thought of as a primitive alternative therapy modality. Its popularity increased after the publication of the gate control theory by Melzack and Wall.[22] In fact, a proposed mechanism of action is that electrical stimulation of A-alpha and A-beta fibers suppresses nociception transmitted by A-delta and C fibers. Many published studies show the efficacy of TENS in the management of a large number of pain syndromes[23] including myofascial, neuropathic and cancer pain.[24] Today, TENS is no longer thought to be an alternative modality and is, in fact, well established as a conventional medical modality for the treatment of chronic pain.[25] Two other variants of TENS that have not been well studied are high-frequency external muscle stimulation (HF) and percutaneous electrical nerve stimulation (PENS).

Acupuncture

Acupuncture has been used for more than 2000 years. It is based on various Chinese scientific principles that are not understood or taught in most Western medical systems, including the United States. Many publications have attested to the efficacy of acupuncture,[26] and it is clear that acupuncture does control pain in selected patients. However, patient selection must be meticulous because some patients are more predisposed to benefit from acupuncture than others. Many other intrinsic factors contribute to the success or failure of acupuncture.[27] The tragedy of acupuncture in an American or Western context is that very few practitioners are adequately trained to use this modality effectively.

Biostimulation Techniques

The various biostimulation techniques include

- Acupressure
- Auriculotherapy
- Vibration therapy
- Magnetic field therapy
- Low-power laser stimulation
- Movement therapy

A major reason for the popularity of these modalities is that they are usually noninvasive and, in appropriate patients, may be beneficial when used as adjuncts to conventional therapy. In a study of 24 patients with chronic pain, Guieu and coworkers[28] demonstrated that TENS therapy and vibration therapy, whether used singly or jointly, were more effective in providing long-lasting analgesia as compared with sham stimulation, or placebo.

Magnetic Field Therapy

First proposed by Franz Mesmer of Austria, magnetic stimuli and magnetic fields have been used medicinally since the 16th century. Mesmer's theories were investigated by a Royal Commission chaired by Lavoisier, whose recommendations were not favorable to the continued use of magnetic therapy. Since that time, magnetic field therapy has been practiced mainly by charlatans.

In the early 20th century, orthopedic surgeons often used magnetic therapy to correct malunion of long bone fractures. At that time, it was safer to use magnetic therapy than orthopedic surgery for long bone fractures, which were usually associated with osteomyelitis. Recently, many claims have been made regarding the efficacy of magnetic field blocks and magnetic fields,[29] but these have not been evaluated scientifically.

To determine the efficacy of magnetic fields, Parris and colleagues[30] investigated the chronic pain animal model (rat) using the sciatic nerve ligation or chronic constriction injury. The objective was to determine whether repeated pulsating magnetic field therapy (PMFT) would affect hyperalgesia and spinal cord, brain, and plasma levels of substance P, met-enkephalin, and dynorphin after chronic constriction injury of the rat sciatic nerve. In this study, the rats were exposed daily to 180 g and 30 Hz for 1 hour. Control rats were exposed to a device in which the magnetic fields were not activated. The magnetic fields significantly increased the delay of hind paw withdrawal and decreased the duration of the evaluation on the side of the chronic constriction injury. Magnetic field therapy did not alter the behavioral pain response in sham rats. The findings also demonstrated that dynorphin levels were greatly elevated in the spinal cord on the side of the constriction injury as compared with the contralateral (unligated) side in animals with chronic constriction injury. No significant changes were noticed in met-enkephalin and substance P levels.

The study showed that magnetic field therapy reduces hyperalgesia induced by chronic constriction injury of the sciatic nerve in the rat model of chronic pain. These basic science studies are important to help investigate purported mechanisms of analgesia in various alternative modalities. Furthermore, this study suggests that magnetic field therapy may be effective in various forms of neuropathic pain.

Low-Power Laser Therapy

Parris and colleagues,[31] using the same animal model described for magnetic field therapy, investigated the effect of low-power laser on neuropathic pain. No biochemical or behavioral changes resulted, illustrating that it is not effective for neuropathic pain; however, low-power laser has been effective for myofascial pain.[32]

SUMMARY

As we approach the start of the new millennium, conventional medicine has taught us that it is reasonable and prudent to reexamine and reutilize old techniques and old drugs for new applications. Examples of these principles include the use of aspirin not only for the prevention of heart disease but also for the management of myocardial infarction; the rejuvenation of gabapentin, an anticonvulsant and antidepressant medication to treat chronic neuropathic pain syndrome is another example of that principle.

As we evaluate new techniques and new drugs, it is also appropriate to evaluate alternative medicine practices, but this needs to be done scientifically and fairly, not in response to commercial interests but in accordance with scientific principles. To accomplish that goal, the Office of Alternative Medicine has been invaluable, not only to the field of pain medicine but also to patients in general. Many aspects of conventional and traditional medicine, if they were subjected to rigorous scientific scrutiny, might be condemned. Nevertheless, the scientific evaluation of alternative medicine may reveal tremendous benefits to patients with chronic pain. It is hoped that just as there are regulations and safeguards for traditional and conventional medicine, there would be similar governmental safeguards and regulations governing alternative and complementary medicine. In this scenario, the appropriate federal, state, and local societies, the different medical organizations, the U.S. Food and Drug Administration, and the various agencies within the Department of Health and Human Services, the Drug Enforcement Agency, and the other centers and divisions of the NIH would help to support the burgeoning field of alternative medicine using their respective expertise, thereby ensuring that patients are not exploited but, instead, are served with some degree of efficiency and integrity. Although practitioners of alternative medicine have no rigid guidelines to follow at present, ideally some regulation will be provided under the leadership of responsible clinical organizations and with direct, or indirect, governmental oversight.

The future appears bright for alternative medicine, and it is hoped that, in the presence of an unbiased, creative, and honest approach to evaluating alternative medicine modalities, beneficial agents and techniques would be promoted so that patients with chronic pain that is unresponsive to conventional therapeutic modalities may have the option of using approved alternative medicine modalities for pain control.

References

1. Murray RH, Rubel AJ: Physicians and healers: Unwitting partners in health care. N Engl J Med 326:61, 1992.
2. Gevitz N, ed: Three perspectives on unorthodox medicine. In Other Healers: Unorthodox Medicine in America. Baltimore, Johns Hopkins University Press, 1988.
3. Eisenberg DM, Kessler RC, Foster C, et al: Unconventional medicine in the United States. N Engl J Med 328:246, 1993.
4. Cook C, Baisen D: Ancillary use of folk medicine by patients in primary care clinics in southwestern West Virginia. South Med J 79:1098, 1986.
5. Superintendent of Documents: GPO Stock No. 052-003-01207-3. Washington, DC, Government Printing Office, 1990.
6. Office of Alternative Medicine Clearing House: Office of Alternative Medicine. Bethesda, Md, National Institutes of Health, 1997.
7. Astin JA: Why patients use alternative medicine: Results of a national study. JAMA 279(11):1548, 1998.
8. Uptake of alternative medicine. Lancet 347(9006):972, 1996.
9. Parris WC, Livengood JM, German D, Wood D: Evaluation of medical school curriculum for management of acute and chronic pain. Anesth Analg 80(2):5370, 1995.
10. Schorr JA: Music and pattern change in chronic pain. ANS Adv Nursing Sci 15(4):27, 1993.
11. Hanser SB: Using music therapy as distraction during lumbar punctures. J Pediatr Oncol Nursing 10(1):2, 1993.
12. McGuire MB: Ritual Healing in Suburban America. New Brunswick, NJ, Rutgers University Press, 1988.
13. Sundblom DM, Haikonen S, Niemi-Pynttari J, Tigerstedt I: Effect of spiritual healing on chronic idiopathic pain: A medical and psychological study. Clin J Pain 10(4):296, 1994.
14. Jacobson E: Progressive Relaxation. Chicago, University of Chicago Press, 1938.
15. Sloman R, Brown P, Aldana E, Chee E: The use of relaxation for the promotion of comfort and pain relief in persons with advanced cancer. Contemp Nurse 3(1):6, 1994.
16. White AH, Derby R, Wynne G: Epidural injections for the diagnosis and treatment of lower back pain. Spine 5:78, 1980.
17. Moret V, Forster A, Laverriere MC, et al: Mechanism of analgesia induced by hypnosis and acupuncture: Is there a difference? Pain 45(2):135, 1991.
18. Cadranel JF, Benhamou Y, Zylberg P, et al: Hypnotic relaxation: A new sedative tool for colonoscopy? J Clin Gastroenterol 18(2):127, 1994.
19. Campion EW: Why unconventional medicine? N Engl J Med 328:282, 1993.
20. Buchko BL, Pugh LC, Bishop BA, et al: Comfort measures in breastfeeding, primiparous women. J Obstet Gynecol Neonatal Nurs 23(1):46, 1994.
21. Whitacre MM: The effect of transcutaneous electrical nerve stimulation on ocular pain. Ophthalmic Surg 22(8):462, 1991.
22. Melzack R, Wall PD: Pain mechanisms: A new theory. Science 150:971, 1965.
23. Jensen H, Zesler R, Christensen T: Transcutaneous electrical nerve stimulation (TNS) for painful osteoarthrosis of the knee. Int J Rehab Res 14(4):356, 1991.
24. Johnson MI, Ashton CH, Thompson JW: Long term use of transcutaneous electrical nerve stimulation at Newcastle Pain Relief Clinic. J R Soc Med 86(8):492, 1993.
25. Sotosky JR, Lindsay SM: Use of TENS in arthritis management. Bull Rheum Dis 40(5):3, 1991.
26. Bossut DF, Mayer DJ: Electroacupuncture analgesia in naïve rats: Effects of brainstem and spinal cord lesions, and role of pituitary-adrenal axis. Brain Res 549(1):52, 1991.
27. Lundenberg T: Peripheral effects of sensory nerve stimulation (acupuncture) in inflammation and ischemia. Scand J Rehab Med Suppl 29:61, 1993.
28. Guieu R, Tardy-Gervet MF, Roll JP: Analgesic effects of vibration and transcutaneous electrical nerve stimulation applied separately and simul-

taneously to patients with chronic pain. Can J Neurol Sci 18(2):113, 1991.
29. Cohen D: Magnetic fields of the human body. Physics Today 28:34, 1975.
30. Parris WC, Janicki PK, Johnson BW, Matthews L: The behavioral and biochemical effect of pulsating magnetic field (PMFT) on chronic pain produced by chronic constriction injury of sciatic nerve in rat. Analgesia 1(1):57, 1994.
31. Parris WC, Janicki PK, Johnson BW, Matthews L: Infrared laser diode irradiation has no behavioral effect or biochemical effect on pain in the sciatic nerve ligation induced mononeuropathy in rat. Anesth Prog 41(4):95, 1994.
32. Waylonis GW, Wilke S, O'Tolle D, et al: Chronic myofascial pain: Management by low-output helium-neon laser therapy. Arch Phys Med Rehabil 69:1017, 1988.

chapter 119

Limitations of Pharmacologic Pain Management

Richard B. Patt

RISK-BENEFIT RATIO

All medical interventions are associated with risks and benefits that, when considered together, compose that intervention's risk-benefit ratio. Alternatives exist for all interventions (including "no intervention"), and these alternatives likewise possess their own risk-benefit ratios. Clinical decision making involves comparing and contrasting the risk-benefit ratios of alternative interventions (relative risk-benefit ratio).

The risk-benefit ratio is multiply determined and is usually inexact. It is, in part, intrinsic to a given therapy, and it is also, in part, dependent on the clinical situation for which treatment is under consideration. How the risk-benefit ratio is determined or interpreted is influenced by numerous factors, some of which are difficult to quantitate (e.g., provider bias, patient preference) or have an ambiguous value (e.g., cost, patient suffering). As a result, the perceived risk-benefit ratio may differ profoundly based on interrelated factors pertinent to the patient (e.g., age, overall health, functional status, ethnocultural and religious background), the physician (e.g., attitudes, beliefs, training, financial incentives), and the system (e.g., regulatory forces, facilities, economic factors). The risk-benefit ratio is not a fixed entity but instead varies as these factors and their relationships with each other change over time. This scenario is further complicated when applied to the treatment of pain because as a result of the subjective nature of pain and the newness of its status as a specialty, there is a paucity of data regarding the outcomes of even accepted interventions. In the past, this has allowed for wide latitude in decision making. However, increased scrutiny of health care costs is likely to be associated with greater constraints on decision making.

PHARMACOLOGIC DICHOTOMY: CANCER PAIN AND CHRONIC NONMALIGNANT PAIN

Cultural and social forces have profound influences on therapeutic decision making regarding the treatment of pain with medications. A curious but contextually understandable dichotomy exists with respect to the treatment of pain of malignant versus nonmalignant origin with opioid analgesics.

Cancer Pain

Until relatively recently, opioids were avoided for all but the most desperate of medical conditions, a stigmatization based more on cultural bias than on medical fact. Initiatives emphasizing the concept of comprehensive cancer care mandate attention to symptom control throughout the course of a cancer illness. Contemporary approaches to managing pain in cancer patients emphasize earlier and more liberal use of opioids, citing a low potential for addiction and a generally favorable risk-benefit ratio. A review of the literature suggests that these principles are grounded firmly in science.

Chronic Pain

Opioids were long considered taboo as treatment for chronic nonmalignant pain. These concerns were mostly grounded in beliefs about the inevitability of addiction and typically reflected not just medical concerns but moral ones as well. In light of data generated by the opioids for cancer pain experience, the prohibition of opioid therapy for noncancer pain has been called into question. A spectrum of opinion currently exists regarding the advisability and proper methodology for prescribing opioids in such patients. Although both proponents and detractors cite data that support opposing views, there is agreement that opioid therapy is more beneficial than harmful in a proportion of patients with chronic, nonmalignant pain. Although there is reasonable scientific support for this general contention, support for guidelines to determine the risk-benefit ratio prospectively in individual cases remains empirical.

ROLE OF INVASIVE PROCEDURES

The role of invasive and regional pain-relieving modalities is even less well-defined than that of drugs, for the treatment of both cancer and noncancer pain. The situation is analogous to that of opioids for nonmalignant pain: although there is fairly widespread agreement that procedures sometimes possess favorable risk-benefit ratios, there is a lack of a uniformly accepted, validated methodology for prospectively determining in what settings certain procedures are valuable.

Cancer Pain

The U.S. Agency for Health Care Policy Research has undertaken the development of treatment guidelines for cancer pain, employing a methodology that used rigorous validation criteria. A robust review of the literature revealed considerably less intense and less valid evidence for the role of procedures than for pharmacologic management. Unfortunately, the validity of this exercise is questionable. Because its methodology is so dependent on the quality of the literature, it more accurately reflects the shortcomings of the available literature than the true risk-benefit ratio. The ill-defined role of invasive procedures relates to many factors including design problems, a historic lack of a mandate for outcome measures, and the relatively recent marriage of academic medicine and pain medicine. Notwithstanding these difficulties, the agency's expert panel still ultimately endorsed a vital role for invasive procedures. Owing to the nature of the process and the quality of data reviewed, however, recommendations for employing procedures are somewhat vague and cite relatively narrow indications.

Chronic Pain

Debate over the role of invasive procedures for chronic nonmalignant pain is, if possible, even more contentious. Evidence has been cited supporting diametrically opposed views, and the quality of such evidence has legitimately been questioned. Factors influencing this debate are as noted previously but also include bias (even rivalry) among specialists, financial stake, and *opiophobia*. There is reasonable agreement regarding when, and in whom, certain procedures provide sufficiently meaningful and durable pain relief to justify their risks and costs. There is agreement that the outcomes for procedures are most favorable when they are "properly" integrated within a multidisciplinary matrix, although the evidence for even this conventional wisdom is questionable.

ADVANTAGES OF PHARMACOTHERAPY FOR CANCER PAIN

Oral opioid therapy is considered the treatment of choice for uncomplicated cancer pain for a variety of reasons. These include the induction of analgesia that is reversible, titratable, and suitable for a variety of types of pain, including multiple topographically distinct pains, generalized pain, and lack of invasiveness. The need for specialized training is modest, and efficacy is maintained when treatment is modified to apply to individuals across cultures and over a range of ages and medical fitness.

LIMITATIONS OF PHARMACOTHERAPY FOR CANCER PAIN

It is well-recognized that in 70% or more of cancer patients, pain relief can be achieved with uncomplicated oral and/or transdermal administration of opioids, especially when combined with nonsteroidal antiinflammatory drugs (NSAIDs) and adjuvant analgesics (e.g., antidepressants, anticonvulsants). Up to 30% of all patients with cancer pain, however, require alternative interventions to achieve comfort. There is widespread acceptance of the construct that opioids should be administered in doses sufficient to either control cancer pain or produce unacceptable side effects. Although the end points of opioid therapy (i.e., comfort and unacceptable side effects) are difficult to quantify, this view recognizes unacceptable side effects as one possible consequence of drug therapy. These side effects constitute the most important limitations of drug therapy for cancer pain.

Several investigators have attempted to identify specific clinical findings that, when identified prospectively, signal that pain relief will be difficult to achieve with pharmacologic means alone. The best validated schema, the Edmonton Staging System, suggests that the presence of a history of alcohol or drug abuse or recent tolerance, neuropathic pain, psychological distress, and movement-related pain predict a relatively poorer prognosis for controlling pain pharmacologically, whereas drug dose and presence of delirium are not predictive. Other investigations suggest that movement-related pain is the only consistent feature predictive of poor outcome for pharmacotherapy. This constitutes an extremely important area for further study, especially with methodologies that target specific clinical pain syndromes. This author's experience suggests that syndromes such as tumor-mediated brachial and lumbosacral plexopathy, abdominopelvic pain, and pain from the skin ulceration that accompanies fungating tumors are among other daunting syndromes in which pain often persists despite aggressive drug therapy. Although no single feature reliably predicts failure of pharmacotherapy, presence of these features should alert the clinician that additional resources may be needed to help manage pain effectively.

LIMITATIONS OF PHARMACOTHERAPY FOR NONCANCER PAIN

The historical view that the use of opioids was prima facie undesirable for the management of chronic pain allowed for a ready determination of risk-benefit ratio, no matter how unscientific. Contemporary views that opioid therapy is sometimes justified call for a general reappraisal of risk-benefit ratio and carefully individualized decision making.

The baseline limitations of drug therapy for nonmalignant pain include the same potential side effects that restrict use in cancer patients. Additional limitations in this population depend on the degree to which a given patient is perceived as being at risk for addiction and the degree to which the practitioner perceives opioid therapy as being potentially effective and appropriate.

Specific Limitations

Dose-Limiting Side Effects

One set of limitations relates to the various collateral (nonanalgesic) effects of the analgesics. The most prominent side effects of the opioids are constipation, nausea, vomiting, cognitive failure (ranging from drowsiness to hallucinations), dysphoria, myoclonus, and pruritus, although other side effects such as respiratory depression occasionally supervene. Similarly, treatment with the NSAIDs and other adjuvants is limited by undesirable pharmacologic side effects such as gastropathy, bleeding, renal insufficiency, masking of fever, and sedation, constipation, dry mouth, dysrhythmias, cognitive failure, ataxia, hepatic insufficiency, and bone marrow depression.

Drug side effects, especially for the opioids, can often be managed effectively. Strategies for managing opioid side effects in cancer patients are depicted in Table 119–1. Side effects from other analgesics may be more problematic and are in many cases less readily reversible. Thus, an important distinction between the opioids and other analgesics is that there are few absolute contraindications to use of the former, whereas the latter often need to be avoided altogether lest complications occur (e.g., aspirin in the patient with an ulcer, hypersensitivity, or bone marrow depression). Paradoxically, for long-term use, the opioids are both the most stigmatized of all analgesics and, on a physiologic basis, arguably the safest.

SPECIFIC SCENARIOS

Besides the general category of dose-limiting side effects, a number of clinical scenarios impose specific limitations or increased risks from pharmacotherapy. Only a few such scenarios are cited here.

Neuropathic Pain

Somatic and visceral nociceptive pain typically responds linearly to escalating doses of opioid analgesics. In contrast, the dose-response relationship for neuropathic pain is often blunted, requiring treatment in higher dose ranges, as a result of which, side effects are more likely to be problematic. Once considered an "opioid-nonresponsive" set of disorders, the range of response observed for neuropathic pain syndromes forms the basis for the concept of relative responsivity to opioids. Increasingly, neuropathic pain syndromes are successfully treated by an approach that uses maintenance therapy with low-dose opioids for the induction of partial analgesia, after which sequential trials of adjuvant analgesics are conducted in an effort to gain more complete analgesia.

Movement-Related Pain (Breakthrough or Incident Pain)

The tempo of chronic pain is most often one of continuous, unrelenting, low-grade basal pain, punctuated by episodic exacerbations that can be unpredictable but that are most often related to activity. These superimposed flares are generally referred to as *breakthrough pain*. The basal component of pain is typically treated with a long-acting opioid administered on a time-contingent basis (by the clock), such as an oral controlled-release formulation of morphine or oxycodone administered every 12 hours, a transdermal preparation of fentanyl applied every 72 hours, or—less commonly—with methadone. Breakthrough pain is then treated with the symptom-contingent administration of a second, short-acting oral opioid administered as needed (immediate-release morphine sulfate, hydromorphone, oxycodone, or oral transmucosal fentanyl citrate). The dose of long-acting medication is then titrated based on the frequency and urgency of the requirement for as-required treatment of breakthrough pain.

Table 119–1

Strategies for Limiting the Side Effects of Opioids

Prophylaxis	Especially for constipation; sometimes for nausea
Patient education	Informed of the potential for side effects, patients are less likely to assume they are allergic and more likely to cooperate with efforts at palliation
Patience	Nausea and sedation are usually transitory and remit with time Slower titration may reduce troublesome side effects
Symptomatic management	Treat with antiemetics, laxatives, psychostimulants, etc.
Trials of alternative (related) analgesics	Efficacy: side effect profile of opioids is often idiosyncratic Trials of alternative opioids are indicated because of incomplete cross-tolerance
Trials of adjuvant analgesics	Side effects may be due to reliance on opioids for a pain syndrome that is relatively nonresponsive to opioids Successful therapy with adjuvants may allow for a reduction in opioid dose with fewer side effects
Alternate treatment modalities	Judicious application of antitumor therapy, procedures, psychotherapy, etc., may permit dose reductions with fewer attendant side effects

Breakthrough pain that occurs with a relatively consistent temporal relationship to specific activities has come to be referred to as *incident pain*. Breakthrough pain that occurs at predictable intervals just prior to the next scheduled dose of an analgesic drug is referred to as *end-of-dose failure*. Breakthrough pain that appears to be idiosyncratic and unrelated to either activity or scheduled doses of analgesics is typically referred to as either *spontaneous* or *idiopathic breakthrough pain*, or simply as *breakthrough pain*.

Pain that is exacerbated with movement is among the most difficult of syndromes to control with analgesics. The pharmacokinetics of currently available drugs, even those administered intravenously, is not well matched to the often unpredictable, rapid, and wide fluctuations in severity of movement-related pain.

When incident pain is relatively unpredictable, rescue doses are provided prophylactically, about 30 minutes in advance of the pain-provoking activity. When unanticipated breakthrough pain occurs, the rescue dose should be taken as soon after onset as possible, independent of the timing of the basal dose. If these strategies are unsuccessful, there should be consideration for a trial of an alternative short-acting opioid or a change in the route of administration. Breakthrough pain that is predictable, infrequent, of mild or moderate intensity, or slow to develop can often be managed effectively with oral analgesics such as immediate-release (IR) morphine, hydromorphone, or oxycodone. Breakthrough pain that is severe or that occurs unpredictably, frequently, or precipitously may not be adequately relieved with currently available oral agents. Although IV and SC opioids are pharmacokinetically well-suited for labile and/or severe breakthrough pain, these advantages are offset by their invasiveness.

Oral transmucosal fentanyl citrate (OTFC), a new formulation of an established opioid analgesic, has been approved specifically for the treatment of breakthrough pain that arises in patients already using around-the-clock opioids. A sweetened fentanyl-impregnated lozenge mounted on a stick, it is a noninvasive means of delivering a potent lipophilic opioid through the oral mucosa, facilitating rapid absorption into the circulation and analgesia of relatively fast onset and short duration. Extensive controlled research has been conducted on the use of OTFC as a specific remedy for breakthrough pain, confirming safety and demonstrating superior efficacy to routine oral agents in cancer patients receiving concomitant therapy with immediate-release and controlled-release oral opioids for basal pain. Onset of meaningful analgesia typically occurs within 5 minutes of beginning consumption of a unit, peaks about 30 minutes later, and usually lasts about 4 hours. The duration of analgesia is slightly prolonged because about one half of each fentanyl dose is inevitably swallowed and subjected to hepatic first-pass effect. The availability of fentanyl in a lozenge form allows for easy self-administration and permits patients to titrate dose to an effective level of analgesia without the need for injections. Given, however, the similarity in its kinetics with intravenous analgesics, it is probably an undesirable choice in patients prone to addictive behaviors.

Even with this addition to our armamentarium, prominent incident pain remains a treatment challenge because opioid requirements vary dramatically over short intervals. Doses of opioids required to treat pain during periods of rest are typically inadequate when activity increases, and, conversely, doses required to ease movement-related pain may produce sedation and other side effects when the provocative activity increases.

Narrow Therapeutic Window: Cachexia and Advanced Age

While a high proportion of patients with cancer are not candidates for curative therapy, palliative and supportive care may extend life. Pharmacologic-based pain control is often more difficult to achieve in patients with advanced cancer because concomitant asthenia and cachexia increase the likelihood of side effects from opioids titrated to therapeutic effect (narrow therapeutic window). The sedative effects of opioids can often be countered by the judicious use of psychostimulants, such as methylphenidate, which are usually administered at starting doses of 10 mg on awakening and 10 mg at the noon meal and can be titrated to effect. While dysrhythmias and anorexia are theoretical concerns, they are rarely problematic, although this approach should be avoided in the presence of an anxiety disorder or brain metastases.

Limited epidemiologic data suggest that chronic pain is about twice as common for geriatric individuals living in residential settings than in their younger counterparts, with incidence ranging from 25% to 50%. Although under-recognition and undertreatment of pain in nursing homes is so rampant that statistics are often misleading, targeted surveys reveal an incidence ranging from 45% to 80%.

Degenerative arthritis and other musculoskeletal disorders compose the most prominent sources of pain in the elderly, although herpes zoster, decubitus ulcers, peripheral vascular disease, temporal arteritis, and polymyalgia rheumatica are disproportionately common with advanced age. Because the incidence of almost all malignancies increases with advancing age, oncologic pain is a particularly common problem in the geriatric population. It is an especially important problem because many of the factors that cause cancer pain to be undertreated in the general population are amplified in aging patients.

Although some degree of age-associated changes in organ function (including the central nervous system) are ubiquitous, with a few exceptions these ordinarily exert little influence on pain threshold or pain tolerance, although pharmacodynamics or pharmacokinetics may be somewhat altered. Loss of neuronal tissue and proliferation of glial cells occur with advancing age, but there is no evidence for impairment in processing pain signals unless dementia or delirium is clinically evident. Clinical lore suggesting that elderly patients do not experience pain as keenly as their younger counterparts is unfounded and is often no more than a rationalization for an unwillingness to spend the added time often required in assessing the elderly patient.

The hospice experience has demonstrated that, when appropriate time and effort are applied, pain can usually be managed effectively even in the frail, elderly patient. However, drug titration should be performed with considerable caution, and, when possible, polypharmacy should be avoided.

Suffering

Pain is multiply determined and often persists as a result of unidentified psychosocial causes. Analgesics per se are

Table 119–2

Potential Limitations of the Pharmacologic Management of Abdominopelvic Pain

Treatment Modality	***Limitations***
NSAIDs	Gastropathy Renal dysfunction Bone marrow depletion Concerns about masking fever
Oral analgesics	Xerostomia Dysphagia Malabsorption Obstruction Nausea Vomiting Coma
Transdermal analgesics	Dose requirements for opioids may exceed limitations of dose form
Parenteral analgesics	Inadequate household or community support to manage infusions
Opioids	Ileus Partial obstruction Intractable constipation Reduced responsivity due to neuropathic component of pain Dose-limiting side effects due to asthenia and cachexia

unlikely to reduce complaints of pain that are rooted in more global suffering. Psychotropic drugs combined with psychotherapy may, however, be effective in this setting.

Abdominopelvic Pain

Factors specific to patients with abdominopelvic pain that reduce the likelihood of attaining adequate pain control with systemic analgesics alone are listed in Table 119–2. NSAIDs, even of the COX-2 selective type, may be poorly tolerated or contraindicated owing to gastropathy and to general factors such as renal insufficiency, coagulopathy, bone marrow suppression, and masking of fever. The oral route may be unreliable in the presence of gastrointestinal dysfunction (e.g., dysphagia, malabsorption, intestinal obstruction, nausea and vomiting, xerostomia, coma). Reduced gastrointestinal motility is a common upshot of tumor encroachment or sequela of surgery or radiation therapy. Even with a strict bowel protocol, opioids may exacerbate ileus or partial obstruction in patients with reduced motility. In such cases, the use of opioids, except in low doses, is undesirable. Although visceral pain is relatively opioid-responsive, patients often present with pain of mixed causes. Typically, pain due to nerve injury (neuropathic pain) is less sensitive to opioids, and thus occult microscopic deposits of perineural tumor invasion may contribute to reduced opioid responsivity.

CONCLUSION

Notwithstanding the opioids-for-chronic-pain controversy, data support the primary role of pharmacotherapy for managing most pain syndromes. Some patients do not, however, derive adequate comfort from systemic drug therapy alone or are not candidates for liberal use of opioids. Even for cancer pain, when addiction is less of a concern and liberal prescribing is widely endorsed, physiologic and psychological features sometimes hinder achieving an adequate pharmacologic remedy.

The most formidable limitations of drug treatment relate to their potential to produce pharmacologic side effects or complications. Careful monitoring and the use of strategies for preventing and managing drug side effects are often all that is required to maintain efficacy. Specific patient-related factors (e.g., neuropathic pain, movement-related pain, psychological distress, cachexia, alterations in gastrointestinal function) are associated with greater likelihood of limitations. The degree to which selected drugs' potential to induce habituation is an impediment to long-term use remains a topic of considerable and heated debate.

Bibliographic References

American Pain Society: Principles of Analgesic Use in the Treatment of Acute Pain and Chronic Cancer Pain, 4th ed. Skokie, IL. American Pain Society, 1999.

Ashby MA, Fleming BG, Brooksbank M, et al: Description of a mechanistic approach to pain management in advanced cancer. Preliminary report. Pain 51:153, 1992.

Bruera E, Chadwick S, Brenneis C: Methylphenidate associated with narcotics for the treatment of cancer pain. Ca Treat Rep 71:120, 1987.

Bruera E, Macmillan K, Hanson J, MacDonald RN: The Edmonton staging system for cancer pain: Preliminary report. Pain 37:203, 1989.

Bruera E, Schoeller T, Wenk R, et al: A prospective multicenter assessment of the Edmonton staging system for cancer pain. J Pain Symptom Manage 10:348, 1995.

Christie JM, Simmonds M, Patt R, et al: Dose-titration, multicenter study of oral transmucosal fentanyl citrate for the treatment of breakthrough pain in cancer patients using transdermal fentanyl for persistent pain. J Clin Oncol 16:3238, 1998.

Ellison NM: Opioid analgesics: Toxicities and their treatments. In Patt RB (ed): Cancer Pain. Philadelphia, JB Lippincott, 1995, p 185.

Ferrell BA: Pain management among elderly persons. In Payne R, Patt RB, Hill CS (eds): Assessment and Treatment of Cancer Pain. Seattle, IASP Press, 1998, p 53.

Galer BS: Opioids and chronic nonmalignant pain. APS J 2:207, 1993.
Getto CJ, Sorkness CA, Howell T: Antidepressants and chronic nonmalignant pain: A review. J Pain Symptom Manage 2:9, 1987.
Hanks GW, Justins DM: Cancer pain: Management. Lancet 339:1031, 1992.
Hogan QH, Abram SE: Epidural steroids and the outcomes movement. Pain Digest 1:269, 1992.
Jacox A, Carr DB, Payne R, et al (eds): Management of Cancer Pain: Clinical Practice Guideline No. 9. Rockville, Md, AHCPR Publication No. 94-0592, March 1994.
Jain S, Patt RB: Complications of invasive procedures. In Patt RB (ed): Cancer Pain. Philadelphia, JB Lippincott, 1995, p 443.
Mercadante S: Predictive factors and opioid responsiveness in cancer pain. Eur J Cancer 34:627, 1998.
Mercandante S, Armata M, Salvaggio L: Pain characteristics of advanced lung cancer patients referred to a palliative care service. Pain 59:141, 1994.
Mercandante S, Maddaloni S, Roccella S, Salvaggio L: Predictive factors in advanced cancer pain treated only by analgesics. Pain 50:151, 1992.
Patt RB: General principles of pharmacotherapy. In Patt RB (ed): Cancer Pain. Philadelphia, JB Lippincott, 1995, p 101.
Patt RB, Jain S: Therapeutic decision making for invasive procedures. In Patt RB (ed): Cancer Pain. Philadelphia, JB Lippincott, 1995, p 275.
Portenoy RK: Chronic opioid therapy for persistent noncancer pain: Can we get past the bias? Am Pain Soc J 1:1, 1991.
Portenoy RK: Chronic opioid therapy in nonmalignant pain. J Pain Symptom Manage 5:S46, 1990.
Portenoy RK: Management of common opioid side effects during long-term therapy of cancer pain. Ann Acad Med 23:160, 1994.
Portenoy RK, Coyle N: Controversies in the long-term management of analgesic therapy in patients with advanced cancer. J Pain Symptom Manage 5:307, 1990.
Portenoy RK, Foley KM: Chronic use of opioid analgesics in non-malignant pain: Report of 38 cases. Pain 25:171, 1986.
Schoefferman J: Long-term use of opioid analgesics for the treatment of chronic pain of nonmalignant origin. J Pain Symptom Manage 8:279, 1993.

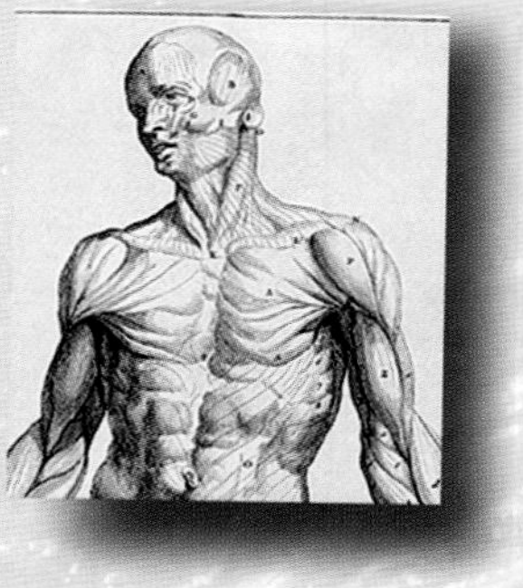

Part B

Psychological and Behavioral Modalities for Pain and Symptom Management

chapter 120

Psychological Interventions

Jennifer B. Levin and Jeffrey W. Janata

A review of the understanding of pain throughout history suggests that theorists have vacillated between definitions that emphasize emotional aspects of pain and definitions that promote a more sensory, physiologic view. Aristotle believed that pain is a "passion of the soul," an affective experience. Aristotle's view was generally embraced until Descartes proposed that pain is a pure sensory phenomenon, a view that has persisted, aided by the rapid advances in medical understanding of sensory systems.[1] Current accepted definitions of pain recognize the emotional and sensory elements; it is almost impossible to read a pain text without being reminded that the International Association for the Study of Pain defined chronic pain as "an unpleasant sensory and emotional experience associated with actual or potential tissue damage."[2]

Current practice often fails to address adequately these psychological aspects of chronic pain. This chapter describes the emotional and behavioral components of chronic pain; reviews the psychotherapeutic strategies that can be combined with rehabilitative, medical, and interventional procedures; describes patient obstacles to engaging in treatment; and presents evidence for the effectiveness of including psychotherapy as an integral part of a comprehensive approach to the management of chronic pain.

PSYCHOLOGICAL ASPECTS OF CHRONIC PAIN

Pain and Depression

Pain and depression are among the most common conditions to confront practitioners. At any given time, it is estimated that 17% of patients seen in primary care complain of persistent pain.[4] Furthermore, approximately 13% of adult Americans lose productive work time as a function of a pain problem with a $61 billion economic impact on productivity alone.[3] Depression often goes undiagnosed or is inadequately treated in this large group of patients and can impede the effective treatment of pain.[5] Experienced pain clinicians attest to the frequency with which patients with chronic pain present with co-occurring depressive symptoms. Studies have shown prevalence rates for depression in chronic pain to range from 10% to 100%,[6] but most find that coexisting depression is at the higher end of probability and is the most frequent psychiatric diagnosis to accompany chronic pain.[7] Depression is more common than anxiety or personality disorders in patients who develop opioid dependency,[8] and depression has been found to play an influential role in the development of chronic pain and disability.[9]

Criteria from the *Diagnostic and Statistical Manual of Mental Disorders, fourth edition, text revision,* for diagnosing depression[10] include marked changes in mood, anhedonia, insomnia or hypersomnia, weight loss or gain, fatigue, psychomotor retardation or agitation, difficulty with concentration or indecisiveness, feelings of worthlessness and guilt, and thoughts of death and suicidal ideation. Anhedonia is the loss of interest in things or activities that previously were pleasurable. Anhedonia often is reported by pain patients, who describe that the pairing of pleasurable activities with pain renders the activities far less pleasurable and, as a result, much less likely to be pursued. Lewinsohn and Gotlib[11] suggested that depression symptoms may be related to the loss of positive reinforcement that pleasurable activities provide. Loss of activities, of interests, and of the often social context in which the activities are enjoyed may contribute to the depression that pain patients experience. Research evidence supports this relationship; a path analysis in an elderly population showed that pain contributes to activity restriction, which contributes to the development of depressive symptoms.[12]

Insomnia is a common complaint in chronic pain patients; studies suggest that insomnia accompanies pain in 50% to 88% of patients with various pain conditions.[13,14] Patients with chronic pain often complain that their pain interferes with the quality of their sleep, and clinicians naturally may attribute sleep dysregulation solely to the painful condition, overlooking the possibility that sleep problems may be symptomatic of depression. Patients with Depression and insomnia experience greater affective distress, reduced sense of control, and greater pain severity. Insomnia without concurrent depression was found to be associated with increased levels of pain,[15] and there is evidence that sleep deprivation produces hyperalgesic changes. Sleep deprivation may impede the analgesic effects of opioids and the serotonin reuptake inhibitor class of antidepressants.[16]

Evidence suggests that although patients complain to clinicians most prominently about pain, often their less emphasized depressive issues are causing patients the greatest distress. A study of patients with facial pain found that depressive symptoms correlate more highly with psychosocial and physical functioning than does pain.[17] This study highlights the concern that clinicians may focus on treating the pain complaints while overlooking the depressive issues. As patient distress persists, clinicians are at risk to escalate the use of analgesics, which are not notably effective at ameliorating depression.

The correlation of pain and depressive symptoms begs the question of which comes first: Does depression increase one's vulnerability to developing chronic pain syndrome, or does the presence of chronic pain increase one's likelihood of becoming depressed? Gamsa,[18] in a review of the literature and study of patients with chronic pain, provided support for the notion that pain is more likely to create than be created by emotional distress. Similarly, a systematic review of the literature yielded evidence that depression is more likely a consequence than an antecedent of chronic pain.[19]

Pain and Anxiety

Studies generally have shown a high incidence of anxiety disorders in patients with chronic pain. Using a structured clinical interview, one study[20] documented an overall prevalence rate of 16% to 28% in a sample of patients with a variety of pain diagnoses. Dersh and colleagues[21] summarized research that suggests studies that have examined lifetime prevalence of anxiety in chronic pain find rates similar to those found in the pain-free population. Current prevalence rates are found to be significantly higher, however, in individuals with chronic pain. Among the anxiety disorders, panic disorder and generalized anxiety disorder seem to be most commonly diagnosed.

A theory of the situational specificity of anxiety in pain was developed by Lethem and colleagues,[22] who articulated the fear-avoidance model, which has been the subject of increased research interest. The model proposes that two factors mediate pain and disability. Fear of pain and hypervigilance to painful stimuli develop as patients attach catastrophic thoughts to the experience of pain. Subsequent avoidance of activity is driven by fear that engaging in activity would worsen pain or cause physical harm. This avoidance of activity serves as negative reinforcement of the patient's fear. Fear-avoidance beliefs and fear of movement and consequent injury have been shown to predict physical performance and disability from pain.[23]

Pain and Personality Disorders

Clinicians often find that their pain populations include a disproportionate share of difficult patients and describe personality difficulties rather than medical complexities. Researchers have examined the prevalence of character pathology in patients who complain of chronic pain. In a study of 200 chronic low back pain patients, 51% met the criteria for one or more personality disorders. Paranoid personality disorder was diagnosed in 33% of the sample; borderline (15%), avoidant (14%), and passive-aggressive traits (12%) also were identified.[24] Gatchel and colleagues[25] reported that 24% of their sample met the criteria for a personality disorder. A study of primary care patients who presented with a range of pain problems found that 25% of the small sample ($n = 17$) met criteria for borderline personality disorder.[26] These studies suggest that Axis II pathology is considerably more prevalent in chronic pain patients than in the population as a whole. Effective pain management in patients with comorbid personality disorders may be possible, but research into the necessary treatment adaptations is lacking.

PSYCHOTHERAPEUTIC APPROACHES

Evidence-based psychotherapeutic approaches that have been shown to be effective for increasing function and decreasing levels of pain and emotional distress include operant conditioning (behavior therapy) developed in the late 1960s[27]; cognitive-behavioral therapy (CBT), which emerged in the early 1980s; and a comprehensive multimodal treatment approach[28] that integrates these treatments into interdisciplinary teams.

Operant Conditioning

The operant conditioning model is based on the principles of Fordyce and colleagues.[29-31] These investigators noted that pain patients exhibit numerous pain behaviors, such as guarding, pain complaints, and grimacing. They also observed that patients with chronic pain exhibit passive, maladaptive behaviors, such as excessive rest, inactivity, a reduction in family and work responsibilities, and an overreliance on pain medications. The operant model assumes that individuals behave in certain ways according to reinforcement patterns. It follows that for chronic pain patients, maladaptive pain behaviors are being positively and negatively reinforced, whereas adaptive, well behaviors are being ignored and extinguished. An example of positive reinforcement is attention from a spouse or coworker; examples of negative reinforcement are avoidance of household or work responsibilities and relief from pain via reliance on as-needed pain medication. As such, the treatment for such maladaptive patterns is to identify the environmental contingencies and restructure them such that the emphasis is on reinforcing active, adaptive coping skills and ignoring maladaptive behaviors until they extinguish or remit. Therapies that rely on the operant conditioning model use graded activity; social reinforcement; time-contingent medication management; and self-control skills training, including self-monitoring, self-reinforcement, and relaxation training.[32]

Studies confirm that operant conditioning has been shown to be effective for increasing activity levels, exercise, and tolerance and for reducing the intake of pain medications. The direct effects on pain are less dramatic, however.[33]

Some researchers note that the efficacy of operant conditioning may have an alternate explanation—that cognition may be an active ingredient in the change process. Specifically, they suggest that the change in environmental contingencies themselves may not be accounting for the improvement, but rather how the patient perceives and interprets the changes that lead to progress.[34] The reconceptualization of the operant conditioning model relies to a large degree on a broader paradigmatic shift in clinical psychology—the shift toward CBT.

Cognitive Behavioral Therapy

Similar to behavior therapy, CBT uses numerous procedures to modify behavior, such as graded practice, relaxation training, homework assignments, and self-reinforcement. In contrast to behavior therapy, CBT acknowledges the relationship between behavior, thoughts, and feelings and places an emphasis on modifying maladaptive thoughts and beliefs to alleviate emotional distress and reinforce behavior change. Although both behavior therapy and CBT manipulate environmental contingencies, the purpose and path toward change differ. In CBT, the goal of these manipulations is to provide the patient with an opportunity to identify, question, reappraise, and restructure thoughts, feelings, behaviors, and physical sensations on which their belief system is built.

CBT for chronic pain management draws to a large degree from the treatment and research literature for depression and anxiety disorders. This affinity stems from the observation that the emotional sequelae of chronic pain often include depressive symptoms related to loss of function, sleep disturbance, and a reduction in pleasurable activities. As such, the treatment of these aspects of pain symptoms employs the same techniques as those used by classic forms of CBT that have been found to be highly efficacious. These include the use of pleasure schedules and identification of negative thought patterns in conjunction with cognitive restructuring. Parallels also may be drawn between the somatic focus, fear-avoidance paradigms, and attention to danger signals central to the development and maintenance of anxiety and chronic pain–based disorders. As such, the behavioral interventions, such as graded exposure and relaxation training, and the cognitive components, such as behavioral experiments, cognitive restructuring, and coping self-statements, that have been found to be efficacious in the treatment of anxiety disorders[34] can be applied effectively in the management of chronic pain.

Comprehensive Multimodal Treatment

It is important to separate the specific procedures and interventions used in CBT from the theory behind the cognitive behavioral approach. The theoretical underpinnings of the approach advocate an active, structured, problem-focused, time-limited, educationally based, scientific methodology that involves a collaboration between the patient and the therapist. The specific CBT multidisciplinary model for pain management as outlined by Turk and Stacey[28] includes an important team rehabilitation approach. Although only the psychological components of the treatment are reviewed here, in the multimodal approach, CBT treatment goals are addressed and reinforced across disciplines. Fear of reinjury would be addressed simultaneously in CBT, physical therapy, and occupational therapy and by the treating physician. In CBT, the focus would be on identifying fear beliefs and understanding the relationship between the beliefs, behavior, and emotions and developing a hierarchy of fears for graded exposure. In physical therapy and occupational therapy, the patient would have the opportunity to carry out the graded exposure. Finally, in the physician-patient treatment relationship, the physician would (1) reinforce the patient taking an active approach to pain management, (2) de-emphasize the role of narcotic and other analgesic medications, (3) eliminate as-needed medication, (4) work to stabilize sleep, and (5) provide information that would contribute to more evidence-based thoughts and expectancies regarding reinjury. In this model, the consistency across modalities accounts for the added efficacy above and beyond that of single modalities.[35] Keeping this idea in mind, this chapter addresses the process of CBT as it relates to pain management.

The main objective of pain management is not pain reduction, but rather to assist patients to learn to live healthier and more satisfying lives, despite the presence of pain and discomfort. Some pain reduction is a natural by-product of the treatment, stemming from increased conditioning and a reduction in focused attention on pain. As such, secondary goals are likely to include taking more responsibility for one's healthcare; decreased dependence on analgesic medication; and increased functioning in occupational, familial, and social settings. The primary CBT objectives in pain management as outlined by Turk and Okifuji[36] include (1) facilitating a change in approach to pain and suffering from being overwhelming and "out of my control" to manageable and "within my control"; (2) teaching coping skills for the pain and problems stemming from the pain; (3) moving from a passive, helpless role to an active, resourceful role; (4) facilitating the understanding of the relationship between thoughts, feelings, and behaviors and being able to identify and modify maladaptive patterns; (5) strengthening self-confidence and taking credit for successes; and (6) facilitating the identification of problems and proactive problem solving to bring about maintenance of gains.

The dominant theme of CBT to be reinforced across disciplines is the paradigm shift from taking a passive role, leading to negative emotional, behavioral, and physical consequences, to taking an active role in finding the wherewithal to confront one's pain and in doing so to "take back their lives." The focus is on (1) developing a more internal rather than external locus of control, as defined by the perception that the individual (internal or self-management), as opposed to outside sources (external or "fix me" approach), has control over the outcomes of his or her actions[37] and (2) increasing self-efficacy, or an individual's belief in his or her ability to influence behavior, thoughts, and feelings[38] as they relate to pain management. These two concepts, although related, are not equivalent. To be successful, patients must maintain the belief that they hold the responsibility for their pain outcomes (internal locus of control) and develop a belief in their ability to carry out what is needed to reach the desired outcomes (self-efficacy).

Although no two CBT protocols would look exactly alike, there is some consistency in the overall conceptualization of pain and appropriate treatment interventions. Turk and Okifuji[36] outlined six phases of CBT treatment, including (1) assessment, (2) reconceptualization, (3) skills acquisition and consolidation, (4) rehearsal and application training, (5) generalization and maintenance, and (6) treatment follow-up. Similarly, Bradley[39] and Johansson and colleagues[40] identified four essential components of CBT: (1) education, (2) skills acquisition, (3) behavioral rehearsal, and (4) generalization. Given that assessment, conceptualization, and skills development are part of an ongoing process in the management of chronic pain, in this chapter we refer to four fundamental treatment components: (1) assessment and initial conceptualization, (2) moving toward a new conceptualization, (3) education and skills development, and (4) generalization and relapse prevention.

Component 1: Assessment and Conceptualization

The initial assessment incorporates information collected from the patient interview, medical records, family interview when available, and validated assessment measures. Areas for assessment include (1) a complete history of the pain, including its location, severity, and duration, what has and has not been effective for the relief of pain, and patterns of pain and well behaviors including activity level and medication intake; (2) degree and type of psychological distress, including depression, anxiety, and relationship between pain and psychological distress; (3) behavioral patterns at home, work, and in social and recreational activities; (4) specific information regarding beliefs surrounding the pain, expectations for recovery, and functional goals; (5) a detailed work history; (6) degree and character of social support, including the possible role of significant others in the maintenance of maladaptive behavior patterns and how to integrate these significant others into the paradigm shift; (7) addiction patterns and risk for addiction; and (8) incentives and disincentives for work, pain, and treatment, including financial consequences of longstanding pain, disability incentives for work-related injury, pending litigation, drug-seeking behavior, and legitimate release from responsibilities. From the information gathered in the assessment phase, the patient-therapist team can begin to develop a conceptualization of the role of the pain for this individual; the way in which pain affects his or her thoughts, feelings, and behavior; and which elements may be maintaining the system.

Component 2: Moving Toward a New Conceptualization

This stage, comparable to Turk and Ofikuji's[36] collaborative reconceptualization of pain, flows directly from the evidence gathered during the assessment phase. During this phase, the focus is on gradually moving the patient from a passive, helpless role in search of pain relief to an active, empowered role of increasing function and satisfaction. This paradigm shift is being reinforced throughout the treatment process, starting as a concept that is discussed to one that is practiced and leads to a change in underlying beliefs about pain and the patient's role in managing it. This reconceptualization is most likely to be gradually internalized by the patient when it is adopted and reinforced by the entire treatment team, including the psychologist, physician, and rehabilitation staff. This attitude can be a particular challenge given that the physician and rehabilitation staff traditionally have approached pain management from a medical and physical perspective. To accomplish this challenging task, the CBT model first must gain acceptance from the team and requires ongoing communication between healthcare providers. This communication is essential because the patient naturally may fall back to the longstanding belief that pain results from purely medical causes whose management must be primarily medical in nature. This is a natural conclusion given that the patient experiences the pain physically, but it must be disproved through the sense of efficacy and control that develops from the mastery of self-management strategies introduced early in treatment.

Component 3: Education and Skills Development

After developing a new conceptualization of pain management, one that places the patient in the driver's seat, it is important to provide the patient with the skills to manage pain successfully. The education and skills development focus on the continuous process of providing information and a forum for the learning and practicing of new skills for pain management. The emphasis is on skills to manage, rather than decrease, pain. These skills fall into the behavioral and cognitive realms. In the behavioral category, elements are likely to include positive coping skills, relaxation training exercises, pacing, graded exposure to feared situations, attention diversion techniques, and pleasant activity scheduling. In the cognitive category, elements are likely to include cognitive restructuring, or the identification and challenging of negative thought patterns that perpetuate negative emotions and subsequent self-defeating behaviors, coping skills such as positive coping self-statements, and behavioral experiments with the goal of gathering evidence to negate unfounded cognitions. Other skills that may be the focus of attention include assertiveness training, development of communication and social skills, and problem solving. These skills are individualized according to the strengths and deficits of each individual patient. Some of these skills may be best introduced and practiced in group settings because role playing and group feedback are likely to enhance the learning experience.

Component 4: Generalization and Relapse Prevention

During the generalization phase, the focus is on practicing the skills developed and reinforced in session and across disciplines in the home and work environments. This practice is essential to the maintenance of treatment gains. Additionally, during this phase, relapse prevention is introduced. Essential elements in this phase include reviewing and integrating material covered during treatment; evaluating and reinforcing treatment gains; identifying areas in need of strengthening; discussing ways to incorporate skills into one's daily routine and how to apply them to unexpected situations, stressors, and flare-ups; and addressing potential pitfalls and how to handle them should they occur. Follow-up booster sessions are carried out with increasingly longer periods between sessions. The goal of these sessions is to let the patients practice their new skills independently between sessions and self-reinforce for their efforts, yet have a place to continue to hone their skills and receive outside feedback and reinforcement. This stage is often a major factor in relapse prevention. It is often the case that the more the patient improves, the more obstacles he or she has to face. Return to work may require more advanced skills than increasing functionality at home. It may only be after taking "a break from treatment" that the patient can really test out how well his or her new skills work in the real world. The application of skills in a real-life situation with limited structure is in stark contrast to the highly structured rehabilitation environment.

TREATMENT EFFECTIVENESS

How effective are these treatments and for whom? We provide a brief overview of the efficacy research in this area. For a more comprehensive review of treatment outcomes, the reader is referred to McCracken and Turk.[41] When reviewing the efficacy data, one should take into consideration the literature's limitations, which include the heterogeneity of pain syndromes studied, and variable inclusion criteria, levels of specificity with regard to treatment components, and outcome measures. Studies also differ in their control of the complexity and variability of medical treatment.

Much of the early efficacy research studied patients with back pain and reported that operant conditioning was successful in increasing activity levels and decreasing medication use in this population.[42-45] In an attempt to tease out which aspects of operant conditioning were effective, Lindstrom and associates[33] reported that graded activity led to a quicker return to work than traditional medical treatment. Similarly, Turner and coworkers[46] found that graded activity was an effective component, contributing significantly to the positive outcomes of behavioral therapy. In McCracken and Turk's[41] review of the literature, they identified five different studies reporting a reduction in pain levels as a function of relaxation training. More recently, Vlaeyen and colleagues[23] studied the effectiveness of graded exposure to feared stimuli, in this case, exposure to particular physical movements previously avoided because of fear of pain, versus an activation intervention. The results indicated that the graded in vivo exposure protocol was more effective in reducing pain-related fear and disability and increasing activity level than the activation intervention. Keefe and coworkers[47,48] provided evidence for the efficacy of spouse-assisted treatment for improvement in pain, self-efficacy, psychological disability, and marital satisfaction.

The clinical efficacy of CBT for the management of chronic pain has been supported in numerous studies with patient populations having headache, arthritis, temporomandibular pain disorders, fibromyalgia, irritable bowel syndrome, low back pain, complex regional pain syndrome, and heterogeneous chronic pain samples, among others.[36] In an early meta-analysis, Malone and Strube[49] reviewed nonmedical treatments, including four studies on cognitive therapy for various chronic pain conditions, and reported effect sizes ranging from 0.55 to 2.74. In a meta-analysis of 25 studies that met inclusion criteria, Morely and colleagues[50] found significant effect sizes on all outcome measures compared with waitlist controls. Compared with other active treatments, CBT produced significantly greater changes on measures of the pain experience, coping, and behavioral expression of pain. Overall, there is strong support that CBT is effective in reducing pain behavior and coping. Results are less clear, however, with regard to work status, medication, or healthcare use given that fewer studies have evaluated these variables.[41]

A meta-analysis of 65 studies of multidisciplinary treatment for chronic pain indicated that such treatments are more efficacious than no treatment; a waitlist control; or componential treatments, made up of an isolated discipline such as medical treatment, physical therapy, psychological treatment, or occupational therapy alone.[51] In Turk's[52] more recent review of the work in this area, he concluded that multimodal rehabilitation programs are comparable to other pain treatments with regard to pain reduction. These programs have significantly better outcomes, however, for decreasing medication and healthcare use and increasing function and activity level, return to work, and closure of disability claims and with significantly fewer adverse events. Turk[52] indicated that such treatment is more cost-effective than some of the more invasive medication interventions, such as spinal cord stimulators and surgery. Despite these positive outcome data, none of the existing treatments are efficacious for all patients. The question remains, what are the obstacles to treatment for patients who are not benefiting, and, ultimately, how to improve treatment options for these patients.

OBSTACLES TO THE TREATMENT OF CHRONIC PAIN

Despite the demonstrated effectiveness of these psychological and behavioral approaches to chronic pain treatment, behavioral issues that may interfere with treatment require attention. Careful clinical assessment can identify the following challenges to successful outcomes and allow clinicians to make informed judgments before proceeding with chronic pain management.

Primary Chemical Dependency

Chronic pain complaints can mask a primary chemical dependency. Addiction affects approximately 10% of the population, and it may be overrepresented in chronic pain populations. Although substance use disorders are beyond the scope of this chapter, clinicians should be aware that pain and addiction have many symptoms in common. Depression, sleep disturbance, anxiety, and disability in work, relationships, and activity are symptoms that are separately typical of pain and addiction.[53] As such, careful addiction assessment should be an integral part of pain management, particularly in patients with a personal or family history of addiction. Although evidence suggests that addiction does not preclude effective pain treatment, practitioners should consider suspending treatment pending a thorough evaluation of any patient whose agenda may include the acquisition of pharmaceutical grade substances. In a study of patients who were otherwise adherent to prescribed controlled substances in a carefully controlled pain practice, 16% were identified through random urine testing to be using illicit drugs.[54]

Primary Psychiatric Disorder

Significant psychological and psychiatric issues accompany chronic pain. Patients with psychotic disorders, with significant dementia, with severe affective disorders, and, particularly, with active suicidal intent are not good candidates for aggressive pain management. Although it is true that "even schizophrenics have bad backs" and should not be cavalierly dismissed from pain treatment, severe psychopathology should be addressed psychiatrically before pain management is reconsidered. Similarly, patients experiencing overwhelming life stresses other than pain are at risk to be emotionally or pragmatically unavailable to take an active role in their treatment.

Ongoing Litigation

It has been axiomatic in chronic pain treatment that practitioners delay treating patients who have ongoing litigation or pending disability until the legal issue is resolved. Although specialty programs and clinics may have the luxury of postponing treatment, most primary care physicians do not. The concern is that patients recognize (or are told) that improvement in pain or in physical function might reduce or eliminate the monetary benefit that drives litigation and disability seeking. Many, if not most, patients who are pursuing legal remedies have honorable and conscientious motives and may cease their legal pursuits if the ability to function is restored. The difficulty the practitioner faces is in determining the motives of any particular patient. The research suggests caution. Blyth and colleagues[55] studied the effect of litigation on pain-related disability and found that past or present pain-related litigation was correlated significantly with higher levels of disability. Long-term follow-up of patients treated with a radiofrequency procedure showed a negative correlation between outcome and litigation status.[56] Factors that mediate the relationship between pain complaints and litigation or pursuit of disability deserve considerable research attention.

Lack of Motivation

A vexing issue for practitioners is to define for individuals experiencing pain the specific behavior changes that would lead to improvement in function and decreases in pain only to have the patient resist making the suggested changes. Despite the evidence supporting the effectiveness of modifying cognitions, exposure to feared stimuli, and increasing productive activity, some patients experiencing chronic pain do not engage successfully with treatment.[57] Prominent among the approaches to addressing this apparent lack of motivation is the application of Prochaska and DiClemente's[58] stages of change model to chronic pain. At its essence, the model proposes that individuals vary in their readiness to engage in behavior change, and that there are a series of stages of readiness. In a typical variant of the model, the stages include precontemplation (in which no change is being considered), contemplation (in which change is considered, but is not likely to occur in the near future), preparation (in which steps are being taken to make changes), action (in which behavior change is attempted), and maintenance (in which one works to sustain change). In addition to developing instruments to quantify readiness to change, researchers have begun to examine the utility of tailoring interventions to match specific stages.[59-61]

CONCLUSION

Chronic pain is maintained by biologic, psychological, and social factors. Conceptual models and treatment strategies that solely emphasize sensory and organic aspects of pain are inadequate in addressing the complex problems presented by many chronic pain patients. Evidence-based interventions require the inclusion of behavioral approaches as a component of a comprehensive interdisciplinary strategy. As treatment strategies have demonstrably become more effective, research efforts are needed to determine which specific interventions tailored to which patients for what particular problems in what social and environmental context are most effective. The research efforts designed to enhance treatment effectiveness for patients who fail to engage are particularly noteworthy. These studies represent important attempts to understand behavioral and psychosocial subgroups of patients within given physical diagnoses.

References

1. Craig K: Emotional aspects of pain. In Wall P, Melzack R (eds): Textbook of Pain, 3rd ed. London, Butler & Tanner, 1994, p 261.
2. Merskey H, Bogduk N: Classification of Chronic Pain. Seattle, IASP Press, 1994.
3. Stewart W, Ricci J, Chee E, et al: Lost productive time and cost due to common pain conditions in the U.S. workforce. JAMA 290:2443, 2003.
4. Gureje O: Persistent pain and well-being: A World Health Organization study in primary care. JAMA 280:147, 1998.
5. Osterweis M, Kleinman A, Mechanic D: Pain and Disability: Clinical, Behavioral and Public Policy Perspectives. Washington, DC, National Academy Press, 1987.
6. Romano J, Turner J: Chronic pain and depression: Does the evidence support a relationship? Psychol Bull 97:18-34, 1985.
7. Fishbain DA, Goldberg M, Meagher B, Rosomoff H: Male and female chronic pain patients categorized by DSM-III diagnostic criteria. Pain 26:181-197, 1986.
8. Strain E: Assessment and treatment of comorbid psychiatric disorders in opioid-dependent patients. Clin J Pain 18(suppl):S14-S27, 2002.

9. Boersma K, Linton S: Psychological processes underlying the development of a chronic pain problem. Clin J Pain 22:160, 2006.
10. American Psychiatric Association: Diagnostic and Statistical Manual of Mental Disorders, 4th ed, text revision. Washington, DC, APA, 2000.
11. Lewinsohn P, Gotlib I: Behavioral theory and treatment of depression. In Beckham E, Leber W (eds): Handbook of Depression, 2nd ed. New York, Guilford Press, 1995, p 352.
12. Williamson G, Schulz R: Pain, activity restriction and symptoms of depression among community-residing elderly adults. J Gerontol 47:367, 1992.
13. Morin C, Gibson D, Wade J: Self-reported sleep and mood disturbance in chronic pain patients. Clin J Pain 14:311, 1998.
14. Pilowsky I, Crettenden I, Townley M: Sleep disturbance in pain clinic patients. Pain 23:27, 1985.
15. Wilson K, Eriksson M, D'Eon J, et al: Major depression and insomnia in chronic pain. Clin J Pain 18:77, 2002.
16. Kundermann B, Krieg J, Schreiber W, Lautenbacher S: The effect of sleep deprivation on pain. Pain Res Manage 9:25, 2004.
17. Holzberg AD, Robinson ME, Geisser ME, Gremillion HA: The effects of depression and chronic pain on psychosocial and physical functioning. Clin J Pain 12:118, 1996.
18. Gamsa A: Is emotional disturbance a precipitator or a consequence of chronic pain? Pain 42:183, 1990.
19. Fishbain DA, Cutler R, Rosomoff HL, Rosomoff RS: Chronic pain-associated depression: Antecedent or consequence of chronic pain? A review. Clin J Pain 13:116, 1997.
20. Fishbain D, Cutler R, Rosomoff H: Comorbid psychiatric disorders in chronic pain patients. Pain Clin 11:79, 1998.
21. Dersh J, Polatin P, Gatchel R: Chronic pain and psychopathology: Research findings and theoretical considerations. Psychosom Med 64:773, 2002.
22. Lethem J, Slade P, Troup J, et al: Outline of a fear-avoidance model of exaggerated pain perceptions. Behav Res Ther 21:401, 1983.
23. Vlaeyen J, de Jong J, Geilen M, et al: The treatment of fear of movement/(re)injury in chronic low back pain: Further evidence on the effectiveness of exposure in vivo. Clin J Pain 18:251, 2002.
24. Polatin P, Kinney R, Gatchel R, et al: Psychiatric illness and chronic low back pain. Spine 18:66, 1993.
25. Gatchel R, Polatin P, Kinney R: Predicting outcome of chronic back pain using clinical predictors of psychopathology: A prospective analysis. Health Psychol 14:415, 1995.
26. Sansone R, Whitecar P, Meier B, Murry A: The prevalence of borderline personality among primary care patients with chronic pain. Gen Hosp Psychiatry 23:193, 2001.
27. Fordyce W, Folswer R, DeLateur B: An application of behavior modification technique to a problem of chronic pain. Behav Res Ther 6:105, 1968.
28. Turk D, Stacey B: Multidisciplinary pain centers in the treatment of chronic pain. In Frymoyer JW, Ducker TB, Hadler NM, et al (eds): The Adult Spine: Principles and Practice, 2nd ed. New York, Raven Press, 1997, p 253.
29. Fordyce WE, Fowler R, Lehmann J, et al: Operant conditioning in the treatment of chronic pain. Arch Physical Med Rehabil 54:399, 1973.
30. Fordyce WE: Behavioural Methods for Chronic Pain and Illness. St. Louis, CV Mosby, 1976.
31. Fordyce WE: Contingency management. In Bonica JJ, Loeser JD, Chapman CR, Fordyce WE (eds): The Management of Pain, 2nd ed. Philadelphia, Lea & Febiger, 1990.
32. Keefe FJ, Lefebvre JC: Behaviour therapy. In Wall P, Melzack R (eds): Textbook of Pain, 3rd ed. Edinburgh, Churchill Livingstone, 1999, p 1321.
33. Lindstrom I, Ohlund C, Eek C, et al: The effect of graded activity on patients with subacute low back pain: A randomized prospective clinical study with an operant-conditioning behavioral approach. Physical Ther 72:279, 1992.
34. Sharp TJ: Chronic pain: A reformulation of the cognitive-behavioural model. Behav Res Ther 39:787, 2001.
35. Okifuji A, Turk D, Kalauokalani D: Clinical outcomes and economic evaluation of multidisciplinary pain centers. In Block A, Kremer E, Fernandez E (eds): Handbook of Pain Syndromes. Mahwah, NJ, Lawrence Erlbaum Publishers, 1999, p 77.
36. Turk DC, Okifuji A: A cognitive-behavioural approach to pain management. In Wall P, Melzack R (eds): Textbook of Pain, 4th ed. London, Butler & Tanner, 1999, p 1431.
37. Rotter JB: Some problems and misconceptions related to the construct of internal versus external control of reinforcement. J Consult Clin Psychol 43:56, 1975.
38. Bandura A: Comments on the crusade against the causal efficacy of human thought. J Behav Ther Exp Psychiatry 26:179, 1995.
39. Bradley LA: Cognitive-behavioral therapy for chronic pain. In Gatchel RJ, Turk DC (eds): Psychological Approaches to Pain Management: A Practitioner's Handbook. New York, Guilford Press, 1996, p 131.
40. Johansson C, Dahl J, Jannert M, et al: Effects of a cognitive-behavioral pain-management program. Behav Res Ther 36:915, 1998.
41. McCracken LM, Turk DC: Behavioral and cognitive-behavioral treatment for chronic pain: Outcome, predictors of outcome, and treatment process. Spine 22:2564, 2002.
42. Linton SJ: A critical review of behavioural treatment for chronic benign pain other than headache. Br J Clin Psychol 21:321, 1982.
43. van Tulder M, Ostelo R, Vlaeyen J, et al: Behavioral treatment for chronic low back pain: A systematic review within the framework of the Cochrane Back Review Group. Spine 26:270, 2001.
44. Turner JA, Chapman CR: Psychological interventions for chronic pain: A critical review: I. Relaxation training and biofeedback. Pain 12:1, 1982.
45. Turner JA, Chapman CR: Psychological interventions for chronic pain: A critical review: II. Operant conditioning, hypnosis, and cognitive-behavioral therapy. Pain 12:23, 1982.
46. Turner JA, Clancy S, McQuade KJ, Cardenas DD: Effectiveness of behavioral therapy for chronic low back pain: A component analysis. J Consult Clin Psychol 58:573, 1990.
47. Keefe FJ, Caldwell DS, Baucom D, et al: Spouse-assisted coping skills training in the management of osteoarthritis knee pain. Arthritis Care Res 9:279, 1996.
48. Keefe FJ, Caldwell DS, Baucom D, et al: Spouse-assisted coping skills training in the management of osteoarthritis knee pain: Long-term followup results. Arthritis Care Res 12:101, 1999.
49. Malone MD, Strube MJ, Sgogin FR: Meta-anaylsis of nonmedical treatments for chronic pain. Pain 34:231, 1988.
50. Morely S, Eccleston C, Williams A: Systematic review and meta-analysis of randomized controlled trials of cognitive behaviour therapy and behaviour therapy for chronic pain in adults, excluding headache. Pain 80:1, 1999.
51. Flor H, Fydrich T, Turk DC: Efficacy of multidisciplinary pain treatment centers: A meta-analytic review. Pain 49:221, 1992.
52. Turk DC: Clinical effectiveness and cost-effectiveness of treatments for patients with chronic pain. Clin J Pain 18:355, 2002.
53. Savage S: Assessment for addiction in pain-treatment settings. Clin J Pain 18(suppl):S28, 2002.
54. Manchikanti L, Vidyasagar P, Damron K, et al: Prevalence of illicit drug use in patients without controlled substance abuse in interventional pain management. Pain Physician 6:173, 2003.
55. Blyth F, March L, Nicholas M, Cousins M: Chronic pain, work performance and litigation. Pain 103:41-47, 2003.
56. McDonald G, Lord S, Bogduk N: Long-term follow-up of patients treated with cervical radiofrequency neurotomy for chronic neck pain. Neurosurgery 45:61, 1999.
57. Turk DC, Rudy T: Neglected topics in the treatment of chronic pain patients—relapse, noncompliance, adherence enhancement. Pain 44:5, 1991.
58. Prochaska J, DiClemente C: The Transtheoretical Approach: Towards a Systematic Eclectic Framework. Homewood, IL, Dow Jones Irwin, 1984.
59. Jensoen M: Enhancing motivation to change in pain treatment. In Gatchel R, Turk D (eds): Psychological Approaches to Pain Management: A Practitioner's Handbook. New York, Guilford Press, 1996.
60. Kerns R, Rosenberg R: Predicting responses to self-management treatments for chronic pain: Application of the pain stages of change model. Pain 84:49, 2000.
61. Habib S, Morrissey S, Helmes E: Preparing for pain management: A pilot study to enhance engagement. J Pain 6:48, 2005.

chapter 121

Biofeedback

Frank Andrasik and Carla Rime

Biofeedback is a process that involves receiving information (*feedback*) about the body or self (*bio*). Applied biofeedback is the monitoring and exerting of influence to produce a change in the incoming information. Individuals receive biofeedback on their physical appearance by looking in a mirror. Applied biofeedback, then, would be altering one's physical appearance and reflection in the mirror. Combing one's hair is an everyday example of applied biofeedback.[1] In a clinical setting, biofeedback is accomplished through specialized equipment that provides information about physiologic responses occurring within the body. These processes may include muscle activity, body temperature, and skin conductance. It would be difficult to obtain accurate information about these processes by simply looking in the mirror. The available feedback provided by proper instrumentation would then allow an individual to monitor and influence these physiologic responses.

The term "applied biofeedback," as it is used in a clinical setting, was introduced by Olson[2] and encompasses the procedural operations and goals of biofeedback. Schwartz and Schwartz[3] made some minor revisions to Olson's definition (indicated by italic words).

As a process, "applied biofeedback" is

1. a group of therapeutic procedures that
2. uses electronic or electromechanical instruments
3. to accurately measure, process, and feed back, to persons *and their therapists*,
4. information with *educational and* reinforcing properties
5. about their neuromuscular and autonomic activity, both normal and abnormal,
6. in the form of analog or binary, auditory, and/or visual feedback signals.
7. It is best achieved with a competent biofeedback professional;
8. the objectives are to help persons develop *greater awareness of, confidence in, and an increase in* voluntary control over their physiologic processes that are otherwise outside awareness and/or under less voluntary control
9. by first controlling the external signal
10. and then by using "*cognitions, sensations, or other cues to prevent, stop, or reduce symptoms*" (p. 35).[3]

Components 1 through 7 of this comprehensive definition depict the key procedures of biofeedback, whereas elements 8 through 10 depict the key goals of biofeedback. The primary goal of biofeedback is the self-management of physiologic responses. This type of treatment emphasizes an active approach on the part of the patient to cope more effectively with pain and its associated symptoms.[4] This active involvement can reduce pain-related disability by increasing a patient's confidence in the ability to prevent, manage, and cope with pain.[5] In fact, patients who attribute improvements in therapy to their own efforts demonstrate better long-term maintenance than do patients who attribute their improvements to others, such as the interventions of healthcare providers.[6] Dr. Bruno Kappes, who has specialized in applied psychophysiology and biofeedback for more than 30 years, stated, "The self-efficacy created by learning to influence our psychophysiological self validates our mind's ability to direct our personal healing of the body."[1]

This chapter on biofeedback outlines the historical considerations of pioneers, research, and other growing fields that have contributed to the development of biofeedback. Treatment indications and the efficacy of biofeedback are then addressed. The techniques section delineates three approaches to biofeedback, practitioner/patient considerations, and typical treatment procedures. Possible complications and side effects are also discussed. It should be noted that biofeedback is often used in conjunction with a host of other self-regulation approaches (such as guided imagery, regulated breathing, autogenic training, and progressive muscle relaxation training, which are discussed in Chapter 123).

HISTORICAL CONSIDERATIONS

Although yogis and other individuals from Eastern cultures have long been exerting voluntary control over their internal states, it was not considered possible in Western science until the 1960s. Previously it had been believed that organisms could not self-regulate visceral functions of the internal organs of the digestive, respiratory, endocrine, and vascular systems. These functions were considered automatic and involuntary. In the 1960s, Dr. Neal E. Miller of Yale University and his colleagues countered this idea by pursuing research on this topic in the animal laboratory.[7] Skeptics believed that so-called volitional control of an involuntary response might well be mediated by slight skeletal movements. To rule out skeletal movement as an explanation for visceral reactions, much of the research was conducted on rats administered curare, which is a paralyzing agent that prevents skeletal movement. The procedure of administering curare was considered too dangerous for human research. Nonetheless, in the name of science a courageous individual offered to undergo curarization.

As recounted by Andrasik and Lords,[1] Lee Birk, who was working with David Shapiro and Bernard Tursky at Harvard University, volunteered for the risky experiment of curarization in 1967. The outcome of such an experiment would determine whether autonomic activity could be operantly conditioned without skeletal muscle movement. The research was conducted safely and the results were successful in indicating that human voluntary control over visceral organs was possible in the absence of skeletal movement. Later, Birk wrote, edited, and published *Biofeedback: Behavioral Medicine* (1973), the first medical book on biofeedback.[1]

The aforementioned pioneers conducted research that was considered unpopular at the time. They were responsible for a paradigm shift regarding potential voluntary control in human physiology. Although these individuals paved the way for biofeedback, other areas of study such as psychophysiology, behavioral therapy, biomedical engineering, and cybernetics also contributed to the development of biofeedback.

Psychophysiology is the study of the interdependent relationships between cognitive and physiologic variables. In 1965, David Shapiro offered the first class in psychophysiology, just 2 years before the pivotal research conducted with Lee Birk. Clinical biofeedback is often considered a form of "applied psychophysiology."[8]

In the 20th century, behavior therapy was a growing field in psychology. This area of study was based on principles of learning and it was contended that a learned maladaptive behavior could be unlearned. Behavioral medicine was a specialized area within behavioral therapy that emerged in light of work on stress management and the physiologic stress response. The emphasis of behavioral medicine is on health behavior associated with medical disorders.[1,8] Many behavioral therapy techniques, such as shaping and reinforcement, are used in biofeedback.

Two other fields that contributed to biofeedback were biomedical engineering and cybernetics. Biomedical engineering supplied instruments that made monitoring physiologic responses possible. With the proper instrumentation, one could detect and monitor muscle activity, cardiac activity, peripheral blood flow, blood pressure, sweat gland activity, and brain electrical activity. Cybernetics involves providing physiologic information, which is otherwise unavailable, to an individual in such a way that learning voluntary control of these responses can be achieved.[1,8]

Miller, Shapiro, and Birk, among many others, were early pioneers in biofeedback. The scientific approaches of psychophysiology, behavioral therapy, biomedical engineering, and cybernetics also assisted in the development of applied biofeedback. The Biofeedback Society of America was formed in 1968 by researchers dedicated to seek out empirical evidence for applied biofeedback. This organization is now called the Association for Applied Psychophysiology and Biofeedback (AAPB). It cosponsors the journal *Applied Psychophysiology and Biofeedback* (previously titled *Biofeedback and Self-Regulation*), in which many studies on biofeedback can be found. The following section addresses the efficacy of biofeedback in terms of medical disorders.

INDICATIONS

The AAPB organized a broad review of evidence-based research for biofeedback applications. The 2003 monograph that resulted used five efficacy levels formulated by La Vaque and associates[9] to evaluate and categorize the research. Level 1 findings are *not empirically supported*. Level 2 indicates biofeedback as *possibly efficacious*. Level 3 findings are *probably efficacious*. Level 4 signifies *efficacious* results, and level 5 consists of *efficacious and specific* findings. Table 121–1 describes the criteria for each level of efficacy. More than 30 conditions were examined and sorted into one of the five levels according to their criteria. In some cases the disorders were not sufficiently investigated, whereas in others research was conducted but some negative results were reported.

Among the disorders investigated by this task force, a number relate to pain management and symptoms that often accompany pain. Of particular interest, with a rating of at least 2 or above in efficacy levels, were anxiety, depressive disorders, arthritis, chronic pain, cystic fibrosis, fibromyalgia, headache, Raynaud disease and phenomenon, repetitive strain injury, and temporomandibular disorders (TMDs). Table 121–2 summarizes the levels of efficacy for the pain disorders discussed in this chapter. Anxiety and depressive disorders are often treated with a general biofeedback approach (the three biofeedback approaches are discussed in the subsequent section on techniques). The other aforementioned conditions are commonly treated with a specific biofeedback approach.

Many studies on biofeedback for anxiety have been comparable, but not superior to relaxation techniques. Roome and Romney,[10] however, found that electromyography (EMG)-assisted biofeedback was better than progressive muscle relaxation training. Other studies have found that biofeedback was effective in decreasing anxiety, but it was not compared with other relaxation techniques.[11,12]

Depressive disorders were rated as level 2 for biofeedback treatment efficacy, and it was noted that this area is not sufficiently investigated. Three preliminary studies[13-15] did indicate that neurofeedback may reduce depressive symptoms. Another study conducted by Corrado and Gottlieg[16] found improved Beck depression scores in chronic pain patients who were treated with biofeedback-assisted relaxation when compared with a waitlist control.

Thermal and EMG biofeedback techniques have been used for the treatment of chronic arthritis. Bradley et al.[17,18] reported a reduction in rheumatoid factor titer, pain behavior, and self-reports of pain intensity with treatment consisting of thermal biofeedback in conjunction with cognitive behavioral therapy. Patients receiving this treatment were compared with participants assigned to a control condition and those who received social support only. Furthermore, another study found that EMG biofeedback decreased the duration, intensity, and quality of arthritis pain.[19] A 2.5-year follow-up of the same participants found that these beneficial effects were maintained.[20]

The literature on biofeedback for chronic pain has often focused on back pain. A meta-analysis of single and combined

Table 121–1

Criteria for Levels of Efficacy

Level 1: Not Empirically Supported
Reports supporting this level are anecdotal or non–peer-reviewed case studies.

Level 2: Possibly Efficacious
Reports supporting this level include at least one statistically sound study but do not include random assignment for a control condition.

Level 3: Probably Efficacious
Reports supporting this level consist of multiple observations, clinical studies, controlled/waitlist conditions, and within-subject replication.

Level 4: Efficacious
Reports supporting this level include studies in which the treatment under examination is statistically significant and superior in comparison to a randomly assigned no-treatment control group, a different treatment group, or a placebo group. The inclusion criteria for a special population are reliable and operationally defined. Outcome measures associated with the problem are valid. The procedures in the study are described in such a way that other independent investigators are able to replicate the study. The superiority of the treatment under examination has been indicated in at least two independent studies.

Level 5: Efficacious and Specific
Reports supporting this level include all the criteria for level 4 in addition to indicating superior statistical significance for the treatment under examination when compared with credible placebo treatment, medication, or a different treatment in at least two independent studies.

From La Vaque TJ, Hammond DC, Trudeau D, et al: Template for developing guidelines for the evaluation of the clinical efficacy of psychophysiological interventions. Appl Psychophysiol Biofeedback 27:273, 2002.

Table 121–2

Efficacy Levels for Biofeedback Treatment of Pain Disorders and Symptoms That Often Accompany Pain

Level 2
Depression
Cystic fibrosis
Fibromyalgia
Raynaud disease/phenomenon
Repetitive strain injury

Level 3
Arthritis
Chronic pain
Pediatric headache

Level 4
Anxiety
Adult headache
Temporomandibular disorders

treatments found moderate evidence for EMG biofeedback as a separate therapy.[21] EMG biofeedback has also shown benefit equivalent to that of cognitive therapy.[22,23] Additionally, Flor and Birbaumer[24] found that EMG biofeedback produced better effects on different aspects of back pain and TMD than cognitive therapy did. These results also remained consistent at a 2-year follow-up.

Biofeedback treatment and the resulting lung function in individuals who have cystic fibrosis have also been examined. One study compared respiratory muscle biofeedback along with breathing retraining and thermal biofeedback–assisted relaxation. The investigators found a significant improvement in forced expiratory volume in 1 second and forced vital capacity in the respiratory EMG biofeedback and breathing retraining groups when compared with the thermal biofeedback group.[25] This area of research has not been sufficiently investigated and received a level 2 efficacy rating.

Fibromyalgia is a mysterious disorder that causes widespread musculoskeletal pain and fatigue. It is often treated with a number of approaches. Biofeedback has a level 2 rating in efficacy, and some negative results have been reported. Nonetheless, biofeedback has been used as part of a treatment package in conjunction with other therapies such as physical exercise, hypnosis, and cognitive behavioral therapy. Improvements have been reported in quality of sleep, pain threshold, and emotional adjustment.[26]

Biofeedback as a treatment of headache, both tension type and migraine, appears to be well validated[27-29] with an efficacy level of 4. One study found a significant reduction in headache after six sessions of EMG.[30] According to a review by Silberstein[31] for the American Academy of Neurology–U.S. Consortium, a recommended treatment option for migraine headache is either thermal or muscle biofeedback (or both). Thermal biofeedback research conducted for the treatment of pediatric headache has been classified as level 3.[32,33] After a review of the literature, Hermann and Blanchard[34] concluded that thermal biofeedback produces clinically significant (at least a 50% reduction in headache) effects in about two thirds of young participants.

Thermal biofeedback for Raynaud disease (a primary condition) and Raynaud phenomenon (a secondary condition) has been investigated. The efficacy is rated at level 2, with some negative results reported. Peterson and Vorhies[35]

conducted a study in which patients with Raynaud disease received biofeedback training. When comparing baseline and recovery measures before and after the patients immersed their hands in ice water, they found that the participants were able to return their hand temperature to baseline about six to seven times faster (an average of 40 minutes before versus 6 minutes after training). Gugliemi, Roberts, and Patterson[36] compared thermal biofeedback with EMG biofeedback and a control group. The investigators found that all three groups had comparable results and suggested that non-specific factors may account for the findings. Although the research is mixed, it is a potential therapy for Raynaud disease and phenomenon.

The AAPB task force concluded that biofeedback treatment has shown some promise in the treatment of repetitive strain injury but has not been sufficiently investigated and is therefore classified as level 2. Research on repetitive strain injury and biofeedback training published after the AAPB review has provided additional support for this treatment approach. Repetitive strain injury is considered a musculoskeletal disorder and can be detected and assessed with EMG.[37-39] Muscle learning therapy (MLT), which involves biofeedback training, was designed to treat work-related musculoskeletal disorders.[40] It has been applied as a primary prevention intervention or as a secondary post-diagnosis intervention. One study that used MLT as a primary intervention reported significant decreases in muscle tension in the trapezius area after 6 weeks of treatment, with the reduction in tension being maintained at 32-week follow-up.[41] In an additional primary intervention investigation involving biofeedback but not specifically MLT, participants who received biofeedback training in conjunction with training in ergonomics for 6 weeks reported an overall decrease in body symptoms and an increase in positive work style habits when compared with participants in the control condition.[42] MLT was also examined as a secondary intervention for individuals in whom work-related upper extremity disorders were diagnosed. After 12 sessions of MLT, participants reported significant reductions in pain and 86% had reported feeling better overall.[43] Although the AAPB rated biofeedback for repetitive strain injury as "possibly efficacious," recent research has lent further support for this approach.

In terms of biofeedback treatment, TMDs have been classified as level 4. Efficacy has been established through research with biofeedback alone[44] or in combination with other treatments.[45,46] Treatment reduces pain and pain-related disability while increasing mandibular functioning. A meta-analysis conducted by Crider and Glaros[47] found that EMG biofeedback was better than no treatment or placebo control for self-reported pain. The mean rate of improvement in the 13 trials in this literature review was 68.6% for biofeedback treatments versus 34.7% for the control conditions. Another meta-analysis, conducted after the AAPB's 2003 broad review, analyzed 14 trials involving biofeedback interventions for TMD. This review concluded that EMG-based treatment and biofeedback-assisted relaxation are probably efficacious whereas EMG in combination with cognitive-behavioral therapy is efficacious.[48]

The research on the preceding conditions described relative to pain management was extensively reviewed by AAPB. The biofeedback levels of efficacy varied. More research is needed in some of these areas to examine biofeedback alone or in combination with other treatments to make more definitive statements.

In addition to the listed disorders in which biofeedback would be a possible treatment, another area of interest is phantom limb pain. Sherman[49] noted that thermal biofeedback may help decrease pain described as burning, throbbing, and tingling whereas EMG biofeedback may help decrease pain described as cramping.

The following section outlines the different approaches to biofeedback and addresses some of the detailed treatments that were discussed for the conditions in this section.

TECHNIQUES

Biofeedback, as a self-management therapy, allows an individual to exert voluntary control over physiologic responses with the use of equipment that provides accurate measures. There is an emphasis on active involvement. In fact, Yucha and Gilbert[50] have advised using the term biofeedback *training* in place of biofeedback *treatment* to portray the active participation necessary for biofeedback therapy. This also stresses the importance of patient education. A certified biofeedback practitioner needs to "coach" patients on what to expect and to assist patients in reaching their goals with biofeedback. There are three approaches to biofeedback: general, specific, and indirect.[4]

The General Approach

The objective of the general biofeedback approach is to decrease overall arousal and to enhance a state of general relaxation. There are three ideas underlying the association between generalized relaxation and pain reduction as described by Andrasik and Thorn.[51] The first is that a decrease in general arousal reduces peripheral sensory input in central processing. The second belief is that relaxation can reduce negative affect. Negative affect is linked to an increase in pain reports and a decrease in pain tolerance.[52] The last view is that the relationship between stress and prolonged cortisol levels with the stress activation response can increase the subjective nature of pain.[53] A decrease in arousal would be beneficial for those experiencing pain. The general biofeedback approach aims to reduce this overall arousal through the three "workhorses" of biofeedback.[1] The three commonly used methods are EMG-assisted relaxation, skin conductance–assisted relaxation, and skin temperature–assisted relaxation. Figure 121–1 shows a therapist explaining biofeedback-assisted relaxation to a child.

EMG-Assisted Relaxation

Areas for placement of the sensors for EMG are generally the forehead, neck, or trapezius. A series of sensors are placed on any of these areas along the muscle fibers. The series of sensors consists of two active electrodes and one ground electrode. The two separate circuits identify electrical activity, and the resultant signal is the difference between each of the two active circuits, with the amount subtracted out being regarded as noise. When a muscle contracts, electrochemical changes occur. The electrodes detect and process the ion exchange across the muscle membrane where the muscle action potential takes place. The raw EMG signal is transformed into an

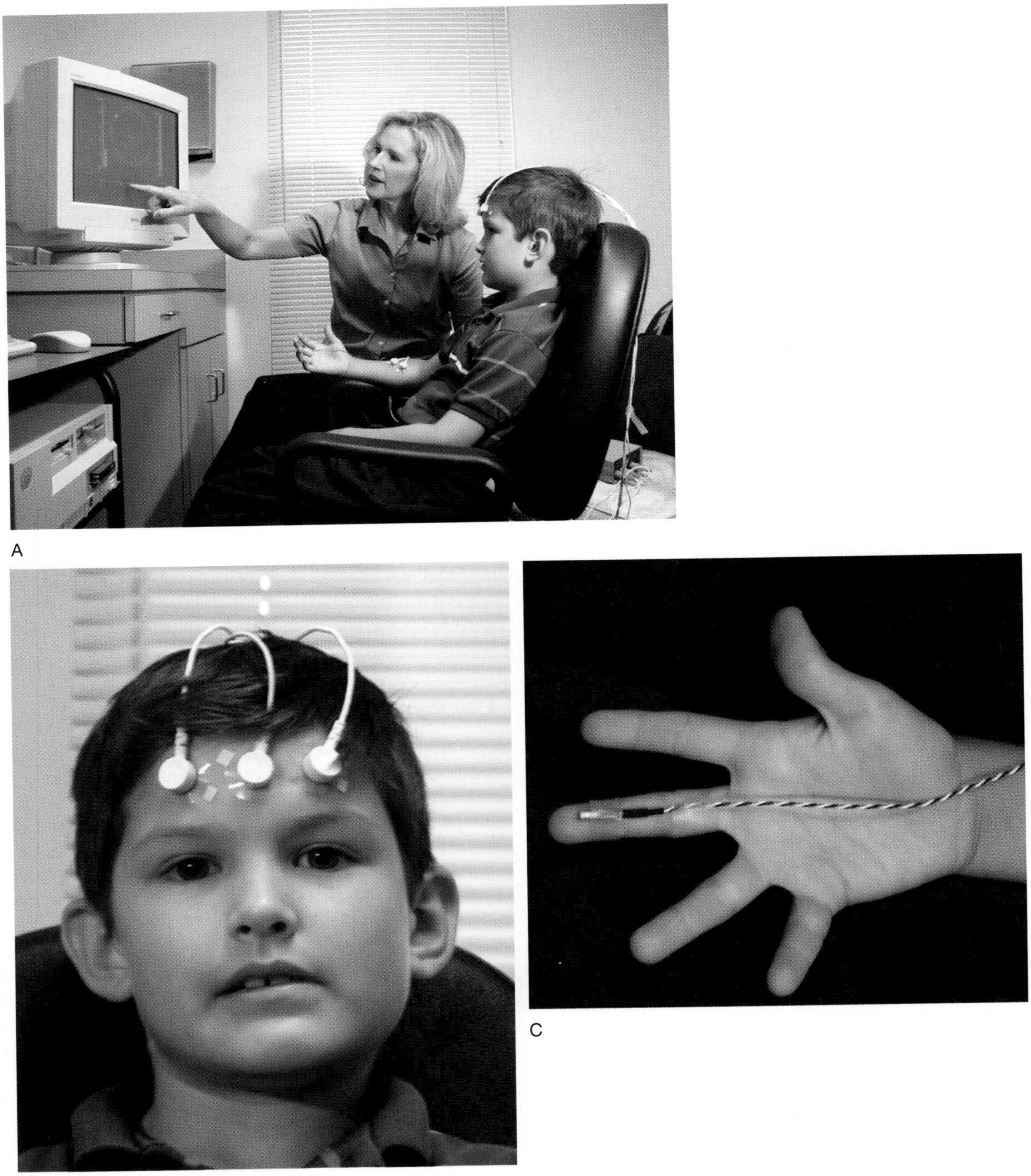

FIGURE 121–1 ■ Child receiving thermal- and EMG-assisted biofeedback training. **A,** The therapist is explaining the feedback modalities to the child. The *vertical bars* on either side of the computer monitor display EMG activity (the one to the *left* presents EMG activity from the forehead, whereas the one to the *right* is monitoring forearm muscle activity). The *circle* in the middle and the *bar* on the bottom of the monitor are providing temperature feedback (in a relative sense). Actual temperature values are provided digitally in the middle of the circle. **B,** Typical EMG electrode array for promoting generalized relaxation. **C,** Typical thermistor placement for monitoring surface skin temperature.

audible or visual presentation with a microvolt value. Modification of the raw signal into average time periods is necessary because EMG activity is too small in its original form and would make such activity difficult to discriminate. To interpret and learn how to influence muscle activity, the signals must be represented in an understandable manner.

The power spectrum of surface EMG can range from 20 to 10,000 Hz. Some of the commercially available biofeedback equipment, however, may have a more limited range, which can result in lower readings overall, so clinicians need to be aware of the "band pass" of their machine. Likewise, a practitioner should know that readings from one machine may

not be equivalent to readings from another machine. Measurements can also be affected by sensor size and type, sensor placement, distance between sensors, and the patient's adiposity because fat can dampen the signal.[54] Practitioners should follow consistent procedures for accurate EMG readings. The goal is to reduce muscle activity and achieve a more relaxed state overall.

Skin Conductance–Assisted Relaxation

Historically, measures of skin resistance were obtained to aid in understanding cases of hysterical anesthesia. Romain Virouroux used this method of measurement in the late 1880s.[54,55] In the 1900s, Carl Jung believed that measuring electrical activity of the skin was a technique that could be used in reading the mind during word association experiments.[1] Electrodermal activity, or sweating, has been long regarded as a measure associated with arousal.

Biofeedback sensors are typically positioned on the palm of the hand or the fingers, which are areas of the body densely populated with eccrine sweat glands. Perspiration is made up of salts that conduct electricity, more so than dry skin. The biofeedback machine sends a small undetectable voltage to the skin and records changes in skin conductivity. The sweat glands are primarily responsive to psychological variables and are associated with the sympathetic division of the autonomic nervous system.[56,57] Changes in autonomic arousal produce changes in dermal activity.

Conductance measures are favored over resistance measures (measured in micro-ohms or micro-siemens) because conductance activity has a linear correlation with the quantity of activated sweat glands. In clinical applications, conductivity measures are more understandable. Skin conductance increases as arousal increases, and as arousal decreases so does skin conductance. The goal of skin conductance–assisted biofeedback is to promote relaxation by reducing skin conductance and arousal.

Skin Temperature–Assisted Relaxation

Skin temperature–assisted relaxation was discovered unexpectedly. During a standard evaluation at the Menninger Clinic, an individual's migraine attack abruptly subsided with a flushing in the hands and a rapid increase in hand temperature.[58] Consequently, the clinicians who observed this event tested hand-warming treatment in migraineurs. Increasing hand temperature became a method of regulating stress and headache activity. Skin temperature is believed to provide an indirect measure of activity in the sympathetic nervous system. A reduction in arousal, or sympathetic outflow, leads to an increase in vasodilation and blood flow to the peripheral areas of the body, which is indicated by an increase in skin temperature. Conversely, an increase in arousal and sympathetic outflow constricts peripheral blood flow and results in a lower skin temperature.

Thermistors containing semiconductors and, occasionally, thermocouples are used to monitor temperature change in the skin. These temperature-sensitive sensors are placed on the fingers. Thermal-assisted biofeedback generally involves aspects of autogenic training[59] in an effort to achieve an increase in peripheral skin temperature. The procedure has been named "autogenic feedback." While recording an individual's skin temperature activity, the practitioner needs to keep in mind that measurements may be influenced by clinic, laboratory, and outdoor temperature and humidity. Heat buildup on the conductive leads and sensors can also affect the accuracy of the measurements.

The primary procedures in the general biofeedback approach are EMG-, skin conductance–, and skin temperature–assisted relaxation, also known as the "workhorses." These therapies promote a decrease in sympathetic arousal and an overall state of relaxation. A common feature of relaxation is distraction, which has been illustrated by functional MRI research to activate areas within the periaqueductal gray region.[60] This brain region has been associated with higher cortical control of pain. General relaxation-assisted biofeedback may be influencing these central mechanisms of pain.[51] For a more detailed description of relaxation therapies, including autogenic training, see Chapter 123. In some instances, a brief psychophysiologic assessment, or psychophysiologic stress profile, is used for biofeedback-assisted relaxation. A more thorough psychophysiologic assessment is used in the specific biofeedback approach, which is described in the ensuing portion of this chapter. (For more information on biofeedback instrumentation, see Peek[54]).

The Specific Approach

Many of the conditions listed in the "Indications" section of this chapter are treated by a specific biofeedback approach. To obtain initial information about a patient's condition, a psychophysiologic assessment is conducted. This preliminary evaluation is designed to identify response modalities and physiologic dysfunction relevant to the pain disorder. Various stimulus conditions, both psychological and physical, that simulate work and rest are examined. These situations may include reclining, bending, stooping, lifting, working a keyboard, and other activities. The information gathered in this assessment guides treatment and gauges progress.

Flor[61] has outlined the utility and advantages of collecting psychophysiologic data for the treatment of chronic pain: (1) provides support for the role of psychological factors in dysfunctional physiologic functioning; (2) justifies the use of biofeedback treatment; (3) facilitates customized therapy for patients; (4) makes it possible to record the efficacy, generalization, and transfer of therapy; (5) assists in predicting treatment response; and (6) serves as a source of motivation for the patient. It can help foster self-efficacy in patients who realize that they are capable of voluntarily controlling physiologic responses with their own cognitions and emotions. Typical phases of the psychophysiologic stress profile consist of adaptation, resting baseline, self-control baseline, reactivity, recovery, muscle scanning, and muscle discrimination.[62,63]

Adaptation

Three objectives for the adaptation phase are to (1) allow patients to become accustomed to the setting, clinician, and monitoring procedure; (2) minimize pre-session effects, such as rushing to the appointment, temperature and humidity differences, and differences between the setting and areas outside the setting; and (3) permit habituation of the orienting response and response stability.

During the adaptation phase, patients are instructed to sit quietly while refraining from any conscious efforts at relaxing. Even though a pre-baseline period is widely accepted, the key parameters and amount of time needed for stability are not well researched. Generally, individuals will adapt to a stable response within 5 to 20 minutes; however, some individuals do not achieve adaptation even after a 60-minute session. Practitioners are advised to extend the adaptation phase until some stability is achieved for the physiologic response of interest. This is defined as a minimal response, no fluctuation in response for a specified period, or a response that is going in a direction opposite that desired. Without an appropriate amount of time for adaptation, a clinician may mistake a habituation effect for a training effect.

Baseline

After the adaptation phase, the baseline phase begins. Data collected from the baseline phase are used as the basis for of comparison with later phases. It also gauges progress within and across subsequent treatment sessions. Again, the parameters and amount of time for collecting information in this phase are not definitive. Considerations such as whether the eyes should be open or closed, whether the patient should recline or sit upright, or whether conditions should be neutral or promote relaxation are at the practitioner's discretion. The baseline duration generally ranges from 1 to 5 minutes, which should provide an adequate, representative sample of the patient's ordinary responses during resting states.

Oftentimes a clinician will obtain a second type of baseline. This is a valuable measure for biofeedback-assisted relaxation. The practitioner instructs the patient to relax with the following sample statements, "I would now like to see what happens when you try to relax as deeply as you can. Use whatever means you believe will be helpful. Please let me know when you are as relaxed as possible." The purpose of the second baseline is to evaluate the patient's preexisting ability to relax and can be used for comparison to future training effects.

Reactivity

The third phase of the psychophysiologic assessment examines simulated stressors that pertain to the patient's condition or similar real-world situations associated with pain onset, exacerbation, or perpetuation. There is no empirically validated procedure, but the following are some common examples:

- Negative imagery, wherein a patient focuses on a personally relevant unpleasant situation (these details are usually obtained during an intake interview)
- Cold exposure (e.g., for Raynaud disease or phenomenon) or a cold pressor test (as a general physical stressor)
- Movement, such as sitting, walking, rising, bending, stooping
- Load bearing, such as lifting or carrying an object
- Operation of a keyboard or other office equipment

Even though baseline differences in EMG have not been reliable in distinguishing pain disorders, certain symptom responses have been found to be more consistent for specific pain conditions (for further discussion see Flor[61]).

Travell and Simons[64] introduced a psychophysiologic model that assesses muscle reactivity. They contended that a large percentage of chronic muscle pain is an effect of "trigger points." Hubbard[65] has extended this view with the following rationale: (1) muscle tension and pain are sympathetically mediated hyperactivity of muscle spindles, or muscle stretch receptors; (2) muscle spindles are encapsulated organs that are composed of their own muscle fibers and are scattered throughout the muscle belly (hundreds of these muscle spindles are present within the trapezius muscle); (3) even though muscle spindles are traditionally thought of as stretch sensors, they are now recognized as organs that can be activated by sympathetic activation and sense pain and pressure; and (4) therefore, the pain associated with trigger points actually arises in the spindle capsule.

This model is supported by research in which careful electrode placement has detected high levels of EMG activity in the trigger point but no activity in non-tender sites just adjacent (only 1 cm away) to the trigger point.[66] Additionally, when an individual is exposed to a stressful stimulus, EMG activity increases at the trigger point but not at any of the nearby sites.[67] These studies demonstrate an association between behavioral and emotional influences on muscle pain. Gervitz, Hubbard, and Harpin[68] designed a treatment program that uses EMG biofeedback to foster awareness of muscle tension in sessions and in daily life activities. This treatment also identifies stressors generating increased EMG activity and assists patients in coping with situations producing tension.

Recovery

After the reactivity phase is the recovery phase, where time is allotted for the patient's physiology to return to a value close to the baseline measure. Most often the responses do not fully return to the values before the reactivity-to-stress phase, and therefore a response is labeled as recovered if it returns to within a certain percentage of its initial value. If a number of stressful stimuli are presented to a patient, a recovery period is suggested after each stimulus.

The preceding phases characterize the progression of a typical psychophysiologic assessment. Though used less frequently, muscle scanning and muscle discrimination are two other approaches that may be useful.

Muscle Scanning

Cram[69] designed an approach that allows a practitioner to quickly evaluate EMG activity from multiple sites but only two channels are required. Two hand-held "post" electrodes are used to acquire brief (about 2 seconds per site) sequential bilateral recordings while the patient is sitting, standing, or moving. A normative database aids the clinician in determining whether any of the measures are abnormally high or low. It also determines whether any asymmetry exists (right versus left side differences), which may suggest bracing or favoring of a particular position or posture. The objective of biofeedback, then, is to return the aberrant recordings to a more normal state.[70] Even though this procedure may seem clear-cut, it is actually more complex. Several factors may affect the measures obtained. For example, the angle and force of the applied sensors, the sensor locations used for the norming sample, and the other variables previously discussed may influence EMG readings.

Muscle Discrimination

Flor and associates[71] found that individuals with chronic pain misperceive muscle tension in both the affected and

non-affected muscles. When the patients were presented with tasks that required the production of muscle tension, they would overestimate physical symptoms, report greater pain, and rate the task as more aversive. Heightened sensitivity may account for the inability to accurately perceive body states. To assess muscle discrimination ability in a clinical setting, Flor[61] recommends the following:

- Present the patient with a bar of varying height on a monitor.
- Instruct the patient to tense a muscle to the level in the height of the presented bar.
- Vary the bar height from low to high.
- Correlate the EMG measures with the actual height of the bars.
- Define correlation coefficients of .80 or greater as "good" discrimination ability.
- Define correlation coefficients of .50 or lower as "bad" discrimination ability.

The psychophysiologic assessment techniques for the specific approach to biofeedback allow a practitioner and the patient to monitor and record progress for areas associated with pain. It may also be used in a more abbreviated manner for the general biofeedback approach. Another style of biofeedback is the indirect approach.

The Indirect Approach

Belar and Kibrick[72] advocated use of the "indirect" approach to biofeedback for certain pain patients based on clinical rather than empirical reasons. Biofeedback may be used as a means of facilitating psychosomatic therapy. Take, for example, a pain patient who has the conviction that the pain is purely somatic while denying the notion that other emotional, behavioral, and environmental factors may be precipitating, perpetuating, and exacerbating the pain. Biofeedback may be considered a "physical" treatment of a "physical" problem, and referral for this type of treatment may be less threatening. Such patients may acquire a "physiologic insight" in which they can see the interactions between psychological and physical factors. It is not uncommon for a patient who denied that psychological factors may be affecting the pain to make a request after a few sessions of biofeedback, such as "How about turning off the biofeedback equipment today. I want to talk to you about a few things." From this point on, treatment sessions may involve time divided between biofeedback and counseling. Some have referred to this as the Trojan horse aspect of biofeedback.

The general, specific, and indirect approaches each have their own unique techniques and objectives. The general approach promotes overall relaxation through EMG, thermal, or skin conductance biofeedback, which can reduce stress, tension, and pain. The specific approach can be used for precise pain sites, such as trigger points. A psychophysiologic assessment, or stress profile, is often used for evaluating the pain symptoms and physiologic responses. The indirect approach to biofeedback may open the door for a patient to recognize the interplay of psychological factors and physiologic responses. Responses to treatment may vary among individual patients. Patient considerations will be discussed next.

Practitioner/Patient Considerations

The emphasis on patient education and treatment progress can establish therapy that is successful. The professional relationship between the clinician and the patient is of great importance. In fact, Taub and School[73] reviewed several experimental variables and reported that the behavior of the practitioner, as well as the practitioner's confidence in the treatment, has the greatest effect on patient progress in biofeedback therapy. In addition to the clinician's expectations, the patient's expectations are also very important. Holroyd et al.[74] found that the greatest predictor of significant improvement in tension-type headache with EMG biofeedback is the patient's expectation of the ability to voluntarily control the onset and course of the condition. Likewise, beneficial treatment outcomes for headache are affected by the individual's perceived self-control.[30]

Individuals referred for biofeedback treatment may be confused about the nature of their pain condition and be uncertain about their chance for improvement. Patient education offered by the practitioner is crucial in alleviating a patient's apprehension of biofeedback treatment. Identification of variables that may be controlled by the patient and are having an impact on the condition is often helpful in alleviating the patient's initial feelings about the therapy. Additionally, a detailed description of the treatment, what to expect, and a live demonstration can give the patient an idea of what to anticipate in therapy (a typical session of biofeedback is described later).

The biofeedback practitioner is regarded as a "coach" guiding patients in treatment. The patient is the active player learning skills of self-management. Coaching involves sharing observations for discussion ("I noticed that your EMG signal suddenly increased. It seemed you might have been clenching your teeth then. How about dropping your lower jaw and moving it a bit forward? I wonder if anything in particular was on your mind then?") The clinician also determines when breaks and encouragement might be needed. Initial attempts to lower EMG activity and skin conductance and increase hand temperature are frequently met with the opposite effect, and this may paradoxically worsen as patients try harder and harder. These situations can be valuable in demonstrating the interaction between psychological and physiologic functioning and illustrate how the patient's current coping strategies are actually "backfiring." The coach explains how and why this happens and can alleviate the patient's frustration to get the patient back on track. In addition, the therapist helps the patient articulate, understand, and consolidate the learning of skills. Other self-management techniques are also imparted to the patient. The discretion of the clinician is important in facilitating progress because if the coach is too overbearing, it can negatively affect treatment.[75]

The U.S. Headache Consortium has described individuals who are good candidates for biofeedback or other behavioral treatments. One or more of the following factors must be present:

- The patient prefers the approach.
- Pharmacologic treatment cannot be tolerated or is medically contraindicated.
- The pharmacologic treatment response is absent or minimal.

- The patient is pregnant, plans to become pregnant, or is nursing.
- The patient has a history of frequent or excessive use of analgesic or acute medications.
- The patient is faced with a number of stressors or has deficient stress-coping skills.

Children often respond especially well to biofeedback.[76,77] Older patients usually need more time to master self-regulation skills.[78,79]

A typical biofeedback session consists of the following components:

- Sensor attachment and time for adaptation
- Initial progress review
- Resting baseline
- "Self-control" baseline (the patient's ability to regulate the target response in the desired direction in the absence of feedback to provide a comparison to the ability to perform skills outside the treatment setting[80])
- 20 to 30 minutes of actual feedback (continuous or with breaks)
- Final resting or self-control baseline (assess learning within the session)
- Final progress review and assigned homework

There is no firm standard for the number of treatment sessions necessary for reaching the appropriate goals of therapy. The duration of treatment depends on the clinical response of relief of symptoms or the patient's adequate control of the target measure. When treatment reaches a point of diminishing returns, such as response plateaus, the practitioner should terminate further treatment. Research on biofeedback-assisted relaxation has shown that the desired goals are typically accomplished in 8 to 12 sessions. Haddock and coworkers[81] found that headache patients respond quicker to treatment when homework assignments consist of detailed manuals and relaxation tapes. The treatment duration is subject to individual differences in treatment response.

Lynn and Freedman[82] have outlined several methods to increase generalization and maintenance of beneficial biofeedback skills: (1) over-learning the response and continuing to practice learned skills; (2) incorporating booster treatments; (3) fading or gradually removing feedback during treatment; (4) training under stressful situations such as during noise, distractions, and physical or mental tasks; (5) using multiple practitioners, which is possible with group treatment; (6) varying the physical setting; (7) providing portable biofeedback devices for homework assignments; and (8) supplementing biofeedback with other procedures such as cognitive and behavioral techniques. Many of these suggestions are based on the learning principles of behavior therapy.

This section has delineated the three approaches to biofeedback, patient considerations, "coach"/practitioner considerations, a typical treatment session, treatment duration, and procedures for improving the durability of the skills learned from biofeedback therapy. The next section addresses some of the side effects and complications of biofeedback treatment.

SIDE EFFECTS AND COMPLICATIONS

Even though biofeedback treatments commonly have positive outcomes, a few difficulties have been reported. A small number of patients may experience initial negative outcomes such as muscle cramps or disturbing sensory, cognitive, or emotional reactions. Other problems may arise that can have an impact on adherence and practice. A small proportion of individuals may experience an abrupt increase in anxiety as they become deeply relaxed because a deep state of relaxation may be foreign to them. This condition is termed *relaxation-induced anxiety,* and symptoms can range from mild to moderate in intensity and may come close to a minor panic attack.[83] If this situation occurs, the practitioner needs to remain calm and reassure the patient that the episode will soon pass. Having the patient sit up or walk around the office usually helps. When patients are at risk for relaxation-induced anxiety, the clinician can instruct them to concentrate on the somatic aspects rather than the cognitive aspects of training.[84] See Schwartz, Schwartz, and Monastra[85] for a discussion of other problems and solutions. A more detailed description of complications associated with relaxation therapies can be found in Chapter 123.

Some medications may act on the central and autonomic nervous systems and complicate biofeedback therapy. For example, muscle relaxants may relax target muscle groups and elicit inaccurate measures for the process of biofeedback training. Other medications, such as asthma inhalers, act on the autonomic nervous system and cause blood vessels to constrict. This may impede thermal biofeedback training by decreasing blood flow to peripheral areas of the body. In some instances, the improvement attained in biofeedback therapy may require medication adjustments. This is one of the many reasons why biofeedback clinicians should maintain a collaborative working relationship with medical associates.

CONCLUSION

Biofeedback treatment is a viable option for several pain disorders and accompanying symptoms. This chapter has summarized historical considerations such as early pioneers, research, and other related fields contributing to the development of biofeedback. A comprehensive AAPB evidence-based review of treatment options for anxiety, depression, arthritis, chronic pain, cystic fibrosis, fibromyalgia, headache, Raynaud disease and phenomenon, repetitive strain injury, and TMD was presented. It was noted that efficacy levels for these conditions varied and that some areas need more research to examine outcomes with biofeedback therapy.

The "Techniques" section addressed the general, specific, and indirect approaches to biofeedback, including the components of psychophysiologic assessment. Furthermore, this section discussed practitioner/patient considerations, a typical biofeedback session, and treatment duration. Side effects and complications of biofeedback therapy are minimal. Relaxation-induced anxiety and medication complications were identified as infrequent occurrences. Throughout the chapter, the patient's active role and education in the therapy process were emphasized.

FURTHER RESOURCES

For more information regarding research, credential programs, or biofeedback in general, visit the following websites:

- Association of Applied Psychophysiology and Biofeedback (*http://www.aapb.org*)
- Biofeedback Certification Institute of America (*http://www.bcia.org*)
- Biofeedback Foundation of Europe (*http://www.bfe.org*)
- International Society for Neuronal Regulation (*http://www.snr-jnt.org*)

References

1. Andrasik F, Lords AO: Biofeedback. In Freeman L (ed): Mosby's Complementary & Alternative Medicine: A Research-Based Approach, 2nd ed. Philadelphia, Elsevier, 2004, p 207.
2. Olson RP: Definitions of biofeedback and applied psychophysiology. In Schwartz MS, et al (eds): Biofeedback: A Practitioner's Guide, 2nd ed. New York, Guilford Press, 1995.
3. Schwartz, NM, Schwartz, MS: Definitions of biofeedback and applied psychophysiology. In Schwartz MS, Andrasik F (eds): Biofeedback: A Practitioner's Guide, 3rd ed. New York, Guilford Press, 2003, p 27.
4. Andrasik F: Relaxation and Biofeedback Self-Management for Pain. In Boswell MV, Cole BE (eds): Weiner's Pain Management: A Practical Guide for Clinicians, 7th ed. Boca Raton, Taylor & Francis, 2006, p 705.
5. French DJ, Holroyd KA, Pineel C, et al: Perceived self-efficacy and headache-related disability. Headache 40:647, 2000.
6. Spinhoven P, Lenssen AC, Van Dyck R, Zitman FG: Autogenic training and self-hypnosis in the control of tension headache. Gen Hosp Psychiatry 14:408, 1997.
7. Dworkin BR, Miller NE: Visceral learning in the curarized rat. In Schwartz GE, Beatty J (eds): Biofeedback: Theory and Research. New York, Academic Press, 1977.
8. Schwartz MS, Olson RP: A historical perspective on the field of biofeedback and applied psychophysiology. In Schwartz MS, Andrasik F (eds): Biofeedback: A Practitioner's Guide, 3rd edition. New York, Guilford Press, 2003, p 3.
9. La Vaque TJ, Hammond DC, Trudeau D, et al: Template for developing guidelines for the evaluation of the clinical efficacy of psychophysiological interventions. Appl Psychophysiol Biofeedback 27: 273, 2002.
10. Roome JR, Romney DM: Reducing anxiety in gifted children by inducing relaxation. Roeper Rev 7:177, 1985.
11. Hurley JD, Meminger, SR: A relapse-prevention program: Effects of electromyographic training on high and low levels of state and trait anxiety. Percept Mot Skills 74:699, 1992.
12. Wenck LS, Leu PW, D'Amato RC: Evaluating the efficacy of biofeedback intervention to reduce children's anxiety. J Clin Psychol 52:469, 1996.
13. Kumano H, Horie H, Shidara T, et al: Treatment of a depressive disorder patient with EEG-driven photic stimulation. Biofeedback Self Regul 21:323, 1996.
14. Rosenfeld JP: An EEG biofeedback protocol for affective disorders. Clin Electroencephalogr 31:7, 2000.
15. Waldkoetter RO, Sanders GO: Auditory brainwave stimulation in treating alcoholic depression. Percept Mot Skills 84:226, 1997.
16. Corrado P, Gottlieb H: The effect of biofeedback and relaxation training on depression in chronic pain patients. Am J Alternative Med 9:18, 1999.
17. Bradley LA: Effects of cognitive-behavioral therapy on pain behavior of rheumatoid arthritis (RA) patients: Preliminary outcomes. Scand J Behav Ther 14:51, 1985.
18. Bradley LA, Young LD, Anderson KO, et al: Effects of psychological therapy on pain behavior of rheumatoid arthritis patients. Treatment outcome and six-month follow-up. Arthritis Rheum 30:1105, 1987.
19. Flor H, Haag G, Turk DC, Koehler H: Efficacy of EMG biofeedback, pseudotherapy, and conventional medical treatment for chronic rheumatic back pain. Pain 17:21, 1983.
20. Flor H, Haag G, Turk DC: Long-term efficacy of EMG biofeedback for chronic rheumatic back pain. Pain 27:195, 1986.
21. Nielson WR, Weir R: Biopsychosocial approaches to the treatment of chronic pain. Clin J Pain 17:S114, 2001.
22. Vlaeyen JW, Haazen IW, Schuerman JA, et al: Behavioural rehabilitation of chronic low back pain: Comparison of an operant treatment, an operant-cognitive treatment and an operant-respondent treatment. Clin Psychol 34:95, 1995.
23. Newton-John TR, Spence SH, Schotte D: Cognitive-behavioural therapy versus EMG biofeedback in the treatment of chronic low back pain. Behav Res Ther 33:691, 1995.
24. Flor H, Birbaumer N: Comparison of the efficacy of electromyographic biofeedback, cognitive-behavioral therapy, and conservative medical intervention in the treatment of chronic musculoskeletal pain. J Consult Clin Psychol 61:653, 1993.
25. Delk KK, Gevirtz R, Hicks DA, et al: The effects of biofeedback assisted breathing retraining on lung function in patients with cystic fibrosis. Chest 105:23, 1994.
26. Berman BM, Swyers JP: Complementary medicine treatments for fibromyalgia syndrome. Baillieres Best Pract Res Clin Rheumatol 13:487, 1999.
27. Arena JG, Bruno GM, Hannah SL, Meader KJ: Comparison of frontal electromyographic biofeedback training, trapezius electromyographic biofeedback training, and progressive muscle relaxation therapy in the treatment of tension headache. Headache 35:411, 1995.
28. McGrady A, Wauquier A, McNeil A, Gerard C: Effect of biofeedback-assisted relaxation on migraine headache and changes in the cerebral blood flow velocity in the middle cerebral artery. Headache 34:424, 1994.
29. Vasudeva S, Claggett AL, Tietjen GE, McGrady AV: Biofeedback-assisted relaxation in migraine headache: Relationship to cerebral blood flow velocity in the middle cerebral artery. Headache 43:245, 2003.
30. Rokicki LA, Holroyd KA, France CR, et al: Change mechanisms associated with combined relaxation/EMG biofeedback training for chronic tension type headache. Appl Psychophysiol Biofeedback 22:21, 1997.
31. Silberstein SD: Practice parameter: Evidence-based guidelines for migraine headache (an evidence-based review): Report of the quality of standards subcommittee of the American Academy of Neurology. Neurology 55:754, 2000.
32. Arndorfer RE, Allen KD: Extending the efficacy of a thermal biofeedback treatment package to the management of tension-type headaches in children. Headache 41:183, 2001.
33. Labbe EE: Treatment of childhood migraine with autogenic training and skin temperature biofeedback: A component analysis. Headache 35:10, 1995.
34. Hermann C, Blanchard EB: Biofeedback in the treatment of headache and other childhood pain. Appl Psychophysiol Biofeedback 27:143, 2002.
35. Peterson LL, Vorhies C: Raynaud's syndrome: Treatment with sublingual administration of nitroglycerin, swinging arm maneuver, and biofeedback training. Arch Dermatol 119:396, 1983.
36. Guglielmi RS, Roberts AH, Patterson R: Skin temperature biofeedback for Raynaud's disease: A double-blind study. Biofeedback Self Regul 7:99, 1982.
37. Clasby RG, Derro DJ, Snelling L, Donaldson S: The use of surface electromyographic techniques in assessing musculoskeletal disorders in production operations. Appl Psychophysiol Biofeedback 28:161, 2003.
38. Donaldson CC, Nelson DV, Skubick DL, Clasby RG: Potential contributions of neck muscle dysfunctions to initiation and maintenance of carpal tunnel syndrome. Appl Psychophysiol Biofeedback 23:59, 1998.
39. Klein BU, Schumann NP, Bradl I, et al: Surface EMG of shoulder and back muscles and posture analysis in secretaries typing at visual display units. Int Arch Occup Environ Health 72:387, 1999.
40. Ettare D, Ettare R: Muscle learning therapy: Clinical EMG for surface recordings. In Cram J (ed): Clinical Resources, vol 2. Nevada City, CA, Cram & Associates, 1990, p 197.
41. Faucett J, Garry M, Nadler D, Ettare D: A test of two training interventions to prevent work-related musculoskeletal disorders of the upper extremity. Appl Ergon 33:337, 2002.
42. Peper E, Gibney KH, Wilson VE: Group training with healthy computing practices to prevent repetitive strain injury (RSI): A preliminary study. Appl Psychophysiol Biofeedback 29:279, 2004.
43. Nord S, Ettare D, Drew D, Hodge S: Muscle learning therapy—efficacy of a biofeedback based protocol in treating work-related upper extremity disorders. J Occup Rehabil 11:23, 2001.
44. Gardea MA, Gatchel RJ, Mishra KD: Long-term efficacy of biobehavioral treatment of temporomandibular disorders. J Orofacial Pain 13:29, 2001.
45. Turk DC, Zaki HS, Rudy TE: Effects of intraoral appliance and biofeedback/stress management alone and in combination in treating pain and

depression in patients with temporomandibular disorders. J Prosthet Dent 70:158, 1993.
46. Turk DC, Rudy TE, Kubinski JA, et al: Dysfunctional patients with temporomandibular disorders: Evaluating the efficacy of a tailored treatment protocol. J Consult Clin Psychol 64:139, 1996.
47. Crider AB, Glaros AG: A meta-analysis of EMG biofeedback treatment of temporomandibular disorders. J Orofacial Pain 13:29, 1999.
48. Crider A, Glaros AG, Gevirtz RN: Efficacy of biofeedback-based treatments for temporomandibular disorders. Appl Psychophysiol Biofeedback 30:333, 2005.
49. Sherman R: Phantom Pain. New York, Plenum Press, 1997.
50. Yucha C, Gilbert C: Evidence-Based Practice in Biofeedback and Neurofeedback for Biofeedback-Assisted Behavioural Therapy. Wheat Ridge, CO, Association for Applied Psychophysiology and Biofeedback, 2004.
51. Andrasik F, Thorn BE: Biofeedback in the treatment of pain. In Schmidt RF, Willis WD (eds): Encyclopedia of Pain. New York, Springer-Verlag (in press).
52. Fernandez E: Anxiety, Depression, and Anger in Pain. Dallas, Advanced Psychological Resources, 2002.
53. Melzack R: Pain and stress: A new perspective. In Gatchel RJ, Turk DC (eds): Psychosocial Factors and Pain: Critical Perspectives. New York, Guilford Press, 1999, p 89.
54. Peek CJ: A primer of biofeedback instrumentation. In Schwartz MS, Andrasik F (eds): Biofeedback: A Practitioner's Guide, 3rd ed. New York, Guilford Press, 2003, p 43.
55. Neuman E, Blanton R: The early history of electrodermal research. Psychophysiology 6:453, 1970.
56. Boucsein W: Electrodermal Activity. New York, Plenum Press, 1992.
57. Stern RM, Ray WJ, Quigley KS: Psychophysiological Recording, 2nd ed. Oxford, Oxford University Press, 2001.
58. Sargent JD, Green EE, Walters ED: The use of autogenic training in a pilot study of migraine and tension headaches. Headache 12:120, 1972.
59. Schultz JH, Luthe W: Autogenic Therapy, vol 1. New York, Grune & Stratton, 1969.
60. Tracey I, Ploghaus A, Gati JS, et al: Imaging attentional modulation of pain in the periaqueductal gray in humans. J Neurosci 22:2748, 2002.
61. Flor H: Psychophysiological assessment of the patient with chronic pain. In Turk DC, Melzack R (eds): Handbook of Pain Assessment, 2nd ed. New York, Guilford, 2001, p 76.
62. Andrasik F, Thorn BE, Flor H: Psychophysiological assessment of pain. In Schmidt RF, Willis WD (eds): Encyclopedia of Pain. New York, Springer-Verlag (in press).
63. Arena JG, Shwartz MS: Psychophysiological assessment and biofeedback baselines for the front-line clinician: A primer. In Schwartz MS, Andrasik F (eds): Biofeedback: A Practitioner's Guide, 3rd ed. New York, Guilford Press, 2003.
64. Travell J, Simons D: Myofascial Pain and Dysfunction: The Trigger Point Manual. New York, Williams & Wilkins, 1983.
65. Hubbard D: Chronic and recurrent muscle pain: Pathophysiology and treatment, and review of pharmacologic studies. J Musculoskel Pain 4:123, 1996.
66. Hubbard D, Berkoff G: Myofascial trigger points show spontaneous EMG activity. Spine 18:1803, 1993.
67. McNulty E, Gevirtz R, Hubbard D, Berkoff G: Needle electromyographic evaluation of trigger point response to a psychological stressor. Psychophysiology 31:313, 1994.
68. Gevirtz RN, Hubbard DR, Harpin RE: Psychophysiologic treatment of chronic lower back pain. Professional Psychol Res Pract 27:561, 1996.
69. Cram JR: EMG muscle scanning and diagnostic manual for surface recordings. In Cram JR (ed): Clinical Resources, vol 2. Nevada City, CA, Cram & Associates, 1990.
70. Sella GE: Neuropathy considerations: Clinical and SEMG/biofeedback applications. Appl Psychophysiol Biofeedback 28:93, 2003.
71. Flor H, Furst M, Birbaumer N: Deficient discrimination of EMG levels and overestimation of perceived tension in chronic pain patients. Appl Psychophysiol Biofeedback 24:55, 1999.
72. Belar CD, Kibrick SA: Biofeedback in the treatment of chronic back pain. In Holzman AD, Turk DC (eds): Pain Management: A Handbook of Psychological Treatment Approaches. New York, Pergamon Press, 1986, p 131.
73. Taub E, School PJ: Some methodological considerations in thermal biofeedback training. Behav Res Methods Instrum 10:617, 1978.
74. Holroyd KA, Penzien DB, Hursey KG, et al: Change mechanisms in EMG biofeedback training: Cognitive changes underlying improvements in tension headache. J Consult Clin Psychol 52:1039, 1984.
75. Borgeat F, Hade B, Larouche LM, Bedwani CN: Effect of therapist's active presence on EMG biofeedback training of headache patients. Biofeedback Self Regul 5:275, 1980.
76. Andrasik F, Blake DD, McCarran MS: A biobehavioral analysis of pediatric headache. In Krasnegor NA, Arasteh JD, Cataldo MF (eds): Child Health Behavior: A Behavioral Pediatrics Perspective. New York, Wiley, 1986, p 394.
77. Attanasio V, Andrasik F, Burke EJ, et al: Clinical issues in utilizing biofeedback with children. Clin Biofeedback Health 8:134, 1985.
78. Arena JG, Hannah SL, Bruno GM, Meador KJ: Electromyographic biofeedback training for tension headache in the elderly: A prospective study. Biofeedback Self Regul 16:379, 1991.
79. Kabela E, Blanchard EB, Appelbaum KA, Nicholson N: Self-regulatory treatment of headache in the elderly. Biofeedback Self Regul 14:219, 1989.
80. Blanchard EB, Epstein LH: A Biofeedback Primer. Reading, MA, Addison-Wesley, 1978.
81. Haddock CK, Rowan AB, Andrasik F, et al: Home-based behavioral treatments for chronic benign headache: A meta-analysis of controlled trials. Cephalagia 17:113, 1997.
82. Lynn SJ, Freedman RR: Transfer and evaluation of biofeedback treatment. In Goldstein AP, Kanfer F (eds): Maximizing Treatment Gains: Transfer Enhancement in Psychotherapy. New York, Academic Press, 1979, p 445.
83. Heide FJ, Borkovec TD: Relaxation-induced anxiety: Paradoxical anxiety enhancement due to relaxation training. J Consult Clin Psychol 51:171, 1983.
84. Arena JG, Blanchard EB: Biofeedback and relaxation therapy for chronic pain disorders. In Gatchel RJ, Turk DC (eds): Psychological Approaches to Pain Management: A Practitioner's Handbook. New York, Guilford Press, 1996, p 179.
85. Schwartz MS, Schwartz NM, Monastra VJ: Problems with relaxation and biofeedback-assisted relaxation, and guidelines for management. In Schwartz MS, Andrasik F (eds): Biofeedback: A Practitioner's Guide, 3rd ed. New York, Guilford Press, 2003, p 251.

chapter 122

Hypnosis

Howard Hall

HISTORICAL CONSIDERATIONS

The origin of hypnosis is associated with an 18th century Viennese physician, Franz Anton Mesmer (1734-1815). He became quite famous in Paris for inducing a type of convulsive seizure he called a "crisis," which was apparently associated with therapeutic effects on the body. The setting for Mesmer's treatments included soft background music, a draped room in which patients would hold on to metal bars extending from a wooden tub filled with water, ground glass, and iron filings (his medium for magnetism). He used magnets for healing purposes, and he developed a theory of animal magnetism, later known as "mesmerism." His theory of disease and healing involved "balancing magnetic fluids,"[1] which today might be termed "energy medicine." Many of the conditions that he treated with mesmerism, however, might now be considered as functional disorders, having a psychological base, such as conversion symptoms of paralyses, seizures, and deafness, or stress-related conditions, such as headaches.[2] Mesmerism generated so much attention that in 1784 Louis XVI of France formed a commission, headed by Benjamin Franklin, to examine the theory of animal magnetism. After running a series of controlled experiments to test the phenomenon, the commission concluded that Mesmer's cures were produced by the patient's imagination and not magnetism.[1] It should be pointed out that the commission did not determine that Mesmer's results were not authentic, just that they were not the results of magnetism. Such a pronouncement during this era of reason and enlightenment, however, was equivalent to saying that the results of magnetism were not real.

One of the most important uses of mesmerism in the early 1800s in France, England, and later the United States was as a benign anesthetic agent for surgical patients. A range of operations were performed with mesmerism, including mastectomies, amputations of legs, removal of glands and jaw tumors, and tooth extractions. In one case of tooth extraction the patient was described as showing no apparent discomfort or reaction to the pain.[2]

Around 1840, English surgeon James Braid (1795-1860) recognized that some mesmeric phenomena were genuine but argued against the doctrine of animal magnetism. Braid put forward his own view that the phenomenon of mesmerism was related to subjective or psychological variables.[3] He employed an eye-fixation induction that he learned from a mesmerist and coined the term "hypnosis" to describe this phenomenon because he believed it was an artificially induced state of sleep (Hypnos is the Greek god of sleep). Today, of course, we know hypnosis has no relationship to sleep in terms of EEG measures.

Some of the most dramatic examples for the application of hypnosis consisted of its use for painless surgery, with work done by Jame Esdaile between 1845 and 1851. Esdaile was a Scottish surgeon who practiced medicine in India and performed several thousand operations with hypnosis used as the sole analgesic technique.[2] Even more impressive was the fact that over 300 of these operations involved major surgery, with a mortality rate of only about 5%, as compared with the 50% death rate for conventional surgical procedures during that time. The use of hypnosis as an anesthetic technique for surgery declined by the third quarter of the 19th century. First, the results with hypnosis were often variable and unpredictable. During this time period, there was a report of one patient suing for assault when she emerged from hypnotic analgesia in the middle of the operation. Second, there was also the development and increasing use of chemical anesthetic agents in 1846 when Liston performed the first operation employing ether in England.[4] Also, unprofessional and fringe practices entered the field of hypnosis, leading to a decline in its use.[2]

Hypnosis for the treatment of children goes back over 200 years, but it was not until the 20th century that it emerged as a subspecialty area with novel training opportunities that put much emphasis on pain management.[5-8] The field of pediatric hypnosis maintains that children are more responsive to hypnosis than are adults, which has important implications for successful pain management. Hypnotic inductions with children also tend to be more permissive, playful, imaginative, and less structured and authoritative than the approaches used with adults. In addition, one has to be mindful of a child's developmental level when using hypnotic approaches.

INDICATIONS

Hypnosis today can be used in an integrative manner as an adjunctive treatment along with traditional medical and pharmacologic treatment, or as an alternative nonpharmacologic traditional treatment. This intervention can be employed before, during, or after painful procedures or operations.

Hypnosis for Preoperative and Postoperative Pain Management

Hypnotic and other psychological interventions before surgery have been associated with faster postoperative recovery, shorter hospital stay, less narcotic use, and less postoperative pain and anxiety.[9] Hypnosis has also been associated with decreased postoperative orthopaedic pain, faster surgeon-rated recovery, and, in one study, no postoperative complications compared to 8 instances in the usual care condition for this quasiexperimental research design (N = 60).[10]

Hypnosis for Management of Acute Pain

There is also good evidence from controlled trials of acute pain reduction that hypnosis is superior to standard care, attention controls, or other viable pain-reduction interventions.[11] Anxiety is a major factor contributing to distress during many painful medical procedures. This becomes clear when children begin crying as soon as a doctor approaches them with a needle or when adults become distressed at the sound of the drill in the dentist chair. Hypnosis has been employed within dentistry, and it can be helpful for both the anxiety and pain perception during many medical procedures.[12] Response to hypnotic interventions for children and adolescents with cancer undergoing bone marrow aspirations varied as a function of the child's age, gender, and hypnotic susceptibility,[13] but the benefit of hypnotic versus other cognitive approaches to pain management in children requires further research.[14] Hypnosis has also provided added benefit to local anesthetics, such as EMLA cream, for lumbar punctures and bone marrow aspirations with young cancer patients. This procedure has an impact on managing both pain and anticipatory anxiety.[15]

Hypnosis for Cancer Pain Management

Hypnosis is employed not only for the management of pain and anxiety of medical procedures associated with cancer, as noted above, but also for the neuropathic pain associated with the disease itself. Often hypnosis can provide added benefits for conditions such as neuropathic cancer pain where opioids and other medical treatments have not been found to be totally effective when used alone. There is now emphasis on integrating hypnosis along with traditional medical treatments for chronic pain conditions.[16]

Hypnosis for Obstetric Pain

Hypnosis has been used during pregnancy for the management of nausea and vomiting, for prevention of premature labor, as an adjunctive treatment for pregnancy-induced hypertension, and as an intervention for pain and discomfort during labor and delivery.[17,18] It is estimated that about 20% to 35% of women are able to use hypnosis as the sole anesthesia during labor or delivery.[19] For everyone else, hypnosis can be used as an adjunctive nonpharmacologic analgesia along with standard care.

Hypnosis for Emergency Treatment of Burns

Case histories of hypnotic interventions for burn victims have reported dramatic results on attenuating the inflammatory response to the burn injury if hypnosis is conducted during the first 2 hours following injury.[20] Controlled studies, however, provide less dramatic outcomes.[21]

Hypnosis for Chronic Pain Conditions: Headaches, Fibromyalgia, Gastrointestinal Disorders, and Sickle Cell Disease

Evidence from controlled trials for chronic pain shows hypnosis to be superior to no treatment, but equivalent to relaxation and autogenic training.[11] Chronic pain is a complex phenomenon and does not respond as robustly to hypnotic interventions as acute pain conditions.[11] Self-hypnosis training, however, was associated with a reduction in pain days, bad sleep, and pain medication for patients with sickle cell disease.[22] Hypnosis is also associated with a substantial reduction of symptoms of irritable bowel syndrome[23] and is considered a well-established and efficacious treatment for recurrent headaches in children.[24]

CLINICALLY RELEVANT ANATOMY

Although there are differing views regarding what hypnosis is and how it works for pain control,[11] it is often described in terms of an altered state of consciousness or awareness.[6] There seems to be some consensus, however, regarding what hypnotic pain control is not. It is not effective because it results in simple relaxation, because hypnosis does not necessarily bring about a relaxed state.[25] Hypnosis does not appear to operate as an opiate receptor based analgesia because the opiate antagonist naloxone has no effect on hypnotic analgesia.[11,26] The adult literature has observed that hypnotic responsiveness can be measured very reliably and that individuals who score very high on these scales are capable of very robust hypnotic analgesia responses in the laboratory.[18] Hypnotic analgesia is not a placebo for individuals who score very high on responsiveness scales because they demonstrate a higher pain threshold and pain tolerance under hypnotic analgesia conditions than under placebo conditions, while those who score very low on these scales demonstrate comparable response levels to pain reduction for hypnosis and placebo conditions.[27]

For highly hypnotizable individuals hypnotic analgesia does appear to be associated with a complex ability to cognitively restructure or dissociate conscious overt pain from covert experiences. In a novel set of experiments, talented hypnotic subjects who reported no overt pain to painful stimulations under hypnosis did indicate pain when a covert or "hidden observer" part of their consciousness was asked about the experience.[18]

TECHNIQUE

Hypnosis Technique for Preoperative and Postoperative Pain Management

The use of language plays an important role in hypnotic work and in clinical practice in general. For children in particular and adults as well, the use of permissive and indirect language is generally preferred to authoritative approaches. For example, direct suggestions that "You will feel no pain" are avoided (especially with adults who are not highly hypnotizable). Instead, the wording to follow might be, "You may be surprised how comfortable you might feel during and after the procedure." Also, permissive suggestions can be given for the preoperative and postoperative periods. For example, the point at which the medication is administered can be a signal for the person to have a pleasant daydream; also, the area being operated on can remain soft, comfortable, and loose during the operation.When the patients awaken in the recovery room the operation will be over, their condition relieved, and healing under way. In addition, suggestions can be made on how surprised they will be at how quickly recovery will occur and how much easier the whole procedure was than they had anticipated.[28] Hypnosis for postsurgical pain management and recovery has included relaxation and suggestions for a smooth recovery, comfort, improved limb mobility, and success with occupational therapy.[10]

Hypnosis Technique for Management of Acute Pain

Techniques of hypnoanalgesia for young patients may include suggestions for feelings of numbness; glove anesthesia and numbing other body parts with that "magic" glove; distancing suggestions such as moving pain away from self, or transferring it to another body part, or moving the self away from the pain; suggestions for feelings antithetical to pain such as comfort, laughter, or relaxation; distraction techniques, directing attention to the pain, time distortion, reframing, and amnesia.[6]

Hypnosis Technique for Cancer Pain Management

Hypnotic suggestions for cancer pain management involve distraction of going to a favorite place, hypnotic analgesia suggestions of numbness or pain switches (i.e., blocking pain), and sensory transformation of either exploring the pain or transforming its intensity, color, or temperature.[16]

Hypnosis Technique for Obstetric Pain

A range of hypnotic processes have been suggested for managing labor and delivery, such as relaxation, trance states, time distortion, redirection of attention, reinterpretation of sensations to familiar and pleasant ones (e.g., ". . . Each contraction can be considered as a pleasing occurrence, drawing you nearer to your goal . . . bringing a new love for your enjoyment."),[28] glove anesthesia, and transferring of numbness, as well as posthypnotic suggestions.

Hypnosis Technique for Emergency Treatment of Burns

Emergency situations are often traumatic and result in trance states as a natural defense against pain and fear. Thus a formal hypnotic induction is not generally needed. When a burn patient is in a natural trance state, he or she can be told to "go to your laughing place" or a similar suggestion and then to allow the health team to take care of the wounds when the hypnotic suggestion is given of being "cool and comfortable."[20] This should be done within 2 hours of the injury to reduce the inflammatory response.

Hypnosis Technique for Chronic Pain

Chronic pain is a complex condition that does not respond as robustly to hypnotic interventions as acute pain conditions.[11] Thus, work with hypnosis needs to be done in an integrative fashion. Self-hypnosis training may also prove helpful in reinforcing the therapeutic effects along with attention to behavioral sleep issues for sickle cell disease.[22]

SIDE EFFECTS AND COMPLICATIONS

In the hands of a practitioner with appropriate background, training, and licensure, hypnosis is generally a safe intervention. When managing pain, however, a good history and physical examination are critical to success. Karen Olness and Patricia Libbey, pioneers in the field of child hypnotherapy, observed that 25% of children referred for hypnotherapy were later found to have some unrecognized organic condition that accounted for their symptoms.[29] Of course, the most important intervention in those cases was not hypnosis, but appropriate medical treatment.

My only negative experience with hypnosis and pain management involved a teenage boy with functional abdominal pain. This was very early in my career, and I made a direct suggestion for the pain to go away (now my approach is more permissive and cautious). After the induction had ended, the boy said that his pain was gone but that everything seemed upside down (i.e., he was disoriented). I had him close his eyes and suggested that when he opened his eyes the room would be back to how it was. This was unsuccessful, and he was becoming somewhat alarmed about how he was feeling (I was becoming concerned as well). Then I had him close his eyes and go back into hypnosis and I had him "bring the pain back." He opened his eyes, said everything was back to normal, but his stomach was hurting again. Our follow-up work involved weekly traditional psychotherapy and learning how to get in contact with feelings he was somatizing. He did well and eventually learned to express his feelings in words instead of somatic complaints. I saw him again about a decade later for a different problem related to the demise of his marriage. We did a lot of talk therapy and some hypnosis with no direct suggestions of symptom removal and no complications.

My first-line approach to chronic pain is a thorough medical, psychological, and life-style assessment, followed by permissive hypnotic approaches and no direct suggestion for pain to go away. If the pain remains despite the lack of obvious physiological cause and active hypnotic work, hypnosis may be used to explore the meaning of the pain. A patient under hypnosis might be asked to describe the pain, ask the pain why it is there, and what the pain is attempting to teach the patient. Some colleagues have children draw pictures to obtain some of this information; one practitioner even has children use a computer word processor to help them gain insight into psychological factors underlying the medical symptoms.[30]

CONCLUSIONS

As noted previously, there is often a discrepancy between modest findings from experimental trials and robust clinical reports for hypnotic pain control. Although this might cast doubts on the clinical reports, it must be kept in mind that clinical and experimental settings are very different and that the standardized protocols are often employed within laboratory settings that would be of limited use in a clinical setting, where one would capitalize on the patient's unique interests, strengths, and preferences.

Some practitioners caution against the use of hypnosis in adolescents who score low on a standard scale of hypnotizability. I find these scales useful in a laboratory setting but not as useful in a clinical setting, because clinically significant improvement can be accomplished if hypnosis is used not as a specific treatment but rather in an integrative manner. Pediatric neurologists often refer children with recurrent headaches to me because they feel that pharmacologic treatments have limited benefit. My approach, after a very careful medical, psychological, and life-style assessment with careful attention to diet and sleep factors, is to teach self-hypnosis as a "skill and not a pill" for headache prophylaxis.[31] My clinical success rates have been excellent, but I look forward to more conventional analyses. In conclusion, it is my opinion that hypnosis can be a valuable component of a comprehensive program for pain management.

Acknowledgments

I would like to thanks Danielle R. Murphy, Case Western Reserve University Senior SAGES Honor Capstone Student, and Belinda Williams, Dwayne Williams, and Barbara Taylor of the Cuyahoga County Community College Bridges to Success in the Sciences for their help in research and preparation of the manuscript for this chapter.

References

1. Bowers KS: Hypnosis for the Seriously Curious. Monterey, CA, Brooks/Cole Publishing, 1976.
2. Gravitz MA: Medical hypnosis: A historical perspective. In Temes R (ed): Medical Hypnosis: An Introduction and Clinical Guide. New York, Churchill Livingstone, 1999, pp 65-78.
3. Shore RE: The fundamental problem in hypnosis research as viewed from historic perspectives. In Fromm E, Shor RE (eds): Hypnosis: Developments in Research and New Perspectives. New York, Aldine Publishing Company, 1979, pp 14-41.
4. Wall PD: Foreword to the 1983 Edition. In Hilgard ER, Hilgard JR (eds): Hypnosis in the Relief of Pain. Levittown, Pa, Brunner/Mazel, 1994, pp xi-xiii.
5. Kuttner L: No fears . . . no tears: Children with cancer coping with pain. Vancouver, BC, Canadian Cancer Society, 1986.
6. Olness K, Kohen DP: Hypnosis and Hypnotherapy with Children, 3rd ed. New York, Guilford Press, 1996.
7. Wester CW, O'Grady DJ: Clinical Hypnosis with Children. New York, Brunner/Mazel, 1991.
8. Zeltzer LK, Schlank B: Conquering Your Child's Chronic Pain: A Pediatrician's Guide for Reclaiming a Normal Childhood. New York, Harper Collins, 2005.
9. Kessler R, Whalene T: Hypnotic preparation in anesthesia and surgery. In Temes R (ed): Medical Hypnosis: An Introduction and Clinical Guide. New York, Churchill Livingstone, 1999, pp 43-57.
10. Mauer MH, Burnett KF, Ouelette EA, et al: Medical hypnosis and orthopedic hand surgery: Pain perception, postoperative recovery, and therapeutic comfort. Int J Clin Exp Hypn 47:144-159, 1999.
11. Patterson DR, Jenson M: Hypnosis and clinical pain. Psychol Bull 65: 60-67, 2003.
12. Berjenke CJ: Painful medical procedures. In Barber J (ed): Hypnosis and Suggestion in the Treatment of Pain: A Clinical Guide. New York, WW Norton & Co., 1996, pp 209-266.
13. Hilgard JR, LeBaron S: Relief of anxiety and pain in children and adolescents with cancer: Quantitative measures and clinical observations. Int J Clin Exp Hypn 30:417-442, 1982.
14. O'Grady DJ: Hypnosis and pain management in children. In Wester WC, O'Grady DJ (eds): Clinical Hypnosis with Children. New York, Brunner/Mazel, 1991.
15. Liossi C, Hatira P, White P: Randomized clinical trial of local anesthetic versus a combination of local anesthetic with self-hypnosis in the management of pediatric procedure-related pain. Health Psychol 25: 307-315, 2006.
16. Syrjala KL, Roth-Roemer S: Cancer pain. In Barber J (ed): Hypnosis and Suggestion in the Treatment of Pain: A Clinical Guide. New York, WW Norton & Co., 1996, pp 121-157.
17. Goldman L: Hypnosis in obstetrics and gynecology. In Temes R (ed): Medical Hypnosis: An Introduction and Clinical Guide. New York, Churchill Livingstone, 1999, pp 43-57.
18. Hilgard ER, Hilgard JR: Hypnosis in the Relief of Pain. Levittown, PA, Brunner/Mazel, 1994.
19. Chiasson SW: Group hypnosis training in obstetrics. In Hammond DC (ed): Handbook of Hypnotic Suggestions and Metaphors. New York, WW Norton & Co., 1990, pp 271-273.
20. Ewin DM: Emergency room hypnosis for the burned patient. Am J Clin Hypn 26:5-8, 1983.
21. Patterson DR, Adcock RJ, Bombardier CH: Factors predicting hypnotic analgesia in clinical burn pain. Int J Clin Exp Hypn 45:377-395, 1997.
22. Dinges DF, Whitehouse WG, Orne DC, et al: Self-hypnosis training as an adjunctive treatment in the management of pain associated with sickle cell disease. Int J Clin Exp Hypn 45:417-432, 1997.
23. Whitehead WE: Hypnosis for irritable bowel syndrome: The empirical evidence of therapeutic effects. Int J Clin Exp Hypn 54:7-20, 2006.
24. Holden EW, Deichmann MM, Levy JD: Empirically supported treatments in pediatric psychology: Recurrent pediatric headache. J Pediatr Psychol 24:91-109, 1999.
25. Barber J: Hypnosis and Suggestion in the Treatment of Pain: A Clinical Guide. New York, WW Norton & Co., 1996.
26. Goldstein A, Hilgard ER: Failure of the opiate antagonist naloxone to modify hypnotic analgesia. Proc Natl Acad Sci USA 72:2041-2043, 1975.
27. McGlashan TH, Evans FJ, Orne MT: The nature of hypnotic analgesia and placebo response to experimental pain. Psychosom Med 31:227-246, 1969.
28. Rodger BP: Outline of hypnotic suggestions in obstetrics. In Hammond DC (ed): Handbook of Hypnotic Suggestions and Metaphors. New York, WW Norton & Co., 1990, pp 273-275.
29. Olness K, Libbey P: Unrecognized biologic bases of behavioral symptoms in patients referred for hypnotherapy. Am J Clin Hypn 30:1-8, 1987.
30. Anbar R: Stressors associated with dyspnea in childhood: Patient's insights and a case report. Am J Clin Hypn 47:93-101, 2004.
31. Kajander R, Andrasik F, Hall H: Integrative approaches to assessment and management of recurrent headaches in children. Biofeedback 31: 18-22, 2003.

chapter 123

Relaxation Techniques and Guided Imagery

Carla Rime and Frank Andrasik

Relaxation therapies are self-management interventions that emphasize active involvement of the patient. Relaxed breathing, progressive muscle relaxation (PMR), autogenic training (AT), and guided imagery (GI) are all forms of relaxation treatment discussed in this chapter. Biofeedback, sometimes referred to as "instrument-aided relaxation" when used in a general sense,[1] and hypnosis are, at times, also considered forms of relaxation therapy and are discussed elsewhere in this volume (Chapters 121 and 122, respectively). It is acknowledged that meditation and yoga practices may also have relaxation properties; however, this chapter will focus on the aforementioned clinical procedures.

Even though the actual mechanism or mechanisms underlying relaxation techniques are unclear,[2] there are theories accounting for their effects. Benson and associates[3] proposed that these types of therapies elicit a general *relaxation response* consisting of a number of physiologic changes, including a reduction in heart rate, respiration, oxygen consumption, carbon dioxide elimination, and arterial blood lactate concentration. Additionally, there is an increase in slow alpha brain waves with intermittent theta brain waves. The *relaxation response*, which is a general reduction in arousal of the autonomic nervous system, competes with Cannon's *fight-or-flight response*, which is a general increase in arousal of the autonomic system.

Davidson and Schwartz[4] believe that relaxation therapies have more pervasive effects and point out the *specific effects* produced by each of the relaxation techniques. These effects are categorized as predominately cognitive, autonomic, or muscular. Lehrer and associates[5] reviewed research on relaxation treatments and found support for the specific effects approach. Despite this controversy between the general relaxation response and the specific effects of relaxation, both may be valid to some extent in that many of the physiologic responses of relaxation are closely interrelated.

With regard to pain, relaxation procedures may be beneficial for a number of reasons. Andrasik[6] outlined the logic of implementing a form of relaxation for those experiencing pain. The first rationale involves the general decrease in arousal, which reduces the central processing of sensory stimulation. Second, depression, anxiety, and fear are implicated in the pain-negative affect cycle,[7] and reducing these secondary symptoms through relaxation can increase pain tolerance. Furthermore, a reduction in the frequent activation of the autonomic stress system can decrease the pain associated with this heightened and prolonged physiologic state.[8] Finally, relaxation may provide a means of distraction (the cognitive effect mentioned earlier). Tracey and colleagues[9] found through functional MRI that distraction activates the periaqueductal gray region, a cortical area related to pain control. Relaxation techniques may operate on the premises of reduced sensory input, competition of the stress response, or distraction.

This chapter on relaxation therapies discusses historical considerations of PMR, AT, and GI. The following section reviews indications for the effectiveness of these therapies in alleviating several pain disorders and their accompanying symptoms. Next, techniques for each of these procedures are addressed. This chapter closes with patient considerations and possible side effects of relaxation techniques.

HISTORICAL CONSIDERATIONS

Progressive Muscle Relaxation

Edmund Jacobson developed PMR. In the early 1900s he had studied reactions to unexpected loud noises known as the startle response. He noted that those who were deeply relaxed did not exhibit this common startle response to sudden noises. This intriguing finding initiated his interest in relaxation effects. He continued to conduct research and found that the strength, or amplitude, of knee jerk reflexes correlated with the individuals' tension levels. For instance, those who displayed muscular tonus, or sustained chronic tension, had less latency and higher amplitude in their knee jerk responses. Those who practiced relaxation demonstrated a decrease in the amplitude of knee jerk reflexes.[10]

The purpose of PMR, as designed by Jacobson, is for an individual to develop an awareness of muscle tension and muscle relaxation through physiologic introspection. Freeman[11] and Lehrer[12] described some of Jacobson's beliefs regarding PMR. First, he did not believe in intentionally tensing muscles in order to perceive the differences between relaxed and tense muscles. Subsequent variations of Jacobson's original PMR have implemented these tension-and-release cycles. Jacobson did, however, incorporate body movements such as raising the arm or bending the hand to create slight tension. Jacobson also avoided the use of suggestion and contended that it is not appropriate to tell individuals that they are relaxed, especially if in actuality they are not relaxed. Individuals are to learn physiologic control of progressively more subtle tension over the course of the program. Jacobson's PMR program involves more than 100 sessions, typically 1 hour in length, while concentrating on certain muscle groups. It could take a number of months or years to acquire the skill to relax.

The extensive time commitment for completing Jacobson's PMR program led some to develop and test more abbreviated forms. Joseph Wolpe incorporated a shortened version of Jacobson's PMR into the counter-conditioning of fear.[13] His therapy, called systematic desensitization, generally takes 10 training sessions or less to complete. In contrast to Jacobson's prescribed methods, Wolpe combined more muscle groups and included suggestions and specific instructions. Over time, others have tailored Jacobson's extensive PMR program and Wolpe's abbreviated form to fit their patients' needs. Examples of these contemporary methods are described in the "Techniques" section of this chapter.

Autogenic Training

Johann Schultz is credited as the founder of AT. Schultz was a German neurologist and psychiatrist who, in 1924, began implementing AT in his private practice. Schultz was disenchanted with psychoanalysis, the prominent school of thought at the time. His private practice gave him the freedom to explore AT as a therapeutic method. His method was derived from his experience with hypnosis and the observations in brain research reported by Oskar Vogt. Vogt had noted that his patients, through mental concentration, could self-hypnotically produce sensations of warmth and heaviness. Based on these principles, Schultz created formulas for AT and, in 1932, published a book titled *Das Autogene Training* in which his standardized method was described.[14]

Literature on AT did not become available in English until the 1960s. Wolfgang Luthe was a physician and follower of Schultz. When Luthe emigrated to Canada, he began writing about AT in English. Luthe, with Schultz's assistance, published *Autogenic Therapy*, Volumes I to VI, which describes the details of AT. This marked the proliferation of AT in English-speaking North American regions.[14]

Guided Imagery

The history of clinical breathing therapies and imagery is not as definitive as the history of PMR and AT. It is difficult to determine who may have been the founder or propagator of these techniques. Imagery can, however, be traced back to the Grecian era where dreams and visions were evaluated in the Asclepian temples for medical purposes. Aristotle, Hippocrates, and Galen were all trained in this method of imagery healing.[15] During the behaviorist movement in the mid-1900s, imagery as a mental process was considered irrelevant for research, let alone for therapeutic purposes. When the cognitive revolution in psychology took place, imagery was reintroduced as a topic for research and treatment.

Edmund Jacobson and Johann Schultz discovered the therapeutic value of PMR and AT, respectively, in the early 1900s. Imagery has a much more dated history. Joseph Wolpe and others have since revised Jacobson's original PMR procedures into abbreviated versions. Wolfgang Luthe pioneered the use of AT in Canada and other English-speaking regions through translated publications of the procedures. The following section discusses the effectiveness of these techniques as they relate to pain management.

INDICATIONS

In 1996, the National Institute of Health organized a non-federal, non-advocate panel of representatives from the fields of medicine, psychiatry, psychology, public health nursing, and epidemiology.[2] This 12-member panel conducted an extensive evaluation of the literature on behavioral and relaxation approaches for the treatment of pain and insomnia. Moreover, 23 experts in the fields of behavioral medicine, pain medicine, psychiatry, psychology, nursing, and neurology presented information to the panel during a conference. After deliberation, the panel concluded that ". . . the evidence is strong for the effectiveness of [relaxation] techniques in reducing chronic pain in a variety of medical conditions" (p. 315). The panel further stated that ". . . the data are insufficient to conclude that one technique is usually more effective than another for a given condition" (p. 315).

Relaxation techniques are often combined into a treatment package in the clinical setting. Investigations of these therapies, either combined or in isolation, have been carried out to determine their effectiveness. Relaxation procedures and GI have been applied to a number of both acute and chronic pain conditions and their secondary symptoms. The following presents a sampling of the literature regarding these techniques as treatments.

Neumann and associates[16] compared pain tolerance between those who received pain-incompatible imagery training and a control group. A pain algometer, which is a cylinder placed on the finger that gradually applies pressure, was used to assess pain thresholds for the participants. Additionally, heart rate and skin resistance measures were obtained. The investigators found that those who had been trained in imagery had higher pain tolerance and lower heart rates than the control group did. There were no differences in skin resistance between the two groups.

Relaxation and imagery are components of the Arthritis Self-Management Program (ASMP) for the treatment of rheumatoid arthritis and osteoarthritis.[17] Other elements of this program include patient education, cognitive restructuring, problem solving, and communication skills. A review of the program indicated that there was an average 15% to 20% reduction from baseline in arthritis-related pain and disability.[18] A study of a modified version of ASMP in which self-efficacy was emphasized reported that the reductions in pain were maintained after 4 years and that there was a 43% decrease in physician visits.[19]

Another study on rheumatic pain compared muscle strength and mobility exercises with an abbreviated form of PMR. The investigators found that PMR was significantly better than strength training with regard to muscle function of the lower extremities. Furthermore, the results suggested that PMR improved health-related quality of life.[20] Likewise, a study using PMR and GI as treatment of osteoarthritis indicated that 12 weeks of this treatment led to a significant decrease in pain and mobility difficulties when compared with a control group.[21]

Other investigations on the use of relaxation techniques for chronic pain have focused on back pain. Turner and Chapman[22] compared PMR, cognitive-behavioral therapy, and a waitlist/attention technique for chronic low back pain. Significant improvements in pain measures for the PMR and cognitive-behavioral groups were reported, and a 1.5- to 2-year follow-up showed that participants in these two groups had a notable decrease in healthcare use. A different study compared a relaxation intervention, an electromyogram (EMG) biofeedback intervention, and a placebo condition for chronic low back pain patients. The relaxation intervention was found to be superior to biofeedback and placebo on measures of reduced pain and increased activity.[23]

Relaxation techniques have also been applied to burn patients. Débridement is a painful procedure that involves scrubbing the dead skin from the burn area. This procedure is performed routinely for weeks or even moths.[15] Achterberg and associates[24] assessed the effectiveness of relaxation, relaxation combined with imagery, and relaxation combined with both imagery and biofeedback for burn victims undergoing débridement. These three interventions were compared with a control group. The study took place in a hospital burn care unit, so the practical implementation of these interventions was also assessed. Even though all three interventions produced improvements in pain and anxiety measures in comparison to the control group, the relaxation/imagery and the relaxation/imagery/biofeedback interventions had superior and nearly equivalent results. The relaxation/imagery intervention was considered the most practical in terms of administration in the busy burn unit of the hospital.

A meta-analysis examining imagery training for cancer pain concluded that this form of treatment significantly decreases the sensory experience of pain, significantly reduces depression and anxiety, but has no effect on the functional status of daily living.[25] Syrjala and colleagues[26] evaluated the following interventions in patients undergoing bone marrow transplantation: (1) relaxation and imagery, (2) cognitive-behavioral treatment combined with relaxation and imagery, (3) therapist support, and (4) treatment as usual, which served as the control condition. This study demonstrated that both the relaxation/imagery and cognitive-behavioral/relaxation/imagery interventions resulted in significant pain reductions on self-report measures but that the inclusion of cognitive-behavioral treatment did not add incremental value. Furthermore, the therapist support group did not significantly reduce pain in comparison to the treatment-as-usual group.

Burish et al.[27] examined the utility of PMR and GI in cancer patients undergoing chemotherapy. The investigators found that patients in the treatment group had significantly less nausea and vomiting than the control group did. Moreover, the intervention group had lower blood pressure, pulse rate, and anxiety.

Several meta-analytic reviews have found that behavioral interventions are effective in preventing and treating tension-type and migraine headaches in both adults and children. The interventions include relaxation training, biofeedback, cognitive-behavioral therapy, and stress management training, either combined or in isolation. The reviews consistently reveal a 35% to 50% improvement in headache activity with the use of these behavioral interventions.[28,29] Other literature reviews have found that behavioral interventions for pediatric headache are also effective treatments.[30,31]

Relaxation techniques and imagery have also been used in a number of pre-surgical and post-surgical settings to reduce both anxiety and pain. For example, Cupal and Brewer[32] randomly assigned individuals who were in rehabilitation for anterior cruciate ligament reconstruction to one of three groups. The first consisted of 10 relaxation and GI sessions, the second consisted of attention and encouragement (placebo group), and the third group did not receive any intervention (control group). The investigators found that participants in the relaxation/imagery group had significantly more knee strength and significantly less pain and re-injury anxiety than did the placebo and control participants at 24 weeks after surgery. The authors of this study offered a few possible explanations for the beneficial results of the relaxation/imagery intervention. The first is that the intervention gave the participants a sense of control of their recovery. Another explanation is that with pain and anxiety reduced, the participants were more able to take part in their knee rehabilitation. Finally, the relaxation/imagery treatment may have facilitated healing through regeneration-repair and immune-inflammatory responses.

Lawlis and associates[33] examined the effects of a 1-hour relaxation intervention the evening before spine surgery. Those who received the relaxation treatment had a significant reduction in hospitalization days and medication use when compared with those in a control group. Furthermore, nurses noted fewer pain complaints from those in the relaxation intervention than in patients in the control group.

Relaxation techniques have also been used to alleviate pain from both ulcerative colitis and peptic ulcers. Shaw and Ehrlich[34] compared the pain ratings of a relaxation intervention group and an attention control group in patients with ulcerative colitis. Immediately after the 6-week intervention, patients in the relaxation group had significant reductions in pain ratings, frequency, and distress. These results were maintained at 6-week follow-up. Brooks and Richardson[35] found a decrease in recurrence of ulcerative symptoms over a period of 3 years after individuals received relaxation and assertiveness training when compared with individuals in a control group.

As this section has demonstrated, there are a number of well-documented studies in which relaxation techniques and GI have produced beneficial outcomes. These therapies can be applied to a variety of medical conditions where pain and anxiety are implicated. Even though relaxation techniques may not be favorable for clinical depression, there is support that relaxation therapies offer relief for secondary depressive symptoms, as may be the case in pain disorders.[5] Pain, as well as its accompanying stress and anxiety, can be combated with relaxation therapy, where the relaxation response replaces the stress response. Relaxation techniques and GI may operate at the emotional and cognitive dimensions of the pain experience, whereas the physical experience may remain the same.[36] These therapies provide cultivated skills in coping that reduce the suffering and distress associated with pain. In some cases (e.g., headaches, ulcers), this skill may prevent the occurrence of a painful episode.

TECHNIQUES

This section describes the commonly used techniques of relaxed breathing, GI, AT, and PMR. Breathing therapy is discussed first because therapists often begin with these techniques. Next, the discussion on GI focuses on pleasant imagery and pain-transforming imagery, techniques often used early in therapy. Then, the six formulas of AT as depicted by Schultz will be addressed. Finally, the abbreviated versions of PMR, as opposed to Jacobson's original version, will be emphasized because the shortened procedures are more frequently used in a clinical setting. A relaxation treatment program generally involves the use of more than one of the procedures by combining and customizing the techniques based on individual needs. An example of a treatment protocol incorporating all of these procedures will be described.

Relaxed Breathing

Slow diaphragmatic breathing is a widely used technique. The patient is instructed to draw air deeply into the lungs by having the diaphragm move downward. This technique minimizes shallow, chest breathing. The following methods demonstrate the use of the diaphragm in breathing: (1) holding the hands straight overhead, (2) lying on the floor with a book placed on the abdomen and lifting and lowering the book while breathing in and out, and (3) while breathing, placing one hand on the chest and the other on the diaphragm area and maximizing movement of the lower hand.[6] On average, people take 12 to 15 breaths per minute. The goal of slow diaphragmatic breathing is usually 6 to 8 breaths per minute.[37] If an individual's respiration is high (30 or more breaths per minute), the decelerated breathing may feel strange. Clients should be reassured that these strange feelings will pass with time.[6]

In addition to diaphragmatic breathing, Gevirtz and Schwartz[37] discuss other breathing therapy techniques, such as paced respiration and pursed-lip breathing. Paced respiration is breathing at a predetermined rate. It usually involves an external pacing device, such as a metronome, to coordinate the rate of respiration. Pursed-lip breathing consists of exhaling slowly while the lips are partially pursed, as though whistling. This type of therapy is generally used with patients who have chronic obstructive pulmonary disease. Gevirtz and Schwartz[37] explain other types of breathing techniques in addition to those described here, such as rebreathing, breath meditation, and breath mindfulness. Furthermore, they discuss the use of instruments to shape breathing, including a nasal airflow temperature gauge, strain gauge, EMG from accessory breathing muscles, and capnometer and oximeter methods, among others.

Nearly every relaxation procedure contains instructions on slower and deeper breathing. Breathing can be easily brought under voluntary control at any time. Clients are encouraged to use diaphragmatic breathing as often as possible and especially in response to stress throughout the day.[38]

Guided Imagery

Imagery can be a powerful experience, and it can be either maladaptive or adaptive. If the images are vivid enough, the body responds as though it were an actual event.[39] In the case of posttraumatic stress, images of an emotional experience can elicit maladaptive responses.[15] In contrast, controlled and pleasant images can be adaptive. Images can have an impact on the immune, endocrine, nervous, cardiovascular, respiratory, and gastrointestinal systems of the body.[39] The physiologic and biochemical changes that occur with imagery have been used to explain the "placebo effect" in untreated individuals.[15,39] The purpose of GI, then, is to induce the healing systems of the body to proceed in the desired direction. The following describes pleasant and relaxing imagery, mental rehearsal, symptom suppression, and symptom substitution.

Clients are often instructed to create an image in the "mind's eye" of a relaxing scene. Examples of pleasant imagery might include lying on the beach or walking in a meadow. It is important to avoid images that may cause arousal (e.g., sexual content, vigorous activity). To enhance the vividness of the image, other sensory modalities (auditory, olfactory, tactile, and gustatory) are included to complement the image.[40] It is suggested that a client have different, personally relevant relaxing scenes to alternate. After practicing a relaxing image, it can be evoked quickly and vividly. Clients are encouraged to recall their relaxing scenes in stressful situations.[6]

Mental rehearsal imagery is often used to prepare a client, emotionally and mentally, for a medical procedure. Freeman[15] explains this technique as a "guided mental imagery trip" for the upcoming procedure and recovery. It is intended to be a factual process in which the medical procedure is reframed in a realistic, yet positive sense. Other relaxation techniques, such as muscle relaxation and diaphragmatic breathing, are frequently used to supplement the imagery trip. This type of imagery fosters a better understanding of what to expect from the medical procedure, and the situation is viewed as less ambiguous and stressful. Mental rehearsal imagery has been used for surgical procedures and childbirth.

Bresler[39] has outlined several Interactive Guided Imagery (IGI) techniques, two of which include symptom suppression imagery and symptom substitution imagery. One example of symptom suppression involves a two-step approach. First, patients are instructed to evoke feelings of numbness in the hand to initiate "glove anesthesia." Once this step has been accomplished, the patient is instructed to place the "anesthetized" hand on painful areas of the body and transfer this numbness to the place where it hurts. Symptom suppression is helpful for patients who are experiencing intense discomfort and are otherwise having trouble concentrating.

Symptom substitution imagery, as described by Bresler,[39] consists of mentally moving pain in the body to another area of the body where it is more tolerable. This technique is not intended to suppress the pain, but instead to move the discomfort to a less threatening area of the body. For instance, a patient may be guided to move a headache to the little finger. Bresler[39] notes that IGI, in general, taps into a patient's inner resources for coping.

Autogenic Training

Schultz and Luthe developed six sequential formulas for AT: (1) the heaviness experience (muscular relaxation), (2) the experience of warmth (vascular dilation), (3) regulation of the heart, (4) regulation of breathing, (5) regulation of visceral organs, and (6) regulation of the head.[41] Each of these stages implements self-suggestion to produce the ideal effect. Key statements are passively focused on, such as a "warm arm."[41] Clinicians generally use the *heaviness* and *warmth* formulas to promote relaxation.[6] A patient is instructed to concentrate on feelings of warmth and heaviness in the extremities. This peripheral warming is believed to increase blood flow and decrease arousal, therefore aiding relaxation. To take full advantage of this technique, patients are advised to personalize their own phrases for warmth and heaviness and to repeat these phrases 50 to 100 times during practice.[42]

Progressive Muscle Relaxation

Bernstein and Borkovec[43] published a book detailing the techniques of relaxation training, derived from Jacobson's method.[10] It was intended to provide consistent procedures to guide both clinical and research endeavors with the use of a much abbreviated approach. Andrasik[44] described a treatment protocol (though discussed for headache patients, it has broad applicability to pain conditions) based on these techniques of relaxation training that incorporates the other allied relaxation procedures of diaphragmatic breathing, GI, and AT. The introduction of relaxation training for a patient, as discussed by Andrasik,[44] is composed of the following points:

- Major muscle groups are systematically tensed and relaxed.
- Production of a broad range of tension levels facilitates discrimination of tension states.
- When tension is released, muscles reflexively go to a lower level (which further enhances discrimination).
- After developing discrimination abilities, applied relaxation, or counteraction of built-up tension during the day, can be skillfully implemented.
- Regular practice is necessary to accomplish the skill of deep relaxation.
- Major muscle groups are the focus in the beginning of the program. Over the course of the program, however, muscle groups are combined for rapid relaxation effects.

After clarification of the procedures, a few practice tension-release cycles of a specified target group are acted out by the patient. The practitioner observes these practice cycles for complete, but not extreme tension levels of the target group only. The formal instruction of this abbreviated version of PMR commences with the sequential tensing and releasing of 14 target muscle groups in 18 distinct steps. Table 123–1 outlines these steps.

The tension-release cycle for each target muscle group consists of 5 to 7 seconds of tensing and 20 to 30 seconds of relaxing. Each step is repeated two times initially (with a third cycle if needed). The patient is instructed to focus on the sensations of both tension and relaxation of the muscles. If it is painful to tense any particular muscles, these muscles are omitted from the procedure (as well as those that might have been injured). While moving through the sequence of target muscle groups, it is important to have the previous muscle group fully relaxed before moving to the next step. After the patient becomes more skilled with the 18 steps of tensing and relaxing, the muscle groups are combined into an even more abbreviated form (Table 123–2).

Relaxation Treatment Regimen

Table 123–3 delineates components of the treatment program, broken down by sessions, as suggested by Andrasik.[44] As illustrated in the table, this program is typically 8 weeks in duration, with fewer than 10 sessions. PMR is an element of each session, whereas the targeted muscle groups are varied. Deepening exercises borrow from the principles of AT, with suggestive self-statements of warmth and heaviness to further the relaxation experience. The clinician may also offer suggestions for deepening exercises, such as counting backward

Table 123–1

The 18 Steps for Tensing the Initial 14 Targeted Muscle Groups

1. Right hand and lower arm (by having the patient make a fist and simultaneously tense the lower arm)
2. Left hand and lower arm
3. Both hands and lower arms
4. Right upper arm (by having the patient bring his/her hand to the shoulder and tense the biceps)
5. Left upper arm
6. Both upper arms
7. Right lower leg and foot (by having the patient point his/her toe and tensing the calf muscle)
8. Left lower leg and foot
9. Both lower legs and feet
10. Both thighs (by pressing the knees and thighs tightly together)
11. Abdomen (draw the abdominal muscles in tightly)
12. Chest (by having the patient take a deep breath and holding it)
13. Shoulders and lower neck (by having the patient "hunch" or draw his/her shoulders toward the ears)
14. Back of the neck (have the patient push his/her head backward against a headrest or chair)
15. Lips (by pressing them together very tightly but not clenching the teeth)
16. Eyes (by closing the eyes tightly)
17. Lower forehead (by having the patient frown and draw the eyebrows together)
18. Upper forehead (by having the patient wrinkle the forehead area)

From Andrasik F: Relaxation and biofeedback for chronic headaches. In Holzman AD, Turk DC (eds): A Handbook of Psychological Treatment Approaches. New York, Pergamon, 1986, p 225.

from 5 to 1 in which the patient imagines descending stairs and becoming more deeply relaxed. These suggestions, either subvocalized by the patient or stated out loud by the clinician, are implemented during the 20 to 30 seconds of the relaxation portion of the tense-and-release cycles. Additionally, slow and deep diaphragmatic breathing is integrated into each session. Pleasant imagery is also incorporated early in the treatment regimen.

Discrimination muscle training can be used for specific muscle groups of interest. Such training involves having the patient complete a tension-release cycle for a target group, then tense only half as much, followed by a quarter and alternations between these values. The patient is instructed to continue tensing with decreased force to discriminate more subtle expressions of tension. The patient is directed to use this differential muscle tensing for problem areas. For instance, it would be suitable for an individual who has tension-type headaches to discriminate among subtle levels of tension in the forehead and neck areas.

As the patient is progressing through the relaxation regimen, more advanced techniques, such as relaxation by recall and cue-controlled relaxation, are introduced. Relaxation by recall consists of having the patient focus on the sensations of relaxation that were produced during the earlier steps. The patient is then directed to replicate these sensations without the tension-and-release cycles. Cue-controlled relaxation involves associating a word with the sensations of relaxation. The cue may be as simple as the word *relax*, and with proficient skills developed through training, the body responds to the cue accordingly. A variation of this approach involves having the patient subvocalize a relaxing word with each exhalation when attention is focused on breathing.

As pointed out in the introduction to this training program, regular practice is crucial in developing the techniques. Patients are instructed to practice at home once or twice a day for 20 minutes from the onset of training. They are also encouraged to continue to practice after the treatment has been completed and to use the techniques for daily coping. Home practice may be supplemented with audiotapes. There is some debate about whether live instruction or self-help audiotapes are more effective.[12,45] Schwartz[45] has listed some advantages of audiotapes, such as conservation of the clinician's time and lower cost. These advantages, however, depend on the quality of the audiotapes and how the patients comply and respond to the tapes. The primary advantage of live instruction is that clinicians can guide the patient through the procedures at an appropriate pace.[12] Coupling of live instruction with either commercial or tailored audiotapes for home practice appears to assist patients in generalizing the skills learned at the clinic to their daily routines. Nevertheless, research on live versus taped instructions is limited, and the research that is available indicates mixed results.[12,45] Individual differences may account for the inconsistent findings.

The treatment protocol illustrated in Table 123–3 provides a format for relaxation training. Many of the components of the training can be modified in the best interest of the

Table 123–2

Abbreviated Target Muscle Groups

Eight-Muscle Groups

1. Both hands and lower arms
2. Both legs and thighs
3. Abdomen
4. Chest
5. Shoulders
6. Back of neck
7. Eyes
8. Forehead

Four-Muscle Groups

1. Arms
2. Chest
3. Neck
4. Face (with focus on eyes and forehead)

From Andrasik F: Relaxation and biofeedback for chronic headaches. In Holzman AD, Turk DC (eds): A Handbook of Psychological Treatment Approaches. New York, Pergamon, 1986, p 228.

Table 123–3

Relaxation Training Regimen

Week	*Session*	*Introduction and Treatment Rationale*	*Number of Muscle Groups*	*Deepening Exercises*	*Breathing Exercises*	*Relaxing Imagery*	*Muscle Discrimination Training*	*Relaxation By Recall*	*Cue-Controlled Recall*
1	1	X	14	X	X				
	2		14	X	X	X			
2	3		14	X	X	X	X		
	4		14	X	X	X	X		
3	5		8	X	X	X	X		
	6		8	X	X	X	X	X	
4	7		4	X	X	X	X	X	
5	8		4	X	X	X	X	X	X
6	9		4	X	X	X	X	X	X
7	None								
8	10		4	X	X	X	X	X	X

From Andrasik F: Relaxation and biofeedback for chronic headaches. In Holzman AD, Turk DC (eds): A Handbook of Psychological Treatment Approaches. New York, Pergamon, 1986, p 225.

patient. Once modifications are made, however, they should be consistently followed throughout the rest of the treatment.[6] The patients are guided to use breathing, imagery, self-suggestion, and cues that are personalized. It is important for patients to discover what techniques and variations are most appropriate to facilitate their own relaxation. Ost[46] devised a muscle relaxation training program similar to the one described in this chapter. He found that 90% to 95% of his participants were able to acquire the skills of relaxation, and he reported that the attrition rate was relatively low (0% to 22%).

Individuals may respond differently to the relaxation techniques. For instance, those who have migraine headaches may find that the AT of peripheral warming is most effective in preventing migraine attacks, whereas those who have tension-type headaches may find beneficial results with PMR.[5] Furthermore, certain types of techniques may induce what Smith[47] has termed "R-states." According to Smith's ABC, or attentional behavioral cognitive, theory on relaxation training, different relaxation states (R-states) are generated from different relaxation techniques. Smith[47] conducted an extensive factor analysis of descriptors related to sensations of relaxation. He found that there are 14 + 1 potential R-states: sleepiness, disengagement, physical relaxation, mental quiet, rested and refreshed, mental relaxation, energized, aware, joy, love and thankfulness, prayerfulness, positive detachment, awe and wonder, timeless, and mystery. Although relaxation procedures may promote a marked decrease in arousal such that there is a generalized *relaxation response*, as proposed by Benson et al.,[3] it appears as though each procedure may also have *specific effects*, as proposed by Davidson and Schwartz.[4] Research carried out by Smith[47] lends support to the specific effects approach as different R-states are experienced, depending on the procedure.

Matsumoto and Smith[48] investigated what R-states might be produced when comparing PMR with breathing exercises over the course of 5 weeks. They found significant differences at weeks 4 and 5: breathing participants had higher levels of strength and awareness (combined R-states energized and aware) and PMR participants had higher R-states of physical relaxation and disengagement. Furthermore, the delayed effects of mental quiet and joy emerged after week 5 in the PMR group. Research has also found gender[49] and ethnic[50] differences in the R-states experienced as a result of different relaxation techniques.

Relaxation techniques and GI can be used in isolation or combined. Individuals may respond differently depending on the type of procedures implemented. In terms of pain, the objective of relaxation is to decrease sympathetic arousal and provide a distraction to reduce suffering.

SIDE EFFECTS

Generally, relaxation techniques lead to beneficial outcomes. However, negative side effects associated with relaxation training have been reported. These negative experiences are infrequent and are usually remedied within a session. Relaxation-induced anxiety (RIA) describes a variety of paradoxical effects from attempting relaxation procedures.[51] Examples of these negative reactions are musculoskeletal activity (tics, spasms, restlessness), disturbing sensory experiences (unusual sensory experiences, feelings of floating), increased sympathetic arousal, and disturbing cognitive/emotional responses (sadness, intrusive thoughts, fear).[52] Heide and Borkovec[51] offer potential explanations for the RIA phenomenon. First, some people may be unfamiliar with relaxation and the novel sensations may be bothersome. Second, the fear of losing control may incite RIA in that many of the procedures emphasize a passive component. Fear of inactivity is another potential explanation for RIA. Sometimes people have a difficult time sitting quietly and relaxing, which can lead to restlessness. Others may find self-focused attention aversive, as is the case with relaxation techniques. Finally, individuals undergoing relaxation training commonly report intrusive thoughts.

Heide and Borkovec[51] also provide solutions for RIA. One solution is to change to an alternate relaxation technique. For instance, if PMR is causing symptoms of RIA, switching to pleasant imagery may be appropriate. "People rarely experience RIA with two different types of relaxation" (p. 255).[52] Another solution would be to approach relaxation training gradually, with shorter sessions.[51] Although RIA is generally uncommon, those who have pervasive or generalized anxiety seem to be the most prone to it. Clinicians should be aware of RIA's occurrence and make accommodations if it develops. Even milder versions of RIA can have an impact on attrition and compliance with relaxation training programs.

Freeman[15] discusses patient considerations for imagery techniques. Because of the change in brain wave activity that can be altered by imagery, clinicians need to carefully monitor those who have epilepsy. Individuals with unstable diabetes should also be carefully monitored because sugar levels can be affected by imagery. Imagery for patients who have chronic severe depression may not be an appropriate technique. It may be suitable if anxiety is an underlying feature, but it would require a well-trained clinician to safely implement this type of technique.

CONCLUSION

In summary, this chapter began with the rationale for the use of relaxation techniques and GI for pain conditions. The section "Historical Considerations" described Jacobson and Schultz as the founders of PMR and AT, respectively, in the early 1900s. The history of breathing therapies and imagery is less definitive and dates much further back. The "Indications" section discussed how relaxation techniques and imagery have been successfully applied to a variety of conditions, including pain tolerance, arthritis, back pain, burn débridement, cancer, tension-type headache, migraine headache, pre-surgical and post-surgical settings, ulcers, and anxiety and depression associated with pain. This chapter then described the techniques of breathing therapies, GI, AT, and PMR. An example of a treatment regimen incorporating many of the techniques was also discussed. The chapter closed with the possible side effect of RIA and other patient considerations.

References

1. Andrasik F, Lords AO: Biofeedback. In Freeman L (ed): Mosby's Complementary & Alternative Medicine: A Research-Based Approach, 2nd ed. Philadelphia, Elsevier, 2004, p 207.

2. NIH Technology Assessment Panel on Integration of Behavioral and Relaxation Approaches into the Treatment of Chronic Pain and Insomnia: Integration of behavioral and relaxation approaches into the treatment of chronic pain and insomnia. JAMA 276:313, 1996.
3. Benson H, Kotch JB, Crassweller KD, Greenwood MM: Historical and clinical considerations of the relaxation response. Am Scientist 65:441, 1977.
4. Davidson RJ, Schwartz GE: Psychobiology of relaxation and related states. In Mostofsky D (ed): Behavior Modification and Control of Physiological Activity. Englewood Cliffs, NJ, Prentice-Hall, 1976.
5. Lehrer PM, Carr R, Sargunaraj D, Woolfolk RL: Stress management techniques: Are they all equivalent, or do they have specific effects? Biofeedback Self-Regulation 19:353, 1994.
6. Andrasik F: Relaxation and biofeedback self-management for pain. In Boswell MV, Cole BE (eds): Weiner's Pain Management: A Practical Guide for Clinicians, 7th ed. Boca Raton, FL, Taylor & Francis, 2006, p 705.
7. Fernandez E: Anxiety, Depression, and Anger in Pain. Dallas, Advanced Psychological Resources, 2002.
8. Melzack R: Pain and stress: A new perspective. In Gatchel RJ, Turk DC (eds): Psychosocial Factors and Pain: Critical Perspectives. New York, Guilford Press, 1999, p 89.
9. Tracey I, Proghaus A, Gati JS, et al: Imaging attentional modulation of pain in the periaqueductal gray in humans. J Neurosci 22:2748, 2002.
10. Jacobson E: Progressive Relaxation. Chicago, University of Chicago Press, 1938.
11. Freeman L: Relaxation therapy. In Freeman L (ed): Mosby's Complementary & Alternative Medicine: A Research-Based Approach, 2nd ed. Philadelphia, Elsevier, 2004, p 145.
12. Lehrer PM: How to relax and how not to relax: A re-evaluation of the work of Edmund Jacobson. Behav Res Ther 20:417, 1982.
13. Wolpe J: Psychotherapy by Reciprocal Inhibition. Stanford, CA, Stanford University Press, 1958.
14. Linden W: Autogenic Training: A Clinical Guide. New York, Guilford Press, 1990.
15. Freeman L: Imagery. In Freeman L (ed): Mosby's Complementary & Alternative Medicine: A Research-Based Approach, 2nd ed. Philadelphia, Elsevier, 2004, p 275.
16. Neumann W, Kugler J, Pfand-Neumann P, et al: Effects of pain-incompatible imagery on tolerance of pain, heart rate, and skin resistance. Percept Motor Skills 84:939, 1997.
17. Lorig K, Laurin J, Gines GE: Arthritis self-management: A five-year history of a patient education program. Nurs Clin North Am 19:637, 1984.
18. Lorig K, Holman H: Arthritis self-management studies: A twelve-year review. Special issue: Arthritis education. Health Educ Q 20:17, 1993.
19. Lorig K, Mazonson P, Holman H: Evidence suggesting that health education for self-management in patients with chronic arthritis has sustained health benefits while reducing health care costs. Arthritis Rheum 36:439, 1993.
20. Stenstrom CH, Arge B, Sundbom A: Dynamic training versus relaxation training as home exercise for patients with inflammatory rheumatic diseases. A randomized controlled study. Scand J Rheumatol 25:28, 1996.
21. Baird CL, Sands L: A pilot study of the effectiveness of guided imagery with progressive muscle relaxation to reduce chronic pain and mobility difficulties of osteoarthritis. Pain Manage Nurs 5:97, 2004.
22. Turner JA, Chapman, CR: Psychological interventions for chronic pain: A critical review. II. Operant conditioning, hypnosis, and cognitive-behavioral therapy. Pain 12:23, 1982.
23. Stuckey SJ, Jacobs A, Goldfarb J: EMG biofeedback training, relaxation training, and placebo for the relief of chronic back pain. Percept Motor Skills 63:1023, 1986.
24. Achterberg J, Kenner C, Lawlis GF: Severe burn injury: A comparison of relaxation, imagery, and biofeedback for pain management. J Mental Imagery 12:71, 1988.
25. Wallace KG: Analysis of recent literature concerning relaxation and imagery interventions for cancer pain. Cancer Nurs 20:79, 1997.
26. Syrjala KL, Donaldson MW, Davis GW, et al: Relaxation and imagery and cognitive-behavioral training reduce pain during cancer treatment: A controlled clinical trial. Pain 63:189, 1995.
27. Burish TG, Carey MP, Krozely MG, Greco FA: Conditioned side effects induced by cancer chemotherapy: Prevention through behavioral treatment. J Consult Clin Psychol 55:42, 1987.
28. Penzien DB, Rains JC, Andrasik F: Behavioral management of recurrent headache: Three decades of experience and empiricism. Appl Psychophysiol Biofeedback 27:163, 2002.
29. Rains JC, Penzien DB, McCrory DC, Gray RN: Behavioral headache treatment: History, review of the empirical literature, and methodological critique. Headache 45(Suppl 2):S92, 2005.
30. Eccleston C, Morley S, Williams A, et al: Systematic review of randomised controlled trials of psychological therapy for chronic pain in children and adolescents, with a subset meta-analysis of pain relief. Pain 99:157, 2002.
31. Holden EW, Deichmann MM, Levy JD: Empirically supported treatments in pediatric psychology: Recurrent pediatric headache. J Pediatr Psychol 24:91, 1999.
32. Cupal DD, Brewer BW: Effects of relaxation and guided imagery on knee strength, reinjury anxiety, and pain following anterior cruciate ligament reconstruction. Rehabil Psychol 46:28, 2001.
33. Lawlis GF, Selby D, Hinnant D, McCoy CE: Reduction of postoperative pain parameters by presurgical relaxation instructions for spinal pain patients. Spine 10:649, 1985.
34. Shaw L, Ehrlich A: Relaxation training as a treatment for chronic pain caused by ulcerative colitis. Pain 29:287, 1987.
35. Brooks GR, Richardson FC: Emotional skills training: A treatment program for duodenal ulcer. Behav Ther 11:198, 1980.
36. Astin JA: Mind-body therapies for the management of pain. Clin J Pain 20:27, 2004.
37. Gevirtz RN, Schwartz MS: The respiratory system in applied psychophysiology. In Schwartz MS, Andrasik F (eds): Biofeedback: A Practitioner's Guide, 3rd ed. New York, Guilford Press, 2003, p 212.
38. Thorn BE, Andrasik F: Relaxation in the treatment of pain. In Schmidt RF, Willis WD (eds). Encyclopedia of Pain. New York, Springer, (in press).
39. Bresler DE: Clinical applications of Interactive Guided Imagery for diagnosing and treating chronic pain. In Boswell MV, Cole BE (eds): Weiner's Pain Management: A Practical Guide for Clinicians, 7th ed. Boca Raton, FL, Taylor & Francis, 2006, p 757.
40. Arena JG, Blanchard EB: Biofeedback training for chronic pain disorders: A primer. In Gatchel RJ, Turk DC (eds): Psychological Approaches to Pain Management: A Practitioner's Handbook, 2nd ed. New York, Guilford Press, 2002, p 159.
41. Schultz JH, Luthe W: Autogenic Therapy, vol 1. New York, Grune & Stratton, 1969.
42. Arena JG, Blanchard, EB: Biofeedback and relaxation therapy for chronic pain disorders. In Gatchel RJ, Turk DC (eds): Psychological Approaches to Pain Management: A Practitioner's Handbook. New York, Guilford Press, 1996, p 179.
43. Bernstein DA, Borkovec TD: Progressive Relaxation. Champaign, IL, Research Press, 1973.
44. Andrasik F: Relaxation and biofeedback for chronic headaches. In Holzman AD, Turk DC (eds): A Handbook of Psychological Treatment Approaches. New York, Pergamon, 1986, p 213.
45. Schwartz MS: The use of audiotapes for patient education and relaxation. In Schwartz MS, Andrasik F (eds): Biofeedback: A Practitioner's Guide, 3rd ed. New York, Guilford Press, 2003, p 265.
46. Ost LG: Applied relaxation: Description of a coping technique and review of controlled studies. Behav Res Ther 25:397, 1987.
47. Smith JC: Advances in ABC relaxation theory: The 14+1 map. In Smith JC (ed): Advances in ABC Relaxation: Applications and Inventories. New York, Springer, 2001, p 3.
48. Matsumoto M, Smith JC: Progressive muscle relaxation, breathing exercises, and ABC relaxation theory. J Clin Psychol 57:1551, 2001.
49. Bowers R, Darner RM, Goldner CL, Sohnle S: Gender differences for recalled relaxation states, dispositions, beliefs, and benefits. In Smith JC (ed): Advances in ABC Relaxation: Applications and Inventories. New York, Springer, 2001, p 111.
50. Smith JC, McDuffie SR, Ritchie T, Holmes R: Ethnic and racial differences in relaxation states for recalled relaxation activities. In Smith JC (ed): Advances in ABC Relaxation: Applications and Inventories. New York, Springer, 2001, p 115.
51. Heide FJ, Borkovec TD: Relaxation-induced anxiety: Mechanisms and theoretical implications. Behav Res Ther 22:1, 1984.
52. Schwartz MS, Schwartz NM, Monastra VJ: Problems with relaxation and biofeedback-assisted relaxation, and guidelines for management. In Schwartz MS, Andrasik F (eds): Biofeedback: A Practitioner's Guide, 3rd ed. New York, Guilford Press, 2003, p 251.

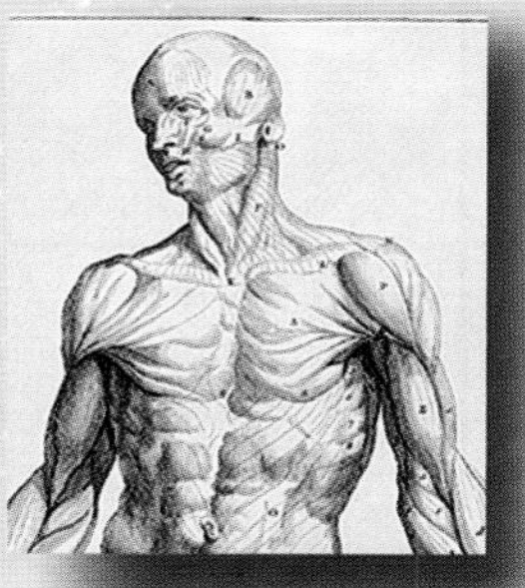

Part C

Physical Modalities in the Management of Pain

chapter 124

Therapeutic Heat and Cold in the Management of Pain

Steven D. Waldman, Katherine A. Waldman, and Howard J. Waldman

Heat and cold have been used in the treatment of pain since the time of Hippocrates. In spite of their widespread use for centuries, it was not until the birth of the specialty of physical medicine and rehabilitation after World War II that a search for the scientific justification for these universally accepted modalities was undertaken. It was the knowledge that was derived from this search that forms much of our rationale for the use of heat and cold in the treatment of pain. This chapter will review common therapeutic heat and cold modalities and provide the clinician with a roadmap for their safe application.

The Physiologic Effects of Therapeutic Heat

The mechanisms by which heat exerts its analgesic effect extend beyond the simple effects of heat locally on the target tissue. Locally, heat elicits the following physiologic responses: (1) increased blood flow; (2) decreased muscle spasm; (3) increased extensibility of connective tissue; (4) decreased joint stiffness; (5) reduction of edema; and most importantly (6) analgesia (Table 124–1).[1] Because the sensation of temperature and pain are both carried to the higher centers via the same neural pathways, it is not unreasonable to imagine that heat exerts a modulating effect at the spinal and supraspinal levels. In addition, the feeling of well being associated with therapeutic heat most likely causes the release of endorphins and other neurotransmitters further modifying the pain response. It should be noted that although the beneficial nature of therapeutic heat cannot be denied, this treatment modality is not without side effects. The relative contraindications to the use of therapeutic heat are summarized in Table 124–2. Although these precautions are not absolute, special care should be taken should a decision be made to use therapeutic heat in these clinical settings.

Table 124–1

Physiologic Effects of Therapeutic Heat

- Increased blood flow
- Decreased muscle spasm
- Increased extensibility of connective tissue
- Decreased joint stiffness
- Reduction of edema
- Analgesia (most important)

Table 124–2

Relative Contraindications to Therapeutic Heat

- Lack of or reduced sensation
- Demyelinating diseases
- Acute inflammation
- Bleeding disorders
- Hemorrhage
- Malignancy
- Inability to communicate or respond to pain
- Atrophic skin
- Ischemia
- Scar tissue

Table 124–3

Therapeutic Heat Modalities

Superficial heat modalities
Modalities that rely on conduction
  Hydrocollator packs
  Circulating water heating pads
  Chemical heating pads
  Reusable microwavable heating pads
  Paraffin baths
Modalities that rely on convection
  Hydrotherapy
  Fluidotherapy

Deep heat modalities
  Modalities that rely on conversion
  Ultrasound
  Short-wave diathermy
  Microwave diathermy

Choosing a Therapeutic Heat Modality

The clinician who is considering therapeutic heat as an adjunct in the treatment of his or her patient's pain has a variety of heating modalities to choose from (Table 124–3). Although the indications for the use of therapeutic heat apply to all therapeutic heating modalities discussed in this chapter, each modality has its own distinct advantages and disadvantages which can influence not only the success or failure of this therapeutic intervention but can also determine the incidence of side effects and complications if the wrong modality is chosen or is used in the incorrect clinical situation (Table 124–4). As a practical consideration, the failure to match the modality to the patient will usually result in a less than optimal outcome.

When matching the modality to the patient, it is essential to understand the underlying physics of each therapeutic heat modality. Each heat modality accomplishes the delivery of heat to the target tissue by a specific physical mechanism of heat transfer. For sake of organization, these mechanisms can be divided into the categories of conduction, convection, and conversion. Whereas conduction and convection provides primarily superficial heating, conversion has the ability to heat deep tissues. Therefore, the first question when choosing a therapeutic heat modality is whether superficial or deep heat is the desired goal.

The next step in matching the modality to the patient is understanding which modalities transfer heat by which mechanism (Table 124–5). Hot packs, the most commonly used heat modality in clinical practice, transfer superficial heat by conduction as do heating pads, circulating water heating pads, chemical heating packs, reusable microwave heating pads, and paraffin baths. Hydrotherapy and fluidotherapy deliver superficial heat to the target tissue by convection. The deep heating modalities of ultrasound, radiant heat, short-wave diathermy, and microwave diathermy deliver heat to the target

Table 124–4

Indications for the Use of Therapeutic Heat Modalities

- Pain
- Muscle spasm
- Bursitis
- Tenosynovitis
- Collagen vascular diseases
- Contracture
- Fibromyalgia
- Induction of hyperemia
- Hematoma resolution
- Superficial thrombophlebitis
- Reflex sympathetic dystrophy

Table 124–5

Indications for Therapeutic Ultrasound

- Tendinitis
- Bursitis
- Non-acutely inflamed arthritis
- Frozen joints
- Contractures
- Degenerative arthritis
- Fractures
- Plantar fasciitis

tissues by conversion. By understanding how each heat modality delivers heat, the clinician can then use the unique characteristics of that modality to best meet the patient's needs. Specific heat modalities are discussed subsequently.

■ SUPERFICIAL HEATING MODALITIES

Modalities That Deliver Heat by Conduction

Hydrocollator Packs

As mentioned earlier, the mechanism by which the various types of hot packs deliver heat to the target tissue is by conduction. The amount of heat delivered by conduction is directly proportional to the following variables: (1) the area of heat delivery; (2) the length of time the heat is delivered; (3) the temperature gradient between the hot pack and the target tissue; and (4) the thermal conductivity of the surfaces.[2] The amount of heat delivered by conduction is inversely proportional to the thickness of the layers of materials and tissue that the heat must be conducted through. By altering any of the above variables, the amount of heat delivered to the target tissue can be increased or decreased as the clinical situation and patient comfort dictate.

Hydrocollator packs are flexible packs that contain a silicate gel product that are heated in a water bath to approximately 170°F (Fig. 124–1). The large surface area and flexible nature make this modality ideally suited for treating low back and dorsal spine pain. Smaller hydrocollator packs are useful in the treatment of neck pain. The packs do not absorb significant amounts of water, but their surface is wet thus increasing conduction. A terry cloth towel is placed between the patient and the hydrocollator pack with the thickness of towels being the easiest way to control the dosimetry and to allow titration of the temperature to patient comfort. The packs maintain a therapeutic temperature for approximately 20 to 30 minutes to allow for superficial heating of large surface areas. To avoid burning the patient, care must be taken to allow excess water to drain from the pack prior to use. The hydrocollator pack should always be placed on rather than under the patient for easy removal should the patient complain that the pad is too hot.

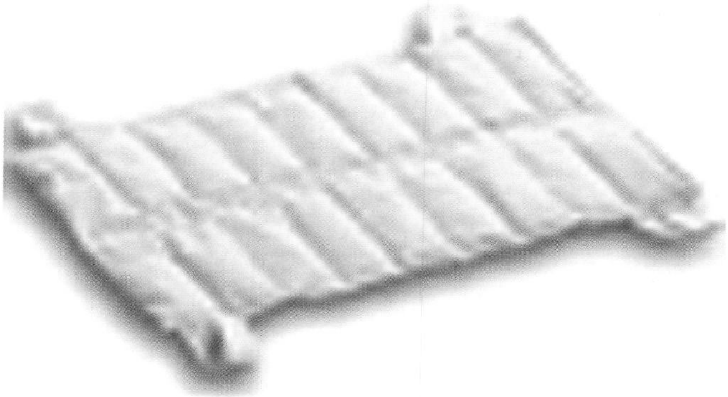

FIGURE 124–1 ■ Hydrocollator packs are flexible silicate gel packs that are heated in a water bath to approximately 170°F.

Circulating Water Heating Pads (K-Pads)

Like the hydrocollator pack, the circulating water heating pad is ideally suited for treating low back and dorsal spine pain. More flexible than hydrocollator packs, the circulating water heating pad can also be used on shoulders and extremities. The circulating water pad is thermostatically controlled so that the water temperature remains constant allowing for superficial heating of relatively large surface areas. This confers two additional benefits to this heat delivery device (1) unlike hydrocollator packs, hot water bottles and microwave heating pads that cool over time, the circulating water heating pad can deliver a constant temperature to the target tissue over time; (2) the thermostatically controlled circulation system greatly decreases the risk of thermal injuries associated with traditional electric pads (Fig. 124–2). In spite of the increased safety of circulating water pads relative to electric heating pads, because they do not cool spontaneously, their use should be closely monitored and carefully timed.

Chemical Heating Packs

Chemical heating packs are readily available in most pharmacies. They consist of a flexible outer layer that contains internally segregated chemicals, which when mixed by squeezing or kneading the package, cause an exothermic reaction that releases heat capable of producing superficial heating of the affected body part. Other chemical heating pads produce heat by oxidation when the chemical heating pack is

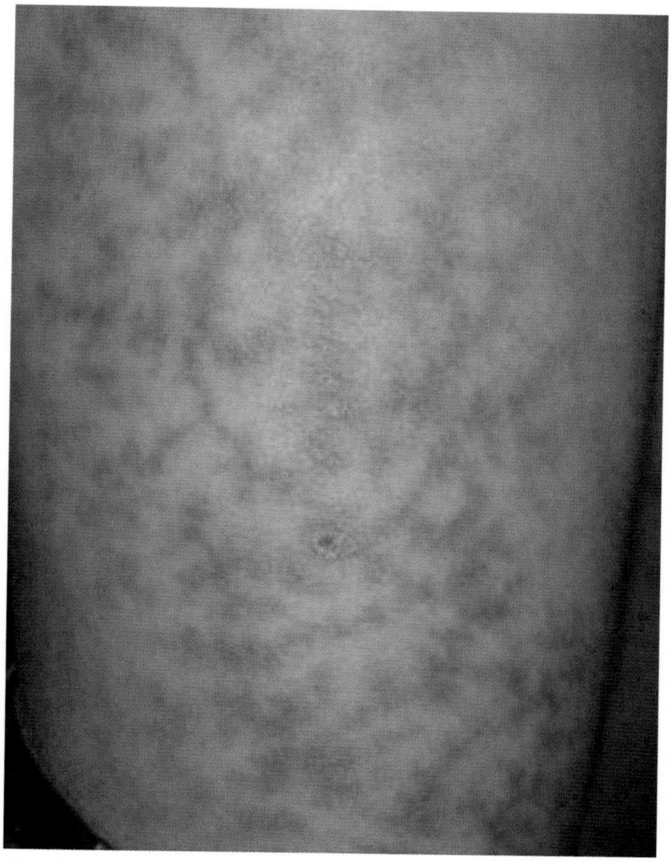

FIGURE 124–2 ■ Thermal injury of the type associated with traditional electric pads.

exposed to air. Most chemical heating packs that rely on oxidation contain iron powder, activated charcoal, sodium chloride, and water. Although inexpensive and convenient to use, the chemical heating packs produce varying degrees of heat and have the potential to cause severe burns even when used properly.[3] The chemicals contained in the packs can cause chemical irritation to the skin if the outer package integrity is compromised. Chemical heating packs have the advantage of being portable and not requiring electricity or external heating.

Reusable Microwavable Heating Pads

The widespread use of microwave ovens has spawned a variety of new reusable heating pad products that are designed to be quickly heated in the microwave oven. These products consist of an outer bag, which may be made of cloth or plastic, with a sealed inner bag containing gel or grains (including rice, corn, or wheat) that delivers heat via conduction to provide superficial heating of the affected tissues (Figs. 124–3 and 124–4). Some products add aromatic substances to provide the added theoretical benefit of aromatherapy. While convenient and easy to use, these products have some serious drawbacks. First, as with microwave popcorn, variations in the heating abilities of microwave ovens can cause over- or under-heating. Additionally, there is no simple way to verify the actual temperature of the product and owing to the nature of microwave ovens, there may be significant inconsistencies of surface temperatures with "hot spots" resulting in serious burns. Like hydrocollator packs and other heat delivery modalities that do not deliver a constant source of heat, cooling can be inconsistent.

Paraffin Baths

Used primarily for the treatment of hand abnormalities associated with rheumatoid arthritis, degenerative arthritis, and the other collagen vascular diseases such as scleroderma, paraffin baths are a useful form of conduction-type heat therapy capable of providing superficial heating of the affected tissues.[4,5] Paraffin baths are reasonably safe as long as the temperature of the liquid paraffin is checked before extremity immersion or application. The paraffin is generally mixed with mineral oil (7 parts paraffin to 1 part of mineral oil) and placed in a thermostatically controlled heater (Fig. 124–5). The affected body part is then dipped into the paraffin bath and then removed to allow the paraffin to solidify. This procedure is repeated up to 10 times. The affected body parts are then placed under an insulating sheet for approximately 20 minutes and then the paraffin is stripped off and returned to the thermostatically controlled heater to re-melt and to be used again. This technique is usually not

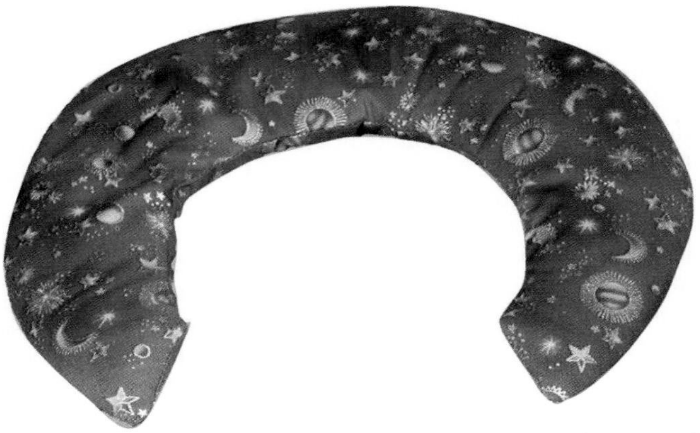

FIGURE 124–3 ■ The widespread use of microwave ovens has spawned a variety of new, reusable heating pad products that are designed to be quickly heated in the microwave oven.

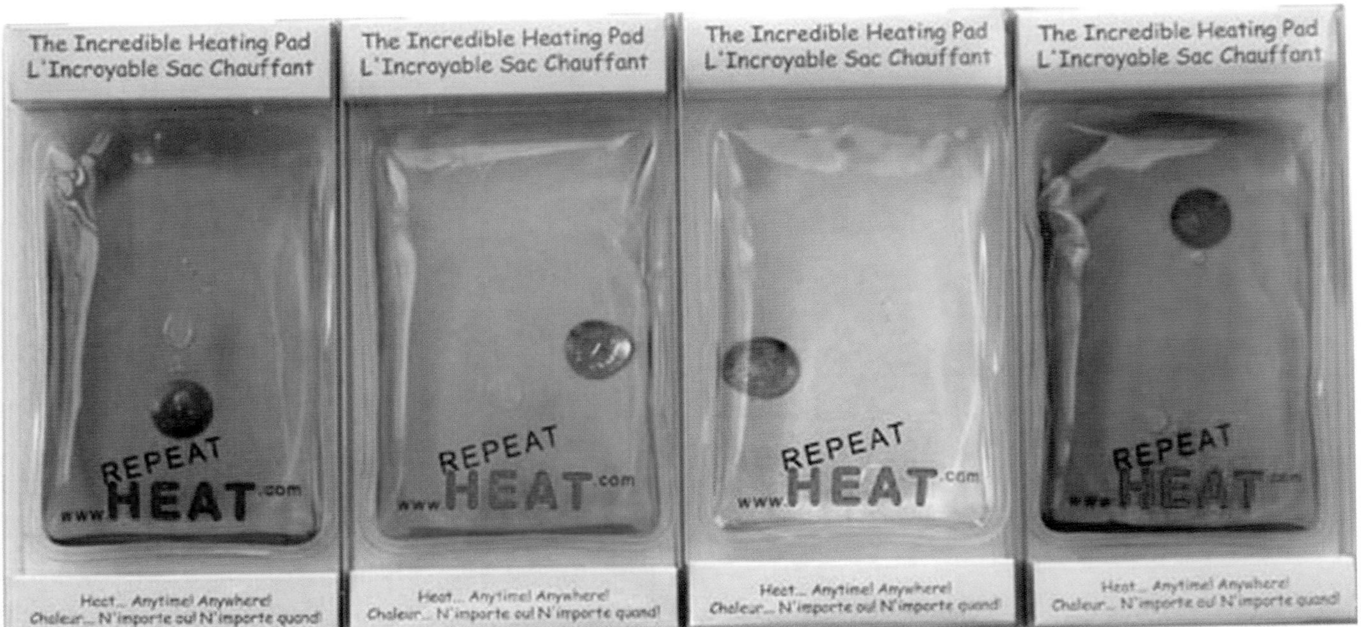

FIGURE 124–4 ■ Reusable microwavable heating pads consist of an outer bag that may be made of cloth or plastic with a sealed inner bag containing gel or grains (rice, corn, or wheat). They deliver their heat via conduction to provide superficial heating of the affected tissues.

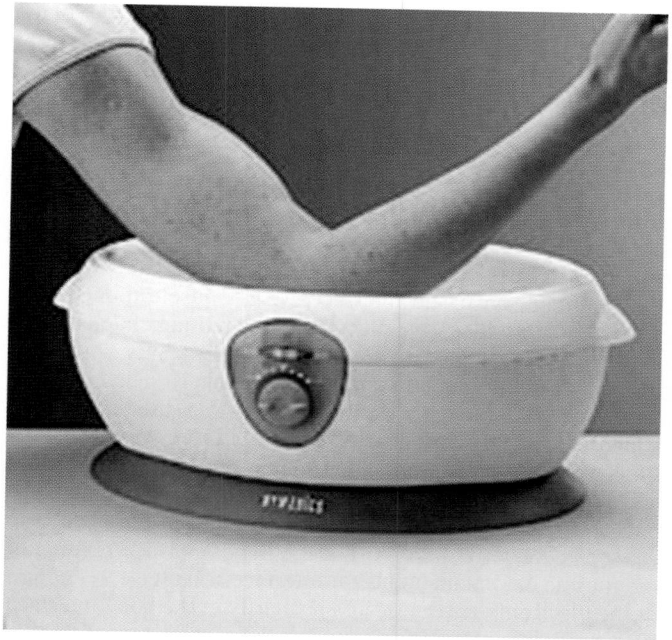

FIGURE 124–5 ■ Paraffin baths are a useful form of conduction-type heat therapy capable of providing superficial heating of the affected tissues.

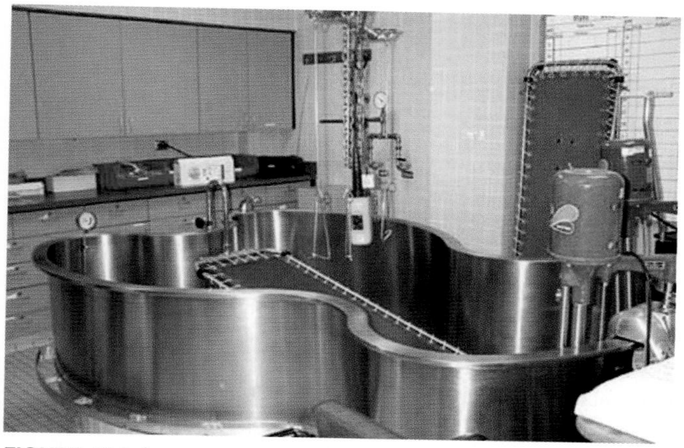

FIGURE 124–6 ■ Immersion of the affected body part or entire body in the case of Hubbard tank therapy allows the high specific gravity of water to partially eliminate the effect of gravity adding another potentially therapeutic sensation to the analgesic milieu.

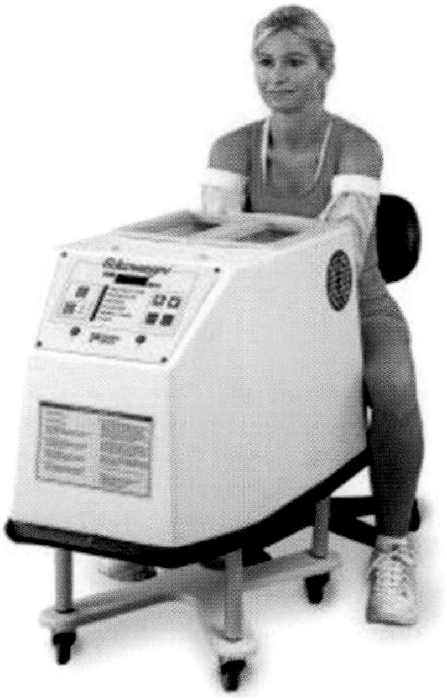

FIGURE 124–7 ■ Fluidotherapy relies on the substances with a low affinity for heat (e.g., glass beads, pulverized corn cobs, etc.) and high temperatures of 116°F.

undertaken if there are acutely inflamed joints, but only after antiinflammatory drugs have begun to treat the acute inflammation.

Modalities That Deliver Heat by Convection

Hydrotherapy

Water is an ideal medium to deliver heat to affected tissues due to its high specific heat. Hydrotherapy uses this physical property to advantage by the agitation of a whirlpool to constantly move the layer of heated water that has cooled after contact with the skin and replacing it with water heated to the correct temperature. In addition to the superficial heat delivery properties of hydrotherapy, immersion of the affected body part or entire body in the case of Hubbard tank therapy allows the high specific gravity of water to partially eliminate the effect of gravity adding another potentially therapeutic sensation to the analgesic milieu (Fig. 124–6). The massaging effect of water can also help reduce muscle spasm as well as provide gentle débridement of wounds. For treatment of single limbs, immersion in waters with temperatures of 115°F are generally well tolerated if careful monitoring is carried out. Temperatures above 102°F should be avoided when using total body immersion to avoid overheating. Total body immersion should not be used in patients with multiple sclerosis to avoid the triggering of neurologic deficits that may sometimes become permanent.

Fluidotherapy

Fluidotherapy uses convection as its mechanism of heat transfer. In contrast with hydrotherapy which relies on the high specific heat of water delivered at lower temperatures, fluidotherapy relies on the substances with a low affinity for heat (e.g., glass beads, pulverized corn cobs, etc.) and high heat temperatures of 116° F (Fig. 124–7). The result is a dry semi-fluid mixture that is heated by thermostatically controlled hot air. The patient is able to immerse the affected hand, foot, or portion of an extremity into the mixture. As the affected body part is heated, sweating enhances heat transfer, producing superficial heating. This treatment modality is useful in the treatment of reflex sympathetic dystrophy in that the medium used (e.g., glass beads) provides gentile tactile desensitization.

DEEP HEATING MODALITIES

Modalities That Deliver Heat by Conversion

The heat delivery modalities just discussed have in common their ability to produce superficial heating of affected tissues. When heating of the deep tissues is desired, the clinician has several modalities at his or her disposal. These include three modalities in common clinical use: (1) ultrasound; (2) shortwave diathermy; and (3) microwave diathermy. These modalities have in common their ability to safely heat deep tissues via the physical property of conversion of physical energy into heat when properly used.

Variables affecting the amount of heat ultimately delivered to deep tissues for each of these modalities include (1) the pattern of relative heating; (2) the specific heat of the tissue being heated; and (3) the physiologic factors affecting the tissues being heated. Each will be discussed individually. Relative heating is the relative amount of energy that is converted into heat at any point in the tissue being heated. For sake of consistency, common reference points for the pattern of relative heating include the subcutaneous fat/muscle interface, the muscle/bone interface, and so on. The pattern of relative heating is different for each of the deep heat modalities currently in common clinical use.

The specific heat of the tissue also influences how deep heat is distributed through affected tissues. Each type of tissue being heated has its own specific heat. As each of these tissues is heated, the thermal conductivity of the tissue changes as the relative temperatures of each type of tissue reaches equilibrium, thus affecting the heat exchange between warmer and cooler tissues.

The physiologic changes induced by deep heating also influence the heat distribution by modifying the physiologic factors that existed before the deep heat was applied. For example, under normal conditions, the skin temperature is generally lower that the deeper muscle tissues. The application of a deep heating modality will further raise the core temperature of the muscle being heated, thereby increasing the temperature gradient between skin and deep muscle. However, as the deep heat is applied to muscle, an increase in blood flow to the heated muscle occurs. The incoming blood is cooler than the heated muscle, so the blood with its relatively high specific heat acts as a cooling agent carrying off excess heat and cooling the muscle.[6] The interplay of these and other physiologic factors ultimately affects the pattern of temperature distribution.

Ultrasound

Ultrasound uses sound waves to deliver energy to affected tissue. These sound waves occur at a frequency well above the upper level of human hearing (which occurs at approximately 20,000 Hz) and are produced by the use of a piezoelectric crystal that converts electrical energy into sound waves. These sound waves produce both thermal and nonthermal therapeutic effects on tissue, and manipulation of the physical properties of these effects can tailor the therapeutic response delivered—for example, high temperature destruction of malignant liver tumors, phonophoresis (the forcing of steroids and antiinflammatories into tissues with sound), lithotripsy, and deep heating of tissues.

Although an extensive discussion of the physics involved in the therapeutic use of ultrasound is beyond the purpose of this chapter, a few general comments are useful for the clinician to understand how the modalities are used to produce deep heat for the treatment of pain and the other conditions listed in Table 124–3. For the purposes of our discussion, it is sufficient to note that the two major variables at play that determine the propagation of ultrasonic energy are (1) the absorption characteristics of the tissues being exposed to the sound waves and (2) the reflection of these sound waves as they impinge on tissue interfaces (e.g., muscle, bone, etc.). These two variables give ultrasound the unique characteristic of being able to heat deep tissues such as joints with little heating of overlying skin and subcutaneous tissues.[7]

Each variable can dramatically affect the amount of sound energy that is converted to heat. For example, absorption: bone absorbs almost 10 times more energy than does skeletal muscle and almost 20 times more energy than subcutaneous fat, which means that much more of the ultrasonic energy is converted into heat at the bone interface relative to the muscle or subcutaneous fat interface. Likewise, reflection of the ultrasonic energy occurs primarily at the bone interface with very little reflection occurring at the subcutaneous fat or muscle interface. This means that most of the sound energy delivered is able to penetrate the subcutaneous tissues and muscle with the reflected sound waves producing much of their heating effect at the muscle-bone interface. This physical property of reflection can produce extremely high temperatures if ultrasound is accidentally used in patients with metal prosthetics or large metal surgical clips because reflection from these artificial interfaces can produce an intense increase in reflected ultrasonic energy that can cause disastrous deep thermal injury. The admonition that ultrasound is contraindicated over metal implants should be heeded.[8]

If sound waves are to be effectively delivered to the intended tissues, coupling between the skin overlying the tissue and the ultrasound wand must be accomplished. This is accomplished by introducing a medium called a *coupling agent*. Gel and degassed water are commonly used coupling agents. Ultrasound is usually delivered by slowly moving the ultrasound wand which has been liberally covered with coupling agent over the affected area for 5 to 10 minutes. For body parts with irregular surfaces such as the ankle, ultrasound can be delivered indirectly by immersing the affected body part in degassed water and placing the ultrasound wand in close proximity to the skin without actually touching it and then slowly moving over the affected areas. This technique is known as indirect ultrasound and will require higher energy levels to offset the absorption of sound waves by the water to achieve similar deep heating effects when compared with direct ultrasound.

Indications for ultrasound are summarized in Table 124–5. Tendinitis and bursitis generally respond well to treatment with ultrasound as does degenerative arthritis.[9] Although the use of ultrasound is generally avoided when a joint is acutely inflamed, it can be beneficial as the joint inflammation is resolving after intra-articular injection of steroids and/or the implementation of antiinflammatory drugs. Ultrasound can be used in concert to enhance the effects of active and passive range of motion and stretching of joints that have lost normal range of motion—as well as in the treatment of plantar fasciitis.[10,11]

Short-Wave Diathermy

Short-wave diathermy uses electromagnetic radio waves to convert energy to deep heat. As with ultrasound, short-wave diathermy is thought to exert its therapeutic effects by both thermal and nonthermal mechanisms. The primary nonthermal mechanism associated with the use of therapeutic short-wave diathermy is via vibration induction of tissue molecules when exposed to radio waves. By changing the characteristics of the short-wave applicator, the clinician can target the specific type of tissue he or she wants to heat. By using an inductive applicator that generates a magnetically induced eddy of radio wave currents in the tissues, selective heating of water-rich tissues, such as muscle, can be obtained (Fig. 124–8). By using a capacity-coupled applicator that generates heat via generation of an electrical field, selective heating of water-poor tissues, such as subcutaneous fat and adjacent soft tissues, can be accomplished.[12] With either type of short-wave diathermy, metal must be avoided; the patient must remove all jewelry and treatment must be carried out on a nonconductive (e.g., wooden) treatment table. Implanted pacemakers, spinal cord stimulators, surgical implants, and copper-containing IUDs should *never* be exposed to short-wave diathermy to avoid excessive heating and thermal injury. Indications for short-wave diathermy mirror those listed for ultrasound, although the ability to heat subcutaneous fat and adjacent soft tissues not reached by superficial heat modalities and less well heated by ultrasound may lead the clinician to choose short-wave diathermy to treat painful conditions and other pathologic processes that are thought to find their nidus in more superficial tissues.[13]

Microwave Diathermy

Microwave diathermy uses electromagnetic radio waves with frequencies of 915 and 2456 MHz.[14] Based on the physical properties of these waves and the corresponding dimensions of the microwave antennae, microwave diathermy has two unique properties that can be used to clinical advantage. The first is that microwaves are selectively absorbed in tissues with high water content, such as muscle.[15] This makes microwave diathermy ideally suited to treat pathologic processes that occur in the muscles and adjacent fat.[16] The second is that microwaves are more easily focused than the short waves used in short-wave diathermy, thereby decreasing energy leakage and making heating more efficient.

Microwave diathermy also has several unique side effects that the clinician must be aware of. First, microwaves can cause cataract formation, so protective eyewear must be worn whenever microwave diathermy is used.[17] Second, in addition to the precautions and contraindications to the use of short-wave diathermy listed earlier, because microwave diathermy has a selective affinity to heat water, this technique should not be used in patients with edema, blisters, or in patients with hyperhidrosis because the sweat beads may become heated and cause burns to the skin.

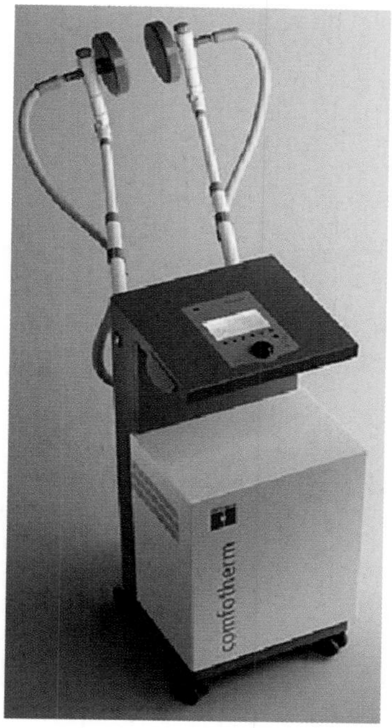

FIGURE 124–8 ■ Short-wave diathermy uses electromagnetic radio waves to convert energy to deep heat.

THERAPEUTIC COLD MODALITIES

The Physiologic Effects of Therapeutic Cold

The application of therapeutic cold exerts both local and remote physiologic effects.[2] Locally, the application of therapeutic cold causes vasoconstriction, which is ultimately followed by a reflex vasodilatation after the vascular smooth muscles are paralyzed from the cold. Therapeutic cold decreases the metabolic activity of the treated part and it decreases muscle tone. As cooling progresses, spasticity will also be decreased.[18] As cooling slows nerve conduction, analgesia will occur. Indications for the use of therapeutic cold are summarized in Table 124–6.

Choosing a Therapeutic Cold Modality

As with the choice of heat modalities, matching the therapeutic cold modality to the patient is paramount to the success of the treatment and to minimizing the side effects and complications associated with its use. The major determinants in the choice of therapeutic cold modalities are based primarily on two categories: (1) the body part being treated and (2) whether the modality will be administered by a qualified health care professional. As with therapeutic heat, improper use of therapeutic cold modalities can cause serious complications (Table 124–7).

Table 124–6

Indications for Therapeutic Cold
■ Pain
■ Muscle spasm
■ Acute musculoskeletal injury
■ Bursitis
■ Tendinitis
■ Adjunct to muscle re-education

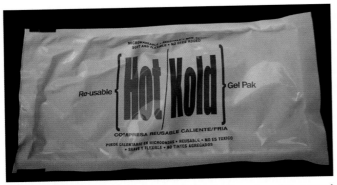

FIGURE 124–9 ■ Commercially available plastic packs, often covered with a soft fabric, which contain gel may be stored in the refrigerator/freezer until use are a convenient way of delivering therapeutic cold.

Table 124–7
Precautions and Contraindications When Using Therapeutic Cold
■ Lack of or reduced sensation
■ Ischemia
■ Raynaud phenomenon
■ Cold intolerance

Ice Packs and Slushes

The high specific heat capacities of ice packs and slushes allow rapid cooling of affected areas. Ice packs can be simply made by placing melting ice and cold water in a Ziploc plastic bag. By using crushed ice and more cold water, a slush pack can be made. Commercially available plastic gel packs, often covered with a soft fabric, may be stored in the refrigerator/freezer and are also a convenient way of delivering therapeutic cold (Fig. 124–9). The flexible nature of both these therapeutic cold modalities allows them to be used over joints or to cool larger areas such as the low back. The rate of cooling of the skin is rapid and the rate of the cooling of deeper tissues is largely a function of the thickness of fat interposed between skin and muscle. When used for periods of 20 minutes or less they are usually safe. The use of a towel between the ice pack or slush and the affected body part will increase tolerance and compliance and decrease the incidence of thermal injury. For home use, a package of frozen peas or corn can serve as an effective and inexpensive ice pack for many painful conditions.

Iced Whirlpools

Used primarily for athletic injuries, the iced whirlpool can rapidly cool an injured extremity by constantly moving water that is warmed by contact with the patient's skin away and replacing it with colder water. Many patients find that the temperatures required to adequately cool muscle are too uncomfortable to tolerate for the time it takes to achieve the intended therapeutic effect. However, some patients find the iced whirlpool more beneficial than similar heated whirlpool treatments.

Ice Rubs

Useful for applying therapeutic cold to larger surface areas such as the low back, ice rubs using water frozen in a plastic or Styrofoam cup can rapidly achieve therapeutic temperatures with cutaneous anesthesia being achieved within 8 to 10 minutes. Additionally, the rubbing action can produce a relaxing effect and aids in tactile desensitization. In healthy patients, ice rubs for periods of 20 minutes or less are usually safe.

Evaporative Cooling Spays

Useful in the treatment of trigger points associated with fibromyalgia and as an adjunct to stretching, the application of evaporative cooling sprays can be quite effective.[19] In the past, ethyl chloride spray was the agent of choice; however the flammability and potential toxicity of the agent has led to the use of the chlorofluormethane compounds. Although effective, these compounds have been criticized as having a negative effect on the environment. To use the evaporative sprays, the trigger point or affected muscle is identified and the agent is aimed at the target area from a distance of approximately 1 meter and applied for approximately 10 seconds. Prolonged cooling of a single point with the evaporative agents can result in thermal injury.

Chemical Ice Packs

There are a large number of disposable ice packs available for home use and for clinical applications. Chemical ice packs are made of a flexible outer layer with a two-compartment inner layer (Fig. 124–10). One inner compartment contains water and the other contains ammonium nitrate that, when combined by squeezing or kneading the package, creates cooling via an endothermic reaction. These products have the advantage of requiring no refrigeration, being easily moldable to joints given their flexibility, and being relatively inexpensive. As with chemical heat packs, the temperature of chemical ice packs is poorly controlled and thermal injuries or inadequate or uneven cooling may occur.[20] Exposure of the skin to the chemicals contained in the pack may cause chemical irritation.

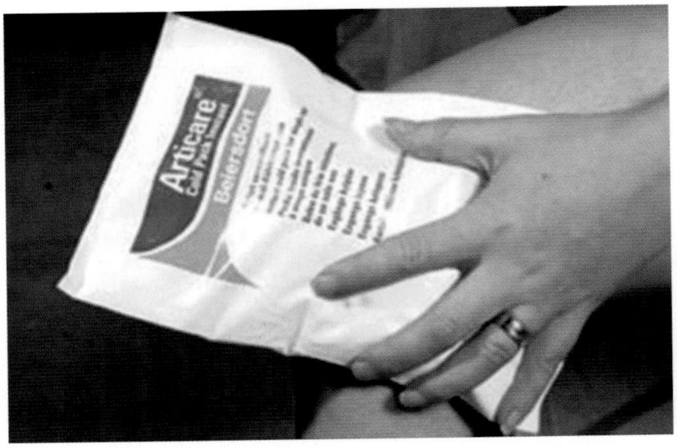

FIGURE 124–10 ■ Chemical ice packs are made of a flexible outer layer with a two-compartment inner layer.

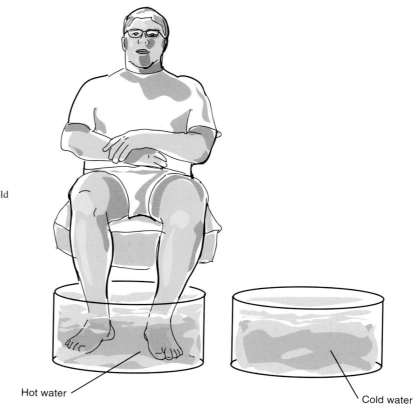

FIGURE 124–11 ■ Contrast baths consist of a hot and a cold bath with temperatures of 110°F and 60°F, respectively.

■ CONTRAST BATHS

A combination of therapeutic heat and cold, contrast baths are useful in the treatment of reflex sympathetic dystrophy and other sympathetically maintained pain syndromes as well as rheumatoid arthritis.[21] Their efficacy is thought to be due to desensitization of nerves by alternating exposure of the affected extremity to heat and cold. Contrast baths consist of a hot and a cold bath with temperatures of 110°F and 60°F, respectively (Fig. 124–11). Therapeutic contrast baths begin with the soaking of the affected extremity in the warm bath for 10 minutes. The extremity is then rapidly transferred to the cold bath for a period of 3 minutes followed by rapid transfer back to the warm bath for 5 minutes. The cycle is repeated four times. For patients with extreme allodynia, less extreme temperatures may be required during initiation of therapy. Contrast baths should be combined with tactile desensitization techniques if optimal results are to be obtained.

■ CONCLUSION

The use of therapeutic heat and cold represents a useful adjunct in the treatment of a variety of painful conditions. Although relatively safe if used properly, severe injury can occur if risk factors are ignored or a specific modality is misused. The correct matching of the modality to the patient is paramount if optimal results are to be achieved and side effects and complications are to be avoided.

References

1. Abramson DI: Physiologic basis for the use of physical agents in peripheral vascular disorders. Arch Phys Med Rehabil 46:216, 1965.
2. Stillwell GK: General principles of thermo-therapy. In Licht S (ed.): Therapeutic Heat and Cold, 2nd ed. Baltimore, Waverly Press, 1965, p. 232.
3. Herman J, Davis C, Mackey M, et al: Clinical trials: Testing of adult chemical heating pad. Sch Inq Nurs Pract 10(2):135, 1996.
4. Robinson VA, Brosseau L, Shea BJ, et al: Thermotherapy for Treating Rheumatoid Arthritis (Cochrane Review) [Update software]. Oxford, The Cochrane Library, The Cochrane Collaboration,1, 2003.
5. Abramson DI, Tuck S, Chu LSW, Augustin C: Effect of paraffin bath and hot fomentations on local tissue temperatures. Arch Phys Med Rehabil 45:87, 1964.
6. Abramson DI, Bell Y, Tuck S Jr, et al: Changes in blood flow, oxygen uptake and tissue temperatures produced by therapeutic physical agents: III. Effect of indirect or reflex vasodilatation. Am J Phys Med 40:5, 1961.
7. Abramson DI, Burnett C, Bell Y, et al: Changes in blood flow, oxygen uptake and tissue temperature produced by therapeutic physical agents: I. Effect of ultrasound. Am J Phys Med 39:51, 1960.
8. Aides JH, Klaras T: Use of ultrasonic radiation in the treatment of subdeltoid bursitis with and without calcareous deposits. West J Surg 62:869, 1954.
9. Gersten J: Effect of metallic objects on temperature rises produced in tissues by ultrasound. Am J Phys Med 37:75, 1958.
10. Gersten JW: Effect of ultrasound on tendon extensibility. Am J Phys Med 34:362, 1955.
11. Glazer JL, Brukner P: Plantar fasciitis. Physician Sports Med 32:11, 2004.
12.. Wilson DH: Comparison of shortwave diathermy and pulsed electromagnetic energy in treatment of soft tissue injuries. Physiotherapy 60:309, 1974.
13. Ginsberg AJ: Pulsed shortwave in the treatment of bursitis with calcification. Int Record Med 174:71, 1961.

14. de Lateur BJ, Lehmann JF, Stonebridge JB, et al: Muscle heating in human subjects with 915 MHz microwave contact applicator. Arch Phys Med Rehabil 51:147, 1970.
15. Rae JW Jr, Herrick JF, Wakim KG, Krusen FH: A comparative study of the temperatures produced by microwave and shortwave diathermy. Arch Phys Med 30:199, 1949.
16. de Lateur BJ, Stonebridge JB, Lehmann JF: Fibrous muscular contractures: Treatment with a new direct contact microwave applicator operating at 915 MHz. Arch Phys Med Rehabil 59:488, 1978.
17. Daily L Jr, Wakim KG, Herrick JF, Parkhill EM: The effects of microwave diathermy on the eye. Am J Physiol 155:432, 1948.
18. Miglietta O: Action of cold on spasticity. Am J Phys Med 52:198, 1973.
19. Schaubel HJ: The local use of ice after orthopedic procedures. Am J Surg 72:711, 1946.
20. Ruane JJ: Identifying and injecting myofascial trigger points. Physician Sports Med 29:12, 2001.
21. Waldman SD: Reflex sympathetic dystrophy. In Waldman SD: Common Pain Syndromes. Philadelphia, Saunders, 2002, p.39.

chapter 125

Hydrotherapy

David A. Soto-Quijano and Martin Grabois

Hydrotherapy is the use of a water environment for therapeutic effects. Aquatic rehabilitation or aquatic therapy refers to the combination of healing and rehabilitation modalities in water.[1] The use of the aquatic environment to help in managing pain and increasing function through rehabilitation is rapidly increasing because of the proven physiologic and biodynamic properties of water, which allow the patient with pain to rehabilitate more rapidly and safely.[2] When used in a comprehensive therapeutic approach, aquatic exercises are designed to aid in pain management and rehabilitation of patients with pain. Aquatic therapy not only promotes modification of pain and increases function, but also accomplishes this in a cost-effective environment.

HISTORICAL CONSIDERATIONS

The use of water as a healing medium dates back many centuries, although its original use does not coincide exactly with the present perception of its use for rehabilitation purposes. The original use of water (dating back to 2400 BC) was closely connected to the mystical and religious worship of water and its perceived power of healing.[3] The Greek civilization in 500 BC began to use water more logically for specific physical treatments, and the Romans expanded the bath system. The Romans added a system of baths at various temperatures and used them not only for rest and recreational activities, but also for health and exercise for healing and treating injuries.[4]

By the early Middle Ages, religious influences had led to the decline of the use of water for its healing power because this use was considered a pagan act.[5] During the period 1600-1800, there was a resurgence of water for healing, but not hygienic purposes, and the term *hydrotherapy* started to take hold.[6] Use of hydrotherapy continued to be primarily passive in nature, however. It was about this time that spas, built around a natural spring and usually surrounded by natural beauty, were developed in Europe and then in the United States.[3]

During the early to mid-1900s, the property of buoyancy began to be used to exercise patients in water with the development of the Bad Ragaz technique and Hallwich method in Europe.[3] During the polio epidemics in the early 1900s, medically supervised exercise in water began to gain popularity in the United States.[3] Finnerty and Corbitt[5] related that a young person with poliomyelitis fell from his wheelchair into a pool. While attempting to keep himself afloat, the young man discovered that he could move his paralyzed legs. This movement had not been possible on land. He continued with a pool exercise program to strengthen his lower extremities and was able to progress from being wheelchair-bound to ambulating independently without braces, using only a cane.

Many European rehabilitation facilities continued to maintain some type of aquatic therapy facility, and it continued to be part of the integrated rehabilitation program that was largely publicly funded. This was not the case in the United States.[3] In the United States, through the 1950s and 1960s,[6] there was a decline in the use of this technique as a result of the control of polio, the limited insurance reimbursement, and the lack of education regarding water as a therapeutic exercise medium.

In the 1980s, although the use of hydrotherapy was increasing in the United States, it still lagged behind Europe because of reimbursement issues, lack of evidence-based efficacy studies, accepted treatment protocols, and education of practitioners.[3] This is also true of other therapeutic treatment techniques that have withstood the test of time but lack significant evidence bases of cost-effectiveness and efficacy. Morris[7] pointed out that there is a shortage of efficacy research in aquatic physical therapy and other therapies that address patient outcomes. Currently, aquatic therapy is being increasingly used in the United States. Its continued acceptance as a highly used modality will depend on continued research on cost-effectiveness and efficacy, protocols of treatment, insurance coverage, and education of healthcare personnel.

PRINCIPLES OF HYDROTHERAPY

The practitioner needs to understand numerous principles of hydrotherapy to appreciate its beneficial effect in pain relief and improvement of function and to prescribe hydrotherapy in a safe, comprehensive, and effective rehabilitation program. All aquatic exercise therapy routines must address two important factors: (1) the body's physiologic response to being immersed in water and (2) the physical properties of water.[1] Nearly all of the biologic effects of immersion are related to the fundamental principles of hydrodynamics, including buoyancy, hydrostatic pressure, and temperature.[2]

Buoyancy is explained by the fact that a body submerged in water is supported by a counterforce that supports the submerged object against the downward pull of gravity. The submerged body seems to lose weight equal to the weight of the water displaced, resulting in less stress and pressure on muscle and connective tissue.[8] Patients exercising in water feel lighter, move more easily, and feel less weight on their joints because of this buoyancy property.[9] On land, the center of gravity of a body is just in front of the sacrum at the S2 level. In the water, the center of gravity is located at the level of the lungs. The degree of partial weight bearing varies with pool depth with buoyancy of 90% when immersed up to the neck.[10] Buoyancy can be used in an assistive, resistive, or supportive manner. This force assists any movement toward the surface of the water and resists any movement away from the surface of the water. These three attributes of buoyancy can be enhanced through the use of flotation devices.

Hydrostatic pressure is pressure exerted by water on a submerged body. The pressure is directly proportional to the depth and the density of the fluid.[12] Hydrostatic pressure opposes the tendency of blood to pool in the lower portions of the body, which helps increase venous return to reduce lower extremity swelling and stabilize unstable joints. Because of the property of hydrostatic pressure, patients with chronic obstructive pulmonary disease may have difficulty breathing because the pressure of water resists chest wall expansion at 85% immersion.[2]

Specific heat is the amount of energy necessary to increase the temperature of a substance by 1°C. Because the specific heat of water is several times that of air, heat loss is 25 times that of air at a given temperature.[12] If more heat is lost to water than is produced by muscle, the patient feels cold.[2] Vigorous exercise performed in warm water (33°C [91°F]) results in an increase in core temperature (39.4°C [103°F]) and premature fatigue.[12] The ideal temperature for vigorous exercise is 28°C (82°F) to 30°C (86°F), but more often for patients with pain, who perform less intense exercise, a higher pool temperature is allowed.[2]

Other properties of water to be considered in the use of hydrotherapy are viscosity and refraction. Viscosity is defined as the frictional resistance presented to a body moving through a fluid. Although resistance in air is negligible, in water, several factors can lead to resistance proportional to effort exerted, and this allows for use of water for strengthening. As water temperature increases, however, the viscosity decreases and can be beneficial for stabilizing small weak muscles.[2] Refraction is the deflectors of light as it passes through air into water. It can affect visual feedback and requires appropriate guidance to patients acquiring new skills and coordination of movements.[1]

Table 125–1

Principles of Hydrotherapy

Buoyancy
Hydrostatic pressure
Specific heat
Viscosity
Refraction

Table 125–2

Physiologic Changes During Warm Water Exercise

Increased respiratory rate
Decreased blood pressure
Increased blood supply to muscle
Increased muscle metabolism
Increased superficial circulation
Increased heart rate
Increased amount of blood returned to heart
Increased metabolic rate
Decreased edema of submerged body parts*
Reduced sensitivity of sensory nerve endings
General muscular relaxation

*Owing to the hydrostatic pressure at the water surface, 14.7 psi plus an increase of 0.43 psi for every 1-ft increase in depth.

Physiologic Effects

Many profound physiologic effects are produced by immersion of the human body in water (Table 125–1). Additionally, the physiologic effects experienced by patients immersed in warm water depend on the posture, with the greatest physiologic changes observed in the upright posture.[13] These effects can be a problem in patients with medical conditions that limit responses to these changes. The physiologic responses experienced by the body during warm water immersion are similar to the responses of localized heat application, but less concentrated.[11]

Wilder and colleagues[2] summarized the physiologic effect of immersion in water. The cardiac effects produced through immersion are profound and probably very salutary for overall health and the rehabilitating heart. Prominent among these effects are the increase in stroke volume and cardiac output resulting from immersion. The effects of immersion of the respiratory apparatus and the pulmonary system have been found to increase respiratory effort and work. A program of regular aquatic exercise should produce a significant training effect and increase pulmonary functioning.

The effects on the circulatory system and the autonomic nervous system and the compressive effect of water pressure dramatically alter muscle blood flow, increasing oxygen delivery and metabolic waste product removal. These effects are salutary on healing and normal exercising muscle and ligament structures.

The aquatic environment produces renal system changes that promote removal of metabolic waste products and produce diuresis, lower blood pressure, and assist the body in regulation of sodium and potassium. These effects persist longer than the period of immersion and may have general applicability in the management of some forms of hypertension. They occur in a medium that also produces an increase in relaxation and in pain threshold.[2]

Therapeutic Effects

The various physiologic changes noted during warm water immersion also can offer therapeutic effects in numerous medical conditions, including chronic pain (Table 125–2).

The relaxation response of muscles depends on how comfortable the patient is in the water. The warmth of the therapeutic pool reduces muscular tension and helps prevent restricted joint movement.[13] Warm water also helps patients with pain relax and feel more comfortable and reduces their pain sensitivity. The water provides support for injured limbs, which allows for comfortable positioning without increased pain. The stimulatory effects of warm water promote the relaxation of "tight" spastic muscles, which reduces muscle guarding. During warm water immersion, the sensory inputs are competing with the pain input; as a result, the patient's pain perception is "gated" or blocked out. This reduction in pain is perhaps the most significant advantage of aquatic therapy. Additionally, body parts immersed in water warmer than 35°C (95°F) begin to increase in temperature toward the temperature of the core.[11] This warmth reduces abnormal muscular tone and spasticity.

The physical properties and the warmth of the water play an important role in improving or maintaining joint range of motion. The buoyancy of the water decreases the compression forces on painful joints and assists movement. The water also provides support and decreases the need for splinting or guarding. The warmth of the water reduces spasticity, promotes relaxation, and helps prepare the connective tissue for stretching. Elongated tissue has a lower risk of injury and of muscle soreness after exercise.[13] The water also provides a greater resistance to movement than air, which allows the joint to move more freely. In the water, movements are more consistent and more easily graded using the principles of buoyancy without the pain of active movement. Warm water promotes the relaxation of the spastic antagonists of a weak, exercising muscle. Strength training often can begin in the water before it is possible on land.[11]

Likewise, after injury, a patient can stand and begin gait training and strengthening exercises earlier on water than on land, without being concerned about causing further damage to the healing structures secondary to the reduction of gravitational forces.[15,16] Walking earlier helps improve balance and increase muscle tone. As time goes on, a gradual reduction in the water level can help retrain for the weight-bearing aspect of gait.

Circulation increases in water temperatures greater than 34°C (>93°F). The redistribution of blood during immersion causes an increase in blood flow to the periphery with exercising causes an increase in the blood supply to the muscles and helps in increasing venous return.[11] Exercising injured limbs in deep water further increases circulation, and as water depth increases, so does the hydrostatic pressure exerted on the submerged body part.[11,16] In chest-deep water, there is an increase in the hydrostatic pressure exerted on the walls of the chest and abdominal muscles during breathing. The neutral warmth provided by the water relaxes spastic respiratory muscles. Aquatic activities that require an increase in respiration (e.g., swimming, aerobic exercise) or help train the breathing component (e.g., blowing bubbles) are beneficial to patients who have respiratory problems.[17]

Warm water stimulates awareness of the moving body parts and provides an ideal medium for muscle re-education. The supportive properties of the water give patients with poor balance time to react when falling by slowing the movement. Stabilization during exercise also can be obtained through the use of railings, parallel bars, underwater benches, submerged chairs, tubes, and other devices.[17] Finally, for patients with pain and patients who cannot exercise yet on land, the water provides a positive medium in which to move and relax. The ease of movement allows the patient to achieve much more in water than on land and provides the patient with confidence to aid rehabilitation. There is less fear of falling or of hurting the injured or painful sites.

Table 125–3

Therapeutic Benefits of Warm Water Exercise
Promotes muscular relaxation
Reduces pain sensitivity
Decreases muscle spasm
Increases ease of joint movement
Increases muscular strength and endurance in cases of excessive weakness
Reduces gravitational forces (early ambulation)
Increases peripheral circulation (skin condition)
Improves respiratory muscles
Improves body awareness, balance, and proximal trunk stability
Improves patient morale and confidence (psychological)

TECHNIQUES

As previously stated, hydrotherapy includes any use of water for healing purposes. Under that definition, hydrotherapy includes hot or cold compresses, sitz baths, steam baths, colonic irrigation, douches, enemas, shower carts, swimming, and saunas. This chapter discusses the hydrotherapy techniques most commonly used for pain management: water-based exercise, Hubbard tank, whirlpool baths, and contrast baths.

Water-Based Exercises

Indications

Water-based exercises are becoming popular in the treatment of musculoskeletal ailments. As previously discussed, the properties of water and the physiologic effects of the water on the body allow a patient with pain to exercise in a safe and controlled environment. Water-based exercises potentially can be used in the treatment and rehabilitation of almost any musculoskeletal problem. Aquatic therapy has been used most commonly for knee osteoarthritis, hip osteoarthritis, low back pain, and obesity.

There are different water-based exercise programs for knee, hip, and back pain, depending on the severity, body characteristics, overall health status, and needs of the patient. Each patient needs to be evaluated by the rehabilitation team before prescribing a specific protocol. Similar to regular physical therapies, there are books of aquatic exercises for the different muscle groups and for therapists who specialize in these types of programs.[18]

For the treatment of joint pain, the goal of the aquatic rehabilitation program is to relieve pain, decrease muscle spasm, maintain or restore muscle strength, maintain or restore range of motion, prevent deformities, promote relaxation, and enforce a normal pattern of movement. Despite the rising popularity of this technique for joint pain, scientific studies to validate its efficacy are lacking. A study that compared the effect of gym versus hydrotherapy exercises for patients with knee or hip osteoarthritis showed a similar beneficial effect on physical function in both groups compared with control subjects, although the gym group gained more leg strength.[8] Another study compared hydrotherapy with land treatment in patients with low back pain and found that both groups improved significantly in functional ability and in decreasing pain levels. Overall, there was no significant difference between the two types of treatment.[19] The consensus of therapists involved in musculoskeletal rehabilitation, based on experience with many patients, is that water-based exercises are helpful in the treatment of joint pain and for patients who have severe pain that precludes any other exercise program.

Obesity is a serious health problem that is difficult to treat, especially in chronic pain patients. Aquatic exercise programs have been used with success as a way to increase activity levels in obese patients. There are no good studies to confirm the effect, but the anecdotal data seem promising. Because of all the previously stated characteristics of the aquatic environments, obese patients who cannot safely tolerate exercises on dry land as part of a weight loss program can benefit from an exercise program in water. Studies on normal populations suggest that exercise in water causes less fat decrease than exercise on dry land.[20,21] Aquatic therapy allows obese patients to exercise without stressing their joints or exacerbating their pain, however. The long-term goal in these patients is that when they build tolerance to exercise, they can be transferred to a regular weight loss exercise program at home or in a gym.

Stroke patients comprise another population that is sometimes difficult to enroll in an exercise program because of residual motor deficits. A relatively short program of water-based exercises, three times a week for 8 weeks, proved to be beneficial for the cardiovascular fitness of a group of patients with stroke with mild to moderate residual motor deficits. The experimental group also improved in maximal workload, gait speed, and paretic lower extremity muscle strength.[22]

Water-based exercises also have been used as part of a comprehensive treatment program for pain syndromes. A group of patients with fibromyalgia received group pool exercises once a week for 6 weeks, combined with an educational program. After 6 weeks, the patients showed improvement in symptom severity, walking ability, and quality of life compared with an untreated control group. A follow-up study found that improvements in symptom severity, physical function, and social function were still present 6 and 24 months after completion of the program.[23,24]

Equipment

Water-based exercises can be performed in any standard pool. Large rehabilitation facilities usually have their own indoor temperature-controlled pool accessible to handicapped patients. The depth of the pool at its deepest point should be enough to cover standard-sized patients up to their necks, although that much water is not needed for getting the benefits from the water environment. Other features, such as ramps, grab bars, seats, or underwater treadmills, also can be included. Some facilities and therapy centers use smaller tanks for water-based exercises. These special tanks can include all the features of a larger pool in a smaller space. Some even include an artificial water flow system that allows the patient to swim without the need of a long pool, similar to running on a treadmill. A hydraulic motor produces an adjustable current that is used for resistance.

Special equipment can be used to enhance the effect of water-based exercises. Some aids include floating balls, web gloves, flippers, and flotation devices of different shapes. Delta bells and barbells are made of foam and consequently weightless outside the pool. When used in water their shape creates resistance that is used in exercise programs. An aqua jogging belt allows a running-like motion and is commonly used in sports rehabilitation to keep an athlete fit while protecting weight-bearing joints.

Prescription

As previously stated, a water-based exercise prescription follows a thorough evaluation by the physician and the therapist. Strengthening exercises are prescribed for weak muscles and stretching and mobilization exercises are recommended for stiff joints, muscles, or segments. The exercises in water differ from similar exercises done on land. A complete discussion of the different exercises is beyond the scope of this chapter. Books and manuals are available that describe the different types of exercises and techniques available.[25] Each patient is unique, and it is impossible to recommend a standard program that fits the needs of every patient. Some common aquatic exercises recommended for diskogenic pain[26] are described here.

Water walking forward (Fig. 125–1) helps strengthen abdominal and ambulatory muscles and promotes a proper posture. *Water walking backward* (Fig. 125–2) helps the same muscles, but emphasizes more the paraspinal muscles. The *wall sit* (Fig. 125–3) is used to strengthen quadriceps and hamstring muscles isometrically. The patient is supported by the pool wall in the vertical position while hips and knees are kept at 90 degrees. The *modified superman* (Fig. 125–4) requires the patient to stand vertical and hold the edge of the pool with both hands. One leg is then flexed 45 degrees at the knee. That same leg is extended to 20 degrees at the hip and brought back to neutral repeatedly. To add difficulty, the knee is flexed to 90 degrees, or a weight or resistance is added to the ankle. This movement trains the ipsilateral hip flexor and extensor muscles, contralateral gluteus medius, and all abdominal and paraspinal muscles. *Supine sculling* (Fig. 125–5) is a more complex exercise that requires the use of a flotation jacket, a flotation collar, and direct assistance from a therapist for the patient to maintain a supine position in the water. Upper extremities perform a sculling motion at the hip level, while the lower extremities execute a flutter kick. This is a good overall exercise that strengthens upper and lower extremities and paraspinal muscles. In the *wall crunch* (Fig. 125–6), the patient stands with back against the pool wall and attempts to flex the hip to 90 degrees with the knee flexed while the ipsilateral hand isometrically resists the movement, maintaining an isometric contraction for 5 seconds at a time. This exercise requires the use of the quadriceps, hamstring, gluteal, ipsilateral hip flexor, rotational abdominal, and paraspinal muscles. *Log roll swim* (Fig. 125–7) is another

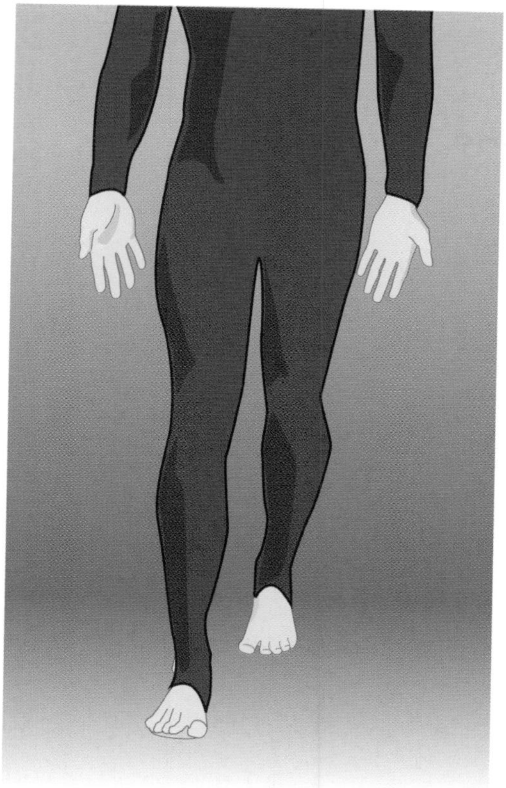

FIGURE 125–1 ■ Water walking forward.

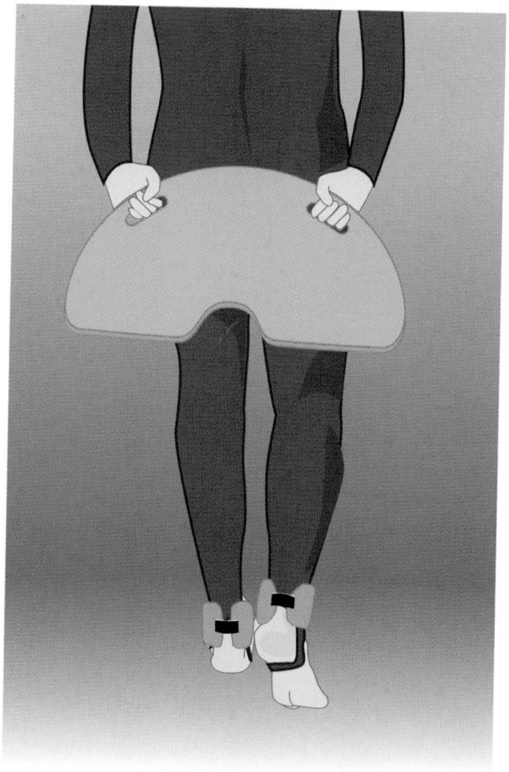

FIGURE 125–2 ■ Water walking backward.

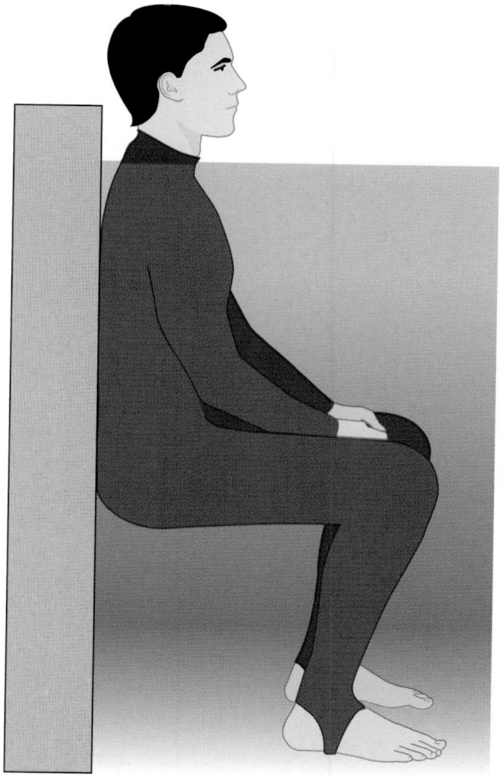

FIGURE 125–3 ■ Wall sit.

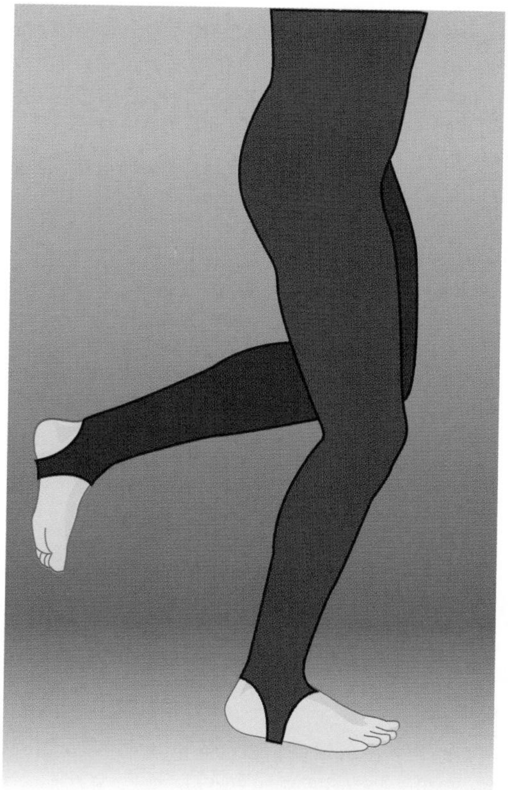

FIGURE 125–4 ■ Modified superman.

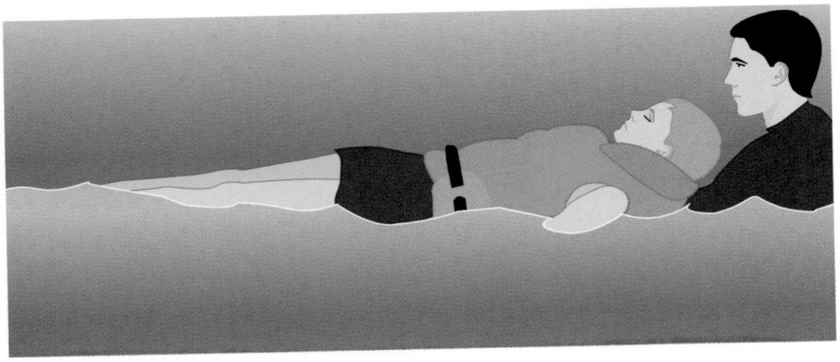

FIGURE 125–5 ■ Supine sculling.

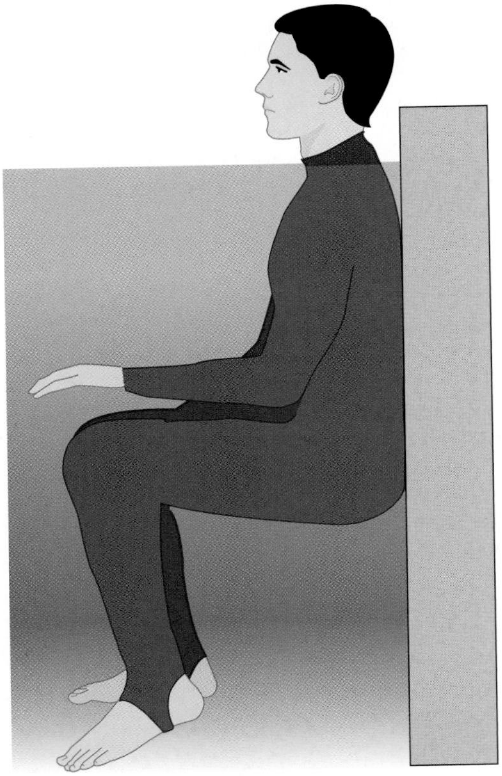

FIGURE 125–6 ■ Wall crunch.

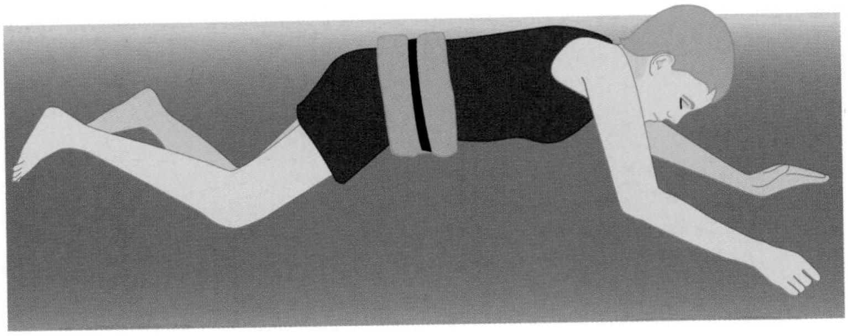

FIGURE 125–7 ■ Log-roll swim.

complex exercise, requiring the use of a mask, a snorkel, a flotation belt, and support from the therapist to keep the body in a prone position. The neck is flexed 20 degrees, knees are flexed 25 degrees, and the patient begins a small rotatory movement of the arms under the chest. With the hips in 25 degrees of flexion, the knees initiate a small flexion-extension propulsion movement. The patient is taught a lateral rocking movement to minimize the segmental stress of the lumbar spine. The whole purpose of the exercise is to promote an appropriate spine movement on ambulation while strengthening upper and lower extremities.

Contraindications

When prescribing water-based exercises, the clinician needs to practice common sense. Under some circumstances, a pool and its surroundings can be a dangerous place. Aquatic therapy should not be ordered for a patient who cannot follow the basic safety rules. Difficult cases always should be discussed with the therapist before the referral. Contraindications for water-based exercises include fear of water, open wounds, bladder or bowel disorders, skin disease, and high fever. Patients with unstable angina, congestive heart failure with symptomatic low ejection fraction, frequent high-grade ectopy, or significant aortic or mitral valve problems should not participate in water programs. A cardiology evaluation and clearance usually is recommended for patients with cardiac conditions.

Whirlpool and Hubbard Tank

Indications

The primary uses of whirlpools and Hubbard tank baths are for adjunctive treatment of degenerative arthritis and acute musculoskeletal injuries and cleansing and débridement of burns or skin ulcerations. Patients with musculoskeletal pain (arthritis, diffuse myalgias, muscle spasm, muscle strains) can benefit from the massage created by water turbulence, the therapeutic effect of water temperature, and the decreased stress on bones and joints that the aquatic environment provides. The massage and heat effects created by the turbulence are helpful for muscle pain and spasm. The agitated water causes a localized and controlled joint movement that is particularly helpful in patients with arthralgias or patients shortly after the removal of a cast. In some cases, the patient also is advised to move the joint actively while receiving the treatment, helping even more to increase the range of motion. Another effect of a whirlpool in musculoskeletal injuries is the resolution of edema and swelling in chronic or acute injuries. The movement and hydrostatic pressure of the water help in the mobilization of fluids.

There also is a relaxation effect of water immersion and a decrease in pain perception. Use of a whirlpool has been mentioned as part of a multi-intervention approach to nonspecific chronic pain patients.[24] A study examined the effects of whirlpool therapy on pain and surgical wound healing in adults having major abdominal surgery. Measures of pain were repeated over a 3-day period. The experimental group response to verbal pain was not significant, but it did reveal an improvement in observable pain behaviors using the Pain Rating Scale. It was concluded that the intervention of whirlpool therapy promoted some degree of comfort and positive signs of wound healing.[27]

Whirlpools and Hubbard tanks are commonly used for wound and burn treatment. The warm, gently agitated water of the whirlpool permits comfortable solvent action and gentle débridement and aids bandage removal. A study of patients with stage III or IV pressure ulcers compared conservative treatment with conservative treatment plus whirlpool 20 minutes per day. Conservative treatment included pressure relief measures and wound care with wet-to-wet dressings using normal saline. When followed up for 2 or more weeks, patients who received whirlpool treatments improved at a significantly faster rate than patients who received the conservative treatment alone.[28]

Equipment

Whirlpool baths and Hubbard tanks possess water pumps or turbines that agitate water and provide connective heating or cooling, massage, and gentle débridement. Whirlpool baths come in different sizes and shapes. Small 120-L tanks are used for treatments to a single extremity or area, whereas big Hubbard tanks are used when the entire body needs to be immersed. These big tanks usually are equipped with a stretcher that may be fitted into an adjustable support bracket. Normally the tank is butterfly-shaped so that the patient can move the extremities through abduction movement if indicated.

Prescription

Whirlpool or Hubbard tank treatments may be given daily or twice daily for acute problems and less often for more chronic problems. The time of treatment is usually 20 to 25 minutes. The water turbulence is directed to the involved area, unless it exacerbates pain. Depending on the affected area, a small whirlpool or a Hubbard tank is recommended. Water temperature is regulated depending on the patient's needs. Temperatures of 33°C (91°F) to 36°C (97°F) are considered neutral. If heat is indicated, water temperature can be increased to 43°C to 46°C in healthy patients receiving localized or single limb treatment. In full body submersion, temperature is limited to 38°C or less if the patient is going to exercise in the tank. Because of the water's constant motion, no insulating layer of cooling water is formed around the patient, and a more vigorous heating is attained. On burns or infected areas, antiseptic conditions are preferred. Although truly sterile conditions are difficult, antibacterial solutions, like sodium hypochlorite or povidone-iodine, may be added to the water. When large wounds or exposed organs are present, sodium chloride should be added to the water to approximate normal saline solution and minimize fluid shift. Cases of severe hyponatremia, hyperkalemia, and prerenal uremia have been described in burn patients after receiving hydrotherapy in tap water.[25]

Contraindications

When using whirlpool or Hubbard tank techniques, extreme temperatures should be avoided in patients with sensory problems, small vessel disease, affected cognition, or inability to communicate. Hot water should not be used in patients with systemic fever or acute inflammatory conditions. Caution should be exercised when using whirlpool with patients with motion sickness because the water movement may cause dizziness.

Epidemiologic studies suggest that the use of a hot tub or whirlpool bath during pregnancy doubles the risk of miscarriage. This risk increases with the frequency of use and use during early gestation. Although there are some groups challenging these findings, this potential complication should be considered when prescribing aquatic therapy to women of childbearing age.[29,30] There is always a chance of drowning in a whirlpool or Hubbank tank. Care should be taken with patients at risk, such as weak patients, cognitively impaired patients, and children.[31]

Contrast Baths

Indications

Contrast baths are indicated for subacute or chronic traumatic and inflammatory conditions and impaired venous circulation and indolent ulcers. Contrast baths also have been used for neuropathic pain, rheumatoid arthritis, chronic pain syndromes, and complex regional pain syndrome. The purpose of this technique is to cause a cyclic vasodilation and vasoconstriction producing neurologic desensitization.[32]

Equipment

Contrast baths use alternate immersion of body parts in baths. Warm water and cold water baths are used, causing alternate dilation and constriction of the local blood vessel. No special equipment is required for this technique. Whirlpool tanks and any other safe water container that can hold water at the required temperatures can be employed.

Prescription

After positioning the patient comfortably, two pails of water of a depth that covers the treated area are prepared. The cold bath is usually 13°C to 18°C (55°F to 65°F), and the hot bath is 38°C to 43°C (100°F to 110°F). The affected area is immersed in the hot bath for about 6 minutes and then in the cold bath for 4 minutes, or at least 1 minute if the patient cannot tolerate it. This process is repeated for about 30 minutes.[26] Similar to in the whirlpool or Hubbard tank, povidone-iodine or sodium hypochlorite can be added to the water to prevent infections.

Contraindications

Contraindications for contrast baths are similar to the contraindications for whirlpools and Hubbard tanks. Extreme temperatures should be avoided in patients with sensory problems, small vessel disease, affected cognition, or inability to communicate. Hot water should not be used in patients with systemic fever or acute inflammatory conditions.

SUMMARY

Hydrotherapy, or use of an aquatic environment for helping to manage pain, has been used since ancient times, and more recently its use has increased again. Reduction of pain and increase in function are accomplished by using the physiologic and biodynamic properties of water. This chapter has presented a basic understanding of hydrotherapy and aquatic exercise. A discussion is presented detailing the use of hydrotherapy since ancient times to the present. The physiologic effects of water are reviewed, including buoyancy, hydrostatic pressure, viscosity, refraction, and specific heat.

The use of water has many physiologic effects. These effects are seen on the cardiopulmonary, circulatory, autonomic, and renal systems. Most appropriate to pain patients is the physiologic and therapeutic effects seen in patients with musculoskeletal pain. The primary therapeutic effects of hydrotherapy are the promotion of muscle relaxation with decreased muscle spasm and increased ease of joint motion. Additionally, decreased pain sensitivity, reduction in gravitational forces, increase in circulation, increase in muscular strength, and improved balance can be helpful in the rehabilitation of patients with chronic pain.

Water-based therapy allows the patient with pain to exercise in a safe and controlled environment and potentially can be used in the treatment and rehabilitation of almost any musculoskeletal problem. Patients who cannot tolerate exercises on dry land can benefit from an exercise program in water. The different water-based exercise programs are prescribed depending on the severity, body characteristics, overall health status, and needs of the patient. Aquatic exercise programs have been used with success in the treatment of hip or knee osteoarthritis, pain syndromes, and back pain. Aquatic exercise also has been proposed for weight loss programs. Scientific studies to validate its efficacy are lacking, however.

Whirlpool and Hubbard tank baths are used for adjunctive treatment of degenerative arthritis and acute musculoskeletal injuries and cleansing and débridement of burns or skin ulcerations. Patients with musculoskeletal pain and spasm can benefit from the massage created by water turbulence, the therapeutic effect of water temperature, and the decreased stress on bones and joints that the aquatic environment provides. It also is useful for resolution of edema and swelling. Antibacterial solutions such as sodium hypochlorite or povidone-iodine may be added to the water when there are concerns about infection. Contrast baths produce neurologic desensitization by alternating heat and cold cyclic vasodilation and vasoconstriction. Contrast baths have been used for subacute or chronic traumatic and inflammatory conditions, impaired venous circulation, indolent ulcers, neuropathic pain, rheumatoid arthritis, chronic pain syndromes, and complex regional pain syndrome.

For patients with pain and patients who cannot exercise on land, the water provides a positive medium in which to move and relax. The ease of movement allows the patient to achieve much more benefit than on land and provides the patient with confidence to aid rehabilitation because there is less fear of falling or of hurting the injured or painful sites.[13]

References

1. Bates A, Hanson N: What is aquatic exercise therapy? Aquatic Exercise Therapy. Philadelphia, WB Saunders, 1996, p 1.
2. Wilder RP, Cole AJ, Becker BE: Aquatic strategies for athletic rehabilitation. In Kibler WB, Herring SA, Press JM (eds): Functional Rehabilitation of Sports and Musculoskeletal Injuries. Gaithersburg, MD, Aspen Publishers, 1998, p 2.
3. Ruoti RG, Morris DM, Cole AJ: Aquatic Rehabilitation. Philadelphia, Lippincott, 1997.
4. Campion MR: Adult Hydrotherapy: A Practical Approach. Oxford, Heinemann Medical Books, 1990.

5. Finnerty GB, Corbitt T: Hydrotherapy. New York, Frederick Ungar Publishing Company, 1960.
6. Wyman JF, Glazer O: Hydrotherapy in Medical Physics I. Chicago, Year Book Medical Publishers, 1944.
7. Morris DM: Is aquatic therapy effective? Aquatic Physical Therapy Report 1:4, 1993.
8. Harrison R, Bulstrode S: Percentage weight bearing during partial immersion in the hydrotherapy pool. Physother Pract 3:60, 1987.
9. Bolton E, Goodwin D: An Introduction to Pool Exercises, 2nd ed. London, E & S Livingstone, 1962.
10. Johnson C: Backstrokes: An Aquatic Rehabilitation Program for People with Back Pain. Haverton, PA, Occupational Therapy Associates, 1989.
11. Skinner AT, Thomson AM: Duffield's Exercise in Water, 3rd ed. London, Bailliere Tindall, 1983.
12. Edlich RF, Towler MA, Goitz RJ, et al: Bioengineering principles of hydrotherapy. J Burn Care Rehabil 8:579, 1987.
13. Bates A, Hanson N: What is aquatic exercise therapy. In: Aquatic Exercise Therapy. Philadelphia, WB Saunders, 1996, pp 294-297.
14. Hall, Bisson D, O'Hare P: The physiology of immersion. Physiotherapy 76:517, 1990.
15. Thomson A, Skinner A, Piercy J: Tidy's Physiotherapy, 12th ed. Toronto, Butterworth-Heinemann, 1991.
16. Duley F: Benefits of aquatic therapy: Part I. American Exercise Association AKWA Newsletter November 1988.
17. Charness A: Physiological and psychological values of pool therapy. Aquatics for the Physically Disabled February 1983.
18. Kiss A: New Techniques in Aqua Therapy. Orlando, Rivercross Publishing, 1999.
19. Sjogren T, Long N, Storay I, Smith J: Group hydrotherapy versus group land-based treatment for chronic low back pain. Physiother Res Int 2:212, 1997.
20. Gwinup G: Weight loss without dietary restriction: Efficacy of different forms of aerobic exercise. Am J Sports Med 15:275, 1982.
21. Kieres J, Plowman S: Effects of swimming and land exercises versus swimming and water exercises on body composition of college students. J Sports Med Phys Fitness 31:189, 1991.
22. Chu KS, Eng JJ, Dawson AS, et al: Water-based trial. Arch Phys Med Rehabil 85:870, 2004.
23. Mannerkorpi K. Ahlmen M, Ekdahl C: Six- and 24-month follow-up of pool exercise therapy and education for patients with fibromyalgia. Scand J Rheumatol 31:306, 2002.
24. Arnoff GM: The use of non-narcotic drugs and other alternative for analgesia as part of a comprehensive pain management program. J Med 13:191, 1982.
25. Said RA, Hussein MM: Severe hyponatraemia in burn patients secondary to hydrotherapy. Burns Incl Therm Inj 13:327, 1987.
26. Foley A, Halbert J, Hewitt T, Crotty M: Does hydrotherapy improve strength and physical function in patients with osteoarthritis—a randomized controlled trial comparing a gym based and a hydrotherapy based strengthening programme. Ann Rheum Dis 62:1162, 2002.
27. Juve Meeker B: Whirlpool therapy on postoperative pain and surgical wound healing. Patient Educ Couns 33:39, 1998.
28. Burke DT, Ho CH, Saucier MA, Stewart G: Effects of hydrotherapy on pressure ulcer healing. Am J Phys Med Rehabil 77:394, 1998.
29. Li DK, Janevic T, Odouli R, Liu L: Hot tub use during pregnancy and the risk of miscarriage. Am J Epidemiol 158:931, 2003.
30. Hertz-Picciott I, Howards PP: Hot tubs and miscarriage—methodological and substantive reasons why the case is weak. Am J Epidemiol 158:938, 2003.
31. Hitosugi M, Kawato H, Matsushima K, et al: Fatal drowning of children in whirlpool baths in Japan. Lancet 361:2248, 2003.
32. Woodmansey A, Collins DH, Ernst MM: Vascular reaction to the contrast bath in health and in RA. Lancet 2:1350, 1932.

chapter 126

Transcutaneous Electrical Nerve Stimulation

Steven D. Waldman

Long before the gate control theory of Melzack and Wall, the use of sensory stimulation as a way to relieve pain had gained widespread acceptance. The modalities of heat and cold, massage, burning, scarification, moxibustion, cupping, and the like were the mainstays of nonpharmacologic pain relief. There are reports from ancient Egypt of the use of electric catfish applied to the area of pain as one means of pain control. One must wonder that given these electric fish could produce a discharge of up to 400 volts whether the patient experienced a miraculous cure just to avoid another treatment.[1]

It was the explanation by Melzack and Wall of how a stimulus could theoretically provide pain relief by modulating or closing a presynaptic gate that allows transmission of pain impulses to the higher centers that finally gave a scientific basis for the use of what heretofore had been highly accepted but largely discounted techniques. It was this impetus that led to renewed interest in the use of electricity as a "counterirritant" or stimulus that could close the gate on pain. The early work by Shealy in dorsal column stimulation spurred a search for less invasive ways to deliver electricity to nerves. One of the results was transcutaneous electrical nerve stimulation (TENS) which was used initially as a noninvasive screening tool to determine if a patient would experience pain relief with implantation of a dorsal column stimulator. The ease of use and noninvasive nature of TENS made it an instant success. It was these same attributes that led to its overuse and, to a certain extent, to its mediocre reputation as a pain relieving modality. This chapter will discuss the scientific rationale behind TENS and provide the clinician with a practical guide to its use.

SCIENTIFIC BASIS OF TENS

As mentioned earlier, the gate control theory was, in essence, the first unified theory of pain. Earlier theories were largely based on the Cartesian view of peripheral nociception carried to the central nervous system could not explain how a peripheral stimulus for counter-irritative techniques (e.g., acupuncture, moxibustion, electric shock, etc.) could produce pain relief. The gate control theory changed everything. For the first time, scientists, psychologists, and physicians were presented with an elegantly simple explanation of how pain could be produced or blocked in the periphery. The theory stated that small fiber afferent stimuli, particularly pain, entering the substantia gelatinosa can be modulated by large-fiber afferent stimuli and descending spinal pathways so that their transmission to ascending spinal pathways is blocked or gated.[2]

It soon became apparent that the gate control theory could not explain many of the clinical observations associated with the use of TENS. Among them, the frequently seen phenomenon of anesthesia persisting hours after stimulation and the delayed onset of analgesia experienced by some patients in pain. The neurophysiologic basis of these clinical observations remains the source of much debate—with alternative explanations such as endorphin or enkephalin release currently the most popular in spite of the fact that TENS analgesia is not reversed by naloxone. This lack of a scientific rationale has not deterred TENS enthusiasts, nor has it been lost on TENS critics, mainly insurance companies trying to avoid paying for this popular pain relieving technique.

INDICATIONS FOR TENS

Practically every known pain syndrome has been treated with TENS due to its ease of use and lack of side effects. The true efficacy of TENS for the painful conditions discussed below is difficult to ascertain because true double-blind placebo-controlled trials are difficult to conduct owing to the patient's ability to perceive whether the TENS unit is delivering stimulation or not. Despite this fact, the following indications fall within the broad category of conditions in which TENS is, at least, worth considering. Table 126–1 summarizes the current clinical applications for TENS.

Acute Pain

TENS has been shown to reduce pain and, in some cases, reduce the need for narcotic analgesics and improve pulmonary function following upper abdominal, thoracic, or orthopedic surgery as well as total hip or knee arthroplasty.[3,4] TENS may also be useful following traumatic rib fracture and

Table 126–1

Clinical Indications for TENS
Acute posttraumatic pain
Acute postoperative pain
Musculoskeletal pain
Peripheral vascular insufficiency
Functional abdominal pain (?)
Neuropathic pain (?)

other acute trauma.[5] Sterile electrodes allow placement of electrodes adjacent to lacerations or surgical incisions theoretically enhancing efficacy.

Musculoskeletal Pain

TENS has been successfully used to reduce pain associated with osteoporosis-induced vertebral compression fractures, arthritis pain, and strains and sprains.[6,7] Anecdotal reports regarding the efficacy of TENS in the management of carpal tunnel syndrome suggest a positive response in some patients who have failed conservative and surgical management of this entrapment neuropathy. The benign nature and flexibility of the modality lend itself to these more chronic pain complaints.

Peripheral Vascular Insufficiency

Early reports suggested that TENS had the ability to not only reduce pain associated with peripheral vascular insufficiency, but to also improve blood flow. Further studies have cast doubt on these claims, although there are many anecdotal reports of improvement in ulcer size and healing with the use of TENS.[8] Given the lack of treatment options for this difficult group of patients, TENS represents a reasonable treatment option if nothing else is working.

Abdominal and Visceral Pain

Most clinicians feel that TENS is not particularly useful in the treatment of chronic abdominal and visceral pain. Some investigators feel that, in spite of less than optimal pain relief, TENS may exert a salutary effect on bowel function and may also improve the obstipation associated with opioid analgesics.[9]

Neuropathic Pain

In general, TENS has been shown to be ineffective in the treatment of most neuropathic pain states. Whether this is due to lack of sensory afferent nerve function to carry the TENS impulses to the spinal cord or due to other changes in the nervous system is unclear. There continue to be anecdotal reports of efficacy in a variety of neuropathic pain states including postherpetic neuralgia and diabetic polyneuropathy.[10]

Behavioral Pain

Beyond the placebo effect, there is very little to recommend TENS in the treatment of pain without an organic basis. Initial patient enthusiasm may be quickly replaced with confounding behavior surrounding the use of TENS in this clinical setting. The use of TENS without a clear clinical indication is in most cases a fruitless endeavor.

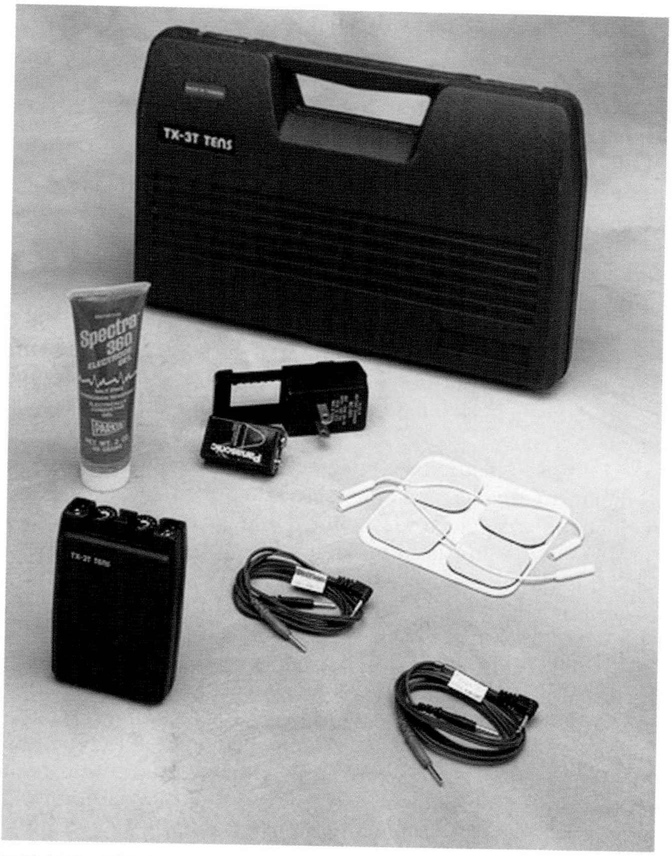

FIGURE 126–1 ■ The transcutaneous electrical nerve stimulation (TENS) apparatus.

■ TENS APPARATUS

The TENS unit consists of a battery-powered pulse generator that is capable of delivering a variety of different pulse characteristics and stimulation frequencies, leads, and a set of electrodes to deliver the stimulus to the affected area (Fig. 126–1). Most investigators prefer a monophasic square wave that is delivered by a pulse generator capable of automatically sensing and compensating for the variation in impedance caused by normal and diseased skin and less than optimal electrode contact. Stimulation frequencies between 30 and 100 Hz are most comfortable for patients. Lower frequencies, which are designed to produce what is thought to be an effect more analogous to acupuncture, are recommended by some clinicians, although many patients find this stimulation frequency too uncomfortable. This discomfort may be decreased by using a pulse generator capable of producing a series of 8 to 10 rapid pulses of a lower-frequency stimulus. Reusable electrodes that require the use of conductive gel and tape have been replaced with disposable pre-gelled self-sticking electrodes.

HOW TO USE TENS

If efficacy is to be achieved, the patient must be thoroughly familiar with the basic operation of the TENS unit and clear on how electrodes are to be placed. Although the placement of electrodes is certainly more of an art than a science, it has been my experience that giving the patient specific parameters for electrode placement works better than telling the patient to experiment with electrode placement. The clinician should generally place the electrodes in the painful area and in most instances place the electrodes within the same dermatome whenever possible. Dual-channel units are currently the norm and allow large painful areas to be treated. A form with an anatomic outline showing where the electrodes should be placed is helpful when instructing the patient on the use of the TENS unit.

Because electricity is involved, it may be useful for the clinician to first demonstrate the TENS unit by having the patient apply the electrodes to the clinician's forearm and then turning on the unit before placing electrodes on the patient. This increases patient confidence and lowers the anxiety regarding getting "shocked."

After proper electrode placement, the patient should be instructed to turn all settings on the pulse generator to zero before turning the unit on. This helps avoid any sudden shock sensation and allows the patient to slowly determine the sensation threshold necessary to feel the first sign of stimulation. In general, a level of 2.5 to 3 times the sensation threshold will be most efficacious for a variety of painful conditions. A stimulus frequency of 90 to 100 Hz is generally a good starting place and the frequency can be adjusted by the patient to comfort and efficacy, thereby giving the patient some control over one portion of his or her treatment. The clinician should demonstrate to the patient what TENS-induced muscle contractions look like and how adjusting the unit can make them stop.

CONTRAINDICATIONS TO TENS

TENS is a remarkably safe treatment modality. Without the risk of thermal injury associated with heat and cold and without the side effects associated with pharmacologic, nerve block, and surgical interventions, it is not surprising that there is a perception among many clinicians and third-party payers that TENS is being over-used. There remains a small group of patients in whom TENS may produce risk (Table 126–2). These include (1) patients with pacemakers; (2) patients with significant sensory impairment (e.g., quadriplegics, due to risk of skin breakdown, patients with implantable drug delivery systems); (3) patients with spinal cord stimulators, and; (4) pregnant patients, due to risk of inducement of labor. Some clinicians caution against placing TENS electrodes near the carotid sinuses or laryngeal nerves, due to the risk of vasovagal syncope and laryngospasm, although this admonition may be more theoretical than real.

Table 126–2

Contraindications to TENS
Patients with pacemakers
Patients with implantable drug delivery systems
Patients with spinal cord stimulators
Patients with significant impairment of sensation
Patients who are pregnant

CONCLUSION

TENS as a pain-relieving modality has appeared to stand the test of time. In spite of the apparent disconnect between the enthusiastic anecdotal clinical reports and lack of demonstrable long-term efficacy of controlled studies, TENS represents a viable alternative for a variety of painful conditions. Given the favorable risk-benefit ratio and cost-benefit ratio of TENS when compared with other pain-relieving options, TENS remains a part of our armamentarium in the treatment of pain.

References

1. Baron VD, Noshnev VM, Olshansky VM, et al: Observations of the electric activity of Silurid catfishes (*Siluriformes*) in Lake Chamo (Ethiopia). J Ichthyol 41:536, 2001.
2. Melzack R, Wall PD: Pain mechanisms: A new theory. Science 150:971, 1965.
3. Benedetti F, Amanzio M, Casadio C, et al: Control of postoperative pain by transcutaneous electrical nerve stimulation after thoracic operations. Ann Thorac Surg 63:773, 1997.
4. Pike PM: Transcutaneous electrical stimulation: Its use in the management of postoperative pain. Anaesthesia 33:165, 1978.
5. Myers RA, Woolf CJ, Mitchell D: Management of acute traumatic pain by peripheral transcutaneous electrical stimulation. S Afr Med J 52:309, 1977.
6. Bushnell MC, Marchand S, Tremblay N, Duncan GH: Electrical stimulation of peripheral and central pathways for the relief of musculoskeletal pain. Can J Physiol Pharmacol 69:697, 1991.
7. Deyo RA, Walsh NE, Martin DC, et al: A controlled trial of transcutaneous electrical nerve stimulation (TENS) and exercise for chronic low back pain. N Engl J Med 322:1627, 1990.
8. Simpson KH, Ward J: A randomized, double-blind, crossover study of the use of transcutaneous spinal electroanalgesia in patients with pain from chronic critical limb ischemia. J Pain Symptom Manage 28:511, 2004.
9. Sylvester K, Kendall GP, Lennard-Jones JE: Treatment of functional abdominal pain by transcutaneous electrical nerve stimulation. Br Med J 293:481, 1986.
10. Cheing GL, Luk ML: Transcutaneous electrical nerve stimulation for neuropathic pain. J Hand Surg [Br] 30:50, 2005.

chapter 127

Exercise and Physical Reconditioning

Donna Bloodworth

When recommending an exercise program or physical therapy to a patient experiencing chronic pain, the health-care professional must establish and disclose realistic and concrete expectations for the patient. A prescription for physical therapy is basically a prescription for strengthening exercise, or endurance exercise, or both. As students of physiology, we know that exercise, performed regularly, may increase strength, muscle bulk, and stamina. Physiologically, the performance of exercise does not directly reduce pain although the literature comments that the performance of exercise modulates pain by a physiologic mechanism that has yet to be fully elucidated. If the patient works with a therapist, the patient will also be more informed about pacing activities, body mechanics, and gauging the need to rest.

HISTORY

The classic physiatrics text, Sidney Licht's *Therapeutic Exercise* provides a detailed history of the therapeutic use of exercise.[1] The oldest, recorded therapeutic use of exercise to relieve pain and other symptoms is the prescription of certain ritualistic positions and motions, Cong Fou, by Taoist priests in China around 1000 BC.[1] In India around 800 BC, exercise and massage were recommended to treat chronic rheumatism.[1] In ancient Greece, three classes of medical practitioners existed: Priest-physicians, philosophers, and gymnasts, who studied the effects of exercise and diet.[1] Similar to practice today, separate from the therapeutic use of exercise, persons who exercised only to win a prize, or *athlon*, were called athletes.[1] The benefits of exercise for weight reduction, improving mental health, the treatment of paralysis and decreasing convalescence were recognized in the time of Hippocrates around 450 BC.[1] Walking, versions of weight lifting, equitation or horseback riding, and movements in water were prescribed for various conditions.[1] Some practitioners recommended exercise for acute conditions such as fever, but debate and dissent existed because other physicians recognized that exercise in acutely ill persons tended to worsen the patient's condition, a recognized fact today.[1]

ACUTE PAIN, ACUTE ILLNESS, AND REST

In distinction to chronic pain, acute pain is usually a sign of tissue injury. Rest, not exercise, has been the traditional initial recommendation. With musculoskeletal injuries, the literature seems to be advocating shorter periods of rest, and earlier introduction of motion, passive or active, depending on the specific diagnosis. However, exercise remains contraindicated for acute cardiopulmonary, febrile, and vascular syndromes.

With sprains, and strains of joints and ligaments, the acronym for the initial activity prescription is RICE: *r*est, *i*ce, *c*ompression, and *e*levation.[2] Kellett explains the duration of this rest and icing phase to be 48 to 72 hours.[2] Thereafter, progressive mobilization, within the limits of pain, is prescribed.[2] More recent work by Green suggests that adding passive range of motion, within the limits of pain, to the RICE treatment of ankle sprains improved ankle range of motion before and after treatment sessions and improved speed of the stride.[3] Acute soft tissue injury should be rested, supported and iced; nonpainful early mobilization is probably beneficial.

Regarding the pervasive condition of low back pain, the benefit of rest is debatable, with a trend toward ever shorter periods of rest or none at all for the condition of acute low back pain. Deyo's article in 1986 showed no difference in clinical outcome for persons who were prescribed 2 versus 7 days of bed rest for acute low back pain.[4] Acute low back pain was defined as that with an onset of less than 30 days and with no neurologic deficits. Persons on 2 days of bed rest were shown to miss fewer days of work.[4] A British article by Wilkinson in 1995 questioned the need for any rest period in persons with acute low back pain of less than 7 days' duration.[5] In this study, 48 hours of strict bed rest was compared to mobility without daytime rest.[5] At 28 days there was no difference between the groups, but at 7 days the mobile group had better disability scores and better, although not significantly, average lumbar flexion.[5] Also in 1995, Finnish researchers found that, in comparison to bed rest or back extension exercises, continuing normal activities after the onset of acute low back pain resulted in more rapid recovery for several end points.[6] These improvements included: time to resolution of pain, pain intensity, lumbar flexion, disability scores, and number of days of work missed.[6] Hagen, searching the Cochrane Musculoskeletal Controlled Trials Register in 2000, deduced that "bed rest compared to advice to stay active will, at best, have small effects, and at worst, might have harmful effects on acute low back pain."[7] Very brief rest or the pursuit of normal nonpainful activities are the evidence-based recommendation after acute low back injury.

Exercise remains contraindicated in severe acute disease states. Exercise is a physiologic stressor and should not be applied to an organism experiencing the physiologic stress of severe acute disease. The American College of Sports Medicine, following the work of Gibbons, has outlined the disease states for which exercise is absolutely or relatively contraindicated (Table 127–1).[8,9] Acute or unstable cardiac, pulmonary, vascular, metabolic, and infectious diseases constitute physiologically stressed states, for which strict bed rest is indicated initially, followed by monitored and assisted mobilization.

INDICATIONS

Physical therapy, or exercise, can be a treatment option for any person with a compensated or treated congenital or acquired, medical or surgical diagnosis that results in functional limitations of mobility or self-care tasks, or vocational or social roles. Examples of diagnoses include spina bifida and cerebral palsy, strokes, arthritis, amputations, and traumatic brain or spinal cord injury. Physical therapy or exercise can also be prescribed for persons with primary goals to increase flexibility or range of motion, or increase strength or stamina and endurance. Prior to prescribing exercise, the physician should confirm that the medical or surgical condition is stable, and the physician should reiterate goals for function, flexibility, strength, or endurance with the patient.

Specific to the diagnosis of chronic pain, physical therapy and exercise probably have more applicability to painful musculoskeletal diagnoses than painful cranial or visceral diagnoses, unless these sufferers are severely deconditioned.

Table 127–1

Contraindications to Exercise

Cardiopulmonary-Vascular

Acute cardiovascular or arrhythmic disease including the symptom of angina
Moderate to severe valve disease including aortic stenosis
Other cardiac dysfunction including myopathy, failure, and pericarditis
Severe peripheral or aortic vascular disease
Severe hypertension
Thromboembolic disease
Acute blood loss

Systemic Diseases

Electrolyte aberrations
Acute infections
Uncontrolled diabetes or other metabolic disease

Neuromusculoskeletal

Conditions with elevated intracranial pressure
Acute fractures
Neuromusculoskeletal conditions worsened by exercise (e.g., multiple sclerosis, myasthenia)
Delirium

TYPES OF EXERCISE, PHYSIOLOGY, ANATOMY

The broad classes of therapeutic exercise include stretching, strengthening, and endurance activities (Table 127–2). Stretching involves the sustained static lengthening of a muscle to increase the flexibility or range of motion of that specific muscle. Strengthening exercise involves the application of weights or resistance to a muscle group for several repetitions of maximal effort in order to increase the force of the muscle. Weight lifting is an example. Endurance exercise involves the application of repeated movements with low resistance to large locomotive muscle groups to increase cardiopulmonary stamina. Examples include jogging and running, "stair stepping," and swimming. Only the application of exercise can directly achieve increased flexibility, increased strength, or increased endurance. Physicians do not prescribe exercise, per se, for the relief of pain—although research outcomes support the ability of exercise participation to modulate pain perception.

Anecdotally, persons who exercise often "feel better." Also, the medical literature documents that the performance of specific exercises results in the relief of pain in certain conditions. Khalil reported that systematic stretching applied to low back pain patients resulted in decreased regional pain.[10] Stretching occurred twice a week and targeted the quadratus lumborum, tensor fascia lata, and hamstring muscles.[10] Lewit reported that contract-relaxation techniques applied to subjects with myalgic pain gave immediate pain relief in 94% of the subjects.[11] Not only does stretching relieve pain in patients with myalgic pain and low back pain, but strengthening exercises may have similar pain-relieving effects in arthritis

Table 127–2

Types of Exercise

Type	*Example*	*Physiologic Result*
Stretching	Yoga, sustained stretch	Increased resting muscle length; increased muscle relaxation; increased tolerance of stretching
Strengthening	Weight lifting	Increased synchrony of muscle fiber firing; increased muscle strength and bulk
Endurance	Swimming, jogging, stair-stepping, cycling	Increased cardiovascular endurance

Table 127–3

Types of Muscle Contraction

Type	*Fixed Property*	*Example*
Isometric	Fixed muscle length	Biceps: Carrying a platter at waist height with the elbows bent
Isotonic	Fixed weight of object lifted	
Concentric		Biceps: Picking up a book by bending the elbow (concentric)
Eccentric		Biceps: Putting a book down by straightening the elbow
Isokinetic	Fixed torque against which contraction is applied	Pushing against a door's hydraulic governor

sufferers. Fisher's summary of the available literature showed that isometric strengthening of the quadriceps reduced pain associated with knee arthritis.[12] Conversely, the presence of weakness, especially in arthritis, has been shown to be associated with increased pain and disability.[13] The mechanism by which strengthening and stretch modulate pain has not been elucidated. The pain-modulating effects of endurance exercises have been postulated. McCain writes that endurance exercise causes predictable increases in serum level of beta-endorphin immunoreactivity.[14] This state of decreased pain sensitivity, called post-run hypoalgesia, is naloxone reversible.[14] Exercise, which has direct cardiac and muscular benefits, effects improvements in pain reporting, possibly through the neurohormonal effects.

Strengthening exercise does result in increased muscle bulk and strength. Muscle contractions can be characterized in three ways, depending on how the length of the muscle changes: isometric, concentric, and eccentric. Three types of strengthening exercises build muscle bulk and force: isometric, isotonic, and isokinetic (Table 127–3).[15]

Isometric contraction and isometric strengthening occur when the length of the muscle is maintained at a fixed length. For example, if a person carries a stack of books to a table, the biceps, triceps, and finger flexors are all at a fixed length, transporting the stack. Isometric strengthening does not have much practicality as an exercise because the muscle is strengthened only at that particular length. Even if more books are added to the stack, thereby increasing the weight, the muscle is only being strengthening at that length, not through full range of motion. A program of isometric strengthening is rarely prescribed and is akin to a person sitting or standing stationary and contracting his muscles. A person might shiver to try to stay warm but the exercise would not have benefit to increase muscle definition or strength. A person in a long leg cast might contract his quadriceps muscle inside the cast, trying to prevent atrophy and maintain some strength. However, strength is not preserved for all lengths of the muscle. Women with compression fractures painful enough to result in a bedfast state can try pressing back the shoulders into the mattress while lying supine to strengthen spinal extensors, and practice the position of optimal posture. Isometric exercise probably has only a limited role in persons with painful movement (e.g., compression fractures) or movement contraindications (e.g., casted long bone fractures).

To review, *isometric* contractions maintain the length of muscle, weight lifted is stable, unless a second party adds more weight. With *isotonic* contractions, the length of the muscle changes and the weight lifted remains constant. Isotonic strengthening involves the remaining two types of muscle contraction: Eccentric and concentric. The muscle shortens and picks up the weight, *concentric* contraction, and then lengthens or puts down the weight, *eccentric* contraction. The act of putting a heavy stack of books on the table causes a controlled lengthening of the biceps; this controlled lengthening is called an eccentric type of isotonic contraction. Often medical and lay persons take for granted the energy-requiring, controllable eccentric contraction; however, if a person put a stack of books on a table without a controlled lengthening contraction, the stack would simply drop down through the atmosphere by the pull of the earth's gravitational field, slamming down on the table. Lay and medical persons alike recognize that they can put down more weight than they can carry, and carry more weight than they can lift. Basic science experiments have demonstrated that eccentric contractions are most forceful, followed by isometric and then concentric contractions.[15] This concept probably has the most applicability in the clinical realm if we postulate that some pain syndromes may arise from imbalance of eccentric and concentric strength. The literature recognizes the imbalance of muscle strength between back extensors and flexors in some back pain syndromes.[16] De Lateur's classic physiatric chapter reminds us that adequate eccentric strength is required for shock absorption.[15] For example, in walking, the calf of the leg in swing phase is slowed down by a controlled lengthening of the hamstrings as the leg is brought forward to contact the floor. In throwing sports, deceleration as opposed to shock absorption is the role of eccentric contraction, and has been studied in the throwing arms of ball pitchers.[17] Isotonic, or variable length-fixed weight contraction has a concentric phase and an eccentric lengthening phase—essential to deceleration, control, and shock absorption.

The last type of strengthening exercise, *isokinetic* contraction, involves shortening or lengthening of a muscle against fixed torque, or fixed rate of rotation. In daily life, one can liken this exercise to pushing closed or pulling open a door attached to a hydraulic governor. No matter how hard one pushes or pulls, the door closes at a fixed rate. In quotidian situations, isometric contractions that occur while carrying things, and concentric and eccentric isotonic contractions that occur while walking or while picking up and placing down objects probably have the most applicability.

The strength of a muscle is proportional to its cross-sectional area.[15] Strengthening exercise, after 3 weeks, increases muscle bulk, or cross-sectional area, and thereby

Table 127–4

Exercise Prescription for Strength and Endurance

Exercise Type	*Examples*	*Prescription*
Strength	Free weight lifting; use of fixed axis weight machines	5 to 10 repetitions of maximally tolerated weight, or of a lesser weight to the point of fatigue; 3 to 5 times per week
Endurance	Biking, jogging, cross-country skiing	20 to 30 minutes, 3 to 5 times per week; to increase heart rate to 70% of age-predicted maximum

increases strength.[15] Strengthening exercise also increases the number of actin and myosin filaments within each myofibril,[18] the number of motor units activated, the rate of activation, and the synchronization of the motor units firing together.[15,19]

The health care professional infers how often and how long to prescribe exercise by understanding what must be done to achieve results. To achieve the results of strengthening, high resistance, low repetition work must be performed to the point of fatigue three to four times per week. DeLateur instructs that adequate weight must be lifted so that the muscle being exercised is "tired" within three to ten repetitions.[15] Weight training for 10 weeks increases muscle strength by 40%.[20] Physical therapy for the goal of strengthening should be prescribed three times per week for 3 to 6 weeks (Table 127–4). Persons who are disciplined exercisers may be given "homework" to do and do not need to come in frequently as long as they have access to strengthening equipment and to a person qualified to "spot" assist with heavier weights. Strength training involves lifting and replacing a heavy weight through several repetitions until the point of fatigue.

Endurance exercise involves no added resistance and maximizes repetitions. Endurance training is the opposite conceptually from strength or weight training. The various forms of human locomotion provide examples of endurance activities: walking, jogging, running, climbing stairs, swimming, and cycling. Endurance activities to build cardiopulmonary stamina must be done, not surprisingly, over a prolonged time period and with adequate vigor. When prescribing endurance exercise, the health care professional asks the patient to exercise vigorously enough to increase heart rate to around 70% of an age-predicted maximum, and then to maintain that intensity of exercise for 20 to 30 minutes (see Table 127–4).[21] The patient's age-predicted maximum heart rate is: 220 minus the patient's age. Multiplying by 0.70 gives the target heart rate for the exercise session. Endurance exercise involves vigorous participation in a jogging or a similar activity for 20 to 30 minutes, three to four times per week.

Participation in an endurance exercise program yields muscular physiologic benefits including increased aerobic capacity, or maximal oxygen uptake, increase in the number and size of muscle mitochondria, increased mitochondrial enzyme activity, and improved efficiency of blood flow shunting to muscles.[22] Physiologic cardiac benefits include increased stroke volume, expanded blood volume, decreased resting heart rate, and decreased resting blood pressure.[22]

Strengthening and endurance exercise have different performance requirements and result in different physiologic effects on muscle and on the cardiovascular systems. Strengthening is a high resistance, low repetition activity whereas endurance is a low resistance but repetitive and vigorous activity. Both need to be done regularly three or more times per week to attain physiologic goals of the exercise.

TECHNIQUES

Preliminary Discussions

Often a patient will respond in one or two predictable ways when exercise is broached as an adjunctive treatment for pain. The patient may respond that he or she gets plenty of exercise "doing his/her normal routine." This type of activity does not condition or strengthen, it simply fatigues. The literature states that mundane activity does not result in adequate flexibility, strength, endurance, or bone density.[21,23] Alternatively the patient may respond that he has already participated in therapy. If this is the case, the physician should explore what exercises were performed and for what duration to assess the adequacy of the program. The patient may express fear that activity will hurt. The physician should not patronize the patient but acknowledge and discuss the patient's concern because exercise can cause discomfort. The literature is mixed. One study showed that, immediately after exercise, patients with knee osteoarthritis have significantly elevated pain, but at 24 hours, pain is significantly lower than after exercise.[24] Another study of arthritis patients and nonarthritic peers reported exercise-related pain in only 2 of the 105 study subjects.[25] Over the 6-month course of the study, fluctuations in reported pain did not differ significantly among experimental exercise groups and nonexercising control groups.[25] The patient should be reassured that pain associated with exercise is transient. Probably specific exercises that reproduce the patient's pain syndrome should be avoided. One of the goals of physical therapy for sciatica is the "centralization" of pain; the "centralization" of pain is practicing positions and performing exercises that move the sciatic pain out of the leg up toward the back. Exercises that increase sciatic pain are avoided. For some conditions, exercise prescriptions need to include work on the strength, endurance, and mechanics of other areas. Reflex sympathetic dystrophy, with its odd associated motor disturbances, provides an example. It is important in these persons not only to restore function of the affected distal limb, but also to maintain function and range of motion in more proximal joints and structures, such as the elbow, shoulder, chest and neck, or knee, hip, lumbosacral spine, and pelvis.

When broaching the subject of exercise in the treatment of chronic pain, remember that mundane activity neither conditions nor strengthens, and that earlier therapy attempts may have been inadequate. It is important to acknowledge that exercise can, in fact, be uncomfortable; however, that sensation has been shown to be temporary. Additionally, the patient should be advised and encouraged to discuss with the therapist not only the exercises that exactly reproduce the pain symptomatology but also the exercises that relieve part or all of the symptomatology.

The patient and doctor, after discussing and agreeing on what the goals of an exercise program are, must elect to exercise in the community on one's own or under the supervision of a therapist. The disciplined patient who has exercised in the past to achieve a goal may not require a therapist and may do well with handout literature and verbal instructions about exercise. The efficacy of a handout information and of verbal instruction from the physician has been evaluated for acute low back pain. Little's group showed that in the first week, supplying the acute back pain sufferer with either a back care book or with specific instruction in exercise improved pain and function.[26] This group was compared to persons told only to mobilize generally and use simple analgesia.[26] The therapist, however, can be invaluable to effect compliance in the less disciplined patient, and they also can help the patient modify exercise techniques to increase efficacy and adjust patient posture to lessen discomfort. The UCLA Low Back Pain study showed that, at 6 months, patients who had physical therapy along with medical intervention had less disability than patients treated with medical or chiropractic intervention alone.[27] A physician who wants to learn about therapeutic exercise may make a sound time investment—spending several mornings or afternoons with a busy therapist.

PRESCRIPTION WRITING

In order to communicate with the therapist, the physician will generate a script, which should include patient identifiers and date, and also the specifics of the exercise prescription. Exercise can affect flexibility, strength, and endurance. Additionally the therapist may educate the patient in body mechanics, or joint conservation, apply thermal or electrical modalities, or instruct the patient in the use of an assistive device, cane, or brace. Collectively, these are the six basic headings of an outpatient therapy script: stretching (flexibility and range of motion), strengthening exercise, endurance exercise, education (joint and back conservation), assistive devices, and modalities (heat and cold packs, ultrasound, iontophoresis, transcutaneous electrical nerve stimulation [TENS]) (Fig. 127–1). The discipline of physical therapy focuses on mobility needs and strength of the spine and lower limbs, and often of the neck and shoulder. The discipline of occupational therapy focuses on the function, strength, and dexterity of the hand, and on the achievement of activity of daily living (ADL) tasks. Depending on the facility, occupational therapists may also work on strength and flexibility of the upper limb and shoulder and neck.

The literature does describe some specific exercise routines for various diagnoses seen in the setting of chronic pain. The literature describes strength and endurance benefits as well as benefits for pain and function of exercise programs applied to persons with many diagnoses. The diagnoses of osteoarthritis, fibromyalgia, axial and radiating back pain, compression fracture, and neck pain are discussed.

HIP AND KNEE ARTHRITIS

Endurance and strengthening exercises have been prescribed for hip and knee osteoarthritis and have been studied in the literature. Quadriceps weakness is known to correlate with the presence of arthritis, and with greater pain and disability, but not with progression of the disease.[13] Both endurance and strengthening programs improve pain and function when prescribed for persons with hip or knee arthritis. Additionally, participation in endurance activities has been shown to decrease depressive symptomatology in this patient group.[13] As discussed, transient increases in pain due to exercise occur and the likelihood of injury as a result of exercise participation is very small.[13] One of the most fundamental exercises in a knee arthritis physical therapy program is the quad set, in

Name: ______________________________	Date: ______________
☐ Physical Therapy (mobility, leg strength and flexibility, spinal strength and flexibility) (Shoulder and neck flexibility and strength) ☐ Occupational Therapy (dexterity, strength, and range of hand, ADLs, upper limb strength and range of motion)	
STRETCH:	ASSISTIVE DEVICE/BRACE:
STRENGTH:	EDUCATION/CONSERVATION:
ENDURANCE:	MODALITIES:
______________________________ Signature line	

FIGURE 127–1 ■ Sample outpatient physical or occupational therapy script.

which the patient lies or sits with the affected knee extended and the shank supported, and isometrically contracts the quadriceps muscle. This exercise has been shown to reduce pain and improve function (Fig. 127–2).[28] Straight leg raises, quadriceps and gluteal strengthening, hamstring stretches, joint conservation instruction and cycling or water aerobics can be added to the script, as well as gait training with a cane (Fig. 127–3).

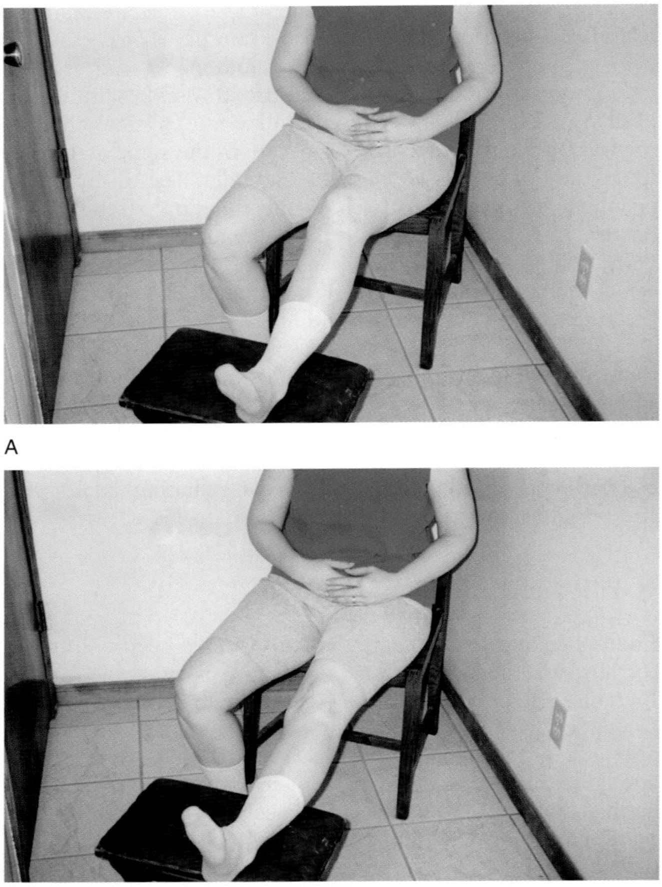

A

B

FIGURE 127–2 ■ "Quad" set. The patient sits with the leg extended (**A**) and "hardens" or contracts the quadriceps muscle (**B**). It is helpful to tell the patient to imagine pressing a sponge with the back of the knee.

■ FIBROMYALGIA

For the treatment of primary fibromyalgia syndrome, the literature has not demonstrated the significant ability of an endurance exercise program to reduce pain in this patient group, but exercise participation in moderate to vigorous aerobic activity does decrease pain thresholds in tender points, and variably improves cardiovascular fitness.[29-32] Improvements in sleep and "number of good days" have been variable, but improvements in pain, anxiety, depression, and self-efficacy have been absent or at best trends.[29,30,33] Examples of previously tested regimens have consisted of cycling 60 minutes three times per week and the other involved walking to increase heart rate to 60 percent of age-predicted maximum three times a week for 8 weeks.[29,30] A recent study by Schachter evaluated whether dividing a 30-minute exercise session into two daily 15-minute sessions improved compliance with exercise; however, dropout rate was increased 33% in the twice-daily exercise group.[33] In this particular study, patients watched a low-impact aerobic exercise video and slowly increased the intensity of the aerobic session over ensuing weeks.[33] Initial target heart rates were 40% to 50% of age-predicted maximum and by 16 weeks were 65% to 75% of age-predicted maximum.[33] Among the twice-daily exercisers who completed the study, their disease severity and self-efficacy scores improved by the end of 16 weeks.[33] The once-daily exercisers showed improvement in pain, physical function, self-efficacy, and disease severity at the midpoint of the study but not at the completion of the study when exercise participation of this group had noticeably declined.[33] The authors questioned whether observing a low-impact aerobic video was the most effective exercise intervention for sufferers of this syndrome, and whether some other aerobic program would have improved the dropout rate.[33] The burden of endurance exercising more than once per day is probably not practicable and the session probably needs to last less than 30 minutes, and closer to 20 minutes (Fig. 127–4). A variety of endurance-type activities may need

Name:____________________	Date:__________
☐ Physical Therapy (mobility, leg strength and flexibility, spinal strength and flexibility)	
STRETCH: Hamstrings	ASSISTIVE DEVICE/BRACE: Gait with cane
STRENGTH: Quadriceps, Gluteals, calves	EDUCATION/CONSERVATION: Joint conservation
ENDURANCE: cycling or water therapy	MODALITIES:
____________________ Signature line	
Evidence-based Goals: Increased flexibility, strength, stamina, decreased pain, decreased disability and decreased depression	

FIGURE 127–3 ■ Sample outpatient physical therapy script for osteoarthritis.

Name:________________	Date:________________
☐ Physical Therapy (mobility, leg strength and flexibility, spinal strength and flexibility)	
STRETCH: Generalized flexibility (control group in McCain's study)	ASSISTIVE DEVICE/BRACE:
STRENGTH: Progressive upper and lower limb strengthening	EDUCATION/CONSERVATION: Pacing, stress management
ENDURANCE: Cycling, water therapy, low-impact aerobic video, walking; target heart rate 40 to 60% age-predicted maximum for 20 to 30 minutes once per day 3 to 4 times per week	MODALITIES:
________________ Signature line	
Evidence-Based Goals: Limited improvements in cardiovascular fitness, tenderness, sleep, self efficacy; questionable improvements in pain	

FIGURE 127–4 ■ Sample outpatient physical therapy script for fibromyalgia.

to be tried before the patient identifies an activity that he can perform regularly.

In contrast to the equivocal results with endurance exercise, work by Geel supported the effectiveness of progressive strengthening exercises in fibromyalgia. Pain and disordered sleep scores, severity of symptoms, and scores of psychological distress all significantly decreased. The subjects exercised twice a week for 8 weeks, starting at 60% of a one-repetition maximum lift, and doing 3 sets of 10 repetitions; upper and lower limbs appeared to have been strengthened.[34]

NONRADIATING AND MYALGIC LOW BACK PAIN

Axial low back pain includes diagnoses of muscular, tendinous, articular, and bony origin. Medical professionals are often under the impression that persons with this diagnosis are less active than persons without the complaint. Recent literature suggests otherwise. Work by Wittink showed that persons with low back pain were not less aerobically fit than persons not complaining of back pain.[35] Verbunt looked at the physical activity in the daily life of persons with low back pain and did not confirm that low back pain sufferers were less active than pain-free controls.[36] These findings suggest that health care personnel should probably avoid pejorative lectures to patients about lack of activity and focus education on meaningful activity to improve the patient's complaint.

The benefit of education in the treatment of low back pain has been supported by the literature. Sikorski prospectively studied 142 patients with acute and chronic low back pain, and showed that patients with chronic low back pain judged education to be the most valuable followed closely by exercise. Both interventions were more useful than manipulation, medication, or bracing.[37]

Studies show the benefit of stretching activity to reduce pain in back pain patients. Khalil, studying patients with myofascial low back pain, showed that stretching plus a multimodality rehabilitation program, compared with only the rehabilitation program, yielded improved measures of muscle function and significantly lowered pain after 2 weeks.[10] Stretch can be added to education and exercise as effective measures to decrease some types of low back pain.

Back braces have not been shown to prevent low back pain or increase lifting or lumbar strength.[30-40] The use of back braces along with education, compared with education alone, leads to less time lost from work for employees who become injured.[41] When patients ask questions about the benefits of bracing, the literature suggests that the expectations for these devices should be low. When a back brace is prescribed, education should also be administered.

The strengthening exercise not only improves strength but also reduces pain. Takemasa's work showed that patients with low back pain had weaker truncal flexors and extensors than normal controls; additionally, extensor muscles in persons with back pain were disproportionately weaker.[16] Patients with back pain and no identifiable lesion (herniated disk, spondylolisthesis, or spondylolysis) who exercised daily for 3 months showed improved strength and reported decreased pain.[16] Several studies have shown that exercise whether flexion biased (with sit-ups and pelvic tilts, Fig. 127–5) or extension biased (with press-ups, Fig. 127–6) improves back pain over only modality-treated groups or no treatment groups.[42,43] The efficacy of aerobic training for 60 minutes twice a week to reduce pain significantly was shown in work by Oldervoll.[44] Oldervoll studied hospital workers with chronic neck, shoulder, and back pain, and compared the efficacy of aerobic training or strength training also done twice a week for 60 minutes against a control group who was not exercised.[44] Maximal aerobic capacity tended to increase

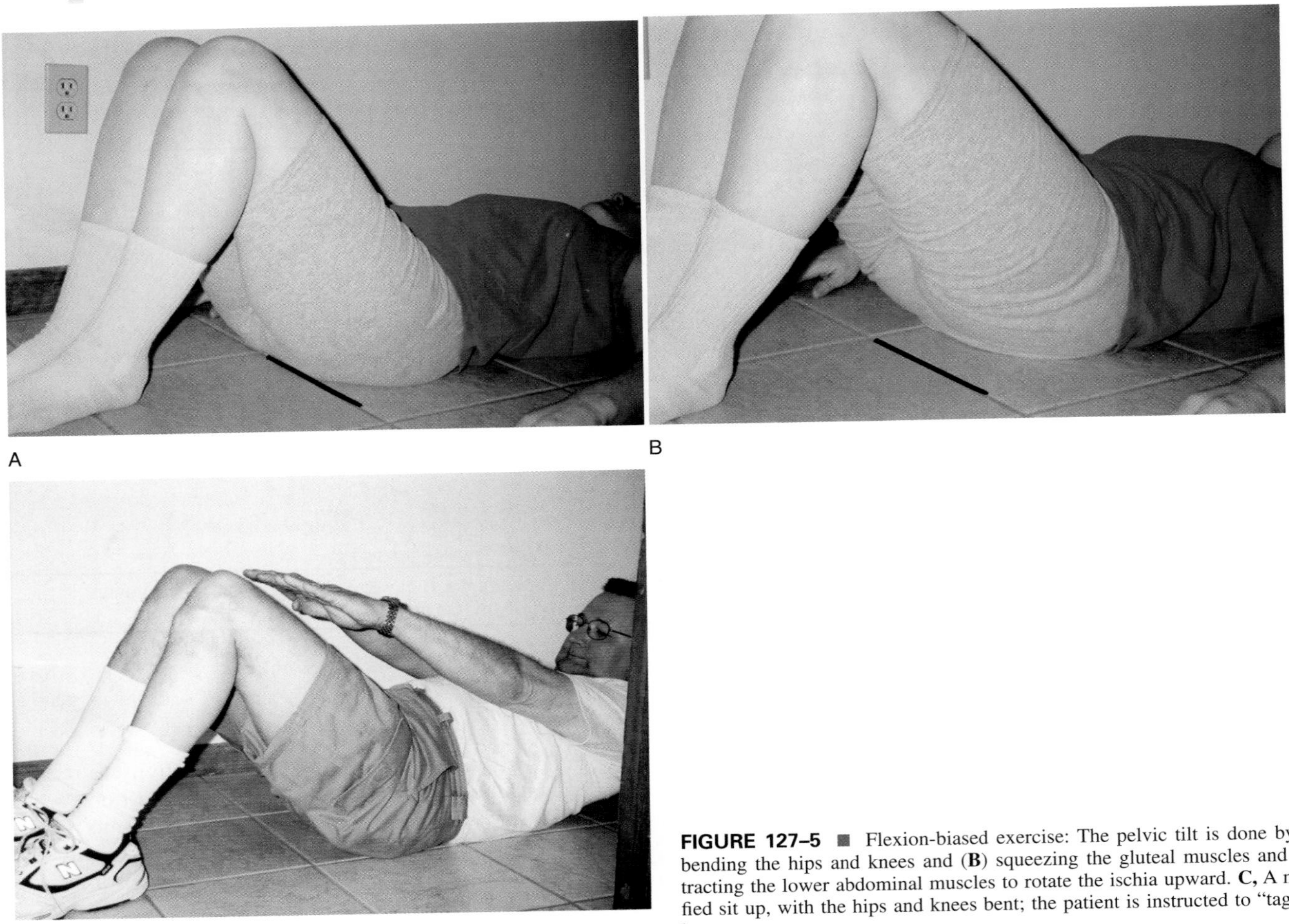

A B C

FIGURE 127–5 ■ Flexion-biased exercise: The pelvic tilt is done by (**A**) bending the hips and knees and (**B**) squeezing the gluteal muscles and contracting the lower abdominal muscles to rotate the ischia upward. **C,** A modified sit up, with the hips and knees bent; the patient is instructed to "tag" the knees.

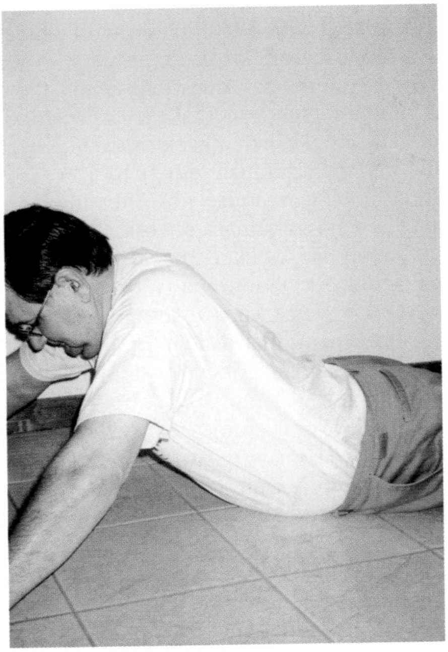

FIGURE 127–6 ■ Extension biased exercise—the press-up. The patient lies prone and presses up on the arms, holding this position while contracting the back muscles.

in both exercise groups but not significantly; in the control group it tended to decrease. Reported pain in both exercise groups decreased significantly, but in the control group pain decreased only minimally.[44] Stretch, flexion, or extension bias strengthening, and aerobic conditioning are all components of an exercise program to relieve nonradiating back pain (Fig. 127–7).

Although strengthening exercise has been shown to help resolve low back pain, the performance of abdominal strengthening has not been shown to prevent the occurrence of low back pain. Similar to the prophylactic use of back braces, abdominal strengthening programs have not been shown to prevent onset of back pain. An exercise group was compared to a nonexercise group for 6 months. Both groups had similar incidences of low back pain, but problems with the study included questions of compliance with exercise regimen.[45]

SPONDYLOLISTHESIS

Specific lumbar pathologies have more specific exercise treatments. Spondylolisthesis treated with flexion-biased truncal strengthening achieves pain reduction as a primary end point. Sinaki retrospectively studied the conservative treatment of spondylolisthesis. After 3 months of flexion-

Name:	Date:
☐ Physical Therapy (mobility, leg strength and flexibility, spinal strength and flexibility)	
STRETCH: Generalized flexibility	ASSISTIVE DEVICE/BRACE: Prescribe only with coincident education
STRENGTH: Abdominal and/or lumbar strengthening, strengthening of arms and legs to promote back conservation	EDUCATION/CONSERVATION: Back conservation
ENDURANCE: Endurance activity 60 minutes twice per week	MODALITIES:
Signature line	
Evidence-based Goals: Limited improvements in cardiovascular fitness, decreased pain after onset; pain may not be prevented by exercise; back bracing used prior to injury with education may decrease lost work days.	

FIGURE 127–7 ■ Sample outpatient physical therapy script for nonradiating low back pain.

biased exercise, only 27% of patients had severe pain; however, 67% of patients treated with extension-biased exercise continued to have pain. For patients with spondylolisthesis, the physician prescribes a lumbar flexion strengthening program.[46]

SCIATICA

Sciatica, or radiating leg pain, due to herniated disk can be treated effectively with an exercise regimen called dynamic lumbar stabilization. Saal and Saal studied a cohort of 64 patients with herniated lumbar disks, sciatic pain, positive electromyograms, and positive straight leg raises. Patients with stable leg weakness could participate in the exercise program. The patient worked with a therapist to find a lumbar-pelvic position that "centralized" or diminished the patient's leg pain. Thereafter, the patient worked on pelvic tilt exercises to hold that "pain-centralized" position. Eighty-five percent of patients had good to excellent relief of pain and 92% of patients returned to work. Only six patients with coexistent foraminal stenosis required surgery.[47]

EXERCISE AFTER DISCECTOMY

Regarding the subset of sciatic patients who had lumbar disk surgery, either standard diskectomy or microdiskectomy, Ostelo reviewed randomized controlled trials of postoperative exercise regimens. His group concluded that there is no evidence that patients should have activities restricted after first time lumbar surgery. Additionally, they found strong evidence that intensive exercise programs started 4 to 6 weeks after surgery led to improved functional status and faster return to work in the short term. At longer follow-up there was no difference between intensive and mild exercise groups. The intensive exercise group did not have a higher repeat surgery rate.[48]

OSTEOPOROSIS AND COMPRESSION FRACTURE

For the condition of osteoporosis and compression fractures an extension-biased strengthening of the thoracic spine and shoulder retracting muscles is recommended. Extension-biased programs, compared to flexion-biased ones, decreased fracture rate and decreased pain.[49] An added benefit of endurance type exercise is increase in bone mineral density.[50-52] In these studies, patients walked 5 miles per week, or 30 to 60 minutes three to five time per week, or jogged or stair-climbed.[51-53] A combination of endurance exercise, including brisk walking, three to five times per week and extension-biased thoracic (Fig. 127–8) and spinal strengthening prevent compression fractures and increase bone mineral density (Fig. 127–9).

CERVICALGIA

Neck pain can be treated with a stabilization program akin to lumbar stabilization. Sweeney reviews the treatment of neck pain by cervicothoracic stabilization training.[54] The author notes the need to correct the "spectator" or "craned neck" posture with the chin thrust forward, and the head carried anterior to the plane of the spine and shoulders (Fig. 127–10).[54] A chin-tucked position is taught, which reduces compression of the facets and stress on ligamentous structures. The position can be practiced lying flat on the floor or standing against a wall (Fig. 127–11). The head and shoulders should touch the planar surface, and then without lifting the head, the chin should be rotated down toward the sternoclavicular notch.

COMPLICATIONS

Except in the acute, unstable, or untreated cardiopulmonary and metabolic conditions already discussed, participation in

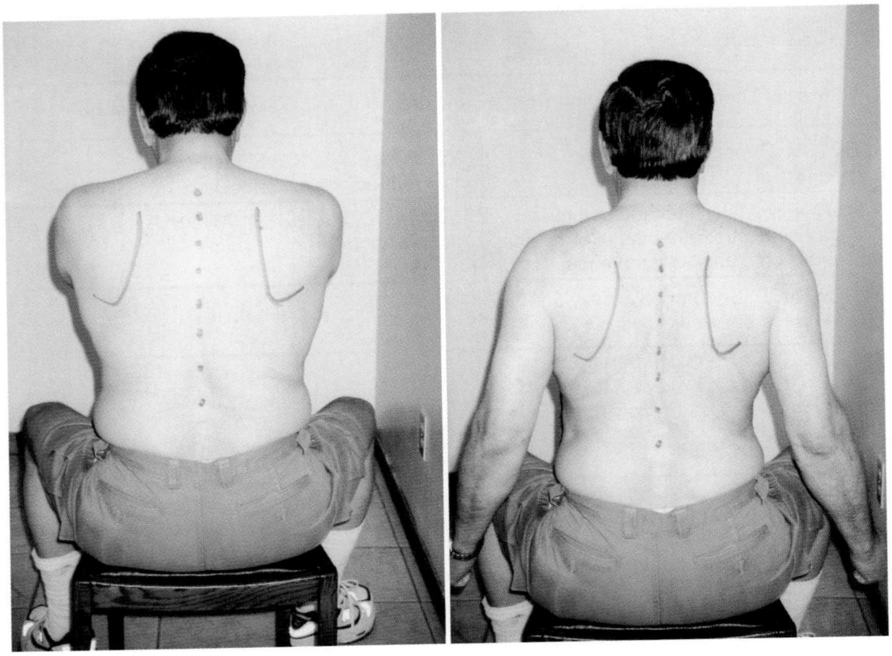

A B

FIGURE 127–8 ■ Thoracic extension exercises: Shoulder retractions can be accomplished isometrically lying supine or isotonically sitting (**A**) or standing; The patient is instructed to pull the shoulder back and down. The subject should feel the shoulder blades move toward each other and down (**B**).

Name:______________________	Date:______________
☐ Physical Therapy (mobility, leg strength and flexibility, spinal strength and flexibility)	
STRETCH:	ASSISTIVE DEVICE/BRACE: Braces to block flexion if severe pain
STRENGTH: Thoracic extension and shoulder retraction exercises	EDUCATION/CONSERVATION: Back conservation
ENDURANCE: Jogging, walking 30 to 60 minutes 3 to 5 times per week	MODALITIES:
______________________ Signature line	
Evidence-based Goals: Decreased fracture rate, decreased pain, increased bone mineral density	

FIGURE 127–9 ■ Sample outpatient physical therapy script for osteoporosis.

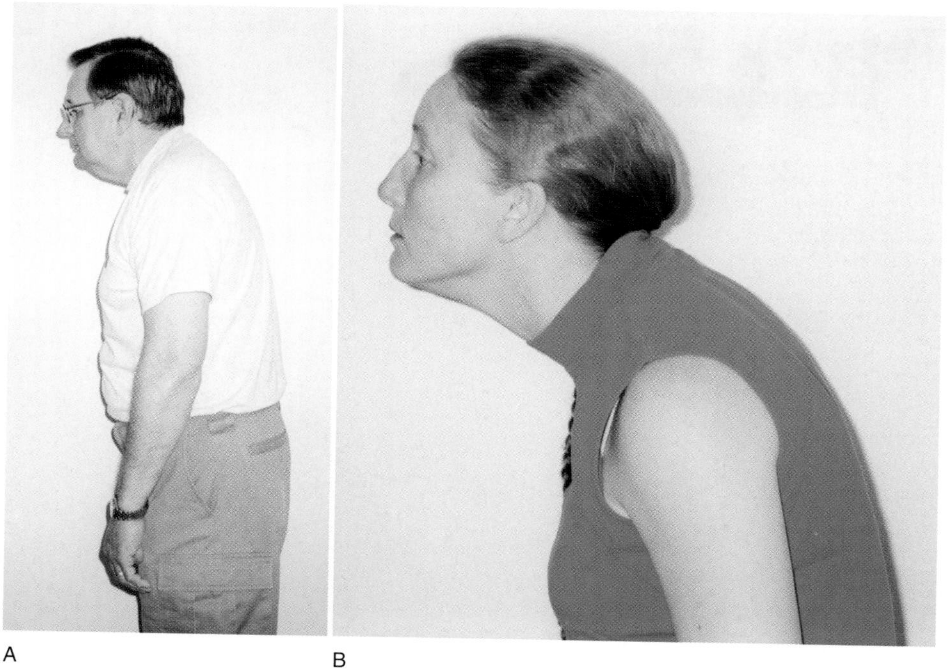

FIGURE 127–10 ■ Craned-neck position. The head is thrust forward beyond the shoulders and center of gravity (**A**). There is upper thoracic kyphosis and exaggerated cervical lordosis (**B**).

exercise can be undertaken without much risk of harm. Range of motion and exercise are also contraindicated with acute fractures; after casting, or internal fixation—the most conservative course of action entails allowing the attending orthopedic surgeon to prescribe activity and exercise.

Before prescribing a moderately vigorous endurance exercise program, for example, brisk walking at 3 to 4 miles per hour, persons at high risk for cardiac disease and some moderate-risk persons first should take an exercise treadmill test.[55] These recommendations come from the American College of Sports Medicine, and they define moderate cardiac risk as men older than 45 years of age or women older than 55 years with two or more risk factors for cardiac disease.[55] Risk factors are well known and include smoking, diabetes, elevated cholesterol, hypertension, inactivity, and strong family history.[55]

In elderly knee arthritis patients who were participating in strength or endurance training, the rate of injury was 2.2 injuries in 1000 exercise hours.[25] The injuries that occurred were considered minor musculoskeletal injuries or exacerbations of previous conditions; no major orthopedic or cardiac events occurred. Reviewing the literature about exercise treatments of knee arthritis, Bischoff cited another study in which two fractures occurred: one due to a falling dumbbell, and the second due to a trip and fall. Studies of moderate distance runners have shown that regular jogging activity does not exacerbate knee arthritis radiographically or clinically.[56] Additionally joint fluid studies of elderly persons participating in 12 weeks of exercise demonstrated no change in the markers of adverse cartilage metabolism.[57] Anecdotally in 14 years of practice, fractures have been rare: one per 5 years and in patients with marked risk factors for osteoporosis. Occurrences of burns have also been rare: One per 7 years. One patient was laid on a hot pack, which is not recommended procedure, and another patient with decreased sensation burned her finger tips on the bottom of a paraffin unit. The use of thermal modalities with altered sensation is strongly contraindicated. One patient reported having a heart attack some time after the completion of a therapy session but the time course and causality were unclear. Patients may trip over hazards on the floor, and meticulous care is needed to keep a tidy work area. Also the therapy gym is no place for unattended children, who may injure themselves on hot or heavy equipment, or create hazards for other patients.

In sum, stretch, strengthening, and endurance activity are activities that may not only build flexibility, strength, and stamina, but may also reduce pain. The type of exercise prescribed is dependent on the specific diagnosis. Activity can be undertaken safely in a tidy gym for persons with stable conditions after any indicated cardiac screening. Acutely ill or fractured persons should not be exercised.

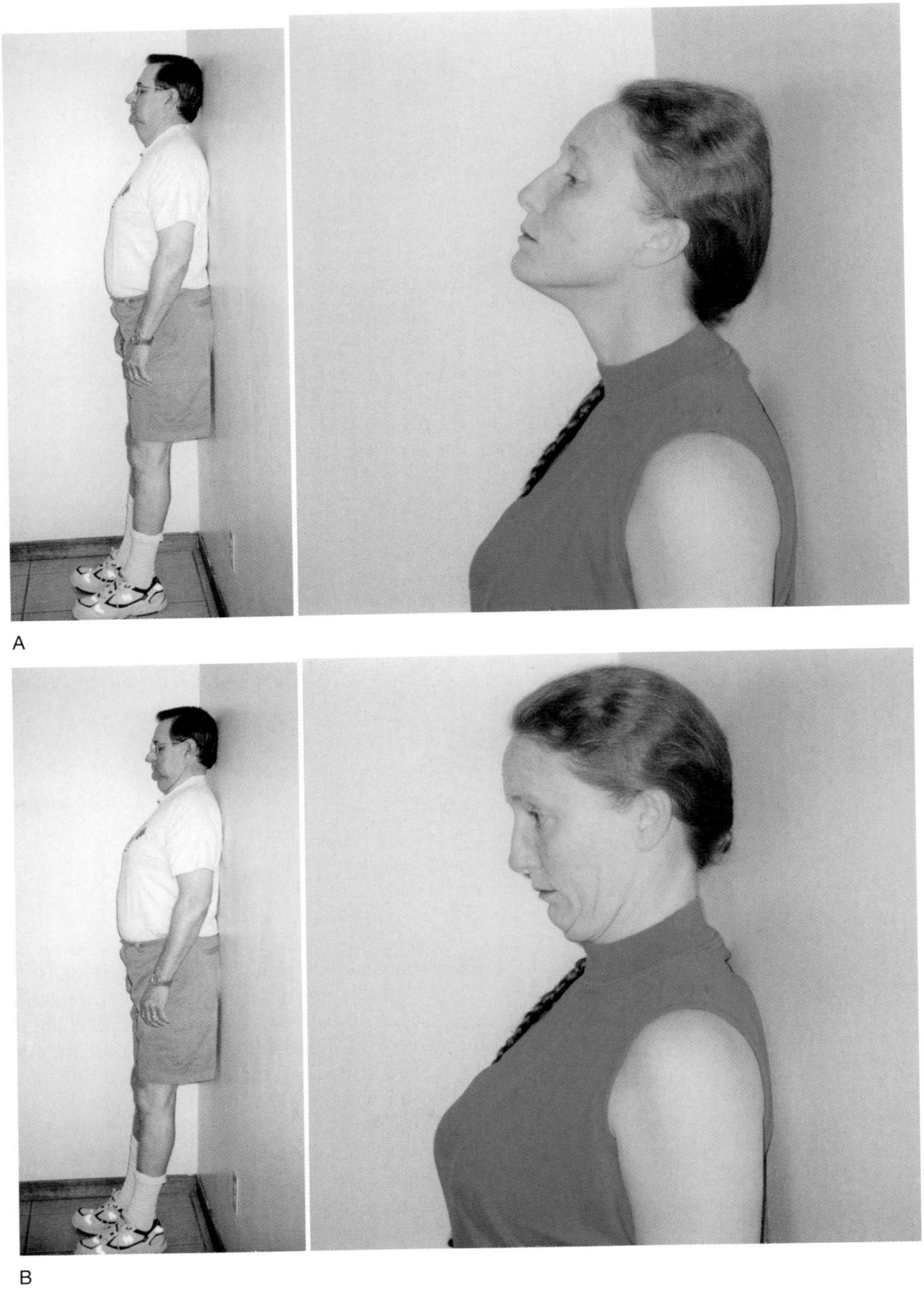

FIGURE 127–11 ■ Chin-tuck. It is easiest to learn the position of the chin tuck standing against a wall with the head and shoulders touching and the feet about 6 to 12 inches out from the wall or lying flat (**A**). Without lifting the head, the entire head, led by the chin is rotated toward the sternoclavicular notch (**B**).

References

1. Licht S: History. In Licht S, Johnson EW (eds): Therapeutic Exercise. New Haven, Conn, Waverly Press, 1965, p 426.
2. Kellett J: Acute soft tissue injuries-A review of the literature. Med Sci Sports Exerc 18(5):489, 1986.
3. Green T, Refshauge K, Crosbie J, et al: A randomized controlled trial of a passive accessory joint mobilization of acute ankle inversion sprains. Phys Ther 81(4):984, 2001.
4. Deyo RA, Deihl AK, Rosenthal M: How many days of bed rest for acute low back pain? A randomized clinical trial. N Engl J Med 315(17):1064, 1986.
5. Wilkinson MJ: Does 48 hours' bed rest influence the outcome of acute low back pain? Br J Gen Pract 45(398):481, 1995.
6. Malmivaara A, Hakkinen U, Aro T, et al: The treatment of acute low back pain—bed rest, exercises, or ordinary activity? N Engl J Med 332(6):351, 1995
7. Hagen KB, Hilde G, Jamtvedt G, et al: Bed rest for acute low back pain and sciatica. Cochrane Database Syst Rev 2:CD001254, 2000.
8. Pretest clinical evaluation. In American College of Sports Medicine Guidelines for Exercise Testing and Prescription, 6th ed. Philadelphia, Lippincott, 2000, p 35.
9. Gibbons RA, Balady JW, Beasely JW, et al: ACC/AHA guidelines for exercise testing. J Am Coll Cardiol 30:260, 1997.
10. Khalil TM, Asfour SS, Martinez LM, et al: Stretching in the rehabilitation of low-back pain patients. Spine 17(3): 311, 1992.
11. Lewit K, Simons DG: Myofascial pain: Relief by post-isometric relaxation. Arch Phys Med Rehabil 65:452, 1984.
12. Fisher NM, Pendergast DR, Gresham GE, et al: Muscle rehabilitation: Its effect on muscular and functional performance of patients with knee arthritis. Arch Phys Med Rehabil 72:3667, 1991.
13. Bischoff HA, Roos EM: Effectiveness and safety of strengthening, aerobic, and coordination exercises for patients with osteoarthritis. Curr Opin Rheum 15:141, 2003.
14. McCain GA: Non-medicinal treatment in primary fibromyalgia. Rheum Dis Clin North Am 15(1):73, 1989.
15. De Lateur BJ: Therapeutic exercise to develop strength and endurance. In Kottke FJ, Stillwell GK, Lehmann JF: Krusen's Handbook of Physical Medicine and Rehabilitation. Philadelphia, Saunders, 1982, p 427.
16. Takemasa R, Yamamoto H, Tani T: Trunk muscle strength in and effect of trunk muscle exercises for patients with chronic low back pain. Spine 20(21):2522, 1995.
17. Milesky AE, Edwards JE, Wigglesworth JK, et al: Eccentric and concentric strength of the shoulder and arm musculature of collegiate baseball pitchers. Am J Sports Med 23(5):638, 1995.
18. Contraction of Muscle. In Guyton AC, Hall JE: Textbook of Medical Physiology, 10th ed: Philadelphia, Saunders, 2000, p 67.
19. Musculoskeletal function. In Pollock ML, Wilmore JH: Exercise in Health and Disease: Evaluation and Prescription for Prevention and Rehabilitation, 2nd ed. Philadelphia, Saunders, 1990, p 202.
20. Hickson RC: Interference of strength development by simultaneously training strength and endurance. Eur J Appl Physiol 12(5):336, 1980.
21. Cardio-respiratory function. In Pollock ML, Wilmore JH (eds): Exercise in Health and Disease: Evaluation and Prescription for Prevention and Rehabilitation, 2nd ed. Philadelphia, Saunders, 1990, p 91.
22. Frontera WR: Exercise in physical medicine and rehabilitation. In Grabois M, Garrison SJ, Hart K, Lemkuhl D: Physical Medicine and Rehabilitation: The Complete Approach. Malden, Mass, Blackwell Science, 2000, p 202.
23. Coupland CA, Cliffe S, Bassey EJ, et al: Habitual physical activity and bone mineral density in postmenopausal women in England. Int J Epidemiol 28:241, 1999.
24. Focht BC, Ewing V, Gauvin L, et al: The unique and transient impact of acute exercise on pain perception in older, overweight, or obese adults with knee osteoarthritis. Ann Behav Med 24(3):201, 2002.
25. Coleman EA, Buchner DM, Cress ME, et al: The relationship of joint symptoms with exercise performance in older adults. JAGS 44:14, 1996.
26. Little P, Roberts L, Blowers H, et al: Should we give detailed advice and information booklets to patients with back pain? Spine 26(19):2065, 2001.
27. Hurwitz EL, Morgenstern H, Harber P, et al: A randomized trial of medical care with and without physical therapy and chiropractic care with and without physical modalities for patients with low back pain: Six-month follow-up outcomes from the UCLA Low Back Pain Study. Spine 27(20):2193, 2002.
28. Fisher NM, Pendergast DR, Gresham GE, et al: Muscle rehabilitation: Its effect on muscular and functional performance of patients with knee arthritis. Arch Phys Med Rehabil 72:3367,1991.
29. McCain GA, Mai FM, Halliday PD: A controlled study of the effects of a supervised cardiovascular fitness-training program on the manifestation of primary fibromyalgia. Arthritis Rheum 31(9):1135, 1988.
30. Nichols DS, Glenn TM: Effects of aerobic exercise on pain perception, affect, and level of disability in individuals with fibromyalgia. Phys Ther 74(4):327, 1994.
31. Van Santen M, Bolwijn P, Landewe R, et al: High or low intensity aerobic fitness training in fibromyalia: Does it matter? J Rheum 29(3):582, 2002.
32. Valim V, Suda A, Silva L, et al: Aerobic fitness effects in fibromyalgia. J Rheum 30(5):1060, 2003.
33. Schachter CL, Busch AJ, Peleso PM, et al: Effects of short versus long bouts of aerobic exercise in sedentary women with fibromyalgia: A randomized controlled trial. Phys Ther 83(4):340, 2003.
34. Geel SE, Robergs RA: The effect of graded resistance exercise on fibromyalgia symptoms and muscle bioenergetics: A pilot study. Arthritis Rheum Arthritis Care Res 47:82, 2002.
35. Wittink H, Michel TH, Wagner A, et al: Deconditioning in patients with chronic low back pain. Fact or Fiction? Spine 25(17):2221, 2000.
36. Verbunt JA, Westerterp KR, van der Heijden GJ, et al: Physical activity in daily life in patients with chronic low back pain. Arch Phys Med Rehabil 82:726, 2001.
37. Sikorski JM: A rationalized approach to physiotherapy for low back pain. Physiotherapy 10(6):571, 1995.
38. Van Poppel MN, Koes BW, Vander Ploeg T, et al: Lumbar supports and education for the prevention of low back pain in industry. JAMA 279(22):1789, 1998.
39. Ciriello VM, Snook SH: The effect of back belts on lumbar muscle fatigue. Spine 20(11):1273, 1995.
40. Reyna JR, Leggett SH, Kenney K, et al: The effect of lumbar belts on isolated lumbar muscle. Spine 20(1):68,1995.
41. Walsh NE, Schwartz RK: The influence of prophylactic orthoses on abdominal strength and low back injury in the workplace. Am J Phys Med Rehabil 69:245, 1990.
42. Davies JE, Gibson T, Tester L: The value of exercises in the treatment of low back pain. Rheum Rehab 18:243, 1979.
43. Detorri JR, Bullock SH, Sutlive TG, et al: The effects of spinal flexion and extension and their associated postures in patients with acute low back pain. Spine 20(21):2103, 1995.
44. Oldervoll LM, Ro M, Zwart J-A, et al: Comparison of two physical exercise programs for the early intervention of pain in the neck, shoulders, and lower back in female hospital staff. J Rehabil Med 33:156, 2001.
45. Helewa A, Goldsmith CH, Lee P, et al: Does strengthening the abdominal muscles prevent low back pain? A randomized controlled trial. J Rheum 26(8):1808, 1999.
46. Sinaki M: Lumbar spondylolisthesis: Retrospective comparison and three year follow up of two conservative treatment programs. Arch Phys Med Rehabil 70:594, 1989.
47. Saal JA, Saal JS: Non-operative treatment of herniated lumbar intervertebral disc with radiculopathy: An outcome study. Spine 14(4):130, 1989.
48. Ostelo RWJG, deVet HCW, Waddell G, et al: Rehabilitation following first time lumbar disc surgery: A systematic review within the framework of the Cochrane collaboration. Spine 28(3):209, 2003.
49. Sinaki M, Mikkelson BA: Postmenopausal spinal osteoporosis: Flexion versus extension exercised. Arch Phys Med Rehabil 65:593, 1984.
50. Coupland CA, Cliffe S, Bassey EJ, et al: Habitual physical activity and bone mineral density in postmenopausal women in England. Int J Epidemiol 28:241, 1999.
51. Smith EL, Reddan W: Physical activity: A modality for bone accretion in the aged. AJR 126:1296, 1976.
52. Dalsky GP, Stocke KS, Ehsani AA, et al: Weight-bearing exercise training and lumbar bone mineral content in postmenopausal women. J Bone Miner Res 7:179, 1992.

53. Bemben DA: Exercise intervention for osteoporosis in postmenopausal women. Ann Intern Med 108:824, 1988.
54. Sweeney T: Neck school: Cervico-thoracic stabilization training. Occup Med: State of the Art Rev 7(1):43,1992.
55. Health screening and risk stratification. In American College of Sports Medicine Guidelines for Exercise Testing and Prescription, 6th ed. Philadelphia, Lippincott, 2000, p 22.
56. Lane NE, Michel B, Bjorkengren A: The risk of osteoarthritis with running and aging: A five-year longitudinal study. J Rheum 20(3):461, 1993.
57. Bautch JC, Clayton MK, Chu Q, et al: Synovial fluid chondroitin sulphate epitopes 3B3 and 7D4, and glycosaminoglycan in human knee osteoarthritis after exercise. Ann Rheum Dis 59(11):887, 2000.

chapter 128

Osteopathic Manipulative Treatment of the Chronic Pain Patient

Kevin D. Treffer

HISTORICAL CONSIDERATIONS

The beginnings of what is now known as *osteopathic medicine* were first developed by Andrew Taylor Still, MD/DO in the mid-1800s (Fig. 128–1). A son of an itinerant preacher/physician, Dr. Still was trained in medicine on the prairies of Kansas by his father. This was not an unusual path of medical education for the time because there were few medical schools at that time in the region. As he began treating patients with the available tools of his day he became dissatisfied with the approach to patients and available treatments believing that there was something else that could be done to help the body help itself. In 1864, three of Dr. Still's children died of meningitis and one of pneumonia, which significantly altered his thoughts on the practice of medicine. He became even more dissatisfied with the treatment methods of the day and their failures and began looking for a better way to approach the human body. He was a student of anatomy and had studied cadaveric specimens very thoroughly looking for the ways in which the musculoskeletal system was integrated into the body and how it could be treated to improve health. As he farmed and practiced medicine he developed his ideas of how the patient should be treated. It was June 22, 1874 that he first expressed his views publicly—thus effectively flinging the banner of osteopathy to the breeze.[1]

The Kirksville consensus report in 1953 perhaps delineates his ideas best for our profession and these have been the standard for the tenets of osteopathic medicine (Table 128–1).[2] Health to Dr. Still is an optimal interaction of all body systems, by communicating via neurologic, vascular, lymphatic, and hormonal means, resulting in a homeostasis (balance) between each, allowing the individual to function at an optimal capacity.[3] By doing so the body would be able to resist environmental noxious influences and compensate for any effects of these influences. Disease then represents the breakdown of this homeostasis between systems—allowing symptoms to be expressed in varied patterns.

Dysfunction within the musculoskeletal system is part of the expression of disease and involves concepts called *viscerosomatic* and *somatovisceral reflexes*. These reflexes involve afferent activity from either the somatic structure or a visceral structure with resulting inhibitory or excitatory effects on motor neurons.[4] The ability to treat the musculoskeletal system effects change throughout the systems of the body by helping the body resolve these inappropriate neural reflexes and aiding in improving neural function to viscera associated with the spinal level.[5]

Osteopathic manipulative medicine then is the ultimate expression of the osteopathic philosophy. By diagnosing and treating the musculoskeletal system, abnormal function of the neurologic, vascular, hormonal, and lymphatic tissues is removed and the body is able to develop a better balance (i.e., homeostasis) between all systems. The result is a reduction of the presenting symptoms and an improvement in function of all systems: a stable state of health for the patient.

Today, osteopathic medicine consists of an integration of the original tenets along with the modern usage of all aspects of medicine (basic sciences and clinical sciences). The chronic pain patient can be effectively treated with osteopathic manipulative treatment (OMT) within the context of the etiology of the pain, to develop an optimal balance of the patient's musculoskeletal mobility and thereby improve functional integration of all body systems.[6,7]

This chapter will describe this author's osteopathic approach to the examination and treatment of the chronic pain patient. The comprehensive evaluation and treatment presented is a unique idea that has evolved out of the osteopathic philosophy. This is not an examination that all osteopathic physicians will do for their patients. The idea of a complete evaluation was first introduced in principle in osteopathic medical schools. While many osteopathic physicians perform manipulation, very few are performing an extensive approach. After several hundred patient visits, I found I did not have great success with chronic pain patients. After much discussion and work with William Brooks, DO, I modified my approach to include the grading of motion patterns and developed my version of this type of examination.[8-10] Since then I have seen a better response in this patient population. This paradigm of evaluation and treatment is still evolving. Treatment modalities will be discussed as well as clinical problems that have responded to OMT.

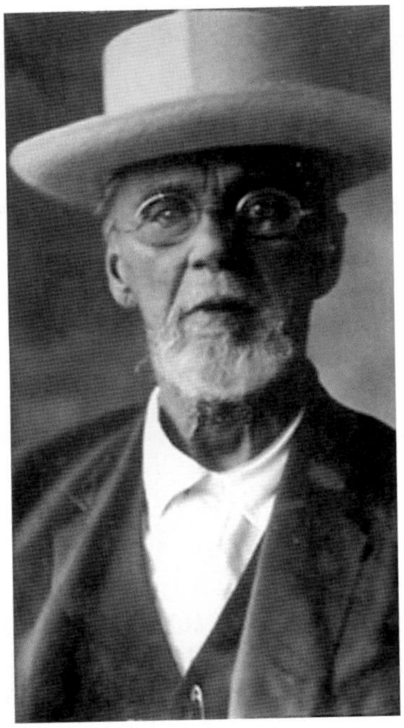

FIGURE 128–1 ■ A. T. Still, MD, DO.

Table 128–1

Principles Emphasized by the Philosophy of Osteopathic Medicine

- The human being is a dynamic unit of function
- The body possesses self-regulatory mechanisms that are self-healing in nature
- Structure and function are interrelated at all levels
- Rational treatment is based on these principles

SOMATIC DYSFUNCTION AND THE NOCICEPTIVE MODEL

In evaluating the musculoskeletal system, the osteopathic physician is looking for what is called *somatic dysfunction*. It is defined as "the impaired or altered function of related components of the musculoskeletal system: skeletal, arthrodial, and myofascial structures, and related vascular, lymphatic, and neural elements."[11] The physician evaluates first for tissue texture changes in all aspects of the musculoskeletal system (Table 128–2). The next aspect is asymmetry of position and motion by palpating bony landmarks for static position and motion by palpating bony landmarks for static position and evaluating dynamic motion (both active and passive motion). By evaluating for motion, the physician assesses for symmetry of the motion pattern noting any restricted motion in one direction and increased motion in the other. Palpation may also elicit tenderness at the site (*t*enderness, *a*symmetry, *r*estricted range of motion, *t*issue texture [TART] changes) (Table 128–3).[11] By finding TART changes in the musculoskeletal palpatory examination, somatic dysfunction can be diagnosed.

It is important to understand how the body develops these TART findings and how they relate to the chronic pain patient. Currently the model for the etiology of somatic dysfunction is via nociceptive pathways. The source of the stimulation of

Table 128–2

Evaluation of Tissue Texture Changes

Tissue Texture Changes	*Acute*	*Chronic*
Texture	Bogginess	Smooth
Temperature	Increased	Decreased (coolness)
Moisture	Increased	Decreased
Tension	Increased	Ropiness, Tissue contraction
Tenderness	Present	Present
Edema	Present	Not generally present
Erythema	Vasodilation in tissues	Minimal

Educational Council on Osteopathic Principles: Glossary of Osteopathic Terminology. Washington, D.C.: American Association of Osteopathic Colleges, 2001.

Table 128–3

TART Examination

T-Tissue texture changes
A-Asymmetry of position
R-Restriction of motion
T-Tenderness

the nociceptor will vary with the variety of injuries and disease processes our patients present with. The stimulus of a peripheral nociceptor must be of sufficient strength and remain for a sufficient time to activate a cascade of events that results in the musculoskeletal effects of somatic dysfunction.[12] As the stimulus (e.g., inflammatory process) continues, the continual afferent activity into the spinal cord level affects interneurons within the cord, lowering their activation thresholds. This facilitates more efferent activity to the motor pathways, including somatic and visceral motor neurons. This is the basis of the facilitated segment concept of Korr and Denslow, developed during the mid-1900s.[6,13] These effects not only reach the somatic structures as evidenced by the TART findings, but have consequences for visceral function (viscerosomatic and somatovisceral reflexes). The result is disruption of the body's homeostasis or system integration. The osteopathic physician recognizes this alteration in integration as a predisposition for disease processes to occur.

The facilitation changes at the spinal cord level can produce short-term effects in neuronal activity that resolve if the stimulus is short lived. If the stimulus is allowed to remain, the effects can become long-term or sometimes permanent and are associated with chronic pain states and central (spinal) sensitization.[14] The nociceptive information (cause of facilitation) is then processed within the cord, brain stem, thalamus, and the cortex. Spinal facilitation processes activate the brain stem arousal system that is coupled to two efferent pathways: sympathetic nervous system (SNS) and the hypothalamic-pituitary-adrenal axis (HPA).[15] These efferent pathways are driven by norepinephrine in the SNS and cortisol in the HPA and alter bodily function (immune and neuroendocrine function) to respond appropriately to a noxious stimulus. This process is referred to as *allostasis* and is a normal response by the body. However, if the stimulus is allowed to continue, the result is an increase in the allostatic load, which is detrimental to reestablishing homeostasis. The continual exposure to an increased allostatic load will decrease the function of feedback loops meant to restore homeostasis—leaving the body "in a chronic compensatory state."[16]

With a chronic, increased allostatic load, the response of the musculoskeletal system is continual motor output to the soma, resulting in the maintenance of somatic dysfunction.[16] From a physical examination standpoint, this means maintenance of restricted ranges of motions within fascial planes, extremity joints, and spinal segments.

Allostatic load also affects visceral function by altering the outflows to the SNS and thereby affects the function of viscera innervated from the spinal segments involved in the somatic dysfunction.[17] The resulting effects involve not just musculoskeletal tissues but potentially affect multiple organ systems and the integration of their functions.

The limbic system of the brain is responsible for the emotional component of the patient and has connections to the brain stem arousal system (SNS and HPA). The spinoreticular tracts of the brain stem arousal system can be affected by limbic system function and emotional feelings become an important part of dealing with chronic somatic dysfunction and its resolution.[18] This reticular system also has connections to postural controls, which may explain persistent postural strain patterns observed in evaluation of chronic pain patients[19-21] How the patient is dealing emotionally with the pain and/or the disease process may play a role in the perpetuation of the severity of the pain and the chronicity of somatic dysfunction.

As a stimulus starts the cascade of effects within the neuroendocrine-immune axis and the spinal cord, the effects are the palpable changes in the tissue texture and the decreased range of motion within the patient's musculoskeletal system. The longer this remains, the more detrimental it will become for the patient by affecting other bodily systems, causing breakdown in function and the possibility of the disease processes to flourish. The osteopathic physician's approach to the chronic pain patient begins by looking at the patient as a whole (all systems) and then using OMT to resolve somatic dysfunction. The result is a reduction in the somatic portion of inappropriate reflexes within the CNS involving the SNS and HPA systems, aiding the body to reestablish a homeostasis (decreased allostatic load). The chronic patient will always have some form of afferent activity and by periodic evaluation and treatment the osteopathic physician helps the patient find health by maintaining the best homeostatic state possible, given the condition and its course.

STRUCTURAL EXAMINATION OF THE CHRONIC PAIN PATIENT

The beginning of all patient interaction is the history and physical examination. A thorough history of the presenting complaint, review of systems, medical history, social history, and surgical history is vital to appropriately guiding the physical examination. From an osteopathic approach this is no different from procedures of our other medical colleagues. The osteopathic physician does emphasize musculoskeletal, neurologic, psychosocial, and trauma histories in the approach to a chronic pain patient but not to the exclusion of any other aspect of the history and physical examination. Because a large percentage of patients have had multiple other evaluations and treatment plans before coming for manipulative evaluation and treatment, the history of these specific evaluations and treatments and their successes/failures are important. Examination of the musculoskeletal (MS) system is of great importance to the osteopathic physician. As the MS system is evaluated, the area(s) of greatest restriction (the primary dysfunction[s]) are of particular clinical significance.

The examination begins with postural evaluation followed by both active and passive motion patterns. How the patient's body responds to gravity may give us clues regarding the regions of the MS system that may have somatic dysfunction. A center of gravity is established to enhance ideal postural alignment because the body responds to forces from within and from without itself (Table 128–4). A failure of establishing ideal posture places a strain on the myofascial and arthrodial tissues generating inappropriate stresses to tissues that are not typically weightbearing.[21] Because the tissues respond to changing forces, the body is observed for symmetry verses asymmetry in the sagittal, coronal, and transverse planes. Surface anatomic landmarks are used to evaluate for asymmetry (Fig. 128–2). Some landmarks require only observation, whereas others require palpation to compare left versus right and anterior versus posterior.

The patient is then put through range of motion involving the entire MS system. As we observe motions actively and passively, we are watching for smooth and sequential motion within the myofascial and arthrodial aspects of the MS system (quantity and quality). Can the patient exhibit full range of motion actively and passively? It is important during passive evaluation to first observe where linkage to other regions of the MS system exists. For example, with the patient in supine position with the knee and hip flexed to 90 degrees, adduction at the hip joint will link into the pelvis and trunk and result in rotation of the pelvis and trunk within the transverse plane (Fig 128–3). To get the best assessment of this hip joint range of motion the physician should block this linkage with one hand while assessing the pattern of motion in question, thereby giving the clinician a truer picture of the available motion. With a restricted pattern of motion, this linkage would be expected to occur early in the range of motion; how much restriction depends on this motion's significance to the overall MS system dysfunction.

Table 128–4

Landmarks for the Sagittal Plane Ideal Postural Line

- External auditory meatus
- Shoulders
- Center of the body of L3
- Greater trochanter
- Lateral condyle of the femur
- Just anterior to the lateral malleolus

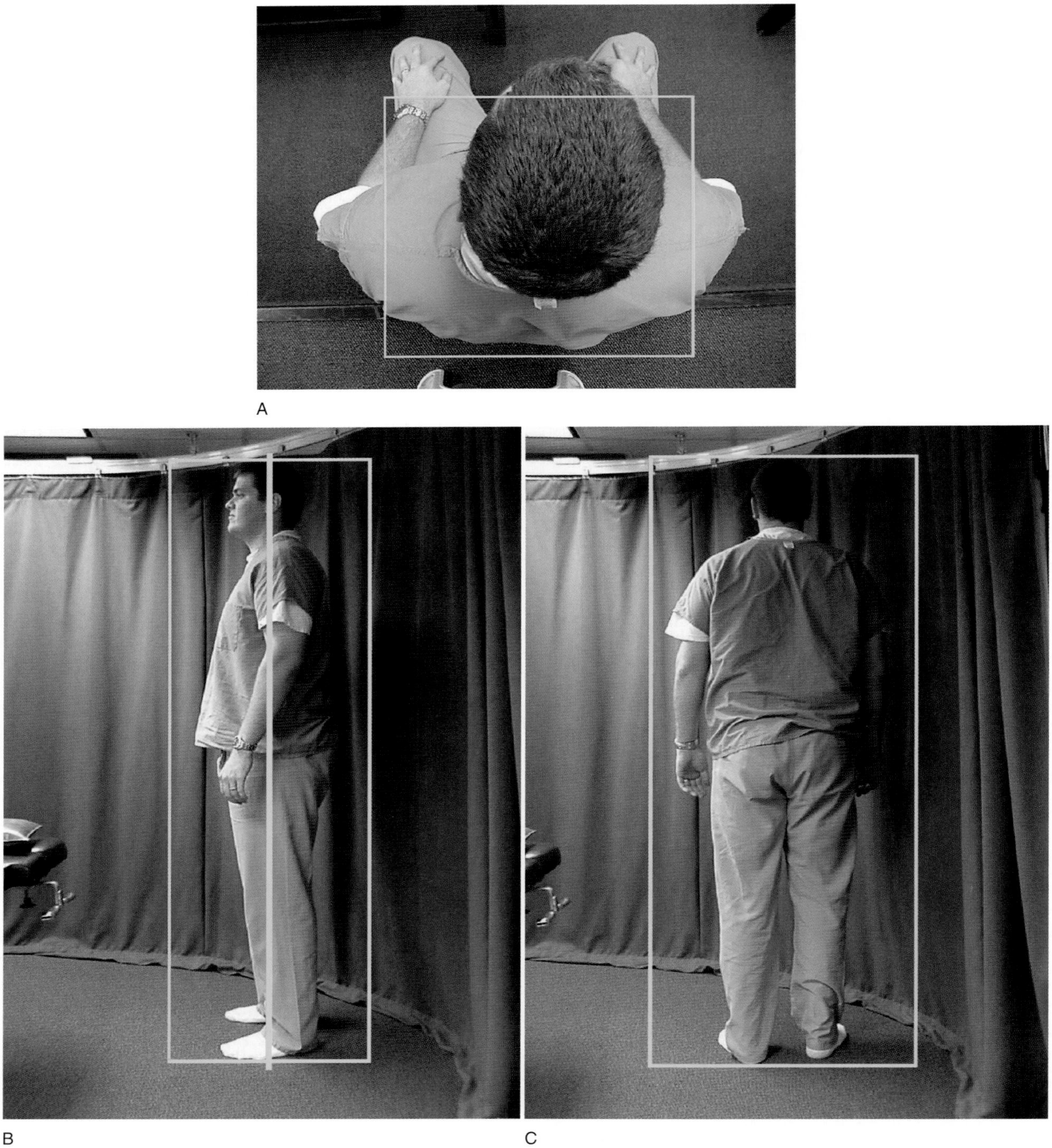

A

B C

FIGURE 128–2 ■ Evaluation of posture is done in three planes: **A,** Transverse plane; **B,** Sagittal plane with ideal postural line; **C,** Coronal plane (anterior and posterior).

As the idea of linkage is applied to each motion pattern, a grade is given for each one. The grading is done during passive motion testing. As one is passively moving part of the MS system in its range of motion, the physician can note the quality of the motion as well as the quantity. A patient may be able to attain the full range of motion (FROM) without causing tissue disruption but may be using a great amount of force to get to FROM. The grade should be applied when the quality of motion changes at the point in which greater force is required to attain the FROM or linkage occurs. The grading system also gives you objective evidence of the available motion within the MS system. If the motion pattern goes from 0% to 25% beyond the FROM, then the grade assigned is a +1. If the motion pattern tested achieves 100% of the expected range of motion then FROM is documented. If the motion attained is between 75% and 100% the grade assigned is −1.

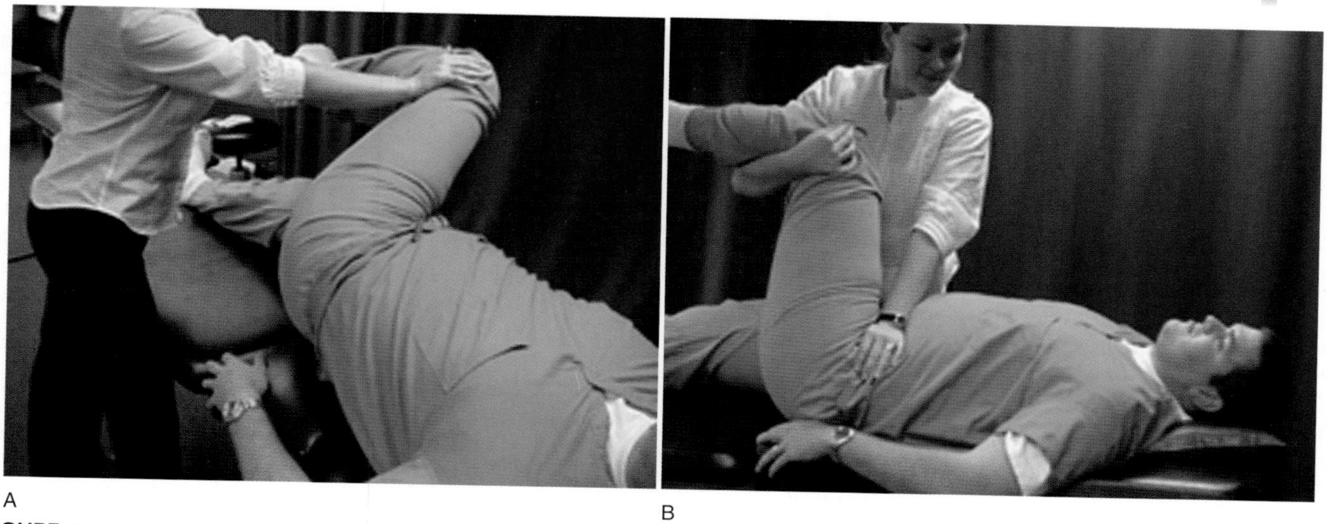

A B

FIGURE 128–3 ■ **A,** With the hip and knee at 90 degrees, linkage within the trunk occurs with abduction at the hip. **B,** By blocking the linkage, the true degree of available motion within the pattern is determined.

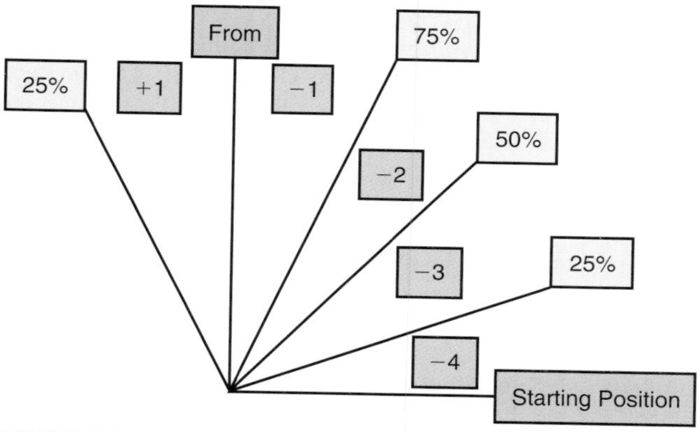

FIGURE 128–4 ■ Graphic representation of motion pattern grading.

If the motion attained is between 50% and 75%, the grade is −2. If the motion is between 25% and 50%, the grade is −3, and if the motion is between starting position and 25% of expected motion, the grade is −4 (Fig. 128–4).[20] This system differs slightly from the American Osteopathic Association standardized outpatient OMT form in which they use a 0 to 3 grading system. Because different postures related to the trunk and the extremities affect symptom expression, repeating the grading of motion patterns in multiple contexts is recommended.[22] The idea is to evaluate motion in the standing, seated, supine, and prone contexts to determine if the greatest restrictions are context dependent. This will become relevant in the planning phase of management because the area of greatest restriction should be treated in the context in which it was found to be the most restricted.[23]

After all motion patterns are graded, the physician identifies the motion pattern that has the greatest restriction. This motion pattern then should be approached by evaluating for functional pathology (i.e., somatic dysfunction) within the joints and myofascial tissues involved with that motion pattern. Once dysfunction is identified, a manipulative treatment plan can be developed and carried out to improve the restriction as much as possible given the chronicity of the cause. Another piece of information available from the grading of motion patterns is total body mobility. If the patient would have a large number of −2s or −3s and very few FROM, then one would note that the patient's system is a very tight system. Contrast this with the patient with a large number of FROM and +1s; this would be considered a loose system. Most patients fall into the range of mostly FROM and a few −1s and/or a few +1s. The motion patterns are reevaluated at each visit and the grades are compared to earlier data. This information can be used at each subsequent visit to evaluate the patient's progress as well as to demonstrate the success of the treatment plan. If the patient was assigned stretching exercises, then the information could be used to show the patient the benefit of the exercises. If the patient is not being compliant, then the information can be used to encourage the patient to do the exercises that are essential to recovery.

The patient's symptomatic complaint may not be associated with those motion patterns with the greatest restriction. If one applies the ideas of biotensegrity, which suggests that the spinal colum is not simply a stack of blocks but a structured systems of continuous tension and discontinuous compression, forces are displaced throughout the MS system to find a balance of tension and force.[24] Levin explains the body as a layer of tensegrity systems within tensegrity systems. The myofascial tissues are analogous to tension trusses and the bony structures are analogous to compression structures. The icosahedral design in this system allows for instantaneous increasing and/or decreasing tensions and compression as loads are placed on the structure without changing overall shape.[24] The loading forces placed on the body are instantaneously displaced through all tissues and allow the body to maintain a posture in relationship to gravity, ideal or not. As disease processes and injury patterns occur in the body, a change in the distribution of force would be expected—thereby changing tension within the MS system to establish a new and/or stable (although abnormal) posture. This would be represented by somatic dysfunction and all its elements that have been discussed so far. Restriction in one motion pattern will have to be compensated by another in order for the posture to balance. The symptomatic expression of this may be in the areas of increased mobility and not in the areas of greatest restriction.[25] For example, McConnell notes that lack of external rotation and extension within the hip will cause an increase in lumbar spine mobility to accommodate for this restriction of motion. Over time, this causes torsional strain in the annulus fibrosus portion of the intervertebral disks. Because there are nociceptors in the outer layers of the annulus fibrosus, this repetitive trauma can cause low back pain. One would expect symptoms to be expressed sooner in patients with preexisting chronic dysfunction and structural pathology in the lumbar spine. The root of the problem exists within the hip muscle restriction and not in the lumbar disks. Manipulative treatment would then provide a way to remove the hip rotation restriction and allow for a release in the tension/compression forces and reestablish a more normal balance in postural control and relief of low back symptoms.

After posture and motion evaluation, it is helpful to evaluate the patient's gait. The patient must be observed for several full-gait cycles watching for symmetry in the stance and swing phases of gait. The patient's postural center of gravity is one of the determinants of how efficient the cycle is. The determinants of gait as noted by Saunders and coworkers are pelvic rotation in the transverse plane toward the stance phase side, downward pelvic tilt in the coronal plane toward the swing phase side, knee flexion during the swing phase side, combined action of the foot, ankle, and knee on the stance phase side, and the constant displacement of the center of gravity during the gait cycle.[26] Optimal mechanics of these determinants will result in an efficient gait cycle. Evaluation of the cycle should be split into the stance and swing phases. Each phase has motions within the MS system that rely on neuromuscular and biomechanical processes to accomplish a normal cycle.

Swing phase begins with toe-off from the stance leg and ends with heel strike of the same leg. During this phase, the pelvis rotates toward the stance leg, the hip and knee are flexing, and the ankle is dorsiflexing. During the later half of the swing phase, the knee extends, and at the end of swing phase, the foot is supinated—which combined with the remaining amount of knee flexion acts as a shock absorption during the heel strike portion of stance phase.[25,26] If there is dysfunction within the knee (e.g., hyperextension) or the subtalar joint, an increase in pelvic rotation and/or coronal plane tilt is noted—resulting in excessive motion within the lumbar spine.[25] Over time, this could lead to strain in the spine and its myofascial structures and further musculoskeletal pain. In individuals who already have significant pathology in the lumbar spine, the added strain can cause exacerbations of their pain (increased allostatic load). Manipulation of the dysfunctions to improve motion will act to decrease the allostatic load and decrease nociceptive input into the system.

Stance phase begins with heel strike and ends with toe-off. During this phase, the hip goes into extension, the knee fully extends, the ankle and foot plantar flex and pronate to allow for toe-off at the end of the cycle[26] The subtalar joint has great clinical significance during stance phase because dysfunction here will result in a disturbance in the shock absorption on heel strike and affect lumbopelvic motion as well.[25] Physical findings are represented by abnormal areas of callus formation on the plantar surface of the foot indicating abnormal weightbearing.[26] Again, manipulative treatment to dysfunctional tissues involved in gait will restore the necessary motions to allow a more efficient gait cycle and lessen nociceptive input. The gait efficiency will show in the stamina of our chronic pain patients in the activities of their daily lives as they try to function with a chronic problem.

The gait cycle is a total body phenomenon. To counterbalance some of the lower extremity and pelvic motions, the upper body will rotate toward the swing leg side and the upper extremities swing anterior on the stance leg side. This also will help minimize head rotation, thus keeping it forward. The physician should be mindful of mobility within the trunk and upper extremities that may have effects on restricting mobility within the gait cycle.

The context the patient is evaluated in includes standing, seated, supine, and prone. Standing context would include the postural examination in three planes. Seated examination begins with simultaneously evaluating passive right and left upper extremity flexion, extension, adduction, and abduction blocking any linkage noted. All of these motions would be done with the elbow in full extension (a so-called *straight upper extremity*). For all of these motions the FROM would be based on the practitioner's favorite reference text for motion mechanics. Hoppenfield's *Physical Examination of the Spine and Extremities* is an excellent resource for the expected ranges of motion (Tables 128–5 and 128–6). Each of these motions should be graded for available motion and documented as discussed earlier.

The scapulothoracic motion is an important component of total shoulder motion and, therefore, the amount of gapping between the scapula and the thoracic cage is noted. By passively retracting the ipsilateral shoulder girdle, the tension around the medial aspect of the scapula is loosened. The free hand then attempts to slide the fingers between the scapula and the thoracic cage. The expectation is that the fingers would be able to slide up to the proximal interphalangeal joint. This would be graded in the same fashion as noted before and documented. Experience in practice reveals that tension within the pectoralis minor muscle and subscapularis muscle commonly restrict this gapping motion, effectively locking the scapula onto the chest cage. Clinical practice has associated tension within these muscles with atypical shoulder pain and restriction of motion of the scapulothoracic joint.

Supine evaluation involves motion of the upper and lower extremity motion patterns noting any linkage and

Table 128–5

Expected Full Range of Motion for Upper Extremity

Seated context	
Abduction	= 180 degrees
Adduction	= 45 degrees
Flexion	= 90 degrees
Extension	= 45 degrees
Supine and seated context	
Internal rotation	= 55 degrees
External rotation	= 40-45 degrees

Hoppenfeld S: Physical Examination of the Spine and Extremities. Norwalk, Conn. Appleton and Lange, 1976, p 1.

Table 128–6

Expected Full Range of Motion for Lower Extremity

Supine context	
Flexion at the hip with knee flexed = 120 degrees	
Flexion at the hip with the knee extended = 90 degrees	
Abduction at the hip with the knee/hip flexed = 45-50 degrees	
Adduction at the hip with the knee/hip flexed = 20-30 degrees	
Internal rotation at the hip with the knee/hip flexed = 35 degrees	
External rotation at the hip with the knee/hip flexed = 45 degrees	
Prone context	
Extension at the hip with the knee flexed = 30 degrees	
External rotation at the hip with the knee flexed = 45 degrees	
Internal rotation at the hip with the knee flexed = 35 degrees	
Flexion at the knee = 135 degrees	

Hoppenfeld S: Physical Examination of the Spine and Extremities. Norwalk, Conn. Appleton and Lange, 1976, pp 143,171.

blocking it appropriately. The lower extremity flexion at the hip is noted with the knee in full extension and then in full flexion. Abduction and adduction at the hip are evaluated with the knee extended and also with the hip and knee flexed to 90 degrees. Internal and external rotation is evaluated with the hip and knee flexed to 90 degrees. The upper extremity is evaluated for internal and external rotation at the shoulder with the elbow flexed 90 degrees and glenohumeral joint abducted 90 degrees. It is important to appreciate the scapulothoracic component of internal rotation at the shoulder, which is a major portion of the normal internal rotation. Restriction within the periscapular muscles will decrease this pattern of motion in combination with a decreased scapular gapping evaluation. Other muscles that cross this region may also produce restriction. The latissimus dorsi muscle takes its origin from the lumbar aponeurosis and inserts into the shoulder, directly linking the shoulder region to the low back. Therefore, restrictions in the shoulder motions may be affected by fascial restrictions within the lumbar spine or may be from the pelvis or lower extremity because the fascial tissue is contiguous through the gluteus medius, into the posterior sacroiliac capsule, into the sacrotuberous ligament and into the origin of the posterior thigh muscles off the ischial tuberosity. This anatomic knowledge lends credence to the idea that the area of greatest restriction may not be in the area of pain expression. It is entirely possible to have significant dysfunction from the lumbar spine or down into the feet that may manifest with upper extremity symptoms due to fascial tethers within the system. It is for this reason that a thorough and comprehensive examination is the best approach to MS system chronic pain issues. For all of these motions, the FROM would be based on the examiner's favorite reference text for motion mechanics.

Prone evaluation of the patient does involve both upper and lower extremity motion patterns. The lower extremity is evaluated for flexion at the knee, external rotation at the hip with the knee flexed, internal rotation with the knee flexed, and extension at the hip with the knee flexed. The upper extremity is evaluated for horizontal extension at the shoulder with the elbow fully extended. Tension with the pectoral muscles of the chest will restrict this motion pattern and is associated with patients with protracted shoulder girdles (rounded shoulders) or slumping postures in today's sedentary society.

After all motion patterns are evaluated and the primary restricted pattern(s) is/are noted the muscles, fascia, and joints involved with each pattern are evaluated specifically for somatic dysfunction. An osteopathic physician is trained to evaluate for dysfunction in all joints and myofascial tissues. The sequence for evaluation is variable using this approach. It may require starting in the foot and ankle or in the head and neck. As the MS system is more specifically evaluated, the areas of greatest restriction are again of high clinical significance. For example, as one palpates for dysfunction of the forefoot, midfoot, and hindfoot, the degree of restriction is noted and documented. This is repeated for the fibula and tibia, hip, innominates, sacrum, lumbar spine, thoracic spine, cervical spine, ribs, shoulders, clavicles, radius, ulna, carpals, and phalanges. Many osteopathic physicians practice osteopathy in the cranial field and would include this portion of the examination as part of the comprehensive examination of the entire musculoskeletal system. The region with the greatest restriction should be addressed manipulatively first. The American Osteopathic Association has a textbook , entitled *Foundations for Osteopathic Medicine* that explains how to diagnose somatic dysfunction in all of the aforementioned areas. This is by no means the only text written on this subject and, indeed, there are many fine texts to choose from.

OSTEOPATHIC MANIPULATIVE TREATMENT AND CHOOSING THE TREATMENT MODALITY

Once a diagnosis of somatic dysfunction is made, then a plan to relieve the restriction and restore motion is produced. The art of practicing manipulative medicine includes knowing when and where to apply a certain modality of manipulation for any given patient. First one must be confident in the diagnosis made and that osteopathic manipulative treatment is indicated for this patient.

During the examination process, one should be determining whether the source of the problem is structural pathology or functional pathology. Structural pathology will generally mean instability within anatomic structures that will need stabilization before applying an OMT modality. Treating unstable structures with manipulation may cause injury and add an acute problem to a chronic one. Most structural instabilities are associated with a hypermobility of the MS segment in question, although not all are hypermobile. For example, degenerative processes such as osteoarthritis and its associated sclerotic changes can give hypomobility to any given segment and still be unstable enough to contraindicate OMT to that segment. However, this may not contraindicate

OMT to other MS segments within the same individual. OMT is best suited for tissues with hypomobility that are capable of responding to treatment.

One caveat should be noted: although an individual may have structural pathology, he or she will possess functional pathology in compensation for the abnormal structure. Somatic dysfunction is a component of functional pathology and is associated with hypomobility within our chronic pain patients.

If OMT is appropriate for the patient, then a decision as to whether one uses a direct or indirect technique needs to be addressed. When evaluating for segmental somatic dysfunction and TART findings, the physician notes the quality of the range of motion end-feel. Does it feel as if a brick wall is being encountered as the segment is being moved into the extremes of motion in one direction or another? If the range of motion for the segment is asymmetrical in one direction versus another, then a restrictive barrier is said to be present, limiting the motion. The quality of the end-feel may determine what modality would be best to use for that dysfunction. A hard end-feel may be better suited for a high-velocity low amplitude (i.e., thrusting) technique indicating the problem is more arthrodial; a softer or tethered end-feel may respond better to a muscle energy or myofascial release modality, indicating the problem is more myofascial. Patient preference of modality may make the decision easier. If a patient does not want a certain modality used then the physician would be well advised not to proceed. Comorbid diagnoses sometime prevent some modalities from being used.

There have been no absolute rules developed for the frequency of manipulative treatments.[27] Therefore, an individualized program should be designed for each patient. Patients with very tight MS systems may require more frequent treatments at first, followed by longer periods of time between treatments. Severely affected patients may require an evaluation and treatment on a weekly basis, whereas others may require only quarterly treatments. As with all patients, it would be ideal if we can treat the patient for a short period of time then release them from care to live a productive life. At times this is a scenario that plays itself out. Given the chronicity of many MS diseases/injuries, these patients will require periodic treatment for them to maintain the homeostasis they have achieved with their disease/injury process. OMT is not a cure for structural changes but is effective for the functional changes related to structural pathology. This author prefers to give the body a chance to adjust to changes made in the MS system and see the patient every 4 to 6 weeks if schedules allow. Few patients require weekly treatment over extended periods of time, although there is always that small percentage who function better with weekly treatments.

MANIPULATIVE MEDICINE MODALITIES

There are multiple treatment modalities available for the osteopathic physician in approaching the chronic pain patient. Each has its pros and cons and the physician must weigh the risk versus the benefit of using the modality. As discussed earlier, it is important to decide if the etiology of restriction originates in the arthrodial or the myofascial tissue. There are times when the problem lies within both aspects and multiple modalities are needed to restore motion. There are times when the patient may have too much tension to allow techniques to be applied to the joints and the clinician must work on the soft tissues to ultimately treat joint motion. Osteopathic texts such as *Foundations for Osteopathic Medicine*, describe each modality well.

Myofascial tissue modalities are very effective at restoring motion restricted by soft tissue strain patterns. These include soft tissue massage, myofascial release (both directly into the restrictive barrier and indirectly or away from the barrier), strain-counterstrain techniques, facilitated positional release, and spray and stretch techniques. These modalities require the physician to concentrate on tissue reaction occurring under his or her hands, such as palpating for tissue relaxation and/or stretch (tissue creep). The physician must have good proprioception skills to be successful with these modalities and be able to respond to changes within the myofascial tissues, as the treatment is applied.

Arthrodial modalities affect joint restriction more than soft tissue restriction. It is important to realize that tissue texture changes occur with all dysfunctions; however some end-feel of motion is harder, requiring different types of treatment modalities. These modalities include muscle energy techniques, high-velocity—low-amplitude or HVLA (i.e., thrusting techniques), articulatory, and Still's techniques. Osteopathy in the cranial field is another modality in that much of the work is done on the sutures, cranial membranes, the sphenobasilar junction, and cranial rhythmic impulse.

Manipulative medicine modalities carry some risk in performing them. Most injuries come from the more forceful modalities. Thrusting techniques are popular and easy to use, however they do have some limitations. Some patients do not care for the techniques due to fear of the popping sound or of injury. Vick and colleagues noted that HVLA techniques are safe given several hundred million treatments done each year and only 185 reported injuries over 68 years.[28] It is realized that the reporting of injuries is probably low during the time frame of the study. Haldeman's recent study did not identify factors in the history and physical that would accurately predict cerebral ischemia after cervical manipulation and, therefore, declared it a rare complication of this treatment approach.[29] Although it would be nice to have a crystal ball, the reasonable conclusion is to examine our patients thoroughly before thrusting and know that there are possible complications that may occur. We must be aware of conditions that carry more risk than benefit from the modality. This then should be communicated to our patients before using a thrusting technique and documented in the record.

POST-PATIENT ENCOUNTER RECOMMENDATIONS

After the examination and the treatment procedure(s) are completed, the patient encounter is not finished without educating the patient about his or her condition. A few minutes spent explaining in simple terms the clinical findings and the plan to manage them will involve the patient in the treatment plan. Recall that the grading of the motion patterns identifies restriction of motion and is useful in demonstrating the need to work on stretching exercises. It is best to actually demonstrate the exercise for them and then give them something in writing. For the chronic low back pain patient, exercises for the abdominal and lumbar multifidus muscles have been noted to decrease pain and increase function.[30,31] As the patient returns for reevaluation the same motion patterns can be reassessed and can be used to show the patient their success of doing the exercises or they may be used to educate and encourage them to perform the exercises if they are not complying. If patients report ache in the muscles for an extended time after the stretch, they potentially are using too much force in the stretch. You may want them to demonstrate how they are doing the exercise. This will allow you to modify the exercise as you see fit. When it comes to stretching exercises, more is better in this situation. Length of time in a stretch as well how often patients perform the stretch is important in overcoming any myofascial recoil that may occur after stretching.

Pharmaceuticals may help the patient tolerate any pain the patient experiences. Medications used with each patient should be individualized. Some may need muscle relaxants and pain medication, whereas some may just need a nonsteroidal antiinflammatory drug. There are those who require short-term narcotics and others who require chronic narcotic usage—including contracts between the doctor and patient while managing their usage. Some patients may benefit from localized epidural injections by a pain management specialist. A multidisciplinary approach is useful in the complicated chronic pain patient. However, it is best to have one physician coordinating the plan and prescribing the narcotics. This physician should keep in contact with other members of the team regarding the response from the patient.

As long as the manipulative evaluations and treatments are helping the patient, they can be continued. If the patient is getting worse, then the manipulative treatments should be stopped and the patient's history and physical examination should be reevaluated. Use the motion pattern grading system to evaluate progress/regression as well as the history. If a plateau is reached and the patient is stable and comfortable, then seeing the patient every 4 to 6 months is appropriate. If there is a flare in symptoms or a new trauma, the patient should be reevaluated sooner. Because chronic pain generally does not go away, expect the patient to return for repeat treatments. Some patients will do better if they are seen on a more frequent basis. Each patient is an individual and the frequency of treatment should be tailored to the point the patient is most functional for the longest amount of time between treatments.

CLINICAL APPLICATIONS

There are many etiologies that may produce chronic pain in our patients. OMT is designed to help treat the functional pathologies that are related to the structural pathologies. Indeed, there are times that only a functional pathology exists and OMT is appropriate for treatment in this case.[32] The general principles presented in this chapter may be applied to any chronic pain patient. Choice of treatment modality should be made in the context of the extent of structural pathologies present and considering the risk versus benefit ratio with each patient individually.

Low Back Pain

Low back pain is one of the most common, if not the most common, problem our patients will face. Furlan notes that 75% to 85% of the population will experience low back pain during their lives with 10% of those developing chronic low back pain accounting for greater than 90% of the costs for back incapacity.[33] Many dollars are spent in this country for low back pain—ranging from $20 to $50 billion annually.[34,35] There are many differing approaches to the treatment of chronic low back pain. The approach that would encompass both structural and functional problems would be the most comprehensive management plan. With the spine resembling a tensegrity tower, a response to treatment is associated with changes in motion and force displacement, thereby integrating this reaction with the rest of the extremities, head, and viscera.[36] Chronic responses as a result of structural and/or functional pathology will result in a repetitive overuse injury with low back pain occurring secondary to an abnormal increase of spinal segmental motion.[37] Therefore, to use the osteopathic approach you must be thorough in your evaluation of the musculoskeletal system to find the primary dysfunction(s).

The chronic pain patient has increased motor output secondary to nociceptive input that maintains the pain-spasm cycle via facilitated segments, thereby sustaining pain.[19] With central descending inhibitory pathways overwhelmed and the convergence of nociceptive and mechanoreceptor stimuli on common spinal pathways, motion can be perceived as pain.[38] Manipulative treatment is designed to decrease the facilitated segments within the cord—allowing a decrease in the motor output. The result would be less muscle spasm, less pain, and more mobility to a segment.

Treatment of the chronic low back pain patient would not be complete without a psychiatric evaluation for anxiety and depression. Depression can affect the function of the descending nociceptive inhibitory pathways in the brain stem, allowing an increase in transmission of nociception.[39] With the central nociceptive connection with the limbic system, an exacerbation of the pain level can fluctuate with the mental state of the patient. Adequate treatment of depression or anxiety can go a long way in helping the patient attain homeostasis in all systems so the patient can find a state of health as defined earlier in the chapter. Early research in the manipulative treatment of psychiatric conditions is not detailed as to specific conditions. However, current research is pending for the role of manipulative treatment in depression. There are studies that demonstrate resolution of psychosomatic back pain after the patient's psychiatric issues have been resolved.[32]

Specific regions to treat depend on the findings of the examination and the associated grade applied to the dysfunctions found. The routine low back pain patient will benefit from manipulation with less medication and physical therapy.[40] In the chronic low back pain patient, McConnell advocates restoring motion to the hips, thoracic spine, and treatment of the subtalar joint motion to help decease the lumbar compensation.[41] This should not be understood as the only regimen for treatment. The chronic patient needs will require more thorough evaluation, increased frequency of treatments, medication, and counseling as needed. Addressing the stabilizing muscles, such as the multifidus, abdominal muscles, and gluteus medius, with endurance exercises aids in appropriate recruitment of muscles during a desired motion pattern and helps your patient rehabilitate to the best possible homeostatic state, given the chronicity of the problem.[41]

Whiplash

Another chronic pain presentation is the whiplash injury patient. The symptoms associated are varied, as is the extent of injury. The typical flexion/extension inertial injury causes an S-shaped curvature in the cervical spine (flexion of upper segments and extension of lower) leading to injury. The soft tissue injury that occurs leads to changes in the mechanical function of the myofascial tissues, which may lead to a significant lowering of the thresholds of nociceptors and mechanoreceptors, resulting in the increased allostatic load and all of its effects over time.[42] If there is rotation of the cervical spine at the time of impact, the tissue trauma may be more extensive with involvement with the scalene muscles and the pectoralis minor muscle—resulting in a thoracic outlet syndrome presentation. The associated headache could be coming from the upper cervical spine owing to common pathways between nociceptive inputs from C1-C3 and the spinal nucleus of the trigeminal nerve.[43] Attention to dysfunctions within the cervical spine may alleviate headache symptoms. Because of the tissue trauma that has occurred, it is not recommended to use modalities that may further traumatize tissue during the early stages of recovery. For example, thrusting techniques may cause further injury to the tissues and direct muscle energy may be more painful to the patient. Indirect myofascial techniques, soft tissue massage, articulatory, facilitated positional release, and Still's techniques are all good choices for treatment in the early stages. Giles found in his comparison study that acupuncture was superior to manipulation for chronic neck pain but spinal manipulation was better for all other chronic spine pain indicating that consideration should be given to alternative modalities in the early course of treatment.[44] As the patient's rehabilitation is progressing, other modalities may be added. Muscle strengthening exercises, along with manipulative treatment, will be beneficial to helping the patient decrease pain and improve neck range of motion as well as muscle function.[45,46]

Migraine Cephalgia

A brief mention of migraine cephalgia and manipulation is appropriate. By addressing the entire musculoskeletal system for dysfunction, this author has seen a decrease in severity and frequency of headache in this patient population. Using cranial manipulation along with all other modalities as needed has been key in seeing this change. Bronfort's review article found studies that show a positive effect for manipulation in tension-type headaches as well as for the management of migraine cephalgia.[47] The connections of the spinal nucleus of the trigeminal nerve and the upper cervical segments may play a role in this effect.

Ankle Sprains

Many chronic pain patients suffer falls and other MS injuries that may cause further problems for their overall homeostasis. Ankle sprains respond to manipulative treatment as long as the modality chosen will not exacerbate tissue trauma. Higher-grade sprains will not be effectively treated with thrusting techniques. Early intervention will help restore lymphatic flow, decrease edema, and help decrease the inflammatory process.[48,49] Pellow looked at a separation thrusting technique for the treatment of lower grade sprains with positive results.[48] Because of compensatory changes, treatment should include a thorough evaluation and treatment of the entire extremity (attention to cuboid and fibular head), pelvis, and lumbar spine. Use the motions of gait with respect to the extremity and low back as a guide for treatment.[49] Low-grade ankle sprains are very common and adding manipulative treatment to the management can decrease healing time for many patients.

Scoliosis

The approach to evaluation and treatment as presented has been applied to scoliotic patients as well. Both direct and indirect modalities can be used effectively in the management of the chronic musculoskeletal pain associated with the curvatures. By using this comprehensive evaluation and treatment approach, Hawes and Brooks demonstrated a decrease in chest circumference inequity by >10 cm, an improvement in the rib cage deformity, and a 40% reduction in the Cobb angle in an idiopathic scoliotic curve that was stable for 30 years.[50] By improving chest wall compliance, the respiratory function and exercise capacity will improve—allowing the patient better overall body function. This may be enough change for the patient to become more active and have improved quality of life.

Fibromyalgia

Fibromyalgia patients benefit from manipulative treatment. Soft tissue massage, myofascial release, muscle energy techniques, and counter-strain techniques are beneficial modalities to use in these patients. Manipulative treatments have been shown to reduce pain at the tender point sites, improve sleep, improve activities of daily living, and decrease depressive symptoms.[51-53] Increased physical activity will increase the nociceptive threshold; therefore, by educating the patient to remain active, the long-term effect would be a decrease in pain.[54]

CONCLUSION

Dr. Still discovered a new way to approach his patients to alleviate their pain by treating the entire body and helping them function at an optimal level. His legacy and philosophy of treatment has grown over the last century. Research is showing the benefits of the addition of manipulative treatment in the management of chronic pain patients. The practitioner must be thorough in the evaluation of the MS system and be mindful of structural and functional pathology. This will require an extended amount of time during the patient encounter; however, the results are well worth the time spent. The patient must be a part of the overall management plan; the success of the treatment plan may hinge on the patient's acceptance of the plan and following through with the post-evaluation instructions and exercises. If medications are used, then close monitoring of usage and effectiveness is required.

If narcotics are used, a contract with the patient is recommended. As the management plan is carried out, the physician should periodically reevaluate the entire patient presentation to see if the patient is responding to treatment and if there is compliance with the plan.

The motion patterns observed for grading can be very numerous especially if all are done in multiple contexts. This author does a more abbreviated version of this examination, saving time in the examination room. Dr. Brooks uses a much more comprehensive evaluation for his patients. I have found that by using a select few motion patterns, I have been able to effectively improve mobility in a majority of my chronic pain patients. In those individuals who do not respond, the full evaluation would then become a better option to guide treatment.

Many chronic pain patients have gone through multiple evaluations over the timeline of their disease process. As a result, many of them have been offered relief from the pain, but many do not get relief. For those who are not responding to medical treatment, the comprehensive evaluation and treatment plan set forth can help these chronic pain patients find health, despite the chronicity of their problems.

References

1. Ward, RC, ed: Foundations for Osteopathic Medicine, 2nd ed. Philadelphia, Lippincott, 2003, p 4.
2. Educational Council on Osteopathic Principles. Glossary of Osteopathic Terminology. Washington, D.C., American Association of Osteopathic Colleges, 2001.
3. Ward RC, ed: Foundations for Osteopathic Medicine, 2nd ed. Philadelphia, Lippincott, 2003, p 5.
4. Ward RC, ed: Foundations for Osteopathic Medicine, 2nd ed. Philadelphia, Lippincott, 2003, p 123.
5. Ward RC, ed: Foundations for Osteopathic Medicine, 2nd ed. Philadelphia, Lippincott, 2003, p 124.
6. Ward RC, ed: Foundations for Osteopathic Medicine, 2nd ed. Philadelphia, Lippincott, 2003, p 129.
7. Ward RC, ed: Foundations for Osteopathic Medicine, 2nd ed. Philadelphia, Lippincott, 2003, p,134.
8. Brooks WJ, William J: Personal Communication.
9. Hawes MC, BrooksWJ: Improved chest expansion after intensive multiple-modality, nonsurgical treatment in an adult. Chest 120:672, 2001.
10. Brooks WJ, William J: The functional pathology of the musculoskeletal system—clinical application of the biomechanical evaluation. In progress, 2006.
11. Educational Council on Osteopathic Principles. Glossary of Osteopathic Terminology. Washington, DC, American Association of Osteopathic Colleges; 2001.
12. Ward RC (ed): Foundations for Osteopathic Medicine, 2nd ed. Philadelphia, Lippincott Williams & Wilkins, 2003, p130.
13. Lehman GJ, Vernon H, McGill SM: Effects of a mechanical pain stimulus on erector spinae activity before and after a spinal manipulation in patients with back pain: A preliminary investigation. J Manipulative Physiol Ther 24:402, 2001.
14. Ward RC (ed): Foundations for Osteopathic Medicine, 2nd ed. Philadelphia, Lippincott, Williams & Wilkins, 2003, pp 145,153.
15. Ward RC (ed): Foundations for Osteopathic Medicine, 2nd ed. Philadelphia, Lippincott Williams and Wilkins, 2003, p 153.
16. Ward RC (ed): Foundations for Osteopathic Medicine, 2nd ed. Philadelphia: Lippincott, Williams & Wilkins, 2003, p 151.
17. Ward RC (ed): Foundations for Osteopathic Medicine, 2nd ed. Philadelphia, Lippincott, 2003, pp 129, 153.
18. Ward RC (ed): Foundations for Osteopathic Medicine, 2nd ed. Philadelphia: Lippincott, Williams & Wilkins, 2003, p146.
19. Lehman GJ, Vernon H, McGill SM, et al: Effects of a mechanical pain stimulus on erector spinae activity before and after a spinal manipulation in patients with back pain: A preliminary investigation. J Manipulative Physiol Ther 24:405, 2001.
20. Brooks WJ: Personal Communication.
21. Ward RC (ed): Foundations for Osteopathic Medicine, 2nd ed. Philadelphia, Lippincott, 2003, p 604.
22. Van Dillen LR, Sahrmann SA, Norton BJ, Caldwell CA: The effect of modifying patient-preferred spinal movement and alignment during symptom testing in patients with low back pain: A preliminary report. Arch Phys Med Rehabil 3:313, 2003.
23. Van Dillen LR, Sahrmann SA, Norton BJ, Caldwell CA: The effect of modifying patient-preferred spinal movement and alignment during symptom testing in patients with low back pain: A preliminary report. Arch Phys Med Rehabil 3:318, 2003.
24. Levin SM: The tensegrity-truss as a model for spine mechanics: Biotensegrity. J Mech Med Biol 3,4:375, 2002.
25. McConnell J: Recalcitrant chronic low back and leg pain—a new theory and different approach to management. Man Ther 7:185, 2002.
26. DiGiovanna EL, Schiowitz S: An Osteopathic Approach to Diagnosis and Treatment, 2nd ed. Philadelphia, Lippincott, 1997, p 240.
27. Licciardone JC, Stoll ST, Carderelli KM, et al: A randomized controlled trial of osteopathic manipulative treatment following knee or hip arthroplasty. J Am Osteopath Assoc 103(5):193, 2004.
28. Vick DA, McKay C, Zengerle CR: The safety of manipulative treatment: Review of the literature from 1925 to 1993. J Am Osteopathic Assoc 2:113, 1996.
29. Haldeman S, Kohlbeck FJ, McGregor M: Unpredictability of cerebrovascular ischemia associated with cervical spine manipulation therapy. Spine 27:49, 2002.
30. Niemisto L, Lahtinen-Suopanki T, Rissanen P, et al: A randomized trial of combined manipulation, stabilizing exercise, and physician consultation compared to physician consultation alone for chronic low back pain. Spine 28(19):2185, 2003.
31. Aure OF, Nilsen JF, Vasseljen O: Manual therapy and exercise therapy in patients with chronic low back pain. Spine 28:525, 2003.
32. Seaman DC: Spinal pain syndromes: Nociceptive, neuropathic, and psychologic mechanisms. J Manipulative Physiol Ther 22(7):458, 1999.
33. Furlan A, Brosseau L, Imamura M., Irvin E: Massage for low back pain: A systematic review within the framework of the Cochrane collaboration back review group. Spine 27(17):1896, 2002.
34. Cherkin D, Sherman K, Deyo R., Shekelle P: A review of the evidence for the effectiveness, safety, and cost of acupuncture, massage therapy, and spinal manipulation for back pain. Ann Int Med 138(11): 898, 2003.
35. Licciardone J, Stoll S, Fulda K, et al:. Osteopathic manipulative treatment for chronic low back pain: A randomized controlled trial. Spine 28(13):1355, 2003.
36. Levin SM: The tensegrity-truss as a model for spine mechanics: Biotensegrity. J Mech Med Biol 375, 2002.
37. Van Dillen LR, Sahrmann SA, Norton BJ, et al: The effect of modifying patient-preferred spinal movement and alignment during symptom testing in patients with low back Pain: A preliminary report. Arch Phys Med Rehabil 84(3):313, 2003.
38. Seaman D, Cleveland C: Spinal pain syndromes: Nociceptive, neuropathic, and psychologic mechanisms. J Manipulative Physiol Ther 22(7):462, 1999.
39. Seaman D, Cleveland C: Spinal pain syndromes: Nociceptive, neuropathic, and psychologic mechanisms. J Manipulative Physiol Ther 22(7):467, 1999.
40. AnderssonG, Lucente J, Davis A, et al: A comparison of osteopathic spinal manipulation with standard care for patients with low back pain. N Engl J Med, 341(19):1426,1999.
41. McConnell J: Recalcitrant chronic low back and leg pain—a new theory and different approach to management. Man Therapy 7:183, 2002.
42. Davis CG: Chronic pain/dysfunction in whiplash-associated disorders. J Manipulative Physiol Ther 24:44, 1998.
43. Seaman D, Cleveland C: Spinal pain syndromes: Nociceptive, neuropathic, and psychologic mechanisms. J Manipulative Physiol Ther 22(7):458, 1999.
44. Giles F, Muller R: Chronic spinal pain: A randomized clinical trial comparing medication, acupuncture, and spinal manipulation. Spine 28(14):1490, 2003.
45. Bronfort G, Evans R, Nelson B, et al: A randomized clinical trial of exercise and spinal manipulation for patients with chronic neck pain. Spine 26(7):788, 2001.
46. Evans R, Bronfort G, Nelson B, Goldsmith C: Two-year follow-up of a randomized clinical trial of spinal manipulation and two types of exercise for patients with chronic neck pain. Spine 27(21): 2383, 2002.

47. Bronfort G, Assendelft WJ, Evans R, et al: Efficacy of spinal manipulation for chronic headache: A systematic review. J Manipulative Physiol Ther 24(7):457, 2001.
48. Pellow J, Brantingham J: The efficacy of adjusting the ankle in the treatment of subacute and chronic grade i and grade ii ankle inversion sprains. J Manipulative Physiol Ther 24(1):17, 2001.
49. Ward RC (ed): Foundations for Osteopathic Medicine, 2nd ed. Philadelphia, Lippincott, 2003, p 543.
50. Hawes M, Brooks W: Reversal of the signs and symptoms of moderately severe idiopathic scoliosis in response to physical methods. Res Spinal Deformities 4:365, 2002.
51. Stotz A, Kappler R: The effects of osteopathic manipulative treatment on tender points associated with fibromyalgia. J Am Osteopathic Assoc 92(9):1177, 1992.
52. Lo KS, Kuchera ML, Preston SC, Jackson R: Osteopathic manipulative treatment in fibromyalgia syndrome. J Am Osteopathic Assoc 92(9): 1183, 1992.
53. Gamber R, Shores J, Russo D, et al: Osteopathic manipulative treatment in conjunction with medication relieves pain associated with fibromyalgia syndrome: Results of a randomized clinical pilot project. J Am Osteopathic Assoc 102(6):321, 2002.
54. Davis CG: Chronic pain/dysfunction in whiplash-associated disorder. J Manipulative Physiol Ther 24:44, 1998.

chapter 129

Nociceptors and Peripheral Sources of Pain

Geoffrey M. Bove and Rand S. Swenson

Pain and its relief are critical to all professions dealing with musculoskeletal injuries and diseases. The approach to a patient in pain requires a strong background in the basic concepts of the neurophysiology underlying pain. The concepts presented in this chapter will aid the reader in understanding some reasons that patients seek care for pain and should help provide rationale for clinical intervention.

NOCICEPTORS

Primary Afferent Nociceptors

Nociceptors serve a primordial function for an organism, providing information about harmful or potentially harmful events that may cause loss of function or life. Even simple organisms essentially have nociceptive function. For example, protochordates display the coiling reflex, a withdrawing from a noxious stimulus.[2] Through evolution, this defense mechanism was conserved and refined, although the basic function of signaling harmful events remained unchanged. The importance of nociceptors is revealed in rare cases in which children have been born without nociceptors. These children are constantly being injured and often die of complications of minor infections or trauma. Similarly, rats whose nociceptors have been destroyed by neonatal treatment with capsaicin have a short life span and are always bruised and incautious.

On a moment-to-moment basis, nociceptors signal that a stone that needs removing is in a shoe, that the time to go to the dentist has arrived, or the time has come to shift from a position that may cause a leg to "go to sleep" (possible beginnings of sciatic or peroneal neuropathy). Inflammation causes pain that is perceived, in part, through activity of nociceptors responding to chemical mediators released by the process. In general, nociceptors exist where it makes sense for them to be, which is anywhere that the organism may be subjected to harmful stimuli.

Nociceptors in the peripheral nervous system are pseudo-unipolar dorsal root ganglion neurons with unmyelinated or thinly myelinated axons (Fig. 129–1A). The unmyelinated axons are referred to as C-fibers, with conduction velocities of less than 2.5 m/s. The thinly myelinated axons are referred to as Aδ-fibers, with conduction velocities of 2.5 m/s to approximately 15 m/s.[3] An unfortunate nomenclature exists regarding cutaneous and noncutaneous nociceptors. Cutaneous nociceptors are called C-nociceptors when they have unmyelinated (C-fiber) axons or Aδ-nociceptors when they have thinly myelinated (Aδ-fiber) axons. Nociceptors innervating deep structures such as muscle and joint are called group IV or group III nociceptors. Group IV nociceptors have unmyelinated axons (C-fibers), and group III nociceptors have thinly myelinated axons (Aδ-fibers; see Fig. 129–1B). To make things slightly more complicated, the centrally and peripherally projecting axons from a nociceptor cell body can be of a different caliber, and an individual A-fiber can thin to a C-fiber caliber as it passes distally.[4,5] This terminology is presented in this text because it will be encountered in the literature.

Cutaneous C- and Aδ-nociceptors are typically discussed as subserving slow and fast pain function, respectively. These functions may have some physiologic and clinical differences, with C-nociceptor activity being more likely to give rise to burning or aching sensations and Aδ-nociceptor activation to better-localized, sharp, stabbing, or pricking pain. However, significant overlap in function occurs. Furthermore, this differentiation was determined from studies of cutaneous innervation, and this distinction may not apply to pain in subcutaneous tissues. Although several subcategories of nociceptors exist, a discussion of these is beyond the scope of this text and the reader is referred to excellent reviews by Cervero, Kumazawa, Mense, and Schaible and Grubb.[6-9] For the purposes of this text, all subcategories of nociceptors are considered together under the heading *nociceptor*.

The distal projection of nociceptive neurons terminates in what has historically been called a free-nerve ending. This unfortunate term implies a nonspecialized structure. The anatomic specialization of these terminals remains elusive, especially for C-fiber nociceptors. However, the terminals are sufficiently specialized to discriminate among mechanical, chemical, and thermal stimuli, or they may respond to all these stimuli, depending on the type of nociceptor. The terminals of cutaneous nociceptors usually split into numerous small branches in the skin, yielding one or more very small (<1 mm^2) points on the skin surface at which they respond most strongly. A zone of lesser sensitivity usually surrounds these points. The receptive fields of nociceptors in subcutaneous tissues have similar properties but branch more freely, thereby having more complex receptive fields.[10] These fields

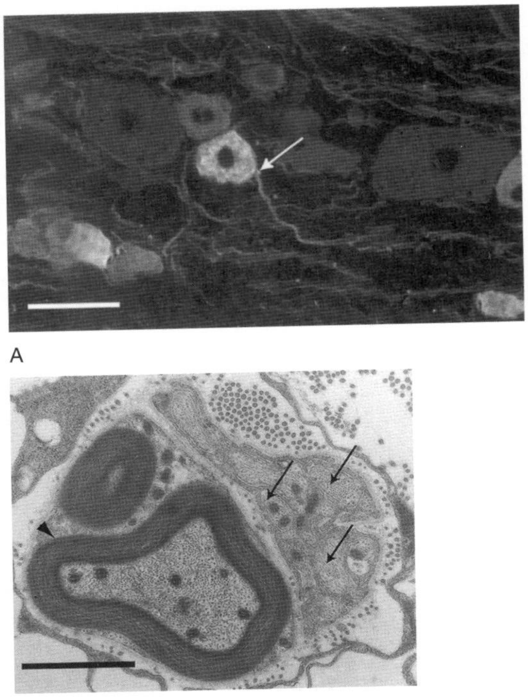

FIGURE 129–1 ■ **A,** Dorsal root ganglion section is labeled with a sodium channel antibody. The single pseudounipolar axon leaves a primary afferent neuron *(arrow)* to branch into peripheral and centrally projecting processes *(not on section).* This axon is approximately 4 mm in diameter and thus classified as an $A\delta$ axon; *scale bar* = 50 mm, section 8 = mm thick. **B,** Electron photomicrograph of a cross section of a nerve branch is demonstrated within the cranial dura mater. Individual C-axons *(arrows)* are less than 1 mm in diameter and are, with their neighbors, combined by one Schwann cell into a Remak bundle. Myelin sheath of an $A\delta$ axon is demonstrated *(arrowhead); scale bar* = 2 mm. (Courtesy of Dr. Andrew Strassman.)

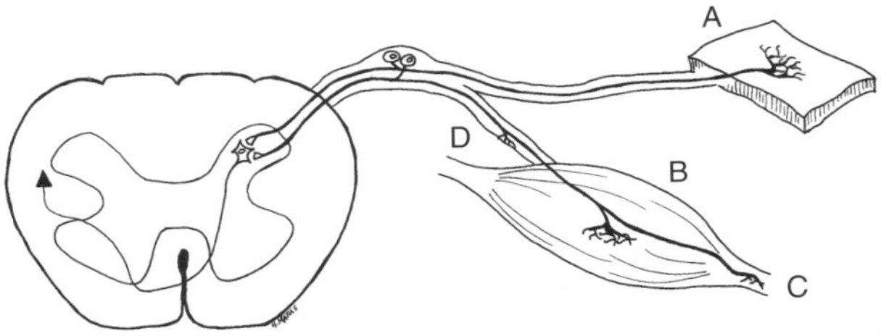

FIGURE 129–2 ■ Schematic of primary afferent neuron innervation pattern. Two neurons are depicted, one innervating skin (A) and the other innervating deep structures. The cutaneous neuron extends to one area of the skin, and the deep neuron branches extend to innervate muscle (B), tendon (C), and even the nerve in which it passes (D). Both neurons are depicted as extending to a single neuron in the dorsal horn, which would be termed a *wide dynamic range neuron.*

could be partially responsible for the relative difficulty in localizing deep, painful stimuli (Fig. 129–2).

As implied by the preceding definitions, the simple anatomic presence of small nerve fibers ending in free-nerve endings does not prove that the structure is a nociceptor; a number of procedures are needed for confirmation, discussed briefly below. It should be kept in mind that axons belonging to the autonomic nervous system are also unmyelinated (C-fiber), but they have purely efferent functions. Afferent fibers that are intermingled with autonomic nerves, such as those accompanying splanchnic nerves, are not part of the autonomic nervous system; they are simply following a convenient path to their innervation target. For the most part, their cell bodies reside in a dorsal root ganglion and they are part of the peripheral nervous system. Some of these neurons are probably nociceptors.

The skin is the largest organ in the body and most subject to external stimuli. It follows that the skin is heavily innervated by nociceptors and by sensory nerve fibers subserving other modalities, such as touch, pressure, and temperature. The densest nociceptive innervation is in the cornea, perhaps pointing to its importance and vulnerability to injury. Muscles, joint capsules, periosteum, and most viscera are also innervated by nociceptors, although less densely. This may be due to the lesser vulnerability of these tissues. Blood vessels are known to have a rich innervation, consisting of somatic afferent and autonomic fibers; indeed, these structures are painful when stimulated.[11] Recently, nerve sheaths and their accompanying blood vessels have been shown to have nociceptive nerve fibers as part of their nervi nervorum (the intrinsic innervation of nerves).[10] Because blood vessels and nerves travel to virtually every tissue in the body, the nervi nervorum may provide a major source of nociceptive input. The paraspinal tissues, including the muscles, joints, and periosteum, are innervated by small-diameter nerve fibers,[12-15] and even small inclusion bodies (intra-articular meniscoids) of the zygapophyseal joint can be innervated.[16]

Small-caliber nerve fibers can be microscopically identified using numerous staining techniques. They can also be labeled using antibodies to various peptide neurotransmitters. Knowledge of the peptide functions provides insight into the function of the cell. However, functional testing using specific stimuli is usually necessary to prove that the nerve fiber or neuron is indeed nociceptive. Knowledge of nociceptors for different tissues varies. For instance, much is known about the nociceptors innervating skin; less is known about subcutaneous and visceral nociceptors. Interestingly, functional information on the innervation of paraspinal tissues is scarce. Only relatively recently have studies shown a substantial nociceptor population, supporting these structures as potential pain sources.[10,12,17]

How Nociceptors Are Studied

Nociceptors can be studied in a variety of ways in humans and animals. In humans, testing can be as simple as applying a stimulus and getting a subjective report from the subject. However, because the stimuli that are known to evoke responses from nociceptors also evoke responses from mechanoreceptors and often thermoreceptors, the results are somewhat nonspecific. Capsaicin, the hot ingredient in peppers, has gained popularity for use in experimental studies because it is fairly specific for activating nociceptors. Numerous studies of the psychophysical parameters of pain have used subdermal injections of capsaicin to activate nociceptor terminals. In animals, the selective response of a nociceptor terminal to application of this chemical has been used as evidence that the receptor is a nociceptor.

Studying the response of individual nociceptors is possible in both animals and humans. In animals, a nerve can be exposed and small nerve filaments (5 to 15 mm) can be carefully teased apart and placed over electrodes connected to amplification and recording devices. This procedure isolates a small population of axons, with the process being repeated until only one neuron or axon is found to be active. The receptive field(s) and sensitivities of this neuron or axon are then determined. In humans, a similar process, called microneurography, can be performed. Fine-needle electrodes are placed into nerves, and the receptive fields of identified axons are characterized. Yet another process in animals uses microelectrodes to record from individual cells in ganglia. In this case, a fine electrode is advanced into the ganglion and used to record the electrical activity of individual cells. Much of the information that follows was gathered using methods similar to these.

Nociceptor Function

In normal, undisturbed tissue, very little (<0.5 Hz) or no activity in nociceptors is usually observed.[18] By definition, nociceptors respond to damaging or potentially damaging stimuli and neurons are characterized as nociceptors if they respond to noxious mechanical, thermal, or chemical stimuli. Various chemical stimuli have been found to activate nociceptors, including components found in the inflammatory milieu, neurotransmitters, and tissue metabolites (Table 129–1).[19] Some of these substances directly activate nociceptors, some only sensitize them to other compounds, and some will only activate nociceptors that have already sustained some injury. These substances have been tested on animal and human nociceptors in a variety of preparations[20] and can evoke discharge from individual nociceptors, cause behavioral changes, and evoke reports of pain. Among the cytokines, the best studied are tumor necrosis factor-α (TNF-α) and interleukin-1b, which are released from numerous cells during immune-mediated inflammation. When injected into the skin, these chemicals are noxious.[21] When TNF-α is placed on a peripheral nerve, nociceptors develop ongoing discharge,[22] and rat feet demonstrate allodynia.[23] Although individual chemicals will elicit responses from varying populations of nociceptors, the combination of mediators found in vivo is most effective.

In diseased or damaged tissue, the properties of nociceptors may change. In a phenomenon called sensitization, they develop ongoing activity, along with a decrease in the thresholds to noxious stimuli and an increase in the size of receptive fields. The effect can occur with even a brief stimulus and can last for hours.[24] In skin, this effect is observed in response to burns, even a small-sized burn. The spontaneous pain and increased sensitivity of the damaged area is mediated by sensitized nociceptors, although other types of receptor may also be active and play a role during injury. Sensitization has been shown to occur in both nociceptors from cutaneous and deep tissues, but the full mechanism of the process remains poorly understood.

Stimulation of sympathetic nerves can affect nociceptors in certain situations. Normally, nociceptors may be sensitized by sympathetic stimulation,[25,26] but they do not directly respond to increased sympathetic activity or to the application of norepinephrine.[27,28] However, during chronic inflammation or after nerve injury, sympathetic stimulation can directly activate C-fiber nociceptors.[29-33] Pain and psychologic stressors increase sympathetic discharge, leading to increased levels of norepinephrine.[34-36] This well-known response provides at least a partial explanation for the clinical observations that reducing psychologic stress responses may decrease pain and facilitate a more rapid recovery.

At the beginning of the 20th century, it was discovered that electrical stimulation of dorsal roots caused cutaneous vasodilation and plasma extravasation whenever the stimulus intensity was high enough to excite unmyelinated fibers.[37] This response was termed the *axon reflex.* Later, this neurally controlled and reflexive release of initiators and inflammatory mediators was termed the *nocifensor system.*[38] More recently, the nerves contributing to the axon reflexes were found to be nociceptors,[39] strongly suggesting that nociceptors have both sensory and efferent functions. Calcitonin gene–related peptide (CGRP) and substance P, which are co-localized in the nociceptor terminal (Fig. 129–3), are the two most important mediators that these nerves release.[40-42] Substance P and CGRP are potent vasodilators, and CGRP potentiates the effects of substance P.[43-48] Moreover, substance P contributes to nociceptor sensitization[49] and is thought to participate in the immune response.[50] Electrical stimulation of nociceptor axons anywhere along their course will cause the release of these peptides from distal terminals, resulting in a focal inflammation, termed *neurogenic inflammation.*

Nociceptors may be essential for an animal to mount an inflammatory response through neurogenic inflammation. For example, it has been shown that the development of peripheral experimental arthritis is at least in part dependent on the presence of afferent innervation.[51] Additionally, the severity of experimental arthritis is reduced in animals depleted of nociceptors through neonatal injection of capsaicin.[52] Finally, the increased cerebral blood flow as a result of meningitis is greatly attenuated by denervation of the primary afferents innervating the intracranial structures.[53] These lines of

Table 129–1

Chemical Sensitivities of Nociceptors

Substance	*Source*	*Effect on Nociceptor*
Acid and potassium	Damaged cells	Activation and sensitization
Prostaglandins	Damaged cells	Sensitization
Leukotrienes	Damaged cells	Sensitization
Bradykinin	Plasma kininogen	Activation
Histamine	Mast cells	Activation
Tumor necrosis factor-α	Immune cells	Activation and sensitization
Serotonin	Platelets (neurotransmitter)	Activation
Substance P	Nociceptors	Sensitization

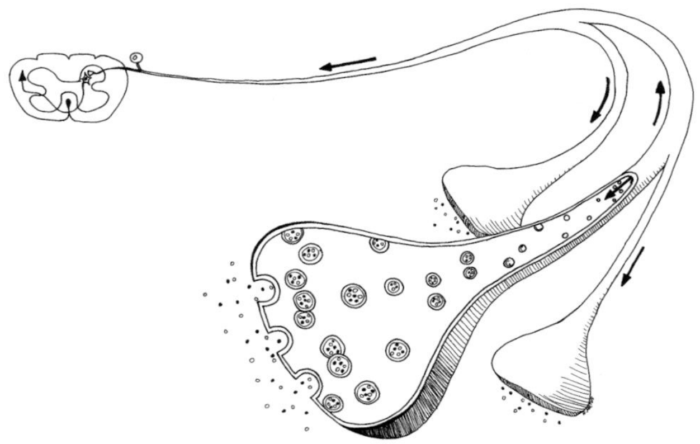

FIGURE 129–3 ■ Release of substance P and calcitonin gene–related peptide (CGRP) by primary afferent nociceptors. When an appropriate stimulation elicits an action potential, the action potential is propagated to the central nervous system and to other branches of the neuron *(arrows)*. Simultaneously, the endings release substance P and CGRP *(small closed and open symbols)* from the terminals, which are co-localized in vesicles that are transported from the cell body. This process is thought to occur in terminals that are invaded by the action potential even when they are not directly stimulated. Substance P and CGRP cause plasma extravasation and vasodilation, respectively, which are necessary components of the inflammatory response. This process is termed *neurogenic inflammation.*

evidence support a critical role of nociceptors in the organism's response to injury.

Although the role of nociceptors in neurogenic inflammation is undisputed, less is known about the role of the sympathetic nervous system in this process. However, sympathetic nerves are clearly important to the generation of experimental immune arthritis. They are also known to participate in the localized edema that occurs in certain models of chronic neuropathic pain. This participation may explain why stressful situations may exacerbate inflammatory conditions and increase pain.

Differences between Deep and Cutaneous Nociceptors

Although most studies of nociceptors have been performed on skin, few clinically important pain conditions exist that primarily affect the skin. Even among conditions felt in the skin, most are neuropathic (the term *neuropathic* refers to a nerve pathology or functional disturbance of a nerve or some axons within a nerve) and may not involve cutaneous nociceptors at all. Cutaneous neuropathic pain is very possibly mediated by sensitization of neurons that are normally not responsive to noxious stimuli, such as neurons that respond to light touch. Recently, we interviewed 25 people with diagnoses of lumbar radiculopathy (i.e., radiating pain due to a pathology of one or more dorsal roots). The participants were asked to identify the perceived location of the radiating leg pain. In every case, the pain at rest and the pain evoked during a straight-leg raising test were reported to be "deep" rather than "on the skin." Thus studies of cutaneous nociceptors may not be fully applicable to deep nociceptors. Indeed, studies that have compared nociceptor sensitivity by innervated structure have shown critical differences. The response to pinch was found to be dramatically greater after a stimulus delivered to a muscle nerve rather than to a cutaneous nerve.[54] Deep nociceptor axons also seem to respond differently to inflammation. During neuritis, or nerve inflammation, axons of deep nociceptors become mechanically sensitive whereas cutaneous nociceptor axons do not.[55] The percentage of deep nociceptors that develop ongoing activity during neuritis is also greater than their cutaneous counterparts. After axonal damage, recordings from nociceptors in muscle nerves reveal ongoing discharge more often than do recordings from cutaneous neurons.[56,57] These data point to fundamental differences in deep versus cutaneous nociceptor physiology.

Neuronal Response to Injury

When their peripheral axons are injured, the central projections of myelinated and unmyelinated dorsal root neurons can sprout into wider territories in the spinal cord.[58,59] The sprouting of presumably nociceptive terminals in the superficial dorsal horn could explain hyperalgesia, because the discharge of an individual sensory axon would be transmitted to more second-order neurons, with their sum predictably leading to an increased perception of pain. The sprouting of larger fibers, usually non-nociceptive, into the laminae (layers) of the spinal cord, which is usually reserved for nociceptor input, may explain allodynia, because their discharge may now activate nociceptive neurons. Indeed, possibly the allodynia that often accompanies chronic regional pain syndromes is mediated by myelinated fibers.[60,61]

Spinal Cord Projections of Nociceptors

Nociceptive dorsal root ganglion neurons project into the dorsolateral portion of the spinal cord where they branch T-wise, sending branches 1 through 5 segments rostral and caudal (1 to 2 for C-fiber nociceptors, 1 through 5 for Aδ-nociceptors).[62] The region of the spinal cord white matter located adjacent to the dorsal horn that contains these ascending and descending fibers has been termed *Lissauer's zone.* C-fiber nociceptors ultimately terminate in the dorsal horn in the most dorsal part of the dorsal horn, termed *laminae I and II,*[63] whereas Aδ-nociceptors additionally project to laminae V and X.[64] Most dorsal horn neurons are classified as wide dynamic range, which means they respond to both noxious and innocuous stimuli, with more intense and widespread stimuli producing greater activation (see Fig. 129–2). A smaller percentage of dorsal horn neurons, particularly located within the most superficial laminae of the dorsal horn, are nociceptive specific. It is believed that the nociceptive-specific neurons are more important to signal the presence of pain and its precise location whereas the wide dynamic range neurons are more important to the recognition of intensity of pain. Nociceptors from the limbs terminate ipsilaterally. However, paraspinal tissue nociceptors project bilaterally to dorsal horn neurons.[65,66] This projection predicts the typically poorly defined nature of back pain and emphasizes the need for bilateral spinal examination.

Molecular Changes in the Spinal Cord Related to Nociception

When nociceptors are stimulated, their central terminals release substance P, CGRP, and glutamate onto spinal cord neurons. Besides transmitting information to these high-order neurons, genes in second- and higher-order neurons increase their expression of some proteins. With even a brief stimulus, some genes are known to be upregulated. The c-*fos* and c-*jun* genes have been intensely studied, and their protein products can be visualized indirectly using immunohistochemical techniques. Studies using these techniques have confirmed the projection of the nociceptive primary afferents, although the stimuli used are not usually specific for nociceptors.[67-69]

The protein products of c-*fos* and c-*jun* initiate a cascade of biochemical reactions in the neurons, resulting in the production of enkephalins and dynorphin (endogenous opiates) in the central nervous system (CNS) (see the following text).[70] Enkephalin is an inhibitor of dorsal horn cells, but dynorphin is known to have variable responses, inhibiting one third of neurons, sensitizing one third of neurons, and increasing the receptive fields of many spinal cord neurons.[71] This effect could also contribute to hyperalgesia and to chronic pain, as well as to their modulation.

The generation of neuronal action potentials requires the opening and closing of numerous ion channels. An electrical charge passing through these channels changes the membrane potential; and if this is changed enough, the neuron will generate an action potential (for details, see any neurophysiology text). Alteration in the number and type of ion channels will change the resting potential and excitability of the neuron. For instance, an increase of tonically open sodium channels or a decrease of tonically open potassium channels would be expected to depolarize the membrane. A depolarized membrane requires less additional depolarization to induce an action potential; a neuron that had such changes in ion channels could be considered facilitated.

Evidence is building that in pathologic states, dorsal root ganglion cells undergo numerous changes in the expression of ion channels, especially sodium channels. Sodium channel expression has been reported to change after axonal injury and during inflammation (reviewed by Waxman and associates[72]), and some of these channels have also been linked to pain.[73-76] Increased cation channel production may lead to increased insertion in axonal membranes and axonal hyperexcitability. Such changes were proposed to account for the recovery of mechanical sensitivity in the tips of previously cut mechanoreceptive axons.[77,78] Increased cation channel production was also proposed to lead to ongoing activity in sensory neurons from muscle, but not from skin, after damage to neighboring axons.[57]

Central Mechanisms Related to Nociception

Nociceptors are not the only neurons active in response to painful stimuli. In a classic study, Adriaensen and colleagues[79] demonstrated that sustained pinch of the skin led to increasing reports of pain with time whereas the neural discharge from nociceptors supplying the area actually decreased. Explaining this paradox is difficult, but other nociceptors are probably recruited and the spinal cord and higher centers are changing their "gain" (i.e., amplifying the signal) in response to the input from the nociceptors.

Substantial evidence suggests that peripheral noxious stimulation leads to changes in the CNS, collectively called spinal cord plasticity (for reviews, see Coderre,[80] Woolf,[81] and Chen and coworkers[82]). These changes lead to sensitization of CNS neurons and may result in hyperalgesia, allodynia, and spontaneous discharge of neurons. Under some conditions, these symptoms may be sustained even if the sensory input from the original source is terminated. All of the characteristics of stimuli that are capable of producing these changes are not yet known, although some experimental models, such as ligating the sciatic nerve, readily produce long-term sensory facilitation. Additionally, because spinal cord neurons have receptive fields that converge from many tissue types (sometimes bilaterally),[65] allodynia and hyperalgesia may be perceived very broadly from uninjured and even rather remote tissues. Indeed, these symptoms are observed among the plethora of acute and chronic back pain presentations; CNS plasticity could help explain these variable presentations.

Concepts of Plasticity

The principal concepts of spinal cord plasticity include wind-up, long-term potentiation (LTP), and long-term depression (LTD). A brief presentation of these processes follows, and further details can be found in a review by Pockett.[83] *Wind-up* is a term that was coined for the phenomenon of increasing the response of a spinal cord neuron to repeated stimuli.[84] When depolarized by the primary afferent neuron, dorsal horn neurons do not always fully recover their resting potential before the arrival of another volley from the primary afferent neuron. Therefore, the threshold for firing of the neuron is lower (facilitated). This process typically lasts seconds to minutes. LTP is similar to wind-up, but it lasts much longer; indeed, some consider LTP to be permanent. This process requires a high-frequency conditioning discharge from the primary afferent neuron[85] and results in increased synaptic efficiency mediated by activation of a specific type of glutamate receptor, the *N*-methyl-D-aspartate (NMDA) receptor. It differs from wind-up in that the increased synaptic efficiency is not related to a change in the resting membrane potential of the postsynaptic cells; rather, it involves complicated changes within the postsynaptic dorsal horn neurons that can best be described as a type of memory. For example, there are changes in postsynaptic receptor properties and possibly numbers.[86] These changes are accompanied by alterations in the expression of messenger RNA, as well as in the expression of specific gene products. Once established, there is nothing known that will reverse LTP except the induction of LTD. LTD can be established by both high- and low-frequency conditioning stimuli, and it involves a long-lasting decrease in synaptic efficacy (thus it is the mirror image of LTP). Repeated episodes of wind-up may possibly induce LTP or LTD, but this response has not been studied.

Hypothetically, LTP is at least partially responsible for chronic pain; and, if so, LTD induction by stimulating an appropriate nerve may relieve it.[83] This mechanism may be behind the anecdotal effectiveness of various forms of clinical electrical stimulation, but it remains to be demonstrated.

Several additional mechanisms may be important to the changes that occur in the sensitivity of spinal cord pathways in pain syndromes. For example, the expression of inflammatory cytokines by the glial cells of the spinal cord increase during an experimental model of nerve injury.[87] Indeed, the interactions between the two great communication systems in the body, the immune system and the nervous system, are substantially more complex and bidirectional than had been previously appreciated.[88,89] However, it must be remembered that the role of long-term changes that occur after experimental injuries and, indeed, whether they occur in clinical problems in humans remains to be determined. However, painful stimuli can have potent and long-lasting effects on the functions in the spinal cord and other levels of the nervous system.

Descending Modulation of Nociception

The ability to perceive pain is critical to the survival and general well-being of the individual. However, it is also important to be able to modulate pain. An example taken from common experience is the ability to "shake off" an injury that produces severe tissue damage until any immediate threat is past. At that time the pain may become severe or even immobilizing, although the injury itself has not changed. What, then, explains this ability to modulate pain transmission and processing?

The earliest hints as to the mechanisms behind pain modulation arose from studies of the most potent pain-suppressing drugs, the opiates.[90] Receptors for opiates have been localized to several brain regions (notably periaqueductal gray [PAG], dorsal horn of the spinal cord, ventral medullary raphe nuclei, and basal ganglia). Electrical stimulation of some of these regions (notably the PAG and raphe nuclei) was found to inhibit nociceptive responses in animals and produce analgesia in humans.[91]

Of course, the presence of these receptors begs the question of why the nervous system would have specific receptors (opiate receptors) for an exogenous compound (opium) derived from a Middle Eastern poppy. Investigation of this question led to the discovery of a group of transmitters contained in small interneurons that bind to these receptors and activate them. These "endogenous opiates" consist of a family of very small peptides (enkephalins) that are synthesized in small neurons of the CNS, as well as a larger compound (endorphin) that is found in the region of the pituitary gland and is released into the circulation. Injection of these compounds into portions of the nervous system that have opiate receptors produces powerful analgesia. As previously discussed, these compounds are also directly produced by spinal cord neurons after intense activity of primary afferent neurons.

It became apparent that some of the enkephalin neurons directly inhibit the pain transmission neurons in the dorsal horn of the spinal cord. For example, intense nociceptive input results in the release of enkephalin from the dorsal horn, providing at least a partial explanation for the inhibition of pain that can occur shortly after the onset of a powerful noxious stimulus. However, that does not adequately explain the role of opiates at the level of the PAG, because the endogenous opiate-containing neurons do not have axons that leave the PAG and also because the PAG does not have direct neuronal connection with the pain pathway. Further investigation revealed that the influence of PAG on pain transmission is rather complex, involving excitatory projections from the PAG to the caudal medulla. These projections, in turn, excite descending projections to the dorsal horn that release norepinephrine and serotonin from their terminals in the spinal cord dorsal horn.

Norepinephrine and serotonin, called monoamine transmitters, have complex effects at the dorsal horn, both by directly affecting the pain transmission neurons and by activating other neurons at the spinal level (e.g., small enkephalinergic interneurons). Of course, in understanding this system the regions that connect with and thereby influence the PAG became important considerations. Many brain regions connect with the PAG, including the frontal and insular cortex, amygdala, hypothalamus, reticular formation, locus ceruleus, and collateral branches of the spinothalamic tract. This connection illustrates the diverse brain regions that can play a part in regulating pain transmission. This descending system, based on the endogenous opiates and monoamines, has become the best-known inhibitory circuit for pain modulation. It defines the analgesic effects of opiates, such as morphine, but it also explains at least some of the role that serotonin and norepinephrine play in pain control. Despite the fact that descending inhibition is the best characterized of all pain-suppression mechanisms (notwithstanding the known effects of various drugs on this system), less well known mechanisms are other physiologic factors that are capable of activating this potent pain-suppression mechanism.

Although, undoubtedly, endogenous opiates play a powerful role in controlling pain, other inhibitory systems are also found in the nervous system. For example, γ-aminobutyric acid (GABA) is the most common inhibitory neurotransmitter in the CNS.[92] Activation of GABAergic interneurons appears to be at least one important mechanism of analgesia provoked by the stimulation of large-diameter sensory nerve fibers (e.g., proprioceptive nerve fibers).[93] Glycine, another neurotransmitter, has a significant inhibitory influence at the spinal cord level with at least some of its effect produced by inhibition of excitatory neurotransmission through NMDA receptors.[94] This effect may be important not only in inhibiting the initial signal but also in preventing the kind of LTP that can accompany activation of NMDA receptors. Recent studies have shown that activation of spinal facet joint receptors can powerfully inhibit the reflex effects of noxious stimulation of the spine.[95] Although the mechanisms of this inhibition are not known, the inhibitory transmitters in the spinal cord represent prime candidates for investigation.

Psychology and Nociception

Why is it that two individuals can be injured in exactly the same manner, with dramatically different results (at least in terms of pain and suffering)? Although, undoubtedly, some of these different results are caused by the differences in the peripheral pain systems and the pain transmission systems in the CNS, the experience of pain goes well beyond the mere activation of a nociceptor and the conduction of an impulse to the cerebral cortex.

Pain is defined as an unpleasant sensory and emotional experience. In addition, the issue of suffering, which is the behavioral and psychologic component that is reflected in the patient's outward affect, is expressed. The patient typically describes his or her suffering as the consequence of the painful disorder. Although all of the mechanisms involved in suffering or in the psychologic ramifications of pain are not understood, several lines of evidence indicate that the frontal lobes of the cerebral cortex are critical in this regard. The first hints of this conclusion arose from the clinical evaluation of patients with frontal lobe injuries and those who had been subjected to frontal lobectomy. Patients with frontal lobe damage can describe the intensity of a painful stimulus, indicating that the principal transmission pathways are intact; however, they do not appear to suffer in proportion to the degree of pain. In such patients, both behavioral and autonomic responses to pain are blunted. Evidence suggests that some of the analgesic effects of some sedatives and antianxiety drugs may have their primary effect at the level of the frontal lobe rather than (or in addition to) affecting pain transmission through nociceptive pathways.

Other lines of investigation have also directed attention to areas of the frontal lobe. These include experimental pain models that have been shown on functional MRI to activate selectively specific portions of the frontal lobes.[96] Additionally, it has been shown that patients with pain who were effectively hypnotized to block the unpleasantness, but not the intensity, of their pain showed changes in the anterior cingulate cortex (i.e., the medial portion of the frontal lobe).[97] It is interesting to note that similar areas of the medial frontal lobes, particularly in the areas of the anterior cingulate and subcallosal gyri, have been shown to be metabolically altered in certain affective disorders, particularly depression. It is well known that a complex interaction between depression and pain exists, and it would appear that at least some physiologic basis for this interaction is evident. Although much has been written about the capacity of depression to magnify pain, some evidence also suggests that effective treatment of chronic pain is capable of ameliorating depression.[98]

Most of the interest in cortical mechanisms of pain has been focused on the issue of suffering rather than pain perception, and there is reason to believe that behavioral factors might have some influence over pain transmission as well. For example, several studies indicate that placebo analgesia is real and is probably mediated via endogenous opiate mechanisms.[99] Certainly, the connections between the frontal cortex and PAG (among other places) might provide the substrate for this effect, although the precise mechanisms remain unknown. Overall, there is good reason to believe that cortical mechanisms play a role in analgesia, and excellent evidence suggests that suffering is a cortical phenomenon that is largely based in the frontal lobes. These findings provide some theoretical underpinning for behavioral interventions in pain management.

SOURCES OF PAIN

Local Tissue Damage

Of course, local tissue damage can lead to pain through direct activation of the peripheral nervous system. Acute activation is usually secondary to direct activation of nociceptor terminals. Persistent pain can be the result of continued direct activation, the result of chemical excitation by inflammatory mediators, or, in some cases, maintained at least in part by the CNS.

A few common sources of somatic pain need mentioning. First, the intervertebral disk has been blamed for most spinal pain, usually secondary to its ability to compress nerve roots when herniated. However, compression alone is not painful, and patients can recover from so-called compressive radiculopathy without resolution of the compression.[100] The source of pain is inflammation induced by the diskal pathology; when the inflammation subsides with healing, the pain also subsides. The inner part of the intervertebral disk is called the nucleus pulposus and contains TNF-α.[101] When released from the disk, this substance promotes an immune-mediated inflammation, which generates more local noxious chemicals. Persistent pain from diskal herniation probably means that the disk is still releasing noxious material, maintaining sufficient inflammation to sensitize the nociceptors in the neighboring tissues. Additionally, in older people the nucleus pulposus dries and therefore cannot herniate; consequently, the prevalence of disk-related pain also decreases with age.

Chronic muscle pain also presents a problem. Two familiar incidences of muscle insult that lead to pain are considered: (1) injury as a result of excessive stretch during a vehicular accident and (2) pain after the overload of muscle during unaccustomed exercise. Although the acute stretch during a vehicular accident is at least transiently painful, pain during unaccustomed exercise is not common. In both cases, symptoms start within 12 to 24 hours and render the muscle allodynic. Why, then, does the pain of an injury often persist whereas the pain after exercise resolves rapidly and without incident? In the case of accidental injury, nerves are damaged through stretch. In the case of normal exercises, nerve injuries are far less likely to occur. This major difference between these two scenarios appears to be the cause of the different results. Afferent activity of damaged or even intact but injured axons would be perceived as coming from the target muscle. This could even be responsible for maintaining a low-grade inflammation in the region through the neurogenic mechanisms previously outlined. We propose that persistent pain probably requires a source of persistent nociceptor activity called a peripheral generator.

Indeed, many cases of persistent severe pain will follow nerve injuries, especially stretch injuries. Although a complicated layering of connective tissues protects the axons within nerves, the nerves can be damaged by direct trauma or stretch. (For further reading, see Sunderland.[102]) Such damage leads to mechanical, chemical, and thermal sensitivity at the cut and regrowing terminal. However, it is not necessary for the axon to be completely interrupted for axonal injury and inflammation to lead to action potential generation.

Radiating Pain Mechanisms

Nerve injury and inflammation result in the perception of radiating pain (radicular pain, if the nerve roots are involved). Neurobiology texts present sensory neurons as having a transducer or receptor in the periphery, an axon, a cell body, another axon, and a synaptic terminal in the spinal cord (Fig. 129–4A). The axons are presented as simple electrical conduits. Normal sensation occurs when the transducer is sufficiently stimulated by touch, generating, for example, an action potential that is propagated to the spinal cord for possible transmission to higher centers. If perceived, the sensation will be in the area of the original transducer.

When the axon has been cut, no possibility of action potential conduction is left from the transducer. The regenerating tip of the severed axon can become chemically and mechanically sensitive. Touching this tip will generate action potentials (see Fig. 129–4C). These action potentials will be perceived as coming from the tissue that contains the now dead transducer, because the signal will follow pathways

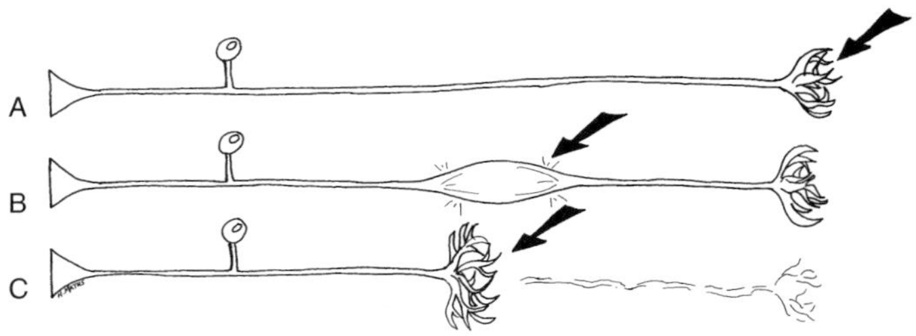

FIGURE 129–4 ■ **A,** Typical representation of primary afferent neuron, with *(right to left)* a receptor, a peripherally projecting axon, the cell body, a centrally projecting axon, and a terminal in the dorsal horn of the spinal cord. Sufficient stimuli of the receptor lead to the generation of action potentials, which are propagated along the axon to the central nervous system. **B,** The axon is an alternate source of action potential generation for slowly conducting neurons innervating deep tissues. Importantly, any sensation arising from stimulation of the axon at such a sensitive site will be perceived as coming from the distal receptive area, not from the site of action potential generation. **C,** A damaged and regrowing axon is another source of action potentials. If numerous axons are cut, the regrowth can cause a mass called a neuroma. Regrowing axons are very sensitive to chemical and mechanical stimuli. As in **B,** sensations arising from such stimuli would also be perceived as coming from the innervated tissue.

that originally conducted impulses from that tissue. This mechanism is the likely cause of "phantom" sensations that often follow limb amputation. The only exception would be if the nervous system reorganizes to accommodate the amputation. More recently, it has been shown that at least some injured axons can develop ongoing activity and mechanical sensitivity without interrupting their normal conduction, secondary to inflammation (see Fig. 129–4B).

Neurons thus have two potential sources of action potential generation: their receptors in the innervated tissue and their axon. It is critical to remember that activity generated at either site will be perceived as coming from the tissue innervated and will probably be difficult or impossible for the patient to distinguish. Such ectopic activity can also arise in injured axons in the dorsal root ganglion and will be similarly perceived as coming from the innervated tissue. For example, inflammation within the intervertebral foramen or TNF-α applied to the dorsal root ganglion causes hyperalgesia of the foot as well as ongoing activity localized to the dorsal root ganglia.[103,104] These data further support that the radiating or projected pain associated with diskal herniation probably arises as a result of ectopic activity of the dorsal roots or ganglia and therefore is not referred.

Referred Pain Mechanisms

A common human experience is the perception of pain radiating into the scapula, posterior head, or upper limb after pressure over so-called trigger points in the muscles of the shoulder girdle. Of course, if this pressure were to be placed on nerve trunks (e.g., upper brachial plexus), the explanation would have to consider radiating pain as described in the preceding section.

However, because most of the stimuli that produce such pain do not directly activate the nerve trunks projecting to these areas, what can explain this perception of pain? Referred pain is the perception of pain in locations other than the site of generation and not localized to the distribution of a damaged nerve.[105] It is a direct result of activation of nociceptive endings in somatic tissues or internal organs. The process depends on the activation of nociceptors that project to the wide dynamic range neurons that receive highly convergent input from the many sites that make input to that particular part of the spinal cord. These projection neurons seem to be primarily designed to relate the intensity rather than the location of a painful stimulus. Typically, the nervous system relies on other clues as to the origin of pain and, in the absence of adequate clues, often "paints" the pain on the body in a manner that may be at some distance from the actual site of pain generation. Because activity in the wide dynamic range neurons is usually perceived as a deep aching or burning sensation, referred pain is rarely sharp, even though it can be both intense and very unpleasant. Additionally, it is not well localized and has indistinct borders that overlap the distribution of several nerves and nerve roots.

■ CLINICAL RELEVANCE

Lumbar Facet Syndrome

The preceding sections have described physiologic mechanisms for the initiation and maintenance of nociception and pain. However, how are these principles relevant to a patient's condition? This section describes how these mechanisms may apply to a common clinical condition, the lumbar facet syndrome.

Lumbar facet syndrome is described as a sprain of the zygapophyseal joints and can be either acute or chronic. The acute form can follow an excessive movement in any plane or combination of planes of motion and more likely involves pinching or excessive stretching of the articular capsule. Although this structure is relatively small, why can the pain be hard to localize and difficult to manage?

Assuming that the injury is restricted to the left L5-S1 joint and is, in fact, from pinching of the joint capsule itself or an intra-articular meniscoid arising from the capsule, the joint capsules are innervated by nociceptors,[17,66] which respond to noxious mechanical stimulation with a high-frequency discharge. This injury leads to mast cell degranulation, releasing histamine that can amplify the neural response and can also lead to the recruitment of macrophages to clear the damaged tissue. Macrophages produce a multitude of proinflammatory cytokines that can directly elicit discharges from nociceptors and their axons.[22] The activated primary afferent neurons release substance P and CGRP into the surrounding tissue. The end result is an inflammatory reaction in the joint and perhaps in other surrounding tissues. Increased concentrations of noxious chemicals and reduced pH, which are also effective stimuli for nociceptors, are also present in the inflammatory milieu.[106]

At the same time, nociceptors that have been damaged or sensitized may now respond to products of increased sympathetic activity; indeed, the inflammation may be affecting the sympathetic axons directly, although no data exist to support this possibility. These pain fibers relay through nociceptive specific neurons in the dorsal horn of the spinal cord (to signal the presence and location of pain) and through wide dynamic range neurons (to signal its intensity). Although the majority of pain will be felt in the region and on the side of the injured facet, the divergence of nociceptive afferent input over several spinal cord segments and the bilateral input of some nociceptors from axial tissues, such as paraspinal muscles and zygapophyseal joints, will mean that the aching component of pain will probably be perceived over a broader area.

The preceding scenario describes the generation of acute pain after a noxious incident. However, in the absence of continued or maintained noxious input, the inflammation is expected to subside and the injury is expected to heal. Indeed, in most cases, the acute injury and pain do resolve. Subsequently, why do many patients have what appears to be chronic facet syndrome with the addition of other typically poorly defined symptoms extending to other areas? Two possible explanations exist, explanations that are not mutually exclusive. First, the symptoms may continue because of continued activity of the nociceptor. This explanation would imply some ongoing mechanical or inflammatory process that continually irritates the nociceptor. In this case, the job of the clinician is to determine the peripheral generator of the afferent discharge and to do whatever is necessary to reduce or terminate the neuronal activity. This might occur if the joint capsule was being intermittently impinged upon by bony structures, with movement reinforcing or worsening the damage. Interventions that remove the impingement would be expected to remove the source of afferent discharge, allowing the inflammation and the pain to subside. One possible mechanism of action of spinal adjustment and manipulation is the removal of such impingements.

Second, and more problematic, would be the persistence of pain symptoms in the apparent absence of afferent discharge. In this case, the practitioner is always urged to continue the search for a peripheral generator, because this represents the more easily correctable problem. Only after a diligent search should it be assumed that the central pain transmission pathways have been facilitated and are now responsible for the prolonged pain. Persistent pain, hyperesthesia, or allodynia would be expected if LTP had resulted in prolonged sensitization. Unfortunately, no available diagnostic tests are currently available to determine the role of such central mechanisms in pain. When all other options have been exhausted, the clinician may have to rely on the previously described (and clinically hypothetical) mechanisms to explain the persistence of symptoms. However, it is proposed that spinal adjustment and manipulation may be an effective source of high-frequency neural discharge that could conceivably reverse LTP.

As previously discussed, nociceptor activity stimulates neurons in the CNS; otherwise, there would be no perception at all. The innervation of the facet joint in question is predominantly through the posterior ramus of the spinal nerve from L4-S1, although there is some evidence from animal studies for even greater spread via sensory fibers that follow lumbar sympathetic nerves. The nociceptive nerve fibers likely synapse with neurons over at least the cord levels L2-S2, with most but certainly not all terminating in the ipsilateral spinal cord dorsal horn. This anatomy has two possible effects: (1) spinal cord neurons receive convergent input from many structures, contributing to poor localization of the pain; and (2) axon reflexes may be propagated to any tissue innervated by these levels. As mentioned, these axon reflexes cause the release of substance P and CGRP by antidromic mechanisms, with the development of at least some degree of neurogenic inflammation. Paraspinal, gluteal, and even leg pain are common and might be explained by these mechanisms in cases in which facet joint syndrome is diagnosed.

These two theories of chronic pain are often regarded as mutually exclusive, and a great deal of controversy remains regarding the relative importance of ongoing nociceptor activation versus plastic changes in pain systems in chronic pain. However, these theories are not mutually exclusive and, even in cases with clear sensitization of the CNS, evidence also typically suggests ongoing peripheral impulse generation.[107] Importantly, until the processes of sensitization are clearly understood and until such time as there are methods for expediting the reversal of such sensitization, therapy will be predominantly directed at the peripheral pain generators. To the extent that central sensitization has occurred, slower improvement in the condition would, of course, be anticipated.

Diagnosis of the facet syndrome is based, at least partially, on orthopedic testing. Orthopedic tests are simple motions that are designed to isolate particular tissues to determine whether these tissues are responsible for the symptom. In the case of pain, the test is considered positive if it reproduces the pain. (*Note:* Production of a new or different pain does not help in the diagnosis.) Unfortunately, in the case of the spine, no motions isolate a single tissue. Therefore, orthopedic tests of the spine must be carefully interpreted. Nonetheless, in the case of the patient with facet syndrome, motions that place a load or a stretch on the injured joint would be likely to reproduce the pain, aiding in diagnosis. However, it must be remembered that if significant facilitation of pain pathways exists, activation of sensory nerve fibers that are not nociceptive may be capable of provoking pain by the mechanisms previously described for allodynia. By this mechanism, the initial injury may have left the patient with hypersensitive tissues and normally innocuous movements could reinitiate or aggravate the processes, which gives further justification for care in interpreting orthopedic tests, particularly in patients with severe or chronic pain.

Despite pain with movement, not all movements are bad. For example, substantial evidence suggests that stimulating mechanoreceptors inhibits nociceptor activity, at least in the acute situation. Therefore, movement may be beneficial to the control of pain. In addition, movements that place normal stresses on an injured tissue are important for directing the proper orientation of collagen tissue during repair. Such interventions could include spinal adjustment and manipulation, mobilization, and exercise.

Neurogenic Inflammation

The issue of neurogenic inflammation as a factor prolonging pain is not settled, particularly in the deeper tissues that are less accessible to direct observation. Nonetheless, neurogenic inflammation is probably important in many cases of prolonged pain, as witnessed by the number of patients who receive at least some relief from powerful antiinflammatory medications. Historically, some changes in tissue texture and consistency and in temperature and sweating patterns associated with various musculoskeletal lesions (e.g., vertebral subluxation complex) have been observed. At least some of these observations could be explained by neurogenic inflammation. However, this process would require significantly more investigation before anything more than speculative explanations could be offered.

UNANSWERED QUESTIONS ABOUT CHRONIC PAIN

The previous sequence of events describes the pain-dysfunction cycles so often used to illustrate musculoskeletal disease processes. It is thought that clinical efforts directed at breaking these cycles will help the patient's recovery. However, most musculoskeletal injuries do get better on their own, probably through the gradual spontaneous resolution of the events described. One major problem with this theory is that it does not explain the significant population of musculoskeletal pain sufferers with chronic pain in the absence of detectable pathology. In many cases these patients are thought to have suffered permanent plastic changes in their CNS, leading to the perception of spontaneous pain thought to be originating from a peripheral site. However, it seems likely that in the majority of cases there is at least some persistent peripheral pathology that has remained undetected and maintains the peripheral noxious input and associated pain. It also seems likely that the persistent peripheral generator is arising from damaged nerve tissue.

CONCLUSION

Pain and nociception are related but different events. The neural events leading to pain usually involve activation of nociceptors innervating a threatened or damaged tissue. Once activated, nociceptors transmit information to the spinal cord for processing and may also participate in the generation of the inflammatory reaction. The response properties of nociceptors are plastic, and they can become sensitized by continued stimulation. This sensitization also occurs in the CNS, evidenced by the development of wind-up and LTP. Several mechanisms in the CNS can suppress pain transmission. These have been best studied at the level of the spinal cord, although similar mechanisms probably exist at higher levels, such as the thalamus. The high degree of convergence of nociceptors from various parts of the body on projection neurons in the spinal cord provides a substrate for referred pain. Additionally, axon reflexes from nociceptive neurons are capable of producing neurogenic inflammation in tissues that are not involved in the initial injury. The neural basis for the affective (emotional) components of pain and suffering are localized to the frontal lobes, in areas known to be affected in depression and anxiety disorders. This is the physiologic substrate for the common and complex clinical interaction between pain and mood.

Acknowledgment

This chapter was excerpted from Bove GM, Swenson RS: Nociceptors, Pain, and Chiropractic. In Redwood D, Cleveland CS III (eds): Fundamentals of Chiropractic. St. Louis, Mosby, 2005, with permission.

References

1. Merskey H, Bogduk N: Classification of Chronic Pain. Seattle, IASP, 1994.
2. Carew TJ, Wallers ET, Candel ER: Classical conditioning in a simple withdrawal reflex in *Aplysia californica*. J Neurosci 1:1426, 1981.
3. Lawson SN: Phenotype and function of somatic primary afferent nociceptive neurones with C- A delta- or A alpha/beta-fibres. Exp Physiol 87:239, 2002.
4. Duclaux R, Mei N, Ranieri F: Conduction velocity along the afferent vagal dendrites: A new type of fiber. J Physiol 260:487, 1976.
5. Morrison JFB: Splanchnic slowly adapting mechanoreceptors with punctate receptive fields in the mesentery and gastrointestinal tract of the cat. J Physiol 233:349, 1973.
6. Cervero F: Sensory innervation of the viscera: Peripheral basis of visceral pain. Physiol Rev 74:95, 1994.
7. Kumazawa T: Functions of the nociceptive primary neurons. Jpn J Physiol 40:1, 1990.
8. Mense S: Nociception from skeletal muscle in relation to clinical pain. Pain 54:241, 1993.
9. Schaible HG, Grubb BD: Afferent and spinal mechanisms of joint pain. Pain 55:5, 1993.
10. Bove GM, Light AR: Unmyelinated nociceptors of rat paraspinal tissues. J Neurophysiol 73:1752, 1995.
11. Bazett HC, McGlone B: Note on the pain sensations which accompany deep punctures. Brain 51:18, 1928.
12. Cavanaugh JM, el-Bohy A, Hardy WN, et al: Sensory innervation of the soft tissues of the lumbar spine of the rat. J Orthop Res 7:378, 1989.
13. El-Bohy A, Cavanaugh JM, Getchell ML, et al: Localization of substance P and neurofilament immunoreactive fibers in the lumbar facet joint capsule and supraspinous ligament of the rabbit. Brain Res 460:379, 1988.
14. Giles LG, Taylor JR, Cockson A: Human zygapophyseal joint synovial folds. Acta Anat 126:110, 1986.
15. Giles LG, Harvey AR: Immunohistological demonstration of nociceptors in the capsule and synovial folds of human zygapophyseal joints. Br J Rheumatol 26:362, 1987.
16. Giles LG, Taylor JR: Intra-articular synovial protrusions in the lower lumbar apophyseal joints. Bull Hosp Jt Dis Orthop Inst 42:248, 1982.
17. Yamashita T, Cavanaugh JM, el-Bohy AA, et al: Mechanosensitive afferent units in the lumbar facet joint. J Bone Joint Surg Am 72:865, 1990.
18. Lundberg LE, Jorun E, Holm E, Torebjork HE: Intra-neural electrical stimulation of cutaneous nociceptive fibres in humans: Effects of different pulse patterns on magnitude of pain. Acta Physiol Scand 146:41, 1992.
19. Reeh P: Chemical excitation and sensitization of nociceptors. In Urban L (ed): Cellular Mechanisms of Sensory Processing. Berlin, Springer-Verlag, 1994.
20. Handwerker HO, Reeh PW: Nociceptors in animals. In Besson JM, et al (eds): Peripheral Neurons in Nociception: Physiopharmacological Aspects. Paris, John Libbey Eurotext, 1994.
21. Watkins LR, Goehler LE, Relton J, et al: Mechanisms of tumor necrosis factor-alpha (TNF-alpha) hyperalgesia. Brain Res 692:244, 1995.
22. Leem JG, Bove GM: Mid-axonal tumor necrosis factor-alpha induces ectopic activity in a subset of slowly conducting cutaneous and deep afferent neurons. J Pain 3:45, 2002.
23. Sorkin LS, Doom CM: Epineurial application of TNF elicits an acute mechanical hyperalgesia in the awake rat. J Peripher Nerv Syst 5:96, 2000.
24. Perl ER, Kumazawa T, Lynn B, Kenins P: Sensitization of high threshold receptors with unmyelinated (C) afferent fibers. Prog Brain Res 43:263, 1976.
25. Sanjue H, Jun Z: Sympathetic facilitation of sustained discharge of polymodal nociceptors. Pain 38:85, 1989.
26. Koltzenburg M, Kress M, Reeh PW: The nociceptor sensitization by bradykinin does not depend on sympathetic neurons. Neuroscience 46:465, 1992.
27. Shea VK, Perl ER: Failure of sympathetic stimulation to affect responsiveness of rabbit polymodal nociceptors. J Neurophysiol 54:513, 1985.
28. Barasi S, Lynn B: Effects of sympathetic stimulation on mechanoreceptive and nociceptive afferent units from the rabbit pinna. Brain Res 378:21, 1986.
29. Devor M, Jänig W: Activation of myelinated afferents ending in a neuroma by stimulation of the sympathetic supply in the rat. Neurosci Lett 24:43, 1981.
30. Sato J, Perl ER: Adrenergic excitation of cutaneous pain receptors induced by peripheral nerve injury. Science 251:1608, 1991.
31. Koltzenburg M, et al: Receptive properties of nociceptors in a peripheral neuropathy. Soc Neurosci Abstr 19:325, 1993.

32. Sato J, Suzuki S, Iseki T, Kumazawa T: Adrenergic excitation of cutaneous nociceptors in chronically inflamed rats. Neurosci Lett 164:225, 1993.
33. Bossut DF, Perl ER: Effects of nerve injury on sympathetic excitation of A delta mechanical nociceptors. J Neurophysiol 73:1721, 1995.
34. Cannon WB: Bodily Changes in Pain, Hunger, Fear, and Rage. New York, D. Appleton, 1929.
35. Ecker A: Norepinephrine in reflex sympathetic dystrophy: An hypothesis. Clin J Pain 5:313, 1989.
36. Selye H: The general adaptation syndrome and diseases of adaptation. In Karsner HT, Sanford AH (eds): The 1950 Year Book of Pathology and Clinical Pathology. Chicago, Year Book Publishers, 1950.
37. Bayliss WM: On the origin from the spinal cord of the vasodilator fibers of the hind limb, and on the nature of these fibers. J Physiol Lond 26:173, 1900.
38. Lewis T: The nocifensor system of nerves and its reactions. BMJ 1:431, 491, 1937.
39. Kenins P: Identification of the unmyelinated sensory nerves which evoke plasma extravasation in response to antidromic stimulation. Neurosci Lett 25:137, 1981.
40. Alvarez FJ, Cervantes C, Blasco I, et al: Presence of calcitonin gene-related peptide (CGRP) and substance P (SP) immunoreactivity in intraepidermal free nerve endings of cat skin. Brain Res 442:391, 1988.
41. Gulbenkian S, Merighi A, Wharton J, et al: Ultrastructural evidence for the coexistence of calcitonin gene-related peptide and substance P in secretory vesicles of peripheral nerves in the guinea pig. J Neurocytol 15:535, 1986.
42. Gibbins IL, Furness JB, Costa M, et al: Co-localization of calcitonin gene-related peptide-like immunoreactivity with substance P in cutaneous, vascular and visceral sensory neurons of guinea pigs. Neurosci Lett 57:125, 1985.
43. Brain SD, Tippins JR, Morris HR, et al: Potent vasodilator activity of calcitonin gene-related peptide in human skin. J Invest Dermatol 87:533, 1986.
44. Holzer P: Peptidergic sensory neurons in the control of vascular functions: Mechanisms and significance in the cutaneous and splanchnic beds. Rev Physiol Biochem Pharmacol 121:49, 1992.
45. Kenins P, Hurley JV, Bell C: The role of substance P in the axon reflex in the rat. Br J Dermatol 111:551, 1984.
46. Le Greves P, Nyberg F, Terenius L, Hokfelt T: Calcitonin gene–related peptide is a potent inhibitor of substance P degradation. Eur J Pharmacol 115:309, 1985.
47. Ishida-Yamamoto A, Tohyama M: Calcitonin gene-related peptide in the nervous tissue. Prog Neurobiol 33:335, 1989.
48. Uddman R, Edvinsson L, Ekblad E, et al: Calcitonin gene-related peptide (CGRP): Perivascular distribution and vasodilatory effects. Regul Pept 15:1, 1986.
49. Cohen RH, Perl ER: Contributions of arachidonic acid derivatives and substance P to the sensitization of cutaneous nociceptors. J Neurophysiol 64:457, 1990.
50. Mantyh PW: Substance P and the inflammatory and immune response. Ann NY Acad Sci 632:263, 1991.
51. Rees H, Sluka KA, Westlund KN, Willis WD: Do dorsal root reflexes augment peripheral inflammation? Neuroreport 5:821, 1994.
52. Levine JD, Dardick SJ, Roizen MF, et al: Contribution of sensory afferents and sympathetic efferents to joint injury in experimental arthritis. J Neurosci 6:3423, 1986.
53. Weber JR, Angstwurm K, Bove GM, et al: The trigeminal nerve and augmentation of regional cerebral blood flow during experimental bacterial meningitis. J Cereb Blood Flow Metab 16:1319, 1996.
54. Wall PD, Woolf CJ: Muscle but not cutaneous C-afferent input produces prolonged increases in the excitability of the flexion reflex in the rat. J Physiol 356:443, 1984.
55. Bove GM, et al: Neuritis induces ectopic mechanical sensitivity in nociceptor axons with deep but not cutaneous receptive fields. Soc Neurosci Abstr 27:928.3, 2001.
56. Li L, Xian CJ, Zhong JH, Zhou XF: Effect of lumbar 5 ventral root transection on pain behaviors: A novel rat model for neuropathic pain without axotomy of primary sensory neurons. Exp Neurol 175:23, 2002.
57. Michaelis M, Liu X, Janig W: Axotomized and intact muscle afferents but no skin afferents develop ongoing discharges of dorsal root ganglion origin after peripheral nerve lesion. J Neurosci 20:2742, 2000.
58. Cameron AA, Pover CM, Willis WD, Coggeshall RE: Evidence that fine primary afferent axons innervate a wider territory in the superficial dorsal horn following peripheral axotomy. Brain Res 575:151, 1992.
59. Woolf CJ, Shortland P, Coggeshall RE, et al: Peripheral nerve injury triggers central sprouting of myelinated afferents. Nature 355:75, 1992.
60. Campbell JN, Raja SN, Meyer RA, Mackinnon SE: Myelinated afferents signal the hyperalgesia associated with nerve injury. Pain 32:89, 1988.
61. Price DD, Bennett GJ, Rafii A: Psychophysiological observations on patients with neuropathic pain relieved by a sympathetic block. Pain 36:273, 1989.
62. Light AR: Normal anatomy and physiology of the spinal cord dorsal horn. Appl Neurophysiol 51:78, 1988.
63. Sugiura Y, Lee CL, Perl ER: Central projections of identified, unmyelinated (C) afferent fibers innervating mammalian skin. Science 234:358, 1986.
64. Light AR, Perl ER: Spinal termination of functionally identified primary afferent neurons with slowly conducting myelinated fibers. J Comp Neurol 186:133, 1979.
65. Gillette RG, Kramis RC, Roberts WJ:: Characterization of spinal somatosensory neurons having receptive fields in lumbar tissues of cats. Pain 54:85, 1993.
66. Gillette RG, Kramis RC, Roberts WJ: Spinal projections of cat primary afferent fibers innervating lumbar facet joints and multifidus muscle. Neurosci Lett 157:67, 1993.
67. Bullitt E: Somatotopy of spinal nociceptive processing. J Comp Neurol 312:279, 1991.
68. Bullitt E: Induction of c-*fos*-like protein within the lumbar spinal cord and thalamus of the rat following peripheral stimulation. Brain Res 493:391, 1989.
69. Menétrey D, Gannon A, Levine JD, Basbaum AL: Expression of c-*fos* protein in interneurons and projection neurons of the rat spinal cord in response to noxious somatic, articular, and visceral stimulation. J Comp Neurol 285:177, 1989.
70. Iadarola MJ, Brody LS, Draisci G, Dubner R: Enhancement of dynorphin gene expression in spinal cord following experimental inflammation: Stimulus specificity, behavioral parameters and opioid receptor binding. Pain 35:313, 1988.
71. Hylden JL, Nahin RL, Traug RJ, Dubner R: Effects of spinal kappa-opioid receptor agonists on the responsiveness of nociceptive superficial dorsal horn neurons. Pain 44:187, 1991.
72. Waxman SG, Dib-Hajj S, Cummins Tr, Black JA: Sodium channels and pain. Proc Natl Acad Sci USA 96:7635, 1999.
73. Akopian AN, Souslova V, England S, et al: The tetrodotoxin-resistant sodium channel SNS has a specialized function in pain pathways. Nature Neurosci 2:541, 1999.
74. Matzner O, Devor M: Hyperexcitability at sites of nerve injury depends on voltage-sensitive Na+ channels. J Neurophysiol 72:349, 1994.
75. Novakovic SD, Tzoumaka E, McGivern JG, et al: Distribution of the tetrodotoxin-resistant sodium channel PN3 in rat sensory neurons in normal and neuropathic conditions. J Neurosci 18:2174, 1998.
76. Tanaka M, et al: SNS Na+ channel expression increases in dorsal root ganglion neurons in the carrageenan inflammatory pain model. Neuro Rep 9:967, 1998.
77. Koschorke GM, Meyer RA, Tillman DB, Campbell JN: Ectopic excitability of injured nerves in monkey: Entrained responses to vibratory stimuli. J Neurophysiol 65:693, 1991.
78. Koschorke GM, Merye RA, Campbell JN: Cellular components necessary for mechanoelectrical transduction are conveyed to primary afferent terminals by fast axonal transport. Brain Res 641:99, 1994.
79. Adriaensen H, Gybels J, Handwerker HO, Van Hees J: Nociceptor discharges and sensations due to noxious mechanical stimulation—a paradox. Hum Neurobiol 3:53, 1984.
80. Coderre TJ, Katz J, Vaccarino AL, Melzack R: Contribution of central neuroplasticity to pathological pain: Review of clinical and experimental evidence. Pain 52:259, 1993.
81. Woolf CJ: Recent advances in the pathophysiology of acute pain. Br J Anaesth 63:139, 1989.
82. Chen R, Cohen LG, Hallett M: Nervous system reorganization following injury. Neuroscience 111:761, 2002.
83. Pockett S: Spinal cord synaptic plasticity and chronic pain. Anesth Analg 80:173, 1995.
84. Mendell LM: Physiological properties of unmyelinated fiber projection to the spinal cord. Exp Neurol 16:316, 1966.

85. Randic M, Jiang MC, Cerne R: Long-term potentiation and long-term depression of primary afferent neurotransmission in the rat spinal cord. J Neurosci 13:5228, 1993.
86. Bliss TVP, Collingridge GL: A synaptic model of memory: Long-term potentiation in the hippocampus. Nature 361:31, 1993.
87. Hunt JL, Winkelstein BA, Rutkowski MD, et al: Repeated injury to the lumbar nerve roots produces enhanced mechanical allodynia and persistent spinal neuroinflammation. Spine 26:2073, 2001.
88. DeLeo JA, Yezierski RP: The role of neuroinflammation and neuroimmune activation in persistent pain. Pain 90:1, 2001.
89. Watkins LR, Maier SF: The pain of being sick: Implications of immune-to-brain communication for understanding pain. Ann Rev Psychol 51:29, 2000.
90. Sandkuhler J: The organization and function of endogenous antinociceptive systems. Prog Neurobiol 50:49, 1996.
91. Fields HL, Basbaum AI: Central nervous system mechanisms of pain modulation. In Wall PD, Melzack R (eds): Textbook of Pain. New York, Churchill Livingstone, 1994.
92. Malcangio M, Bowery NG: GABA and its receptors in the spinal cord. Trends Pharmacol Sci 17:457, 1996.
93. Lundeberg T, Nordemar R, Ottoson D: Pain alleviation by vibratory stimulation. Pain 20:25, 1984.
94. Dickenson AH, et al: The pharmacology of excitatory and inhibitory amino acid-mediated events in the transmission and modulation of pain in the spinal cord [Review]. Gen Pharmacol 28:633, 1997.
95. Indahl A, Kaigle AM, Reikeras O, Holm SH: Interaction between the porcine lumbar intervertebral disc, zygapophysial joints, and paraspinal muscles. Spine 22:2834, 1997.
96. Rainville P: Brain mechanisms of pain affect and pain modulation. Curr Opin Neurobiol 12:195, 2002.
97. Rainville P, Duncan GH, Price DD, et al: Pain affect encoded in human anterior cingulate but not somatosensory cortex. Science 277:968, 1997.
98. Wallis BJ, Lord SM, Bogduk N: Resolution of psychological distress of whiplash patients following treatment by radiofrequency neurotomy: A randomised, double-blind, placebo-controlled trial. Pain 73:15, 1997.
99. ter Riet G, De Craen AJ, de Boer A, Kessels AG: Is placebo analgesia mediated by endogenous opioids? A systematic review. Pain 76:273, 1998.
100. Garfin SR, Rydevik BL, Brown RA: Compressive neuropathy of spinal nerve roots: A compressive or biological problem? Spine 16:162, 1991.
101. Olmarker K, Larsson K: Tumor necrosis factor-alpha and nucleus-pulposus-induced nerve root injury. Spine 23:2538, 1998.
102. Sunderland S: Nerve Injuries and Their Repair. Edinburgh, Churchill Livingstone, 1991.
103. Song XJ, Hu SJ, Greenquist KW, et al: Mechanical and thermal hyperalgesia and ectopic neuronal discharge after chronic compression of dorsal root ganglia. J Neurophysiol 82:3347, 1999.
104. Homma Y, Brull SJ, Zhang JM: A comparison of chronic pain behavior following local application of tumor necrosis factor-alpha to the normal and mechanically compressed lumbar ganglia in the rat. Pain 95:239, 2002.
105. Lundeberg T, Ekholm J: Pain—from periphery to brain. Disabil Rehabil 24:402, 2002.
106. Steen KH, Steen AE, Reeh PW: A dominant role of acid pH in inflammatory excitation and sensitization of nociceptors in rat skin, in vitro. J Neurosci 15:3982, 1995.
107. Gracely RH, Lynch SA, Bennett GJ: Painful neuropathy: Altered central processing maintained dynamically by peripheral input. Pain 51:175, 1992.

chapter 130

Acupuncture

M. Kay Garcia and Joseph S. Chiang

Public interest in complementary and alternative therapies, both for the maintenance of wellness and the treatment of disease, has grown rapidly in the United States in recent years.[1-5] Integrating complementary and alternative treatment approaches shown to be effective into the current mainstream healthcare system in a well-regulated environment is an important step toward achieving goals set forth by the U.S. Department of Health and Human Services in *Healthy People 2010.*[6] Unfortunately, putative mechanisms of many such therapies remain unclear, and the need for quality research evaluating integrative clinical practice remains. In this chapter we discuss complementary and integrative medicine with a focus on traditional Chinese medicine (TCM) and, more specifically, acupuncture for pain control.

HISTORICAL CONSIDERATIONS

With the arrival of the 21st century, a multibillion dollar industry in complementary and alternative medicine (CAM) has emerged.[7] Overall estimates of CAM use in the United States range from 28.9% to 42%.[1-5] To maximize the benefit to public health and ensure quality of care, in 1998, the U.S. Congress established the National Center for Complementary and Alternative Medicine (NCCAM) at the National Institutes of Health (NIH). The purpose of the NCCAM is to stimulate, develop, and support CAM-related research.[8] Furthermore, in response to public demand for more information and guidance, the White House Commission on Complementary and Alternative Medicine Policy was created in March, 2000. Among the recommendations made by the commission were (1) federal agencies should receive increased funding for clinical, basic science, and health services research of CAM therapies; (2) the federal government should consider enacting legislative and administrative incentives to stimulate private sector investment in CAM research of products that may not be patentable; (3) federal, private, and nonprofit sectors should support research of CAM modalities and approaches designed to improve self-care and promote wellness; and (4) these sectors should support innovative CAM research of core questions posed by new areas of scientific study that might expand our understanding of health and disease.[9]

Additionally, the World Health Organization (WHO) established specific objectives regarding CAM use that address policy; safety, efficacy and quality; access; and rational use.[10] The challenges of meeting these objectives are many, but considering the global economic and public health impact of CAM, they are challenges that must be addressed. Efforts by the WHO and the US government to establish meaningful healthcare policies regarding CAM are extremely important for ensuring the safe and appropriate use of these therapies.

History of Acupuncture

TCM is a complete system of healthcare that has been practiced in China for thousands of years. According to the WHO, TCM is used to treat at least 200 million people annually and accounts for nearly 40% of all healthcare provided in China. The primary disciplines within TCM include acupuncture, herbs, and food therapy; Tui na, or Chinese bodywork; Tai chi (therapeutic exercise); and Qi gong (meditative/energy therapy). Acupuncture is among the most popular of these therapies and is used in at least 78 countries worldwide.[10]

In the West, acupuncture therapy has grown substantially more common over the past few decades. In 1971, James Reston, a journalist for the *New York Times,* wrote a front-page article describing how his postoperative pain from an emergency appendectomy was relieved by acupuncture while traveling in Beijing.[11] Three months later, a group of US physicians visiting hospitals in China observed acupuncture for surgical analgesia and reported their observations in the *Journal of the American Medical Association.*[12] Growing public interest ensued, and in 1972, President Richard Nixon, accompanied by his personal physician, witnessed several surgeries using acupuncture-assisted anesthesia.[13] The NIH subsequently sponsored a team of physicians to study the healthcare system in China; as a result, several studies attempting to elucidate the underlying mechanisms of action for acupuncture were initiated, textbooks of TCM were translated into English, and training programs were established.[14]

Before President Nixon's visit to China, little information about acupuncture was available in the United States. There is documented evidence, however, of acupuncture being used in clinical practice as early as 1826, when Franklin Bache, a Philadelphia physician and grandson to Benjamin Franklin, concluded in a published report that he had found acupuncture to be an effective treatment for pain due to rheumatism and neuralgia among prisoners at the Pennsylvania state penitentiary.[15] Sir William Osler also endorsed acupuncture as an effective treatment for lumbago and sciatica in *The Principles and Practice of Medicine*[16]; and, interestingly, brief passages on acupuncture appeared in an American Civil War surgeon's manual and in two medical treatises written in 1876 and 1880.[17]

In the late 1970s and early 1980s, researchers demonstrated acupuncture analgesia was associated with the stimulation of endogenous opioid peptides and biogenic amines through the central nervous system[18-23]; although later work has revealed multiple underlying mechanisms, these findings helped give acupuncture scientific credibility in the minds of medical professionals.[24] As a result, clinical training programs in acupuncture techniques and guidelines for education, practice, and regulation have been developed and programs in integrative medicine are beginning to appear in medical schools, nursing schools, and hospitals throughout the United States.

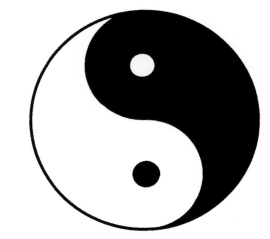

FIGURE 130–1 ■ Yin-yang symbol.

BASIC PRINCIPLES

Acupuncturists use many different models and approaches to understand and apply treatment. These models range from a metaphysical paradigm used by those traditionally trained to a strictly neurophysiologic approach incorporated by physicians who use acupuncture exclusively for pain control. Although the former may seem untenable to the Western scientific community, it is useful in treating problems that are not well described by the latter. Acupuncture sometimes has effects on the body that are difficult to explain in purely scientific terms, and a symptom-complex that does not easily fit a given set of diagnostic criteria may elucidate a meaningful clinical pattern when analyzed using a different model. In TCM, emphasis is placed on function, not structure. As a result, certain aspects of human physiologic functional relationships are emphasized that are not directly addressed by Western biomedicine.

In TCM, it is more important to understand the relationships between variables and the functional "whole" of the patient than it is to identify the specifics of a single pathology. Diagnoses in TCM are made according to manifestations of the root cause, as opposed to the sequelae of illness, as in Western biomedical practice.[25] This contrasts sharply to the Western allopathic medical approach of attempting to change or remove a precise underlying cause to an isolatable illness or injury.

Yin-Yang Theory

Although there are many theoretical foundations underlying the practice of TCM and acupuncture, basic to all approaches is yin-yang theory (Fig. 130–1). The constructs within this framework are relatively simple, but yin-yang thinking is substantially different from the classical Aristotelian dogma underlying Western medicine. Within yin-yang conceptualization, qualities may be simultaneously opposite and complementary. Yin always possesses characteristics of yang and vice versa. So while being opposites, yin and yang are also interdependent, can transform into each other, and can consume each other. Physiology and pathology represent variations along a continuum of health and illness. Thus, a state of good health is determined by the dynamic balance between opposing yin-yang forces.[25]

In TCM, acupuncture is based on the premise that there are well-defined patterns of Qi (pronounced "chee") flow throughout the body. The concept of Qi has been discussed by Chinese philosophers throughout time, and the symbol representing Qi in the Chinese language indicates something that is simultaneously material and immaterial. Some authors define Qi as matter + energy or "mattergy," thus expressing the same continuum of matter and energy explained by modern particle physics.[26]

In ancient Chinese thought, Qi was believed to be a fundamental and vital substance of the universe, with all phenomena being produced by its changes. There are many types of Qi classified according to source, function, and distribution. It is considered one of the human body's fundamental substances, helping to maintain normal activities, permeating all parts of the body, and flowing along organized pathways known as acupuncture channels, or meridians. TCM practitioners believe that a balanced flow of Qi throughout the system is required for good health, and imbalances can be corrected by acupuncture stimulation.[25,26]

It is also important to recognize that the Blood of Chinese medicine has broader characteristics and functions than blood in Western medicine. (*Note:* Blood is capitalized here to distinguish the TCM concept from the concept of blood in biomedicine). In TCM, Blood is a yin substance and is a dense and material form of Qi, which is relatively more yang. Blood circulates continuously throughout meridian pathways as well as through blood vessels, although the meridians carry relatively more Qi while the latter carries relatively more Blood. The primary functions of Blood are to nourish, maintain, and moisten various parts of the body and to provide the material foundation for mental, emotional, and spiritual activities. Qi and Blood are inseparable, and without Qi, Blood would be an inert fluid.[25,26]

Since the late 1950s, numerous studies have been published in the Peoples' Republic of China hypothesizing the underlying mechanisms of action for acupuncture; and by the mid 1990s, compelling evidence describing a neurohumoral model for acupuncture analgesia could be found in the English literature. More recently, basic scientific research has revealed that bioelectromagnetic, as well as neurohumoral, mechanisms are responsible for the effects of acupuncture on various types of health problems. The stimulation of acupuncture points is believed to cause biochemical changes that affect the body's natural healing abilities. The primary mechanisms of these changes include enhanced conduction of bioelectromagnetic signals, activation of opioid systems, and activation of the autonomic and central nervous systems, causing the release of various neurotransmitters and neurohormones.[24]

Neurohumoral Mechanisms of Acupuncture

Awareness that acupuncture analgesia was at least partially mediated through endogenous opioids was first demonstrated in 1976. Shortly after opiate receptors were discovered in the periaqueductal gray matter, the limbic system, and the periventricular gray matter of the CNS, it was discovered that acupuncture analgesia could be reversed by naloxone, a pure antagonist at all known opioid receptors.[27] Acupuncture can change concentrations of serotonin and biogenic amines, including opioid peptides, met-enkephalin, leu-enkephalin, β-endorphin, and dynorphin. These are involved in the activation of descending tracts that inhibit transmission of nociceptive information in the spinal cord and also inhibit ascending tracts transmitting nociceptive information. When large, unmyelinated Aδ-fibers that sense touch and pressure are stimulated with an acupuncture needle, impulses from small, unmyelinated C-fibers transmitting ascending nociceptive information are blocked by a gate of inhibitory interneurons in the substantia gelatinosa of the spinal cord, releasing neurotransmitters such as γ-aminobutyric acid and enkephalins and resulting in the inhibition of transmission of pain impulses to the brain. There is also a regional effect, since Aδ-fibers transmit cranially and caudally in the dorsolateral funiculus before entering the substantia gelatinosa to stimulate inhibitory interneurons.[28-30]

Functional magnetic resonance imaging (fMRI) studies suggest stimulation of acupuncture points can initiate multiple endogenous pathways of analgesia by the neuromodulation and integration of neurotransmitter and pain control systems at various levels. The release of serotonin, endogenous opioids, and other neurotransmitters leads to an alteration of nociceptive processing and perception, and quantifiable changes in specific areas of the human brain have been observed with fMRI after acupuncture. In patients who experienced *De Qi* sensation, unilateral needling has been shown to activate structures of the descending antinociceptive pathways and cause deactivation of multiple limbic areas subserving pain perception (i.e., activation of the hypothalamus and nucleus accumbens and deactivation of the rostral part of the anterior cingulate cortex, amygdala formation, and hippocampal complex). Superficial tactile stimulation caused a signal increase in the somatosensory cortex but did not cause signal decreases in deeper structures as was observed with true acupuncture. When combined with fMRI studies in which brain function is localized, observations suggest that stimulation of specific points can initiate multiple endogenous pathways of analgesia through neuromodulation and integration of neurotransmitter and pain control systems at various levels of the CNS.[28,31]

Acupuncture points have also been found to have a higher temperature and a higher metabolic rate and to release more carbon dioxide than surrounding tissues.[32,33] Needle stimulation at an acupuncture point causes erythema and heat to develop, and patients often report a feeling of warmth at the site. Furthermore, unilateral stimulation can cause cutaneous skin temperatures to rise bilaterally. Local vasodilation, decreased sympathetic tone, and increased cholinergic efferent impulses may all contribute to this effect and may play an important role in relieving chronic pain.[34] Vasodilation is also mediated by the physical irritation of the needle and stimulates the release of histamine and other vasodilators.

Although acupuncture has been most widely recognized for pain control, stimulation of certain points can also affect the viscera and immune system, partially through the multifaceted role of opioids. Acupuncture promotes neuroendocrine modulation of the hypothalamus-pituitary axis, which interacts with the immune system to modulate cellular function.[28,35-39] Because opioid receptors are found on neurons and lymphocytes, they provide communication between the CNS and the immune system.

Morphogenetic Singularity Theory

A speculative but compelling theory regarding acupuncture involves developmental biology and suggests the meridian system is related to the bioelectric field in morphogenesis and growth control. According to the morphogenetic singularity theory, acupoints originate from organizing centers in morphogenesis and channel distribution is not solely determined by nerves, muscles, or blood vessels but is the result of the morphogenesis of both internal and external structures. Although compatible with neurohumoral constructs, this theory explains several long-standing puzzles that the neurohumoral model cannot. For example, the theory helps explain indications for specific acupoints and meridians, such as the Du channel (also called Governing vessel), whose distributions do not follow any major nerve, lymphatic, or blood vessels.[40]

CLINICALLY RELEVANT ANATOMY

Acupuncture Points

Many studies have described acupuncture point morphology,[28,41-55] relating the so-called "acupoints" to areas on the skin surface with decreased electrical resistance and increased conductance. Most acupoints are palpable as a surface depression located along the cleavage between muscles. They generally correspond to peripheral, cranial, and spinal nerve endings and are often hypersensitive. According to Bossy and Sambuc,[43] they have a surface area of 1 to 5 mm^2.

In 1979, Senelar used statistical evaluation of a large number of histologic sections from rabbits, cats, mice, and human cadavers to describe acupoint morphology as a lymphatic trunk coupled to a large arteriole accompanied by a satellite vein. This lymph-arteriole-venous system creates a passageway between the skin and deeper tissue and is located in a vertical column of loose connective tissue surrounded by the thick, dense connective tissue of skin.[44] This sleeve of connective tissue, through which neurovascular, lymphatic, and tendinomuscular structures pass enhances the conduction of bioelectric energy.[28] Approximately 80% of traditional

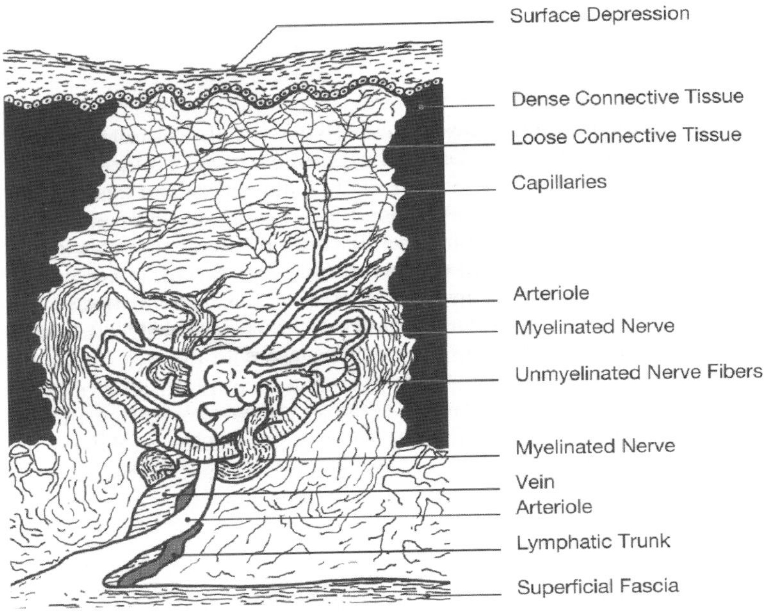

FIGURE 130–2 ■ Acupuncture point diagram. (From Helms JM: Acupuncture Energetics: A Clinical Approach for Physicians. Berkeley, CA, Medical Acupuncture Publishers, 1997, p 26, with permission.)

acupuncture points have this morphologic organization (Fig. 130–2),[45] which may partially explain the effects of acupuncture in soft tissue disease.

In the 1980s, observations from both conventional light microscopy and electron microscopy confirmed a high concentration of microvesicles and perineural cells situated at the contact zones of sympathetic nerve terminations at the walls of large vessels.[45] Other studies in the 1980s described these thin-walled vascular structures as sinuous, organized in a series of closed loops, and surrounded by a web of unmyelinated cholinergic nerve fibers from the autonomic nervous system. Nerves are located proximal to the vasculature, with additional myelinated nerves woven among the blood and lymph vessels leading to superficial levels of the dermis. The epidermis thins at the acupuncture point and has a corresponding modification of collagen fibers.[46]

Types of Acupuncture Points

Acupuncture points can be categorized in various ways.[28,41] One approach separates points according to their relationship with known neural and tendinomuscular structures. For example, type I acupoints correspond to motor points located where a nerve enters muscle. Maximal muscle contraction with minimal electrical stimulation is achieved at these points. Type II points are located on superficial nerves in the sagittal plane at dorsal and ventral midlines. Type III points are located in areas with a high density of superficial nerves and nerve plexi, and type IV points are found where tendons join muscles.

Several studies have investigated the correlation between acupuncture points, motor points, and trigger points. In 1977, one group of researchers reported a 71% correlation between trigger points and acupuncture points.[56] Trigger points are hypersensitive regions in muscle tissue that can be palpated as taut bands. They are similar to acupuncture points in that they may lie within areas where referred pain is experienced or be located some distance away. The increased sensitivity of acupuncture points is not fully understood; however, hyperalgesia may arise spontaneously from local irritation or from excitation of somatic or visceral structures distant from the painful point. Stimulation of trigger points can provide long-lasting analgesia similar to that achieved through acupuncture. The high correlation between acupuncture points used to treat pain and myofascial trigger points suggests similar underlying mechanisms for analgesia.[26]

With greater pain intensity, both the number of sensitive acupuncture points and the diameter of the sensitive area increase. In the presence of underlying pathology (i.e., yin-yang imbalance), points become tender in a predictably progressive order, and the tenderness disappears in reverse order as healing occurs.[57] Mann described the general mechanism by which diseased organs are able to refer pain, sensitivity, or muscle contraction to acupuncture or trigger points as a viscerocutaneous reflex and stated the pathways of referred pain appear to follow autonomic and sensorimotor, myotomal, and dermatomal distributions for each spinal segment. Acupuncture may cause excitation of a cutaneovisceral reflex, allowing stimulation of a point on the skin to influence the neurologic excitation of corresponding organs.[58] The characteristics of acupuncture point morphology and related tissues allow for the transmission and integration of bioelectromagnetic and neurohumoral information between systems.[28]

Channels and Collaterals

According to TCM theory, specific pathways known as meridians or channels carry Qi and Blood throughout the body. These pathways differ from neurovascular systems as defined by modern anatomy and physiology and comprise an infinite network linking all fundamental substances and organs. There are 12 regular channels and 8 extra channels, each with divergent branches and numerous divisions known as collaterals. Channel/meridian theory assumes that blockage or disorder within the system can be identified using a systematic method of differential diagnosis and treatment strategies can be developed based on restoring orderly flow.[25]

Several attempts have been made to explain acupuncture channels in modern scientific terms, and most, but not all, channels follow the pathways of major nerves, vessels, and fascial cleavage planes.[24] During acupuncture treatment, patients frequently describe a sensation of numbness, aching, heaviness, or warmth along the channel pathway.[59] Many TCM clinicians consider this phenomenon, sometimes called *De Qi* sensation, to be essential for effective therapy and suggest it carries the therapeutic signal to the target area.[24,25,60] After needling a point on the Stomach channel in one study, fluoroscopic imaging revealed peristalsis was different among patients who experienced *De Qi* as compared with those who did not. Furthermore, gastrographs registered decreased frequency and increased amplitude in gastric contractions when the sensation was felt in the abdominal area.[61] Some studies have shown surgical analgesia is also more effective when *De Qi* is felt.[62]

De Qi sensation has been shown to travel along channel pathways at 1 to 10 cm/sec. This rate varies depending on the subject and the type of needle stimulation but is considerably slower than visceral or somatic nerve conduction.[63,64] *De Qi* appears to be primarily a peripheral phenomenon, because it can be blocked by chilling, local anesthetic, and mechanical pressure.[65,66] Some investigators, however, have stated it can travel to phantom limbs, implying participation by the CNS.[67]

Darras and colleagues[68] attempted to identify the network of acupuncture channels and collaterals by comparing the trajectory of a radioactive tracer, technetium-99m, injected into real acupuncture points with the trajectory of the tracer injected into sham points. The tracer was observed with a scintillation camera that revealed that diffusion patterns from the real acupuncture points corresponded to classically described channels, whereas a centrifugal diffusion pattern without linearity was observed at the sham points. Furthermore, radioisotope diffusion moved beyond a tourniquet that blocked surface peripheral blood circulation. Tracer injected into lymphatic vessels showed they also were distinct from acupuncture channels. Since the migration rate of the tracer did not correspond to vascular or lymphatic circulation rates, the authors concluded diffusion did not appear to be via either the vascular or lymphatic system.

Mussat evaluated the electrical propagation along traditionally defined acupuncture pathways. He concluded acupuncture channels carry a measurable charge, due to lower resistance and increased conductance, that is relatively independent from surrounding tissue and propagation of an electrical current between acupuncture points follows the organization of classical channel theory. He demonstrated that (1) placing a barrier needle between needles placed at two points along the same channel can increase the resistance of the channel; (2) electrical current introduced into a channel on the upper extremity can be captured in its corresponding channel on the lower extremity; and (3) current introduced into one channel can be captured in the internally-externally related channel, according to TCM theory, of the same extremity after a 5-minute latent period.[69]

Ancient Chinese scholars were unable to identify electro-ionic migration patterns or discuss electron flow between needles. They were, however, able to recognize patterns and qualities of response and subjectively quantify the distribution and actions of a phenomenon they referred to as "Qi." Although no single discipline can definably illustrate the presence or absence of acupuncture channels and collaterals according to classical theory, combined evidence from many different approaches can provide a basic scientific explanation for ancient Chinese conceptualizations.

In brief, the mechanical act of needling an acupuncture point stimulates a bioelectric response initiating polarization and ionizing tissues along preferential pathways, in part because of the piezoelectrical characteristics of collagen (i.e., the property of a material that results in polarization when subjected to mechanical strain and a change in conformation when subjected to an electric field).[70] Adding an electrical stimulus (i.e., electroacupuncture) causes further morphologic changes and alterations in the alignment of collagen fibers.[28] Increased conductance along the meridian system is further supported by a high density of gap junctions at the epithelia of acupuncture points. Gap junctions facilitate intercellular communication and increase electric conductivity through hexagonal protein complexes that form channels between adjacent cells.[71,72]

The exploration of bioelectromagnetic phenomena in living systems is an emerging area of study, and speculative theories have been proposed regarding the manipulation of the body's endogenous electromagnetic fields through acupuncture. As research in this area continues, a more comprehensive and dynamic explanation of the effects of acupuncture on physiologic functional relationships will become apparent.

TECHNIQUE

Electroacupuncture

The most common acupuncture technique for pain control involves the penetration of the skin by thin, solid, metallic needles that are stimulated either manually or electrically. In the United States, the manufacture and use of acupuncture needles is regulated by the Food and Drug Administration (FDA) and compliance with Good Manufacturing Practices and single-use standards of sterility is required. Guidelines and standards for the clean and safe clinical practice of acupuncture have been established by the National Acupuncture Foundation. This nationally accepted protocol reflects Occupational Safety and Health Administration (OSHA) requirements, and successful completion of a certification examination in clean-needle technique is required by most states before licensure to practice is granted.[73]

Electroacupuncture involves the passage of electrical energy through acupuncture points by attaching battery-operated electronic devices to the needles. This technique allows for more accurate and uniformly regulated stimulation than can be achieved using manual stimulation of the needles alone.[74] According to Han, specific frequencies of electrical stimulation induce the gene expression of specific neuropeptides in the CNS. A frequency of 2 Hz induces the gene expression of endorphins in the diencephalons, which act on anxiolytic μ receptors. A frequency of 2 to 15 Hz causes the release of β-endorphin and met-enkephalin in the brain and dynorphin in the spinal cord and is more effective in relieving deep and chronic pain than is higher-frequency stimulation (100 Hz), which causes the release of dynorphin alone. In the periaqueductal gray matter, the effects of acupuncture may be predominantly mediated by the enkephalins and β-endorphin. In the spinal cord, effects are predominantly due to enkephalins and dynorphin.[75-78] A synergistic effect from these three types of opioids is likely to occur in response to simultaneous stimulation from acupuncture as they bind to their respective receptors.[28] Furthermore, combined or alternating low- and high-frequency electrical stimulation may facilitate synaptic remodeling to pre–pain-activated microanatomy.

Although some authors state the frequency of stimulation may be of greater importance than classical rules for needle placement,[78] pain relief achieved through acupuncture treatment cannot be explained by this mechanism alone because the analgesic effect is much longer than the half-life of endorphins.

Auricular Acupuncture

Auricular acupuncture is a commonly practiced technique involving the stimulation of specific points on the ear. Although it has long been used in China for a variety of conditions, auricular diagnosis and treatment has become a unique branch of TCM throughout other parts of the world since the late 1980s. When internal disorders occur, changes such as tenderness, decreased cutaneous electrical resistance, morphologic changes, or discoloration may appear at specific ear points.[79]

In classical TCM literature, there are many references to stimulating specific points on the ear with needles, moxibustion, and massage to both prevent and treat disease. Ancient Chinese clinicians classified and recorded information about the ear on silk scrolls discovered in the excavation of the No. 3 Han Tomb at Mawangdui, Changsha City, in 1973. Two of these scrolls, entitled *Moxibustion Classic with Eleven Yin-Yang Channels,* discuss the "ear meridian." Other descriptions of auricular acupuncture appear in the earliest existing classic of TCM, the *Huang Di Nei Jing.*[80] Citations of treatments using points on the ear are also found in Egyptian tomb paintings and in ancient Persian medical references.[81]

In France in the early 1950s, Paul Nogier systematically mapped the auricular/body correspondences. His teachings spread from France to Germany, Japan, and finally to China, where his charts were screened, verified, and refined in clinical practice.[82-84] In 1960, Xu Zuolin, a physician at the Beijing Pingan hospital, published a paper summarizing the application of auricular therapy for 255 cases; and in 1970, the *Hanging Wall Chart of Acupoints*, published by the Peoples' Liberation Army (PLA) hospital in Gang Zhou illustrated 107 auricular acupoints. Since that time, the number used in clinical practice has expanded to include points on both anterior and posterior portions of the ear.[80]

More recently, authors have discussed auriculotherapy as a reflex somatotropic microsystem.[85] Many such systems have been described in the human body and range from the very simple to quite complex. In TCM, three primary somatotropic microsystems involve the tongue, radial pulse, and ear. The first two are used for diagnostic purposes only. Theorists have speculated that reflex somatotropic systems behave as bioholographic phenomena, with each cell containing information about the whole organism. This view reflects ancient Chinese beliefs that man is a microcosm expressing harmony of a natural order within the overall universe.[25]

In his text, *Acupuncture Energetics: A Clinical Approach for Physicians*, Helms states afferent excitation arriving at a modulating center in the brain may trigger efferent impulses that change the sensitivity of the skin on surface reflex zones. This may involve the reticular formation in the brainstem, which functions as a modulating intersection activating and inhibiting cranial, spinal, somatic, visceral, and autonomic neurologic impulses. This reticular unit may respond to input by patterning topographic regions of the body and subsequently activating the thalamic reticular formation involved in pain modulation, influencing somatic motor and sensory functions, and regulating viscera through the autonomic nervous system.[24]

Scalp Acupuncture

Although ancient Chinese clinicians needled acupuncture points on the scalp, Jiao Shunfa first described treatment of various diseases using a systematic approach to scalp acupuncture in the early 1970s.[86] Like auriculotherapy, scalp acupuncture is considered to be a microreflex system that involves needling areas directly above corresponding nerve centers.[24] It has been used to treat problems such as chronic headaches, facial paralysis, cerebrovascular disease, enuresis, vertigo, cerebral palsy, and epilepsy.[86] To date, few controlled studies evaluating the use of scalp acupuncture have been conducted in the United States.

CONCOMITANT THERAPIES

In China and many parts of the world, other therapies are used as adjuncts to acupuncture. These include moxibustion, cupping, gua sha or scraping, Tui na, Qi gong, Tai chi, and herbal and food therapy. The same diagnostic paradigm and treatment strategies used for acupuncture are used to develop a treatment plan utilizing these techniques.

Moxibustion

Moxibustion (moxa) is an ancient technique that uses heat from burning preparations of the herb *Artemisia vulgaris* (mugwort) to stimulate the circulation of Qi and Blood. Ancient clinicians believed moxa was effective in treating a variety of disorders and regular use could prevent illness. Today, many TCM practitioners use moxa to treat pain or strengthen the immune system.[79]

Moxa can be applied using a variety of direct and indirect methods. Direct moxa was used in ancient times and is still used in some cultures today. It involves placing a moxa cone directly on the skin at specified acupuncture points and allowing it to burn to completion. Blistering and scarring occur at the site. A nonscarring method is also used in which the moxa cone is removed and replaced with a new one before burning to completion. With indirect moxa, the cone is insulated from the skin with slices of ginger, garlic, or salt. The type of insulating material chosen depends on the specific indication. With indirect moxa, the cones may also be placed directly on the acupuncture needles. Finally, the indirect method may be applied using a cigar-like stick of tightly rolled moxa held near the skin at acupuncture sites. The patient is instructed to indicate when he or she feels warmth, and individual acupoints may be heated or groups of points warmed in succession along the channel being treated to stimulate Qi and Blood flow.[79]

Indirect moxa is most often used to treat chronic pain conditions. Although a few recent studies from China and Japan have evaluated the effects of moxa on the immune system, with one reporting moxa smoke induces cytotoxicity by its pro-oxidant action,[87-90] its use for pain control has not been systematically evaluated. Furthermore, fire safety concerns and the potential for allergic reactions limit its usefulness as an adjunctive treatment modality.

Cupping and Scraping (Gua Sha)

Cupping is another treatment often combined with acupuncture therapy for pain control. In this technique, the inside of a small jar or cup is heated to create negative pressure. The cup is then attached to the surface of the skin using the vacuum created by the heat. In ancient times, bamboo jars were used; today, glass or plastic cups are most common. The cups may be left in place for 5 to 10 minutes or may be continuously applied and removed along the meridian pathway. Experienced clinicians may also be able to carefully slide the cup along the chosen meridian. The cups are removed by placing a finger at its edge on the skin to release the vacuum. After removal, the area is massaged lightly for patient comfort and to further stimulate Qi and Blood flow. The suction from the cups may leave a painless mark on the skin,[79] and informed consent should be obtained before using this adjunctive therapy. Although it has not been systematically evaluated, cupping is frequently combined with acupuncture to treat various pain syndromes, including myofascial pain and fibromyalgia.[24,79]

Another therapeutic approach used by TCM clinicians is scraping or gua sha. In gua sha, some form of oil or lubricant is placed on the skin, followed by scraping with a smooth-edged instrument such as a coin or porcelain spoon. Again, this is done to stimulate circulation to specific areas and is used to treat chronic pain. The procedure is somewhat uncomfortable, and a mark or bruise is left on the skin surface for 3 to 5 days. There have been reports in the literature of marks left from this procedure being mistaken for abuse. Physicians should be aware that it is a common practice in Asian culture and can be recognized by the pattern of the mark. Although there are no published randomized trials evaluating the use of gua sha for pain, there is considerable anecdotal evidence that it mobilizes stagnant blood and body fluid, thereby relieving pain.[24] It should not be used in areas where tissue is fragile or near skin lesions of any type.

Tui Na

Tui na (Chinese bodywork) is based on the theory of meridians and collaterals and is a special form of massage that utilizes techniques specific to Chinese medicine. It involves stimulation of areas along specific pathways and is considered a major area of specialty within TCM.[91] In the United States, examination and certification in Chinese bodywork is provided through the National Certification Commission for Acupuncture and Oriental Medicine. In order to be eligible for the national board examination, applicants must demonstrate the successful completion of an educational program or apprenticeship documenting at least 500 contact hours. A significant portion of those hours must be dedicated to direct patient care.[92]

Qi Gong and Tai Chi

Very few randomized controlled trials evaluating the use of Qi gong or Tai chi for pain control have been published to date. Three key elements of these exercises, however, are to physically relax the body, focus the mind, and control the breath. Anecdotally, many patients have reported using these simple, inexpensive, behaviorally based techniques for painful conditions with good results, and further investigation is most definitely warranted.

Qi gong is a form of mental and physical exercise that has been practiced in China for thousands of years.[93] It is mentioned in ancient Chinese books such as the *I Ching* (Book of Changes) and the *Huang Di Nei Jing* (Yellow Emperor's Classic of Internal Medicine). The *I Ching* was written in 2852 BC by Fu Xi. The *Huang Di Nei Jing* was written around 2697-2597 BC. Its authorship is attributed to the great Huang Di (Yellow Emperor) who ruled during the middle of the third millennium BC and who symbolizes the vital spirit of Chinese civilization.[94,95] The book provides the accumulated knowledge of many generations underlying the philosophy and foundation of acupuncture, Qi gong, and Tai chi and is used in colleges and universities of TCM even today.

Although there are different schools of Qi gong, in general, the practice involves meditation, special breathing techniques, and physical exercises that can be either static or dynamic. Buddhist and Taoist monks practice many ancient Qi gong techniques, and masters believe the practice enables them to accumulate, store, and consume energy in a controlled manner, strengthens their resistance to illness and injury, and can be used as an aid in healing others.[94,95] Although the underlying mechanisms of Qi gong are not well understood, it partially blocks sympathetic activity and it may be effective in treating certain types of sympathetic-related chronic pain syndromes caused either by disease or biomedical treatment.

Tai chi, a form of Qi gong, was originally developed by Chang San Feng in the 13th century. Involving slow, controlled movements coordinated with special breathing techniques, Tai chi is based on a defensive form of martial arts. The original form of Tai chi included 12 movement sequences known as the 12 Chi Disruption Forms. It later evolved into the Wu Dang Mountain Tai chi style. During the 19th century, it was further developed by Yang Lu Chan and became known as the Old Yang Style of Tai chi. Today, many forms of Tai chi are practiced in China,[95,96] and practitioners believe it is an effective form of exercise to promote Qi and Blood flow, maintain balance, and promote longevity.

Herbal and Food Therapy

TCM practitioners often combine acupuncture with the use of herbal or food therapy. It is not the purpose of this chapter to discuss the topic of herbs or therapeutic dietary guidelines, but the same diagnostic paradigm and treatment strategies used in acupuncture therapy are used to select herbal supplements and foods intended to correct imbalances that cause illness and/or pain. Many Chinese herbs have analgesic properties,[97] and further research is greatly needed to understand mechanisms and interactions.

In TCM, single herbs are rarely given. Rather, formulas containing many plant, mineral, or animal substances are given in pill, tincture, powder, or loose herb form. Loose herbs are decocted into teas and taken in divided doses over a 24-hour period.[97] Because of the vast interest in and use of herbal supplements by the public and especially by pain patients, it is important that research to explore herb-drug interactions be conducted and that physicians familiarize themselves with this growing area. Because patients are often reluctant to discuss the use of herbal supplements with their doctor, asking questions in an open-ended, nonjudgmental way during history taking is imperative.

OUTCOMES

Hundreds of clinical trials evaluating the efficacy of acupuncture for various conditions have been conducted since the 1970s. Yet, many studies have been poorly designed, and even today, studies evaluating acupuncture as it is applied in actual clinical practice are few. Nevertheless, evidence of efficacy has reached a sufficient critical mass to draw conclusions in some areas. Strong evidence exists that acupuncture is effective in treating postoperative dental pain and postoperative or chemotherapy-related nausea and vomiting, and two recent meta-analyses found acupuncture is an important adjunct in the treatment of chronic low back pain.[98,99]

In the mid 1990s, the Cochrane Collaboration established a field for reviewing complementary medicine trials. As a result, guidelines and methods for conducting meta-analyses and systematic reviews of acupuncture have become more standardized. While most authors agree methodologic rigor has been weak and further research with stronger study design is needed, properly performed acupuncture seems to be a safe procedure and an important adjunct in the treatment of various conditions. Table 130–1 provides a list of systematic reviews[98-108] and meta-analyses of acupuncture for pain control published since 2000.

One systematic review published in 2005 evaluated 35 randomized clinical trials within the framework of the Cochrane Collaboration. Authors concluded acupuncture and dry needling may be useful adjuncts in the treatment of chronic low back pain but emphasized data are too sparse to evaluate efficacy for acute back pain.[98] A second study[99] published that same year compared 33 randomized, controlled trials of needle acupuncture, sham acupuncture, other sham treatments, no additional treatment, and other active therapies. Again, authors concluded data are too sparse to evaluate acute low back pain but found acupuncture effectively relieves chronic low back pain. For a number of other conditions such as headaches, temporomandibular disorders, neck pain, shoulder pain, tennis elbow, fibromyalgia, and osteoarthritis of the knee, evidence is considered promising but difficult to interpret in many cases. There is a consensus that more and better research is needed.

Acupuncture for Cancer Pain

Several studies have evaluated acupuncture for cancer pain. A randomized, blinded, controlled trial conducted in France investigated the use of auricular acupuncture for cancer pain. Ninety patients were randomly divided into three groups: one group received two courses of auricular acupuncture, one received acupuncture at placebo auricular points, and one group received auricular seeds at placebo points. Efficacy was based on a decrease in pain intensity 2 months after random-

Table 130–1

Systematic Reviews and Meta-Analyses of Acupuncture for Pain Control

Condition	*Authors/Year*	*No. of Studies Included*	*Conclusions*
Chronic pain	Ezzo et al, 2000	51 RCTs	Inconclusive, poor methodology
Low back pain	Ernst et al, 2002	12 RCTs	Data imply acupuncture is superior to various control interventions
	Furlan et al, 2005	35 RCTs	Acupuncture and dry needling may be useful adjuncts for the treatment of chronic low back pain. Data are too sparse to evaluate efficacy for acute back pain.
	Manheimer et al, 2005	33 RCTs	Acupuncture effectively relieves chronic low back pain, but no evidence suggests it is more effective than other active therapies.
Low back + neck pain	Smith et al, 2000	13 RCTs	Negative
Osteoarthritis, knee	Ezzo et al, 2001	7 RCTs	Somewhat positive, poor methodology
	Fernandez et al, 2002	4 RCTs	Insufficient evidence
Inflammatory rheumatic disease	Casimiro et al, 2005	2 RCTs	Inconclusive/negative, poor methodology
Tennis elbow	Green et al, 2002	4 RCTs	Insufficient evidence
Dysmenorrhea	Proctor et al, 2002	2 RCTs	Insufficient evidence
Procedural pain, oocyte aspiration	Stener-Victorin, 2005	12 RCTs	No consensus found on optimal method for pain control during oocyte retrieval

ization using the Visual Analog Scale. At 2 months, pain intensity decreased by 36% from baseline among the treatment group versus 2% among patients in the two placebo groups ($P < 0.0001$).[109] A nonrandomized preliminary study of 20 subjects conducted by the same authors had also revealed a significant decrease in pain intensity after receiving auricular acupuncture. All patients had a chronic pain syndrome related to their cancer diagnosis. The authors reported improvement was not limited to a reduction in pain because some patients stated they felt better in general and wanted to interrupt analgesic treatment.[110]

In 1999, a German study reported positive findings for the use of acupuncture to treat pain in breast cancer patients. Forty-eight patients (group I) who received acupuncture after ablation and axillary lymphadenectomy were compared with 32 patients (group II) who had the same surgical procedure but no acupuncture. Group I showed greater improvement in terms of the maximum abduction angle reached without pain and the maximum tolerable pain barrier after the first treatment, on postoperative days 5 and 7, and at the time of discharge ($P < 0.001$ in each situation). Pain in the operative field at rest was significantly lower in the treatment group on day 5 ($P < 0.01$) but not on day 7 or at discharge ($P > 0.05$). Pain during arm movements was significantly less in the treatment group on days 5 and 7 ($P < 0.01$) and at discharge ($P < 0.001$). The authors concluded acupuncture was effective in this study population for reducing pain and improving arm mobility.[111]

Another randomized clinical trial conducted in China studied pain control in patients with stomach cancer. The results showed similar outcomes in the acupuncture and Western medicine groups at 2 months. According to the authors, long-term outcome measures were superior for the acupuncture group.[112]

Issues in Acupuncture Research

Identifying research methodologies that are scientifically sound yet sensitive to the TCM paradigm is difficult. Often, we find ourselves guilty of comparing the proverbial apples to oranges, and, in many instances, it may be inappropriate to apply an Eastern treatment to a Western diagnosis without first understanding the relationships between Eastern and Western diagnoses. The subset of signs and symptoms deemed clinically relevant often differs between Eastern and Western perspectives even though the patient may have a single chief complaint. For example, in TCM, the prescribed treatment for someone with a migraine headache varies from one patient to another. Thus, a research protocol designed to study migraine headaches must give consideration to the process of TCM differential diagnosis and cannot be based simply on the Western diagnosis of "migraine headache." While the scientific community is unwilling to accept the outcome of studies that are not well designed, TCM practitioners are just as unwilling to accept the outcome of studies that ignore current standards of clinical practice.[113] Although the fact that TCM has been used as a primary source of healthcare by millions of people for thousands of years provides some degree of pragmatic validity, if it is to be integrated into a Western model of healthcare, the two systems must merge so that the strengths of one overcome the weaknesses of the other.

Designing and conducting valid and reliable acupuncture research presents many challenges. Because standard TCM clinical practice calls for individualized treatment, studies from which meaningful results can be drawn have been relatively few. Misleading conclusions, either false negative or false positive, occur for a variety of reasons, including inadequate treatment regimens as well as inappropriate controls.

Determining an adequate study design and optimal treatment plan is extremely complex, and a number of factors must be considered beyond symptomatology and patient characteristics. For example, the specific points selected and number of points used, type of needle, depth of needle insertion, method of stimulation, duration of treatment, and number and frequency of sessions may all affect outcome. Seemingly, the art and science of practice are both important aspects of care, but this poses many problems from a researcher's perspective. Although the specific question under study determines the choice of controls, the use of sham points and/or the use of penetrating sham procedures and nonpenetrating methods such as mock transcutaneous electrical nerve stimulation (TENS) or inactivated laser to either real or sham point locations and blinding of patients, assessors, investigators, analysts, acupuncturists, and other participants are all important considerations for ensuring the accuracy of findings. Recommendations for optimizing treatment and controls have been developed,[114] but debate in this area continues.

COMPLICATIONS AND PITFALLS

Safety and Adverse Events

When compared with other treatments, acupuncture is considered to be relatively safe. Several publications have investigated the safety of acupuncture treatment.[115-119] One prospective survey following 34,000 consultations with professional acupuncturists (members of the British Acupuncture Council) reported no serious adverse events; serious adverse events were defined as requiring hospital admission, prolonging hospital stays, permanently disabling, or resulting in death (95% CI: 0 to 1.1 per 10,000 treatments). Only 43 significant minor adverse events were reported (1.3 per 1000 treatments; 95%CI: 0.9 to 1.7), including severe nausea, fainting, aggravation of symptoms, pain, bruising, and psychological and emotional reactions.[115]

Another large-scale project investigated all first-hand case reports of complications and adverse effects of acupuncture identified in the English language between 1965 and 1999. Over the 35-year period, only 202 incidents were identified in reports from 22 countries. Complications from acupuncture included infections (primarily hepatitis) and organ, tissue, and nerve injury. Other minor adverse effects included cutaneous disorders, hypotension, fainting, and vomiting. Fewer adverse events have been reported since 1988 because of improvements in clinical practice, standardization of clean-needle techniques, and better training of practitioners.[116] A recent multicenter survey conducted in Norway reported that, like any treatment intervention, acupuncture has adverse effects but is safe when performed according to established guidelines.[117]

Most serious adverse events associated with acupuncture treatment occur as a result of improper needle placement secondary to inadequate training of personnel, of not using single-use disposable needles, or of poor technique when cleaning the area before needling. In other words, most adverse events from acupuncture are due to a lack of education or negligence on the part of the practitioner and are not due to the treatment itself. The side effects reported when acupuncture is performed correctly by properly trained personnel are relatively minor and most commonly include fainting, nausea, vomiting, bruising, and mild pain.[115-118] For higher-risk patients (i.e., those with valvular heart disease or neutropenic patients), semipermanent needles should not be used owing to the risk of infection.[119] Finally, electroacupuncture should not be used in patients with cardiac pacemakers or other electronic devices and should be used with caution in patients with metal implants.

Provider Credentialing

Selecting a qualified practitioner is an important decision, and guidelines have been recommended by the NIH/NCCAM.[120] Specific requirements for credentialing acupuncturists vary from state to state, but training programs in the United States have a standardized, clinically based curriculum and are formally accredited by the Accreditation Commission for Acupuncture and Oriental Medicine.[121] In addition, a nonprofit organization, the National Certification Commission for Acupuncture and Oriental Medicine (NCCAOM), was established in 1982 to promote nationally recognized standards of competence and safety. The primary mission of NCCAOM is to protect the public interest in quality care by examining and certifying competence in the practice of acupuncture, Chinese herbology, and Asian bodywork (Tui na) through national board examinations. The first comprehensive written examination administered by NCCAOM for acupuncture was given in March, 1985. Beginning in 2004, testing for competency in basic principles of biomedicine was added. Most states now require successful completion of the NCCAOM board examination for licensure to practice acupuncture.[92]

Guidelines for Patients

Patients should be encouraged to gather as much information about CAM therapies as possible from reputable sources and share that information with their doctor. Patients also should be instructed to bring a list of questions and a complete list of all dietary supplements, including dosage, to follow-up visits and to promptly report any changes to the list. It is particularly important for physicians to inform patients of the risks involved in delaying or foregoing conventional treatment. Asking informed and appropriate questions can help patients to recognize fraudulent claims and avoid potential illness or injury. Table 130–2 provides patients and physicians with a list of questions to ask to ensure that CAM treatments are being provided by a reputable practitioner or group.

Table 130–2

Guidelines for Patients

- What are the provider's credentials and experience?
- Is the provider willing to answer any and all questions you may have regarding his/her background as well as other treatment options and likely outcomes?
- What claims are made for the treatment (i.e., cure, symptom reduction, or to help conventional treatment work better)?
- What are the costs, risks, and potential side effects of treatment?
- Is the provider encouraging you not to use conventional medical care?

CONCLUSION

With an explosion of interest in CAM therapies in recent years,[1-5] several steps have been taken to ensure the quality of care and safety to public health. Healthcare policy has been developed in the United States, and the NCCAM was established at the NIH to stimulate, develop, and support CAM-related research.[8] Specific objectives addressing policy; safety, efficacy, and quality; access; and rational use were also set forth in the *WHO Traditional Medicine Strategy 2002-2005*.[10]

The history of acupuncture spans thousands of years, but its popularity in the United States has grown substantially since the early 1970s. Interest continued to grow after President Richard Nixon's visit to China in 1972, and since that time, programs in training and research have been developed.[13,14]

Acupuncture practitioners use many different approaches for diagnosing and treating patients, ranging from the purely metaphysical to the strictly neurophysiologic. Although integrating ancient concepts into a healthcare delivery system relying solely on modern scientific methods is difficult, it is an endeavor worthy of exploration as certain aspects of human physiologic functional relationships are emphasized in TCM that are not directly addressed by Western biomedicine. Thus, integrating therapies that have been demonstrated to be empirically effective, such as acupuncture, into mainstream healthcare in a well-regulated environment could lead to a dramatic medical paradigm shift, benefiting the general health of the public.[113]

When properly performed, acupuncture is considered a safe procedure. The most common adverse reactions are mild pain or discomfort, fainting, nausea, and bruising. Semipermanent needles should not be used in vulnerable neutropenic patients or in patients with valvular heart disease,[119] and, as a precaution, electroacupuncture should be avoided in patients with cardiac pacemakers or other implanted electronic devices.

Several promising studies are beginning to elucidate the mechanisms and efficacy of acupuncture in a variety of areas. As our understanding improves of how this ancient tradition works, our ability to optimize treatment regimens will also improve. As we endeavor to learn more about therapies such as acupuncture, our focus should not be limited to clinical medicine. Future research should also consider the social, cultural, political, and economic contexts of traditional Chinese medicine.

References

1. Eisenberg DM, Kessler RC, Foster C, et al: Unconventional medicine in the United States: Prevalence, costs and patterns of use. N Engl J Med 328:246, 1993.

2. Eisenberg DM, Davis RB, Ettner SL, et al: Trends in alternative medicine use in the United States, 1990-1997: Results of a follow-up national survey. JAMA 280:1569, 1998.
3. Astin JA: Why patients use alternative medicine: Results of a national study. JAMA 279:1548, 1998.
4. Ni H, Simile C, Hardy AM: Utilization of complementary and alternative medicine by United States adults: Results from the 1999 national health interview survey. Med Care 40:353, 2002.
5. Barnes PM, Powell-Griner E, McFann K, et al: Complementary and alternative medicine use among adults: United States, 2002. Advance Data from Vital and Health Statistics. CDC 343:1, 2004.
6. U.S. Department of Health and Human Services (DHHS): Healthy People 2010. McLean, VA, International Medical, 2000.
7. Bodeker G, Kronenberg F: A public health agenda for traditional, complementary, and alternative medicine. Am J Public Health 92:1582, 2002.
8. National Institutes of Health (NIH): National Center for Complementary and Alternative Medicine (NCCAM). Available at http://www.nccam.nih.gov
9. White House Commission on Complementary and Alternative Medicine Policy: Final Report. Washington, DC, DHHS, 2002. Available at http://www.whccamp.hhs.gov
10. World Health Organization: WHO Traditional Medicine Strategy 2002-2005. Geneva, World Health Organization, 2002.
11. Reston J: Now about my operation in Peking. New York Times, July 26, 1971, pp 1, 6.
12. Dimond EG: Acupuncture anesthesia: Western medicine and Chinese traditional medicine. JAMA 218:1558, 1971.
13. Tkach W: I have seen acupuncture work. Today's Health 50:50, 1972. Cited in Helms JM: Acupuncture Energetics: A Clinical Approach for Physicians. Berkeley, CA, Medical Acupuncture Publishers, 1997, p 3.
14. Chen JYP: Medicine and Public Health in the People's Republic of China. In Quinn JR (ed): U.S. Department of Health, Education and Welfare: National Institutes of Health, John S. Fogarty International Center, 1972, pp 65-90. Cited in Helms JM: Acupuncture Energetics: A Clinical Approach for Physicians. Berkeley, CA, Medical Acupuncture Publishers, 1997, p 3.
15. Bache F: Cases illustrative of the remedial effects of acupuncture. North Am Med Surg J 2:311, 1826. Cited in Helms JM: Acupuncture Energetics: A Clinical Approach for Physicians. Berkeley, CA, Medical Acupuncture Publishers, 1997, p 5.
16. Osler W: The Principles and Practices of Medicine. New York, Appleton, 1892, pp 282, 820. Cited in Helms JM: Acupuncture Energetics: A Clinical Approach for Physicians. Berkeley, CA, Medical Acupuncture Publishers, 1997, p 4.
17. Warren E: An Epitome of Practical Surgery. Richmond, VA, West and Johnston, 1863, p 228. Cited in Helms JM: Acupuncture Energetics: A Clinical Approach for Physicians. Berkeley, CA, Medical Acupuncture Publishers, 1997, p 4.
18. Mayer DJ, Price DD, Rafii A: Antagonism of acupuncture analgesia in man by the narcotic antagonist naloxone. Brain Res 121:368, 1977.
19. Pomeranz B, Cheng R: Suppression of noxious responses in single neurons of cat spinal cord by electroacupuncture and its reversal by the opiate antagonist naloxone. Exp Neurol 64:327, 1979.
20. Clement-Jones V, McLoughlin L, Tomlin S, et al: Increased beta-endorphin but not met-enkephalin levels in human cerebrospinal fluid after acupuncture for recurrent pain. Lancet 2:946, 1980.
21. Pert A, Dionne R, Ng L, et al: Alterations in rat central nervous system endorphins following transauricular electroacupuncture. Brain Res 224:83, 1981.
22. Han JS, Terenius L: Neurochemical basis of acupuncture analgesia. Annu Rev Pharmacol Toxicol 22:193, 1982.
23. Han JS, Xie GX: Dynorphin: Important mediator for electroacupuncture analgesia in the spinal cord of the rabbit. Pain 18:367, 1984.
24. Helms JM: Acupuncture Energetics: A Clinical Approach for Physicians. Berkeley, CA, Medical Acupuncture Publishers, 1997.
25. Kaptchuk T: The Web That Has No Weaver: Understanding Chinese Medicine. Chicago, Congdon & Weed, 1983.
26. Maciocia G: The Foundations of Chinese Medicine: A Comprehensive Text for Acupuncturists and Herbalists. New York, Churchill Livingstone, 1998.
27. Pomeranz B, Chiu D: Naloxone blockade of acupuncture analgesia: Endorphin implicated. Life Sci 19:1757, 1976.
28. Mittleman E, Gaynor JS: A brief overview of the analgesic and immunologic effects of acupuncture in domestic animals. J Am Vet Med Assoc 217:1201, 2000.
29. Kendall DE: A scientific model for acupuncture: II. Am J Acupunct 17:343, 1989.
30. Melzack R, Wall PD: Pain mechanisms: A new theory. Science 150:971, 1965.
31. Wu MT, Hsieh JC, Xiong J, et al: Central nervous system pathway for acupuncture stimulation: Localization of processing with functional MR imaging of the brain—preliminary experience. Radiology 212:133, 1999.
32. Zhang D, Fu W, Wang S, et al: Displaying of infrared thermogram of temperature character on meridians. Zhen Ci Yan Jiu 21:63, 1996.
33. Eory A: In-vivo skin respiration (CO_2) measurements in the acupuncture loci. Acupunct Electrother Res 9:217, 1984.
34. Lee MH, Ernst M: The sympatholytic effect of acupuncture as evidenced by thermography: A preliminary report. Orthop Rev 12:67, 1983.
35. Petti F, Bangrazi A, Liguori A, et al: Effects of acupuncture on immune response related to opioid-like peptides. J Tradit Chin Med 18:55, 1998.
36. Matthews PM, Froelich CJ, Sibbitt WL, et al: Enhancement of natural cytotoxicity by beta-endorphin. J Immunol 130:1658, 1983.
37. Bianchi M, Jotti E, Sacerdote P, et al: Traditional acupuncture increases the content of beta-endorphin in immune cells and influences mitogen induced proliferation. Am J Chin Med 19:101, 1991.
38. Moss CS: Acupuncture stimulation of endogenous opioids and effects on the immune system. Clin Ecol 88:140, 1987.
39. Sin YJ, Sedgewick AR, Mackay MB, et al: Effect of electric acupuncture on acute inflammation. Am J Acupunct 11:359, 1983.
40. Shang C: Mechanism of acupuncture: Beyond neurohumoral theory. 2003. Available at www.acupuncture.com
41. Gunn CC: Type IV acupuncture points. Am J Acupunct 5:51, 1977.
42. Huang YC: Anatomy and classification of acupoints. Probl Vet Med 4:12, 1992.
43. Bossy J, Sambuc P: Acupuncture et système nerveaux: Les acquis. Acupuncture et Médecine Traditionnelle Chinoise. Paris, Encyclopédie des Médecines Naturelles, IB-1, 1989. Cited in Helms JM: Acupuncture Energetics: A Clinical Approach for Physicians. Berkeley, CA, Medical Acupuncture Publishers, 1997, p 26.
44. Senelar R: Caractéristiques morphologiques des points chinois. In Niboyet JEH (ed): Nouveau Traité d'Acupuncture. Moulins-lès-Metz, Maisonneuve, 1979, pp 247. Cited in Helms JM: Acupuncture Energetics: A Clinical Approach for Physicians. Berkeley, CA, Medical Acupuncture Publishers, 1997, p 26.
45. Senelar R, Auziech O: Histophysiologie du point d'acupuncture. Acupuncture et Médecine Traditionnelle Chinoise. Paris, Encyclopédie des Médecines Naturelles, IB-2C, 1989. Cited in Helms JM: Acupuncture Energetics: A Clinical Approach for Physicians. Berkeley, CA, Medical Acupuncture Publishers, 1997, p 27.
46. Auziech O: Étude Histologique des Points Cutanés de Moindre Résistance Électrique et Analyse de Leurs Implications Possibles Dans la Mise en Jeu des Mécanismes Acupuncturaux. Montpellier, Thèse de Médecine, 1984. Cited in Helms JM: Acupuncture Energetics: A Clinical Approach for Physicians. Berkeley, CA, Medical Acupuncture Publishers, 1997, p 27.
47. Dung HC: Anatomical features contributing to the formation of acupuncture points. Am J Acupunct 12:139, 1984.
48. Kendall DE: A scientific model for acupuncture: I. Am J Acupunct 17:251, 1989.
49. Dolson AL: Acupuncture from a pathologist's perspective: Linking physical to energetic. Med Acupunct 10:25, 1998.
50. Becker RO, Reichmanis M: Electrophysiologic correlates of acupuncture points and meridians. Psychoenergetic Systems 1:195, 1976.
51. Reichmanis M, Marino AA, Becker RO: DC skin conductance variation at acupuncture loci. Am J Chin Med 4:69, 1976.
52. Still J: Relationship between electrically active skin points and acupuncture meridian points in the dog. Am J Acupunct 16:55, 1988.
53. Niboyet JEH, Mery A: Compte-rendu recherches expérimentales sur les méridiens; chez le vivant et chez le cadavre. Actes des IIlème Journées Internationales d'Acupuncture, 1957, pp 47-51. Cited in Helms JM: Acupuncture Energetics: A Clinical Approach for Physicians. Berkeley, CA, Medical Acupuncture Publishers, 1997, p 20.
54. Grall Y: Contribution à l'Étude de la Conductibilité Électrique de la Peau. Algiers, Thèse de Médecine, 1962. Cited in Helms JM:

Acupuncture Energetics: A Clinical Approach for Physicians. Berkeley, CA, Medical Acupuncture Publishers, 1997, p 21.
55. Human Anatomy Department of Shanghai Medical University: A relationship between points of meridian and peripheral nerves. Acupuncture Anesthetic Theory Study. Shanghai, Shanghai Peoples Publishing House, 1973. Cited in Helms JM: Acupuncture Energetics: A Clinical Approach for Physicians. Berkeley, CA, Medical Acupuncture Publishers, 1997, p 27.
56. Melzack R, Stillwell DM, Fox EJ: Trigger points and acupuncture points for pain: Correlations and implications. Pain 3:3, 1977.
57. Dung HC: Three principles of acupuncture points. Am J Acupunct 12:263, 1984.
58. Mann F: Acupuncture: The Ancient Chinese Art of Healing and How it Works Scientifically. New York, Random House, 1971, pp 5-16.
59. Deng L, Gan Y, He S, et al: Acupuncture techniques. In Cheng Y (ed): Chinese Acupuncture and Moxibustion. Beijing, Foreign Languages Press, 1997, pp 325-326.
60. Cooperative Group of Investigation of PSAC: Advances in Acupuncture and Acupuncture Anesthesia. Beijing, The Peoples' Medical Publishing House, 1980.
61. Meng Z, et al: New development in the researches of meridian phenomena in China during the past five years. Zhen Ci Yan Jiu 9:207, 1984.
62. Cooperative Group in Research of PSC, Fujian Province: Studies of relation between propagated sensation along channels and effectiveness of clinical acupuncture analgesia. In Zhang XT (ed): Research on Acupuncture, Moxibustion, and Acupuncture Anesthesia. Beijing, Science Press, 1986.
63. Eckman P: Acupuncture and science. Int J Chin Med 1:3, 1984.
64. Xuetai W: Research on the origin and development of Chinese acupuncture and moxibustion. In Zhang XT (ed): Research on Acupuncture, Moxibustion, and Acupuncture Anesthesia. Beijing, Science Press, 1986, p 791.
65. Xiao YJ, Su DG: Effect of local refrigeration on ECG changes of EA in Neiguan acupoint. In Second National Symposium of Acupuncture and Moxibustion and Acupuncture Anesthesia. Beijing, 1984, p 291. Cited in Helms JM: Acupuncture Energetics: A Clinical Approach for Physicians. Berkeley, CA, Medical Acupuncture Publishers, 1997, p 23.
66. Research Group of Acupuncture Anesthesia, Fujian: Studies of phenomenon of blocking activities of channels and collaterals. In Zhang XT (ed): Research on Acupuncture, Moxibustion, and Acupuncture Anesthesia. Beijing, Science Press, 1986, pp 653-667.
67. Xue CC: The phenomenon of propagated sensation along channels (PSAC) and the cerebral cortex. In Zhang XT (ed): Research on Acupuncture, Moxibustion, and Acupuncture Anesthesia. Beijing, Science Press, 1986, pp 668-683.
68. Darras JC, et al: Visualisation isotopique des méridiens d'acupuncture. Cahiers de Biothérapie 95:13, 1987. Cited in Helms JM: Acupuncture Energetics: A Clinical Approach for Physicians. Berkeley, CA, Medical Acupuncture Publishers, 1997, p 23.
69. Mussat M: Les Réseaux d'Acupuncture: Étude Critique et Expérimentale. Paris, Librairie le Francois, 1974, pp 255-300. Cited in Helms JM: Acupuncture Energetics: A Clinical Approach for Physicians. Berkeley, CA, Medical Acupuncture Publishers, 1997, pp 24-25.
70. Shamos MH, Lavine LS: Piezoelectricity as a fundamental property of biological tissues. Nature 213:267, 1967.
71. Fan JY: The role of gap junctions in determining skin conductance and their possible relationship to acupuncture points and meridians. Am J Acupunct 18:163, 1990.
72. Zheng JY, Fan JY, Zhang YJ, et al: Further evidence for the role of gap junctions in acupoint information transfer. Am J Acupunct 24:291, 1996.
73. National Acupuncture Foundation: The theory and practice of clean needle technique. In Mitchell B, Davis E, McCormick J, et al (eds): Clean Needle Technique Manual for Acupuncturists: Guidelines and Standards for the Clean and Safe Clinical Practice of Acupuncture. Washington, DC, National Acupuncture Foundation, 1997, pp 10-22.
74. Altman S: Techniques and instrumentation: Electroacupuncture. In Schoen AM (ed): Veterinary Acupuncture—Ancient Art to Modern Medicine. St. Louis, Mosby, 1994, pp 95-102.
75. Han JS: Physiologic and neurochemical basis of acupuncture analgesia. In Han JS (ed): The Neurochemical Basis of Pain Relief by Acupuncture. Beijing, Beijing Medical University, 1987, pp 589-597.
76. Pomeranz B: Electroacupuncture and transcutaneous electrical nerve stimulation. In Stux G, Pomeranz B (ed): Basics of Acupuncture, 2nd ed. Berlin, Springer-Verlag, 1991, pp 250-260.
77. Han JS: The Neuro-chemical Basis of Pain Control by Acupuncture. Beijing, Hu Bei Technical and Science Press, 1998.
78. Ulett G: Acupuncture: Archaic or biologic? Am J Public Health 93:1037, 2003.
79. Deng L, Gan Y, He S, et al: Acupuncture techniques. In Cheng Y (ed): Chinese Acupuncture and Moxibustion. Beijing, Foreign Languages Press, 1997, pp 491-512.
80. Huang LC: Auriculotherapy: Diagnosis and Treatment. Bellaire, TX, Longevity Press, 1996, p 3.
81. Nogier P: Treatise of Auriculotherapy. Moulins-lès-Metz, Maisonneuve, 1972. Cited in Helms JM: Acupuncture Energetics: A Clinical Approach for Physicians. Berkeley, CA, Medical Acupuncture Publishers, 1997, p 135.
82. Nogier P: Introduction Pratique à l'Auriculothérape. Moulins-lès-Metz, Maisonneuve, 1978. Cited in Helms JM: Acupuncture Energetics: A Clinical Approach for Physicians. Berkeley, CA, Medical Acupuncture Publishers, 1997, p 135.
83. Nogier P: From Auriculotherapy to Auriculomedicine. Moulins-lès-Metz, Maisonneuve, 1983. Cited in Helms JM: Acupuncture Energetics: A Clinical Approach for Physicians. Berkeley, CA, Medical Acupuncture Publishers, 1997, p 135.
84. Nogier P, Nogier R: The Man in the Ear. Moulins-lès-Metz, Maisonneuve, 1985. Cited in Helms JM: Acupuncture Energetics: A Clinical Approach for Physicians. Berkeley, CA, Medical Acupuncture Publishers, 1997, p 135.
85. Taillandier J: Réflexothérapies et microsystèmes en acupuncture. Bases physiologiques et thérapeutiques. Acupuncture et Médecine Traditionnelle Chinoise. Paris, Encyclopédie des Médecines Naturelles, II-1, 1989. Cited in Helms JM: Acupuncture Energetics: A Clinical Approach for Physicians. Berkeley, CA, Medical Acupuncture Publishers, 1997, p 132.
86. Jiao S: Scalp Acupuncture and Clinical Cases. Beijing, Foreign Languages Press, 1997.
87. Chen Y, Zhao C, Chen H, et al: Effects of "moxibustion serum" on proliferation and phenotypes of tumor infiltrating lymphocytes. J Tradit Chin Med 23:225, 2003.
88. Liu J, Yu RC, Tang WJ: Influence of combined therapy of guben yiliu III, moxibustion and chemotherapy on immune function and blood coagulation mechanism in patients with mid-late stage malignant tumor. Zhongguo Zhong Xi Yi Jie He Za Zhi 22:104, 2002.
89. Liu J, Yu RC, Rao XQ: Study on effect of moxibustion and guben yiliu III combined with chemotherapy in treating middle-late stage malignant tumor. Zhongguo Zhong Xi Yi Jie He Za Zhi 21:262, 2001.
90. Hitosugi, N, Ohno, R, Hatsukari I, et al: Induction of cell death by pro-oxidant action of Moxa smoke. Anticancer Res 22:159, 2002.
91. Wang G, Fan Y, Guan Z, et al: Chinese massage. In Zhang E (ed): A Practical English-Chinese Library of Traditional Chinese Medicine. Shanghai, Publishing House of Shanghai University of Traditional Chinese Medicine, 1988.
92. National Certification Commission for Acupuncture and Oriental Medicine: General Information Brochure. NCCAOM, 2003. Available at http://www.nccaom.org/om_first.htm
93. Bi YS, Sun H, Guo Y, et al: Chinese qigong. In Zhang E (ed): A Practical English-Chinese Library of Traditional Chinese Medicine. Shanghai, Publishing House of Shanghai University of Traditional Chinese Medicine, 1988.
94. Ni M: The Yellow Emperor's Classic of Medicine: A New Translation of the Neijing Suwen with Commentary. Boston, Shambhala, 1995.
95. Brecher P: Secrets of Energy Work. London, Dorling Kindersley, 2001, pp 16-17.
96. Yang JM: Advanced Yang Style Tai Chi Chuan Martial Applications. Jamaica Plain, MA, YMAA Publication Center, 1996.
97. Bensky D, Barolet R: Chinese Herbal Medicine: Formulas & Strategies. Seattle, WA, Eastland Press, 1990.
98. Furlan AD, van Tulder M, Cherkin D, et al: Acupuncture and dry-needling for low back pain: An updated systematic review within the framework of the Cochrane collaboration. Spine 30:944, 2005.
99. Manheimer E, White A, Berman B, et al: Meta-analysis: Acupuncture for low back pain. Ann Intern Med 142: 651, 2005.
100. Ezzo J, Berman B, Hadhazy VA, et al: Is acupuncture effective for the treatment of chronic pain: A systematic review. Pain 86:217, 2000.

101. Ernst E, White AR, Wider B: Acupuncture for back pain: Meta-analysis of randomized controlled trials and an update with data from the most recent studies. Schmerz 16:129, 2002. In German.
102. Smith LA, Oldman AD, McQuay HJ, et al: Teasing apart quality and validity in systematic reviews: An example from acupuncture RCTs in chronic neck and back pain. Pain 86:119, 2000.
103. Ezzo J, Hadhazy V, Birch S, et al: Acupuncture for osteoarthritis of the knee: A systematic review. Arthritis Rheum 44:819, 2001.
104. Fernandez IA, Garcia OL, Gonzalez GA, et al: Effectiveness of acupuncture in the treatment of pain from osteoarthritis of the knee. Aten Primaria 30:602, 2002.
105. Casimiro L, Barnsley L, Brosseau L, et al: Acupuncture and electroacupuncture for the treatment of rheumatoid arthritis. The Cochrane Database of Systematic Reviews (4): CD003788, 2005.
106. Green S, Buchbinder R, Barnsley L, et al: Acupuncture for lateral elbow pain. The Cochrane Database of Systematic Reviews (1):CD003527, 2002.
107. Proctor ML, Smith CA, Farquhar CM, et al: Transcutaneous electrical nerve stimulation and acupuncture for primary dysmenorrhea (Cochrane Review). In The Cochrane Library, Issue 3. Oxford, Update Software, 2002.
108. Stener-Victorin E: The pain-relieving effect of electroacupuncture and conventional medical analgesic methods during oocyte retrieval: A systematic review of randomized controlled trials. Hum Reprod 20:339, 2005.
109. Alimi D, Rubino C, Pichard-Leandri E, et al: Analgesic effect of auricular acupuncture for cancer pain: A randomized, blinded, controlled trial. J Clin Oncol 21:4120, 2003.
110. Alimi D, Rubino C, Leandri EP, et al: Analgesic effects of auricular acupuncture for cancer pain. J Pain Symptom Manage 19:81, 2000.
111. He JP, Friedrich M, Ertan AK, et al: Pain-relief and movement improvement by acupuncture after ablation and axillary lymphadenectomy in patients with mammary cancer. Clin Exp Obstet Gynecol 26:81, 1999.
112. Dang W, Yang J: Clinical study on acupuncture treatment of stomach carcinoma pain. J Tradit Chin Med 18:31, 1998.
113. Giordano J, Garcia MK, Boatwright D, et al: Complementary and alternative medicine in mainstream public health: A role for research in fostering integration. J Altern Complement Med 9:441, 2003.
114. White AR, Filshie J, Cummings TM, et al: Clinical trials of acupuncture: Consensus recommendations for optimal treatment, sham controls and blinding. Complement Ther Med 9:237, 2001.
115. MacPherson H, Thomas K, Walters S, et al: A prospective survey of adverse events and treatment reactions following 34,000 consultations with professional acupuncturists. Acupunct Med 19:93, 2001.
116. Lao L, Hamilton GR, Fu J, et al: Is acupuncture safe? A systematic review of case reports. Altern Ther Health Med 9:72, 2003.
117. Ernst G, Strzyz H, Hagmeister H: Incidence of adverse effects during acupuncture therapy—a multicentre survey. Comp Ther Med 11:93, 2003.
118. Chung A, Bui L, Mills E: Adverse effects of acupuncture: Which are clinically significant? Can Fam Physician 49:985, 2003.
119. Filshie J: Safety aspects of acupuncture in palliative care. Acupunct Med 19:117, 2001.
120. National Center for Complementary and Alternative Medicine: Selecting a complementary and alternative medicine (CAM) practitioner. NIH/NCCAM, 2003. Available at http://nccam.nih.gov/health/practitioner/index.htm
121. Accreditation Commission for Acupuncture and Oriental Medicine: Handbook. Greenbelt, MD, ACAOM, 2003. Available at http://acaom.org/handbook.htm

chapter 131

Prolotherapy: Regenerative Injection Therapy

K. Dean Reeves

Prolotherapy is injection of growth factors or growth factor production stimulants to grow normal cells or tissue.[1] Growth factors are powerful (hormone-like) polypeptides that induce wide-ranging effects including cell migration, proliferation, and protein synthesis. These powerful proteins may be produced by the cell affected or may be produced in other cells. To be effective, these growth factors (GFs) must avoid the binding proteins that could cause their inactivation, find their way to the area needing growth, and hook onto an appropriate receptor protein.

GROWTH FACTOR INJECTION PROLOTHERAPY AND GROWTH FACTOR PRODUCTION PROLOTHERAPY: REVIEW OF THE LITERATURE

There are two major methods of prolotherapy. The first such method is growth factor injection in which already-produced growth factors are injected. Examples of this include injection of blood, and injection of mass-produced recombinant growth factors. The second method is growth factor production stimulation in which there is the injection of a solution that initiates production of growth factors. Examples of this method include injection of dextrose, injection of inflammatory agents that initiate an inflammatory cascade to produce growth factors, and injection of plasmid DNA that produces growth factors.[1-2]

Non-musculoskeletal Prolotherapy

Non-musculoskeletal prolotherapy is a very large area of research, with examples of current use including erythropoietin (erythrocyte growth factor) injection for treatment of anemia[3] and injection of megakaryocyte growth factor injection for platelet production in aplastic anemia patients.[4] Other examples of growth factor injection uses in humans that are in process of study include injection of non-graftable heart muscle with fibroblast growth factor (FGF),[5] or injection of vascular endothelial growth factor in the heart muscle of inoperable patients with coronary artery disease.[6] Clinically significant benefit has been demonstrated in animal work in a variety of areas, such as in hepatocyte growth factor (HGF) injection to reverse renal failure after injury,[7] femoral artery infusion of vascular endothelial growth factor in intermittent claudication,[8] intravenous infusion of FGF-18 in acute middle cerebral artery occlusion,[9] or injection of growth factors to treat induced diabetic neuropathy.[10]

Although the primary object of this chapter is to summarize research and describe methods for musculoskeletal prolotherapy, there are several key points to learn from non-musculoskeletal prolotherapy that apply to musculoskeletal prolotherapy. The first is that the names of growth factors do not correspond to their effects and that some growth factors affect a variety of cells. For example, erythrocyte growth factor has recently been found to have potent neural cell protective effects.[11] The growth factors are usually named by the cell in which they were first found to have an effect. A second key point is that injection needs to be in the correct area, as non-discriminant IV injection of growth factor can make a variety of cells grow that are bathed by the circulation, rather than the one desired. An example of this is the creation of proteinuria by IV administration of fibroblast growth factor that affects renal cells rather than the cell intended.[12] A third key is that the presence of a growth factor can be brief and still create a substantial clinical effect. Lederman and coworkers provided an example in their femoral artery infusion study of FGF-2 in which a single intra-arterial infusion of FGF-2 with a short half-life led to an increased walking time 90 days later.[8]

Animal Research in Musculoskeletal Prolotherapy

Animal research in prolotherapy has predominantly looked at one of the following areas: Collagen fiber diameter, ligament/tendon thickness/mass, tendon strength, or cartilage growth.

1. Collagen fiber diameter: Liu and coworkers demonstrated a highly significant 56% increase in collagen fiber diameter in rabbit medial collateral ligaments after injection of an inflammatory solution (sodium morrhuate) compared to normal saline control.[13]
2. Ligament/tendon thickness/mass: Liu and coworkers also demonstrated a mass increase of 47% in medial collateral ligaments injected by sodium morrhuate. The ligaments

were removed and weighed to determine this increase (or change).[13]

3. Ligament/tendon strength: Growth factor injection (cartilage-derived morphogenetic protein-2, CDMP-2) was performed in the Achilles tendon equivalent in rats within 6 hours of an induced injury to that tendon.[14] Eight days later those rats injected with CDMP-2 were 39% stronger to the point of rupture than controls. More recently, injection of TGF beta 1 immediately post-repair of transected Achilles tendon in rats increased force to rupture 4 weeks postoperatively.[15] Blood contains platelets that have a variety of growth factors such as platelet-derived growth factor (PDGF), transforming growth factor beta (TGF beta) and epidermal growth factor (EGF). Autologous platelet concentrate has been injected in the postsurgical hematoma after Achilles transection and repair with resultant increase in tendon strength of 30%.[16] The ability of whole blood injection to strengthen even normal tendons was demonstrated by Taylor and associates when they injected normal rabbit patellar tendon equivalent just once with 0.15 mL of autologous blood.[17] Twelve weeks after injection, the tendon was normal in morphology under the microscope but was 15% stronger. ($P < .014$) .
4. Cartilage growth: Exposure of full-thickness defects in the medial femoral condyle in immature rabbits to a collagen sponge impregnated with insulin-like growth factor-1 led to full-thickness repair of hyaline cartilage.[18] However no studies designed to demonstrate full-thickness hyaline cartilage repair in mature animals using injection of multiple growth factors simultaneously have been reported.

Human Research in Musculoskeletal Prolotherapy

Human studies have primarily been in four areas: low back pain, arthritis, ligament tightening, and sports.

Low Back Pain

In the treatment of low back pain there are four treatment-comparison studies.[19-22] They are published as placebo-controlled studies, but the control group in all back studies involved needle contact with attachments of ligaments and tendons. By injecting ligaments and tendons, there is needle contact with cell membranes of connective tissue cells. Disrupting cell membranes releases lipids, which in turn cause signaling of fibroblasts. In addition, microbleeding from needle contact is expected, and Edwards and colleagues have demonstrated the potential healing effect of whole blood injection in patients with recalcitrant tennis elbow.[23]

Despite better-than-placebo improvement in the control group, the first two blinded studies of chronic low back pain (using phenol/dextrose/glycerin as active solution) demonstrated significant ($P < .001$)[19] and near significant ($P = .056$)[20] evidence for superior effect of the inflammatory proliferant solution over saline needling (study one) and anesthetic needling (study two). These two studies were weakened somewhat by multiple simultaneous treatments, although the injection solution was the only significant difference between the two groups. Unfortunately the third[21] and fourth[22] blinded studies were hampered by technique issues, especially the third. Study three was led by a chief investigator who did not know referral patterns for ligaments, excluded patients with leg pain, and arranged for prolotherapy from another physician who was allowed to treat only areas that would treat leg pain rather than back pain.[21] Study results clearly demonstrated the importance of examination and knowledge of ligament referral patterns, in that these patients who were injected in the incorrect areas with inflammatory proliferant did worse than the controls. Study four showed an excellent design in general and showed substantial benefit to needling with proliferant (dextrose) and without proliferant both, even at 1-year follow-up, with no significant difference for the inclusion of proliferant solution.[22] However, incomplete injection method in this study was also present and likely affected the ability to demonstrate a difference between inclusion of proliferant and simple needling.

The hope is that future studies on low back pain will include a near-placebo arm that avoids connective tissue contact or blood effects and that standard injection methods will be used. In the treatment of low back pain, standard treatment methods are now taught in cadaver courses offered by the American Academy of Orthopedic Medicine. An example of such a near-placebo would be needle insertion through skin without contacting bone or ligament. Meanwhile consecutive patient studies with complete technique continue to support a high percentage of response to proliferant injection in chronic back pain patients.[24]

Arthritis

Simple dextrose injection has been researched in several double blind studies on arthritis. The reason dextrose is of interest as a potential growth stimulant is related to the effects of serum (and related tissue) dextrose (glucose) elevation in humans with the diagnosis of diabetes. A variety of cell growth occurs in diabetic humans, and this includes retinal proliferation of blood vessels, mesangial cell proliferation in kidneys, and endothelial cell proliferation in blood vessels. Table 131–1 lists major growth factors for both ligament, tendon, and cartilage.[25] Cells in the animal or human body either produce the growth factors necessary for their own repair and multiplication or nearby cells do. In vitro studies on human fibroblasts and chondrocytes show that glucose elevation to 0.5% to 0.6% (normal cell concentration is 0.1%) results in prompt and powerful stimulation of growth factor production by a variety of human cells, including fibroblasts and chondrocytes, within 2 hours.[26-29] Table 131–1 demonstrates that the growth factors produced by glucose elevation are the same as those that stimulate ligament, tendon, and cartilage repair. It is important to note that glucose elevation is not associated with production of disrepair factors or bone growth factors. Glucose elevation, in fact, appears to elevate gremlin, an inhibitor to bone growth factor[30] and to decrease levels of disrepair factors such as collagenase and tissue inhibitor of matrix metalloproteinase.[31]

Double-blind placebo-controlled studies on glucose injection in arthritis have been conducted on large and small joints. A large joint study was conducted on patients with knee osteoarthritis.[32] At 0, 2, and 4 months, 9 mL of 10% dextrose was injected in 111 knees. Knee pain had been present an average of >8 years, <3 mm of cartilage remained on average, and 35/111 knees were bone on bone in at least one compartment. The treatment amounted to injection of less than one ounce of 10% dextrose total, over the 6-month period, and resulted in 35% reduction of pain, 45% improvement in

Table 131–1

Growth Factors Associated with Ligament and Tendon Healing and Those That Elevate with Cellular Exposure to Dextrose 0.5%

Growth Factor (GF)	*Ligament and Tendon GFs*	*Cartilage GFs*	*Dextrose GF Effects*
PDGF	Yes	Yes	Yes
TGF-β	Yes	Yes	Yes
bFGF	Yes	Yes	Yes
IGF	Yes	Yes	Yes
CTGF		Yes	Yes

bFGF, basic fibroblast growth factor; CTGF, connective tissue growth factor; IGF, insulin-like growth factor; PDGF, platelet-derived growth factor; TGF-beta, tumor growth factor-beta.

swelling, and a 67% improvement in knee buckling. Treatment solution was superior to placebo solution ($P = 0.015$). Knee flexion improved 13.2 degrees ($P < 0.0001$) from baseline.

A small joint double-blind placebo-controlled study was conducted on finger osteoarthritis (OA).[33] Subjects were patients with OA of fingers by standard radiographic criteria[34] and had pain for more than 5 years. In this study, symptomatic finger joints were injected with ¼ to ½ mL of 10% dextrose on both sides of each joint at 0, 2, and 4 months. This resulted in a 42% improvement in pain and an 8-degree improvement in range of motion, with dextrose superior to bacteriostatic water in pain improvement ($P = 0.027$) and flexibility of joints ($P = 0.003$). Note that in these studies, a 10% concentration of dextrose was chosen—a concentration not shown to cause any inflammation—thus helping to ensure that clinical benefit was an effect of elevated dextrose, not from elevation of the inflammatory cascade. This also ensured blinding accuracy because no post-injection inflammation occurred.

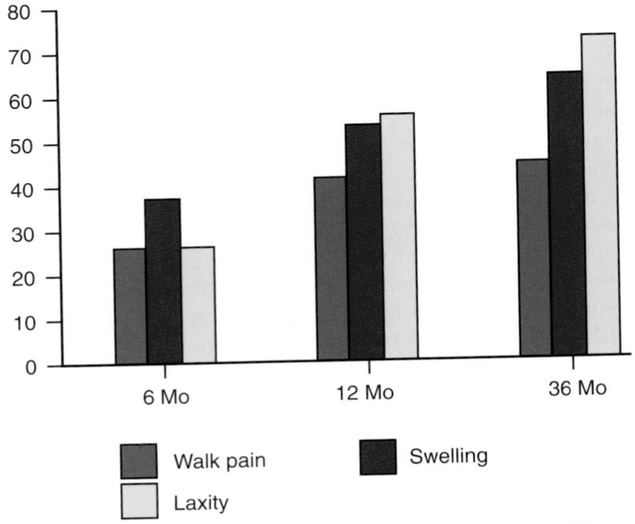

FIGURE 131–1 ■ Percentage improvement in walking pain, swelling, and measurable joint laxity (KT1000 anterior displacement) difference at 6, 12, and 36 months.

Ligament Tightening

A pilot study on ligament tightening in humans was conducted by Ongley in which a Genucom knee apparatus was used to measure knee laxity in anterior drawer fashion.[35] Although this was a small study, objective measurement of ACL excursion decreased from a mean of 9.4 mm to a mean of 6.2 mm. A 3-year follow-up study of patients with ACL laxity treated with simple dextrose injection was published in 2003.[36] All but 2 of the 16 patients also had symptomatic osteoarthritis with minimal or no residual cartilage. All knees were machine measured on both sides with a KT-1000 arthrometer to determine a side-to-side difference (termed ADD or anterior displacement distance), which is the definitive way to objectively determine laxity. They were injected bimonthly with 10% to 25% dextrose solution for 1 year and then on an as-needed basis for knee looseness or pain complaints until 3-year follow-up. Ten out of 16 knees were no longer loose by machine measurement at time of follow-up. In addition, despite advanced osteoarthritis, data showed a gain of range of motion of 10.5 degrees over the course of the study without other intervention, and a continuing improvement in pain, feeling of swelling and in knee laxity measures over the 3-year follow-up period (Fig. 131–1).

Sports

The ability to objectively demonstrate radiographic healing of sprain and strain is now available via high-resolution CT scan and high-resolution ultrasound. The first case study has been published, demonstrating healing of a complete Achilles tendon rupture in a soccer athlete.[37] Topol published a consecutive patient prospective study involving 24 elite athletes (22 rugby and 2 soccer players) with >6 months of chronic groin pain preventing full sports participation, unresponsive to therapy, and graded sports reintroduction.[38] Patients received monthly injection of 12.5% dextrose/0.5% lidocaine in adductor and abdominal insertions and symphysis pubis, depending on palpation tenderness. Injections were given until complete resolution or lack of improvement for two consecutive treatments. A mean of 2.8 treatments were given. Reduction in visual analog pain scale (for pain with sports) was from a mean of 6.3 to 1.0 ($P < 0.0001$) and reduction in Nirschl pain phase scale was from 5.25 to 0.79. ($P < 0.0001$) 22 of 24 athletes were unrestricted with sports at an average 17 months of follow-up, and 20 of 24 patients had no pain in the groin.

Needling: A Cousin of Prolotherapy

The power of traumatic needling was illustrated by Altay when he published a double blind study of steroid injection versus anesthetic in lateral epicondylosis in which 56/60 patients in the anesthetic group had excellent results defined as no pain, no loss of grip strength, and no pain with resisted dorsiflexion at 1-year follow-up.[39] Also powerfully illustrated was that steroid did not blunt the healing response to traumatic needling; the group that received traumatic needling with steroid included did just as well. Needling is not technically prolotherapy because the solution itself does not contain growth factors or growth factor stimulants. However, earlier in this chapter we considered the effects of nontraumatic injection of blood to strengthen rabbit tendon even without trauma[17] and the ability to benefit patients with lateral epicondylosis without trauma with blood injection.[23] With trauma of tapping, bleeding would be expected and thus traumatic tapping would be similar to injecting with blood. One may ask why bother to include a proliferant in the solution if traumatic needling is so effective? The answer is found in practicality. Areas that are larger in size may require sedation for aggressive tapping to be tolerated. Also, if small nerve branches are touched in the process of injection, additional trauma can occur if tapping is under way and not stopped at the first indication of an electrical response.

Specificity of Response of Ligaments and Tendons to Growth Factors

Chun and colleagues published a critical observation that showed differences in fibroblast cell response in rabbit MCL and ACL ligament.[40] Specifically rabbit MCL fibroblast cells respond substantially faster in terms of growth than do ACL fibroblasts when exposed to TGF-β. Tang and coworkers illustrated the cooperative nature of injectants by demonstrating that in culture hyaluronic acid plus basic fibrublast growth factor (bFGF) together had an additive effect on growth of both ACL and MCL ligament cells.[41] These observations are critical as we look to the future because we are treating a complex human body in which one treatment may work best for certain ligaments and not for others and in which combinations may be more effective than single components. Inexpensive approaches currently available such as dry needling and dextrose injection stimulate a variety of growth factors simultaneously.

GENERAL INDICATIONS FOR MUSCULOSKELETAL PROLOTHERAPY

Sprain and Strain

A *sprain* by definition is damage to a ligament and a *strain* is damage to a tendon. The poor results from steroid injection in chronic sprain and strain are consistent with lack of evidence of inflammation as the primary or even a critical secondary pathology in most cases. Thus, many of the recommendations for the use of local corticosteroid injections in chronic sprain/strain do not rely on sound scientific basis.[42] Prolonged administration of nonsteroidal antiinflammatory drugs (NSAIDs) is a common practice following musculoskeletal injuries, but there is a lack of scientific data on the effect of NSAIDs on tendon healing. Many cellular and subcellular events occurring during the inflammatory response lead to the release of a variety of growth factors that appear critical in the healing phase. Thus, with respect to acute sprain/strain, there may be reason to avoid interfering with the body's natural inflammation-induced fibroblast activation. Traditional and COX-2-specific nonsteroidal antiinflammatory drugs have been shown to significantly inhibit tendon-to-bone healing in a study of rotator cuff repair in rats.[43] The use of nonsteroidal antiinflammatory drugs (NSAIDs) to treat most muscle, ligament, and tendon injuries should be limited until further scientific data are available. NSAIDs have, at best, a mild effect on relieving symptoms and are potentially deleterious to tissue healing.[44]

In chronic sprain/strain, the connective tissue has lost strength and may be stretched out as well. The usual best result of a completed natural repair process after significant injury is a return to normal connective tissue length but only 50% to 70% of preinjury tensile strength.[45] Load bearing on an area of connective tissue which has insufficient tensile strength because of acute or degenerative change will stimulate pain mechanoreceptors.[46] As long as connective tissue remains functionally insufficient, the pain mechanoreceptors can continue to malfunction.[47] When connective tissue becomes weaker, symptoms can unpredictably be noted, even with a little additional weakness. The term for this change in tendon and ligament and joint capsule in which tissue becomes weaker and/or stretched out is *connective tissue insufficiency*.

Myofascial Syndrome

The relationship of connective tissue insufficiency to myofascial syndrome is potentially critical. Myofascial syndrome has been defined as "pain and/or autonomic phenomena referred from active myofascial trigger points."[48] A trigger point is defined as "a small, exquisitely tender area in soft tissue, including muscles, ligaments, periosteum, tendons, and pericapsular areas"[49] "Mechanoreceptors in connective tissue are not only capable of triggering nociception but also can trigger myotendinous reflexes."[47] These myotendinous reflexes would clinically be termed *twitch contractions*. Also, because tendons fail fiber by fiber much as a frayed rope, and each fiber connects to a section of a muscle, connective tissue insufficiency can easily explain taut bands by reflex effects. A twitch contraction from trigger points in ligaments or tendons can only be seen in nearby contractile tissue (muscle). This is why myofascial pain research has ignored connective tissue, with virtually all biopsy studies addressing muscular changes rather than looking at connective tissue pathology. Because triggers in muscle may largely be secondary to primary triggers in connective tissue, trigger injection of muscles or myofascial release will often have temporary benefit.

Arthritis

Arthritis pain does not come from interarticular cartilage, which is aneural, but rather it originates from the joint surface, which has a thin cartilage layer, or the joint capsule, or other peri- or intra-articular soft tissue structures. Growth factors critical for cartilage growth have been previously described in Table 131–1. One aspect unique to synovial joints, however, is that the levels of disrepair factors may be elevated and this may serve as a blocking effect to growth factors injected in such joints. Indeed, studies have shown an elevation of collagenase up to 100 times normal and elevation of binding proteins up to 24 times normal in synovial joints.[50-51] Injection to elevate growth factor levels appears to be likely to benefit arthritis, depending on levels of interarticular binding proteins and collagenase.

PATIENT SELECTION

An 8-week delay after injury before prolotherapy treatment is recommended to allow the body time to self-repair. If the patient is severely affected after sprain/strain, stopping the pain cycle before development of secondary complex pain syndromes has merit, and prolotherapy effectiveness in aborting conversion to chronic pain syndrome will be an important area of future research. Reasons for intervention earlier than 8 weeks may include previous chronic sprain/strain in a region such that spontaneous healing is not expected to be efficacious, or patient's inability to work.

Pregnant patients are not generally treated during the first trimester (except for focal peripheral joint issues) and during the last trimester due to positioning issues. Before initiating proliferation therapy, if inflammatory prolotherapy methods are to be performed, it is preferable to discontinue all nonsteroidal anti-inflammatory drugs (NSAIDs) 2 days before treatment and 10 days subsequent to treatment. However clinical benefit occurs in patients taking routine prednisone, so taking antiinflammatories does not preclude treatment.

SOLUTION PREPARATION

Syringes or bags can be prepared using ¼ volume of 50% dextrose (i.e., 3 mL in a 12-mL syringe) to make 12.5% soft tissue solution, or ½ volume for 25% joint injection solution. Xylocaine percentage varies from 0.4% to 0.075%, depending on how large an area is injected. Bacteriostatic water is recommended for the diluent. Discarding single-use containers at day's end is recommended. Solution made in advance should be refrigerated. Benzyl alcohol can be obtained from the manufacturer for large-volume solution preparation if other than bacteriostatic water is used as diluent.

Phenol is obtainable in bottles from the manufacturer, allowing for small amounts to be added with precision to 12.5% dextrose to convert solution to phenol/dextrose. Concentrations of 0.5% to 0.75% are alternatives to the 1.25% phenol concentration in the Ongley solution, remembering to keep the volume of injection low. The glycerin component function has not been studied individually. Sodium morrhuate can be obtained, and comes as a 5% solution. Adding 1 to 2 mL of this per 10-mL syringe makes a 0.5% to 1% concentration. Again, low volumes should be used in each injection aliquot if sodium morrhuate is in the solution.

Except for the most experienced practitioner, phenol use should be avoided and usually for the first treatment it is best to establish how the patient handles low-grade inflammation (dextrose 12.5%) before more inflammatory solutions are used. In patients with central hypersensitivity who will misinterpret post-injection soreness, a gentle proliferant is recommended. In extreme cases, the noninflammatory 10% dextrose solution used in double-blind studies on arthritis may be preferable.

COMPLICATIONS

The most common complication is an exacerbation of pain that lasts 2 to 7 days following the injection session. If pain persists beyond this time, residual ligament or tendon trigger points may be present, excess volume injection may have occurred, or a stronger proliferant may have resulted in an overreaction in central hypersensitivity. A superimposed inflammatory process may also be present that would potentially benefit from NSAID use and/or rarely from steroid injection. Avoiding anaphylaxis is imperative. The risk of this is real with sodium morrhuate even when shellfish allergy is not recalled by the patient.. Methylparaben-free lidocaine and methylparaben-free bacteriostatic water are recommended as diluents, and the usual caution should be observed with latex allergies. Epinephrine should be readily available, preferably predrawn. Injections around the thorax can lead to pneumothorax, although with proper technique this is rare (estimated at 1 in 10,000 insertions over ribs). Injection into a vertebral artery is avoided by aspiration with lateral neck injection and with injection about the base of the skull in the deepest row. However, injection in a vertebral artery is safe when dextrose solution contains the equivalent of less than ¾ mL of 1% lidocaine.[52] Inadvertent intrathecal injection of phenol greater than 1% concentration can cause inflammation of the spinal cord. This appears to be very rare, and symptoms are primarily temporary. Note that intrathecal infiltration in the cases in question occurred despite fluoroscopy and is another reason to avoid phenol about the facet ligaments unless limiting concentration to 1.25% and very small volume at a time (0.5 mL) and only with the most experienced physicians. Other local nerve trauma may occur despite good technique, because of the nearly ubiquitous presence of nerve fibers, but no cases of permanent dysesthesia have been reported, even from mixed somatic nerve block with phenol.[53] However, to minimize dysesthesia time and preserve good range of motion, aggressive treatment of any neuralgia is recommended.

The risk of joint infection with proliferant injection appears to be no more than that with steroid injection, which is generally regarded as approximately between 1/10,000 and 1/50,000.[54-55] This compares to a postarthroscopic joint sepsis risk of as much as 1/200,[56] and a rate of joint sepsis after a total joint replacement as much as 1/100.[57-58] Skin prep is advised, either with chlorhexidine or Betadine or alcohol. Trigger injection of multiple locations, with or without proliferant included, is typically given using a single needle. If the needle and syringe are to be set down between injections, it is recommended that a bacteriostatic or bacteriocidal surface be available.

Another issue, due to interventionalists performing prolotherapy more often and their preference for fluoroscopic guidance, is whether fluoroscopic guidance is necessary. Because the proliferant solution spreads, it is not necessary to use fluoroscopy for prolotherapy pinpoint precision. In addition, for more extensive cases, especially when conscious sedation is given, fluoroscopy will slow the treatment enough that conscious sedation time would be prolonged, which is inadvisable. With or without fluoroscopy, the injector needs to be aware of the anatomy of the bony skeleton and practice appropriate depth injection for the bony landmarks in question. Fortunately, prolotherapy is often a regional treatment in which one bony landmark assists in recognition of the next.

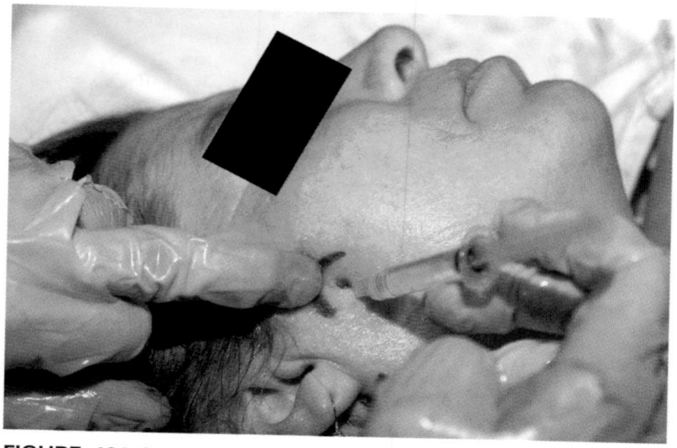

FIGURE 131–2 ■ Temporomandibular joint (TMJ) injection with 30-gauge, 1-inch needle.

The common guiding factor is that one never injects unless one touches bone first, unless one is injecting into a joint. Other than the spinal cord, loci of internal structures must be learned anatomically rather than avoided by fluoroscopy. The most serious complications this author has seen were those that occurred from the treating physician assuming the needle was in a safe location by fluoroscopy and then injecting more than the recommended dosage of a phenol-containing solution in one location.

COMMONLY RESISTANT PAIN CONDITIONS AMENABLE TO PROLOTHERAPY

Temporomandibular Joint Syndrome

This condition in isolation is addressed very simply with interarticular injection. Bruxism is considered by this author to be a reflexive phenomenon. This opinion is bolstered by a typical immediate elimination of bruxism after injection at least for a period of time, likely as a result of neurologic (reflex) effects of the distention itself. The goal, however, is to tighten ligaments and joint capsule to allow the jaw to find a position of rest. With the patient's mouth closed and teeth not clenched (closed-mouth approach), the physician palpates the zygomatic arch adjacent to the condylar process of the mandible with a finger of the injecting hand. A 1-inch, 30-gauge needle or $1\frac{1}{4}$-inch, 27-gauge needle is inserted $\frac{1}{4}$-inch inferior to the apex of this palpable structure, felt as a semicircle (Fig. 131–2). The needle is advanced about $\frac{3}{4}$ to 1 inch, and $\frac{1}{2}$ mL of 25% dextrose solution is injected unless the sensitivity is severe—in which case as little as 12.5% dextrose may be preferable.

Arthritis of Shoulder

Interarticular injection is with a typical posterior approach (Fig. 131–3). The needle insertion point is 1 full cm inferior to the posterior angle of the acromion, with needle directed superiorly at about 30 degrees and on line mediolaterally with the coracoid process or medial to that with a $1\frac{1}{2}$-inch needle. Five milliliters of 10% to 25% dextrose is sufficient here. If needle contact with bone is felt, this is usually because the needle is not aimed far enough medially.

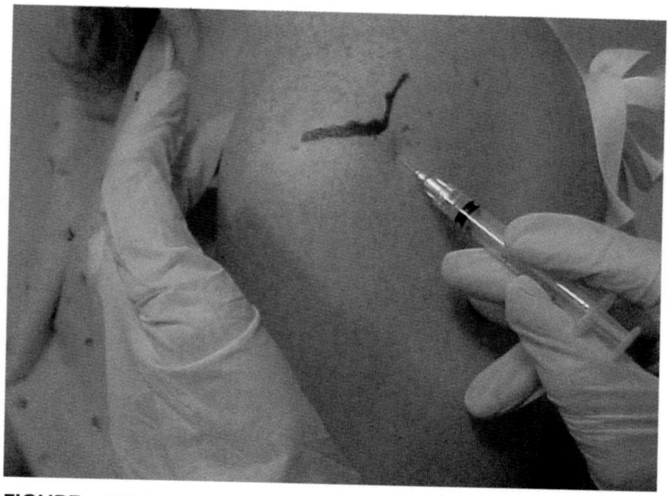

FIGURE 131–3 ■ Glenohumeral injection with 25-gauge, $1\frac{1}{2}$-inch needle.

Rotator Cuff Injury

Symptoms can be minimized, even with a full tear, by interarticular 10% to 25% dextrose, but definitive surgical repair should not be delayed with a complete tear if patient is a candidate. Sprain without tear is another matter and is quite amenable to prolotherapy. Injection of the posterior cuff starts with outlining the palpable scapulae with arm in internal rotation, resting at the patient's side (Fig. 131–4). The teres major and minor origins are injected along the lateral edge, injecting medially to be certain to touch bone and then redirecting the needle by coming out nearly to skin surface and redirecting to the very edge of the scapula (also described as "walking off the bone"), but the needle must come out mostly before redirection to avoid having the needle follow the previous tract (Fig. 131–5). If painful to palpation, the posterior humeral attachments of the infraspinatus and teres minor are addressed (Fig. 131–6). The infraspinatus bulk commonly requires injection, with numbness or pain radiating as far as the hand (Fig. 131–7). The supraspinatus insertion can be injected from a superior approach or a lateral approach, with the lateral approach most critical, injecting areas of tenderness over the proximal lateral humerus (at the condylar level). Anteriorly the pectoralis and subscapularis insertions are injected in several rows along the anterior humerus, typically with hand palm up (Fig. 131–8).

Biceps Tendinitis (Tendinosis)

The subscapularis, coracobrachialis, and pectoral insertions are often sources of anterior shoulder pain mimicking bicipital tendinosis. The subscapularis and pectoralis major insertion sites are injected with the shoulder in external rotation to expose the anterior insertions as above (see Figure 131–8). Injections are given in two to three rows over the proximal 3 to 4 inches of the anterior humerus. Coracobrachialis and pectoralis minor insertions are injected vertically down onto the coracoid process.

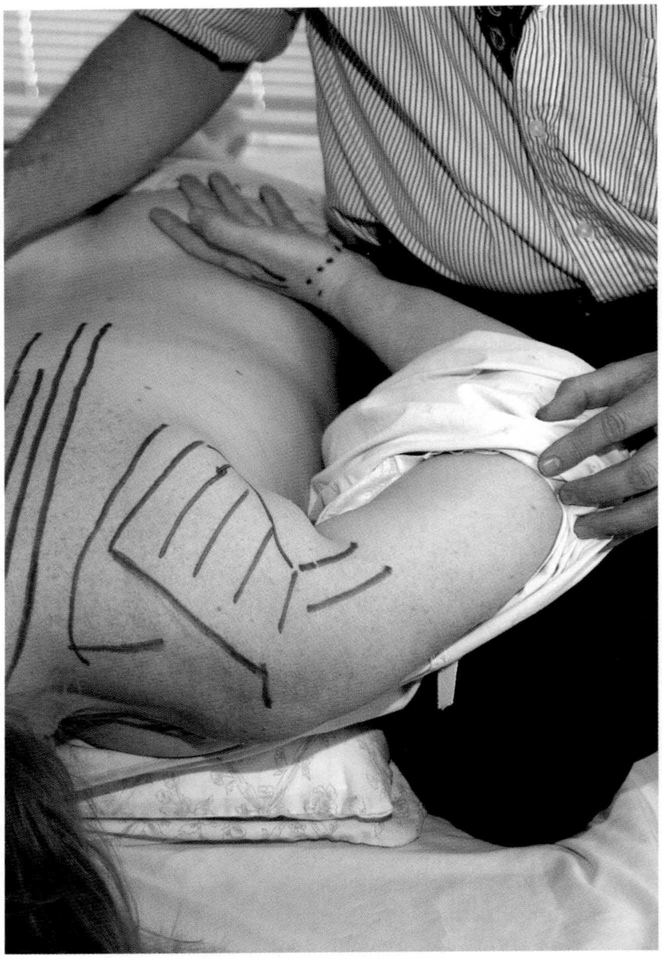

FIGURE 131–4 ■ Positioning from rhomboid and levator scapulae injection.

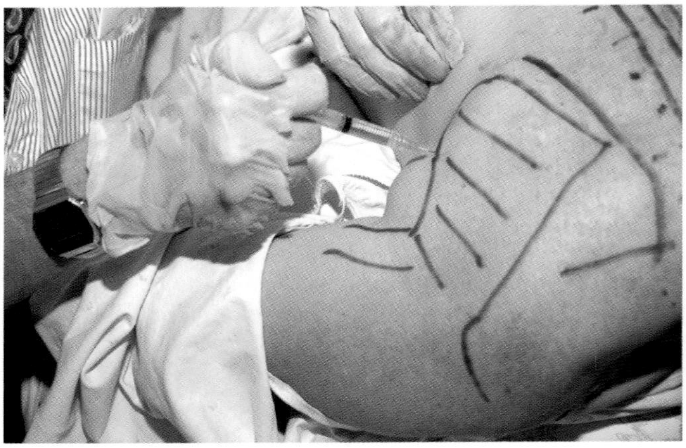

FIGURE 131–5 ■ Injection of teres major/minor origin with 25-gauge, 1½-inch needle.

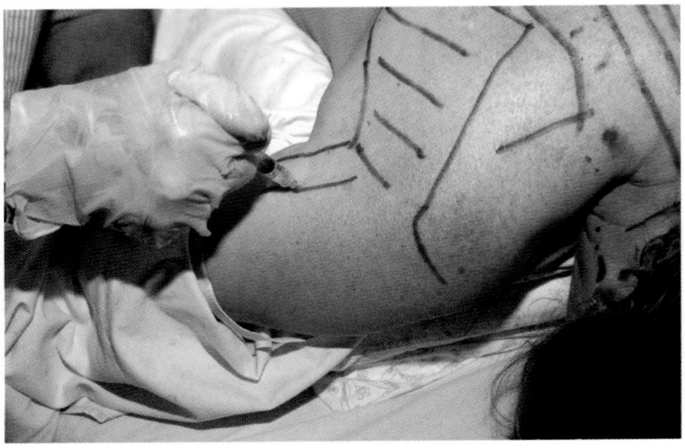

FIGURE 131–6 ■ Injection of infraspinatus/teres minor insertion with 25-gauge, 2-inch needle.

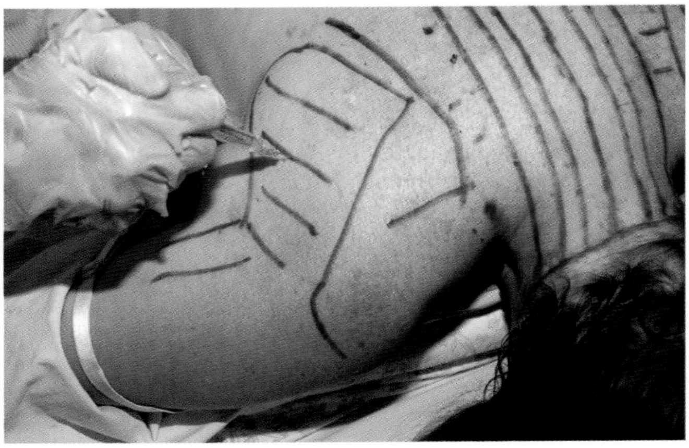

FIGURE 131–7 ■ Origin of infraspinatus injection with 25-gauge, 2-inch needle.

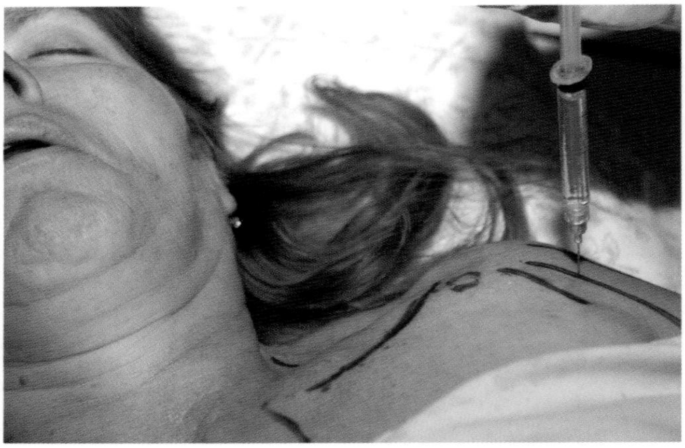

FIGURE 131–8 ■ Injection of pectoralis/subscapularis insertions with 25-gauge, 2-inch needle.

Shoulder Bursitis/Shoulder Laxity

Injection into the subacromial bursa is accomplished with needle entry ¼ inch below the acromion and with a slightly cephalad angulation (Fig. 131–9). As long as fluid goes in easily, fluid will effectively enter into the space. This space is one where inflammation is the underlying cause of pain in a number of cases, and steroid injection is a reasonable initial choice for the injectant. However, with recurrent symptoms, the key is finding the source of subacromial dysfunction. If

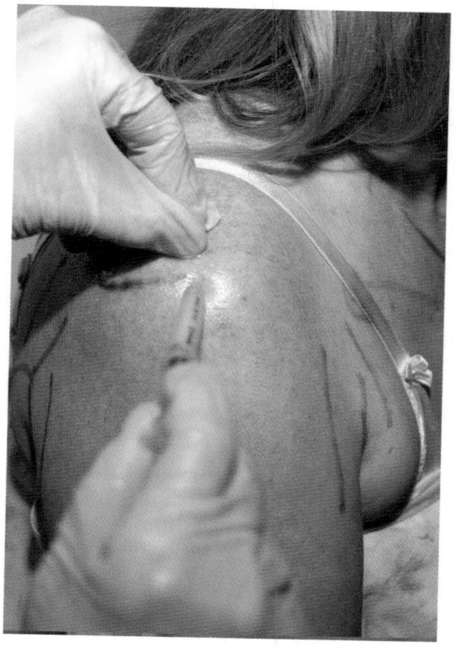

FIGURE 131–9 ■ Subacromial bursa injection with 27-gauge, 1¼-inch needle.

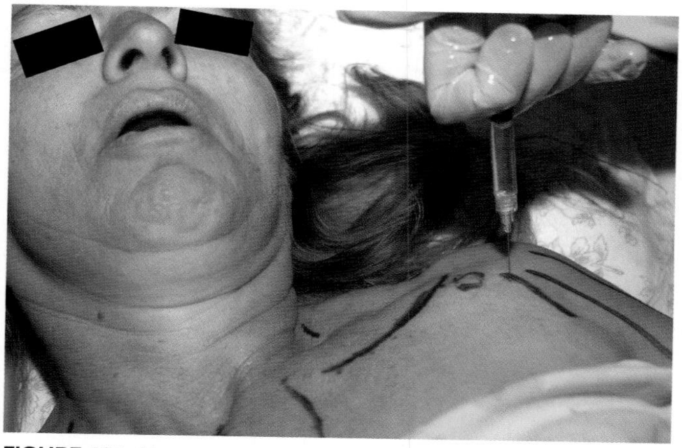

FIGURE 131–10 ■ Anterior shoulder capsule injection with 25-gauge, 2-inch needle.

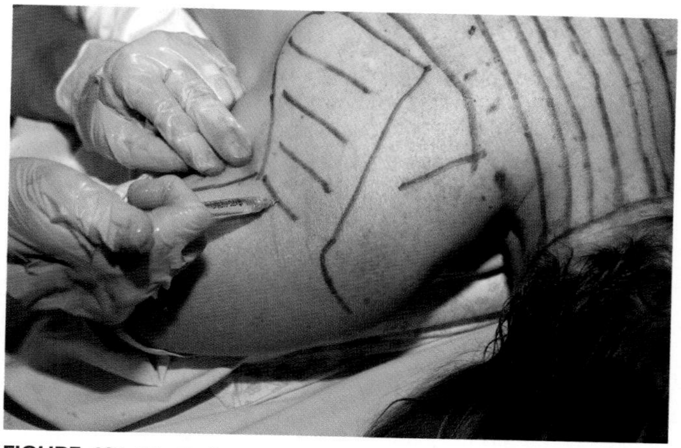

FIGURE 131–11 ■ Posterior shoulder capsule injection with 25-gauge, 2-inch needle.

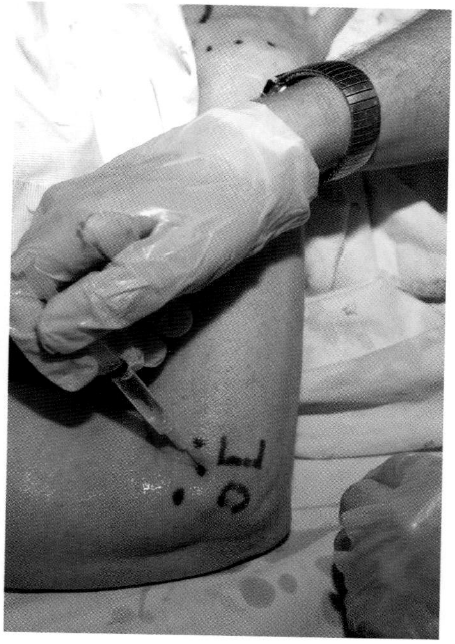

FIGURE 131–12 ■ Common wrist extensor injection with 27-gauge, 1¼-inch needle.

the shoulder capsule is lax in either anterior or posterior portions, abnormal motion with use will lead to impingement, perpetuating the syndrome. Therefore, the anterior capsule is infiltrated from the anterior aspect, inserting the needle 1 cm lateral and 1 to 2 cm inferior to the coracoid process tip and injecting several times in a vertical line (Fig. 131–10). This is best done with the palm up to keep the arm in external rotation. The posterior capsule is easily addressed by injecting the rotator cuff posteriorly (Fig. 131–11). Typically ½ mL each is injected in 4 to 6 locations.

Tennis Elbow

Proliferation treatment of medial and lateral epicondylosis is preferable to use of steroids, and is best performed early, prior to the development of prominent disorientation of tissue common with this disorder. Abundant tapping and low volume (3 to 4 mL total) gentle proliferant are recommended to avoid excess inflammatory effect, particularly with the first treatment. In lateral epicondylosis, the common extensors are injected starting at the supracondylar ridge, with injections also medial to the condyle (Fig. 131–12), down onto the radial head ligament and directly onto the condyle as tender. Exercise caution to position needle prior to injection when injecting medial to the condyle and in the supracondylar region, as temporary radial nerve palsy can be created via nerve trauma. The usual precaution of waiting to inject until bone contact is made is recommended. A pronation position of the forearm is advised to minimize any potential nerve contact issues.

Golfer's Elbow

Similar spread of fluid about the medial epicondyle is recommended for medial epicondylosis with three insertion points, but the distal insertion aiming back toward the condyle must not go too far posteriorly to avoid traumatizing the ulnar nerve (Fig. 131–13).

Pseudo de Quervain's/Sprained Wrist

In this author's experience, a chronic wrist sprain of the radial wrist is often misdiagnosed as de Quervain stenosing tenosynovitis. If results are not excellent with first dorsal compartment infiltration with steroid, a switch to connective tissue treatment is recommended. In typical chronic wrist sprain treatment, injection is usually not just in the vicinity of the radial collateral ligament (Fig. 131–14), but also is across the dorsal aspect of the wrist where tenderness is palpable with ligament stretch by finger pressure (Fig. 131–15).

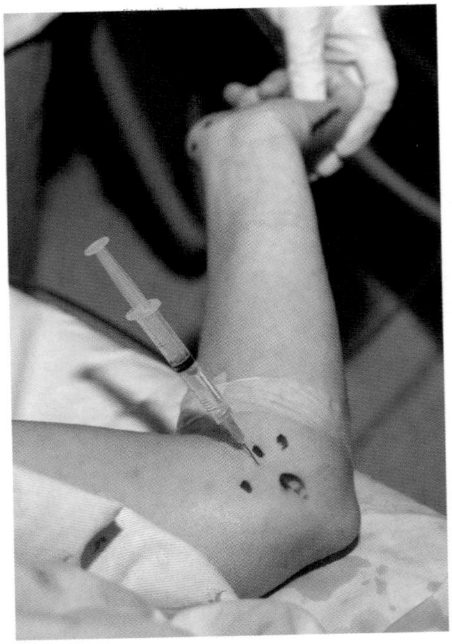

FIGURE 131–13 ■ Common wrist flexor injection with 25-gauge, $1\frac{1}{2}$-inch needle.

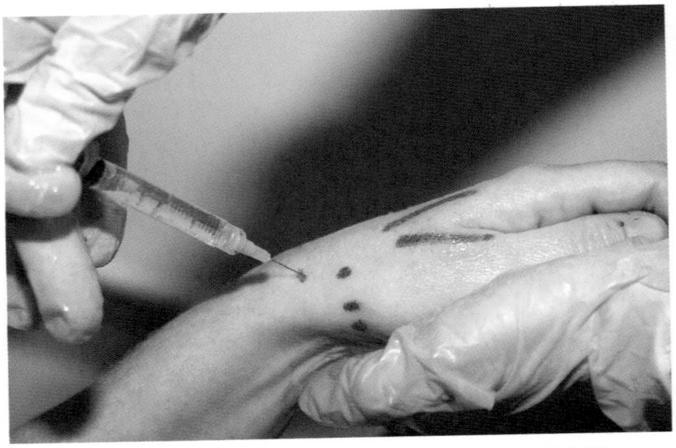

FIGURE 131–14 ■ Radial collateral ligament injection with 27-gauge, $1\frac{1}{4}$-inch needle.

Finger Joint Sprain/Finger Arthritis

Metacarpophalangeal (MCP) joint injection for painful function is performed by entering over the palpable joint line with the MCP in about 70 degrees of flexion, applying a little distal traction for joint separation and entering with about a 20-degree distal inclination (Fig. 131–16). Proximal and distal interphalangeal injections are from a lateral approach and medial approach, approximating the joint line (Fig. 131–17). This results in capsular infiltration rather than joint infiltration which is quite adequate and results in diffusion into collateral ligaments which is productive as well because painful joints often have mediolateral laxity. Injection slightly above midline (slightly dorsal) is better to minimize contact with digital nerves. A special joint to consider is the trapeziometacarpal (CMC) of the thumb, which tends to have some inflammation baseline, and a small amount of steroid

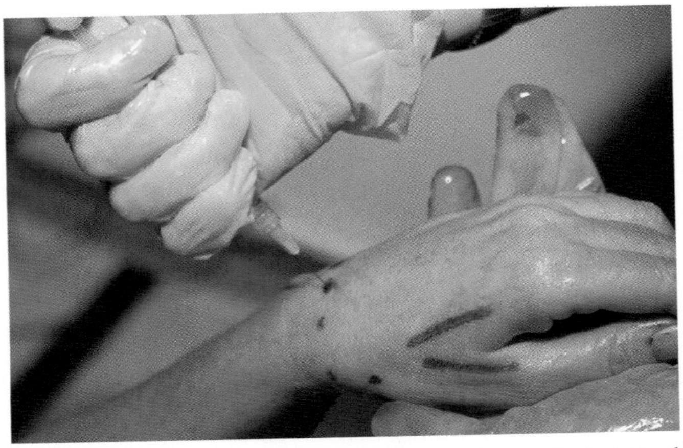

FIGURE 131–15 ■ Injection of radioulnar articulation with first carpal row using 27-gauge, $1\frac{1}{4}$-inch needle.

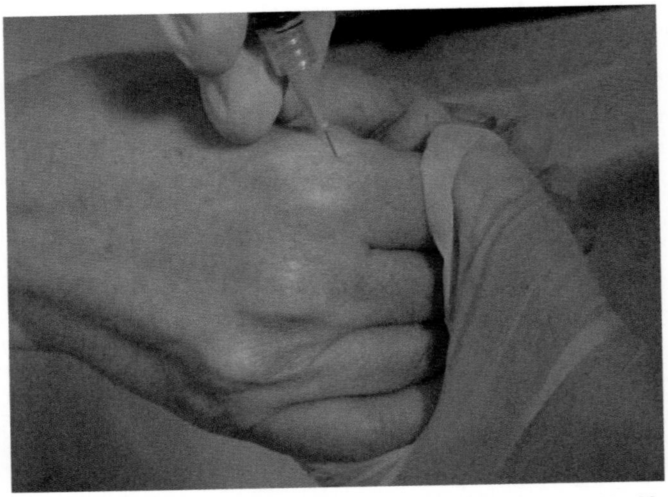

FIGURE 131–16 ■ Metacarpophalangeal (MCP) injection with 30-gauge, 1-inch needle.

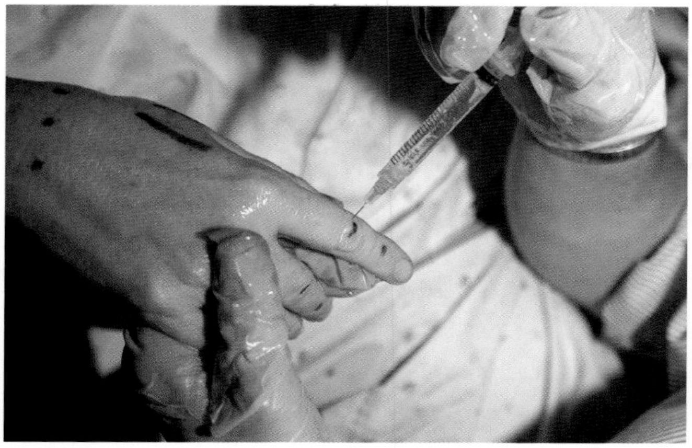

FIGURE 131–17 ■ Proximal interphalangeal (PIP) injection with 27-gauge, $^{1}/_{2}$-inch needle

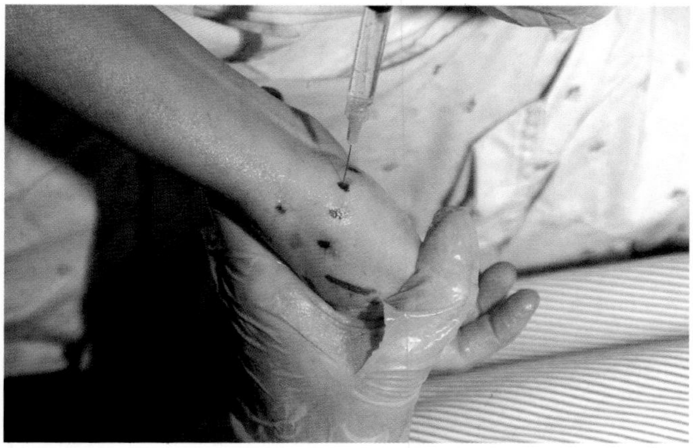

FIGURE 131–18 ■ Thumb CMC injection with 27-gauge, $1^{1}/_{4}$-inch needle.

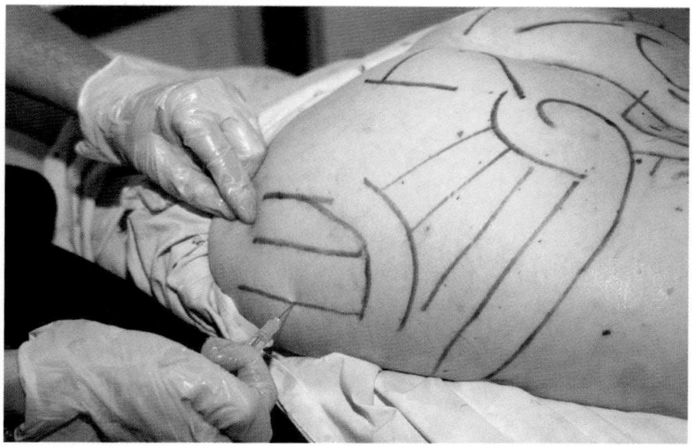

FIGURE 131–19 ■ Tensor/gluteal injection with 22-gauge, 3-inch needle.

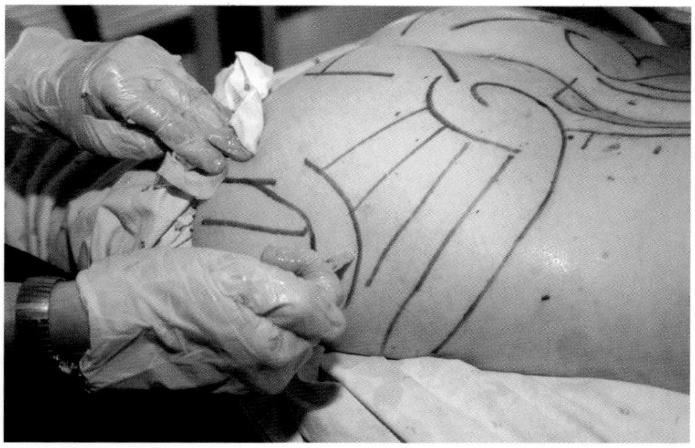

FIGURE 131–20 ■ Hip capsule/hip injection with 22-gauge, $3^{1}/_{2}$-inch needle.

may need to be included in the injection for patients in whom a small amount of 25% or 12.5% dextrose flares their pain. Thumb orthoses are used as necessary to minimize repetitive stresses as needed. Injecting in circle about the CMC may be more effective (Fig. 131–18), and is advocated by some to address capsular attachments more thoroughly, but the total load within the joint should be limited to 1 mL maximum to minimize post-injection discomfort.

Hip Bursitis

Although again this area has an inflammatory mediation of pain and may benefit from an initial steroid injection (Fig. 131–19) shows marks in several lines about the trochanter, going down the leg. Treating the entheses to strengthen them addresses the bursitis, which is probably secondary to muscle dysfunction.

Hip Arthritis

Injection of the hip is conducted from entries along a semicircle about an inch away from the trochanter (Fig. 131–20). Injection is conducted both vertically and proximally and distally, altering angle of attack to inject proximal attachments of hip ligaments and distally for distal portion, and infiltrating the hip capsule in between.

Leg Cramping/Medial Knee Pain/ Anserine Bursitis/Feeling of Unstable Knee

Sensory input from medial attachments about the knee appear to be critical for a feeling of knee stability. Irritation of adductors or hamstrings appears to result in a feeling of untrustworthiness on weight bearing, and results in cramping in the thigh or calf at rest and can contribute to restless legs syndrome. Injection of steroid in the anserine bursa is rarely used by this author, because injecting the hamstring insertion injection with dextrose resolves the medial pain without need for steroid in more than 90% of cases. The thigh adductor insertions and vastus medialis insertions are injected from a semicircle about the medial condyle of the femur (Fig. 131–21) and the hamstring insertions from several rows oriented vertically below the knee articular line (Fig. 131–22). This can most easily be done with the knee bent and leg in external rotation resting on the examiner's bent leg.

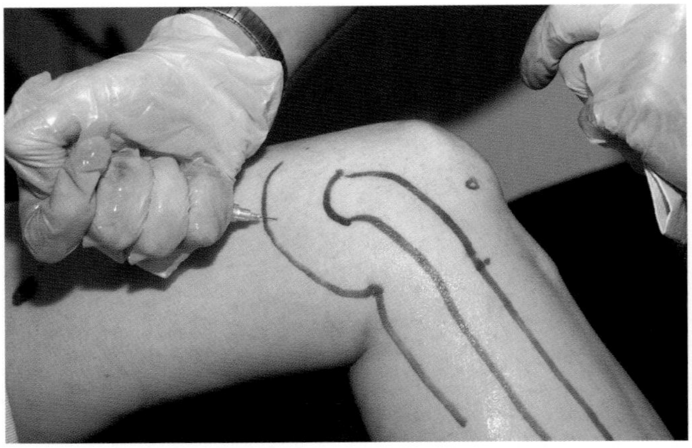

FIGURE 131–21 ■ Distal adductor/medial collateral ligament origin injection with 22-gauge, 2-inch needle.

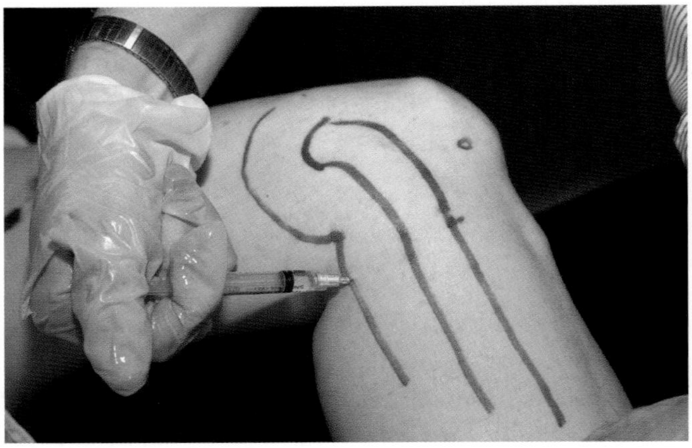

FIGURE 131–22 ■ Hamstring insertion and soleus origin injection with 22-gauge, 2-inch needle.

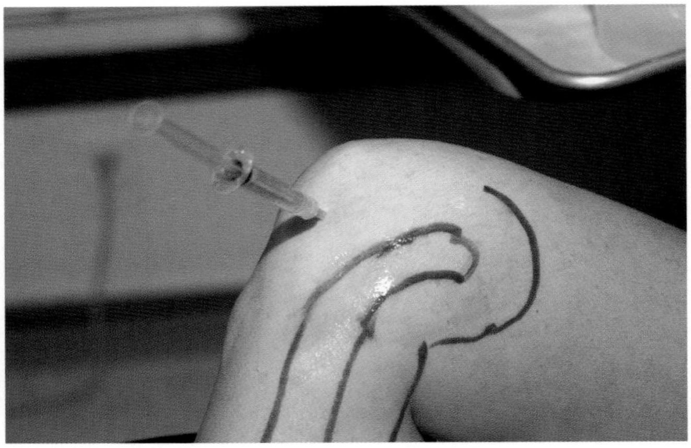

FIGURE 131–23 ■ Medial tibiofemoral joint injection with 27-gauge, 1¼-inch needle.

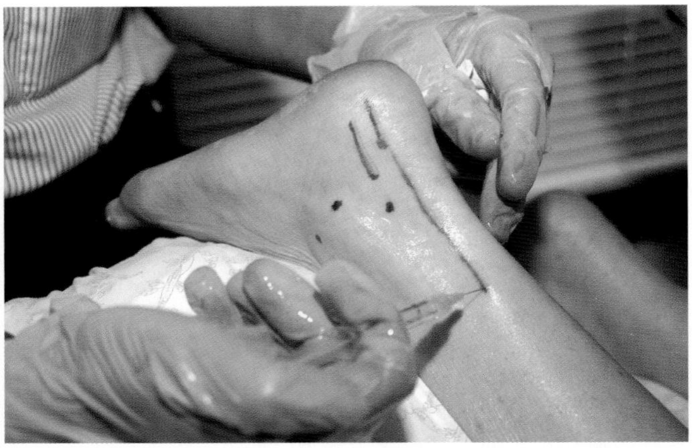

FIGURE 131–24 ■ Achilles tendon sheath injection with 27-gauge, 1¼-inch needle.

Knee Laxity/Knee Arthritis/Knee Pain

The collateral ligament origins and insertions are injected when painful and the coronary ligaments are injected as well. Most knee interarticular ligaments will respond nicely to a simple interarticular approach either inferomedially or inferolaterally with 4 to 6 mL of 12.5% to 25% dextrose (Fig. 131–23). The latter dextrose concentration is stronger, but if interleukins/metalloproteinases are high in the joint, a steroid injection may be needed or follow-up of 10% dextrose used with a small amount of steroid (i.e., one tenth the usual dose). Insertion is along the line of the femur superoinferiorly and the mediolateral direction aims for what would be the estimated joint center. In some patients, there may be a membrane separating the tibiofemoral from infrapatellar joint—such that chondromalacia patients or anterior compartment patients may merit infrapatellar injection of 3 mL of 12.5% to 25% dextrose. This injection is about ¼ inch off edge of patella with patella pushed away if feasible to open the space underneath, using a 45-degree angle from vertical to table and entry depth of about ¾ inch due to the rhomboid shape of the patella.

Achilles Tendinosis

Achilles tendinosis is injected if painful over the entire length from calcaneus to muscle belly (Figs. 131–24 and 131–25). Proliferants with no inflammation or low-grade inflammation (10% to 12.5% dextrose) are recommended for this injection because there is a low-grade inflammatory component in some cases. Injection is from both medial and lateral aspects, inserting gently through the skin and advancing until slight resistance to inject about the peritendinous area. Entering the tendon is not an issue, as with steroid injection, because proliferation, not weakening, is the expected result.

Repetitive Ankle Sprain/Chronic Pain After Ankle Sprain

Nociceptive limits from excess connective tissue length appear to be related to a repetitive tendency to roll the ankle in, predisposing to repetitive sprain/strain. Injection of the distal tibiofibular, anterior talofibular, calcaneofibular and posterior talofibular ligaments is performed via a semicircle about the lateral malleolus, aiming superiorly and inferiorly to infiltrate both the origins and insertions (Fig. 131–26). The

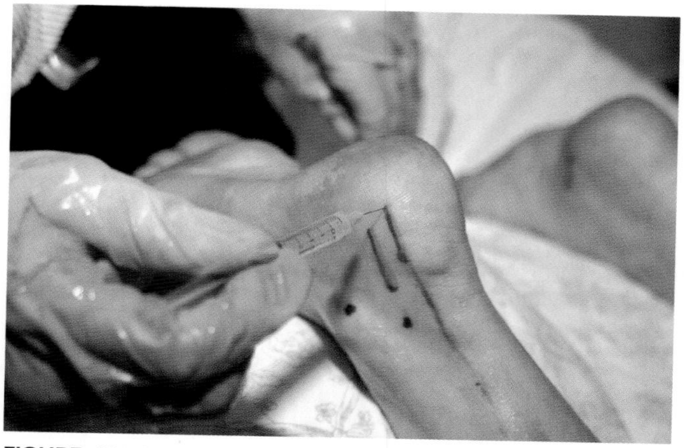

FIGURE 131–25 ■ Distal Achilles tendon insertion injection with 27-gauge, $1\frac{1}{4}$-inch needle.

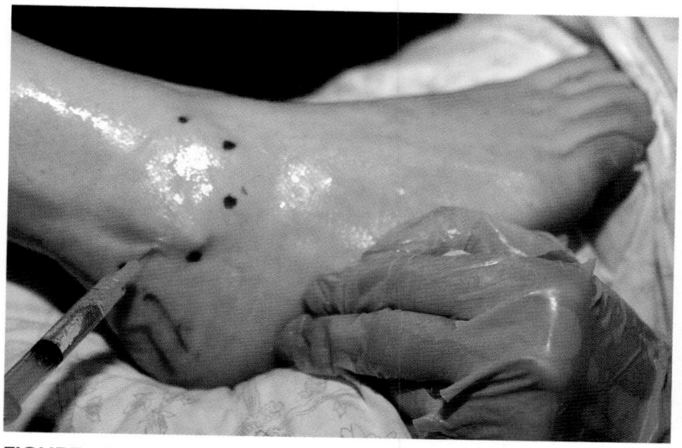

FIGURE 131–26 ■ Posterior calcaneofibular ligament injection with 27-gauge, $1\frac{1}{4}$-inch needle.

subtalar joint is helpful to inject as well because its interosseous ligaments appear to be of significant importance in chronic pain. The injector will drop into the subtalar joint almost invariably during the above semicircle injection (Fig. 131–27). Injection of the medial ankle is similar, with palpation revealing tenderness in the tibionavicular, tibiotalar, and tibiocalcaneal portions.

Plantar Ligament Sprain/Posterior Tibialis Strain

Arch sprain typically involves both spring and plantar ligaments. Although single medial insertion techniques are available, it is more reliable for the usual injector to use a 27-gauge, $1\frac{1}{4}$-inch needle and separately inject the spring and plantar ligaments (Figs. 131–28 and 131–29). It is a common experience that some patients benefit from steroid injection initially, but if a patient presents with recurrent pain, staying with a gentle proliferant such as 10% dextrose may be best to help weight bearing, not to be unfavorably affected post-injection, and to avoid the need to go back in with steroid. A medial arch support is recommended to avoid overuse post-injection. The posterior tibialis is usually injected vertically onto its primary insertion on the navicular (Fig. 131–30).

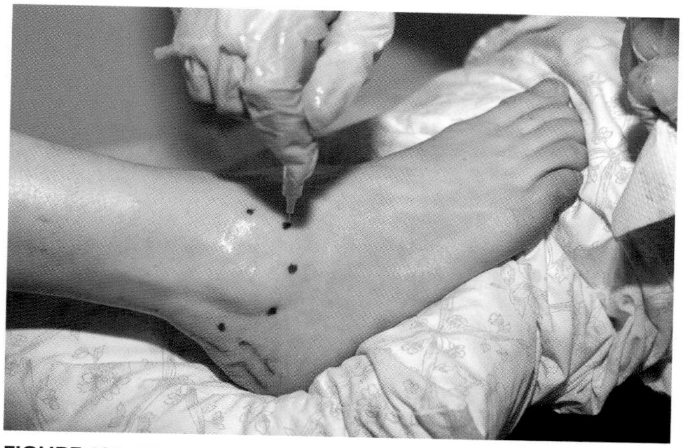

FIGURE 131–27 ■ Anterior talofibular ligament/sinus tarsi injection with 27-gauge, $1\frac{1}{4}$-inch needle.

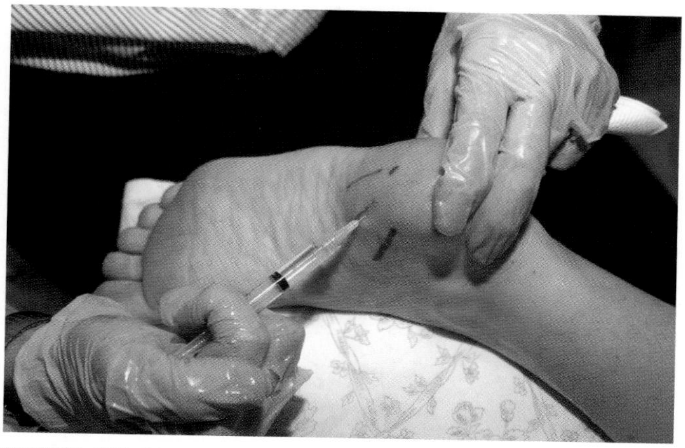

FIGURE 131–28 ■ Spring ligament injection with 27-gauge, $1\frac{1}{4}$-inch needle.

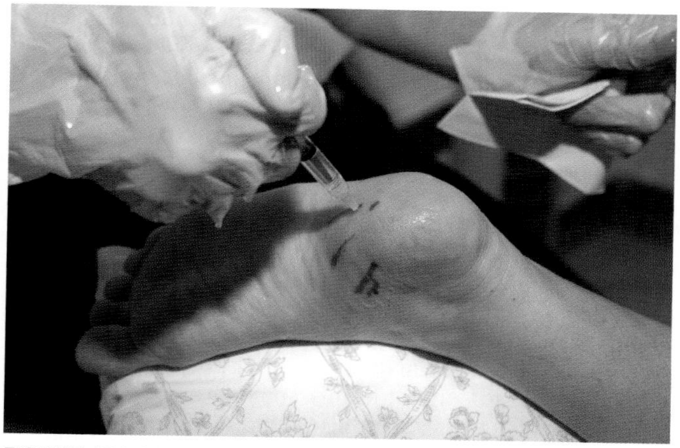

FIGURE 131–29 ■ Proximal plantar ligament injection with 27-gauge, $1\frac{1}{4}$-inch needle.

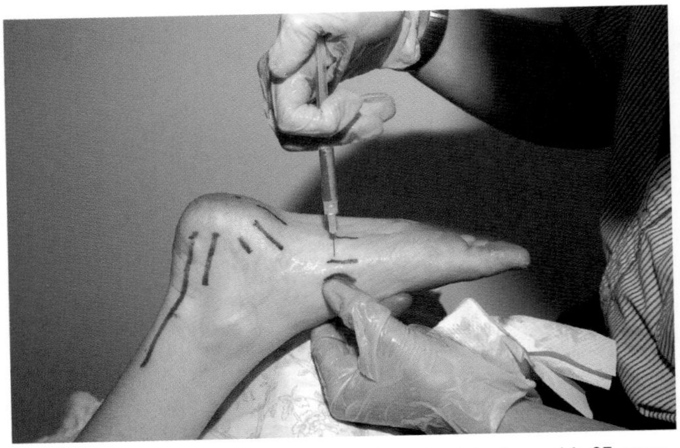

FIGURE 131–30 ■ Posterior tibialis insertion injection with 27-gauge, 1¼-inch needle.

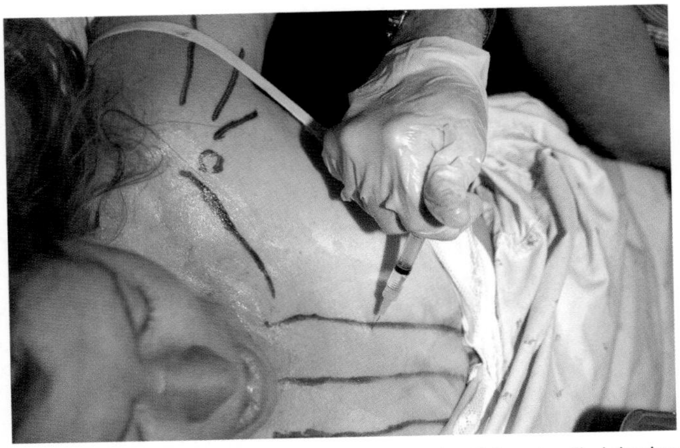

FIGURE 131–32 ■ Chondrosternal ligament/medial pectoralis injection with 27-gauge, 1¼-inch needle.

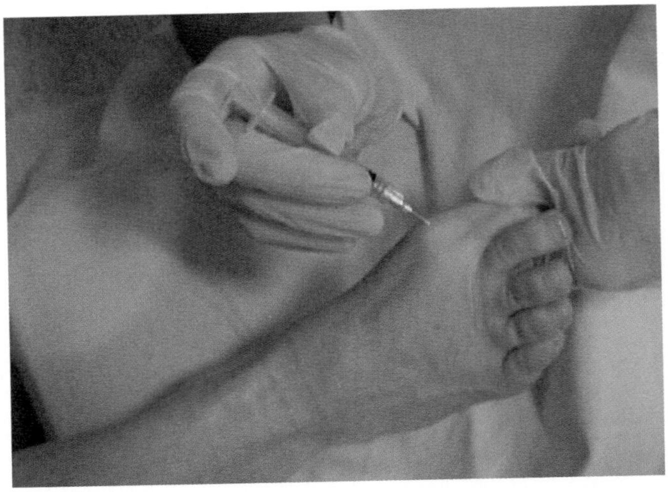

FIGURE 131–31 ■ Metatarsophalangeal (MTP) injection with 27-gauge, 1¼-inch needle.

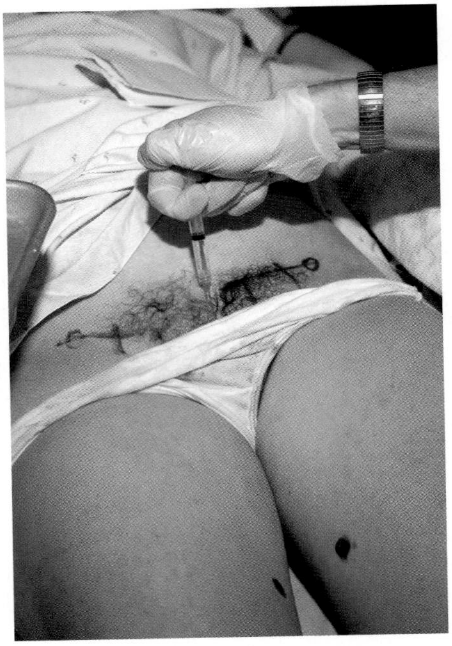

FIGURE 131–33 ■ Injection abdominal attachments/symphysis pubis capsule with 25-gauge, 1½-inch needle.

Metatarsalgia/Morton Neuroma/ Arthritis of Toes/Hallux Valgus

Metatarsalgia relief by footwear is recommended, of course, but elimination of symptoms appears to require addressing connective tissue insufficiency about the metatarsophalangeal joints. Injection for this is from the dorsum of the foot with the toes flexed. Injection can be both distal to the bony prominence felt with toe flexion and proximal because both joint and capsule injections are beneficial. A 27-gauge needle is typically used, although as little as ½ inch of needle length may be adequate (Fig. 131–31). Entering the joint is not critical because injection under the joint capsule appears to give equivalent results. Morton's neuroma appears to relate to irritation from instability of the metatarsal row, and simple metatarsal injection from the dorsum relieves pain that would otherwise lead to surgery in this author's experience. Injection over hallux valgus can also address pain from a commonly associated mediolateral laxity but does not correct the valgus.

Pseudocostochondritis

For medial chest pain, palpation typically localizes pain over an entire row of chondrosternal ligaments or medial pectoralis origins (Fig. 131–32). Injecting that row with a 27-gauge, 1¼-inch needle starting 1 inch from midline and aiming 30 degrees toward midline of body from vertical, addresses the entire row.

Groin Pain/Osteitis Pubis/Dyspareunia

These common maladies are addressed from an anterior approach only, except for the latter. Anteriorly the symphysis pubis and adductor insertions are treated, depending on palpation tenderness (Fig. 131–33). The symphysis pubis is injected vertically at a depth of 2 to 4 cm, and then the top of the pubic

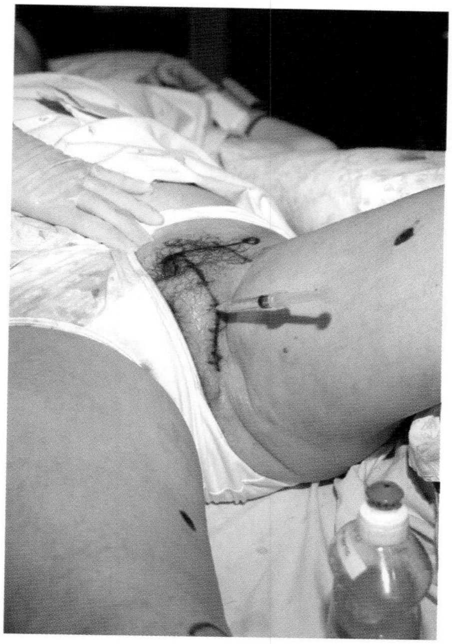

FIGURE 131–34 ■ Adductor origin injection with 25-gauge, 2-inch needle.

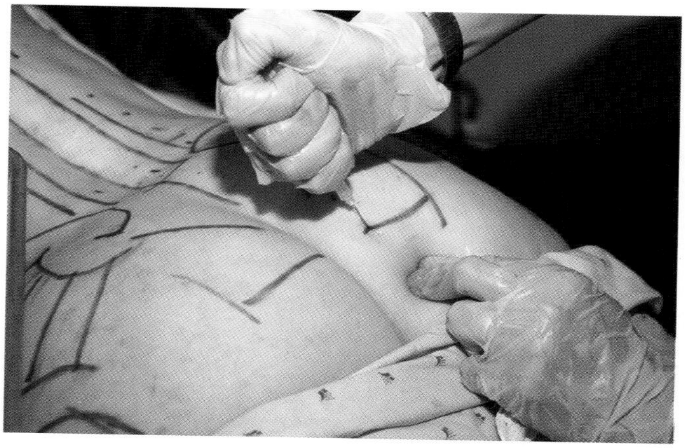

FIGURE 131–35 ■ Posterior pelvic floor injection with 22-gauge, 3½-inch needle.

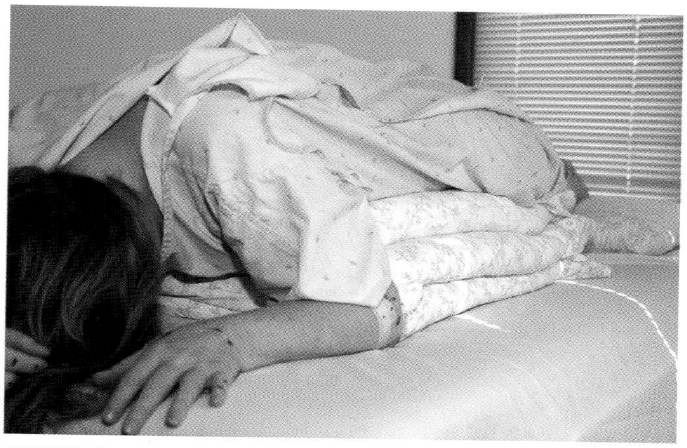

FIGURE 131–36 ■ Positioning for back injection, optimal for neck, upper and lower back injections.

crest is injected as painful at 1-cm intervals, covering pectineus and pyramidalis insertions and abdominal muscle insertions. For ischiopubic ramus injection (adductor origins), the patient lies supine with their opposite leg extended and the injected leg-foot touching the medial border of the other knee (Fig. 131–34). The needle insertion is at 90 degrees to skin surface and starts at the palpable ischial tuberosity. Insertion sites follow essentially a straight line in ventral direction but the needle direction is altered medially as needed to contact bone since the bony target is circular. Typically this injection method uses a 1½- to 2-inch, 25-gauge needle. These injections address adductors magnus, brevis, and longus origins, and the insertion for the rectus abdominis (on pubic tubercle). In addition, the gracilis and obturator externus origins are close enough to the adductor attachments to expect solution spread to affect them as well. When pain with intercourse is a complaint of the patient, the posterior pelvic floor is the common source and is addressed effectively by using good antisepsis, and injecting in a vertical/lateral direction along the ischiopubic ramus from a posterior direction (Fig. 131–35). Injections begin at the ischial tuberosity and then with more medial entry points, the needle is directed in a somewhat lateral direction to contact the ramus more easily.

Pseudo-carpal Tunnel Syndrome/ Pseudo-radiculopathy/Pseudo-reflex Sympathetic Dystrophy

In the absence of corroborating reflex changes, motor changes, or dermatomal findings of radicular nature with MRI correlation, connective tissue should be suspected as a very frequent source of radiating numbness of unclear mechanism, but it should be noted that not only referred numbness but also autonomic changes can occur as a result of trigger activity in connective tissue. Chief culprits for radiating numbness into the hand include the infraspinatus and teres, common wrist extensors at the elbow, pectoralis and subscapularis, cervical paraspinals, and sometimes even costotransverse ligaments.

Upper Back Pain

Positioning for injection is important to allow comfort for upper back, neck, and base of head and shoulder injections (Fig. 131–36). Note many prefer positioning the arm down at the patient's side to make palpation easier and rib depth about ¼ inch shallower. However, this author trusts careful needle search more than palpation and finds tissue depth about ¾ inch for the most shallow ribs more ideal for a 1-inch needle. Injection begins at about T5-6 where the ribs are most superficial (Fig. 131–37). Use of a short (i.e., ½- to 1-inch) needle is recommended, palpating, inserting, and searching at ½-inch depth with 5- to 10-degree angulation changes of the needle. Redirection is performed by coming out nearly fully to avoid bending of the needle and then reinserting at a different angle. If the rib is not found, repalpate if rib is palpable, and then reinsert and search again with a ⅛- to ¼-inch increase in depth. Repeat the process until the rib is found. Because of the many reangulations attempted at each depth, it appears very difficult to pass the rib. Then observe bony depth without indenting, which provides a basic guideline for depth of subsequent rib injections. Key ligaments are costotransverse and

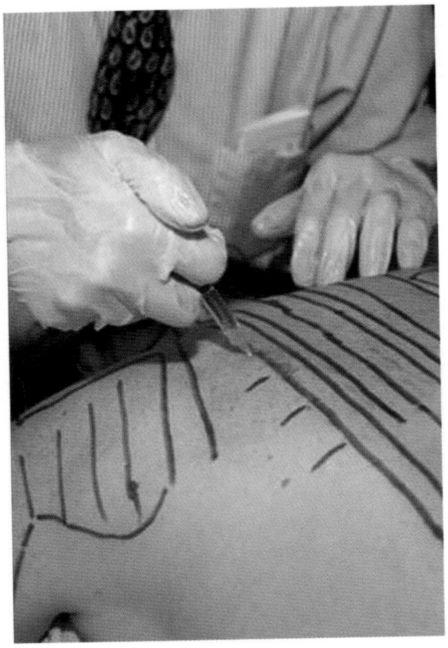

FIGURE 131–37 ■ Costotransverse ligament injection using 25-gauge, 1-inch needle

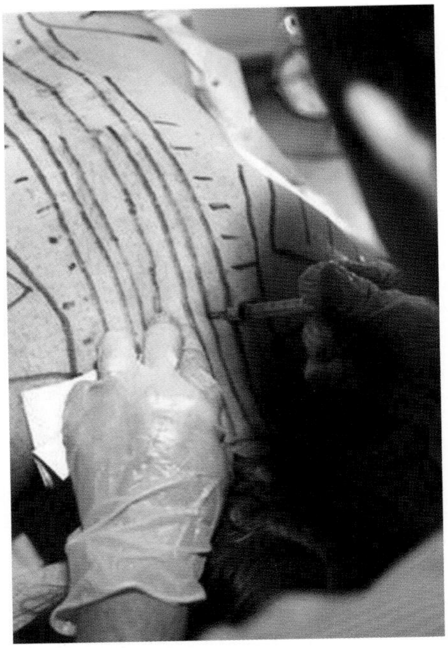

FIGURE 131–38 ■ Facet ligament injection using 25-gauge, 1½-inch needle.

facet ligaments for interscapular pain. A non-indenting injection is preferred by this author as this method allows the treating physician to know exactly how far from the skin surface the needle is going, which is vital for ribs that cannot accurately be palpated, and works for patients in excess of 300 pounds.

When the most superficial costotransverse ligament (CTL) is found, mark that rib, and use that depth to find the other levels. Note that depth increases about ¼ inch at about T1 level and similarly at about T12 level in an average-sized patient. Slowly increasing the length of the needle may be helpful to the physician. At each level, insert to a level known to be safe from previous rib, and if the rib is not touched, search in a similar manner to that described earlier. This method is used for both costotransverse ligaments and iliocostalis thoracis, commonly involved in upper back pain and with referred pain as far as the hand or up into the head. Note in this picture there is an additional line present. Thoracic facet ligament injection depth is usually about ½ inch deeper with needle directed slightly medially (Fig. 131–38). Note the inner row is the multifidi injection row which may not be used unless facet ligament and costotransverse ligament injections are inadequate. The multifidi can also be easily injected from the same row as the facet ligament row, but aiming more medially. For each injection, a finger is on the spinous process, ensuring that the distance from midline stays at about an inch and ruling out or compensating for scoliosis. Injection of interspinous ligaments at thoracic levels is often reserved for initial lack of adequate response to more lateral injection (Fig. 131–39). Supraspinous injection is similar and often both inter- and supraspinous ligaments are addressed along with multifidi insertions for patients with clearly medial more than lateral pain.

Injection of the posterior superior trapezius is facilitated by bringing the arm up such that the elbow is even with the shoulder. This elevates the clavicle such that the posterior superior trapezius insertion can be injected safely. Insertion can be at 90 degrees to the plane of the table but then angling

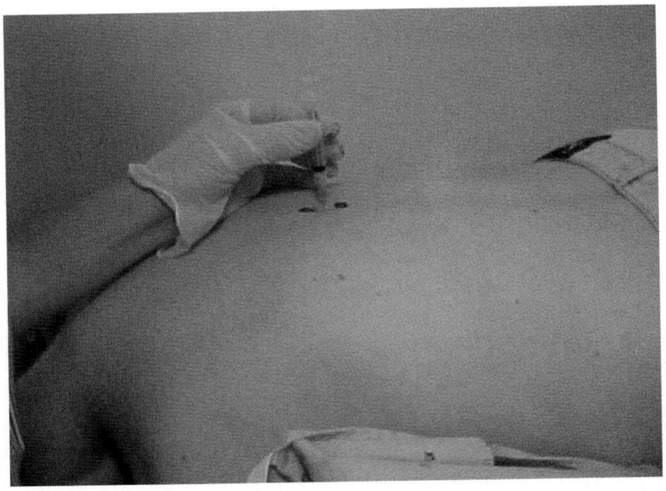

FIGURE 131–39 ■ Interspinous ligament injection with 25-gauge, 1½-inch needle.

laterally is advised to find the clavicle with the least distance traveled, aiming just under a palpating finger on top of the clavicle (Fig. 131–40). Approximately three insertion points are used to cover the lateral 2 inches of the lateral clavicle. For the rhomboid and levator scapulae injection, the patient's arm is either resting on the back with shoulder in internal rotation, or on the leg of the examiner, and usually both (Fig. 131–41). If this position is uncomfortable, the arm can be injected with arm down by the patient's side or even off the side of the table. The reason the scapula appears lateral compared to the line of needle insertion is that when the arm is laid down to the side after rhomboid/levator injection, the scapula moves and needs to be re-marked. Levator scapulae injections are above the spine of the scapula, traveling up medially to the scapular tip (Fig. 131–42). Depth for this is about ½ inch deeper than that for the rhomboid injection.

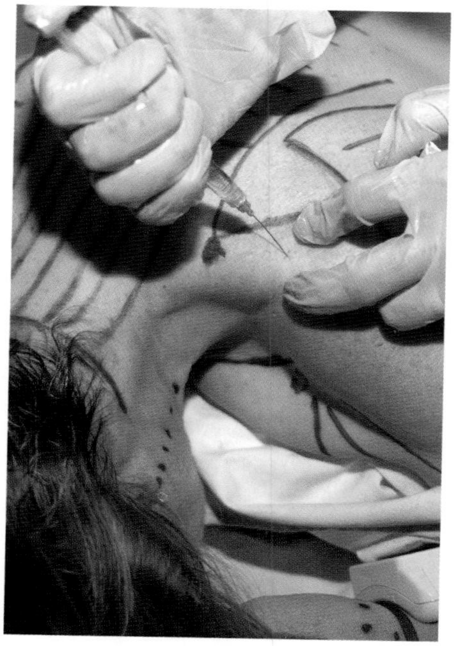

FIGURE 131–40 ■ Posterior superior trapezius injection with 25-gauge, 2-inch needle.

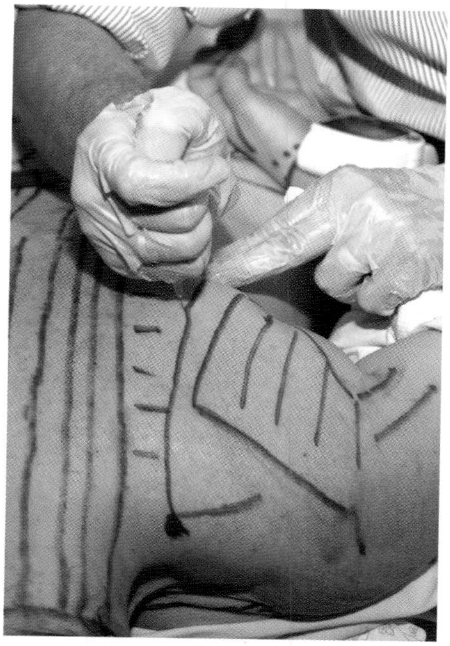

FIGURE 131–41 ■ Injection of rhomboid insertion with 25-gauge, 1-inch needle. Note scapular markings are made with arm at side, but for this injection patient's arm is elevated on examiner's leg so the medial border of the scapula will be medial to marks made with arm at side.

Neck Pain

The depth of the costotransverse ligament at T1 approximates the depth for injection of the posterior cervical vertebral body at C7 laterally and medially (Fig. 131–43). Injections are typically along a line to evenly distribute the proliferant. At cervical levels the needle is directed about 10 to 20 degrees inferiorly to avoid any possibility of passing between verte-

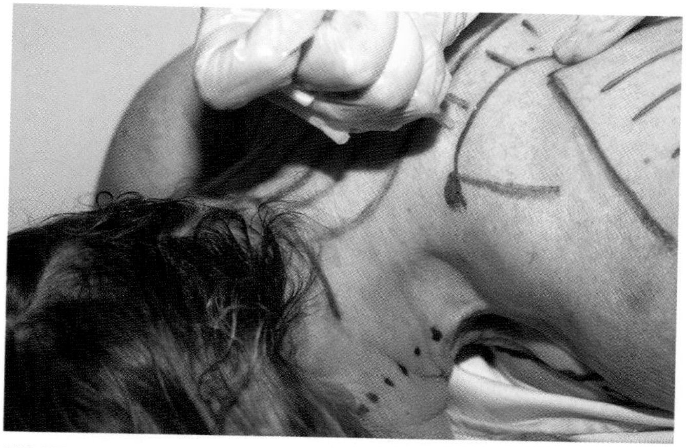

FIGURE 131–42 ■ Levator scapulae injection with 27-gauge, $1\frac{1}{4}$-inch needle.

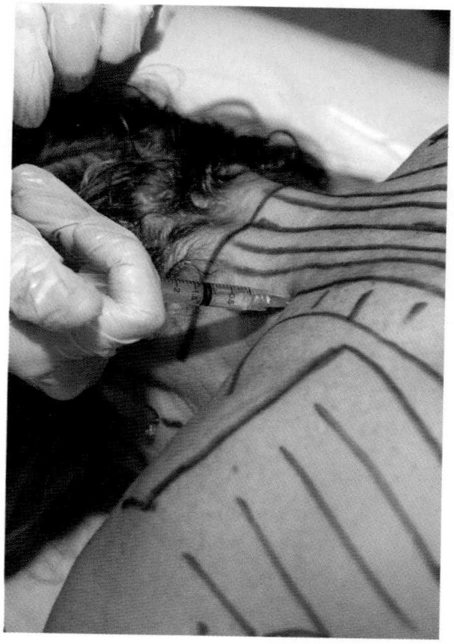

FIGURE 131–43 ■ Cervical intertransversarii injection using 25-gauge, $1\frac{1}{2}$-inch needle.

bral bodies. The top level injected is C2. This is recognized by palpating the posterior spinous process of C2, which is palpated about 1 cm below the base of the skull.

Attachments of the scalenes to the cervical tubercles appear critical in patients with lateral neck pain or autonomic dysfunction symptoms (posterior cervical sympathetic syndrome or Barré-Liéou syndrome) with symptoms previously labeled as hysterical—such as intermittent blurry vision, intermittent hearing loss, ringing in ears, dysphagia, vague off-balance sensations, or tendency to fainting. A simple technique for lateral injection is available that appears to be as effective as touching each tubercle. This is done by starting at C5 on a line between the most anterior portion of the ear and midline in the neck (Fig. 131–44). Needle entry is typically about $\frac{3}{4}$ inch or until an electricity sensation is felt with needle insertion or bony contact is made. (Bony contact and electricity both indicate that the needle is at least at tubercle

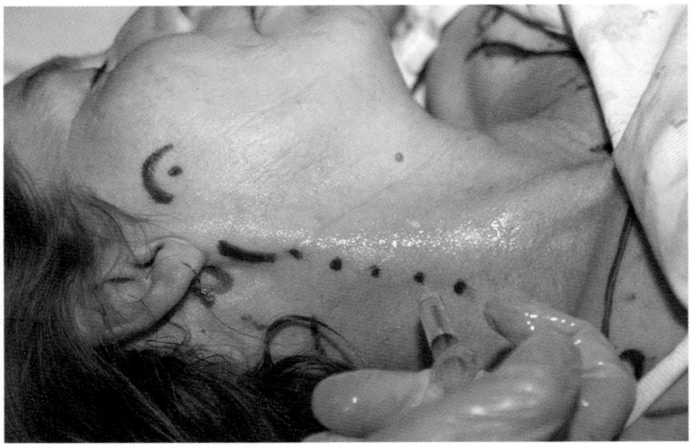

FIGURE 131–44 ■ Scalene insertion infiltration with 27-gauge needle.

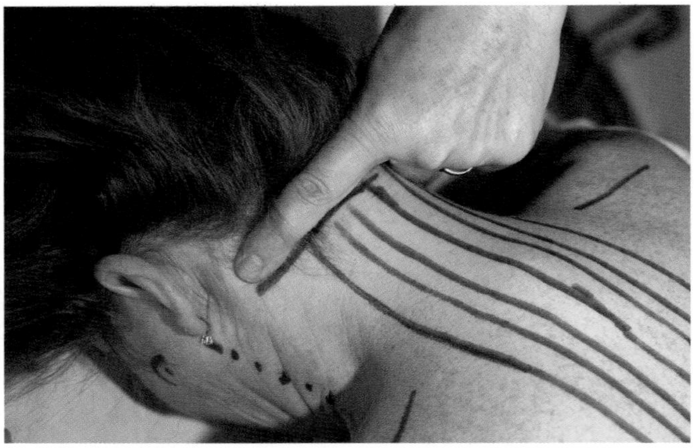

FIGURE 131–45 ■ Marking base of head for base of head injection sites (C2 level for skin puncture).

level). The injections are then made at that same depth in four total locations on a line starting two finger-breadths between the mastoid process and three finger-breadths above the clavicle. This then amounts to an exception to the "inject only when bone is felt" rule, which is used for all injections except into joints with proliferant. Aspiration is recommended before injection at each level. This injection does require that anesthetic concentrations be kept low because bony contact is not necessarily made and intravascular infiltration can still occur.

Headaches

Multiple sources of headache pain have been described already, including those of the trapezii, temporomandibular joint, scalenes, levator scapulae, or cervical paraspinals. Chief among causes of musculoskeletal headache, however, are the entheses at the base of the skull, including rectus capitis, semispinalis, and splenius capitis. Marks for insertion are made on a line across the width of the neck about 1 finger-breadth inferior to the base of the skull (Fig. 131–45). Entry at that level is about C2 spinous process level, with needle directed superiorly to touch the skull at about 1 inch. The physician then redirects caudally to feel the needle deepen to about 1½ inches to touch the rectus capitis insertion area (Fig. 131–46). An injection here may inadvertently get the vertebral artery, so aspiration is recommended prior to injection, and/or use of a low concentration of anesthetic (0.1% to 0.25%) so that intravascular infiltration is of little concern. The rectus capitis row should not be missed. Four insertion points are typically used on each side, beginning about ½ inch from midline to avoid midline injection. The more rostral base-of-head insertions are then in two rows about ½ and 1 inch above the first row, with a 1-inch needle typically being satisfactory (Figs. 131–47 and 131–48).

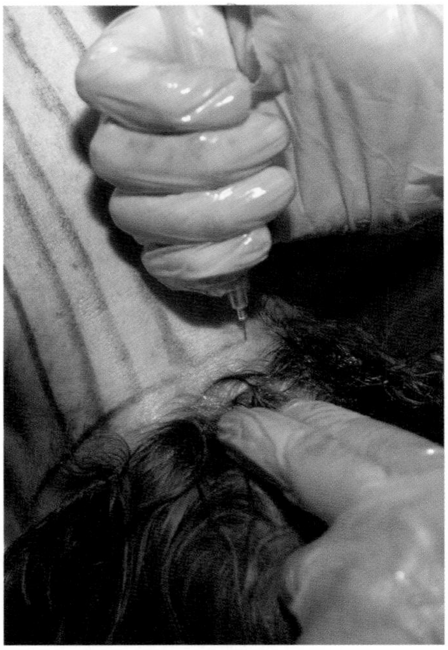

FIGURE 131–46 ■ Injection of deep attachments at the base of the skull with 25-gauge, 2-inch needle.

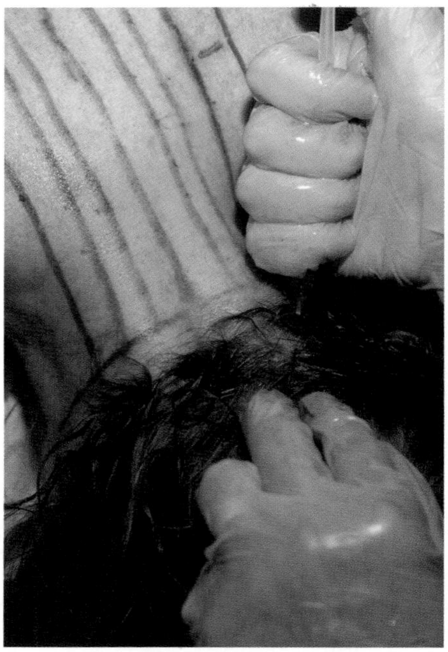

FIGURE 131–47 ■ Base of head second-row injection with 25-gauge, 1-inch needle.

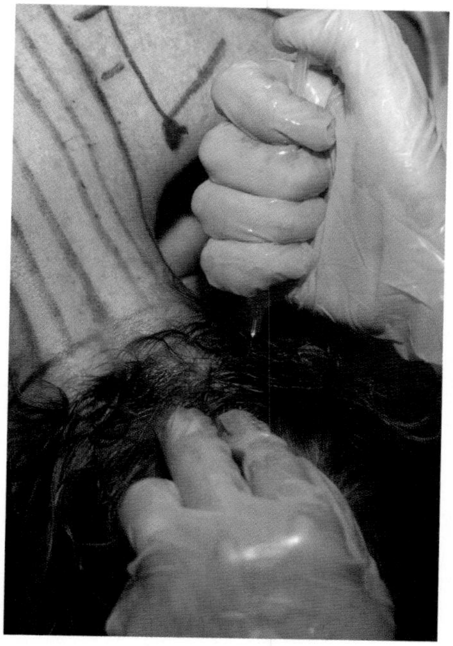

FIGURE 131–48 ■ Top base of head injection with 25-gauge, 1-inch needle.

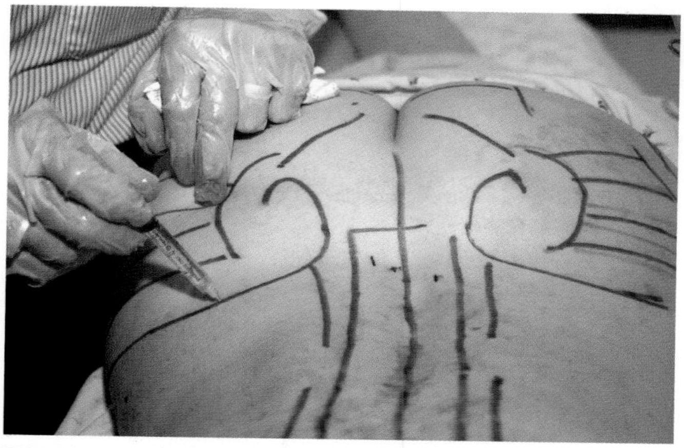

FIGURE 131–49 ■ Finding top of iliac crest for orientation to lumbar spine using 25-gauge, 2-inch needle.

Low Back Pain

Acute and chronic back, hip, buttock, and lower extremity pain can often be attributed to referred pain from trigger points within ligaments or tendon structures around the sacrum or lumbar spine. Failed back syndrome from surgery may be due to instability of ligament and tendon structures. Chronic pain from osteoporotic fractures can be due to traumatic laxity of spinal ligaments with pain from the facet and costotransverse ligaments or longissimus muscle attachments. Thorough palpation is necessary to identify abnormal ligaments that appear to be painful, keeping in mind that the sacroiliac ligament is deeply situated and may not be palpably painful.

For injections in this area, anatomic localization can be difficult. For that reason, placement of a needle vertically is helpful (Fig. 131–49) because the most common error is misjudging the top of the iliac crest, thinking it is up to 2 to 3 cm higher than it actually is. Also injected commonly is the iliac crest (not depicted) when tender due to the large amount of fascial attachments there. However, slight withdrawal (i.e., ⅛ inch) of the needle from the bony contact point is preferred by this author to avoid irritation of the cluneal nerves. Once the top of the iliac crest is localized, keeping in mind that the tip of the L5 transverse process is below the top of the iliac crest, vertically place the needle to a depth of about ¼ to ¾ inch deeper than the iliac crest height and ¼ inch below the marked top of the iliac crest (Fig. 131–50). This will touch or be close to the L5 transverse process. Then, depending on tenderness, the transverse processes of L4 through L2 are injected (Fig. 131–51). This author prefers to inject fairly vertically for L4 and L3 to get a good idea of distance from midline, using the same depth as for the L5 transverse process and entering about 1½ inch from midline. L2 does not protrude as far and 20 to 30 degrees medial angulation will allow it to be contacted. Depth is the same for L5 and L4, with transverse process depth of L3 and L2 becoming more shallow by about ¼ inch or more. However, with medial angulation of the needle, they may not appear to be more shallow. It may be wiser to depend on solution spread to travel from L2 to L1 to avoid any pneumothorax risk, due to a not-infrequent error by novices of misjudging the top of the crest. The facet

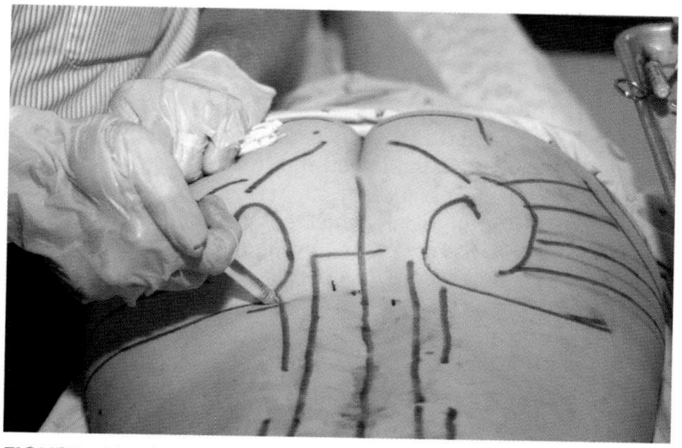

FIGURE 131–50 ■ L5 transverse process midportion injection with 25-gauge, 2-inch needle.

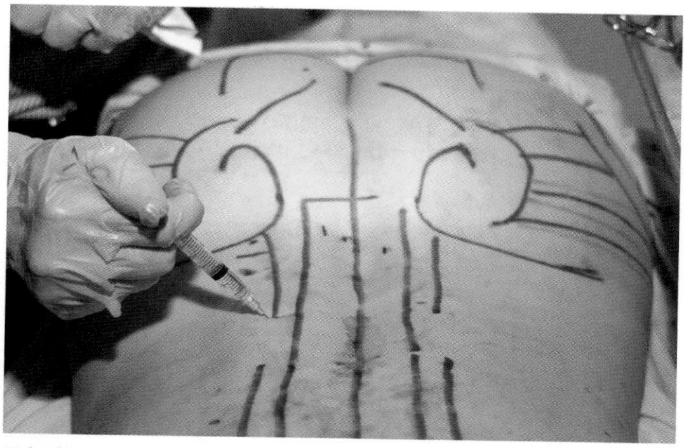

FIGURE 131–51 ■ L3 transverse process injection with 25-gauge, 2-inch needle.

ligament regions are injected similarly to those in thoracic and cervical regions with a slight inferior and medial direction of needle (Fig. 131–52)—entering from 1 inch lateral to spinous processes. The point of contact is typically medial to the facet joints with this, and diffusion is used to reach the facet joints themselves. It is not established that fluoroscopy with direct facet injection is necessary. After facet ligament injection, the top of the sacrum is usually injected and a needle is chosen that is short enough (i.e., 1½ inch) such that the epidural space cannot be entered (Fig. 131–53). The medial sacrum is part of the origin of the sacroiliac ligament and can be injected in areas of tenderness (Fig. 131–54). However, these injections enter ¾ inch from midline and angulate 30 degrees medially to avoid entering a sacral foramina. Sacroiliac and iliolumbar ligament attachments are injected entering about 1½ inches away from the iliac crest, which by now has been localized by needle superiorly and by palpation medially (Fig. 131–55). Several redirections are needed to cover thoroughly the medial ilium and deep sacroiliac and iliolumbar ligaments, but as long as the needle is directed laterally, these injections are quite safe (Fig. 131–56). The physician will often feel the needle slip into the SI joint and that area is beneficially 3½-inch needle injected as well. Depth of injection varies from 1½ to 3 inches (depending on SI entry) using a 3- to 3½-inch needle. The volume of injection is typically 2 cm with each needle insertion but that is spread three to four individual areas with needle redirection.

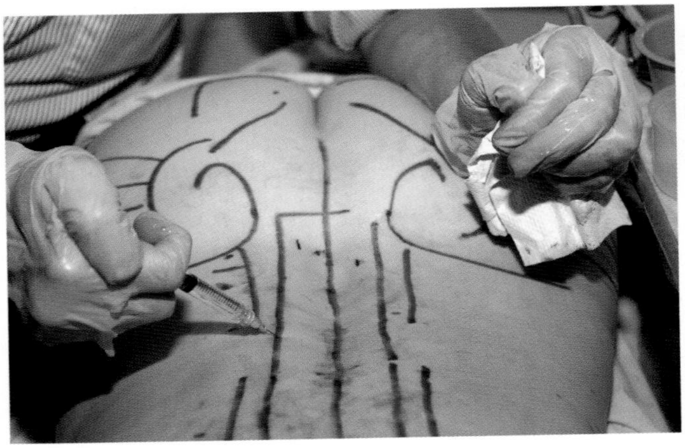

FIGURE 131–52 ■ Lumbar facet ligament injection with 25-gauge, 2-inch needle.

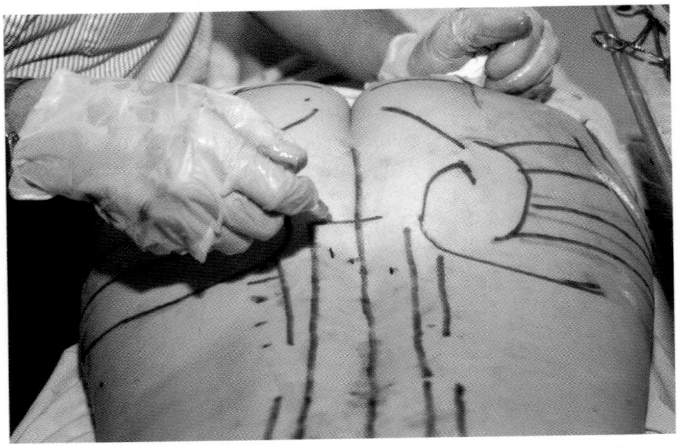

FIGURE 131–53 ■ Top of sacrum injection with 25-gauge, 1½-inch needle.

Sciatica

In the posterior gluteal region, multiple ligaments and muscular attachments are potential radiating pain generators. Groin or inferior abdominal pain is often from the iliolumbar ligament, pain to the great toe is often from the hip articular ligament, and SI ligament and gluteal attachments can refer pain in a variety of directions into the leg. The lower portion of the SI ligament under the posterior superior iliac spine (PSIS) is injected commonly, and this area is often

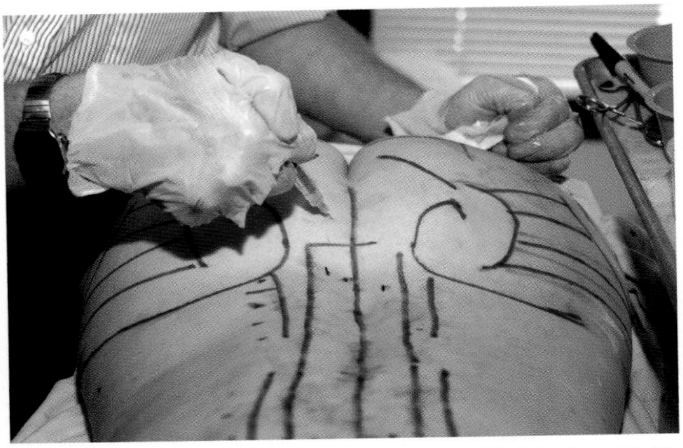

FIGURE 131–54 ■ Medial sacroiliac ligament origin injection with 25-gauge, 1½-inch needle.

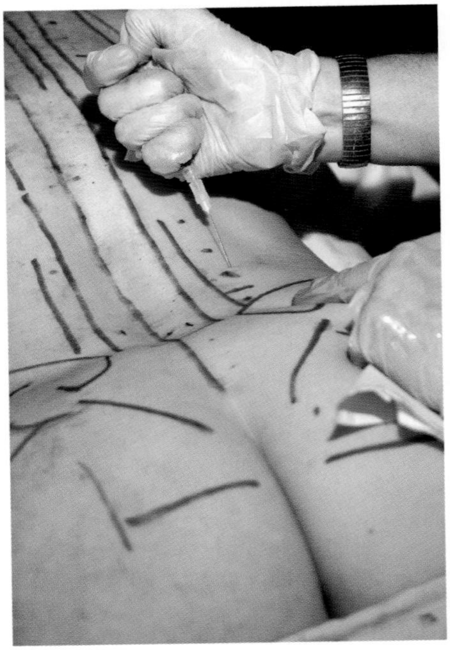

FIGURE 131–55 ■ Injection at top of ilium using 22-gauge, 3½-inch needle, anticipating diffusion to iliolumbar ligament.

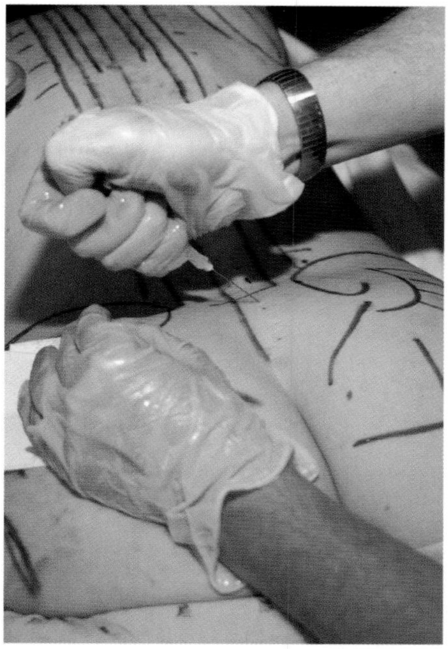

FIGURE 131–56 ■ Medial posterior sacroiliac (SI) ligament injection using 22-gauge, 3½-inch needle.

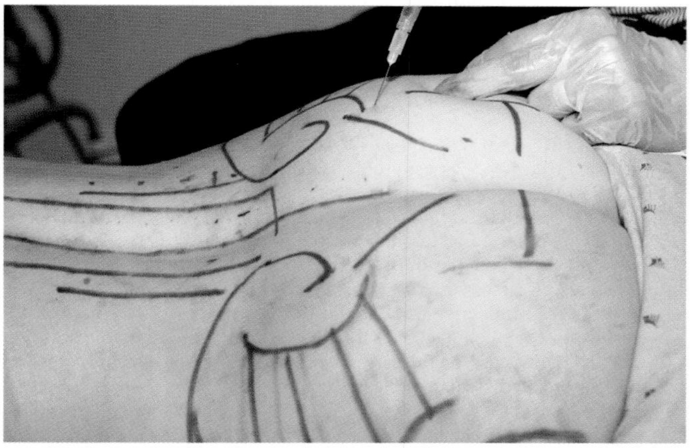

FIGURE 131–57 ■ Interior posterior sacroiliac (SI) ligament injection with 22-gauge, 3½-inch needle.

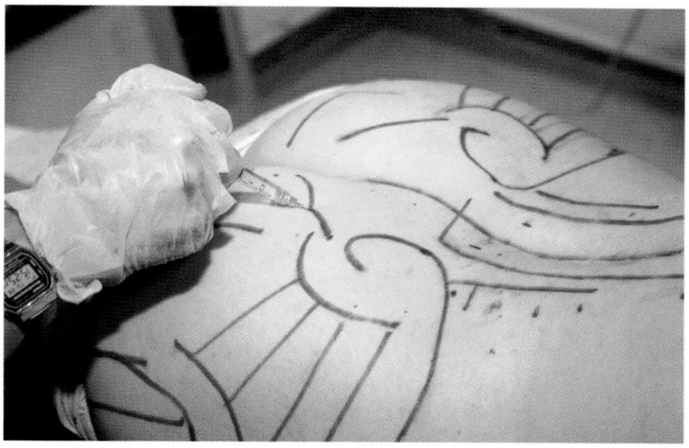

FIGURE 131–58 ■ Sacrospinous/sacrotuberous ligament injection with 22-gauge, 2-inch needle.

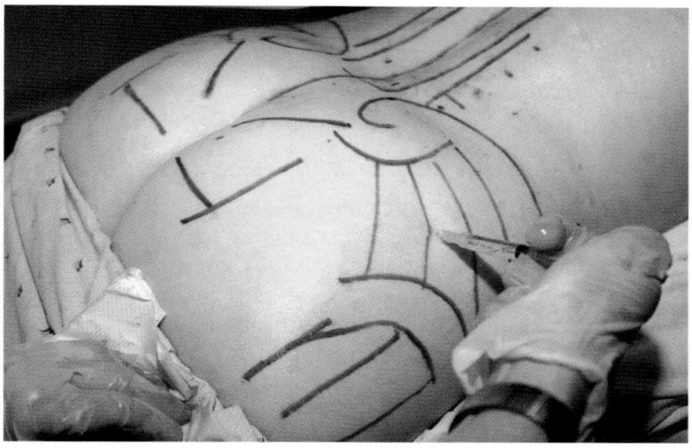

FIGURE 131–59 ■ Midgluteal insertions on ilium with 22-gauge, 3½-inch needle.

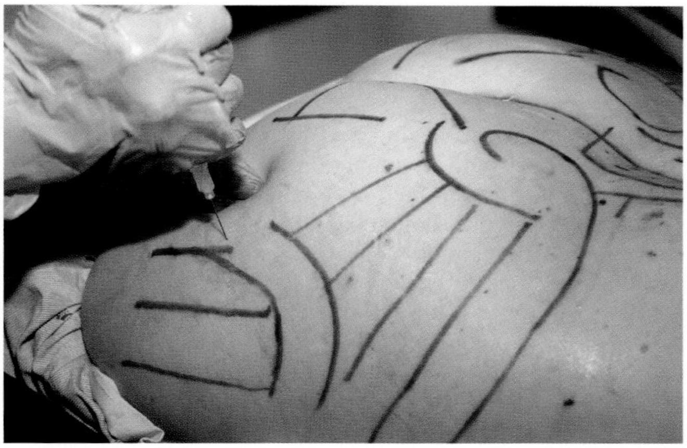

FIGURE 131–60 ■ Posterior trochanter injection using 22-gauge, 3½-inch needle.

responsible for posterior leg pain (Fig. 131–57). This injection covers the area between the tip of the lower PSIS and the point of bone fall off in the sciatic foramen. Posterior leg pain is also commonly from sacrospinous and sacrotuberous ligament attachments to the edge of a sacrum, which are injected with an emphasis on being sure to touch bone before walking off the edge of the sacrum (Fig. 131–58). Keep in mind that this needle can be 1½ inches long or less, with an emphasis on *less* for thin patients. One must make sure the needle first is on the sacrum before walking off the edge of the sacrum. Bowel puncture, although never reported, should be avoided by first starting medially to be certain of bone contact and depth needed. Insertion in the gluteal bulk over the entire gluteal origin can be helpful, and is typically along several lines to ensure somewhat even coverage (Fig. 131–59). For piriformis syndrome, the critical enthesis is, thankfully, the attachment on the posterior trochanter, injected vertically, keeping in mind to not inject until bone contact because the sciatic nerve passes fairly close to the lesser trochanter in its route down the leg (Fig. 131–60). For success, the inferior SI

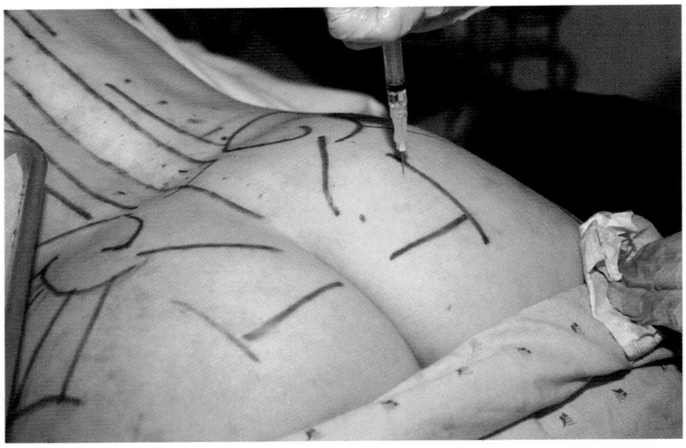

FIGURE 131–61 ■ Gemellar origin injection using 22-gauge, 3½-inch needle.

ligament is usually addressed, and often the SI joint proper because it can imitate posterior leg pain. Note also that if patients still have pain when sitting, the gemelli can be culprits. Both chronic hamstring sprain and gemellary sprain/strain are addressed proximally by direct vertical injection down onto the ischial tuberosity posteriorly (Fig. 131–61). Then several injections are given, moving rostrally, with entry points along the back of the ischium toward the ischial spine. Bone touch before injection is again particularly critical here because the sciatic exits the pelvis through the greater sciatic foramen just above the ischial spine.

CONCLUSION

Needle contact of connective tissue may cause proliferation from cell membrane disruption or bleeding, but prolotherapy is specifically injection to create growth of normal cells or tissue. The literature on low back pain treatment with proliferant injection is complicated by multiple simultaneous treatment methods, technique issues, and control groups that were actually active treatment groups only due to injection effects, with substantial and lasting benefit in all groups injected as long as history and examination by an experienced prolotherapist are performed to help determine candidacy. Double-blind studies have occurred in arthritis with significant results; tightening of loose ligament (ACL) has been demonstrated; initial sports studies look favorable; and a variety of growth factor-based proliferants are being studied and other basic science and clinical studies are underway. The use of current high-intensity ultrasound imaging will soon provide many radiographic demonstrations of sequential healing from simple dextrose injection and will be applied to other proliferant solutions as well. Future studies on growth factor use should include low-cost (growth factor stimulation) options as well as high-cost (primary growth factor application) options to determine cost efficacy factors. Prolotherapy is expected to offer a unique, vital, and inexpensive role in the field of sprain and strain, arthritis, and chronic pain. For further information the web site of the American Academy of Orthopedic Medicine is particularly useful (www.aaomed.org).

References

1. Reeves KD: Prolotherapy: Basic science, clinical studies, and technique. In Lennard TA(ed): Pain Procedures in Clinical Practice, 2nd ed. Philadelphia, Hanley and Belfus, 2000, p172.
2. Yang LW, Zhang JX, Zeng L, et al: Vascular endothelial growth factor gene therapy with intramuscular injections of plasmid DNA enhances the survival of random pattern flaps in a rat model. Br J Plast Surg 58(3):339, 2005.
3. Price S, Pepper JR, Jaggar SI: Recombinant human erythropoietin use in a critically ill Jehovah's witness after cardiac surgery. Anesth Analg 101(2):325, 2005.
4. Yonemura Y, Miyake H, Asou N, Mitsuya H: Long-term efficacy of pegylated recombinant human megakaryocyte growth and development factor in therapy of aplastic anemia. Int J Hematol 82(4):307, 2005.
5. Grines CL, Watkins MW, Mahmarian JJ, et al: A randomized, double-blind, placebo-controlled trial of Ad5FGF-4 gene therapy and its effect on myocardial perfusion in patients with stable angina. J Am Coll Cardiol 42(8):1339, 2003.
6. Lathi KG, Vale PR, Losordo DW, et al: Gene therapy with vascular endothelial growth factor for inoperable coronary artery disease: Anesthetic management and results. Anesth Analg 92(1):19, 2001.
7. Nagano T, Mori-Kudo I, Kawamura T, et al: Pre- or post-treatment with hepatocyte growth factor prevents glycerol-induced acute renal failure. Ren Fail 26(1):5, 2004.
8. Lederman RJ, Mendelsohn FO, Anderson RD, et al: Therapeutic angiogenesis with recombinant fibroblast growth factor-2 for intermittent claudication (the TRAFFIC study): A randomized trial. Lancet 359(9323):2053, 2002.
9. Ellsworth JL, Garcia R, Yu J, Kindy MS: Fibroblast growth factor-18 reduced infarct volumes and behavioral deficits after transient occlusion of the middle cerebral artery in rats. Stroke 34(6):1507, 2003.
10. Leinninger GM, Vincent AM, Feldman EL: The role of growth factors in diabetic peripheral neuropathy. J Peripher Nerv Syst 9(1):26, 2004.
11. Bartesaghi S, Marinovich M, Corsini E, et al: Erythropoietin: A novel neuroprotective cytokine. Neurotoxicology (Netherlands) 26(5):923, 2005.
12. Cooper LT, Hiatt WR, Creager MA, et al: Proteinuria in a placebo-controlled study of basic fibroblast growth factor for intermittent claudication. Vasc Med (England) 6(4):235, 2001.
13. Liu YK, Tipton CM, Matthes RD, et al: An in-situ study of the influence of a sclerosing solution in rabbit medial collateral ligaments and its junction strength. Conn Tissue Res11:95,1983.
14. Forslund C, Aspenberg P: Tendon healing stimulated by injected CDMP. Med Sci Sports Exerc 33(5):685, 2001.
15. Kashiwagi K; Mochizuki Y; Yasunaga Y; et al: Effects of transforming growth factor-beta 1 on the early stages of healing of the Achilles tendon in a rat model. Scand J Plast Reconstr Surg Hand Surg (Sweden) 38(4):193, 2004.
16. Aspenberg P; Virchenko O: Platelet concentrate injection improves Achilles tendon repair in rats. Acta Orthop Scand (Norway) 75(1):93, 2004.
17. Taylor MA, Norman TL, Clovis NB, Blaha JD: The response of rabbit patellar tendons after autologous blood injection. Med Sci Sports Exerc 34(1):70, 2002.
18. Tuncel M, Halici M, Canoz O, et al: Role of insulin-like growth factor-I in repair response in immature cartilage. Knee (England) 12(2):113, 2005.
19. Ongley MJ, Klein RG, Dorman TA, et al: A new approach to the treatment of chronic low back pain. Lancet 2:143, 1987.
20. Klein RG, Bjorn CE, DeLong B, et al: A randomized double-blind trial of dextrose-glycerine-phenol injections for chronic low back pain. J Spinal Disord 6:23, 1993.
21. Dechow E, Davies RK, Carr AJ, et al: A randomized, double-blind, placebo-controlled trial of sclerosing injections in patients with chronic low back pain. Rheumatolgy 39:1255, 1999.
22. Yelland MJ, Glasziou PP, Bogduk N, et al: Prolotherapy injections, saline injections, and exercises for chronic low-back pain: A randomized trial. Spine 29(1):9, 2004.
23. Edwards SG, Calandruccio JH: Autologous blood injections for refractory lateral epicondylitis J Hand Surg [Am] 28(2):272, 2003.
24. Hooper RA, Ding M: Retrospective case series on patients with chronic spinal pain treated with dextrose prolotherapy. J Altern Complement Med 10(4):670, 2004.

25. Hickey DG, Frenkel SR, Di Cesare PE: Clinical applications of growth factors for articular cartilage repair. Am J Orthop 32(2):70, 2003.
26. Roos MD, Han IO, Paterson AJ, et al: Role of glucosamine synthesis in the stimulation of TGF-alpha gene transcription by glucose and EGF. Am J Physiol 270(3 Pt 1):C803, 1996.
27. Di Paolo S, Gesualdo L, Ranieri E, et al: High glucose concentration induces the over expression of transforming growth factor-beta through the activation of a platelet-derived growth factor loop in human mesangial cells. Am J Pathol 149(6):2095, 1996.
28. Pugliese G, Pricci F, Locuratolo N, et al: Increased activity of the insulin-like growth factor system in mesangial cells cultured in high glucose conditions. Relation to glucose-enhanced extracellular matrix production. Diabetologia 39(7):775, 1996.
29. Ohgi S, Johnson PW: Glucose modulates growth of gingival fibroblasts and periodontal ligament cells: Correlation with expression of basic fibroblast growth factor. J Periodontal Res (Denmark) 31(8):579, 1996.
30. Kane R, Stevenson L, Godson C, et al: Gremlin gene expression in bovine retinal pericytes exposed to elevated glucose. Br J Ophthalmol 89(12): 1638, 2005.
31. Singh R, Song RH, Alavi N, et al: High glucose decreases matrixmetalloproteinase 2 activity in rat mesangial cells via transforming growth factor-beta1. Exp Nephrol 9(4):249, 2001.
32. Reeves KD, Hassanein K: Randomized prospective double-blind placebo-controlled study of dextrose prolotherapy for knee osteoarthritis with or without ACL laxity. Alt Ther Hlth Med 6(2):68, 2000.
33. Reeves KD, Hassanein K: Randomized prospective placebo-controlled double-blind study of dextrose prolotherapy for osteoarthritic thumbs and fingers (DIP, PIP and trapeziometacarpal joints) : Evidence of clinical efficacy. Jnl Altern Compl Med 6(4):311, 2000.
34. Altman RD, Hochberg M, Murphy WA, Jr, et al: Atlas of individual radiographic features in osteoarthritis. Osteoarthritis Cartilage 3(Suppl A):3, 1995.
35. Ongley MJ, Dorman TA, Eek BC, et al: Ligament instability of knees: A new approach to treatment. Manual Med 3:152, 1988.
36. Reeves KD, Hassanein K: Long term effects of dextrose prolotherapy for anterior cruciate ligament laxity: A prospective and consecutive patient study. Altern Ther Health Med 9(3):58, 2003.
37. Lazzara MA: The non-surgical repair of a complete Achilles tendon rupture by prolotherapy: Biological reconstruction. A case report. J Orthop Med 27(3):128, 2005.
38. Topol GA, Reeves KD, Hassanein K: Efficacy of dextrose prolotherapy in elite male kicking-sport athletes with chronic groin pain. Arch Phys Med Rehabil 86(4):67, 2005.
39. Altay T, Gunal I, Ozturk H: Local injection treatment for lateral epicondylitis. Clin Orthop 398:127, 2002.
40. Chun J, Tuan TL, Han B, et al: Cultures of ligament fibroblasts in fibrin matrix gel. Connect Tissue Res 44(2):81, 2003.
41. Tang Y, Chen HH, Li SM. [The influence of hyaluronic acid and basic fibroblast growth factor on the proliferation of ligamentous cells] Zhongguo Xiu Fu Chong Jian Wai Ke Za Zhi (China) 15(3):158, 2001.
42. Paavola M, Kannus P, Jarvinen TA, et al: Treatment of tendon disorders. Is there a role for corticosteroid injection? Foot Ankle Clin 7(3):501, 2002.
43. Cohen DB, Kawamura S, Ehteshami J, Rodeo SA: Indomethacin and celecoxib impair rotator cuff tendon-to-bone healing. Am J Sports Med Online: 0363546505280428, 2005.
44. Paoloni JA, Orchard JW: The use of therapeutic medications for soft-tissue injuries in sports medicine. Med J Aust 183(7):384, 2005.
45. Frank C, Amiel D, Woo SL-Y, et al: Normal ligament properties and ligament healing. Clin Orthop Rel Res 196:15, 1985.
46. Leadbetter WB: Soft tissue athletic injury. In Fu FH (ed): Sports Injuries: Mechanisms, Prevention, Treatment. Baltimore, Williams & Wilkins, 1994, p 736.
47. Biedert RM, Stauffer E, Freiderich NK: Occurrence of free nerve endings in the soft tissue of the knee joint. Am J Sports Med 20(4):430, 1993.
48. Travell JG, Simons DG: Myofascial Pain and Dysfunction. The Trigger Point Manual. Baltimore, Williams and Wilkins,1983, p 3.
49. Fischer AA: Trigger point injection. In Lennard TA (ed): Pain Procedures in Clinical Practice, 2nd ed. Philadelphia, Hanley and Belfus, 2000, p 153.
50. Tsuchiya K, Maloney WJ, Vu T, et al: Osteoarthritis: Differential expression of matrix metalloproteinase-9 mRNA in nonfibrillated and fibrillated cartilage. J Orthop Res 15(1):94, 1997.
51. Olney RC, Tsuchiya K, Wilson DM, et al: Chondrocytes from osteoarthritic cartilage have increased expression of insulin-like growth factor I (IGF-I) and IGF-binding protein-3 (IGFBP-3) and -5, but not IGF-II or IGFBP-4. J Clin Endocrinol Metab 81(3):1096, 1996.
52. Bonica J: Anatomic and physiologic basis of nociception and pain. In Bonica JJ (ed): The Management of Pain, 2nd ed. Philadelphia, Lea & Febiger, 1990, p 28.
53. Reeves KD: Mixed somatic peripheral nerve block for painful or intractable spasticity: A review of 30 years of use. Am Pain Mgt 2:205, 1992.
54. Pal B, Morris J: Perceived risks of joint infection following intra-articular corticosteroid injections: A survey of rheumatologists. Clin Rheumatol 18(3):264, 1999.
55. Gray RG, Gottlieb NL: Intra-articular corticosteroids. An updated assessment. Clin Orthop 177:235, 1983.
56. Yang K, Yeo SJ, Lee BP, et al: Total knee arthroplasty in diabetic patients: A study of 109 consecutive cases. J Arthroplasty 16(1):102, 2001.
57. Lazzarini L, Pellizzer G, Stecca C, et al: Postoperative infections following total knee replacement: An epidemiological study. J Chemother 13(2):182, 2001.
58. Miyasaka KC, Ranawat CS, Mullaji A: 10- to 20-year followup of total knee arthroplasty for valgus deformities. Clin Orthop 345:29, 1997.

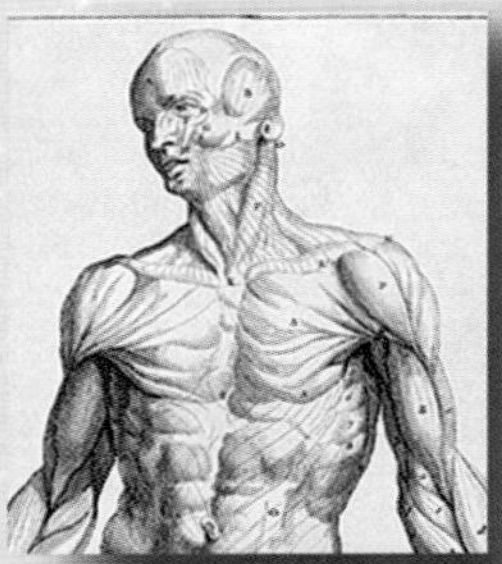

Part D

Neural Blockade and Neurolytic Blocks in the Management of Pain

chapter 132

Atlanto-occipital Joint Injections

Luminita Vladutu and Gabor Racz

HISTORICAL CONSIDERATIONS

Cervicogenic headaches cannot be diagnosed on clinical grounds alone. The term itself is used in a generic sense to apply to any form of headache arising from the neck.[1] The data in the early literature were not scientific. The main diagnostic criterion for cervicogenic headaches was tenderness in the neck, and the treatment recommended was injection of local anesthetic in the tender site. At no time was there discussion of attempts to define the true etiology of the pain.

Interest in cervicogenic headaches can be traced back to Gordon Holmes in 1913 when he reported that headaches could arise from the neck.[1] In 1949, Hunter and Mayfield proposed that occipital neuralgia could be caused by compression of the occipital nerve between the posterior arch of the atlas and the lamina of C2. Baree introduced another concept stating that headaches could be caused by irritation of the vertebral nerves by arthritis of the cervical spine. Pawl suggested the theory by which irritation of the vertebral nerves by cervical disk lesions could result in spasm of the vertebrobasilar system, producing pain in the head by causing ischemia of the vessel walls. This theory was soon refuted. Another concept is that headaches can be caused by cervical spondylosis. An additional view is that cervicogenic headaches represent referred pain from the upper cervical joints.

Multiple etiologies exist; therefore, it is important to identify by a thorough history and physical examination, potential pain generators so that proper treatment, including diagnostic blocks, can be performed.

INDICATIONS

Atlanto-occipital block is useful in the diagnosis and treatment of painful conditions involving trauma or inflammation of the atlanto-occipital joint. These problems manifest clinically as neck pain or suboccipital headache pain and occasionally as suboccipital pain that radiates into the temporomandibular joint region.

Any structure with nociceptive innervation in the upper three cervical segments is capable of causing upper cervical complex pain and cervicogenic headaches. Pathology may be located in the joints, ligaments, or other soft tissues of the neck.[2] Diagnosis is confounded by contributions from the autonomic nervous system, dura mater, adjacent vertebral arterial system, and activity in cervical cranial nerve ganglia to upper cervical symptoms.[3] The cervical joints potentially responsible for the upper cervical pain and headache include the atlanto-occipital (AO), lateral atlanto-occipital, atlanto-axial, and C2-3 synovial joints. An efficient therapeutic approach to neck pain and cervical headaches necessitates isolation of specific anatomic pain generators.

Atlanto-occipital-mediated joint pain has been reported in those affected by rheumatoid arthritis; some of the earliest destructive cervical changes occur in the joint and result in occipital-cervical headaches.[4] Additional causes of AO-mediated joint pain include other inflammatory spine disorders, such as ankylosing spondylitis, trauma, and osteoarthritis.[1] Recently, via provocative intra-articular injections in five asymptomatic subjects, the AO joint was shown to be a potential source of neck and head pain.[5]

CLINICALLY RELEVANT ANATOMY

The upper cervical spine is distinctly different from segments in the lower cervical spine.[3] Anatomically, C0-C1, C1-C2 differ from the cervical disk segments in their architecture: they lack both intervertebral disks and uncinate processes. The joint is not a true facet joint because it lacks posterior articulations characteristic of a true zygapophyseal joint. The atlanto-occipital joint allows the head to nod forward and backward with an isolated range of motion of approximately 35 degrees. This joint is located anterior to the posterolateral columns of the spinal cord.

Neither the atlas nor the axis has an intervertebral foramen to accommodate the first or second cervical nerves. These nerves are primarily sensory and after leaving the spinal canal travel through muscle and soft tissue laterally and then superiorly to contribute fibers to the greater and lesser occipital nerves. The atlas (C1) is unique in that it lacks a vertebral body and, instead, functions as a disk, or "relay center," between the occiput and C2.[3] The cranial articular surfaces for the occiput are large and biconcave, complementing the occipital articular surfaces. The posterior arch lies deep under the skin, hence palpation is challenging. The anterior and posterior arches form the triangular spinal foramen that accommodates the brain stem. The transverse processes are long and perforated, accommodating the passage of the vertebral arteries through the transverse foramina. After exiting these transverse foramina, they course through grooves that can be observed posterior to the lateral masses. Theses grooves, or occasional tunnels, accommodate the vertebral arteries as they loop for a second time in the upper cervical region. Bone changes can occur here that have the potential to compromise vertebral artery function and promote symptoms associated with vertebral basilar insufficiency. The architecture of these grooves is different in men and in women; as a consequence, women may be more susceptible to arterial compromise.[6]

Functionally, the upper cervical spine demonstrates several distinctive uses. The muscle and joint receptors from these segments play a vital role in providing information on the orientation of the body in space.[3] C0-C3 acts as a relay station, where the information on head position is harmonized with afferents from positions and movements of the trunk and extremities. These afferent interactions become vital to maintaining balance and improving coordination between head, trunk, and limbs. Disturbances in motion and control of the upper cervical spine not only may produce pain and dysfunction but may also alter balance and coordination.

The atlanto-occipital joint is susceptible to arthritic changes and trauma secondary to acceleration-deceleration injuries. Such damage to the joint results in pain secondary to synovial joint inflammation and adhesions.

PRE-PROCEDURE WORK-UP

Any patient being considered for atlanto-occipital nerve block should undergo magnetic resonance imaging (MRI) of the head to rule out unsuspected intracranial and brain stem pathology. Furthermore, cervical spine radiographs should be considered to rule out congenital abnormalities such as Arnold-Chiari malformations that may be the hidden cause of the patient's headache symptomatology.

TECHNIQUE

The atlanto-occipital block can be safely performed under fluoroscopic guidance. Although some pain specialists perform this procedure without fluoroscopy, we believe that, because of the proximity of the joint to the spinal cord and vertebral artery, it is not a safe practice, and we recommend the use of fluoroscopy. Contradictions are local infection, coagulopathy, cervical vertebrae/spine instability, patient refusal.

Equipment: 25-gauge, ¾-inch infiltration needle, 22- or 25-gauge, 3½-inch spinal needle, 3-mL syringe, 1-mL syringe, T-piece extension.[3]

Drugs: 1.5% lidocaine for infiltration, 2% lidocaine preservative-free, 0.5% levo-bupivacaine/ropivacaine, Omnipaque (iohexol) 240 radiographic contrast, 40 mg methylprednisolone and either 40 mg triamcinolone diacetate/acetonide or 6 mg betamethasone.

The patient is placed in a prone position with the neck slightly flexed. Pillows are placed under the chest to allow the cervical spine to be moderately flexed without discomfort to the patient. The forehead is allowed to rest on a folded blanket.

With fluoroscopy the beam is rotated in a sagittal plane from an anterior to a posterior position, which allows identification and visualization of the foramen magnum. Just lateral to the foramen magnum is the atlanto-occipital joint. A total of 3 mL of contrast medium suitable for intrathecal use is drawn up in a sterile 3-mL syringe. Then, 3 mL of preservative-free local anesthetic is drawn up in a separate 5-mL sterile syringe. When treating pain thought to be secondary to an inflammatory process, corticosteroid is added to the local anesthetic.

After preparation of the skin with antiseptic solution, a skin wheal of local anesthetic is raised at the site of needle insertion. An 18-gauge, 1-inch needle is inserted at the insertion site to serve as an introducer. The fluoroscopy beam is aimed directly through the introducer needle, which will appear as a small point on the fluoroscopy screen. The introducer needle is then repositioned under fluoroscopic guidance

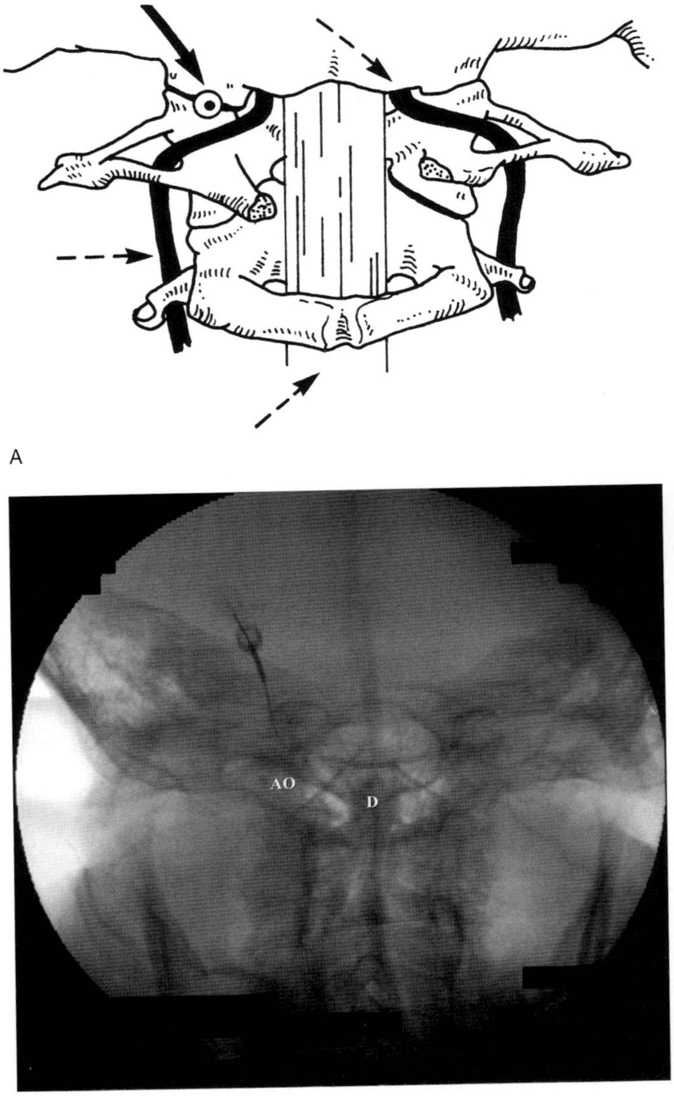

FIGURE 132–1 ■ **A,** A drawing of posteroranterior (oblique) view of the atlanto-occipital joint showing the needle insertion in a tunneled view. (From: Raj, et al: Radiographic Imaging for Regional Anesthesia and Pain Management, Philadelphia, Churchill Livingstone, 2003, p 83. Fig. 13-3b.) **B,** Posteroanterior radiographic image with a 25-gauge spinal needle in the atlantooccipital joint. The dens (D) is labeled and the atlantooccipital joint (AO) is just above its label.

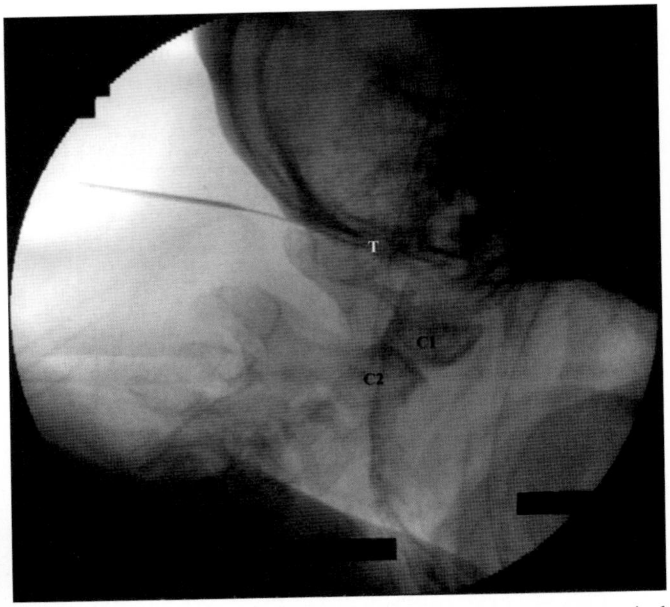

FIGURE 132–2 ■ Lateral radiographic image of the 25-gauge spinal needle in the posterior portion of the atlanto-occipital joint. T, tip of needle.

until this small point is visualized over the posterolateral aspect of the atlanto-occipital joint (Figs. 132–1 and 132–2). This lateral placement avoids trauma to the vertebral artery, which lies medial to the joint at this level.

A 25- or 22-gauge, 3½-inch stylet spinal needle is then inserted through the 18-gauge introducer. If bony contact is made, the spinal needle is withdrawn and the introducer needle is repositioned over the lateral aspect of the joint. The 25-gauge spinal needle is then re-advanced until a pop is felt, indicating placement within the atlanto-occipital joint (see Fig. 132–1A and B). It is essential to then confirm that the needle is actually in the joint, which is anterior to the posterior lateral aspect of the spinal cord. This is accomplished by rotating the C-arm to the horizontal plane and confirming needle placement within the joint (see Fig. 132–2). If intra-articular placement cannot be confirmed, the needle should be withdrawn.

After confirmation of needle placement within the atlanto-occipital joint, the stylet is removed from the 25-gauge spinal needle, and the hub is observed for blood or cerebrospinal fluid. If neither is present, gentle aspiration of the needle is carried out, and if no blood or cerebrospinal fluid is seen, 0.5 to 1 mL of contrast medium is slowly injected under fluoroscopy. An arthrogram of the normal atlanto-occipital joint reveals a bilateral concavity representing the intact joint capsule (Fig. 132–3A and B). However, if the joint has been traumatized, it is not unusual to see contrast medium flow freely from the torn joint capsule into the cervical epidural space. If the contrast medium is seen to rapidly enter the venous plexus rather than outline the joint, the needle is almost always outside the joint space. If this occurs, the needle should be repositioned into the joint prior to injection. If the contrast medium remains within the joint or if it outlines the joint and a small amount leaks into the epidural space, 1 to 1.5 mL of the local anesthetic and steroid is slowly injected through the spinal needle.

SIDE EFFECTS AND COMPLICATIONS

The proximity to the brain stem and spinal cord makes it imperative that this procedure be carried out only by those well versed in the regional anatomy and experienced in performing interventional pain management techniques. Fluoroscopic guidance is recommended for most practitioners because neural trauma is a possibility even in the most experienced hands.

Complications of atlanto-occipital blocks include epidural and intrathecal injections, intravascular injections, and brain stem/spinal cord injury.[7] The proximity to the vertebral artery combined with the vascular nature of this

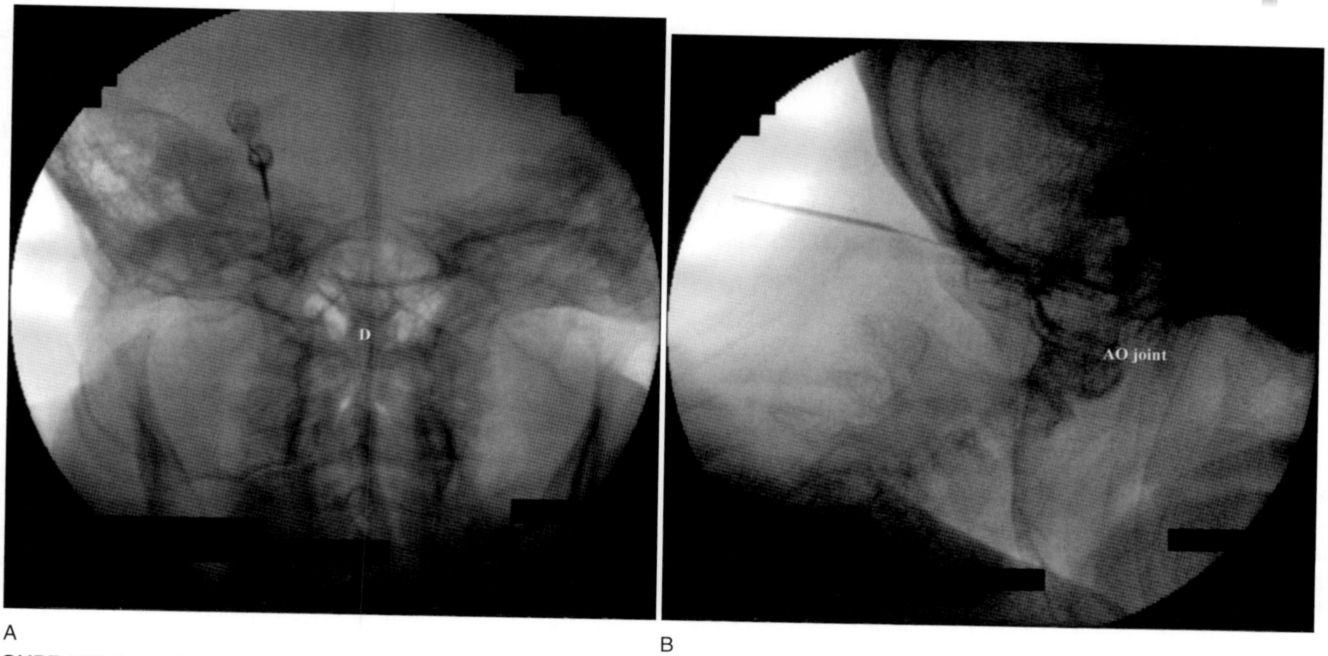

A

B

FIGURE 132–3 ■ **A,** Posteroanterior (PA) view of the atlanto-occipital joint after injection of 0.5 mL of contrast. The image is not a true PA image because two lines of contrast in the joint can be seen. **B,** Lateral view showing filling of the contrast in the atlanto-occipital (AO) joint.

anatomic region makes the potential for intravascular injection high. Despite the "perfect" anatomical drawings in medical textbooks, the vertebral artery can be tortuous and while the path of the placed needle may be "textbook," vascular injuries can happen.[8] Even small amounts of local anesthetic injected into the vertebral arteries will result in seizures. Neural blockade at the atlanto-occipital joint is a very technically demanding technique. The physician doing the procedure must avoid placing the needle into the brain stem or the vertebral artery and avoid injecting either air or particulate matter such as precipitated or particulate steroids.[9] Given the proximity of the brain and brain stem, ataxia after atlanto-occipital block due to vascular uptake of local anesthetic is not an uncommon occurrence.

■ CONCLUSION

The definitive criterion for the diagnosis of cervicogenic headache is complete relief of pain after controlled diagnostic blocks of a cervical structure or its nerve supply. This is the one means of establishing a cervical source of the pain. The blocks required are not office procedures. They require special skills and special facilities that are not within the province of most practitioners, and they may not be available readily to most practitioners.

The atlanto-occipital block is often combined with an atlanto-axial block when treating pain in the previously mentioned areas. Although neither joint is a true facet joint in the anatomic sense of the word, the block is analogous to the facet joint block technique used commonly by pain practitioners and it may be viewed as such. Many pain specialists believe that these techniques are currently under-used in the treatment of "post-whiplash" cervicalgia and cervicogenic headaches. These specialists believe that both techniques should be considered when cervical epidural nerve blocks and/or occipital nerve blocks fail to provide palliation of these headache and neck pain syndromes. Efficacy can be based on individual anecdotal patient pain relief. No randomized controlled double-blind studies can be found.

References

1. Bogduk N: The neck and headache. Neurol Clin North Am 22:151, 2004.
2. Mueller L: Cervicogenic headache: A diagnostic and therapeutic dilemma. Headache & Pain: Diagnostic Challenges. Curr Ther 14(1):29, 2003.
3. Racz G, Anderson S, Sizer P, Phelps V: Atlantooccipital and atlantoaxial injections in the treatment of headache and neck pain. In Waldman S (ed): Interventional Pain Management 2nd ed. Philadelphia, WB Saunders, 2001, p 295.
4. Dreyfuss P, Rogers J, Dreyer S, Fletcher D: Atlanto-occipital joint pain: A report of three cases and description of an intra-articular joint block technique [abstract]. Reg Anesth 19:344, 1994.
5. Dreyfuss P, Michaelson M, Fletcher D: Atlanto-occipital and lateral atlanto-axial joint pain patterns. Spine 19:1125, 1994.
6. Ebraheim N, Xu R, Ahmad M, Heck B: The quantitative anatomy of the vertebral artery groove of the atlas and its relation to the posterior atlantoaxial approach. Spine 23:320, 1998.
7. Silverman S: Cervicogenic headache: Interventional, anesthetic, and ablative treatment. Curr Pain Headache Rep 6:308, 2002.
8. Oga M, Yuge I, Terada K, et al: Tortuosity of the vertebral artery in patients with cervical spondylotic myelopathy: Risk factor for the vertebral artery injury during anterior cervical decompression (case report). Spine 21:1085, 1996.
9. Raj P, Lou L, Erdine S, et al (eds): Radiographic Imaging for Regional Anesthesia and Pain Medicine, Philadelphia, Churchill Livingstone, 2003, p81.

chapter 133

Atlantoaxial Injection

Jonathan Barry, Miles Day, and Gabor Racz

HISTORY

Injections of the atlantoaxial joints and atlanto-occipital joints have been recognized for some time as having a role in care of patients with neck and head pain.[1] Diagnostic blockade of the lateral atlantoaxial joints has been used to implicate this joint as a source for occipital headaches.[2] Techniques for a posterior approach and a lateral approach to the atlantoaxial joint have been described.

INDICATIONS

Atlantoaxial injection is frequently combined with atlanto-occipital injections for the diagnosis and treatment of neck pain and headache. Specifically, headaches that are suboccipital or occipital in distribution and irritated by flexion, extension, or rotation frequently have a component related to the atlantoaxial joint.[3] This statement is complicated by the lack of a strong correlation between physical signs at the C1-C2 level or specific pain distributions and positive relief from atlantoaxial injections.[2] Contraindications to this procedure include: infection, presence of surgical hardware, presence of metastatic disease, and coagulopathy.

CLINICALLY RELEVANT ANATOMY

The anatomy of the C1-C2 junction is unique for the cervical vertebrae. The most characteristic feature of C2 is the dens. This tooth-like prominence functions as a pivot point on which C1 rotates. A normal distance of 2 to 3 mm between the arch of C1 and the odontoid process of C2 should be maintained through all motions. If this distance is exceeded, this is indicative of dislocation of the dens or damage to other elements of the joint.

The interaction between the dens and the arch of the axis is maintained by the transverse ligament of the atlas (TLA). The TLA runs between the lateral masses of the axis, and acts to secure C1 to C2. Laxity of this ligamentous bony relation due to whiplash injury or other mechanism places the brain stem in danger of compression by the dens during flexion.

The vertebral artery courses through the transverse foramen of C1 and C2. Consequently, this important vascular structure lies lateral to the atlantoaxial joint. This fact is vitally important to remember in order to avoid the disastrous complications associated with an intra-arterial injection. Avoiding the artery is complicated by the observation that in some patients with cervical spondylosis, the course of the artery is more medial than expected.[4]

TECHNIQUE

The following equipment is needed:

- 18-gauge needle to be used as "introducer"
- 22- or 25-gauge spinal needle (modified by a bend approximately 5 mm from the tip)
- Local anesthetic (0.2% ropivacaine or 0.25% bupivacaine)
- Steroid (preferably water soluble such as dexamethasone)
- Fluoroscopy equipment

Descriptions have been made for a lateral technique of atlantoaxial injection.[1] For posterior access, clear visualization of the foramen magnum and the atlas is necessary using AP fluoroscopy. Next, identify the atlantoaxial joint. Point of entry for the introducer needle is the middle aspect of the joint. This is critical, given that the vertebral artery lies lateral to the joint. It is important to ensure that the introducer is placed using a true "gun-barrel" view. Once this is achieved, the spinal needle is placed in the introducer with stylet in place. Advancement is performed with frequent AP and lateral views to ensure appropriate location and depth. Entry into the joint is usually marked with a "pop." A lateral view is then used to confirm that the needle is in the joint. Having done this, the stylet is removed and observed for blood or cerebrospinal fluid.

Confirmation within the joint is next made with a nonionic, water-soluble radiographic dye. First, careful aspiration on the spinal needle is performed. Injection of a small volume of dye (0.5 to 1.0 mL) is performed. Ideally the bilateral convexity of the joint should be outlined. Frequently, some of the dye leaks from the joint because of capsule penetration and resultant epidural run off. However, a pattern of venous runoff is usually experienced if the needle is outside of the joint due to the presence of an extensive venous plexus. Once appropriate dye spread is noted, 1 mL of local anesthetic and steroid solution is injected. The use of nonparticulate water-soluble steroid deserves special attention in this block because particulate emboli in the vertebral arteries could have disastrous consequences for the brain stem.

For the lateral injection technique, the patient is positioned in a lateral decubitus position with the side to be injected up. Fluoroscopy is used to confirm that the C2 and C3 segments overlap in a lateral view. The atlantoaxial joint space is maximized by angling the fluoroscopy C-arm in a cephalad to caudad direction. The anterior one third of this joint lucency is identified and marked with a radiopaque marker. The skin and subcutaneous tissues are then anesthetized. A 25-gauge spinal needle is then advanced in a gun barrel fashion. It is important to avoid the midpoint of the joint as well as the posterior aspect of the joint because these correspond to the location of the vertebral artery. Similarly, placement too anterior in the joint risks injection into the internal carotid artery. Osseous contact with the superior or inferior aspect of the joint is made. Then an anterior-posterior view is used to guide the needle into the atlantoaxial joint cavity. Injection of dye is made in the same fashion as described earlier.[1]

SIDE EFFECTS AND COMPLICATIONS

It is important to prepare patients for the possibility that headache may transiently increase following this technique. Ataxia has been noted for a period following this procedure. For this reason, it is mandatory to monitor the patient postprocedure for at least 30 minutes and note resolution of this effect. Additional complications can be predicted by the anatomic structures in close proximity. These include epidural injections; intrathecal injections; injuries to the surrounding venous plexus; carotid artery injury; and vertebral artery injections. Obviously with the proximity to the central nervous system, even low concentration and low volumes of local anesthetic intravascularly can have significant effects. Use of nonparticulate water-soluble contrast is extremely important, given the potential for runoff of vascular structures to the brain stem, where occlusion secondary to large steroid particles could be devastating.

CONCLUSION

Blockade at the C1-C2 atlantoaxial joint is a technically challenging procedure requiring familiarity with the surrounding anatomy; the ability to assimilate two-dimensional information into a three-dimensional format; and skill with interventional techniques and equipment. Despite its challenges, it does have a role in the armamentarium of appropriately trained interventional pain specialists for the management of neck pain.

References

1. Dreyfuss P, Michaelson M, Fletcher D: Atlanto-occipital and lateral atlantoaxial joint pain patterns. Spine19:1125, 1994.
2. Aprill C, Axinn MJ, Bogduk N: Occipital headaches stemming from the lateral atlanto-axial (C1-C2) joint. Cephalgia 22:15, 2001.
3. Racz GB, Sanel H, Diede JH: Atlanto-occipital and atlantoaxial injections in the treatment of headache and neck pain. In Waldman S, Winnie AP (eds): Interventional Pain Management. Philadelphia, WB Saunders, 1996, p 220.
4. Oga M, Yuge I, Terada K: Tortuosity of the vertebral artery in patients with cervical spondylotic myelopathy: Risk factor for the vertebral artery injury during anterior cervical decompression. Spine 21(9):1085, 1996.

chapter 134

Sphenopalatine Ganglion Block

Lawrence Kropp, Miles R. Day, and Gabor B. Racz

Facial pain is one of the most demanding and difficult to treat syndromes encountered by pain physicians. Confusing histories and variable symptomatology are the norm, and patients have a difficult time describing what they are experiencing. In addition, most patients may have had extensive work-ups and questionable treatments for years before being referred to a qualified pain interventionalist. This is due mostly to the lack of knowledge of these very complicated pain syndromes by the general medical community. Even practitioners with some experience with facial pain will most likely not be up to date on the advances that have made treatments in this area far more effective than in previous years.

HISTORY

The medical history of treatments of the sphenopalatine ganglion (SPG) really breaks up into two categories: those approaches done before the advent of real-time fluoroscopy and radiofrequency and those done after. There is no smooth continuum connecting the two.

Blocking the SPG with local anesthetics was first published by Sluder in 1908.[1,2] Done mainly for the treatment of headaches and using limited technology, it is not hard to understand why these early procedures were met with inconsistent results. Complicating matters further was the push to implicate the SPG in pain syndromes ranging from headaches to dysmenorrhea. The greater medical community for the most part abandoned the SPG as a possible target for facial pain for many decades. There are scattered papers throughout the 20th century that re-explored this area, but most with limited numbers and variable results. For an excellent review of this history, the reader is referred to Waldman's article on the history of SPG blockade.[3]

The approach that was the most widely used from 1940 through 1960 was a blind paranasal needle approach using 10 mL of local anesthetic. Eventually this technique fell out of favor owing to the rare but dangerous complication of retrograde injection into the maxillary artery causing seizures, loss of consciousness, and even death. Today, it appears that virtually every medical specialist feels qualified to do these blocks owing to the recent technologic advances—such as fluoroscopic guidance. The authors, though, warn all practitioners of the dangers in this area. Intravascular injections, although rare, can and still do happen, and they require that a resuscitative expert be in attendance. No one should attempt these blocks without full resuscitative equipment, and ideally all procedures in the face, head, and neck should be performed in the operating room with a board-certified anesthesiologist in attendance.[4]

INDICATIONS

Blockade of the SPG has been used to treat syndromes of complex facial pain, cluster headaches, and numerous other pain syndromes in the head and neck area. The modern indications for the procedure have narrowed somewhat from its very broad use in early times.[5] The current indications are listed in Table 134–1.

DIAGNOSIS

The diagnostic approach should include categorization of the pain by location, intensity, quality, and frequency. If these features can be ascertained, the puzzle becomes clearer. The face has a complicated innervation with many overlying distributions, but several pain patterns can be established. The differential diagnoses can be extensive, and entire textbooks are devoted to the neural innervation of the face. Despite this complexity, several guidelines are generally followed by experienced practitioners. The list in Table 134–2 will serve as a useful guide, although it is not exhaustive.

The quality of the pain is also important. Most facial pain is a balance between somatic and sympathetically maintained pain. Symptoms of burning or anesthesia dolorosa (painful numbness), along with hyperpathia (prolonged response to painful stimulus) are good indicators of sympathetically maintained pain, but the most important indicator is allodynia (pain with light touch). Allodynia is a reliable sign of sympathetic reflexes causing release of pain mediators such as substance P and bradykinin, which can also cause discoloration. Sympathetically maintained pain is most often constant and dull without sharp character. A sharp pain is more associated with tic douloureux or Bell's palsy and can be associated with nerve compressions from tumors, sinus swelling, or trauma.

Frequency of pain can indicate several things. Lancinating intermittent pain is consistent with tic douloureux or

Bell's palsy. Intermittent pain around the eye can also be caused by cluster headaches or migraines. Pain that is worse in the morning is often associated with nighttime sinus swelling. Pain that worsens throughout the day can be more headache related. These generalizations are by no means rigid, which is what makes facial pain so difficult to accurately diagnose. Certainly, every interventional procedure is aimed at healing pain, but for complex facial pain the diagnostic benefit of these blocks is extremely valuable, and often is the only way to make a diagnosis.

When the above issues are taken into consideration, and a patient's pain cannot be attributed to known causes, it is reasonable to address a more central therapeutic target. One last consideration is whether the pain fibers are more attributed to the trigeminal ganglion or the SPG. Trigeminal neuralgia is another frequent cause of atypical facial pain and has been implicated as an agonist for sphenopalatine neuralgia by Sluder's contemporary, Ruskin, in the 1920s.[7] Both somatic sensory and sympathetic fibers travel through the trigeminal ganglion, so it would be assumed that trigeminal neuralgia would be more distinct and follow one of the three branch distributions (V1/V2/V3). Although no good study exists on this, it is the authors' experience that trigeminal neuralgia does not follow discrete distributions, and can be responsible for vague and complex facial pain syndromes. That said, if the facial pain is in a discrete distribution, then the trigeminal ganglion may be a better target, but the approach of the authors is to address the SPG first for signs and symptoms of atypical facial pain. This may be due, in part, to the increased risk associated with the trigeminal ganglion and its close proximity to the brain. It is also interesting to note that these two ganglions are not completely separate. The trigeminal ganglion communicates with the SPG by its maxillary division.

Table 134–1

Indications for Sphenopalatine Ganglion Block

- Atypical facial pain
- Migraine headaches
- Cluster headaches
- Sympathetically maintained pain of the face
- Trigeminal neuralgia: typical (tic douloureux) and atypical
- Sphenopalatine neuralgia

CLINICALLY RELEVANT ANATOMY

The SPG resides in the pterygopalatine fossa. Other names include Meckel ganglion, the nasal ganglion, and the sphe-

Table 134–2

Differential Diagnosis for Pain in the Face, Head, and Neck Region

Type of Pain	*Clinical Pearls*
Tumors of the parotid gland and neck	These lesions can compress the facial nerve, posterior auricular, anterior auricular, and the mandibular nerves. Palpate this area extensively to see if the pain can be reproduced. Any swelling on the lateral face in the presence of pain should be worked up with needle aspiration and appropriate imaging.
Zygomatic arch tenderness	Make note of all previous traumas in this area, especially those that fit the time course. LeFort fractures can impinge the maxillary nerve.
Dental involvement	Dental pain can masquerade as atypical facial pain, but facial pain can also radiate to the teeth. The mandibular nerve travels down the jaw and emerges through the inferior alveolar foramen to become the submental nerve and innervate the inferior alveolar ridge. The maxillary nerve innervates the superior alveolar ridge.
Lacrimation	This is usually a sign of direct sphenopalatine involvement through parasympathetic fibers.
Ear pain	This needs to be further characterized by inner versus outer ear and canal pain—the former requiring a detailed ENT examination. Pay special attention to any audio disturbances. Outer ear pain is often associated with geniculate neuralgia.*
Sinus pain	Sinus pain is probably the most common form of facial pain, and can sometimes be elucidated by tapping over the maxillary or frontal sinuses, or by having the patient place his/her head inferiorly to increase vascular congestion and test for pain.
Temporomandibular joint dysfunction	Physical examination should elucidate this. Pain on palpation with jaw opening and audible clicks should warrant a complete work-up. This pain does not respond well to SPG blockade.
Pain on the lateral aspect of the tongue	This can be a sign of glossopharyngeal neuralgia and should be considered as a possibility other than SPG neuralgia.

ENT, ear, nose, and throat; SPG, sphenopalatine ganglion.
*Pulec J: Geniculate neuralgia: Long-term results of surgical treatment. Ear Nose Throat J 81:30, 2002.

nomaxillary ganglion. It is the large collection of neurons outside the cranial cavity and the second largest nerve center in the head. It resides in the pterygopalatine fossa just lateral to the lateral nasal wall at the level of the middle turbinate. This is a small pyramidal space that is approximately 2 cm high and 1 cm wide. The borders of the fossa are the maxillary sinus on the anterior side, the medial plate of the pterygoid process to the posterior, the perpendicular plate of the palatine bone on the medial side and the sphenoid bone superiorly. The foramen rotundum is on its superior-lateral side and from it emerges the second branch of the trigeminal nerve. The pterygoid canal just inferior to that transmits the vidian nerve. The fossa also contains the internal maxillary artery.

The SPG carries autonomic parasympathetic and sympathetic fibers. Parasympathetic fibers synapse with postganglionic fibers at the SPG. These autonomic pathways then emerge from the SPG and innervate nasal mucosa, secretory glands, and sympathetic vasomotor structures. The pterygopalatine fossa itself has an opening that is actually anterior and lateral instead of the lateral opening that may seem to appear on lateral fluoroscopic view (Fig. 134–1).

TECHNIQUES

Anesthesia Considerations

When doing blocks in the head and neck, the practitioner, regardless of background and specialty, must temporarily become an anesthesiologist. This requires that the airway be assessed with regard to the anatomic constraints of intubation. A full anesthetic history must be obtained in addition to a cardiovascular and pulmonary examination. The room must contain resuscitation equipment, which may include an anesthesia machine. If bupivacaine is injected intravascularly in the head, it will take more than an Ambu Bag to recover this patient. The resulting neuro- and cardiotoxicity requires the availability of monitoring equipment fully compliant with the American Society of Anesthesiologists (ASA) guidelines, as well as medications to abort seizures, support contraction of the heart, treat arrhythmias, sedate, and sometimes paralyze. Code doses of epinephrine may not accomplish these complex therapeutic goals. If the practitioner performing this procedure is not an anesthesiologist and is untrained in any of these areas, it is the opinion of the authors that this block should be scheduled in the operating room with a board-certified anesthesiologist in attendance.

Any signs of tinnitus, perioral numbness and tingling, visual disturbances or dizziness are early signs of local anesthetic toxicity or intravascular injection. If this occurs, monitor the patient closely with ASA monitors for at least 90 minutes and make sure these symptoms have resolved before discharging the patient.

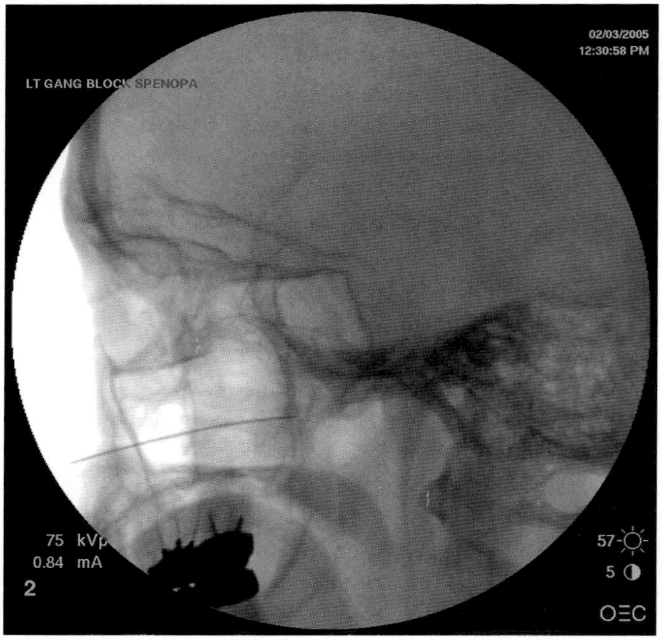

FIGURE 134–1 ■ Lateral fluoroscopic view showing a transnasal approach using a hollow-shaft Q-Tip with a Frazier stylet inserted.

Transnasal Approach

The SPG can be treated using a transnasal approach and a medication that can cross the nasal mucosa. Cocaine is a local anesthetic that has been used for years with good success. Cocaine is an ester local anesthetic that crosses mucous membranes quickly. Viscous lidocaine can also be used, and other anesthetics have also been tried.

After a history, physical examination, and consent are obtained, the patient is placed in a supine position and a semisterile technique is used. No preparation is required in the nares. The authors perform this block in the operating room, but it can be done in any environment that has an ASA-compliant monitoring set-up. If cocaine is to be used, a 4% solution works well, but care must be taken to watch the patient closely for signs of tachycardia, chest pain, palpitations, or any cardiovascular abnormalities. If lidocaine is to be used, a 4% viscous or regular solution can be used.

Two long cotton-swabs are soaked in the anesthetic solution and introduced into the naris on the side affected. It is advisable to do one side and not do a bilateral procedure. As mentioned earlier, the diagnostic benefit is critical, and bilateral techniques are less revealing. Even if the pain is bilateral, a unilateral relief of pain that corresponds to the one-sided procedures will be more diagnostic. The other side can then be done at another time. The cotton swab should be advanced slowly in a perpendicular plane to the face. There is a natural tendency to follow the angle of the nose, but the nasal cavity is directly posterior to the inferior opening of the naris. Placing the swab superiorly can perforate the ethmoid sinus and create a CSF leak, which is not easily fixed. The swabs are advanced to the rear of the nasal cavity. If the patient feels discomfort with the advancement of the swab, stop and wait momentarily for the anesthetic to numb the surrounding tissues before proceeding. There is a characteristic resistance once the swab is at the posterior of the nasal cavity. This is the correct position. A second swab should then be placed in a similar fashion in the same naris. The patient should then be monitored for 35 to 45 minutes to allow the medication to cross the nasal mucosal barrier and reach the SPG. Adequate monitoring includes a heart monitor that has an ECG display screen. Early signs of cocaine or local anesthetic toxicity are premature ventricular contractions (PVCs), peaked T waves or depressed ST segments. If the procedure was done in an operating room, the patient can be transferred after 5 minutes of intraoperative monitoring, and if no abnormalities exist, can then be taken to the recovery room for an additional 30 to 40 minutes of monitoring. After this time has passed the swabs can be removed. Tearing is a good sign of SPG block and is a result of sympathetic/parasympathetic imbalance caused by the local anesthetic. Tearing is not a requirement for successful block and may not occur even in the best blocks.

Another method can be used for the transnasal approach that involves using a hollow swab applicator. A Frazier suction stylet can be introduced into the hollow shaft to make this swab radio-opaque. The swab is then soaked in the anesthetic solution and introduced in a similar fashion but under fluoroscopic guidance on lateral view. The pterygopalatine fossa can be seen as indicated in Figure 134–1 and the swab can be seen just medial to this structure. This technique, although more expensive, ensures that the swab is in the correct location, and the authors have found it gives a better block.

Infrazygomatic Approach

If the transnasal block is unsuccessful in reducing pain, the next step is to attempt an infrazygomatic approach. This will deliver medications in a more potent way and also allow the delivery of steroid to this area. This block is more technically demanding and takes some experience to perform well. The pterygopalatine fossa opens in a medial/anterior direction, and does not open directly laterally. This should be kept in mind on the approach, and the best method for entering in exactly the correct location is to use a curved, blunt Coudé block needle. The coronoid process is then palpated and a location is palpated just anterior to this over the mandibular notch. A lidocaine wheal is raised and a 16-gauge Angiocath is introduced about 1 to 2 cm. The Coudé blunt block needle is then introduced and advanced under fluoroscopic guidance toward the pterygopalatine fossa, which resembles the letter "V" on a lateral fluoroscopic image. Once the needle tip is in the fossa, ½ mL of nonionic, water-soluble contrast in introduced, which should fill the contours of the fossa. Care should be taken not to introduce too much contrast because it is common for the needle not to be in position on the first attempt. Too much contrast may obscure the area and require the procedure to be rescheduled. When advancing the needle, frequent checks of anteroposterior (AP) and lateral views should be taken to make sure the needle is advancing correctly in all planes.[8] On an AP image, the tip of the needle should be at the level of the middle turbinate. It is not uncommon to take 5 or 10 minutes to carefully place this needle. Care must also be taken not to advance too far and breach the nasal mucosa. The cartilaginous and bony structures bordering the nasal cavity from this approach are thin and fragile. A breach in this area can lead to the introduction of bacteria into an otherwise sterile area that has indirect communication with the cranial cavity. Contrast injection in the nasal nares on AP view confirms breach of the nasal mucosa. The treatment for this complication is prophylactic antibiotics and education of the patient to watch for fevers, visual disturbances, headaches, and dizziness.

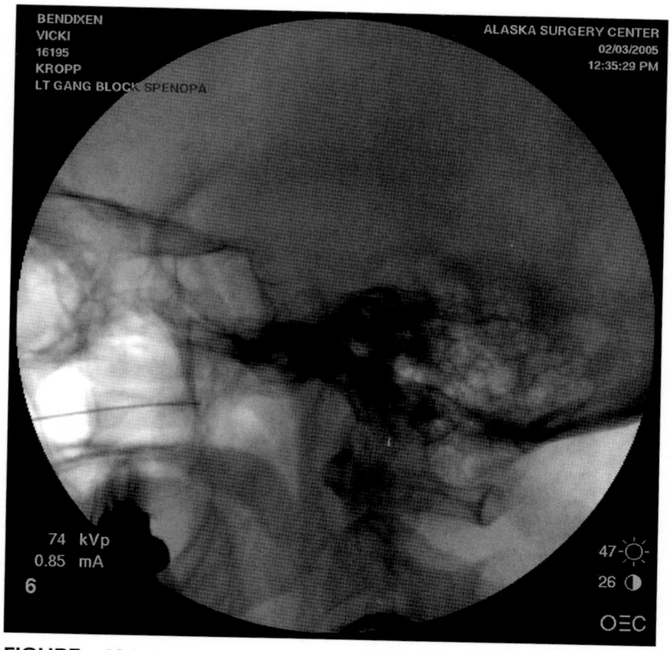

FIGURE 134–2 ■ Fluoroscopic view showing an infrazygomatic approach with the needle located in the inferior aspect of the pterygopalatine fossa.

Once in position, as shown in Figure 134–2, the aspirates are checked for CSF, blood, and air, and then an anesthetic solution is injected containing 2 mL of local anesthetic and 1 mL of 4 mg/mL dexamethasone. The particulate steroids such as triamcinolone and Celestone can also be used, but are more problematic if injected into the internal maxillary artery and can cause infarction. Dexamethasone has minimal mineralocorticoid activity, and it is nonparticulate.

After the block, the area is inspected for hematoma formation. The facial artery sends a branch near the mandibular notch that may be transected during needle placement. This will usually stop bleeding with constant pressure for 5 minutes.

Radiofrequency Ablation

If the transnasal and lateral needle blocks are successful, radiofrequency ablation (RFA) can be considered to prolong the relief. This technique is really better termed a *neuromodulation* instead of an ablation, although the other fibers of the nerve and the myelin in this area are affected. Several theories exist as to the mechanism of RFA and why it works. Authors have proposed theories from up-regulation of the *C-FOS* gene, which has been shown to play an important role in pain transmission mechanisms[9] to direct fenestration of myelin creating a disorganized conduction.[10] There are several books on this subject that cover this in greater detail.[11,12] The needle is positioned in exactly the same method as described earlier, but this blunt Coudé needle is a 10-mm active tip RF needle. Sensory stimulator is performed at 50 Hz with a 20 ms pulse width and a voltage between 0.1 and 1.0 V. The patient will feel a paresthesia at the root of the nose (i.e., where the nose joins the face) when the SPG is being stimulated. Stimulation sensed in the hard palate (palatine nerves) or in the upper teeth (maxillary nerve) requires redirection of the needle. Reproduction of the painful symptoms or at least radiation of the sensory stimulation into the area that is usually painful is optimal. The author has watched practitioners take 60 minutes to attempt to get a perfect stimulation pattern; this increases the chance of injury to surrounding structures and infection. If the fluoroscope shows the needle in good position on AP and lateral views and the diagnostic blocks are positive, sensory stimulation patterns should be attempted but should give way to common sense if not exactly reproductive of the patient's usual pain. Motor stimulation should then be performed using a 2-Hz cycle and a voltage between 0.1 and 2.0 V. Motor stimulation can produce a broad distribution of symptoms. Sensations can be felt in the superior alveolar ridge, the buccal surface of the cheek, or in the lateral face. Any of these patterns are good indicators of position. Twitching of the paranasal skin usually indicates stimulation of the maxillary nerve. If this happens, the needle is in the fossa, but a slightly more inferior position will more accurately target the SPG itself. Once in position, RF lesions can be delivered at 80°C for 90 seconds. It is generally accepted practice to deliver no more than two lesions at a specific location.[11]

Pulsed Radiofrequency Ablation

Pulsed lesions differ from continuous mode RF in that the energy is pulsed in a 20-ms scale square wave pulse. This method of delivering energy accomplishes several goals. The temperature of the lesion is now only 42° C, whereas with a continuous RF, the temperature is allowed to rise to 80° C. Because of the lower temperature, longer treatment times up to 120 seconds repeated three times have been found to be safe and provide significant relief. The theory is to expose the nerve to the electrical and magnetic fields and minimize the effects of the thermal fields. Thermal fields reach further into tissues and expose nontargeted neural tissues to potentially damaging heat. This technique also nearly eliminates the very common phenomeon of post-radiofrequency neuritis, which in the face can be significant. Thermal fields reach further into tissues and expose nontargeted neural tissues to potentially damaging heat. The authors feel that a pulsed RF ablation should be chosen in favor of full temperature RF at least initially to gauge the patient's response. There are several justifications for this. It is true the full temperature RF will more deeply treat the SPG, but it will also introduce more injury to motor nerves in this area. The SPG hangs from the vidian nerve, which if injured can cause vasodilatation, hypersecretion, and chronic sneezing through deregulation of the parasympathetic system.[13] Pulsed lesioning makes this complication much more remote. Sluijter also believes that the pulsed lesion is more directed out the tip of the needle and has a narrower cone of energy than that created by a high-temperature RF.[12]

Recovery includes postoperative monitoring and close inspection for hematoma near the needle entry site. As mentioned earlier, medications delivered into this area can track back along the nerves into the cranial cavity. Signs of tinnitus, dizziness, perioral numbness, or visual disturbances are early signs of local anesthetic toxicity. If these occur, increase the monitoring time to 90 minutes and make sure these symptoms are resolved before the patient is discharged or removed from monitoring.

COMPLICATIONS AND PITFALLS

The most serious complication is intravascular injection that tracks back through the maxillary artery into the brain. This can result in a very quick loss of consciousness and cessation of respirations. The treatment for this is to intubate the patient, place all necessary monitors, and monitor cardiovascular parameters. If seizures ensue, the patient should be intubated and abortive therapy initiated using benzodiazepines, propofol or nondepolarizing paralytics if indicated. The patient can be extubated usually within 1 hour, but should be admitted for 24 hours for observation and laboratory testing carried out the morning of discharge to make sure that liver function and renal function are within normal limits.

There are case reports of oculocardiac reflexes occurring as well. This reflex can cause profound bradycardia that needs medical intervention. Glycopyrrolate can reverse mild bradycardia but atropine is more definitive. The proposed mechanism is medication tracking back through the SPG, through V2 to the dorsal vagal nucleus. Alternate pathways proposed include medication tracking back along the vidian nerve to the geniculate ganglion and nervus intermedius to reach the solitary tract nucleus that connects to the dorsal vagal nucleus.[14]

Perforation of the nasal mucosa is a real consideration. This happens most often with the infrazygomatic technique but can happen with infranasal approaches. The concern here is introducing an infection into the SPG that can track back into the brain. Any suspicion of this complication should warrant prophylactic oral antibiotics and one dose of intravenous antibiotics while the patient is still at the procedure center. Contrast injection into the nasal nares, or drainage of liquid from the nasal cavity at the moment of injection are both presumed to prove breach of the nasal mucosa.

RESULTS

As the field of pain medicine grows, third-party payers and other skeptics have increased efforts to decrease reimbursements for these techniques. The authors receive frequent requests from insurers for double-blind, controlled studies, which cannot be performed because it is unethical to give placebo to a patient in pain, and anyone who has ever had to appear before an internal review board will confirm that the first concern is that no patient will suffer because of a scientific study. That provision is a primary directive of all review boards. It is for this reason that only rare trials in the field of pain medicine use a double-blind control. The field is largely limited to case and cohort studies and will likely remain so. In the authors' experience, the efficacy of SPG block for facial pain is about 50%, and the efficacy in cluster headaches is about the same. Several studies quantify these results more scientifically.

Sanders and colleagues[15] followed 66 patients in a 12- to 70-month study and report that complete relief was achieved in 34% of patients. In that study, 34% of patients never experienced the return of pain and they were cured for all practical purposes. This number may appear low, but it is actually quite high when one considers that this condition had a 0% cure rate using medications alone. Despite the small number of patients in the study, it is one of the largest to date. Cepero and associates[16] found that in 12 patients—if the pain returned, it was much more responsive to medications after the blocks.

CONCLUSION

When performed properly and in appropriately selected patients, the sphenopalatine block can be an effective treatment modality for facial pain and cluster and other headaches.

References

1. Sluder G: The role of sphenopalatine ganglion in nasal headaches. New York Med J 87:989, 1908.
2. Sluder G: Etiology, diagnosis, prognosis and the treatment of sphenopalatine ganglion neuralgia. JAMA 61:1201, 1913.
3. Waldman SD: Sphenopalatine ganglion block—80 years later. Reg Anesth 18:274, 1993.
4. Barash PG, Cullen BF, Stoelting RK (eds): Clinical Anesthesia, 4th ed. Philadelphia, Lippincott Williams & Wilkins, 1999.
5. Byrd H, Byrd W: Sphenopalatine phenomena: Present status of knowledge. Arch Intern Med 46:1026, 1930.
6. Pulec J: Geniculate neuralgia: Long-term results of surgical treatment. Ear Nose Throat J 81:30, 2002.
7. Ruskin S: Techniques of sphenopalatine therapy. Eye Nose Throat Monthly 30:28, 1951.
8. Day M: Sphenopalatine ganglion analgesia. Curr Rev Pain 3:342, 1999.
9. Higuchi Y: Exposure of the dorsal root ganglion in rats to pulsed radiofrequency currents activates dorsal horn lamina I and II neurons. Neurosurgery 50:850, 2002.
10. Van Zundert J, de Lame L, Louw A, et al: Percutaneous pulsed radiofrequency treatment of the cervical dorsal root ganglion in the treatment of chronic cervical pain syndromes: A clinical audit. Neuromodulation 6:6, 2003.
11. Sluijter M: Radiofrequency: Part 1. Meggen, Switzerland, FlivoPress, 2001.
12. Sluijter M: Radiofrequency: Part 2. Meggen, Switzerland, FlivoPress, 2001.
13. Kirtane M, Rajaram D, Merchant S: Transnasal approach to the vidian nerve: Anatomical considerations. J Postgrad Med 30:210, 1984.
14. Konen A: Unexpected effects due to radiofrequency thermocoagulation of the sphenopalatine ganglion: Two case reports. Pain Digest 10:30, 2000.
15. Sanders M, Zuurmond W: Efficacy of sphenopalatine ganglion blockade in 66 patients suffering from cluster headache: A 12- to 70-month follow-up evaluation. J Neursurg 87:876, 1997.
16. Cepero R, Miller R, Bressler K: Long-term results of sphenopalatine ganglioneurectomy for facial pain. J Otolaryngol 170, 1987.

chapter 135

Greater and Lesser Occipital Nerve Block

David L. Brown and Gilbert Y. Wong

HISTORICAL CONSIDERATIONS

Occipital nerve block is most often used to diagnose or treat occipital pain. There are many causes of occipital pain, and they are frequently grouped as *occipital neuralgia.* This categorization was first used in 1821, when Beruto y Lentijo and Ramos made reference to an occipital neuralgic syndrome.[1] Early in this century, Luff[2] and Osler and McRae[3] reemphasized the importance of attempting to identify the causes of occipital pain. Other investigators suggested that, in addition to the neuropathic changes that lead to occipital headaches, the pain characteristic of occipital neuralgia may also be related to arthritis of the cervical spine (cervicogenic headache) and other rare but serious conditions (Table 135–1).[4-8] After the development of safe injectable local anesthetics, occipital nerve block was commonly used in the diagnosis and treatment of pain originating in the occipital region. Occipital nerve block also provides scalp anesthesia for surgical procedures when local infiltration techniques alone do not suffice.

INDICATIONS AND CONTRAINDICATIONS

Occipital nerve block is most often used to diagnose and treat pain in the occipital region. When it is used for diagnosis, a careful history and thorough physical examination are necessary to minimize the chance that serious causes of occipital pain will be missed or diagnosis delayed (see Table 135–1). By International Headache Society definition, occipital neuralgia is relieved by local anesthetic blockade of the involved occipital nerve; thus, the principal indication for occipital block is diagnosis.[9] Another indication is the treatment of chronic occipital neuralgia, often with a series of therapeutic blocks combining local anesthetic and depot corticosteroid. Because of the preservatives included in depot corticosteroid preparations, it is suggested that a minor degree of neurolysis may result and contribute to prolonging pain relief.[10]

If occipital nerve block is used to differentiate occipital neuralgia from pain of other causes, one must remember that potential interneuronal connections within the upper spinal cord may allow occipital nerve (C2) pain to be referred to the trigeminal distribution (Fig. 135–1).[11] This referred pain is due to the proximity of the C2 root to the trigeminal spinal nucleus. Thus, block of the occipital nerve may relieve pain outside the typical C2 distribution but within the trigeminal distribution.[12]

CLINICALLY RELEVANT ANATOMY

The cutaneous innervation of the posterior head and neck comes from the cervical spinal nerves. The dorsal rami of C2 end in the greater occipital nerve, which provides cutaneous innervation to the major portion of the posterior scalp (Fig. 135–2). Based on cadaver studies, the topographic anatomy of the occipital nerve can vary.[13] After following a winding course as the medial branch of the dorsal ramus of C2, the greater occipital nerve ascends in the posterior neck from its origin lateral to the lateral atlantoaxial joint and deep to the oblique inferior muscle. At this point, a communicating branch from C3 may join the greater occipital nerve (Fig 135–3).[14,15] The greater occipital nerve ascends in the posterior neck over the dorsal surface of the rectus capitis posterior major muscle, and, approximately at the midpoint of this muscle, the greater occipital nerve turns dorsally to pierce the fleshy fibers of the semispinalis capitis, after which it runs a short distance rostrolaterally, lying deep to the trapezius. The nerve becomes subcutaneous slightly inferior to the superior nuchal line, not by piercing the trapezius, as is often suggested, but by passing above an aponeurotic sling. This sling is composed of a blending of the aponeurotic insertions of the trapezius and sternocleidomastoid muscles medially and laterally, respectively.[15]

As the occipital nerve emerges via this aponeurotic sling, it is close to the occipital artery. At this point, the greater occipital nerve is immediately medial to the occipital artery, and the artery is lateral to the inion (Fig. 135–4A). Again, the ventral rami of C2 through C4 provide the majority of cutaneous innervation to the anterior and lateral portions of the neck, with C2 providing innervation to the scalp through both the lesser occipital and posterior auricular nerves (see Fig. 135–2).

Table 135–1

Possible Causes of Occipital Pain Syndrome

Relatively Common	***Relatively Rare***
Headache	Arnold-Chiari malformation
Tension	Tumor
Vascular	Primary
Cervicogenic	Secondary
Occipital neuralgia	Infection
Cervical arthritis	Mastoid
Myofascial pain	Intraspinal

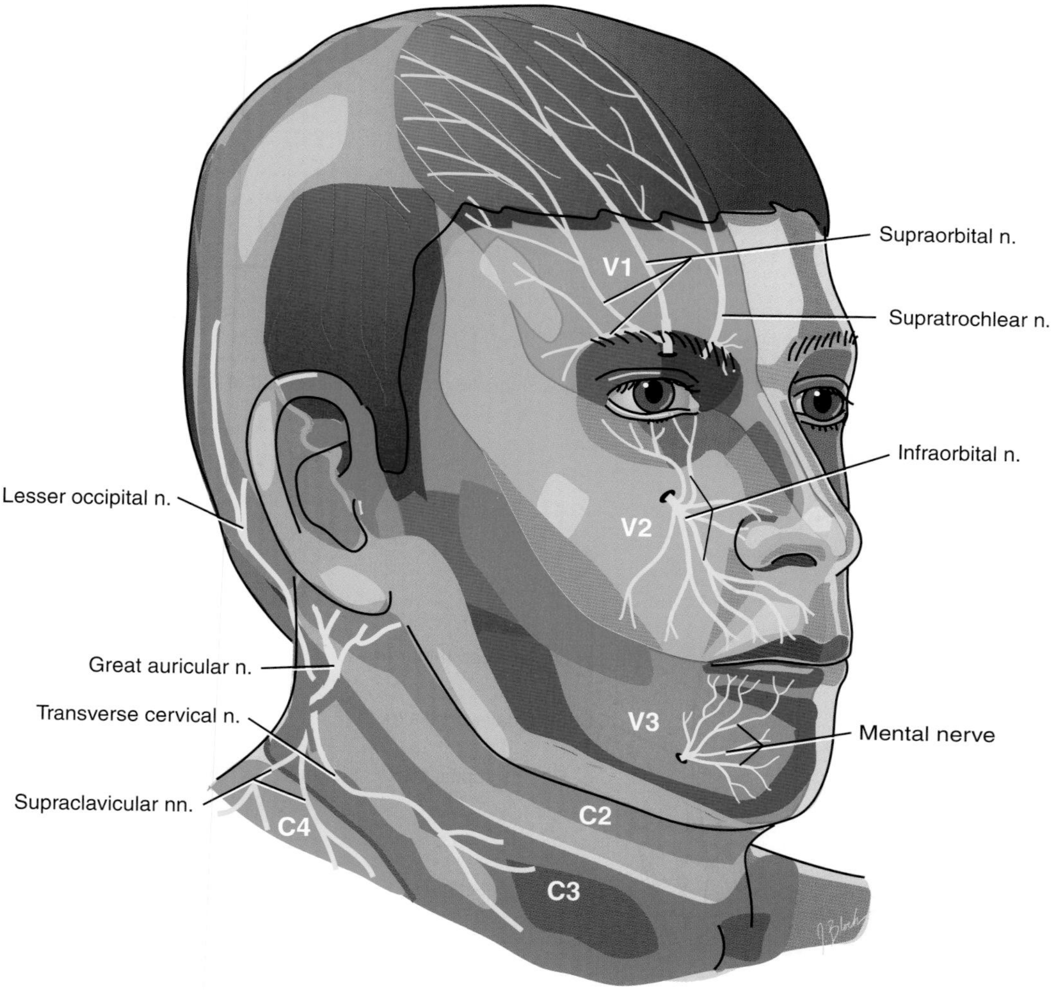

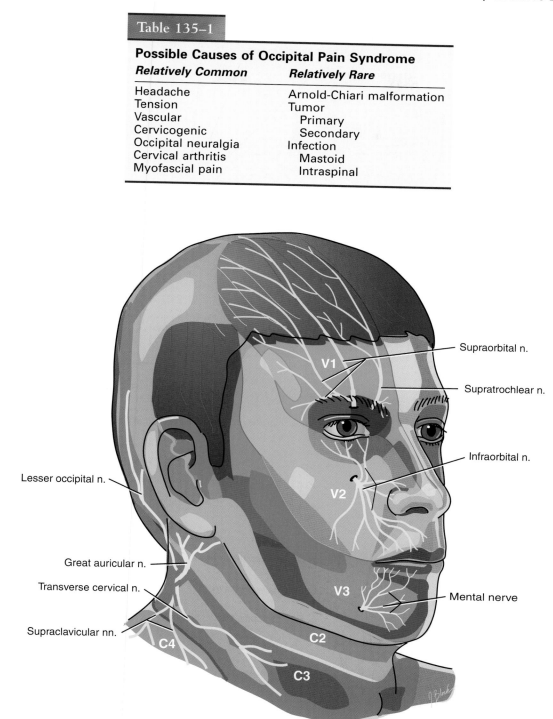

FIGURE 135–1 ■ The cervico-trigeminal interneuronal relay. A potential overlap of central neuronal connections occurs between the spinal nucleus of the trigeminal nerve and the upper cervical cord neurons. The trigeminal nucleus develops from the pyramidal decussation and descends to the level of C2, and perhaps as far caudad as C4, as the nucleus caudalis, which principally subserves pain and temperature information to the head and neck. This trigeminal nucleus is associated, both morphologically and functionally, with the upper cervical segments, and its cells form a column continuous with the column of cells forming the posterior horn in the cervical cord.

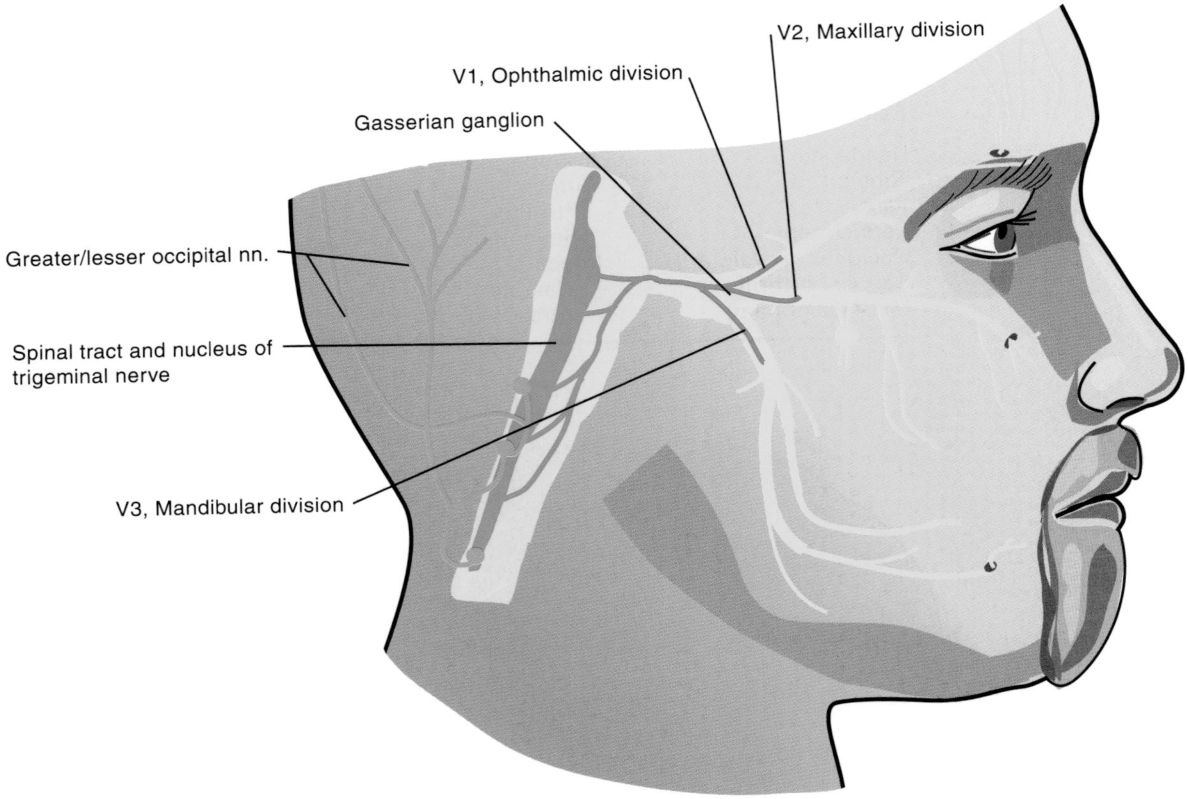

FIGURE 135–2 ■ Peripheral sensory and dermatomal innervation of greater and lesser occipital nerves and of other head and neck nerves.

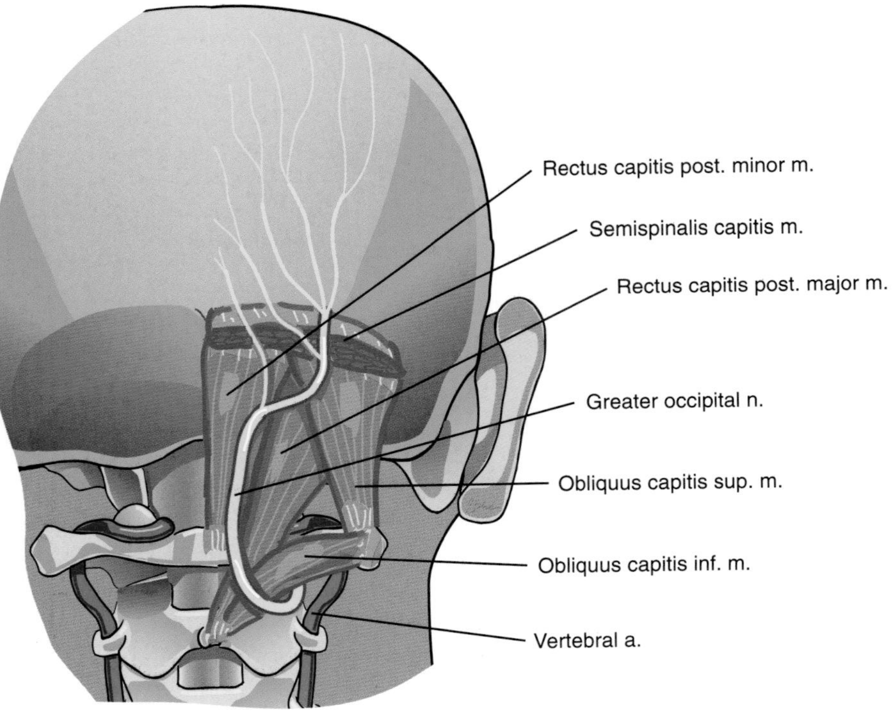

FIGURE 135–3 ■ Anatomic schematic of the greater occipital nerve in the neutral position as it arises from the medial branch of the dorsal ramus of the second cervical nerve, on its way to its eventual subcutaneous position, lateral to the inion (external occipital protuberance).

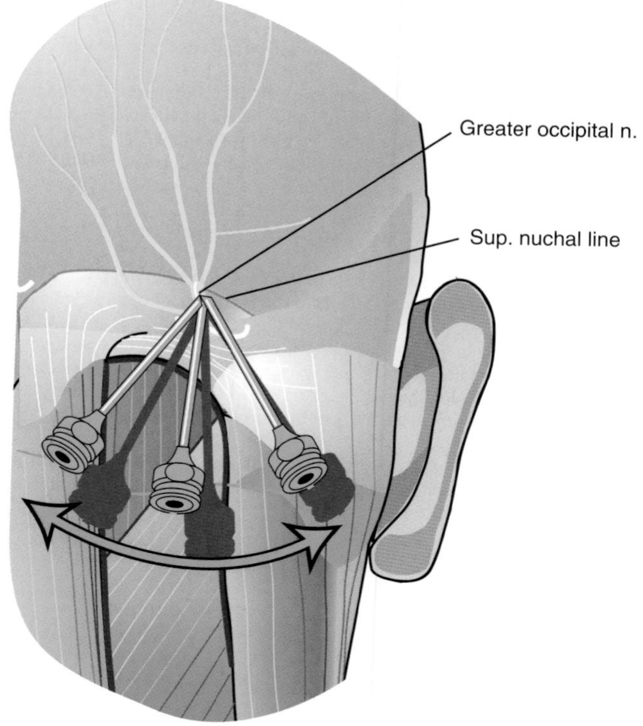

FIGURE 135–4 ■ Posterior view of the course of the greater occipital nerve and artery as they course cephalad in the neck, via the aponeurotic sling on their way to the posterior scalp. Note the "wall" of local anesthetic (*curved arrow*) developed in a mediolateral sequence to ensure adequate block of the greater occipital nerve.

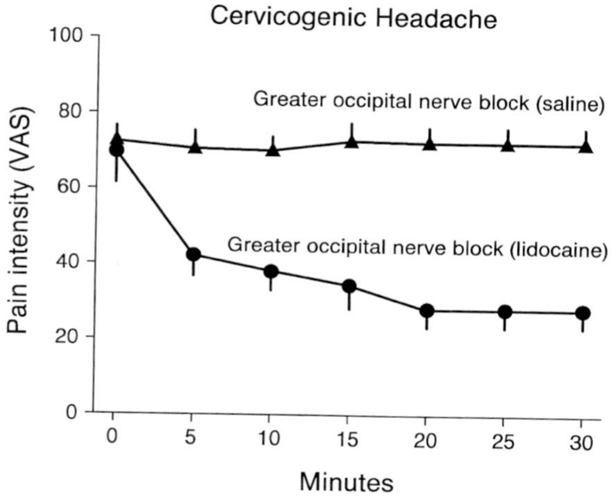

FIGURE 135–5 ■ Pain relief measured by visual analog scale (VAS) in patients with cervicogenic headache when 1.5 to 2.0 mL of saline or lidocaine was used during greater occipital nerve block. Measurements of pain intensity (pi) were made every 5 minutes for 70 minutes. There were no major changes from 30 to 70 minutes. The bars indicate standard error of the mean (SEM). *P* <pi>l1.05 from the 5th minute onward. (Modified from Bovim G, Sand T: Cervicogenic headache, migraine without aura and tension-type headache: Diagnostic blockade of greater occipital and supraorbital nerves. Pain 51:43, 1992. Copyright 1992, with permission from Elsevier Science.)

■ CLINICAL PEARLS AND TRICKS OF THE TRADE

The most effective patient position for the greater or lesser occipital block is sitting with the neck in a flexed position. The selection of the nerve(s) to be blocked may depend, in part, on the pain distribution and the ability to reproduce the pain with palpation. The occipital artery is the most useful landmark for locating the greater occipital nerve, which lies immediately medial to the artery. A short (1- to 1.5-inch), 25-gauge needle is inserted through the skin at the level of the superior nuchal line. The artery is commonly found at a point approximately one third of the distance from the external occipital protuberance to the mastoid process on the superior nuchal line. The lesser occipital nerve is commonly found at a point two thirds of the distance from the external occipital protuberance on the superior nuchal line. Injection of 3 to 5 mL of local anesthetic produces satisfactory greater or lesser occipital nerve anesthesia in the corresponding area. If a diagnostic block is planned, the dose should be limited to 1 to 2 mL to minimize confusion with relief of myofascial pain when larger volumes are injected (see Fig. 135–4B). Bovim and Sand[16] reported that greater occipital nerve block reduced pain in 19 of 135 patients with cervicogenic headache (Fig. 135–5). Cervical epidural nerve block with local anesthetic and corticosteroid could be considered for cervicogenic headache that is refractory to occipital nerve block.

■ PITFALLS

When a diagnostic block is planned, it is important to keep the dose of local anesthetic small to avoid confounding results with relief of myofascial pain. Likewise, relief of ipsilateral retro-orbital or temporal pain does not rule out occipital neuralgia as the cause of an occipital pain syndrome because pain relief is produced outside the "typical" sensory distribution of the occipital nerve.[12] Because of the brain stem and spinal cord interneuronal connections between the trigeminal nucleus and C2, it is common to find retro-orbital pain relieved by greater occipital nerve block.[12] Failure to obtain successful occipital nerve block can be due to an anatomic variation. Patients whose occipital pain is complicated by confounding economic variables, especially those who have sustained flexion-extension neck injuries in motor vehicle accidents and are involved in litigation for compensation, are difficult for us to manage until the confounding economic variables are resolved or removed.

■ COMPLICATIONS

The superficial location of this block should make complications uncommon. In spite of the close relation between the occipital artery and nerve, intravascular injection is uncommon. The small volume of local anesthetic and corticosteroid injected makes systemic toxicity a rare event. Some patients who have undergone posterior suboccipital cranial surgery are referred for evaluation of an occipital pain syndrome. One needs to be cautious about the occipital nerve block in such patients because subcranial injections producing total spinal anesthesia have been reported.

FUTURE DIRECTIONS

The development of long-acting local anesthetics may allow prolonged relief of occipital neuralgia. Depot formulations of local anesthetics may, indeed, be more useful than intermittent blocks. Nevertheless, proof of such a theory needs further study.

References

1. Perelson HN: Occipital nerve tenderness: A sign of headache. South Med J 40:653, 1947.
2. Luff AP: The various forms of fibrositis and their treatment. Br Med J 1:756, 1913.
3. Osler W, McRae T: The Principles and Practice of Medicine, 10th ed. New York, Appleton, 1925, p 1117.
4. Horton BT, Macy D, Jr: Treatment of headache. Med Clin North Am 30:811, 1946.
5. Nielsen JM: Textbook of Clinical Neurology. New York, Paul B. Hoeber, 1941, p 509.
6. Pollock LJ: Head pain: Differential diagnosis and treatment. Med Clin North Am 25:3, 1941.
7. Echni G, Benner B: Occipital neuralgia and the C1-2 arthrosis syndrome. J Neurosurg 61:961, 1984.
8. Sjaastad O, Federiksen JA, Pfaffenrath V: Cervicogenic headache: Diagnostic criteria. Headache 30:725, 1990.
9. Headache Classification Committee of the International Headache Society: Classification and diagnostic criteria for headache disorders, cranial neuralgias and facial pain. Cephalgia 9(Suppl 7):1, 1988.
10. Selby R: Complications of Depo-Medrol. Surg Neurol 19:393, 1983.
11. Kerr FWL: A mechanism to account for frontal headache in cases of posterior fossa tumour. J Neurosurg 18:605, 1961.
12. Anthony M: Headache and the greater occipital nerve. Clin Neurol Neurosurg 94:297, 1992.
13. Becser N, Bovim G, Sjaastad O: Extramural nerves in the posterior part of the head. Anatomic variations and their possible clinical significance. Spine 23(13):1435, 1998.
14. Vital JM, Grenier F, Dautheribes M, et al: An anatomic and dynamic study of the greater occipital nerve (n. of Arnold): Applications to the treatment of Arnold's neuralgia. Surg Radiol Anat 11:205, 1989.
15. Bogduk N: The clinical anatomy of the cervical dorsal rami. Spine 4:319, 1982.
16. Bovim G, Sand T: Cervicogenic headache, migraine without aura and tension-type headache: Diagnostic blockade of greater occipital and supra-orbital nerves. Pain 51:43, 1992.

chapter 136

Gasserian Ganglion Block

Steven D. Waldman

HISTORICAL CONSIDERATIONS

On December 6, 1884, Halsted and Hall reported their success in blocking the branches of the trigeminal nerve with local anesthetic in the *New York Medical Journal.*[1] Shortly after this landmark publication, these distinguished New York surgeons showed the utility of "nerve blocks" when Hall had Halsted remove a lipoma from his forehead under "painless" nerve block anesthesia.[2] One can only imagine the tremendous benefit that this clinical discovery afforded surgeons and their patients at a time when, in the absence of endotracheal intubation, muscle relaxants, and sophisticated monitoring, head and neck surgery was, at best, an extremely risky undertaking.

The effectiveness of nerve blocks was rapidly exploited for pain management. Blockade of the gasserian ganglion and distal trigeminal nerve were among the first applications of nerve blocking for pain. By 1900, blockade of these neural structures was considered one of the primary means of alleviating the pain of trigeminal neuralgia and pain secondary to cancers of the face and head.[3] These techniques remained the mainstays of the nonsurgical treatment of trigeminal neuralgia until the introduction of carbamazepine in 1960.

The shift to the managed care paradigm has led pain management specialists to seek the most efficacious, safe, and cost-effective treatments for headache and facial pain.[4,5] This paradigm shift has led to renewed interest in gasserian ganglion block for the management of a variety of painful conditions. This chapter reviews the current indications, contraindications, and technique for blockade of the gasserian ganglion.

INDICATIONS AND CONTRAINDICATIONS

Blockade of the gasserian ganglion with local anesthetics and steroids and destruction of this neural structure by freezing, radiofrequency lesioning, neurolytic agents, compression, and other means have many applications in contemporary pain management.[6] Advances in radiographic imaging, electronics, and needle technology have improved the efficacy and reduced the cost, complications, and adverse side effects of these useful pain management procedures.

Indications for gasserian ganglion block are summarized in Table 136–1. In addition to applications for surgical anesthesia, gasserian ganglion block with local anesthetics can be used as a diagnostic tool when performing differential neural blockade on an anatomic basis for evaluation of head and facial pain.[7] This technique also is useful as a prognostic indicator of the degree of motor and sensory impairment that the patient might experience when destruction of the gasserian ganglion is being considered.[3] Gasserian ganglion block with local anesthetic may be used to palliate acute pain emergencies, including trigeminal neuralgia and cancer pain, while waiting for pharmacologic, surgical, and antiblastic methods to become effective.[8]

Destruction of the gasserian ganglion is indicated for palliation of cancer pain, including the pain of invasive tumors of the orbit, maxillary sinus, and mandible.[9] This technique also is useful in the management of the pain of trigeminal neuralgia that has been refractory to medical management or for patients who are not candidates for surgical microvascular decompression.[10] Gasserian ganglion destruction also has been used successfully in the management of intractable cluster headache and in the palliation of ocular pain secondary to persistent glaucoma.[3,11,12]

Contraindications to blockade of the gasserian ganglion are as follows:

- Local infection
- Sepsis
- Coagulopathy
- Significantly increased intracranial pressure
- Disulfiram therapy (if alcohol is used)
- Significant behavioral abnormalities

Local infection and sepsis are absolute contraindications to gasserian ganglion block.[13] Coagulopathy and markedly increased intracranial pressure are strong contraindications. Owing to the desperation of many patients with aggressively invasive head and face malignancies, however, ethical and humanitarian considerations dictate use of this procedure despite the increased risks of bleeding or CSF leak secondary to coagulopathy or increased intracranial pressure.

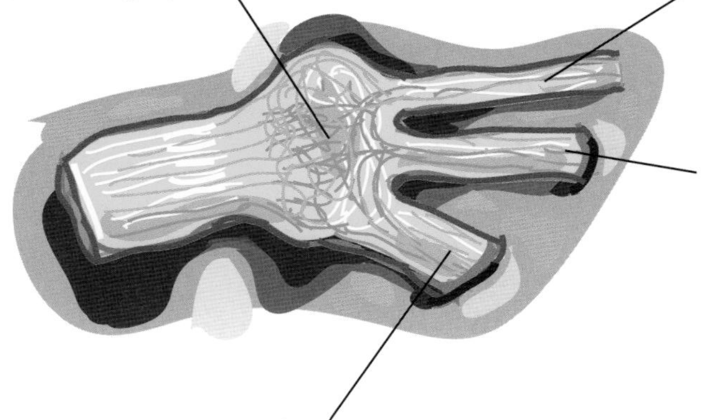

FIGURE 136–1 ■ Gasserian ganglion and Meckel's cave.

Table 136-1

Indications for Gasserian Ganglion Block

Local Anesthetic Block	*Neurolytic Block or Neurodestructive Procedure*
Surgical anesthesia	Palliation of cancer pain
Anatomic differential neural blockade	Management of trigeminal neuralgia
Prognostic nerve block before neurodestructive procedures	Management of cluster headache
Palliation in acute pain emergencies	Management of intractable ocular pain

CLINICALLY RELEVANT ANATOMY

Role of the Trigeminal System

The trigeminal nerve is the largest and the most complex of the cranial nerves, containing sensory and motor fibers.[14] Somatic afferent impulses carried by the trigeminal nerve transmit pain, light touch, and temperature sensation. Information is transmitted to the central nervous system via the trigeminal nerve from the skin of the face, the mucosal lining of the nose and mouth, the teeth, and the anterior two thirds of the tongue.[15] The trigeminal nerve also carries proprioceptive impulses and afferent impulses from stretch receptors of the teeth, oral mucosa, muscles of mastication, and temporomandibular joint to aid in mastication.

In addition to the sensory innervation just described, visceral efferent fibers help to innervate a variety of muscles of facial expression, the tensor tympani, and some muscles of mastication. Communications exist between the trigeminal nerve and the autonomic nervous system, including the ciliary, sphenopalatine, otic, and submaxillary ganglia and the oculomotor, facial, and glossopharyngeal nerves. Because of the complex structure of the trigeminal nerve, a thorough understanding of the clinically relevant anatomy is crucial to obtaining optimal results with neural blockade.

Gasserian Ganglion

The gasserian ganglion is formed from two roots that exit the ventral surface of the brain stem at the midpontine level (Fig. 136–1).[16] These roots pass forward and lateral in the posterior cranial fossa across the border of the petrous temporal bone. They enter a recess called *Meckel's cave,* which is formed by an invagination of the surrounding dura mater into the middle cranial fossa. The dural pouch that lies just behind the ganglion, called the *trigeminal cistern,* contains CSF. The gasserian ganglion is canoe-shaped and has three sensory divisions, the ophthalmic (V_1), maxillary (V_2), and mandibular (V_3) nerves, which exit on the anterior convex aspect. A smaller motor root joins the mandibular division as it exits the cranial cavity via the foramen ovale.

Ophthalmic Division

The ophthalmic branch, the smallest division of the trigeminal nerve, is purely sensory in function (Fig. 136–2).[17] It enters the orbit via the superior orbital fissure. The branch is divided into the frontal, nasociliary, and lacrimal nerves. The terminal cutaneous branches of the frontal nerve consist of the supraorbital and supratrochlear nerves. These terminal branches exit the orbital cavity anteriorly and provide innervation to the upper eyelid, forehead, and anterior scalp. The terminal cutaneous branches of the nasociliary nerve consist of the infratrochlear and external nasal branches, which provide cutaneous and mucosal innervation to the apex and ala of the nose and anterior nasal cavity. The lacrimal nerve continues, without any additional major branches, to innervate the lacrimal gland and outer canthus of the eye.

Maxillary Division

The maxillary division is a pure sensory nerve. It exits the middle cranial fossa via the foramen rotundum and crosses the pterygopalatine fossa (Fig. 136–3).[17] Passing through the inferior orbital fissure, it enters the orbit, emerging on the face via the infraorbital foramen.

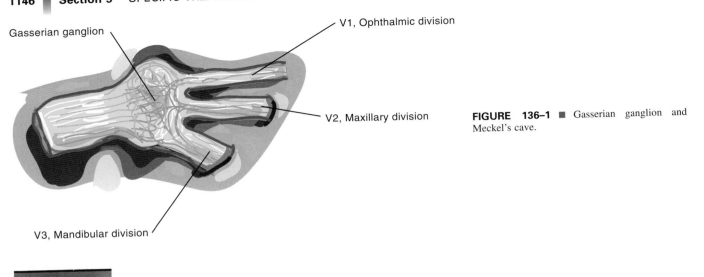

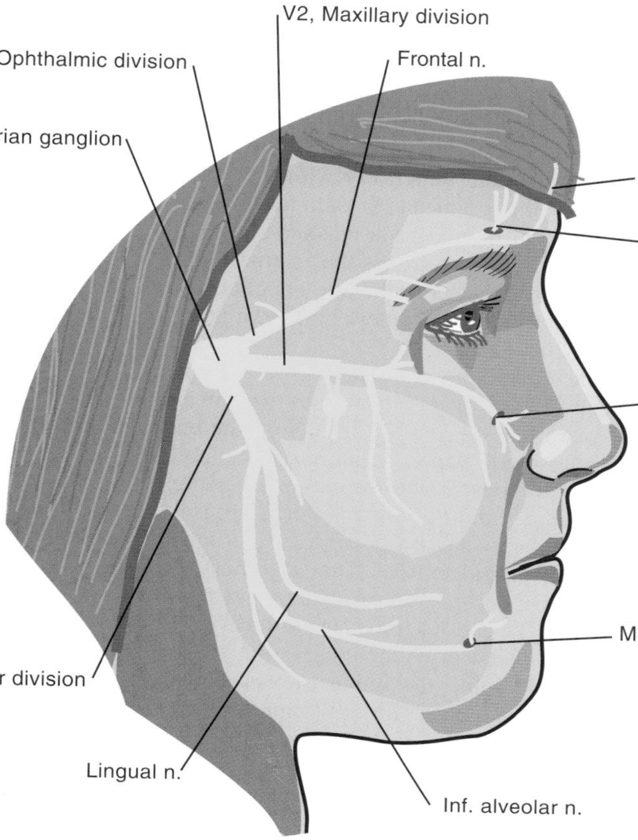

FIGURE 136–2 ■ Trigeminal nerve and its branches.

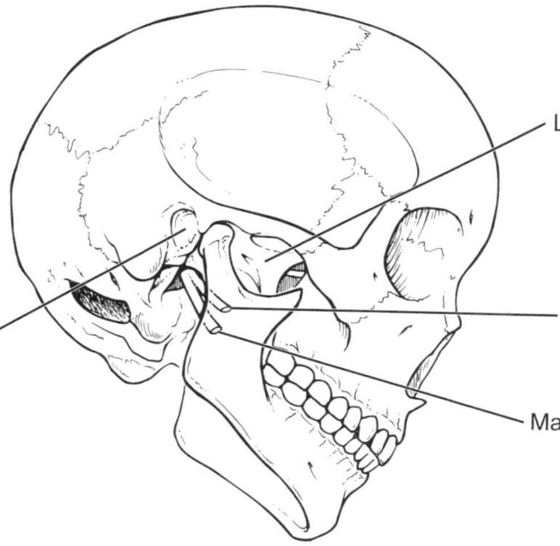

FIGURE 136–3 ■ Major branches of the trigeminal nerve.

The branches of the maxillary nerve are divided into four regional groups: (1) The intracranial group includes the middle meningeal nerve, which innervates the dura mater of the medial cranial fossa. (2) The pterygopalatine group includes the zygomatic nerve, which provides sensory innervation to the temporal and lateral zygomatic region, and the sphenopalatine branches, which help to innervate the mucosa of the maxillary sinus, upper gums, upper molars, and mucous membranes of the cheek. (3) The infraorbital canal group comprises the anterior-superior alveolar branch, which innervates the incisors and canines, the anterior wall of the maxillary antrum, and the floor of the nasal cavity, and the middle superior branch, which supplies the premolars. (4) The infraorbital facial group consists of the inferior palpebral branch, which innervates the conjunctiva and skin of the lower eyelid; the external nasal branch, which supplies the side of the nose; and the superior labial branch, which supplies the skin of the upper lip and part of the oral mucosa (see Fig. 136–2).

Mandibular Division

The large sensory root and smaller motor root of the mandibular division leave the middle cranial fossa together via the foramen ovale.[17] They join to form the mandibular nerve (see Fig. 136–3). This combined trunk gives off two branches: (1) the nervus spinosus, which runs superiorly with the middle meningeal artery through the foramen spinosum to supply the dura mater and the mucosal lining of the mastoid sinus, and (2) the internal pterygoid, which supplies the internal pterygoid muscle and gives off branches to the otic ganglion. The mandibular nerve divides into a small anterior and a large posterior trunk (see Fig. 136–2).

Branches from the small anterior trunk are the buccinator nerve, which is purely sensory and innervates the skin and mucous membrane overlying the anterior portion of the buccinator muscle; the masseteric nerve, which provides motor innervation to the masseter muscle; the deep temporal nerves, which provide motor innervation to the temporalis muscle; and the external pterygoid nerve, which provides motor innervation to the external pterygoid muscle. The large posterior trunk comprises primarily sensory fibers, but a few motor fibers as well. Branches of the posterior trunk are (1) the auriculotemporal nerve, which provides innervation to skin anterior to the tragus and helix, the lining of the acoustic meatus, the tympanic membrane, the posterior temporomandibular joint, the parotid gland, and the skin of the temporal region; (2) the lingual nerve, which provides sensory innervation to the dorsum and lateral aspects of the anterior two thirds of the tongue and the lateral mucous membranes of the mouth and the sublingual gland; and (3) the inferior alveolar nerve, which provides sensory innervation to the lower teeth and mandible. The terminal branch of the inferior alveolar nerve is the mental nerve, which exits the mandible via the mental foramen and provides sensory innervation to the chin and to the skin and mucous membrane of the lower lip.

TECHNIQUE

The patient lies supine with the cervical spine extended over a rolled towel. Approximately 2.5 cm lateral to the corner of the mouth, the skin is carefully prepared with povidone-iodine solution, and sterile drapes are placed.[7] The skin and subcutaneous tissues are anesthetized with 1% lidocaine with epinephrine. A 13-cm 20-gauge Hinck needle is advanced through the anesthetized area, traveling perpendicular to the pupil of the eye (when the eye is in midposition) in a cephalad trajectory toward the auditory meatus (Fig. 136–4).[13] The needle is advanced until contact is made with the base of the skull (Fig. 136–5). The needle tip is withdrawn slightly and "walked" posteriorly into the foramen ovale (Fig. 136–6). Paresthesia of the mandibular nerve may occur as the needle enters the foramen ovale.[7]

After the foramen ovale is entered, the stylet of the Hinck needle is removed. The operator carefully aspirates for blood. Free flow of CSF is typical. Failure to observe free flow of CSF does not mean that the needle tip does not lie within the central nervous system close to the gasserian ganglion, but simply that the needle tip rests, not within the trigeminal cistern, but more anteriorly, within Meckel's cave.[13]

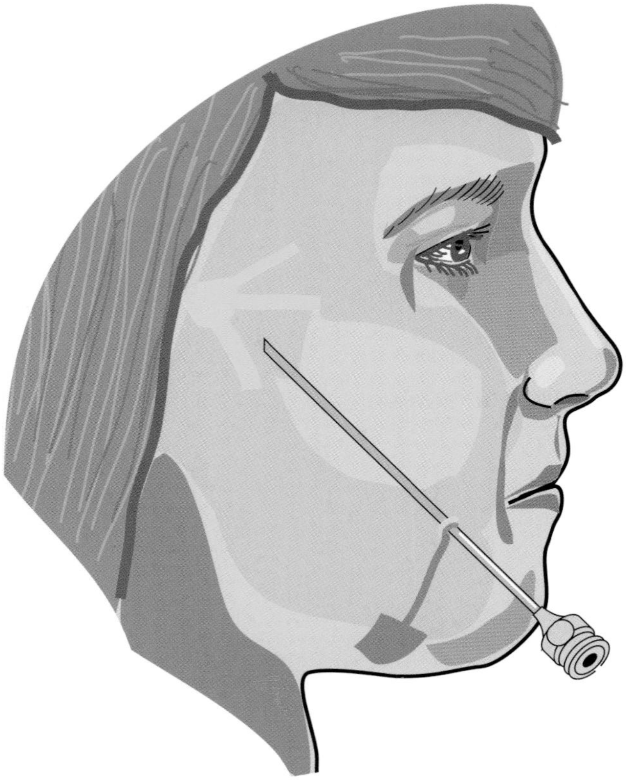

FIGURE 136–4 ■ Needle trajectory for gasserian ganglion block.

The needle position should be confirmed by radiography before any local anesthetic or neurolytic substance is injected (Figs. 136–7 and 136–8). After needle position is confirmed, 0.1-mL aliquots of a preservative-free local anesthetic, such as 1% lidocaine for diagnostic blocks and 0.5% bupivacaine for therapeutic blocks, or of sterile glycerol, 6.5% phenol in glycerin, or absolute alcohol may be injected.[7] An average volume of 0.4 mL of neurolytic solution is usually adequate to provide long-lasting pain relief. Owing to significant interpatient variability in the size of Meckel's cave, however, careful titration of the total injected volume is indicated.

If hyperbaric neurolytic agents are used, the patient should assume a sitting position with the chin on the chest before the injection, to ensure that the solution is placed primarily around the maxillary and mandibular divisions (Fig. 136–9) and avoids the ophthalmic division. The patient should remain in the supine position when absolute alcohol is used. This approach to the gasserian ganglion may be used to place radiofrequency needles, cryoprobes, and stimulating electrodes.

Practical Considerations

Because of the densely vascular nature of the pterygopalatine and its proximity to the middle meningeal artery, significant hematoma of the face and subscleral hematoma of the eye are common sequelae. The patient should be warned of the probability of these complications before institution of the block. Because the ganglion lies within the CSF, small amounts of

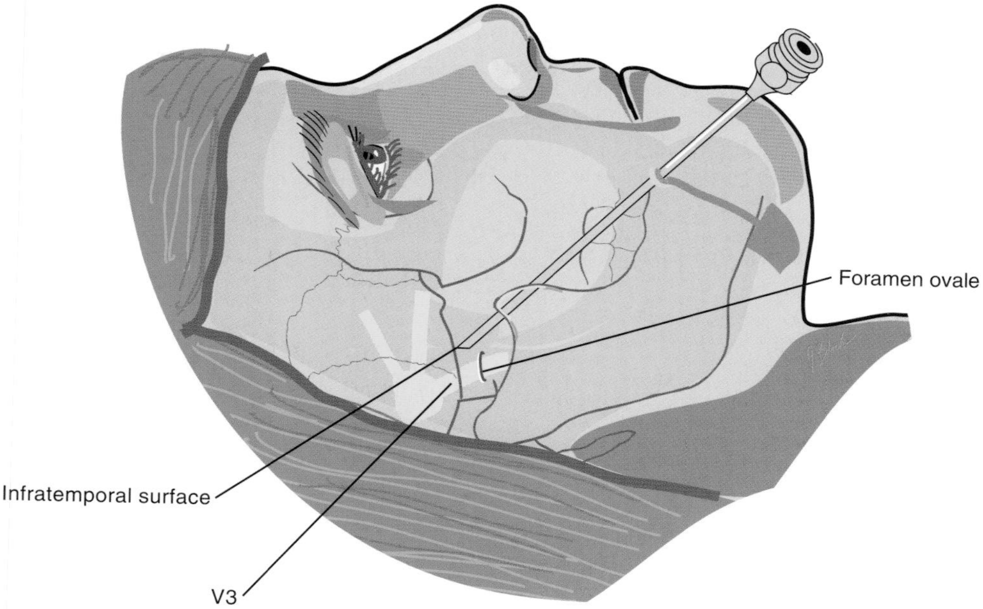

FIGURE 136–5 ■ Needle against roof of infratemporal surface.

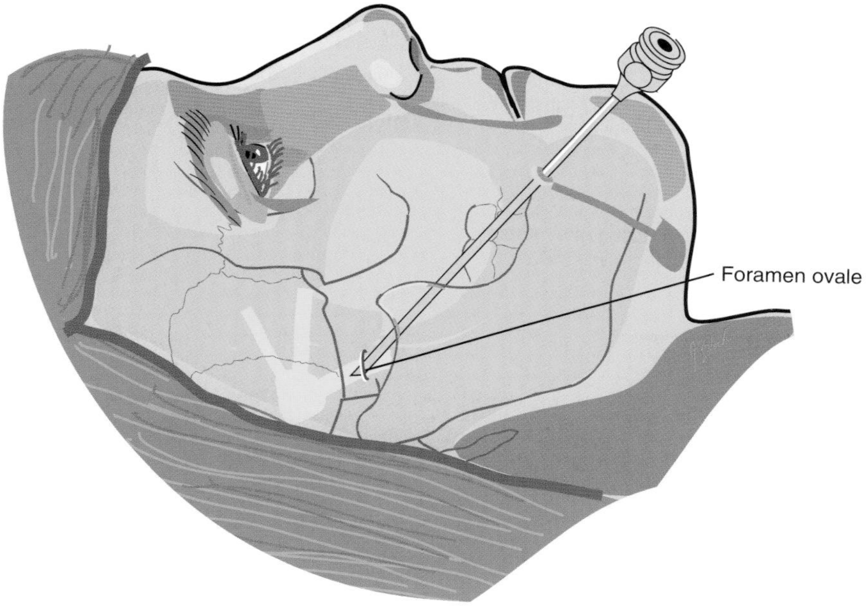

FIGURE 136–6 ■ Needle "walked" into foramen ovale.

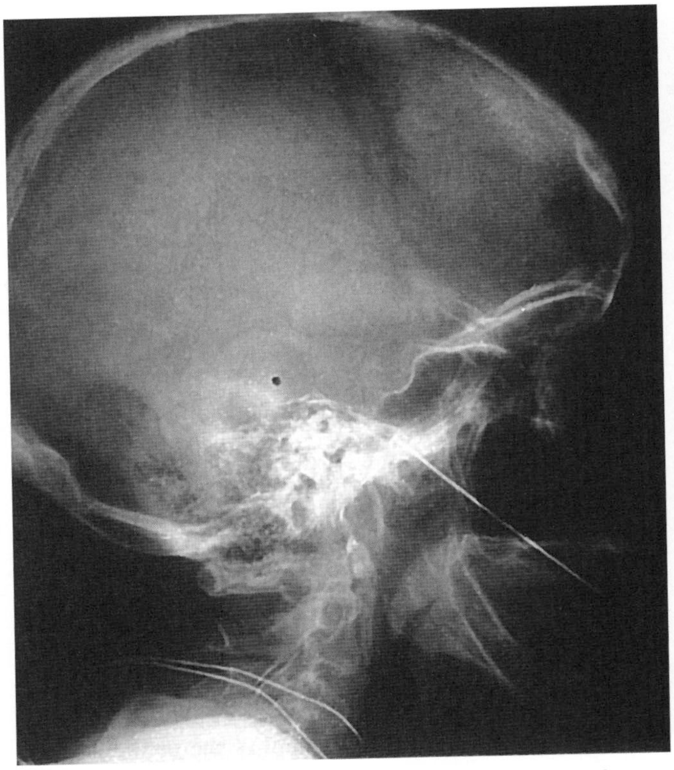

FIGURE 136–7 ■ Lateral view of the needle placed through the foramen ovale. (From Waldman SD: Gasserian ganglion block. In Interventional Pain Management, 2nd ed. Philadelphia, WB Saunders, 2001, p 320.)

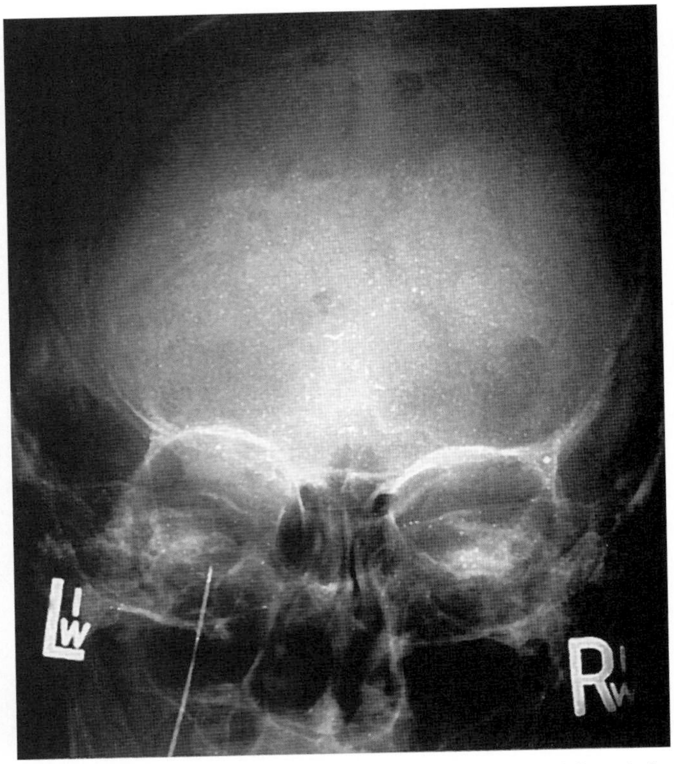

FIGURE 136–8 ■ Anteroposterior view of the needle placed through the foramen ovale. (From Waldman SD: Gasserian ganglion block. In Interventional Pain Management, 2nd ed. Philadelphia, WB Saunders, 2001, p 320.)

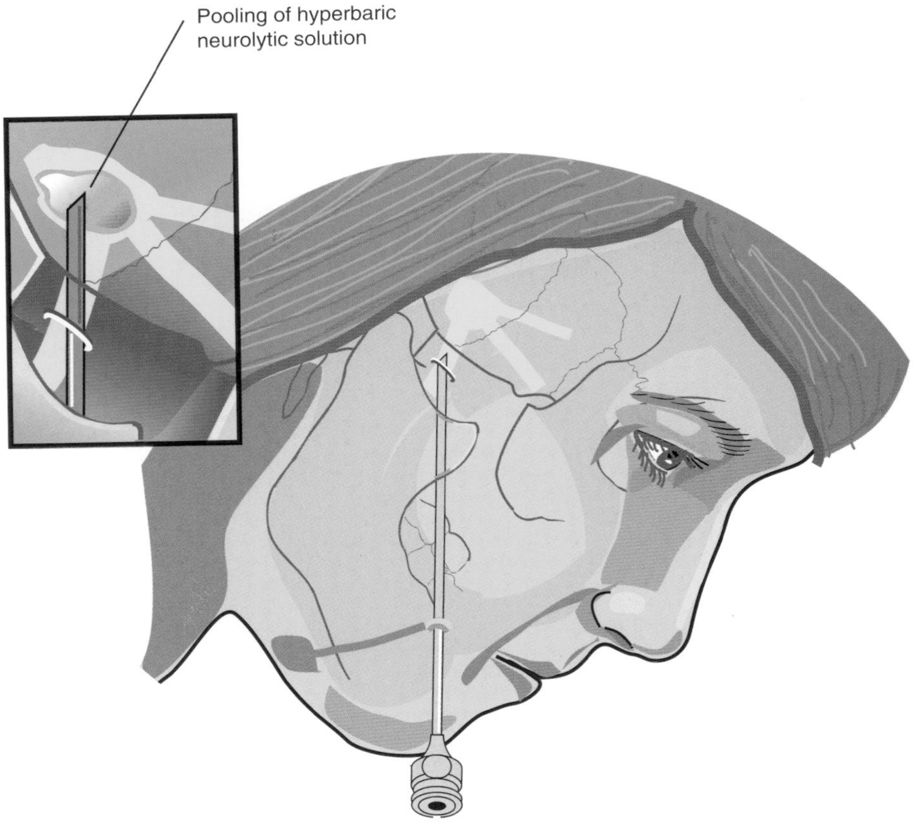

FIGURE 136–9 ■ Patient positioning for gasserian ganglion block with hyperbaric solution.

local anesthetic injected through the needle may produce total spinal anesthesia.[13] For this reason, it is imperative that small doses of local anesthetic be injected incrementally, allowing time after each dose to observe its effect.[3] Chemical neurolysis and neuroablative procedures on the gasserian ganglion should be performed only by individuals familiar with the anatomy and the technique of gasserian ganglion block, and only under radiographic guidance.

CONCLUSION

Gasserian ganglion block is a straightforward technique with a favorable risk-to-benefit ratio when careful attention is paid to the functional anatomy, indications, and contraindications. Given the cost-effective nature of this technique, gasserian ganglion block is a reasonable next step for patients with facial pain and cluster headache who have not responded to more conservative therapy.

References

1. Hall RJ: Hydrochlorate of cocaine. N Y Med J 40:643, 1886.
2. Winnie AP: The early history of regional anesthesia in the United States. In Scott DB, McClure J (eds): Regional Anesthesia, 1884-1984. Sodertalje, Sweden, ICM Press, 1984, p 35.
3. Bonica JJ: Neurolytic blockade and hypophysectomy. In Bonica JJ (ed): The Management of Pain. Philadelphia, Lea & Febiger, 1990, p 584.
4. Waldman SD: Medical staff credentialing—physician constitutional rights and remedies: Part I. The law and public policy of medical staff credentialing. Am J Pain Manage 7:100, 1997.
5. Waldman SD: Medical staff credentialing—physician constitutional rights and remedies: Part II. The law and public policy of medical staff credentialing. Am J Pain Manage 7:146, 1997.
6. Waldman SD: Gasserian ganglion block. In Hahn MB, McQuillan PM, Sheplock GJ (eds): Regional Anesthesia. St. Louis, CV Mosby, 1996, p 41.
7. Waldman SD: Gasserian ganglion block. In: Atlas of Interventional Pain Management Techniques. Philadelphia, WB Saunders, 1998, p 136.
8. Waldman SD: Management of acute pain. Postgrad Med 87:15, 1992.
9. Lipton S: Neurolysis: Pharmacology and drug selection. In Patt RB (ed): Cancer Pain. Philadelphia, JB Lippincott, 1993, p 354.
10. Waldman SD: Trigeminal neuralgia. Intern Med 13:45, 1992.
11. Waldman SD: Cluster headache. Intern Med 13:31, 1992.
12. Waldman SD: Evaluation and treatment of common headache and facial pain syndromes. In Raj PP (ed): Practical Management of Pain. St. Louis, CV Mosby, 1992, p 217.
13. Feldstein G: Percutaneous retrogasserian glycerol rhizotomy. In Racz G (ed): Techniques of Neurolysis. Boston, Kluwer, 1989, p 126.
14. Brown DL: Trigeminal (gasserian) ganglion block. In Brown DL (ed): Atlas of Regional Anesthesia, 2nd ed. Philadelphia, WB Saunders, 1999, p 137.
15. Raj PP, Gesund P, Phero J: Rationale and choice for surgical procedures. In Raj PP (ed): Clinical Practice of Regional Anesthesia. New York, Churchill Livingstone, 1991, p 200.
16. Katz J: Gasserian ganglion. In Katz J (ed): Atlas of Regional Anesthesia. Norwalk, CT, Appleton & Lange, 1994, p 4.
17. Neill RS: Head, neck and airway. In Wildsmith JAW, Armitage EN (eds): Principles and Practice of Regional Anesthesia. New York, Churchill Livingstone, 1987.

chapter 137

Blockade of the Trigeminal Nerve and Its Branches

Steven D. Waldman

INDICATIONS AND CONTRAINDICATIONS

Blockade of the trigeminal nerve and its branches with local anesthetics, steroids, or neurolytic agents and destruction of these structures by freezing, radiofrequency lesioning, and other means have many applications in contemporary pain management. Technologic advances in radiographic imaging, electronics, and needle technology have improved the efficacy and decreased the cost, complications, and adverse side effects of these procedures.

The indications for blockade of the trigeminal nerve and its branches are summarized in Table 137–1. In addition to applications for surgical anesthesia, trigeminal nerve block with local anesthetic can be used as a diagnostic and prognostic maneuver when performing differential neural blockade on an anatomic basis.[1] This technique can be used to treat trismus secondary to tetanus and as an aid in awake endotracheal intubation.[2] Trigeminal nerve block with local anesthetic or steroids is an excellent adjunct to pharmacologic treatment of trigeminal neuralgia.[3] The use of this technique allows rapid palliation of pain while oral medications are being titrated to effective levels; it also may be valuable in patients with atypical facial pain.[4] Other indications for trigeminal nerve block with local anesthetic or steroids are acute pain secondary to trauma, neoplasms of the head and face, cluster headaches refractory to sphenopalatine ganglion block, and the pain of acute herpes zoster in the distribution of the trigeminal nerve that is not controlled by stellate ganglion block.[5,6]

Indications for destruction of the distal trigeminal nerve and its branches are similar to the indications for gasserian ganglion block.[2] Because more peripheral destruction of the trigeminal nerve results in lower incidences of unwanted motor and sensory disturbance than destruction of the gasserian ganglion (especially corneal anesthesia), this approach may be the preferred course when it is efficacious for the pain syndrome being treated.

Contraindications to blockade of the trigeminal nerve and its branches are as follows:

- Local infection
- Sepsis
- Disulfiram therapy (if alcohol is used)
- Significant behavioral abnormalities

Local infection and sepsis are absolute contraindications to all procedures.[2,7] Coagulopathy is a relative contraindication to blockade of the trigeminal nerve and its branches. Owing to the desperation of many patients with aggressively invasive head and face malignancies, however, ethical and humanitarian considerations dictate the use of this procedure despite the increased risk of bleeding. If there are strong clinical indications, blockade of the distal trigeminal nerve and its branches using a 25-gauge needle may be done in the presence of coagulopathy, albeit with increased risk of ecchymosis and hematoma formation.

CLINICALLY RELEVANT ANATOMY

Role of the Trigeminal System

The trigeminal nerve, the largest and the most complex of the cranial nerves, contains sensory and motor fibers.[8,9] Somatic afferent impulses carried by the trigeminal nerve transmit pain, light touch, and temperature sensation. Information is transmitted to the central nervous system via the trigeminal nerve from the skin of the face, the mucosal lining of the nose and mouth, the teeth, and the anterior two thirds of the tongue.[8] The trigeminal nerve also carries proprioceptive impulses and afferent impulses from stretch receptors of the teeth, oral mucosa, muscles of mastication, and temporomandibular joint to aid in mastication.

In addition to the sensory innervation just described, visceral efferent fibers help to innervate a variety of muscles of facial expression, the tensor tympani, and some muscles of mastication. Communications exist between the trigeminal nerve and the autonomic nervous system, including the ciliary, sphenopalatine, otic, and submaxillary ganglia and the oculomotor, facial, and glossopharyngeal nerves. Because of the complex nature of the trigeminal nerve, a thorough understanding of the clinically relevant anatomy is crucial to obtaining optimal results of neural blockade of these structures.

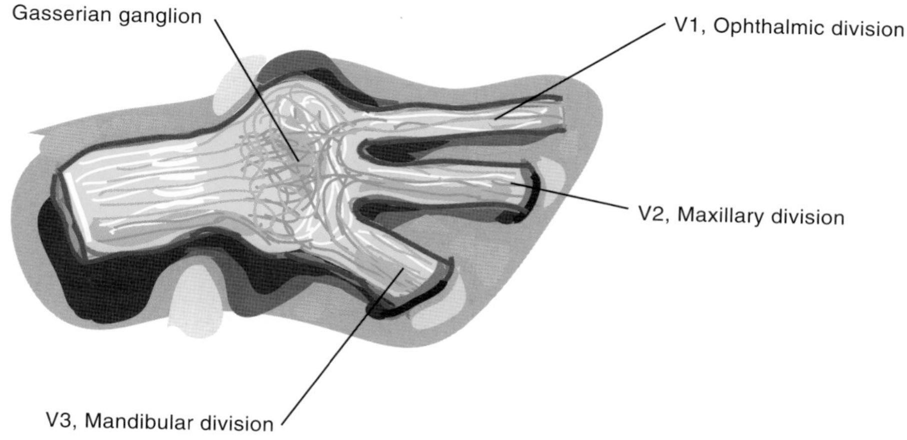

FIGURE 137–1 ■ Gasserian ganglion and Meckel's cave.

Table 137-1

Indications for Blockade of the Trigeminal Nerve and Its Branches

Local Anesthetic Block	***Neurolytic Block or Neurodestructive Procedures***
Surgical anesthesia	Palliation of cancer pain
Anatomic differential neural blockade	Management of trigeminal neuralgia
Prognostic nerve block before neurodestructive procedures	Management of cluster headache
Treatment of trismus	
Aid to awake endotracheal intubation	
Palliation in acute pain emergencies	
Palliation of acute herpes zoster	

Gasserian Ganglion

The gasserian ganglion is formed from two roots that exit the ventral surface of the brain stem at the midpontine level (Fig. 137–1).[10] These roots pass in a forward and lateral direction in the posterior cranial fossa across the border of the petrous temporal bone. They enter a recess called *Meckel's cave,* which is formed by an invagination of the surrounding dura mater into the middle cranial fossa. The dural pouch that lies just behind the ganglion, called the *trigeminal cistern,* contains CSF.

The gasserian ganglion is canoe-shaped. Its three sensory divisions, the ophthalmic (V_1), maxillary (V_2), and mandibular (V_3) nerves, exit the anterior convex aspect of the ganglion. A smaller motor root joins the mandibular division as it exits the cranial cavity via the foramen ovale.

Ophthalmic Division

The ophthalmic branch, the smallest division of the trigeminal nerve, is purely sensory in function (Fig. 137–2).[11] It enters the orbit via the superior orbital fissure. The branch is divided into the frontal, nasociliary, and lacrimal nerves. The terminal cutaneous branches of the frontal nerve consist of the supraorbital and supratrochlear nerves. These terminal branches exit the orbital cavity anteriorly and provide innervation to the upper eyelid, forehead, and anterior scalp. The terminal cutaneous branches of the nasociliary nerve consist of the infratrochlear and external nasal branches, which provide cutaneous and mucosal innervation to the apex and ala of the nose and anterior nasal cavity. The lacrimal nerve continues, without additional major branches, to innervate the lacrimal gland and outer canthus of the eye.

Maxillary Division

The maxillary division is a pure sensory nerve. It exits the middle cranial fossa via the foramen rotundum and crosses the pterygopalatine fossa (Fig. 137–3).[8] Passing through the inferior orbital fissure, it enters the orbit, emerging on the face via the infraorbital foramen.

The branches of the maxillary nerve are divided into four regional groups. (1) The intracranial group includes the middle meningeal nerve, which innervates the dura mater of the medial cranial fossa. (2) The pterygopalatine group includes the zygomatic nerve, which provides sensory innervation to the temporal and lateral zygomatic region, and the sphenopalatine branches, which help to innervate the mucosa of the maxillary sinus, upper gums, upper molars, and mucous membranes of the cheek. (3) The infraorbital canal group comprises the anterior-superior alveolar branch, which innervates the incisors and canines, the anterior wall of the maxillary antrum, and the floor of the nasal cavity, and the middle superior branch, which supplies the premolars. (4) The infraorbital facial group consists of the inferior palpebral branch, which innervates the conjunctiva and skin of the lower eyelid; the external nasal branch, which supplies the side of the nose; and the superior labial branch, which

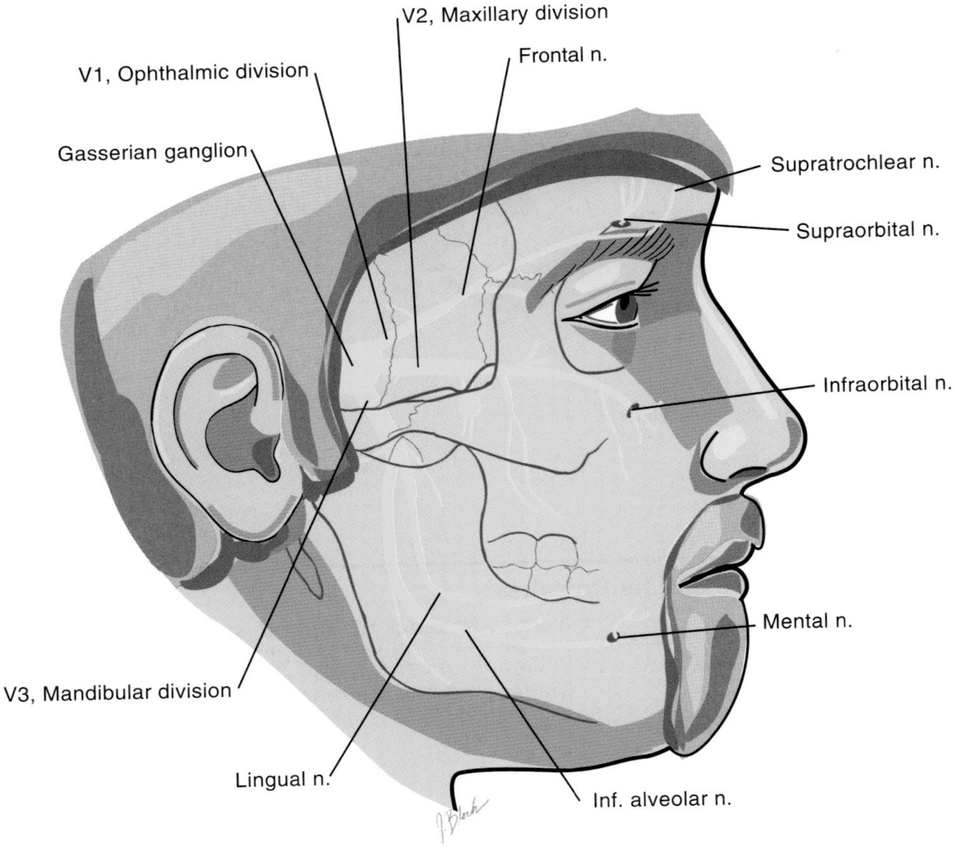

FIGURE 137–2 ■ Trigeminal nerve and its branches.

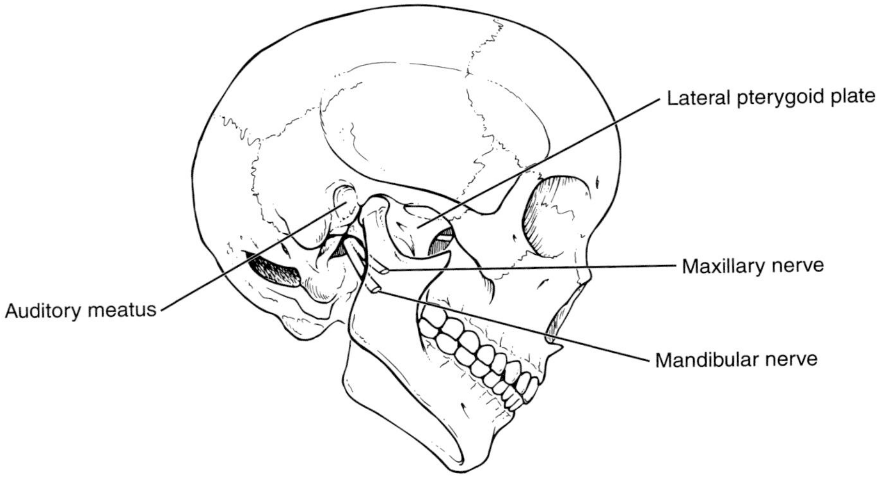

FIGURE 137–3 ■ Major branches of the trigeminal nerve.

supplies the skin of the upper lip and part of the oral mucosa (see Fig. 137–2).

Mandibular Division

The large sensory root and smaller motor root of the mandibular division leave the middle cranial fossa together via the foramen ovale.[8] They join to form the mandibular nerve (see Fig. 137–3). This combined trunk gives off two branches: the nervus spinosus, which runs superiorly with the middle meningeal artery through the foramen spinosum to supply the dura mater and the mucosal lining of the mastoid sinus, and the internal pterygoid, which supplies the internal pterygoid and gives off branches to the otic ganglion. The mandibular nerve divides into a small anterior and a large posterior trunk (see Fig. 137–2).

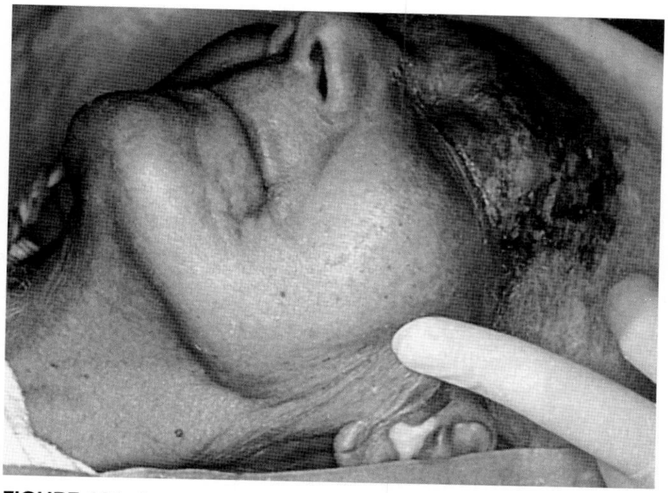

FIGURE 137–4 ■ Palpation of the coronoid notch. (From Waldman SD: Interventional Pain Management, 2nd ed. Philadelphia, WB Saunders, 2001, p 323.)

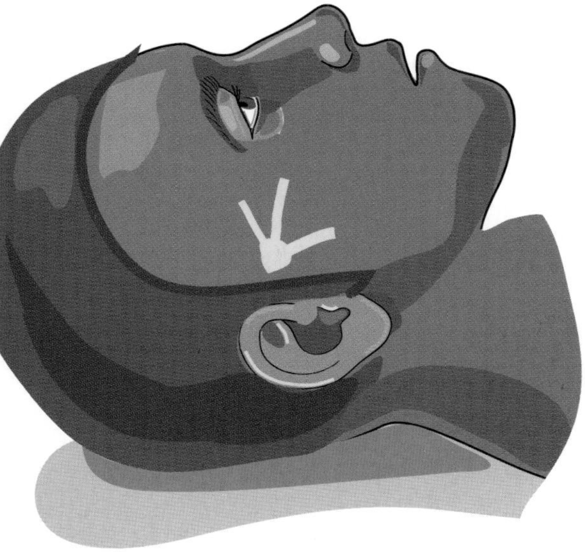

FIGURE 137–5 ■ Patient position for maxillary and mandibular nerve block.

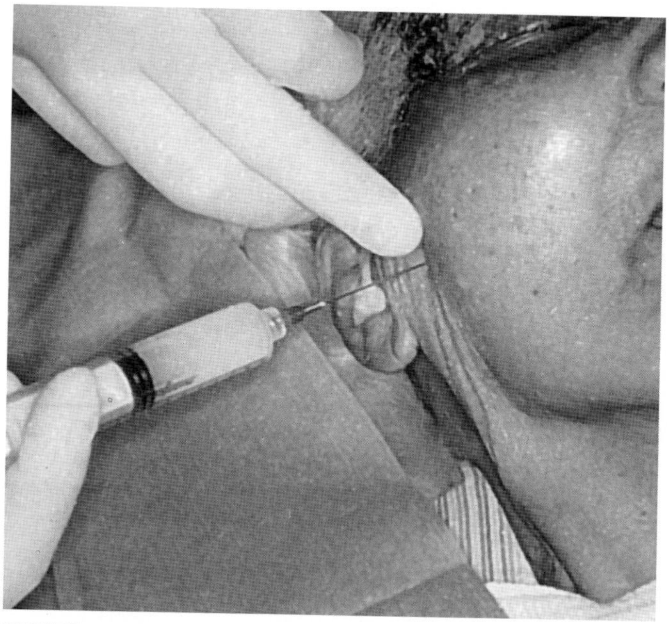

FIGURE 137–6 ■ Correct needle position for the trigeminal nerve block via the coronoid notch. (From Waldman SD: Interventional Pain Management, 2nd ed. Philadelphia, WB Saunders, 2001, p 324.)

Branches from the small anterior trunk are the buccinator nerve, which is purely sensory and innervates the skin and mucous membrane overlying the anterior portion of the buccinator muscle; the masseteric nerve, which provides motor innervation to the masseter muscle; the deep temporal nerves, which provide motor innervation to the temporalis muscle; and the external pterygoid nerve, which provides motor innervation to the external pterygoid muscle. The large posterior trunk comprises primarily sensory fibers, but also contains a few motor fibers. Branches of the posterior trunk are the auriculotemporal nerve, which provides innervation to skin anterior to the tragus and helix, lining of the acoustic meatus, tympanic membrane, posterior temporomandibular joint, parotid gland, and skin of the temporal region; the lingual nerve, which provides sensory innervation to the dorsum and lateral aspects of the anterior two thirds of the tongue and the lateral mucous membranes of the mouth and the sublingual gland; and the inferior alveolar nerve, which provides sensory innervation to the lower teeth and mandible. The terminal branch of the inferior alveolar nerve, the mental nerve, exits the mandible via the mental foramen and provides sensory innervation to the chin and to the skin and mucous membrane of the lower lip.

TECHNIQUE OF BLOCKADE OF THE MAXILLARY AND MANDIBULAR DIVISIONS OF THE TRIGEMINAL NERVE VIA THE CORONOID APPROACH

The patient is placed in the supine position. The coronoid notch is palpated by asking the patient to open and close the mouth several times. The level of the coronoid notch is at the external auditory meatus (Figs. 137–4 and 137–5). After the notch is identified, the patient is asked to hold the mouth in the neutral position.[2,8]

A 3½-inch 22-gauge styletted spinal needle is inserted just beneath the zygomatic arch, at the midpoint of the coronoid notch (Fig. 137–6). The needle is advanced approximately 1½ to 2 inches perpendicular to the base of the skull, until the lateral pterygoid plate is encountered (Fig. 137–7). At this point, if maxillary and mandibular nerve blocks are desired, the needle is withdrawn approximately 1 mm. After careful aspiration for blood, 7 to 10 mL of preservative-free local anesthetic is injected in small increments (Fig. 137–8).[2] During the injection procedure, the patient must be observed carefully for signs of local anesthetic toxicity. For selective maxillary nerve block, the styletted spinal needle is withdrawn and reinserted to slip just above the anterior margin of the lateral pterygoid plate (Fig. 137–9).[2] A maxillary paresthesia generally is produced approximately 1 cm deeper than the level at which the pterygoid plate was first encountered. After careful aspiration, 3 to 5 mL of preservative-free local anesthetic may be injected in increments.

If selective blockade of the mandibular division of the trigeminal nerve is desired, the lateral pterygoid plate is identified, and the needle is withdrawn and directed slightly farther posteriorly and inferiorly. A paresthesia in the mandibular distribution is elicited in most cases (Fig. 137–10).[2]

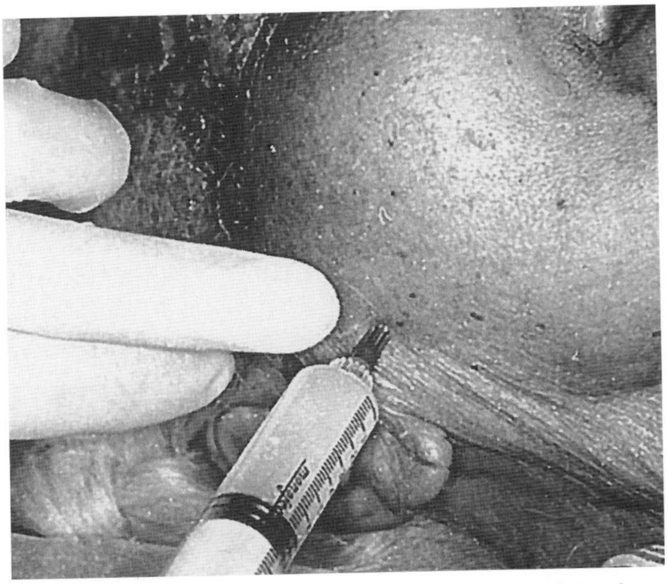

FIGURE 137–7 ■ Needle tip positioned in the pterygopalatine fossa. (From Waldman SD: Interventional Pain Management, 2nd ed. Philadelphia, WB Saunders, 2001, p 324.)

After careful aspiration, 3 to 5 mL of preservative-free local anesthetic is injected in incremental doses.

For diagnostic and prognostic blocks, 1% preservative-free lidocaine is a suitable local anesthetic.[12] For therapeutic blocks, 0.5% preservative-free bupivacaine in combination with 80 mg of depot methylprednisolone (Depo-Medrol) is injected.[2] Subsequent daily nerve blocks are done in a similar manner, substituting 40 mg of methylprednisolone for the initial 80-mg dose. Five to six trigeminal nerve blocks daily may be required to treat the painful conditions listed earlier.[4] If selective neurolytic block of the mandibular or maxillary nerve is desired, incremental 0.1-mL injections of sterile glycerol, 6.5% phenol in glycerin, or alcohol to a total volume of 1 mL may be used after adequate pain relief with local anesthetic blocks is confirmed.[13]

Practical Considerations

The pterygopalatine space is densely vascular. The possibility of intravascular uptake of local anesthetic is significant with this nerve block. Careful aspiration of blood and incremental dosage with local anesthetic are important to allow early detection of local anesthetic toxicity. Careful observation of the patient during and after the nerve block is mandatory.[2]

■ TECHNIQUE OF NEURAL BLOCKADE OF THE SUPRAORBITAL AND SUPRATROCHLEAR BRANCHES OF THE OPHTHALMIC DIVISION OF THE TRIGEMINAL NERVE

The patient is placed supine with the head in neutral position. The supraorbital notch is identified by palpation. The skin is

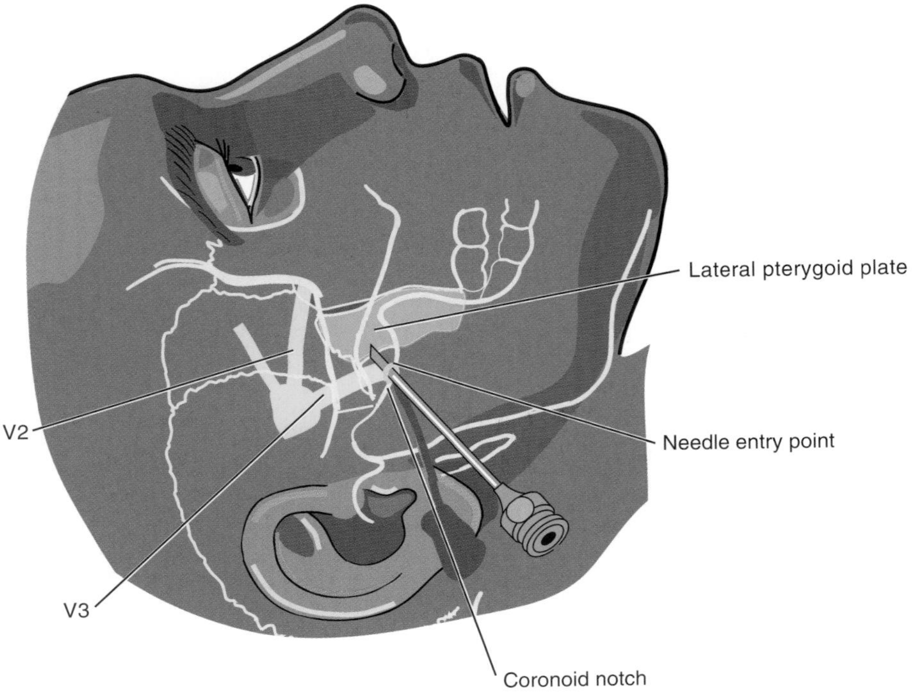

FIGURE 137–8 ■ Nonselective trigeminal nerve block.

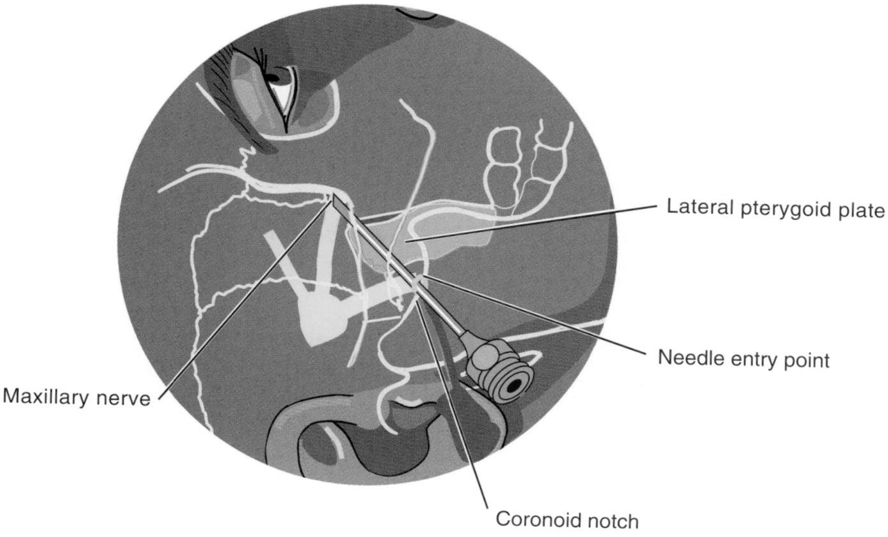

FIGURE 137–9 ■ Selective maxillary nerve block.

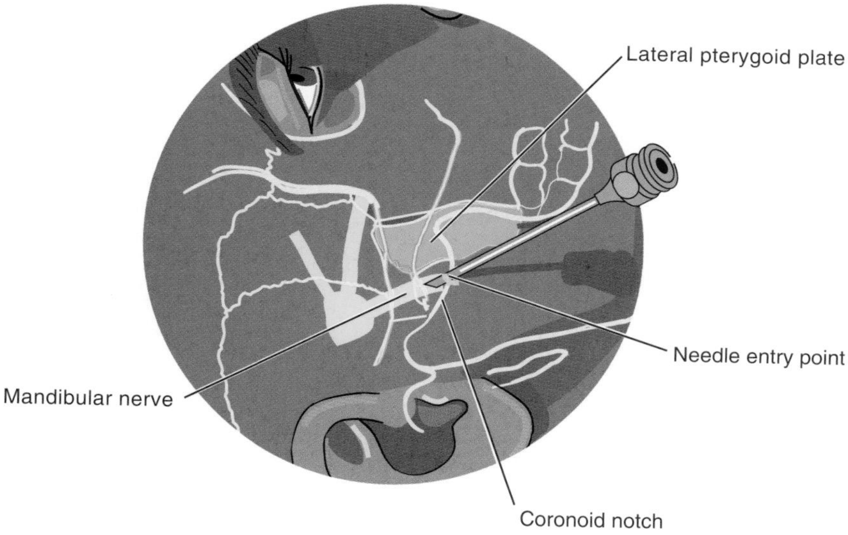

FIGURE 137–10 ■ Selective mandibular nerve block.

prepared with povidone-iodine solution, with care being taken to avoid spilling solution into the eye.

A 1½-inch 25-gauge needle is advanced perpendicularly to the skin at the level of the supraorbital notch. To anesthetize the peripheral branches of the nerve, 3 to 4 mL of preservative-free local anesthetic is injected in a fanlike configuration (Fig. 137–11).[14] To block the supratrochlear nerve, the needle is directed medially from the supraorbital notch toward the apex of the nose.[8] Paresthesias are occasionally elicited.[7] If neurolytic block of the supraorbital and supratrochlear branches is desired, incremental 0.1-mL injections of sterile glycerol or 6.5% phenol in glycerin, to a total volume of 0.5 mL, may be used after adequate pain relief with local anesthetic blocks is confirmed.[13]

Practical Considerations

Because of the loose alveolar tissue of the eyelid, a gauze sponge should be used to apply gentle pressure on the eyelids and supraorbital tissues to keep the local anesthetic from dissecting into the eyelid and supraorbital tissues. This pressure is maintained after the nerve block to avoid periorbital hematoma and ecchymosis.

■ TECHNIQUE OF NEURAL BLOCKADE OF THE INFRAORBITAL BRANCH OF THE MAXILLARY NERVE

Intraoral Approach

The upper lip is folded backward, and a cotton ball soaked with 10% cocaine solution or 2% viscous lidocaine is placed in the alveolar ridge, just inferior to the intraorbital foramen (Fig. 137–12). After adequate topical anesthesia is obtained, a 1½-inch 25-gauge needle is advanced through the anesthetized area superiorly toward the infraorbital foramen.[2] A paresthesia may be elicited.[2] After careful aspiration, 2 to

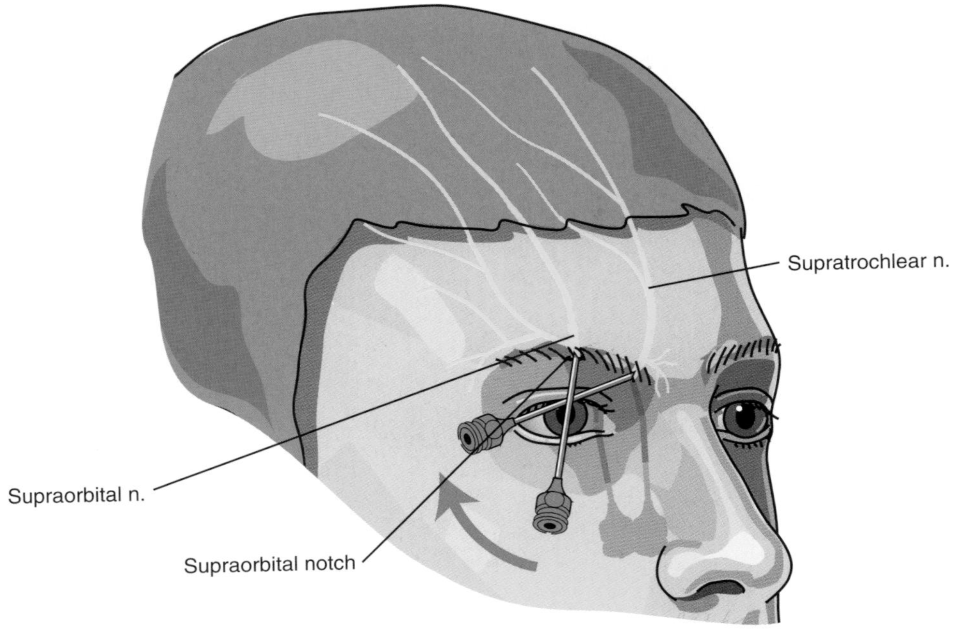

FIGURE 137–11 ■ Supraorbital and supratrochlear block.

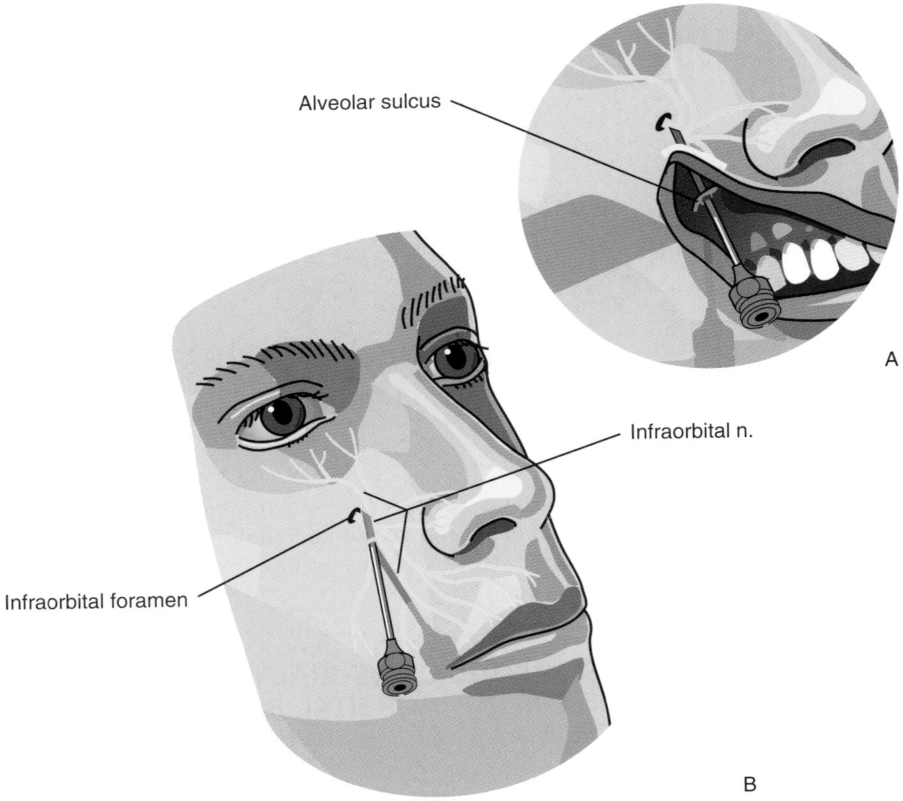

FIGURE 137–12 ■ Intraoral **(A)** and extraoral **(B)** approaches to infraorbital nerve block.

3 mL of preservative-free local anesthetic is injected.[3] If neurolytic block of the infraorbital nerve is desired, incremental 0.1-mL injections of sterile glycerol or 6.5% phenol in glycerin may be used after adequate pain relief with local anesthetic block is confirmed.[3]

Practical Considerations

As with the supraorbital nerve block, pressure over the inferior periorbital tissues limits dissection of the local anesthetic superiorly into the periorbital region and avoids ecchymosis and hematoma formation. The intraoral route is particularly suited to pediatric patients.

Extraoral Approach

The infraorbital ridge of the maxillary bone is identified, and the infraorbital foramen is palpated. The skin is prepared with povidone-iodine solution, with care being taken to avoid spillage of the solution into the eye. A ½-inch 25-gauge needle is advanced at a 45-degree angle toward the foramen (see Fig. 137–12).[15] A paresthesia may be elicited. After careful aspiration of blood, 2 to 3 mL of preservative-free local anesthetic is injected. Percutaneous neurolytic block of the infraorbital nerve is performed as for the intraoral route.

Practical Considerations

Similar to the intraoral approach, pressure must be applied to the infraorbital tissues to avoid dissection of local anesthetic. When the infraorbital branch is blocked using the extraoral approach, if the needle enters the infraorbital foramen, it should be withdrawn to avoid hematoma, injection-induced compressive neuropathy, and damage to the contents of the orbit.

TECHNIQUE OF NEURAL BLOCKADE OF THE MENTAL BRANCH OF THE MANDIBULAR NERVE

Intraoral Approach

The lower lip is pulled downward and away from the face. A cotton ball soaked in 10% cocaine or 2% viscous lidocaine is placed in the alveolar ridge against the mucosa, just superior to the mental foramen.[2] After topical anesthesia is obtained, a ½-inch 25-gauge needle is advanced via the anesthetized area in a perpendicular plane (Fig. 137–13). Paresthesia occasionally develops. After careful aspiration of blood, 2 to 3 mL of preservative-free bupivacaine is injected.[2] If neurolytic block of the mental nerve is desired, successive 0.1-mL injections of sterile glycerol or 6.5% phenol in glycerin may be used after adequate pain relief with local anesthetic blocks is confirmed.

Extraoral Approach

An area approximately 2 cm from the midline in a plane parallel with the supraorbital and infraorbital foramina is identified. Careful palpation generally allows identification of the mental foramen. The skin is prepared with povidone-iodine solution. A ½-inch 25-gauge needle is advanced toward the foramen (see Fig. 137–13).[16] If the needle enters the mental foramen, it should be withdrawn to avoid injection-induced compressive neuropathy. After careful aspiration of blood, 2 to 3 mL of preservative-free local anesthetic is injected. If neurolytic block of the mental nerve is desired, incremental 0.1-mL injections of sterile glycerol or 6.5% phenol in glycerin, to a total volume of 0.5 mL, may be given after adequate pain relief with local anesthetic blocks is confirmed.

Practical Considerations

Because of the acute angle at which the mental branch exits the mental foramen, it is susceptible to compression neuropathy. For this reason, it is advisable to avoid advancing the needle into the canal because theoretically hematoma forma-

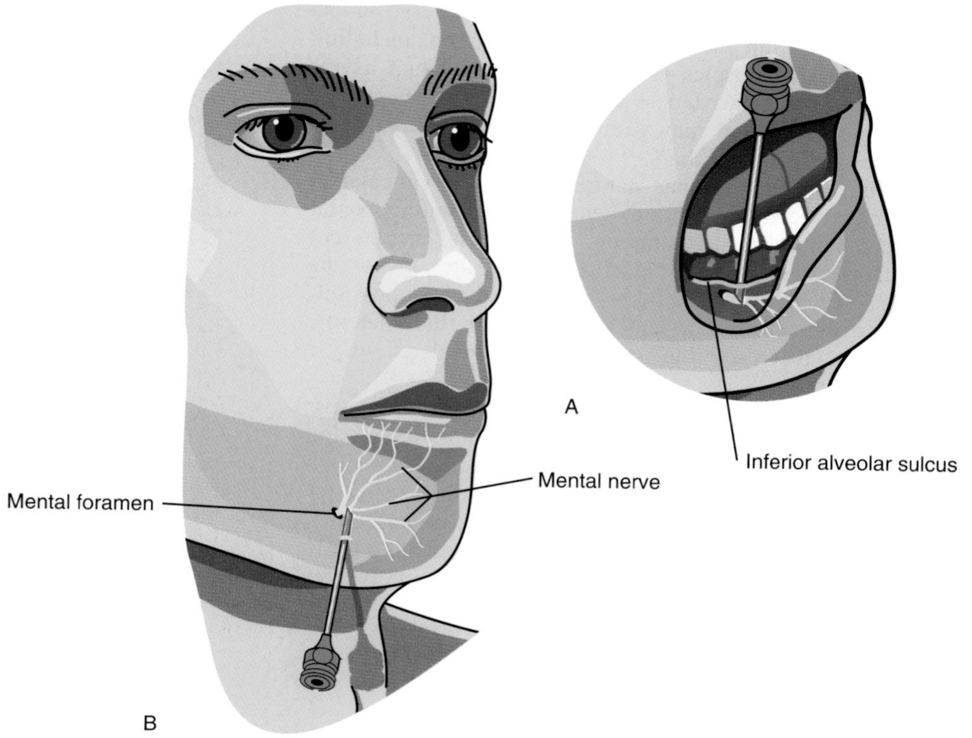

FIGURE 137–13 ■ Mental nerve block. **A,** Intraoral approach. **B,** Extraoral approach.

tion or increased pressure during injection can cause compression neuropathy.

COMPLICATIONS AND UNWANTED SIDE EFFECTS

The potential complications and unwanted side effects of blockade of the trigeminal nerve and its branches are as follows:

- Activation of herpes labialis and herpes zoster
- Postprocedure dysesthesias, including anesthesia dolorosa
- Abnormal motor function, including weakness
- Facial asymmetry
- Horner syndrome
- Facial ecchymosis and hematoma
- Ocular subscleral hematoma
- Local anesthetic toxicity
- Trauma to nerves
- Infection
- Sloughing of skin and subcutaneous tissue

Although it is associated more often with procedures involving the gasserian ganglion, blockade of the trigeminal nerve and its branches may activate herpes labialis and occasionally herpes zoster in the distribution of the trigeminal nerve.

A few patients who undergo chemical neurolysis or neurodestructive procedures of the trigeminal nerve and its branches have postprocedure dysesthesias in the area of anesthesia.[17] These symptoms range from mild, uncomfortable burning or pulling sensations to severe pain. Severe postprocedure pain, called *anesthesia dolorosa,* may be worse than the patient's original pain complaint and often is harder to treat. Sloughing of skin and subcutaneous tissue has been associated with anesthesia dolorosa.

In addition to disturbances of sensation, neurolytic block or neurodestructive procedures of the trigeminal nerve and its branches may result in abnormal motor function, including weakness of the muscles of mastication and facial asymmetry secondary to weakness and altered proprioception.[13] Horner syndrome also may occur from block of the paratrigeminal sympathetic fibers.

Owing to the vascular nature of the pterygopalatine space, facial ecchymosis, and hematoma, including ocular subscleral hematoma, are common.[8,18] Although generally not harmful, these unwanted side effects are distressing to the patient, so each patient should be forewarned of the possibility before the procedure. The vascularity of this anatomic region also increases the potential for local anesthetic toxicity.[18]

The terminal branches of the trigeminal nerve are susceptible to trauma from needle, hematoma, and compression during injection procedures.[2] These complications, although usually transitory, can be quite upsetting to the patient. Infection, although also uncommon, is always a possibility, especially in immunocompromised cancer patients. Early detection of infection is crucial to avoiding potentially life-threatening sequelae.

FUTURE DIRECTIONS

Continuing advances in the understanding of the basic science of pain will improve management of patients with pain. Research on the serotoninergic system and its role in the pathogenesis of headache has led to the development of a whole new class of drugs that have revolutionized the way clinicians manage acute migraine and cluster headache.[19] The search for safer local anesthetics yielded ropivacaine, which seems to have less cardiotoxicity than bupivacaine.[20] In view of the relatively high incidence of local anesthetic toxicity associated with this technique, such a characteristic would offer a great advantage for neural blockade of the trigeminal system. Microencapsulation of local anesthetics with lecithin seems to increase the duration of action fourfold; this advance would be beneficial for trigeminal nerve block when the lesion responsible for the pain is self-limited.

References

1. Waldman SD: Trigeminal nerve block. In Weiner RS (ed): Innovations in Pain Management, vol I. Orlando, PMD Press, 1990, p 10.
2. Waldman SD: Trigeminal block. In: Atlas of Interventional Pain Management Techniques. Philadelphia, WB Saunders, 1998, p 30.
3. Waldman SD: Trigeminal neuralgia. Intern Med 13:45, 1992.
4. Waldman SD: The role of neural blockade in the management of headaches and facial pain. Curr Rev Pain 1:346, 1997.
5. Waldman SD: Cluster headache. Intern Med 13:31, 1992.
6. Waldman SD: Evaluation and treatment of common headache and facial pain syndromes. In Raj PP (ed): Practical Management of Pain. St. Louis, CV Mosby, 1992, p 217.
7. Feldstein G: Percutaneous retrogasserian glycerol rhizotomy. In Racz G (ed): Techniques of Neurolysis. Boston, Kluwer, 1989, p 126.
8. Hahn MB: Trigeminal nerve block. In Hahn MB, McQuillan PM, Sheplock GJ (eds): Regional Anesthesia. St. Louis, CV Mosby, 1996, p 41.
9. Brown DL: Trigeminal (gasserian) ganglion block. In Brown DL (ed): Atlas of Regional Anesthesia. Philadelphia, WB Saunders, 1999, p 149.
10. Katz J: Gasserian ganglion. In: Atlas of Regional Anesthesia. Norwalk, CT, Appleton & Lange, 1994, p 4.
11. Neill RS: Head, neck and airway. In Wildsmith JAW, Armitage EN (eds): Principles and Practice of Regional Anesthesia. New York, Churchill Livingstone, 1987.
12. Raj PP: Prognostic and therapeutic local anesthetic blocks. In Cousins MJ, Bridenbaugh DO (eds): Neural Blockade. Philadelphia, JB Lippincott, 1988, p 900.
13. Bonica JJ: Neurolytic blockade and hypophysectomy. In Bonica JJ (ed): The Management of Pain. Philadelphia, Lea & Febiger, 1990, p 587.
14. Katz J: Supraorbital nerve. In: Atlas of Regional Anesthesia. Norwalk, CT, Appleton & Lange, 1994, p 25.
15. Katz J: Infraorbital nerve. In: Atlas of Regional Anesthesia. Norwalk, CT, Appleton & Lange, 1994, p 14.
16. Katz J: Mental nerve. In: Atlas of Regional Anesthesia. Norwalk, CT, Appleton & Lange, 1994, p 27.
17. Lipton S: Neurolysis: Pharmacology and drug selection. In Patt RB (ed): Cancer Pain. Philadelphia, JB Lippincott, 1993, p 354.
18. Waldman SD: Complication of trigeminal nerve block. Pain Clin 7:211, 1994.
19. Waldman SD: Recent advances in analgesic therapy: Sumatriptan. Pain Digest 3:260, 1993.
20. Waldman SD: Recent advances in analgesic therapy: Ropivacaine. Pain Digest 4:42, 1994.

chapter 138

Glossopharyngeal Nerve Block

Steven D. Waldman

HISTORICAL CONSIDERATIONS

The early use of glossopharyngeal nerve block in pain management centered around two applications (1) the treatment of glossopharyngeal neuralgia; and (2) the palliation of pain secondary to head and neck malignancies. In the late 1950s, the clinical use of glossopharyngeal nerve block as an adjunct to awake endotracheal intubation was documented.

Weisenburg first described pain in the distribution of the glossopharyngeal nerve in a patient with a cerebellopontine angle tumor in 1910.[1] In 1921, Harris reported the first idiopathic case and coined the term *glossopharyngeal neuralgia*.[2] He suggested that blockade of the glossopharyngeal nerve might be useful in palliating this painful condition.

Early attempts at permanent treatment of glossopharyngeal neuralgia and cancer pain in the distribution of the glossopharyngeal nerve consisted principally of extracranial surgical section or alcohol neurolysis of the glossopharyngeal nerve.[3] These approaches met with limited success in the treatment of glossopharyngeal neuralgia but were useful in some patients who were suffering from cancer pain mediated via the glossopharyngeal nerve. Intracranial section of the glossopharyngeal nerve was first performed by Adson in 1925 and was subsequently refined by Dandy. The intracranial approach to section of the glossopharyngeal nerve appeared to yield better results for both glossopharyngeal neuralgia and cancer pain but was a much riskier procedure.[4] Recently interest in extracranial destruction of the glossopharyngeal nerve by glycerol or by creation of a radiofrequency lesion has been renewed.

INDICATIONS AND CONTRAINDICATIONS

Indications for glossopharyngeal nerve block are summarized in Table 138–1. In addition to applications for surgical anesthesia, glossopharyngeal nerve block with local anesthetics can be used as a diagnostic tool when performing differential neural blockade on an anatomic basis in the evaluation of head and facial pain.[5] Glossopharyngeal nerve block is used to help differentiate geniculate ganglion neuralgia from glossopharyngeal neuralgia. If destruction of the glossopharyngeal nerve is being considered, this technique is useful as an indicator of the extent of motor and sensory impairment that the patient will likely experience.[6] Glossopharyngeal nerve block with local anesthetic may be used to palliate acute pain emergencies, including glossopharyngeal neuralgia and cancer pain, until pharmacologic, surgical, and antiblastic methods take effect.[7] This technique is also useful for atypical facial pain in the distribution of the glossopharyngeal nerve[8] and as an adjunct for awake endotracheal intubation.[9]

Destruction of the glossopharyngeal nerve is indicated in the palliation of cancer pain, including invasive tumors of the posterior tongue, hypopharynx, and tonsils.[10] This technique is useful in the management of the pain of glossopharyngeal neuralgia for those patients who have failed to respond to medical management or those who are not candidates for surgical microvascular decompression.[11]

Contraindications to blockade of the glossopharyngeal nerve, are summarized in Table 138–2. Local infection and sepsis are absolute contraindications to all procedures. Coagulopathy is a strong contraindication to glossopharyngeal nerve block, but owing to the desperate nature of many patients' suffering from invasive head and face malignancies, ethical and humanitarian considerations dictate its use, despite the risk of bleeding. When clinical indications are compelling, blockade of the glossopharyngeal nerve using a 22-gauge needle may be carried out in the presence of coagulopathy, albeit with increased risk of ecchymosis and hematoma formation.

CLINICALLY RELEVANT ANATOMY

The glossopharyngeal nerve contains both motor and sensory fibers.[10] The motor fibers innervate the stylopharyngeus muscle. The sensory portion of the nerve innervates the posterior third of the tongue, palatine tonsil, and the mucous membranes of the mouth and pharynx. Special visceral afferent sensory fibers transmit information from the taste buds of the posterior third of the tongue. Information from the carotid sinus and body, which help to control blood pressure, pulse, and respiration are carried via the carotid sinus nerve, a branch of the glossopharyngeal nerve.[10] Parasympathetic fibers pass via the glossopharyngeal nerve to the otic ganglion. Postganglionic fibers from the ganglion carry secretory information to the parotid gland.[12]

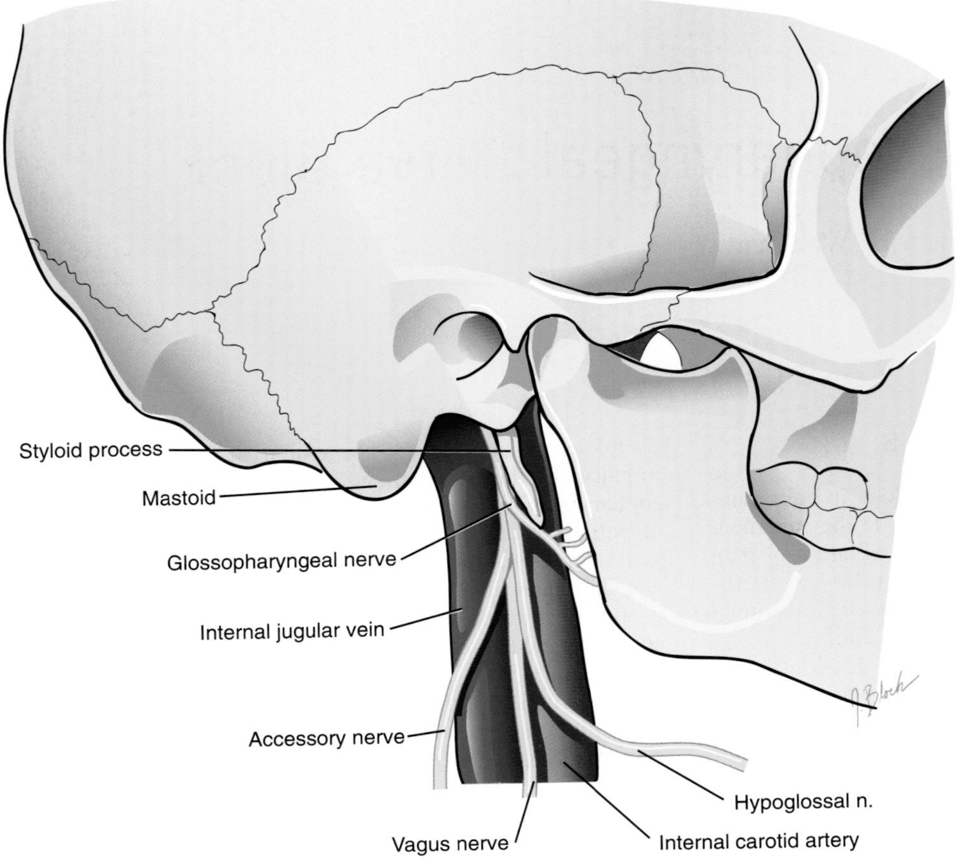

FIGURE 138–1 ■ Relationship of glossopharyngeal, vagus, and hypoglossal nerves to artery and vein in context with skull and mandible. (From Waldman SD: Atlas of Interventional Pain Management, 2nd ed. Philadelphia, Saunders, p 69, Figure 19–2.)

Table 138–1

Indications for Glossopharyngeal Nerve Block

- Local anesthetic block
- Surgical anesthesia
- Anatomic differential neural blockade
- Prognostic nerve block before neurodestructive procedures
- Acute pain emergencies (palliation)
- Adjunct to awake intubation
- Neurolytic block or neurodestructive procedure
- Cancer pain (palliation)
- Management of glossopharyngeal neuralgia

Table 138–2

Contraindications to Glossopharyngeal Nerve Block

Local infection
Sepsis
Coagulopathy
Disulfiram therapy (if alcohol is used)
Significant behavioral abnormalities

The glossopharyngeal nerve exits the jugular foramen near the vagus and accessory nerves and the internal jugular vein.[13] All three nerves lie in the groove between the internal jugular vein and internal carotid artery (Fig. 138–1). Inadvertent puncture of either vessel during glossopharyngeal nerve block can result in intravascular injection or hematoma formation. Even small amounts of local anesthetic injected into the carotid artery at this site can produce profound local anesthetic toxicity.[11]

One landmark for glossopharyngeal nerve block is the styloid process of the temporal bone. This structure is the calcification of the cephalad end of the stylohyoid ligament. Although usually easy to identify, when ossification is limited, it may be difficult to locate with the exploring needle.

TECHNIQUE

The Extraoral Approach

The patient is placed in the supine position. An imaginary line is visualized running from the mastoid process to the angle of the mandible (Fig. 138–2).[14] The styloid process should lie just below the midpoint of this line. The skin is "prepped"

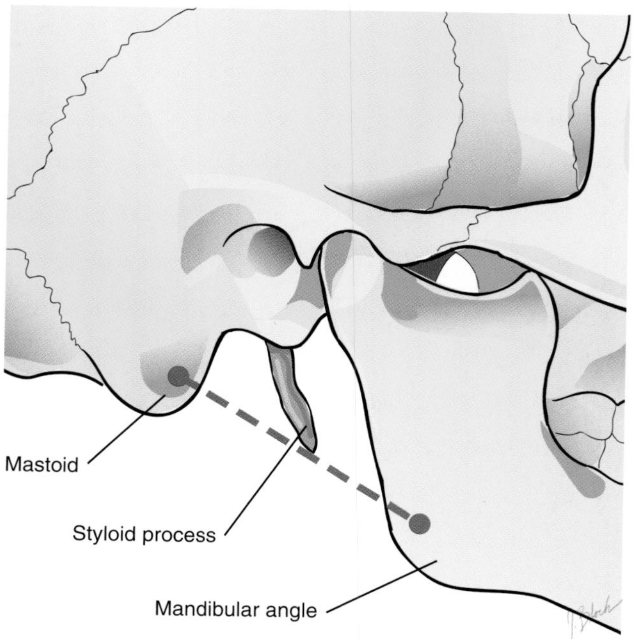

FIGURE 138–2 ■ Close-up view of the line from mastoid to styloid. (From Waldman SD: Atlas of Interventional Pain Management, 2nd ed. Philadelphia, Saunders, p 70, Figure 19–3.)

with antiseptic solution. A 22-gauge, 1.5-inch needle attached to a 10-mL syringe is advanced at this midpoint location in a plane perpendicular to the skin (Fig. 138–3). The styloid process should be encountered within 3 cm. After contact is made, the needle is withdrawn and walked off the styloid process posteriorly. As soon as bony contact is lost and careful aspiration reveals no blood or cerebrospinal fluid, 7 mL of 0.5% preservative-free lidocaine combined with 80 mg of methylprednisolone is injected in incremental doses. Subsequently, daily nerve blocks are performed in the same manner but substituting 40 mg of methylprednisolone for the first 80-mg dose. This approach may also be used for breakthrough pain in patients who previously experienced adequate pain control with oral medications.[11]

The Intraoral Approach

The tongue is anesthetized with 2.0% viscous lidocaine. With the patient's mouth open wide, the tongue is retracted downward with a tongue depressor or laryngoscope blade (Fig. 138–4). A 22-gauge, 3.5-inch spinal needle that has been bent approximately 130 degrees is inserted through the mucosa at the lower lateral portion of the posterior tonsillar pillar. The needle is advanced approximately 0.5 cm. After careful aspiration for blood and cerebrospinal fluid, local anesthetic or steroid or both are injected in a manner like that for the extraoral approach to glossopharyngeal nerve block.

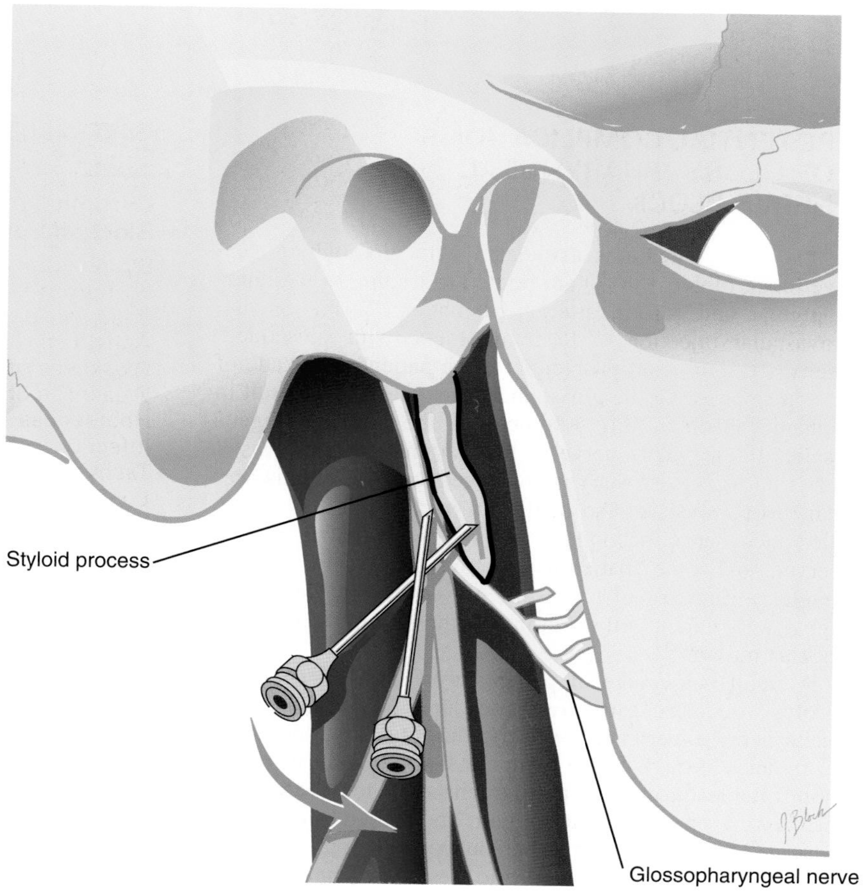

FIGURE 138–3 ■ Needle placement for glossopharyngeal nerve block. Needle is in contact with styloid process. Needle is redirected posteriorly to the glossopharyngeal nerve. (From Waldman SD: Atlas of Interventional Pain Management, 2nd ed. Philadelphia, Saunders, p 70, Figure 19-4.)

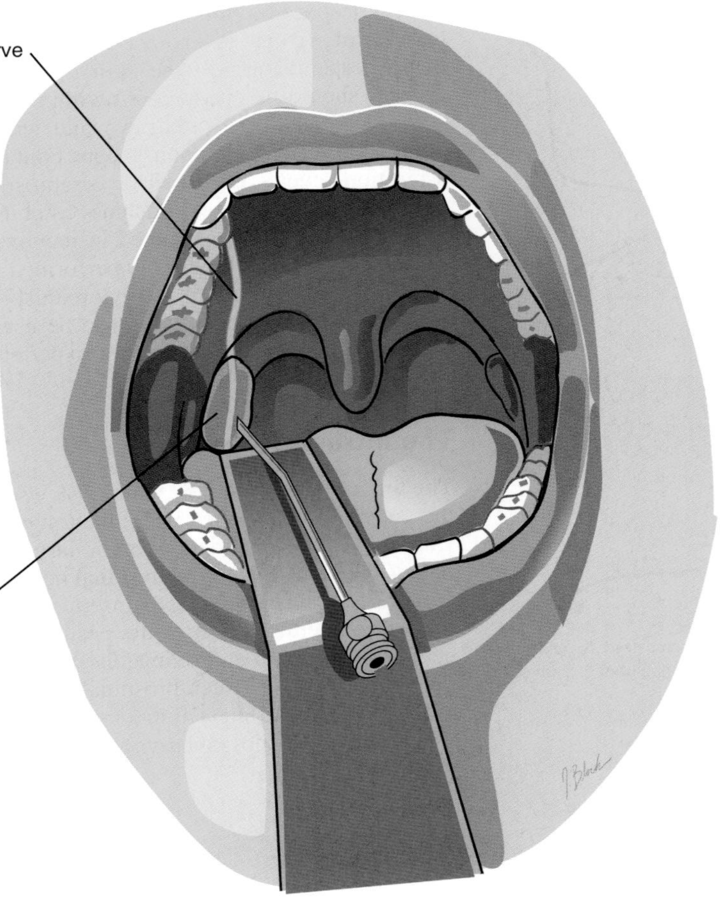

FIGURE 138–4 ■ Intraoral approach to glossopharyngeal nerve block. (From Waldman SD: Atlas of Interventional Pain Management, 2nd ed. Philadelphia, Saunders, p 80, Figure 20–1.)

POTENTIAL COMPLICATIONS OF GLOSSOPHARYNGEAL NERVE BLOCK

The major complications associated with glossopharyngeal nerve block (Table 138–3) are related to trauma to the internal jugular and carotid artery.[10] Hematoma formation and intravascular injection of local anesthetic with subsequent toxicity are significant problems for the patient. Blockade of the motor portion of the glossopharyngeal nerve can result in dysphagia secondary to weakness of the stylopharyngeus muscle.[9] If the vagus nerve is inadvertently blocked, as it often is during glossopharyngeal nerve block, dysphonia secondary to paralysis of the ipsilateral vocal cord may occur. Reflex tachycardia secondary to vagal nerve block is also observed in some patients.[10] Inadvertent block of the hypoglossal and spinal accessory nerves during glossopharyngeal nerve block will result in weakness of the tongue and trapezius muscle.[15]

A small percentage of patients who undergo chemical neurolysis or neurodestructive procedures of the glossopharyngeal nerve experience post-procedure dysesthesias in the area of anesthesia.[16] These symptoms range from a mildly uncomfortable burning or pulling sensation to severe pain. Such severe post-procedure pain is called *anesthesia dolorosa*. Anesthesia dolorosa can be worse than the patient's original pain and is often harder to treat. Sloughing of skin and subcutaneous tissue has been associated with anesthesia dolorosa.

The glossopharyngeal nerve is susceptible to trauma from needle, hematoma, or compression during injection procedures. Such complications, although usually transitory, can be quite upsetting to the patient. Although uncommon, risk of infection is ever present, especially in immunocompromised

Table 138–3

Complications and Unwanted Side Effects of Blockade of the Glossopharyngeal Nerve
Dysphagia
Ecchymosis and hematoma
Postprocedure dysesthesias
Anesthesia dolorosa
Weakness of trapezius muscle
Weakness of tongue
Hoarseness
Infection
Tachycardia
Local anesthetic toxicity
Trauma to nerves
Sloughing of skin and subcutaneous tissue

cancer patients.[6] Early detection of infection is crucial to avoiding potentially life-threatening sequelae.

NEURODESTRUCTIVE PROCEDURES

The injection of small quantities of alcohol, phenol, and glycerol into the area of the glossopharyngeal nerve often provide long-term relief from glossopharyngeal neuralgia and cancer-related pain that has been refractory to optimal trials of the therapies discussed earlier.[10,13] Destruction of the glossopharyngeal nerve can be carried out by creating a radiofrequency lesion under biplanar fluoroscopic guidance.[17] This procedure is reserved for patients in whom all the treatments discussed here for intractable glossopharyngeal neuralgia have failed and whose physical status precludes more invasive neurosurgical treatments.

MICROVASCULAR DECOMPRESSION OF THE GLOSSOPHARYNGEAL ROOT

Microvascular decompression of the glossopharyngeal root (Jannetta procedure) is the neurosurgical procedure of choice for intractable glossopharyngeal neuralgia.[18] The rationale for this operation is the theory that glossopharyngeal neuralgia is, in fact, a compressive mononeuropathy. In this operation, the glossopharyngeal root is identified close to the brain stem and the compressing blood vessel is isolated. A sponge is interposed between the vessel and nerve, effecting a cure. Intracranial section of the glossopharyngeal nerve is indicated for intractable cancer pain in the distribution of the glossopharyngeal nerve that does not respond to more conservative treatment approaches.[10]

CONCLUSION

The pain specialist should be aware of the clinical utility of glossopharyngeal nerve block. Correctly used, pharmacologic therapy combined with glossopharyngeal nerve block should control the pain of glossopharyngeal neuralgia and cancer-related pain in the distribution of the glossopharyngeal nerve in the majority of cases. Surgical therapy should be considered when conservative therapy fails to provide long-lasting relief from pain mediated via the glossopharyngeal nerve.

References

1. Weisenburg TH: Cerebello-pontine tumour diagnosed for six years as tic douloureux. JAMA 54:1600, 1910.
2. Harris W: Persistent pain in lesions of the peripheral and central nervous system. Brain 44:557, 1921.
3. Doyle JB: A study of four cases of glossopharyngeal neuralgia. Arch Neurol Psychiatr 9:34, 1923.
4. Dandy WE: Glossopharyngeal neuralgia: Its diagnosis and treatment. Arch Surg 15:198, 1927.
5. Waldman SD: The role of neural blockade in the management of headaches and facial pain. Curr Rev Pain 1:346, 1997.
6. Waldman SD: The role of nerve blocks in pain management. In Weiner R (ed): Comprehensive Guide to Pain Management. Orlando, Fla, PMD Press, 1990, p 10-1.
7. Waldman SD: Management of acute pain. Postgrad Med 87:15, 1992.
8. Waldman SD. The role of nerve blocks in the management of headache and facial pain. In Diamond S (ed): Practical Headache Management. Boston, Kluwer, 1993, p 99.
9. Brown DL: Glossopharyngeal nerve block. In Brown DL (ed): Atlas of Regional Anesthesia. Philadelphia, WB Saunders, 1999, p 203.
10. Bonica JJ: Neurolytic blockade and hypophysectomy. In Bonica JJ (ed): The Management of Pain. Philadelphia, Lea & Febiger, 1990, p 1996.
11. Waldman SD, Waldman KA: The diagnosis and treatment of glossopharyngeal neuralgia. Am J Pain Manage 5:19, 1995.
12. Pitkin GP: The glossopharyngeal nerve. In Southworth JL, Hingson RA (eds): Conduction Anesthesia. Philadelphia, JB Lippincott, 1946, p 46.
13. Bajaj P, Gemavat M, Singh DP: Ninth cranial nerve block in the management of malignant pain in its territory. Pain Clin 6:153, 1993.
14. Murphy TM: Somatic blockade of the head and neck. In Cousins MJ, Bridenbaugh PO (eds): Neural Blockade, 2nd ed. Philadelphia, JB Lippincott, 1988, p 546.
15. Katz J: Glossopharyngeal nerve block. In Katz J (ed): Atlas of Regional Anesthesia. Norwalk, Conn, Appleton & Lange, 1994, p 52.
16. Brisman R: Retrogasserian glycerol injection. In Brisman R (ed): Neurosurgical and Medical Management of Pain. Boston, Kluwer, 1989, p 51.
17. Arbit E, Krol G: Percutaneous radiofrequency neurolysis guided by computerized tomography for the treatment of glossopharyngeal neuralgia. Neurosurgery 29:580, 1991.
18. Fraioloi B, Esposito V, Ferrante L, et al: Microsurgical treatment of glossopharyngeal neuralgia. Neurosurgery 138:630, 1989.

chapter 139

Vagus Nerve Block

Steven D. Waldman

HISTORICAL CONSIDERATIONS

Early in the history of regional anesthesia, vagus nerve block was used to treat a variety of conditions that included both pain and cardiac arrhythmias. Often combined with stellate ganglion block, blockade of the vagus nerve was a mainstay in the treatment of intractable angina and pain emanating from the esophagus, trachea, and other mediastinal structures.[1] Many of the early indications for vagus nerve block now are treated medically or surgically, but vagus nerve block remains useful for management of cancer pain in structures innervated by this nerve.

INDICATIONS

Vagus nerve block with local anesthetics can be used as a diagnostic tool when performing differential neural blockade on an anatomic basis to evaluate head and facial pain.[2] When destruction of the vagus nerve is being considered, this technique is a useful indicator of the degree of motor and sensory impairment the patient may experience. Vagus nerve block with local anesthetic can be used to palliate acute pain emergencies, including vagal neuralgia and cancer pain, while waiting for pharmacologic, surgical, or antiblastic methods to take effect.[3] Vagus nerve block is used as a diagnostic and therapeutic maneuver when vagal neuralgia is suspected. Destruction of the vagus nerve is indicated for palliation of cancer pain, including that associated with invasive tumors of the larynx, hypopharynx, and pyriform sinus, and, occasionally, intrathoracic malignancies.[3,4]

Owing to the desperate situation of many patients suffering from aggressive head and neck malignancies, blockade of the vagus nerve using a 25-gauge needle may be carried out in the presence of coagulopathy or anticoagulation, albeit with increased risks of ecchymosis and hematoma formation.

CLINICALLY RELEVANT ANATOMY

The vagus nerve contains both motor and sensory fibers.[5] The motor fibers innervate the pharyngeal muscle and provide fibers for the superior and recurrent laryngeal nerves. The sensory portion of the nerve innervates the dura mater of the posterior fossa, the posterior aspect of the external auditory meatus and inferior aspect of the tympanic membrane, and the mucosa of the larynx below the vocal cords. The vagus nerve also provides fibers to the thoracic contents, including the heart, lungs, and major vessels.

The vagus nerve exits from the jugular foramen close to the spinal accessory nerve (Fig. 139–1). The vagus lies just caudad to the glossopharyngeal nerve and is superficial to the internal jugular vein. The vagus courses downward from the jugular foramen within the carotid sheath along with the internal jugular vein and internal carotid artery.

The technique of blockade of the vagus nerve is much like that of glossopharyngeal nerve block.[3] The key landmark for vagus nerve block is the styloid process of the temporal bone. This osseous process represents the calcification of the cephalad end of the stylohyoid ligament. Although usually easy to identify, if ossification is limited, the styloid process may be difficult to locate with the exploring needle.

TECHNIQUE

The patient is placed in the supine position. An imaginary line is visualized running from the mastoid process to the angle of the mandible. The styloid process should lie just below the midpoint of this line. The skin is "prepped" with antiseptic solution. A 22-gauge, 1.5-inch needle attached to a 10-mL syringe is advanced at this midpoint in a plane perpendicular to the skin. The styloid process should be encountered within 3 cm (Fig. 139–2). After contact is made, the needle is withdrawn and "walked" off the styloid process posteriorly and slightly downward. The needle is advanced approximately 0.5 cm past the depth at which the styloid process was identified. If careful aspiration reveals no blood or cerebrospinal fluid, 5 mL of 0.5% preservative-free lidocaine combined with 80 mg of methylprednisolone is injected in incremental doses. Subsequent daily nerve blocks are carried out in a similar manner, substituting 40 mg of methylprednisolone for the initial 80-mg dose. This approach may also be used for breakthrough pain in patients who previously experienced adequate pain control with oral medications.

SIDE EFFECTS AND COMPLICATIONS

The major complications of vagus nerve block are related to trauma to the internal jugular and carotid arteries.[2,3] Hematoma formation and intravascular injection of local

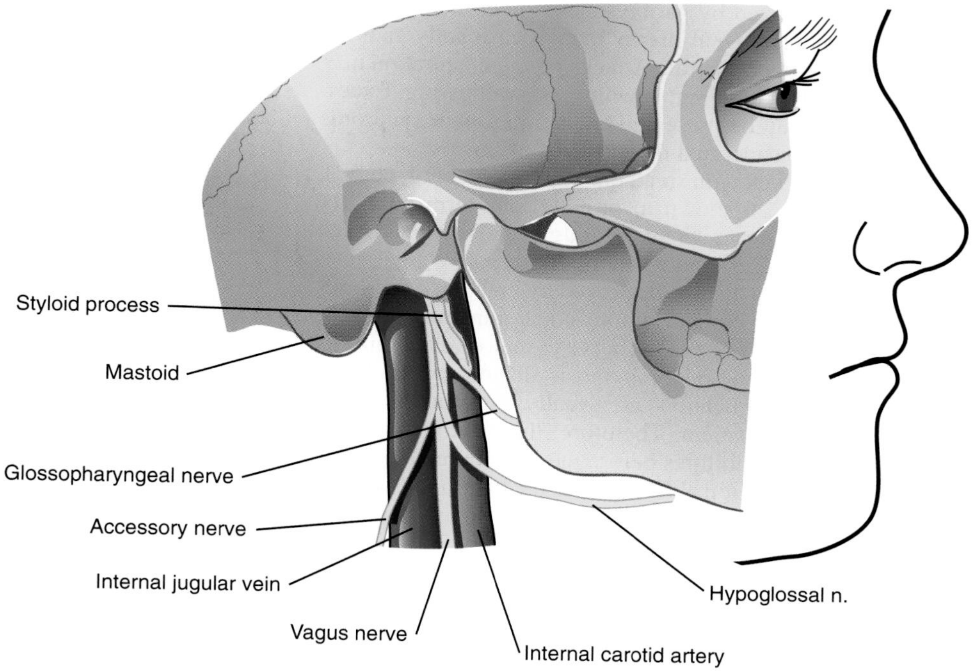

FIGURE 139–1 ■ The vagus nerve and surrounding structures.

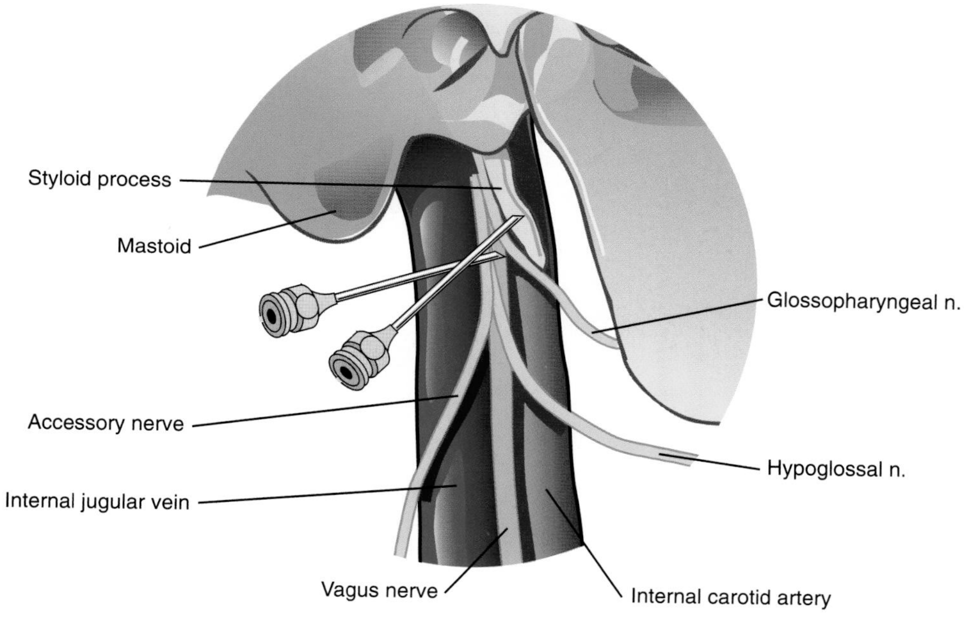

FIGURE 139–2 ■ Positioning of needle for vagus nerve block.

anesthetic (with subsequent toxicity) are not uncommon after vagus nerve block. Blockade of the motor portion of the vagus nerve can result in dysphonia and difficulty coughing secondary to blockade of the superior and recurrent laryngeal nerves. Reflex tachycardia secondary to vagal nerve block is also observed in some patients. Inadvertent block of the glossopharyngeal, hypoglossal, and spinal accessory nerves during vagus nerve block will result in weakness of the tongue and trapezius muscle and numbness in the distribution of the glossopharyngeal nerve. Although uncommon, the risk of infection is ever present, especially in immunocompromised cancer patients. Early detection of infection is crucial to avoiding potentially life-threatening sequelae.

■ CLINICAL PEARLS

Vagus nerve block should be considered in two clinical situations: (1) for vagal neuralgia, and (2) for persistent, ill-defined pain related to the cancers discussed earlier that fails to respond to conservative measures. Vagal neuralgia is clinically analogous to trigeminal and glossopharyngeal neuralgia. It is characterized by paroxysms of shock-like pain into the thyroid and laryngeal areas. Pain occasionally radiates into the jaw and upper thorax. Attacks of vagal neuralgia may be precipitated by coughing, yawning, or swallowing. Excessive salivation may be present. This is a rare pain syndrome that should be considered a diagnosis of exclusion.

Neurolytic block with small quantities of alcohol, phenol, or glycerol has been shown to provide long-term relief for patients suffering from vagus neuralgia and cancer-related pain that does not respond to more conservative treatment. The vagus nerve can also be destroyed by creating a radiofrequency lesion under biplanar fluoroscopic guidance.

The proximity of the vagus nerve to major vessels makes post-block hematoma and ecchymosis distinct possibilities. Although these complications are usually transitory, they can be upsetting to the patient. Therefore, the patient should be warned of these possibilities before the procedure. The dense vascularity of this region also increases the likelihood of inadvertent intravascular injection. Even small amounts of local anesthetic injected into the carotid artery at this level will result in local anesthetic toxicity and seizures. Incremental dosing and careful monitoring of the patient for signs of local anesthetic toxicity help to avoid these complications.

References

1. Harris W: Peripheral pain in lesions of the peripheral and central nervous systems. Brain 44:557, 1921.
2. Katz J: Vagus nerve block. In Katz J (ed): Atlas of Regional Anesthesia. Norwalk, Conn, Appleton, 1995, p 52.
3. Waldman SD: Vagus nerve block. In Waldman SD (ed): Atlas of Interventional Pain Management Techniques. Philadelphia, WB Saunders, 1998, p 76.
4. Bonica JJ: Neurolytic blockade. In Bonica JJ (ed): The Management of Pain, 2nd ed. Philadelphia, Lea & Febiger, 1990, p 1996.
5. Bonica JJ: General considerations of pain in the head. In Bonica JJ (ed): The Management of Pain, 2nd ed. Philadelphia, Lea & Febiger, 1990, p 660.

chapter 140

Phrenic Nerve Block

Mark A. Greenfield

The pain management consultant may be asked to evaluate a patient for phrenic nerve block. Blockade of the phrenic nerve, like other nerve blocks, is but one component of a multifaceted approach to the patient with acute or chronic pain syndromes. It may become a very useful treatment modality for patients who do not respond to other therapeutic interventions.

CLINICAL ANATOMY

The phrenic nerve, the most important branch of the cervical plexus, comprises the ventral roots of C3-C5—the principal component being the anterior primary ramus of C4. The three nerve roots join at the lateral border of the scalenus anterior muscle, and the phrenic nerve passes inferiorly between the omohyoid and sternocleidomastoid muscles. In 20% to 84% of patients, an accessory phrenic nerve arises from C5 and contributes to the phrenic nerve, joining the main nerve in the root of the neck or behind the clavicle.[1] In the phrenic nerve's course distally, it lies close to the internal mammary artery, the root of the lung, the pericardium, and the peritoneum. The superior and inferior sympathetic ganglia, the spinal accessory nerve, and the hypoglossal nerve also have communications with the phrenic nerve as it courses through the chest.

INDICATIONS

Phrenic nerve block can be useful in the diagnosis and treatment of intractable singultus (Latin for *sob* or *speech broken by sobbing*), or hiccups. Hiccups, while ubiquitous, serve no known physiologic function. *Persistent* hiccups are defined as an episode that lasts less than 1 month; *intractable* hiccups last longer than 1 month. Table 140–1 describes some of the complications of intractable hiccups.[2] Benign and persistent or intractable hiccup have different causes (Table 140–2).[3] Chronic idiopathic hiccups are believed to be attributable to central and peripheral mechanisms. It has been suggested that chronic hiccups may result from chronic stimulation of a central nervous system "hiccup center." The afferent limb of the hiccup reflex includes not only the phrenic nerve but also the vagus nerve and the sympathetic chain from T6-T12.[4] This hiccup center is believed to comprise a complex association between several areas of the central nervous system. This includes the phrenic nerve nuclei, the brain stem, the respiratory center, the hypothalamus, and the medullary reticular formation. The primary efferent limb of this reflex is mediated by motor fibers of the phrenic nerve. Interestingly, the majority of hiccup spasms are unilateral and usually confined to the left hemidiaphragm.[5]

The ill-defined supraclavicular or scapular pain of diaphragmatic or subdiaphragmatic cancers may be elucidated or ameliorated by phrenic nerve block. This referred pain is known as the *Kerr sign* and often does not respond to direct tumor treatments.[6]

The pain management specialist must try to establish an underlying cause to guide therapeutic intervention. A targeted history and physical examination are essential first steps, followed by laboratory studies. The work-up would also be expected to include magnetic resonance imaging (MRI) studies of the head, especially the posterior fossa and brain stem.[2,7,8] Imaging of the diaphragmatic and subdiaphragmatic regions should also be performed.

After identification and treatment of underlying causes, different therapies may be entertained. In 1932, Dr. C. W. Mayo said, in reference to the myriad remedies and treatments for hiccups, "The amount of knowledge on any subject such as this can be considered as being in inverse proportion to the number of different treatments suggested and tried for it."[9] After nonpharmacologic, noninvasive therapies have been tried and found unsuccessful, drug therapy may be used. Table 140–3 lists several medications that have been used to treat hiccups.[7,10-12]

PROCEDURE

The patient is placed supine with the head turned away from the side being blocked and is then asked to lift his or her head against resistance to identify the sternocleidomastoid muscle. The groove between the posterior border of the sternocleidomastoid muscle and the anterior scalene muscle then becomes palpable (Fig. 140–1).[13,14] At a level 1 inch above the clavicle, sterile preparation is performed. A 22-gauge, 1.5-inch block needle is inserted parallel to the scalene muscle with a slightly anterior trajectory (Fig. 140–2). At a depth of approximately 1 inch, and after gentle aspiration to identify blood or cerebrospinal fluid, 8 to 10 mL of local anesthetic is incrementally injected (infiltrated) along the anterior surface of the anterior scalene muscle. This nerve block is often done in a fan-like manner. Phrenic nerve block with local anesthetic may be used in a prognostic manner to evaluate the possibility of neurodestruction of the phrenic nerve by chemical neurolysis, cryoneurolysis, radiofrequency lesioning, phrenic nerve stimulation (diaphragmatic pacing), or surgical crushing of the nerve.[15] A depot steroid may be added to the local anesthetic for inflammation-associated pain that is mediated via the phrenic nerve.[6] A nerve stimulator with stimulation as low as 0.75 mA may be useful in this block to observe diaphragmatic contraction (via fluoroscopy or ultrasound).[16] The patient is then monitored closely for changes in vital signs (especially signs of respiratory compromise) and signs of local anesthetic toxicity and of inadvertent subarachnoid injection.

SIDE EFFECTS AND COMPLICATIONS

The proximity of several major blood vessels to the phrenic nerve may produce local anesthetic toxicity from intravascular uptake or inadvertent intravascular injection.[17] In addition, the vascularity of this region may result in hematoma and/or ecchymosis. While many of these vessels may be available by direct pressure to control bleeding, bleeding of the subclavian vessels may be difficult to control. Manual pressure to the area blocked and application of ice packs after the nerve block is performed decrease bleeding or ecchymosis. Ice packs applied at 20-minute intervals may also be useful in limiting these side effects or complications.

With injection of the phrenic nerve, unilateral diaphragmatic paralysis is expected. Unilateral paralysis of the diaphragm may lead to a 37% reduction in total lung capacity. Maximal voluntary ventilation and vital capacity may be decreased by 20%.[18] This reduction in lung function may be exacerbated by spread of the local anesthetic solution to the recurrent laryngeal nerve and difficulty in clearing

Table 140–1

Complications of Intractable Hiccups

- Malnutrition
- Cardiac dysrhythmias
- Insomnia
- Fatigue/exhaustion/dehydration
- Gastroesophageal reflux
- Weight loss
- Death

Table 140–2

Causes of Persistent or Intractable Hiccups

- Idiopathic psychogenic
  - Conversion reaction
  - Malingering
  - Hysterical neurosis
  - Personality disorder
- Organic
  - Central nervous system
    - Neoplasm
    - Multiple sclerosis
    - Cerebrovascular accident
    - Trauma
  - Peripheral nervous system (secondary to phrenic or vagus nerve irritation)
    - Renal (uremia) or hepatic disorders
    - Cancer (gastric, pancreatic, pulmonary)
    - Pericarditis
    - Intestinal obstruction/gastric distention
    - Tumors or cysts of neck
    - Hiatal hernia
- Drug-induced/metabolic
  - Intravenous steroids
  - Benzodiazepines, barbiturates
  - General anesthesia
  - Infection (sepsis, malaria, tuberculosis, influenza)
  - Electrolyte disturbances (hypocalcemia, hyponatremia)

Table 140–3

Pharmacologic Management of Hiccups

Drug	*Class*	*Action*
Chlorpromazine	Phenothiazine	Central
Haloperidol		Central
Amitriptyline	Tricyclic antidepressant	Central
Diphenylhydantoin		Central
Valproic acid	Anticonvulsant	Central
Carbamazepine		Central
Baclofen	GABA mimetic	Central
Gabapentin	Anticonvulsant	Central
Nifedipine	Calcium channel blocker	Central, peripheral
Nimodipine		Central, peripheral
Metoclopramide	Dopamine antagonist	Gastric emptying
Midazolam	Benzodiazepine	Central
Omeprazole	Proton pump inhibitor	Suppresses gastric acid
Cisapride	Myenteric plexus activity	Facilitates gastric emptying

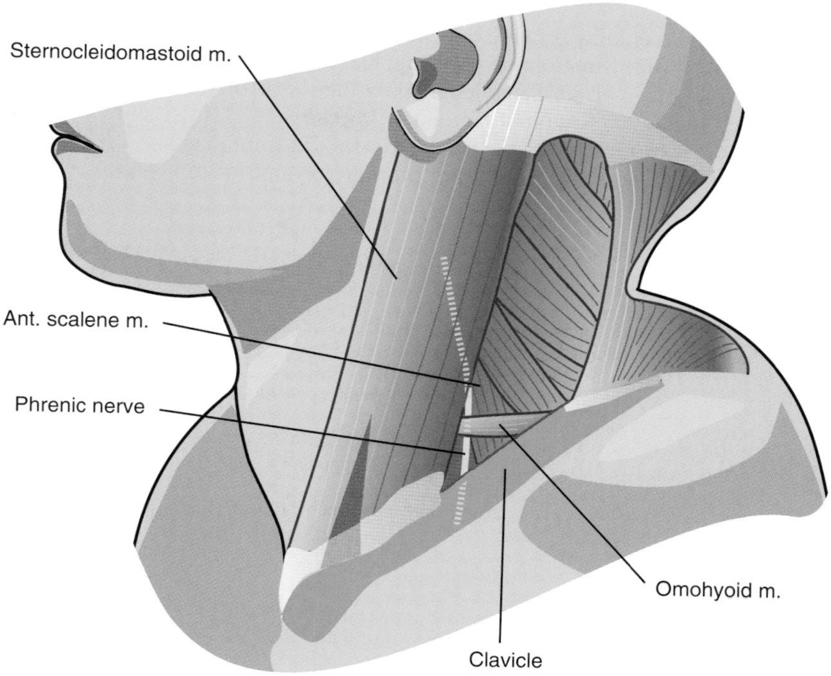

FIGURE 140–1 ■ Relation of the phrenic nerve to the muscles of the neck.

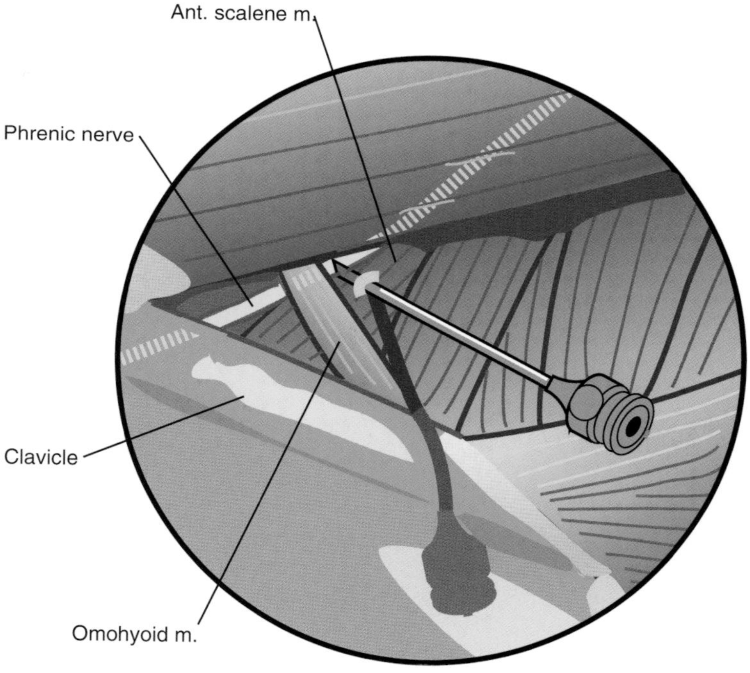

FIGURE 140–2 ■ Needle placement for phrenic nerve block.

secretions secondary to vocal cord paralysis and associated hoarseness.

The phrenic nerve also lies close to central neuraxial structures. Should the needle be placed too deep, unintended subarachnoid or epidural block could result. The consequences of either block could be significant sensory and motor block and marked respiratory compromise, or even cardiopulmonary arrest. Other possible complications of phrenic nerve block are infection and pneumothorax. Horner syndrome may be produced by spread of local anesthetic to the sympathetic ganglia. Left phrenic nerve block carries a risk of injury to the thoracic duct and, possibly, formation of a chylothorax.

CONCLUSIONS

Phrenic nerve block is a useful diagnostic and therapeutic tool. The primary indications are chronic hiccups refractory to other nonpharmacologic and pharmacologic interventions. Phrenic nerve block may provide the pain management physician with useful information for the diagnosis and treatment of chronic shoulder or supraclavicular pain that is mediated by diaphragmatic or subdiaphragmatic processes. Careful attention to the clinically relevant anatomy should minimize side effects and complications and promote symptomatic relief.

References

1. Fodstad H, Nilsson S: Intractable singultus: A diagnostic and therapeutic challenge. Br J Neurosurg 7:255, 1993.
2. Rousseau P: Hiccups. South Med J 2:175, 1995.
3. Petroianu G: Idiopathic chronic hiccup (ICH): Phrenic nerve block is not the way to go. Anesthesiology 5:1284, 1998.
4. Lewis JH: Hiccups: Causes and cures. J Clin Gastroenterol 7:539, 1985.
5. Kolodzik PW, Eilers MA: Hiccups: Review and approach to management. Ann Emerg Med 20:565, 1991.
6. Waldman SD: Atlas of Interventional Pain Management. Philadelphia, WB Saunders, 1998, p 83.
7. Petroianu G, Hein G, Petroianu A, et al: ETICS study: Empirical therapy of idiopathic chronic singultus. Z Gastroenterol 36:559, 1998.
8. Williamson BW: Management of intractable hiccup. Br Med J 2:501, 1977.
9. Mayo CW: Hiccup. Surg Gynecol Obstet 55:700, 1932.
10. Friedman NL: Hiccups: A treatment review. Pharmacotherapy 6:986, 1996.
11. Hernandez JL, Fernandez-Miera MF, Sampedro I, et al: Nimodipine treatment for intractable hiccups. Am J Med 106:600, 1999.
12. Quigley C: Nifedipine for hiccups. J Pain Symptom Manage 13:313, 1997.
13. Walker P, Watanabe S, Bruera E: Baclofen, a treatment for chronic hiccup. J Pain Symptom Manage 16:125, 1998.
14. Wilcock A, Twycross R: Midazolam for intractable hiccup. J Pain Symptom Manage 12:59, 1996.
15. Fodstad H, Blom S: Phrenic nerve stimulation (diaphragm pacing) in chronic singultus. Neurochirurgia (Stuttg) 140:115, 1984.
16. Okuda Y, Kitajima T, Asai T: Use of a nerve stimulator for phrenic nerve block in treatment of hiccups. Anesthesiology 88:525, 1998.
17. Bonica JJ: Regional analgesia with local anesthetics. In Bonica JJ (ed): The Management of Pain. Philadelphia, Lea & Febiger, 1990, p 1903.
18. Baum GL: Neurologic diseases. In Baum GL, Wolinsky PMD (eds): Textbook of Pulmonary Diseases. Orlando, Fla, 1994, p 1673.

chapter 141

Cervical Plexus Block

John L. Pappas and Carol A. Warfield

HISTORY

Cervical plexus blocks were first performed by Halsted at Bellevue Hospital in New York in 1884.[1-3] Halsted performed many experiments with the new anesthetic cocaine, including one that showed excellent surgical anesthesia could be obtained by injecting the nerve trunks in the neck. The first description of cervical plexus block for surgical anesthesia was published in Germany in 1912 by Kappis,[4] who advocated a posterior approach. Two years later, Heidenhein[5] introduced the lateral approach to cervical plexus block. These techniques were popularized in France by Pauchet and in the United States by Labat.[1]

The posterior approach has never achieved widespread acceptance except as an alternative to the lateral approach. Through the years, many modifications of the lateral approach have been described. Most modifications have altered the position of the primary line that connects the tip of the mastoid process to the anterior tubercle of C6. The change in position is intended to place the primary line more precisely over the tips of the cervical transverse processes.[2] Other methods of cervical plexus block have included a single-injection technique and a technique that uses the angle of the mandible and the thyroid notch as topographic landmarks to improve the success rate of the block.[1,3,6-8] The lateral and posterior approaches to cervical plexus blockade are described here.

INDICATIONS

Cervical plexus block has a variety of indications. Because it can be performed easily in a supine patient, almost any patient is a candidate. Surgical procedures in the anterior and lateral neck and supraclavicular fossa can be performed using superficial or deep cervical plexus blocks.[3,7]

Superficial cervical plexus block provides surface anesthesia of the neck, but not muscle relaxation. Superficial cervical plexus block provides the same sensory (dermatome) anesthesia as deep cervical plexus block, which simply incorporates the motor component of the cervical plexus at the nerve roots before the sensory and motor aspects separate.[9] It is useful in procedures in which retraction of the major muscles of the neck is not required, such as cervical fat pad biopsy, lymph node biopsy, plastic procedures, and superficial surgical procedures in the neck.[8,9] Some workers have advocated superficial cervical plexus blocks for carotid artery surgery to avoid the potential complications of deep cervical plexus block.[10-12] For adequate anesthesia, however, it also may be necessary to inject local anesthetic under the carotid sheath, under the adventitia of the carotid bifurcation, and into the superior angle of the incision.

Deep cervical plexus block provides anesthesia of the deep and superficial branches of the cervical plexus because the nerve roots are anesthetized before the motor and sensory components separate. The deep block anesthetizes not only all the sensory components of the cervical plexus, but also the muscles that arise and insert on the corresponding cervical vertebrae and transverse processes of C2-4.[9]

Practically any procedure involving the anterior or lateral aspect of the neck may be performed with this technique, including dissections of the neck; excision of masses, tumors, thyroglossal cysts, or branchial cysts; operations on the thyroid, parathyroid, or lymph glands; operations on the trachea and larynx; and operations on the blood vessels, including ligations of the carotid and lingual arteries and carotid endarterectomy.[1,6] Most of these procedures require only unilateral block of the deep cervical plexus. Bilateral block is advocated, however, for any operative procedure that extends to within ½ inch of the midline of the neck.[1] Such procedures include thyroidectomy and excision of the lymphatic glands of the neck. During thyroidectomy, despite the depth of anesthesia after bilateral blockade, traction on the gland is felt as choking, so intravenous sedation is required.[6] In addition, bilateral blockade causes bilateral phrenic nerve paresis and carries the potential for respiratory compromise.

Carotid endarterectomies are perhaps the most common procedures performed with cervical plexus block. Most clinicians who use regional anesthetic techniques for these procedures advocate performing superficial and deep cervical plexus block to ensure a high success rate, owing to the difficulties of establishing general anesthesia and endotracheal intubation with an open wound in the neck. Several studies have compared general anesthesia with regional anesthesia for carotid endarterectomy. Most cited the value of direct assessment of central nervous system function in the awake patient and the ability to assess the need for vascular shunting as the major advantages of regional anesthesia.[13-19]

Cervical plexus blocks also are performed for relief of pain in the neck and occiput secondary to pharyngeal cancer and metastatic lesions and for occipital and posterior auricular neuralgias associated with acute inflammation or compression of the cervical plexus by tumors or aneurysms.[3,17-21] Deep cervical plexus blockade, especially bilateral blockade of the fourth cervical nerve, is useful for relief of hiccups. The success of the block may be determined during fluoroscopy, which should show bilateral diaphragmatic paresis. Although the paresis is temporary, permanent relief may be afforded by breaking the hiccup cycle.[3,6]

CONTRAINDICATIONS

There are no specific contraindications to cervical plexus block aside from contraindications to regional blocks in general, such as coagulopathy, infection at the site of the block, history of allergy to local anesthetics, and patient refusal.[7] Significant respiratory disease is a relative contraindication, especially to bilateral cervical plexus block, because of the potential for blockade of the phrenic nerve, which can cause diaphragmatic paralysis.

ANATOMY OF THE CERVICAL PLEXUS

The cervical plexus is formed by the anterior primary division of the first four cervical nerves. The anterior and posterior roots of cervical nerves C2-4 emerge from the spinal canal through their respective intervertebral foramina. The first cervical nerve, the suboccipital nerve, emerges between the occipital bone and the posterior arch of the atlas. The posterior sensory root of this nerve is much smaller than the anterior motor root and may be entirely absent (Fig. 141–1).[1]

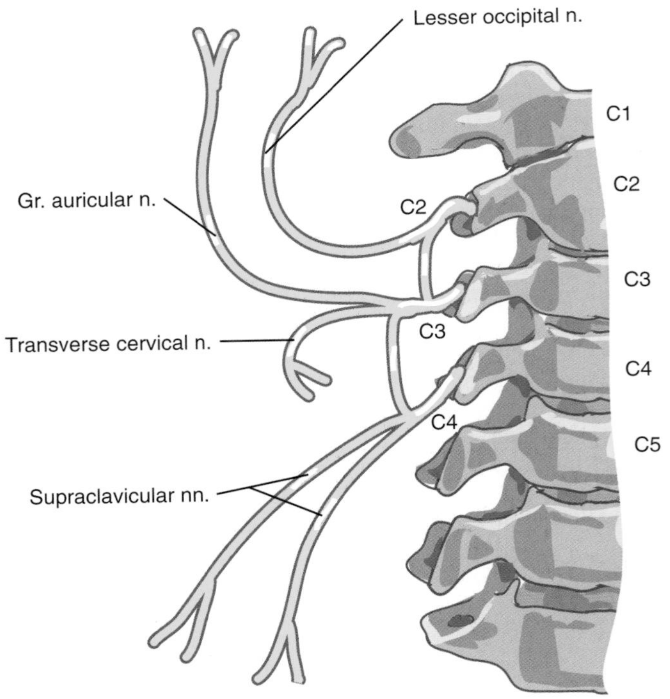

FIGURE 141–1 ■ Formation of the cervical plexus and its branches.

After the mixed nerves are formed by the union of the anterior and posterior roots, they divide into anterior and posterior primary divisions. The exception is the first cervical nerve, which seldom has an anterior division. Because the first cervical nerve is composed almost exclusively of motor fibers to the muscles of the suboccipital triangle and only rarely has any significant sensory component, it is usually unnecessary to block this nerve.

After exiting the intervertebral foramina, the anterior primary rami of C2-4 pass in an anterocaudolateral direction behind the vertebral artery and vein, in the gutter formed by the anterior and posterior tubercles of the corresponding transverse processes of the cervical vertebrae (Fig. 141–2).[3,22] The tubercles of the transverse processes lie ½ inch (1.3 cm) to 1¼ inches (3.2 cm) below the skin, depending on the size of the patient and the cervical level. The lower cervical tubercles are more superficial than the tubercles of the upper cervical transverse processes.[23] The anterior tubercles are located farther cephalad and medial than the posterior tubercles.[1]

The first cervical nerve passes under the vertebral artery in its relationship to the posterior arch of the atlas and is held in place by a fibrous tunnel.[1] The anterior primary rami of C2-4 also are held firmly on the transverse process by a fibrous tunnel. After leaving the transverse processes, these nerves are enclosed in a perineural space formed by the muscles and tendons attached to the anterior and posterior tubercles of their respective cervical vertebrae. The muscles and tendons of the anterior tubercles are the longus colli, the longus capitis, and the scalenus anterior. The muscles and tendons attached to the posterior tubercles are the scalenus medius, the scalenus cervicis, and the longissimus cervicis.[1,2] As the prevertebral fascia moves laterally and splits to invest these muscles and tendons, it forms a closed fascial space that is a superior extension of the interscalene space (Fig. 141–3).[2] The fascia investing the muscles and tendons that lie anterior and posterior to the cervical plexus provides an envelope around the plexus, which can serve as a perineural sheath and provides the basis for a single-injection technique to block the cervical plexus.[2]

Within the perineural sheath, the anterior primary rami of C2-4 divide into ascending and descending branches forming a series of three loops known as the *cervical plexus* (Fig. 141–4).[2,3,23,24] The cervical plexus, which lies lateral to the upper four cervical vertebrae and anterior to the levator scapulae muscle and the middle scalene muscle, is covered by the sternocleidomastoid muscle. Each loop gives rise to a superficial and a deep branch. This anatomic separation enables the sensory branches of the cervical plexus, via the superficial branches, to be blocked selectively without any motor blockade in the neck.

The superficial branches of the cervical plexus pierce the deep fascia of the neck approximately at the middle of the posterior margin of the sternocleidomastoid muscle, just below the emergence of the accessory nerve. Then they curve around the posterior border of the muscle and proceed to supply the skin and superficial fasciae of the head, neck, and shoulder (Figs. 141–5 and 141–6). The ascending branches (small occipital and great auricular nerves) supply the occipitomastoid region of the head, the auricle of the ear, and the parotid gland; the transverse branch (superficial cervical) innervates the anterior part of the neck between the lower border of the jaw and the sterum; and the descending branches

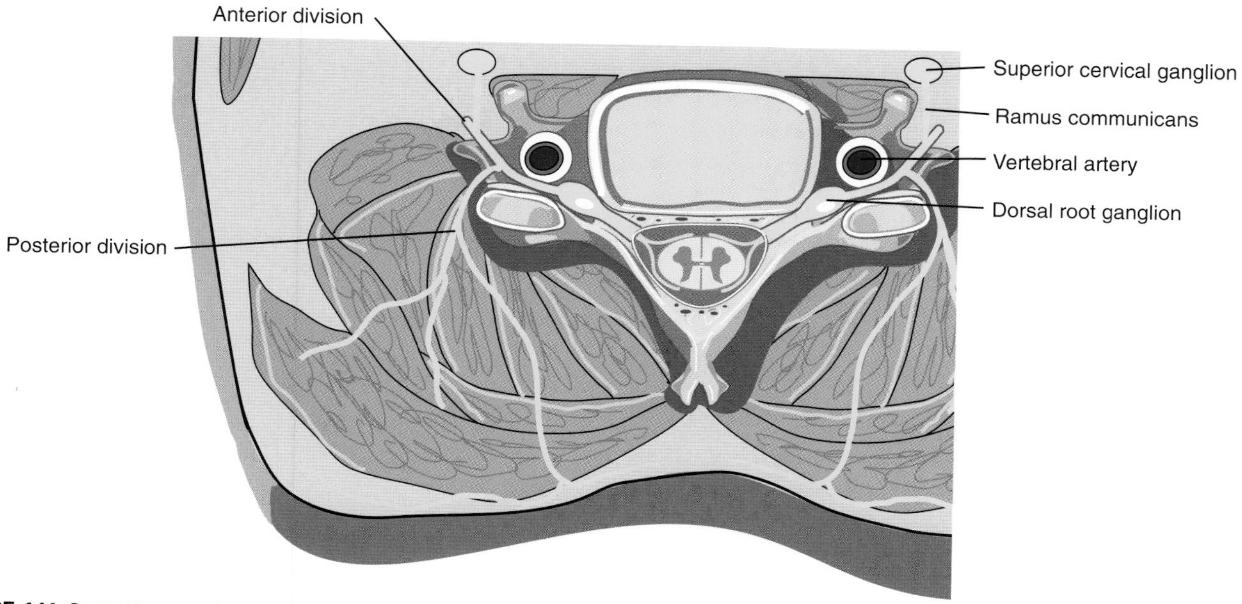

FIGURE 141–2 ■ Cross-section of the third cervical segment showing the course and distribution of the posterior primary division with its medial branch passing posteriorly to supply the skin and subcutaneous structures and the lateral branch supplying the muscles. Also shown is a cross-section of the superior cervical ganglion and its connection to the nerve by the white ramus communicans. Note the vertebral vessels just anterior to the nerves.

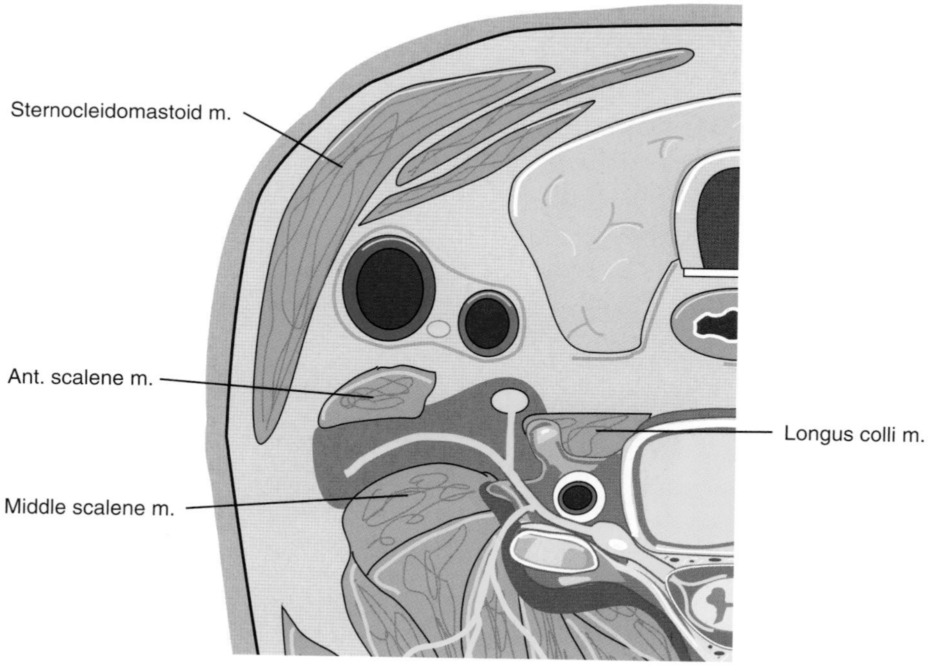

FIGURE 141–3 ■ After leaving the intervertebral foramina, the anterior primary rami of the cervical nerves pass laterally behind the vertebral artery and vein in the gutter formed by the anterior and posterior tubercles of the corresponding transverse processes of the cervical vertebrae. In this short course, each ramus actually lies in a short fibrous tunnel formed by the transverse processes superiorly and inferiorly and by the anterior and posterior intertransverse muscles (not shown here), which extend, respectively, between the anterior and posterior tubercles of the transverse processes of the contiguous cervical vertebrae. The posterior primary division leaves the anterior division just before the latter passes between the two tubercles so that injected anesthetic solutions must move centrad into this tunnel to block the posterior division.

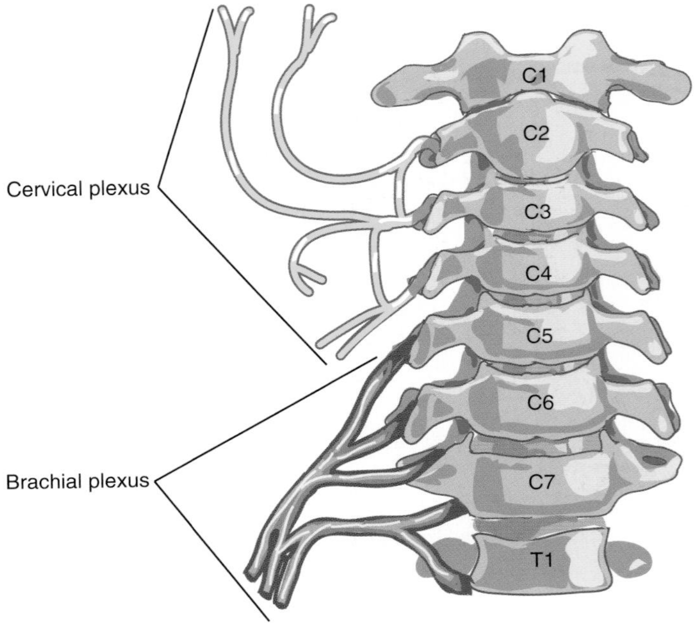

FIGURE 141–4 ■ Cervical and first thoracic spinal nerves. Anterior view showing the formation of the cervical and brachial plexus.

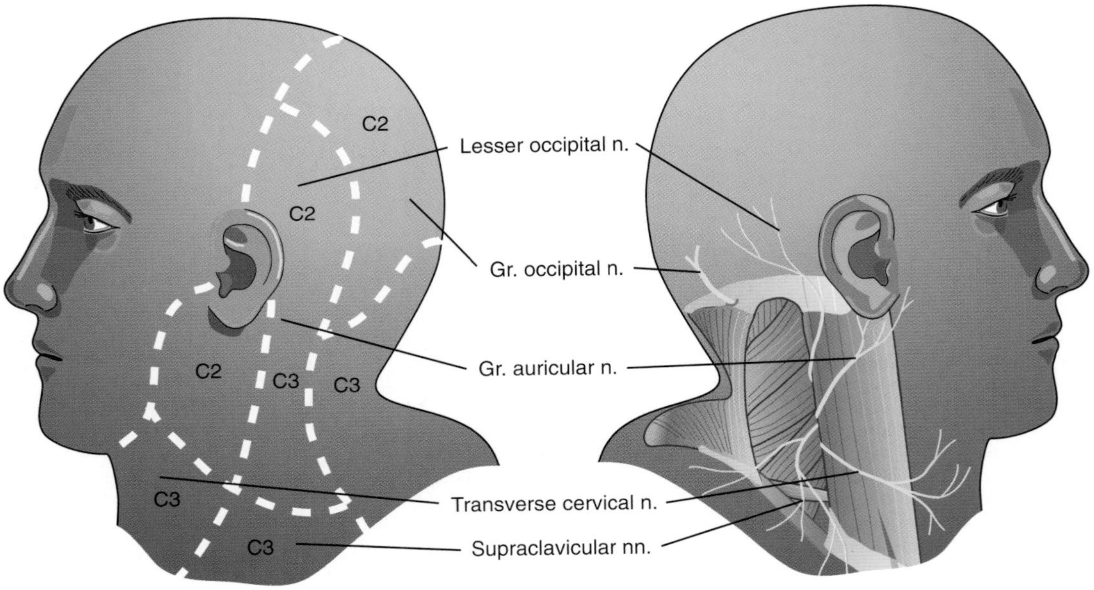

FIGURE 141–5 ■ Cutaneous nerves derived from the cervical plexus.

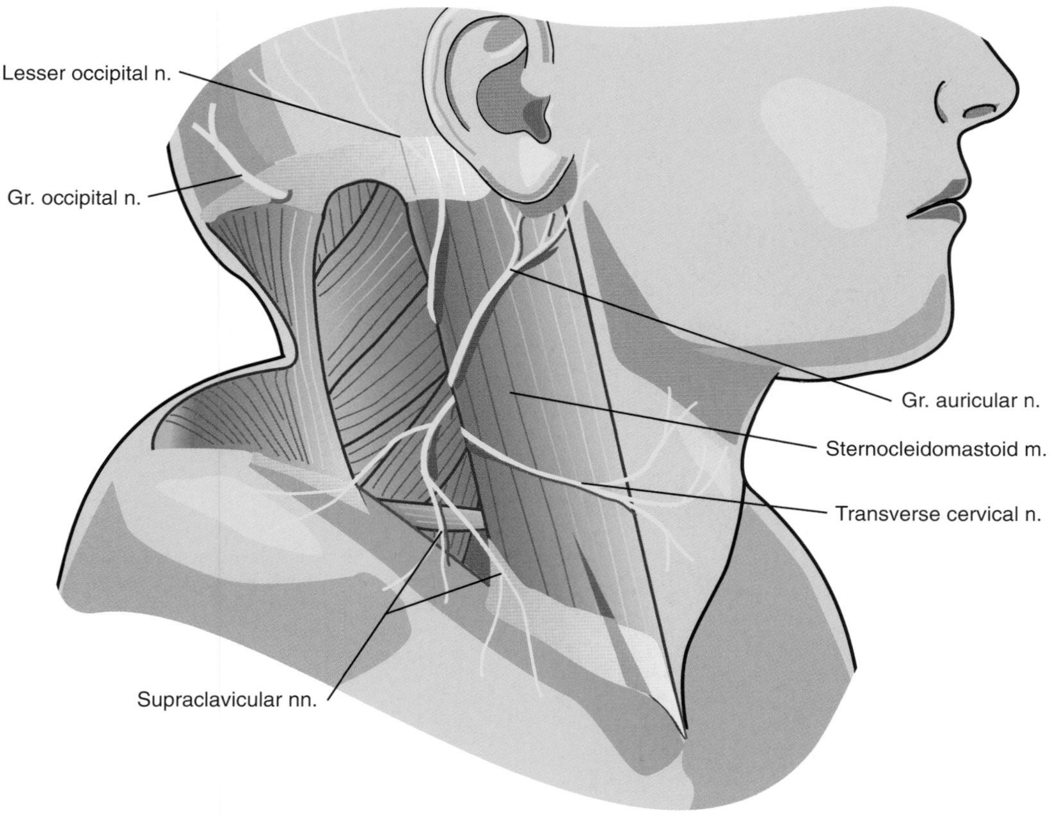

FIGURE 141–6 ■ Superficial branches of the cervical plexus at their points of emergence on the posterior margin of the sternocleidomastoid muscle.

(suprasternal, supraclavicular, and supra-acromial) supply the shoulder and upper pectoral region (Fig. 141–7).[6,7,21,24]

The deep cervical plexus supplies mainly the deep structures of the anterior and lateral neck and sends branches to the phrenic nerve (Fig. 141–8). It also contributes to the hypoglossal loop.[3,6] One group of nerve branches, the lateral (external) group, proceeds from beneath the sternocleidomastoid muscle in a posterolateral direction toward the posterior triangle. This group provides muscular branches to the scalenus medius, sternocleidomastoid, trapezius, and levator scapulae muscles. The medial (ventral) group runs medially and forward to the anterior triangle. It provides muscular branches to the rectus capitis lateralis and rectus capitis anterior, longus capitis, and longus colli muscles and to the diaphragm via the phrenic nerve. By means of the ansa hypoglossi, it also innervates the thyrohyoid, geniohyoid, omohyoid, sternothyroid, and sternohyoid muscles (Fig. 141–9).[3,6,24]

The cervical plexus communicates with the sympathetic chain in the neck by means of rami communicantes. Sympathetic fibers do not accompany the spinal nerves from their origin in the cord. Instead, they are derived from the superior, middle, and inferior (stellate) cervical ganglia (Fig. 141–10).[6,24] The cervical plexus also communicates with the vagus, hypoglossal, and accessory cervical nerves.[24] These communications may explain some of the side effects often seen with cervical plexus block.

CLINICAL PEARLS AND TRICKS OF THE TRADE

The choice of a superficial or deep cervical plexus block, or both, is based on the surgical procedure and the desired extent of anesthesia. Only one technique has been described for superficial block, whereas multiple techniques are available for deep block.

Technique of Superficial Block

Superficial cervical plexus block provides the same sensory (dermatome) anesthesia as deep cervical plexus block, which also incorporates the motor component of the cervical plexus at the nerve roots before the sensory and motor branches separate.[9] The patient is placed in the supine position with the head turned away from the side to be blocked. The patient may be asked to raise the head slightly to outline better the border of the sternocleidomastoid muscle midway between its origin on the clavicle and its insertion on the mastoid. This is also the point where the external jugular vein crosses the posterior border of the sternocleidomastoid muscle (Fig. 141–11).

Superficial cervical plexus blockade requires a sufficient volume of local anesthetic to be effective. A 4-cm, 22-gauge or a 1-inch, 25-gauge needle is inserted subcutaneously immediately posterior and deep to the midpoint of the

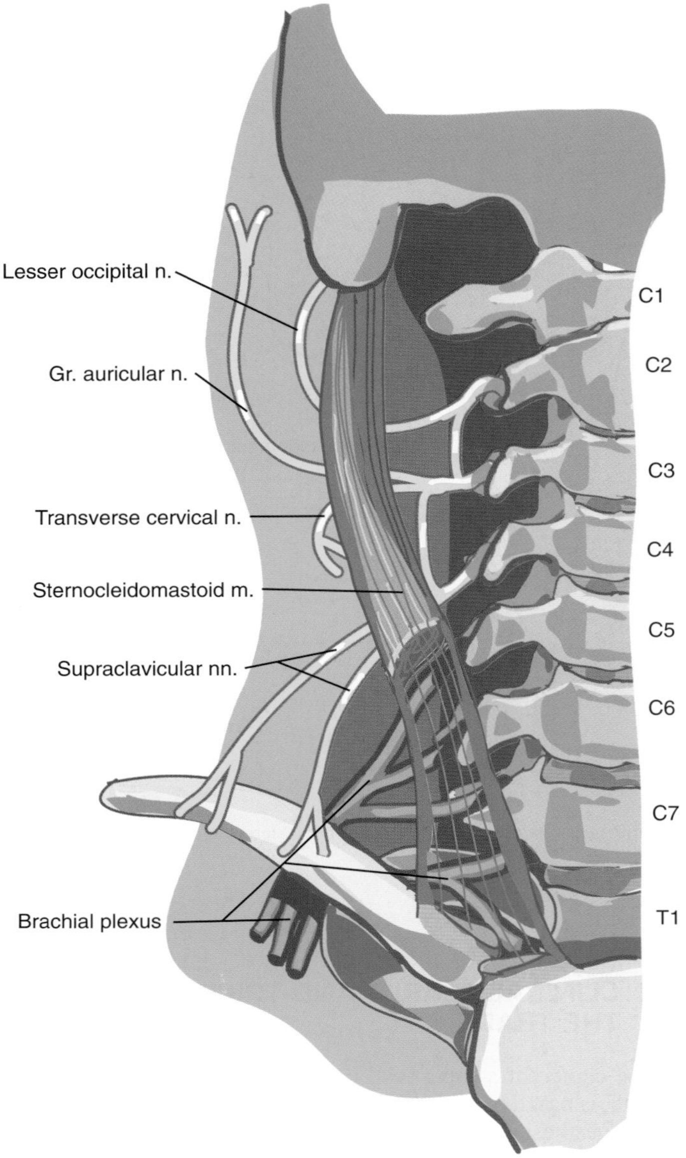

FIGURE 141–7 ■ Semischematic representation of the cervical plexus and the phrenic nerve shown in relation to the transverse processes, which are threaded by the vertebral blood vessels.

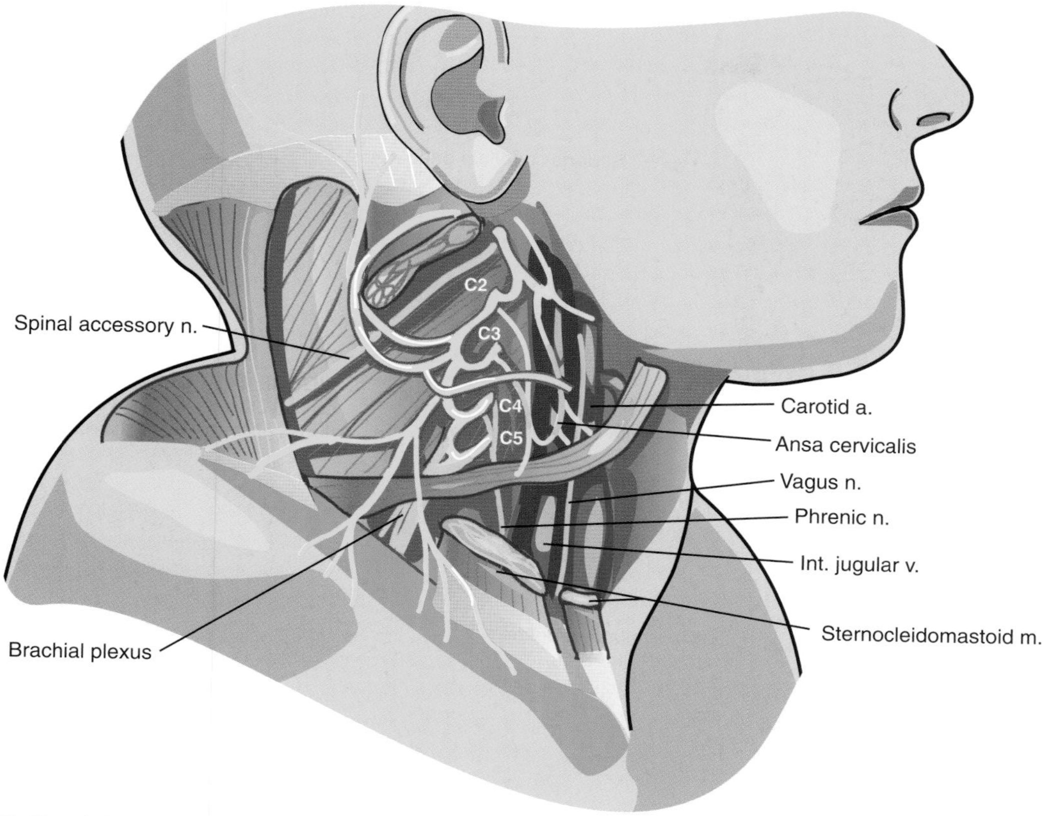

FIGURE 141–8 ■ The relationship of the cervical plexus and the phrenic nerve.

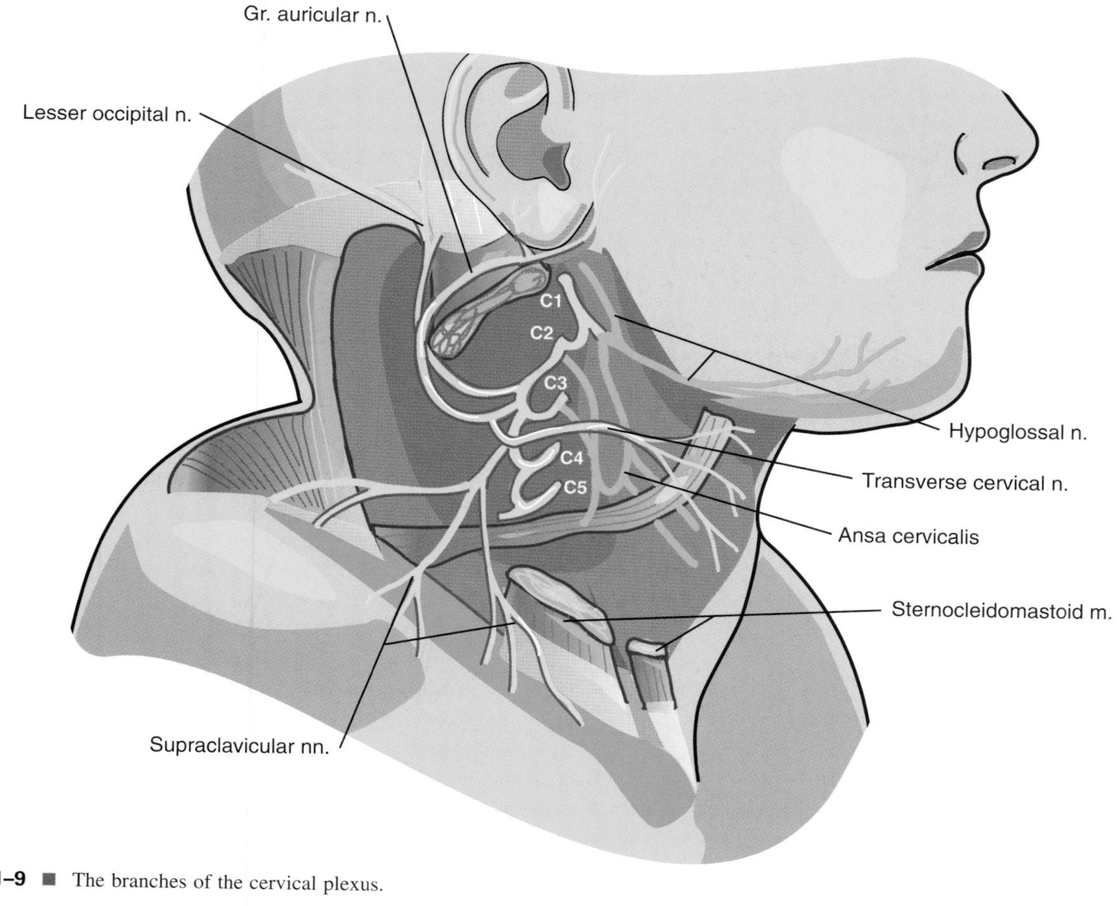

FIGURE 141–9 ■ The branches of the cervical plexus.

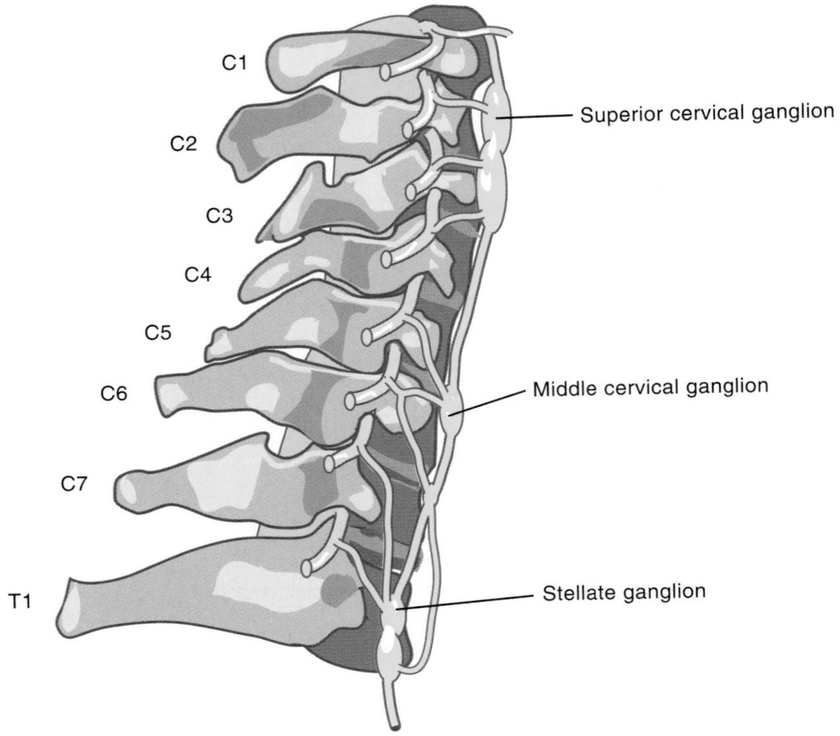

FIGURE 141–10 ■ Cervical and first thoracic spinal nerves. Lateral view showing the course and relation of the cervical nerves and the cervical sympathetic chain.

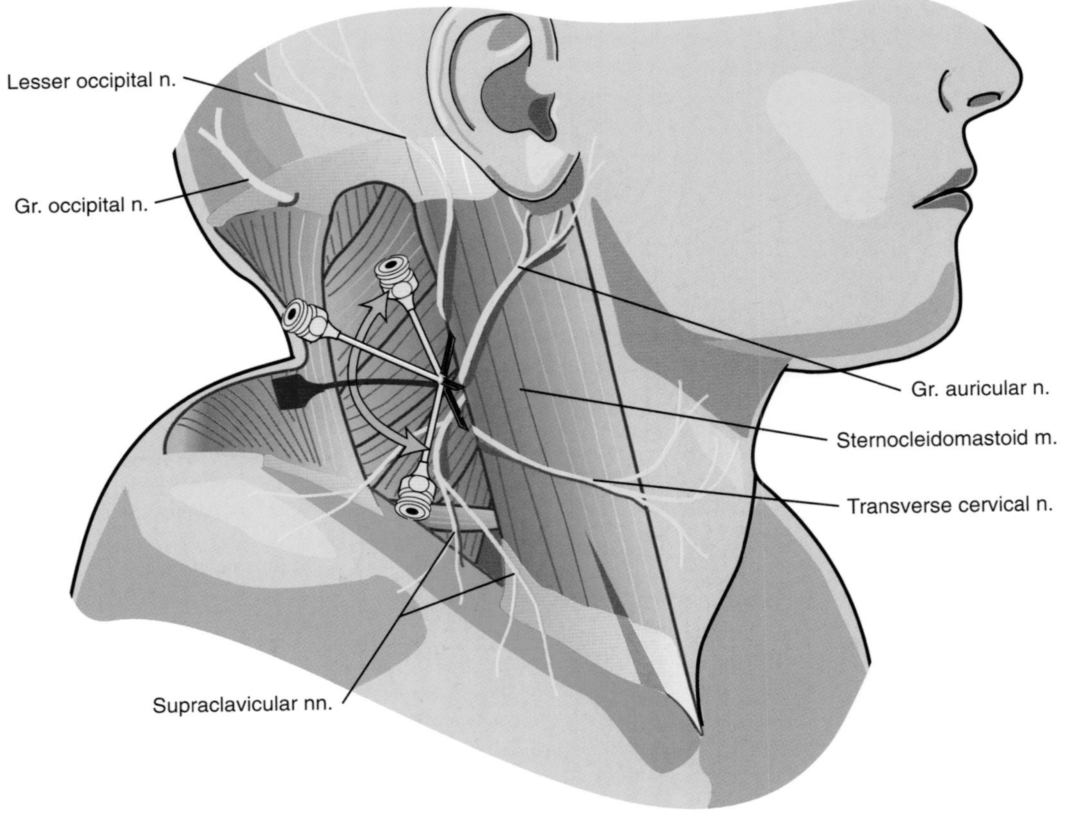

FIGURE 141–11 ■ The technique of superficial cervical plexus block.

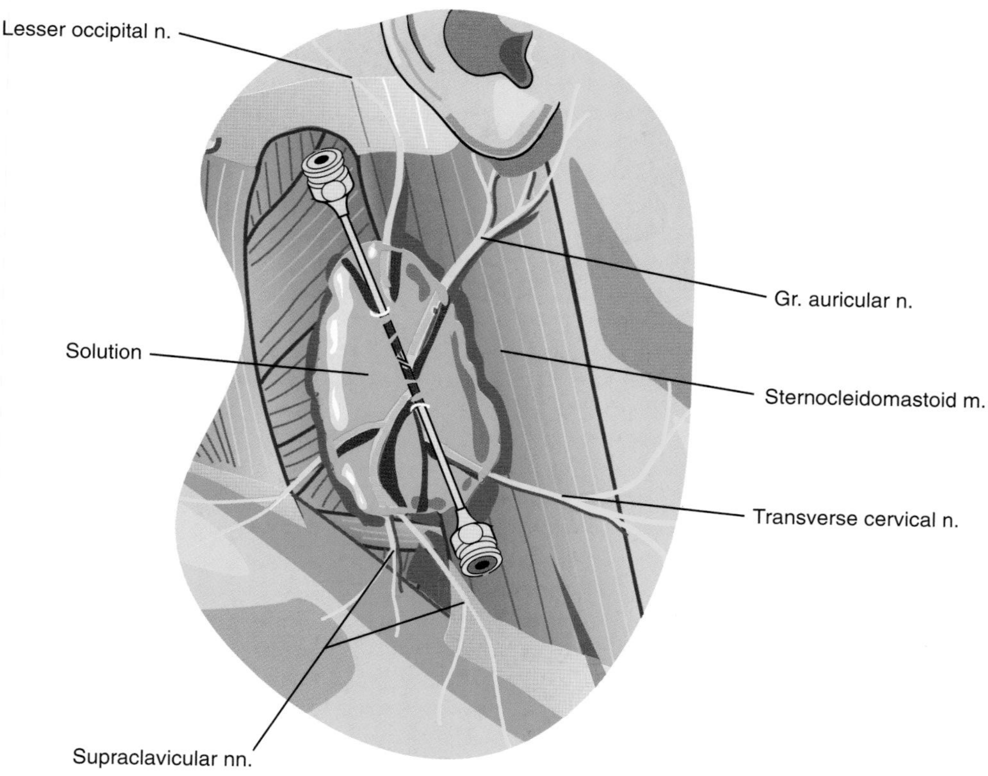

FIGURE 141–12 ■ The technique of superficial cervical plexus block.

sternocleidomastoid muscle. Approximately 5 mL of local anesthetic is injected at this midpoint. The needle is redirected superiorly and inferiorly along the posterior border of the sternocleidomastoid muscle, and approximately 5 mL of local anesthetic is injected along each of these sites for a total of 15 mL of local anesthetic (Fig. 141–12).[8,21,22,25] Paresthesias are not sought. This injection produces cutaneous analgesia of the neck from the mandible to the clavicle anteriorly and laterally (Fig. 141–13).[21]

Technique of Deep Block

Deep cervical plexus block anesthetizes all of the sensory components of the cervical plexus and the muscles that arise and insert on the corresponding cervical vertebrae and transverse processes of C2-4. If this deep cervical plexus is blocked close to the lateral edges of the transverse processes, the nerve roots are anesthetized before the motor and sensory components separate. This is one of the primary differences between deep and superficial cervical plexus blocks.[9] A deep cervical plexus block is a paravertebral nerve block of C2-4 as the nerves emerge from the foramina in the cervical vertebrae. The patient is in the same position as for superficial cervical plexus block.

The lateral route, also known as the Heidenhein or Labat method, is most often described because the superficial landmarks for this technique are numerous and reliable. A mark is placed on the tip of the mastoid process of the temporal bone behind the ear. A second mark is placed on the anterior tubercle of the C6 transverse process, Chassaignac's tubercle, at the level of the cricoid cartilage. The most prominent cervical transverse process, C6, may be felt by deep palpation between the trachea and carotid sheath at the level of the cricoid cartilage. A straight line, known as the *primary line*, is drawn between these two marks to indicate the position of the cervical transverse processes. Some authors advocate drawing this line parallel and 1 cm posterior to the first line to produce a more accurate superficial indicator of the cervical transverse processes below.[22] Other authors construct the primary line by connecting the mastoid process with the suprasternal notch.[25]

On this line, the transverse processes of C2-4 are palpated. The transverse process of C2 is approximately 1.5 cm caudad to the tip of the mastoid process. Points marked 1.5 and 3 cm below this first point on the primary line indicate the transverse processes of C3 and C4. The transverse process of C3 can be found at the level of the body of the hyoid bone, and the C4 transverse process is located at the level of the upper border of the thyroid cartilage (Figs. 141–14 and 141–15).

Skin wheals are raised at these three points with a 27-gauge needle. A 5-cm, 22-gauge or a 1-inch, 25-gauge, short beveled block needle is inserted medially and caudad to a depth of 1.5 to 2 cm, until the tip of the transverse process is contacted at the three designated points. The needle is walked laterally until it slips off the most lateral aspect of the bone, and the tip is identified again. It is important to locate the transverse processes as far laterally as possible to avoid injection into the vertebral artery.[26] It is important to maintain a caudad direction to avoid unintentional entry into the intervertebral foramen, which would result in epidural or subarachnoid injection (Fig. 141–16). Paresthesias may or may not be elicited. After careful aspiration for blood and CSF, 3 to 5 mL of local anesthetic is injected through each

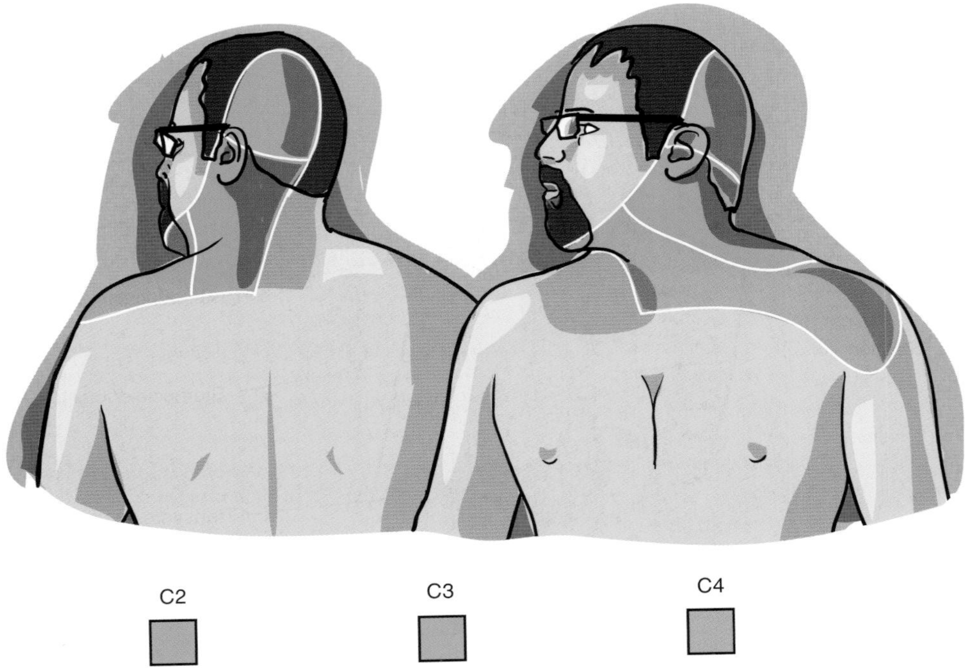

FIGURE 141–13 ■ The technique of superficial cervical plexus block.

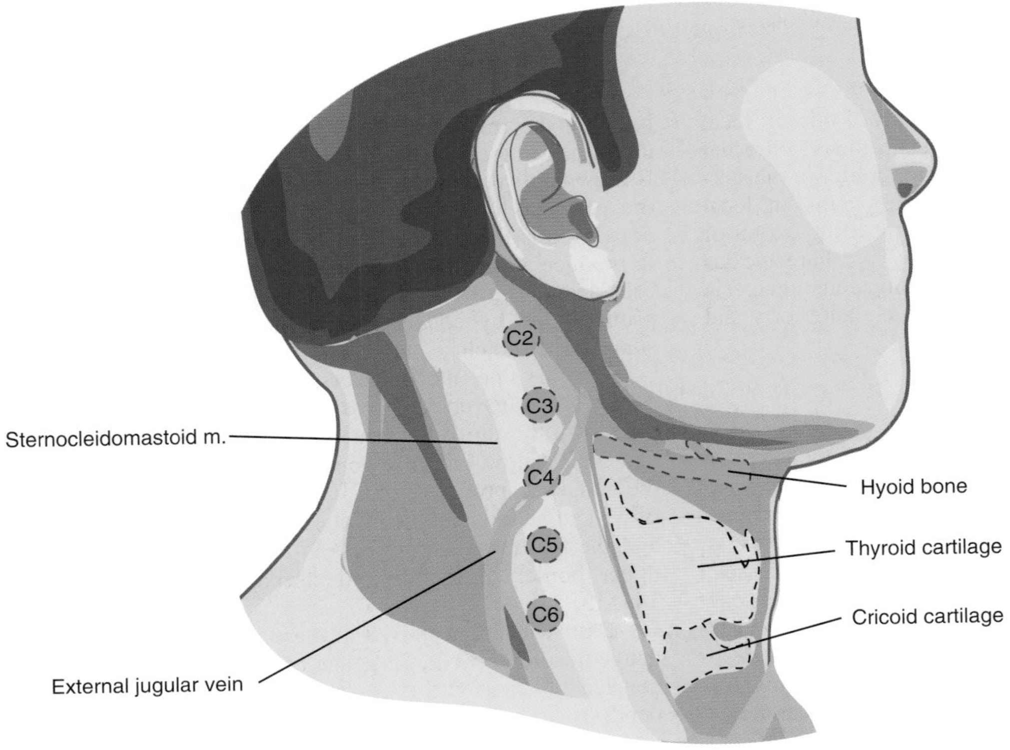

FIGURE 141–14 ■ Position and surface landmarks for performing deep cervical plexus block. (From Pai U, Raj P: Peripheral nerve blocks: Cervical plexus. In Raj P (ed): Handbook of Regional Anesthesia. New York, Churchill Livingstone, 1985, p 163.)

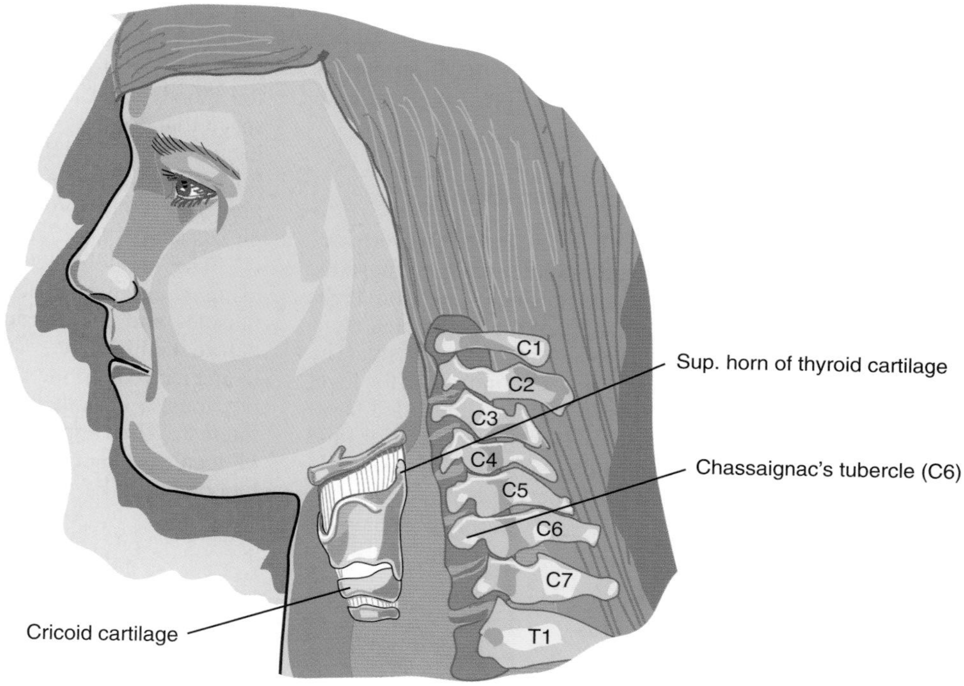

FIGURE 141–15 ■ Bony landmarks for performing deep cervical plexus block.

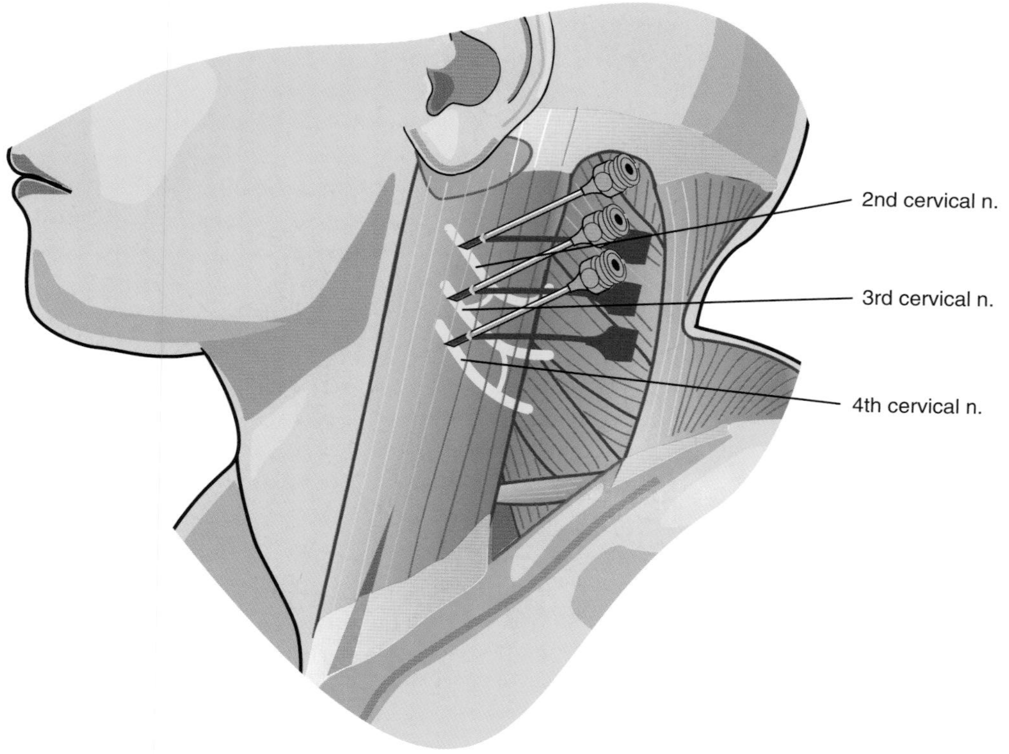

FIGURE 141–16 ■ Needle placement for deep cervical plexus block. The needles are noted at the sulci of the transverse processes of C2, C3, and C4.

needle. If the needles are properly placed, the onset of analgesia occurs within 5 minutes, regardless of what agent is used. The area of cutaneous anesthesia is the same as for superficial cervical plexus block, but deeper structures also are anesthetized.[3,6-8,21-23,25]

Alternative Techniques for Deep Block

Because the cervical plexus is invested in the prevertebral fascia between the anterior and middle scalene muscles, Winnie and colleagues[2] advocated a single-injection technique for neural blockade. Positioning of the patient and identification of bony landmarks are as noted previously. The posterior border of the sternocleidomastoid muscle at the level of C4 is identified, and the clinician's fingers are rolled laterally until the groove between the scalenus anterior and scalenus medius muscles is palpated. A 5-cm, 22-gauge or 1-inch, 25-gauge, short, beveled block needle is inserted medially and caudally at this point until either paresthesia is elicited or the transverse process of C4 is encountered. Local anesthetic, 10 to 25 mL, is injected after aspiration to check for blood and CSF.[2,11,27] The perineural sheath provides a space that communicates freely in the cervical region, so the local anesthetic solution can spread easily to adjacent levels.[21] Finger pressure at the C5 transverse process can be used to prevent caudad spread of the anesthetic toward the brachial plexus (Fig. 141–17).

The single-injection technique also can be performed using a nerve stimulator to produce twitches of the neck muscles and paresthesias over the shoulder and upper arm before the blockade.[28] An 18-gauge Venflon needle connected to an electrode of the nerve stimulator is inserted as described previously; the other electrode is placed on the shoulder of interest. When appropriate twitches are obtained, 10 to 15 mL of local anesthetic is injected after aspiration to check for blood and CSF.

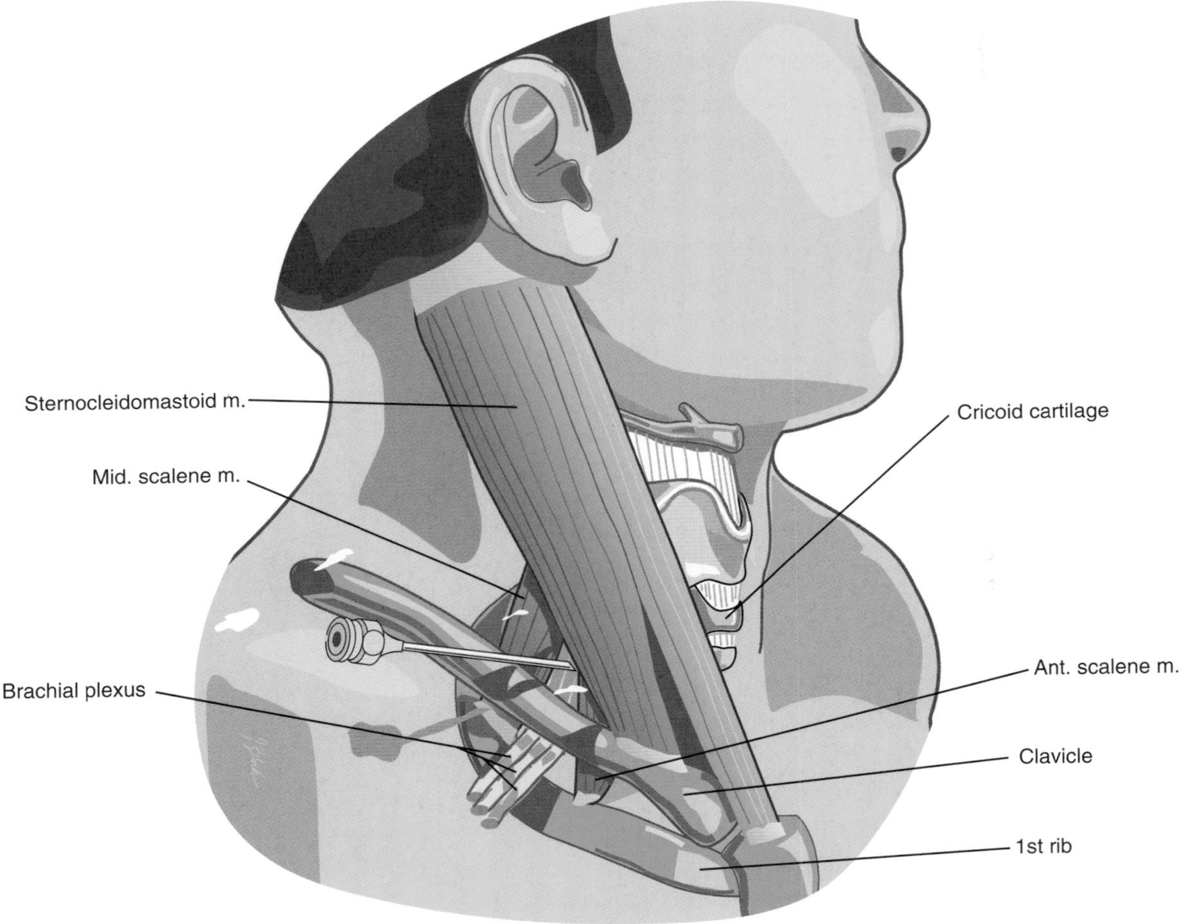

FIGURE 141–17 ■ The technique of interscalene cervical plexus block. The patient is supine with the head turned slightly to the side opposite that to be blocked. The level of C4 is determined by noting the level of the upper margin of the thyroid cartilage. While the patient elevates the head to bring the sternocleidomastoid muscle into prominence, the anesthetist places the index and middle fingers behind (posterior to) the latter muscle at the level of C4, and the patient is asked to relax. The palpating fingers now lie upon the anterior surface of the belly of the anterior scalene muscle. The anesthetist now carefully rolls the fingers laterally until the groove between the anterior and middle scalene muscles is palpated. When two fingers are utilized for palpation, digital pressure indents the skin and decreases the distance between the skin and cervical transverse processes. An immobile needle is inserted at the level of C4 between the palpating fingers as they depress the skin over the interscalene groove. The needle is advanced perpendicular to the skin in all planes; that is, the direction is mostly mesiad but slightly dorsad and caudad. The caudal direction is critical to the safety of the technique, because the advancing needle, properly directed, encounters the next cervical transverse process if paresthesias are not produced. A horizontal direction would allow a needle that has missed the cervical roots to enter the vertebral vessels or the epidural or subarachnoid space.

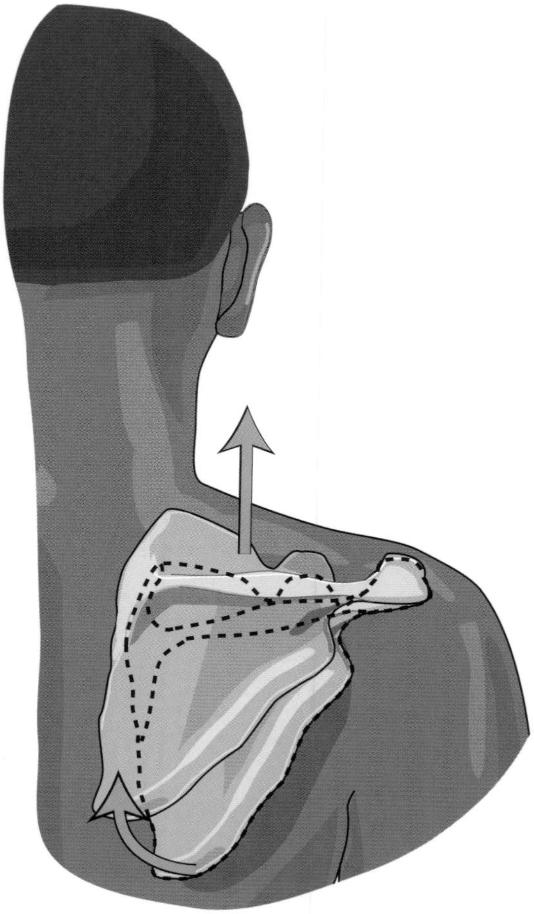

FIGURE 141–18 ■ Movement of the scapula elicited by stimulation of the cervical plexus.

Another method of using a nerve stimulator with the single-injection technique was described more recently.[29] A short, beveled needle (Stimuplex cannulas; Braun, Melsungen, Germany) is connected to a nerve stimulator and directed in the interscalene groove at the level of the upper margin of the thyroid cartilage (C4-5). The needle is directed caudad and medially until elevation and internal rotation of the scapula is elicited (Fig. 141–18). This muscle-evoked response occurs because of stimulation of the levator muscle of the scapula. The tip of the needle is positioned correctly when a current intensity of less than 0.5 mA elicits this muscle response. While digital pressure is applied below the needle, 40 mL of local anesthetic is injected slowly. The use of a nerve stimulator may increase the success rate of the block and improve the quality of anesthesia.

Another alternative route of deep cervical plexus block was described by Wertheim and Rovenstine (Fig. 141–19).[1,6] The patient is placed supine with the head midline and the chin pointing upward. The landmarks are the condyle of the mandible, the surface of the second lower molar, and the transverse processes of the cervical vertebrae. A vertical line is drawn through the condyle of the mandible, perpendicular to the operating line. The transverse processes of the cervical vertebrae are palpated, and a horizontal line is drawn along them, making right angles with the vertical line. A second perpendicular line is drawn that passes over the surface of the second molar. The point of intersection of this line with the horizontal line is marked, as is a point 1 cm caudad to the first point on the horizontal line. This latter point corresponds to the top of the transverse process of the second cervical vertebra. Points 2.5 and 3.5 cm caudad to the first point are marked on the skin. These correspond to the tips of the transverse processes of C3 and C4. Four points are drawn on the horizontal line, the upper point serves only as a reference point, and the three lower points indicate sites of injection. Injection of local anesthetic for deep cervical plexus block is carried out as described for the lateral approach (Fig. 141–20).

Posterior Approach

A posterior approach for deep cervical plexus block also has been described. The patient lies in the lateral position with the side to be blocked superior. The head is supported with cushions to prevent distortion of the structures of the neck and to render the landmarks more accessible. The cervical spinous processes are identified, C7 being most prominent. If they are difficult to palpate, the spinous process of C6 can be identified by drawing a line from the cricoid cartilage to the back of the neck. The transverse processes of C5-2 are located 1.5, 3, 4.5, and 6 cm above C6.

Skin wheals are raised opposite the spinous processes of C2-4 approximately 2 cm from the midline (Fig. 141–21). An 8-cm, 22-gauge needle is passed through these points parallel to the sagittal plane of the neck, until its point reaches the lateral transverse processes of the vertebrae. The needle is withdrawn into the subcutaneous tissue and redirected obliquely and outward. When the needle point rests along the lateral aspect of the vertebral arch, it is advanced 1 cm farther, and local anesthetic is injected as for the lateral approach.[6]

The posterior approach is technically difficult, and results of blockade using it have been poor. The landmarks are difficult to identify accurately, and the depth of needle insertion is greater with this technique. It is used only in cases in which the lateral approach is technically impossible (e.g., because of a tumor in the neck at the site of injection).[2]

Anesthetic Agents

A variety of local anesthetic agents have been used for surgical procedures under cervical plexus block.[29-35] For short-duration procedures, 1% to 2% lidocaine or mepivacaine can be used.[32,34] For prolonged block, a 50 : 50 mixture of 1% to 2% lidocaine and 0.5% to 0.75% bupivacaine can be used.[35-38] Other authors use various concentrations of plain bupivacaine, 0.375% to 0.5%, for deep and superficial blocks.[11,27,30] Newer local anesthetics, such as ropivacaine, are used in similar volumes and concentrations and offer similar anesthesia, perhaps with a better safety profile.

Epinephrine, 1 : 200,000 solution, also can be used to prolong block. Because this block is used most often for carotid endarterectomies in a high-risk group of patients, addition of epinephrine may produce undesirable cardiovascular effects.[9,39]

A total volume of 10 to 15 mL of local anesthetic usually is used for superficial cervical plexus block, and a total volume of 9 to 15 mL is used for deep cervical plexus block. The single-injection deep cervical plexus block usually

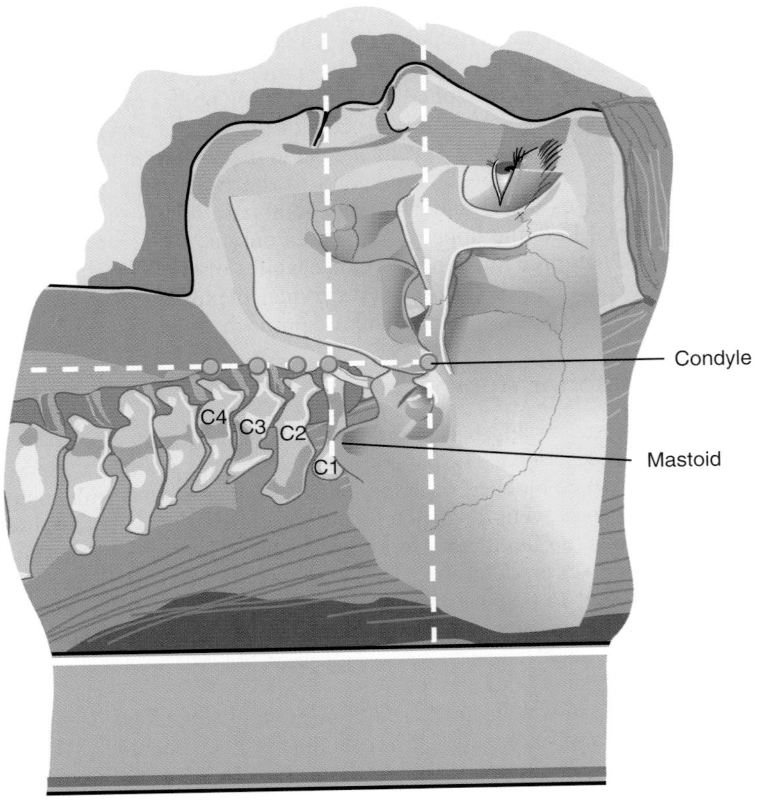

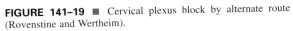

FIGURE 141–19 ■ Cervical plexus block by alternate route (Rovenstine and Wertheim).

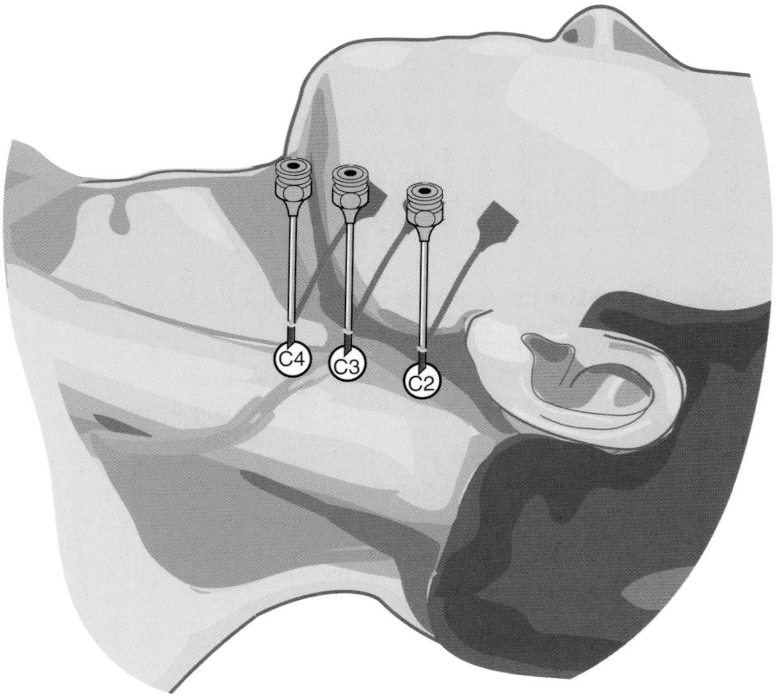

FIGURE 141–20 ■ Cervical plexus block; site of injection by alternate route.

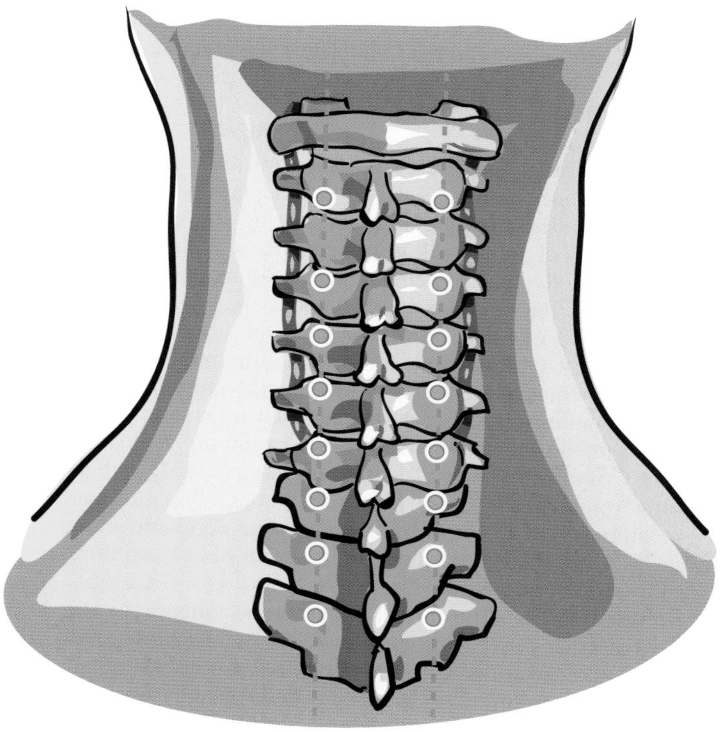

FIGURE 141–21 ■ Cervical plexus block by the posterior route. Superficial landmarks as viewed on the skeleton. The wheals are raised opposite the spinous processes, at a distance of 2 cm from the midline. These landmarks apply to the cervical area only.

requires 10 to 25 mL of local anesthetic, although greater volumes have been used.[2,11,27,29,31]

In addition to local anesthetic alone, neurolytic block using equal parts of 0.5% bupivacaine with absolute alcohol has been used to block the cervical plexus for neck pain secondary to metastatic lesions. Methylprednisolone (Depo-Medrol), 40 mg, also has been added to local anesthetics for its antiinflammatory actions.[20]

Several studies have measured the blood levels of local anesthetic and monitored side effects after cervical plexus block and found no significant degree of toxicity. One study using lidocaine 1.5% with epinephrine 1 : 200,000 at 6 mg/kg found that symptoms of lidocaine toxicity did not occur.[41] Another study using a mixture of lidocaine and bupivacaine for cervical plexus blockade at commonly used concentrations and volumes also failed to elicit toxic systemic effects.[33] Bupivacaine levels also were measured in a study in which patients received a combination of general anesthesia and cervical plexus block. The mean total bupivacaine dose was 3.4 mg/kg, higher than the manufacturer's recommendation of 2 mg/kg. Nevertheless, there were no signs of systemic bupivacaine toxicity during the procedure or in the postoperative period.[42] Although cervical plexus block is safe, the usual recommendations of multiple aspirations, slow injection, and careful needle placement must be observed.

PITFALLS

Cervical plexus block fails for many reasons. When the landmarks have been located, care should be taken to ensure that the patient does not move; otherwise, the landmarks may be misleading, and the block may fail.[23] The needle should not be inserted too deep. The depth of the tips of the transverse processes from the skin varies from approximately 1.3 to 3.2 cm, depending on the pressure of palpation, the build of the patient, and the location of the injection. The transverse processes become more superficial as they descend.[22,23]

The needle also should be directed slightly caudad to avoid entry into the epidural or subarachnoid space. The neck is a densely vascular area, so aspiration before injection is mandatory. Injection of a 1-mL test dose of anesthetic is prudent to detect any systemic effect. Placement of the needle should be at the lateral surface of the transverse processes before injection. If the needle lies too far posteriorly, analgesia is poor. If the needle tip is placed too far anteriorly, puncture of the carotid artery, internal jugular vein, or vertebral vessels may occur, with subsequent hematoma formation. This may make operating conditions difficult. Injection too far anteriorly also may cause sympathetic ganglion blockade, resulting in Horner syndrome.[6]

If the cervical plexus block is unsuccessful and if time permits, the block may be repeated. The total dose of local anesthetic should be calculated to avoid injection of a toxic dose.[40] If partial blockade is obtained, supplementation with intravenous agents can be considered. If these techniques fail, a means providing general anesthesia should be used.[7]

COMPLICATIONS

A variety of complications can occur with cervical plexus block. The block is occasionally inadequate and has to be supplemented by infiltration of additional local anesthetic. This complication is more common when the site of operation extends beyond the midline of the neck during unilateral blockade.[16] Surgical traction high in the neck wound, where glossopharyngeal innervation occurs, commonly requires supplementation of anesthesia.[14] Discomfort also can occur because of retraction onto the mandibular periosteum, which is innervated by branches of the mandibular division of the trigeminal nerve. Supplementation of anesthesia also may be necessary in this area.[35]

Because the neck is richly vascular, intravascular injections of local anesthetic may occur. Accidental injection into the internal and external jugular veins during superficial cervical plexus block may result in systemic toxicity, tears in the wall of the vein leading to hematoma formation, and possibly air embolism if the needle is not attached to the syringe. Accidental injection of even 0.2 mL of local anesthetic into the vertebral artery, which travels through the foramina transversaria in each transverse process, can produce profound toxic effects, including convulsions, apnea, total reversible blindness, and unconsciousness. This is due to the direct flow of the artery to the brain stem.[27,40] If colloidal materials, such as depot steroids, are added to local anesthetics for pain management, injection of this material into the vertebral artery can result in Wallenberg syndrome or occlusion of the posterior inferior cerebellar artery (Fig. 141–22).[21-23,25,39] In addition, injecting a large volume of local anesthetic anterior to the transverse processes during deep cervical plexus block may compress the carotid sheath. This compression could impair blood flow to the brain, which would be especially deleterious to patients with preexisting carotid artery disease.

Local anesthetic injection into the epidural or subarachnoid spaces also is possible through penetration into dural sleeves or through the intervertebral foramina.[21,23,25,39,43,44] There is also the potential complication of injury to the spinal cord. Careful aspiration is required for any evidence of CSF. Epidural injection, in contrast to subarachnoid injection, cannot spread into the cranium. An epidural block at the cervical level results in anesthesia of the upper limbs and thorax and can cause bilateral phrenic nerve block with subsequent bilateral diaphragmatic paralysis.[9]

The recurrent laryngeal nerve is blocked in 2% to 3% of cases during unilateral cervical plexus block. It occurs when local anesthetic is injected too deep along the posterior border of the sternocleidomastoid muscle. Sequelae are hoarseness, aphonia, and difficulty breathing. Blockade of the vagus nerve also may occur, which causes increased heart rate and loss of phonation. Bilateral hypoglossal nerve denervation with resultant total upper airway obstruction has been described.[37]

The phrenic nerve, arising mainly from C4 with small branches from C3 and C5, can be blocked (50% of cases) during deep cervical plexus block, causing transient diaphragmatic paresis and mild hypercapnia.[45,46] If only one hemidiaphragm is paralyzed, only patients with chronic obstructive pulmonary disease seem to be at risk for significant changes in carbon dioxide concentration. Most patients describe only a "heavy chest" sensation[9]; this is usually treated by providing reassurance, administering supplemental oxygen, and elevating the patient's head.

Bilateral phrenic nerve block can be a serious hazard, especially in patients with concurrent respiratory compromise, and endotracheal intubation may be required.[31] If respiratory compromise from a paralyzed diaphragm could be a risk to a given patient, bilateral cervical plexus blocks should be avoided. If such blocks are carried out, dilute concentrations and small volumes of local anesthetic agents should be used.[21] Alternatively, the use of a superficial cervical plexus block alone may lower the risk of respiratory complications.[53]

Blockade of cranial nerves IX and X or a combination of both through the pharyngeal plexus also can occur during deep cervical plexus block. This can cause dysphagia, and patients usually complain of a sensation of fullness in the back of the throat, which dissipates with time.[9]

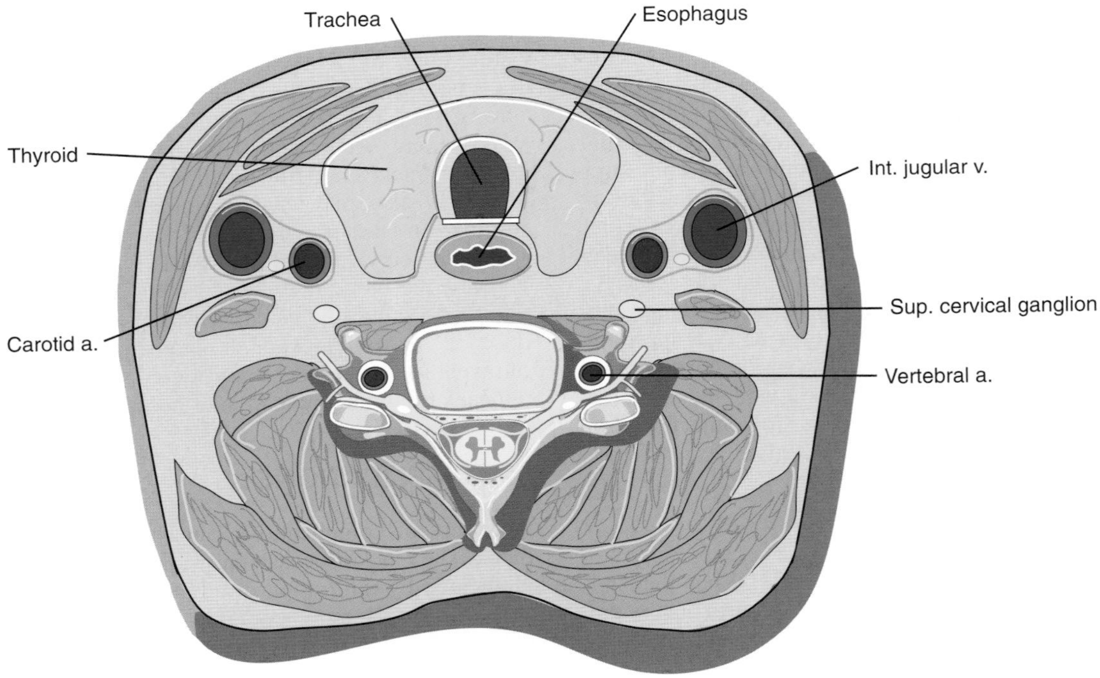

FIGURE 141–22 ■ Cervical plexus cross-sectional anatomy—midpoint of sternocleidomastoid muscle.

Because the deep cervical plexus lies below the deep cervical fascia, spread of anesthetic to the cervical sympathetic chain, including the stellate ganglion, should not occur. If infiltration has spread anterior to the prevertebral fascia, the cervical sympathetic chain can be blocked, with resultant Horner syndrome. This can be manifested as ptosis, constricted pupil, unilateral anhidrosis, nasal congestion, and sometimes respiratory compromise.[37] These symptoms should be noted before surgery, to avoid any confusion in the neurologic examination later. This complication in a failed block indicates that the injection was placed too far anteriorly and too superficially.[21] Bilateral stellate ganglion block may result in profound bradycardia that is due to interruption of the cardioaccelerator fibers.[25]

Finally, occipital headaches have been described after some surgical procedures under cervical plexus block.[9] The cause seems to be hyperextension of the neck muscles, however, and not the block itself. Headaches also can occur after carotid endarterectomy secondary to reperfusion of the cerebral circulation.

FUTURE TRENDS

Although cervical plexus block has been widely described in the literature, the use of this technique for surgical procedures has been limited. From the surgeon's standpoint, the potential for a delay in surgery because of the time required to perform the block and the potential for unsatisfactory anesthesia that would require further supplementation are deterrents to performing cervical plexus block. From the standpoint of the anesthesiologist, inexperience with performing the block and fear of complications reduce the use of this technique.[36]

The most common surgical procedure performed under cervical plexus block is carotid endarterectomy. Because enormous progress in the past decade has validated the efficacy of this procedure, its use may increase.[47] A newer technique, percutaneous carotid angioplasty and stenting performed via direct common carotid access, has been done successfully with cervical plexus block.[48] This technique may broaden the indications further for this type of nerve block. As the surgical population grows older and presents with more severe systemic illnesses, regional anesthesia may prove to be the safest form of anesthesia. Carotid endarterectomy performed under cervical plexus block has many benefits over general anesthesia, among them the opportunity to monitor the patient's neurologic status during the operation. Periodic examinations of the awake patient have proved to be more accurate than electroencephalography or any other form of monitoring in assessing neurologic status. Another advantage is that regional anesthesia allows for a trial of carotid clamping and carotid stump pressure measurements while neurologic status is monitored with the patient awake. Routine shunting, which carries its own risks of morbidity and mortality, is avoided.[49]

Perioperative complications occur during carotid endarterectomy under cervical plexus block and general anesthesia. Cervical plexus block seems to be associated with greater activation of the sympathetic nervous system, which is manifested as hypertension and tachycardia, whereas general anesthesia is associated with a greater incidence of hypotension.[50,51] Postoperative blood pressure instability is less common in patients who have had cervical plexus block for the procedure.[13,16,17] A report from Corson and colleagues[52] showed a statistically significant difference in neurologic complications between regional and general anesthesia during carotid endarterectomy—0.6% versus 4%.

In recent years, growing emphasis has been placed on cost containment by the government, third-party payers, and the public. A study by Godin and colleagues[49] confirmed that cervical plexus block is a safe, reliable, and less costly alternative to general anesthesia in patients undergoing carotid endarterectomy. As evidence accumulates to support the use of regional anesthetic techniques for carotid endarterectomy and other procedures and conditions, facility in performing cervical plexus blocks should be encouraged. Cervical plexus block should be considered an important regional technique in the armamentarium of any anesthesiologist.

References

1. Wertheim HM, Rovenstine EA: Cervical plexus block. N Y State J Med 39:1311, 1939.
2. Winnie AP, Ramamurthy S, Durrani Z, Radonjic R: Interscalene cervical plexus block: A single-injection technique. Anesth Analg 54:370, 1975.
3. Collins VJ: Blocks of cervical spinal nerves. In: Fundamentals of Nerve Blocks. Philadelphia, Lea & Febiger, 1960, p 234.
4. Kappis H: Uber Leitunganasthesie am Bauch, Brust, Arm, und Hals durch Injection ans Foramen intervertebrale. Munchen Med Wschr 59:794, 1912.
5. Heidenhein L: Operations on the neck. In Braun H (ed): Local Anesthesia. Philadelphia, Lea & Febiger, 1914, p 268.
6. Adriani J: Labat's Regional Anesthesia: Techniques and Clinical Applications, 3rd ed. Philadelphia, WB Saunders, 1967, p 180.
7. Pai U, Raj P: Peripheral nerve blocks: Cervical plexus. In Raj P (ed): Handbook of Regional Anesthesia. New York, Churchill Livingstone, 1985, p 163.
8. Katz J: Cervical plexus. In Katz J (ed): Atlas of Regional Anesthesia, 2nd ed. Norwalk, CT, Appleton & Lange, 1994, p 40.
9. Masters RD, Castresana EJ, Castresana MR: Superficial and deep cervical plexus block: Technical considerations. AANA J 63:235, 1995.
10. Rainer WG, McCrory CB, Feiler EM: Surgery on the carotid artery with cervical block anesthesia: Technical considerations. Am J Surg 112:703, 1966.
11. Stoneham MD, Doyle AR, Knighton JD, et al: Prospective, randomized comparison of deep or superficial cervical plexus block for carotid endarterectomy surgery. Anesthesiology 89:907, 1998.
12. Stoneham MD: Correspondence-applied anatomy of cervical plexus blockade. Anesthesiology 90:1791, 1999.
13. Castresana MR, Balser JS, Newman WH, Stefansson S: Cervical block for carotid endarterectomy followed immediately by general anesthesia for coronary artery bypass and aortic valve replacement. Anesth Analg 77:186, 1993.
14. Davies MJ, Murrell GC, Cronin KD, et al: Carotid endarterectomy under cervical plexus block: A prospective clinical audit. Anaesth Intensive Care 18:219, 1990.
15. Jopling MW, deSanctis CA, McDowell DE, et al: Anesthesia for carotid endarterectomy: A comparison of regional and general techniques. Anesthesiology 59:A217, 1983.
16. Pick MJ, Taylor GW: Selective shunting on the basis of carotid clamping under regional anesthesia. Int Anesthesiol Clin 22:1141, 1984.
17. Fried KS, Elias SM, Raggi R: Carotid endarterectomy under local anesthesia. N J Med 87:795, 1990.
18. Muskett A, McGreevy J, Miller M: Detailed comparison of regional and general anesthesia for carotid endarterectomy. Am J Surg 152:691, 1986.
19. Andersen CA, Rich NM, Collins GJ, McDonald PT: Carotid endarterectomy: Regional versus general anesthesia. Am Surgeon 46:323, 1980.
20. Owitz S, Koppolu S: Nerve blocks: An anesthesiologist's approach to the relief of cancer pain. Mt Sinai J Med 53:550, 1986.
21. Cousins MJ, Bridenbaugh PO: Neural Blockade in Clinical Anesthesia and Management of Pain, 2nd ed. Philadelphia, JB Lippincott, 1988.

22. Brown DL: Cervcal plexus block. In: Atlas of Regional Anesthesia, Philadelphia, WB Saunders, 1992, p 165.
23. Moore DC: Regional block. In: A Handbook for Use in the Clinical Practice of Medicine and Surgery: Block of the Cervical Plexus, 2nd ed. Springfield, IL, Charles C Thomas, 1957, p 88.
24. Bonica JJ: General considerations of pain in the neck and upper limb. In: The Management of Pain, 2nd ed. Philadelphia, Lea & Febiger, 1990, p 823.
25. Carron H: Cervical plexus blocks. In: Regional Anesthesia: Techniques and Clinical Applications. New York, Grune & Stratton, 1984, p 10.
26. Mulroy MR: Peripheral nerve blockade. In Barash PG, Cullen BF, Stoelting RK (eds): Clinical Anesthesia, 2nd ed. Philadelphia, JB Lippincott, 1992, p 847.
27. Stoneham MD, Bree SEP: Epileptic seizure during awake carotid endarterectomy. Anesth Analg 89:885, 1999.
28. Mehta Y, Juneja R: Regional analgesia for carotid artery endarterectomy by Winnie's single injection technique using a nerve detector. J Cardiothorac Vasc Anesth 6:772, 1992.
29. Merle JC, Mazoit JX, Desgranges P, et al: A comparison of two techniques for cervical plexus blockade: Evaluation of efficacy and systemic toxicity. Anesth Analg 89:1366, 1999.
30. Allen BT, Anderson CB, Rubin BG, et al: The influence of anesthetic technique on perioperative complications after carotid endarterectomy. Vasc Surg 19:834, 1994.
31. Stoneham MD, Wakefield TW: Acute respiratory distress after deep cervical plexus block. J Cardiothorac Vasc Anesth 12:197, 1998.
32. Davies MJ, Murrell GC, Cronin KD, et al: Anaesthesia and intensive care: Carotid endarterectomy under cervical plexus block—a prospective clinical audit. Anaesth Intensive Care 18:219, 1990.
33. Tissot S, Frering B, Gagniew MC, et al: Plasma concentrations of lidocaine and bupivacaine after cervical plexus block for carotid surgery. Anesth Analg 84:1377, 1997.
34. Davies MJ, Mooney PH, Scott DA, et al: Neurologic changes during carotid endarterectomy under cervical block predict a high risk of postoperative stroke. Anesthesiology 78:8141, 1993.
35. Burke DL, Thomas P: Mandibular nerve block in addition to cervical plexus block for carotid endarterectomy. Anesth Analg 87:1034, 1998.
36. Levelle JP, Martinez OA: Airway obstruction after bilateral carotid endarterectomy. Anesthesiology 63:220, 1985.
37. Satyanarayana T, Ali M, Ramanathan S, et al: Cervical plexus block for carotid endarterectomy. Anesthesiology 55:A170, 1981.
38. Dawson AR, Dysart RH, Amerena JV, et al: Arterial lignocaine concentrations following cervical plexus blockade for carotid endarterectomy. Anaesth Intens Care 19:197, 1991.
39. Neill RS, Watson R: Plasma bupivacaine concentrations during combined regional and general anaesthesia for resection and reconstruction of head and neck carcinomata. Br J Anaesth 56:485, 1984.
40. Goldberg MJ: Complications of cervical plexus block of fugue state. Anesth Analg 81:1108, 1995.
41. Paul RS, Abadir AR, Spencer FC: Resection of an internal carotid artery aneurysm under regional anesthesia: Posterior cervical block. Ann Surg 168:147, 1968.
42. Kumar A, Battit GE, Froese AB, Long MC: Bilateral cervical and thoracic epidural blockade complicating interscalene brachial plexus block: Report of two cases. Anesthesiology 35:650, 1971.
43. Huang KC, Fitzgerald MR, Tsueda K: Bilateral block of cervical and brachial plexuses following interscalene block. Anaesth Intensive Care 14:87, 1986.
44. Winnie AP: Regional anesthesia. Surg Clin North Am 54:880, 1975.
45. Emery G, Handley G, Davies MJ, Mooney PH: Incidence of phrenic nerve block and hypercapnia in patients undergoing carotid endarterectomy under cervical plexus block. Anaesth Intensive Care 26:377, 1998.
46. Castresana MR, Masters RD, Castresana EJ, et al: Incidence and clinical significance of hemidiaphragmatic paresis in patients undergoing carotid endarterectomy during cervical plexus block anesthesia. J Neurosurg Anesthesiol 6:21, 1994.
47. Gelb AW, Herrick IA: Anesthesia for carotid endarterectomy. In: IARS 1999: Review Course Lectures. New York, Elsevier, 1999, p 45.
48. Alessandri C, Bergeron P: Local anesthesia in carotid angioplasty. J Endovasc Surg 3:31, 1996.
49. Godin MS, Bell WH, Schwedler M, Kerstein MD: Cost effectiveness of regional anesthesia in carotid endarterectomy. Am Surgeon 55:656, 1989.
50. Forssell C, Takolander R, Bergqust D, et al: Local versus general anaesthesia in carotid surgery: A prospective, randomised study. Eur J Vasc Surg 6:503, 1989.
51. Takolander R, Bergqust D, Hulthen UL, et al: Carotid artery surgery: Local versus general anaesthesia as related to sympathetic activity and cardiovascular effects. Eur J Vasc Surg 4:265, 1990.
52. Corson JD, Chang BB, Karmody AM: The influence of anesthetic choice on carotid endarterectomy outcome. Arch Surg 122:807, 1987.
53. Weiss A, Isselhorst C, Gahlen J, et al: Acute respiratory failure after deep cervical plexus block for carotid endarterectomy as a result of bilateral recurrent laryngeal nerve paralysis. Acta Anaesthesiol Scand 49:715-719, 2005.

chapter 142

Stellate Ganglion Block

P. Prithvi Raj

INDICATIONS

Stellate ganglion block is useful in the treatment of a variety of painful conditions, including Raynaud disease, arterial embolism in the area of the arm, accidental intra-arterial injection of drugs, and Meniere syndrome. Although stellate ganglion block for treatment of Meniere syndrome is controversial, several clinicians have had success with it. Stellate ganglion block is beneficial in the treatment of acute herpes zoster of the face and lower cervical and upper thoracic dermatomes. The technique also may be used for palliation of postherpetic neuralgia involving this anatomic area.

The posttraumatic syndrome, which is often accompanied by swelling, cold sweat, and cyanosis, is an ideal indication for stellate ganglion block. Several clinical syndromes fall into this category, including complex regional pain syndromes type I (reflex sympathetic dystrophy) and type II (causalgia) and Sudeck disease. Stellate ganglion block also is useful in the treatment of facial reflex sympathetic dystrophy.

For patients requiring vascular surgery on the upper extremities, stellate ganglion block has diagnostic, prognostic, and, in some cases, prophylactic value. Simultaneous bilateral blocks are not advisable. Nevertheless, in cases of pulmonary embolism, bilateral stellate ganglion block is absolutely indicated as immediate therapy.

CONTRAINDICATIONS

Absolute contraindications of stellate ganglion block are (1) anticoagulant therapy because of the possibility of bleeding if there is vascular damage during insertion of the needle, (2) pneumothorax and pneumonectomy on the contralateral side because of the danger of additional pneumothorax on the ipsilateral side, and (3) recent myocardial infarction because stellate ganglion block cuts off the cardiac sympathetic fibers (accelerator nerves) with possible deleterious effects in this condition. Glaucoma can be considered a relative contraindication to stellate ganglion block because provocation of glaucoma by repeated stellate ganglion blocks has been reported. Marked impairment of cardiac stimulus conduction (e.g., atrioventricular block) also is to be regarded as a relative contraindication because blockade of the upper thoracic sympathetic ganglia aggravates bradycardia.

EQUIPMENT, DRUGS, AND PATIENT PREPARATION

Necessary equipment includes a 25-gauge local infiltration needle; 22-gauge, 1-inch of 1½-inch block needle; 5-cm or 10-cm (2-mm or 5-mm tip) sharp Sluijter Mehta or Racz, Finch, Kit needle (Radionics Burlington, MA) for radiofrequency; and the radiofrequency machine. Drugs used for local anesthetic blocks include 0.5% bupivacaine/ropivacaine 0.5% total = 8 mL or 0.2% to 5% ropivacaine, 1% to 2% lidocaine, and steroids (optional). Phenol preparations require 3% phenol in iohexol (Omnipaque 240) (total 6 mL) and 0.9% normal saline (total 2 mL). Radiofrequency thermocoagulation uses the same local anesthetics as for block with steroids.

Physical examination should include checks for neck extension mobility, prior radical neck surgery, infection at injection site, prior thyroid surgery, and any anatomic variations related to surgery. In terms of preoperative medications, I recommend following the standard American Society of Anesthesiologists conscious sedation protocol.

CLINICALLY RELEVANT ANATOMY

Cell bodies for preganglionic nerves originate in the anterolateral horn of the spinal cord. Fibers destined for the head and neck originate in the first and second thoracic spinal cord segments, whereas preganglionic nerves to the upper extremity originate at segments T2-8 and occasionally T9. Preganglionic axons to the head and neck exit with the ventral roots of T1 and T2, then travel as white communicating rami before joining the sympathetic chain and passing cephalad to synapse at the inferior (stellate), middle, or superior cervical ganglion. Postganglionic nerves follow the carotid arteries (external or internal) to the head or integrate as the gray communicating rami before joining the cervical plexus or upper cervical nerves to innervate structures of the neck.

To achieve successful sympathetic denervation of the head and neck, the stellate ganglion should be blocked because all preganglionic nerves synapse here or pass through

---

Some portions of this chapter have been excerpted from Raj PP, Lou L, Erdine S, et al: Radiographic Imaging for Regional Anesthesia and Pain Management. Philadelphia, Churchill Livingstone, 2003, pp 72-80, with permission.

on their way to more cephalad ganglia. Blockade of the middle or superior ganglion would miss the contribution of sympathetic fibers traveling from the stellate ganglion to the vertebral plexus and, ultimately, to the corresponding areas of the cranial vault supplied by the vertebral artery.[1]

Sympathetic nerves to the upper extremity exit T2-8 through ventral spinal routes, travel as white communicating rami to the sympathetic chain, then pass cephalad to synapse at the second thoracic ganglion, first thoracic or interior cervical (stellate) ganglion, and occasionally the middle cervical ganglion. Most postganglionic nerves leave the chain as gray communicating rami to join the anterior divisions at C5-T1, nerves that form the brachial plexus. Some postganglionic nerves pass directly from the chain to form the subclavian perivascular plexus and innervate the subclavian, axillary, and upper part of the brachial arteries.[2]

In most humans, the inferior cervical ganglion is fused to the first thoracic ganglion, forming the stellate ganglion. Although the ganglion itself is inconstant, it commonly measures 2.5 cm long, 1 cm wide, and 0.5 cm thick. It usually lies in front of the neck of the first rib and extends to the interspace between C7 and T1. When elongated, it may lie over the anterior tubercle of C7; in persons with unfused ganglia, the inferior cervical ganglion rests over C7, and the first thoracic ganglion rests over the neck of the first rib. From a three-dimensional perspective, the stellate ganglion is limited medially by the longus colli muscle, laterally by the scalene muscles, anteriorly by the subclavian artery, posteriorly by the transverse processes and prevertebral fascia, and inferiorly by the posterior aspect of the pleura. At the level of the stellate ganglion, the vertebral artery lies anterior, having originated from the subclavian artery. After passing over the ganglion, the artery enters the vertebral foramen and is located posterior to the anterior tubercle of C6 (Fig. 142–1).

Because the classic approach to blockade of the stellate ganglion is at the level of C6 (Chassaignac's tubercle), the needle is positioned anterior to the artery. Other structures posterior to the stellate ganglion are the anterior divisions of the C8 and T1 nerves (inferior aspects of the brachial plexus). The stellate ganglion supplies sympathetic innervation to the upper extremity through gray communicating rami of C7, C8, T1, and occasionally C5 and C6. Other inconstant contributions to the upper extremity are from the T2 and T3 gray communicating rami, which do not pass through the stellate ganglion, but join the brachial plexus and ultimately innervate distal structures of the upper extremity. These fibers sometimes have been implicated when relief of sympathetically mediated pain is inadequate despite evidence of a satisfactory stellate block.[3]

PROCEDURE

Patient Preparation

Ideally, proper patient preparation for the stellate ganglion block begins at the visit before the procedure. The patient is much more likely to remember discharge instructions and expected side effects if they are explained during a visit when the patient is not apprehensive about the imminent procedure, what side effects may be expected, and potential complications. Discussions of the realistic expectations of sympathetic blockade should be held before any procedure. The goals of blockade and the number of blocks in a given series differ with each pain syndrome, and these variables should be discussed, when possible, at visits before the actual blockade. Patients are much less likely to experience frustration or despair if they understand beforehand what can be expected. If the cause of pain is unclear, and the intended block is considered diagnostic, a complete explanation allows the patient to record valuable information on the effectiveness of the procedure.

Informed consent must be obtained. Potential risks, complications, and possible side effects should be explained in detail. The patient should share responsibility for decision making and must understand the risks and the fact that complications do occur.

Placement of an intravenous line before the block is not mandatory at all pain clinics, but it facilitates use of intravenous sedation, when indicated, and provides access for administration of resuscitative drugs should a complication occur. In skilled hands, a stellate ganglion block can be performed quickly and relatively painlessly, so an intravenous line may not be necessary. All standard resuscitative drugs, suction apparatus, oxygen delivery system, cardiac defibrillators, and equipment for endotracheal cannulation need to be readily accessible. For anxious patients and in teaching institutions when the operator is inexperienced or when "hands-on" teaching is expected, preblock sedation through an intravenous line is beneficial.

Paratracheal Approach

The patient is placed in the supine position with the head resting flat on the table without a pillow. A folded sheet or thin pillow should be placed under the shoulders of most patients to facilitate extension of the neck and accentuate landmarks. The head should be kept straight with the mouth slightly open to relax the tension on the anterior cervical musculature. Hyperextension of the neck also causes the esophagus to move midline, away from the transverse processes on the left.

To ensure proper needle positioning, the operator must identify the C6 tubercle correctly. Identification is accomplished most easily using firm pressure with the index finger (Fig. 142–2). In either a left-handed or a right-handed stellate ganglion block, the operator's nondominant hand should be used for palpating landmarks. Patients do not tolerate jabbing; gentle but firm probing can easily define the borders of the tubercle. A single finger, the index finger, relays the most specific tactile information. An alternative approach traps the tubercle between the index and middle fingers.[4]

The skin is antiseptically prepared, and the needle is inserted posteriorly, penetrating the skin at the tip of the operator's index finger. Making a skin wheal with local anesthetic is rarely necessary except in some teaching situations or in patients with obese necks (in both situations, a 5-cm needle [or a 22-gauge B-bevel needle] is used and should puncture the skin directly downward [posterior], perpendicular to the table in all planes). Although a smaller (e.g., 25-gauge) needle can be used, the added flexibility and smaller caliber make it more difficult to ascertain reliably when bone is encountered and then maintain the proper location for injection.

The needle passes through the underlying tissue until it contacts the C6 tubercle or the junction between the C6 vertebral body and the tubercle. The depths of these structures

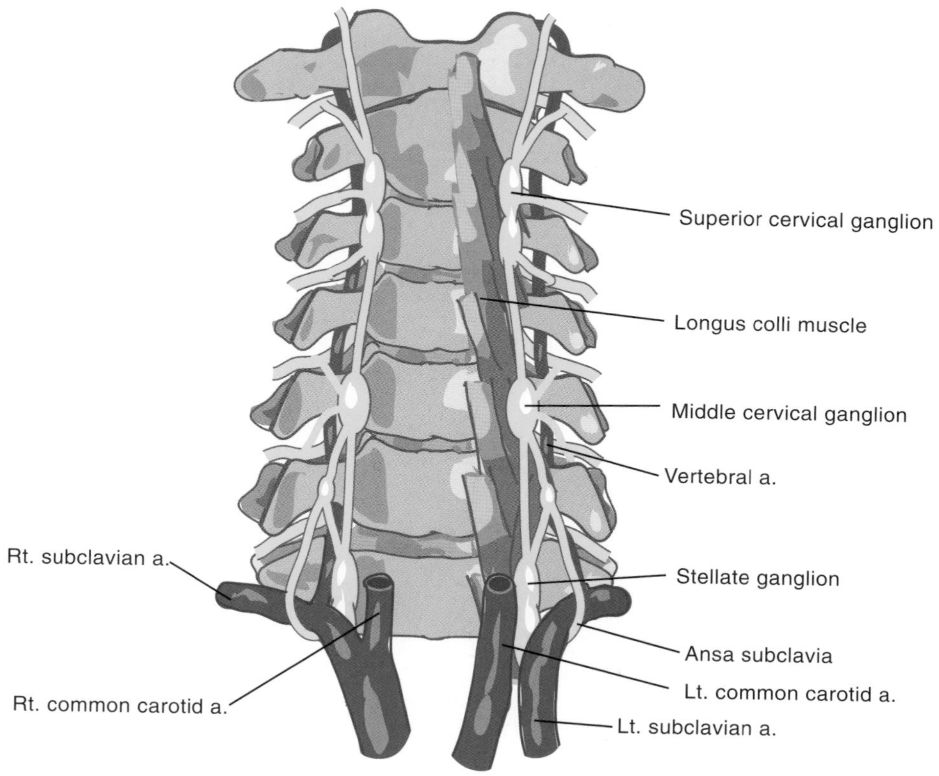

A

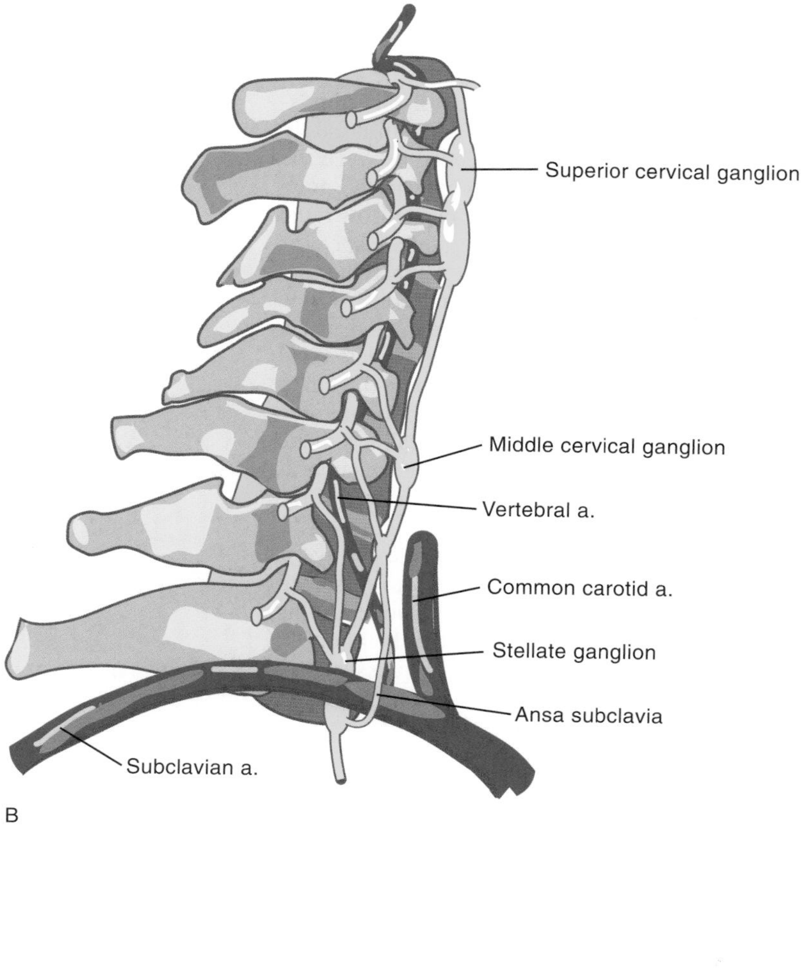

B

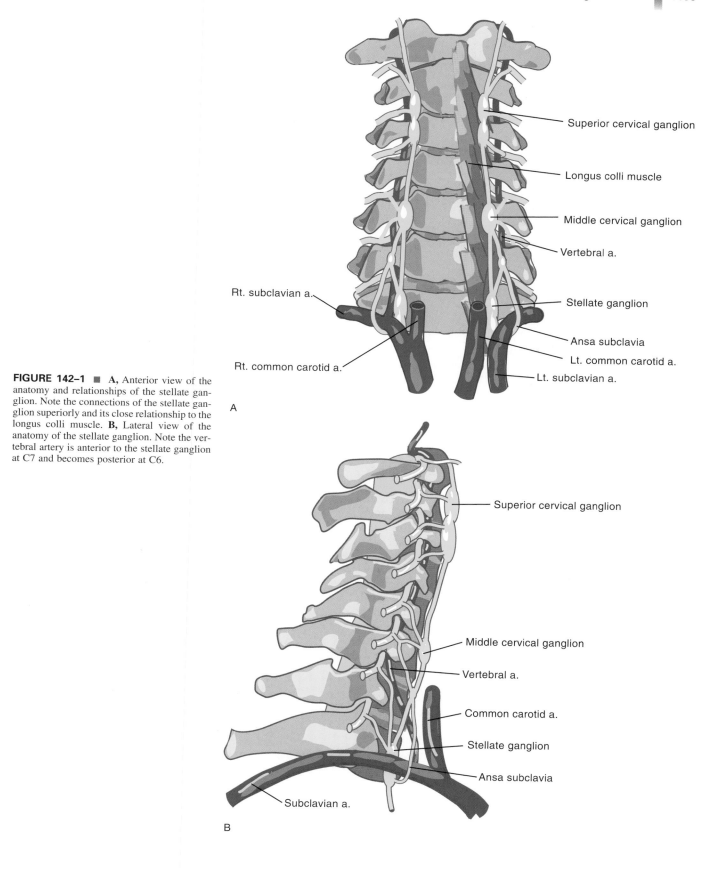

FIGURE 142–1 ■ **A,** Anterior view of the anatomy and relationships of the stellate ganglion. Note the connections of the stellate ganglion superiorly and its close relationship to the longus colli muscle. **B,** Lateral view of the anatomy of the stellate ganglion. Note the vertebral artery is anterior to the stellate ganglion at C7 and becomes posterior at C6.

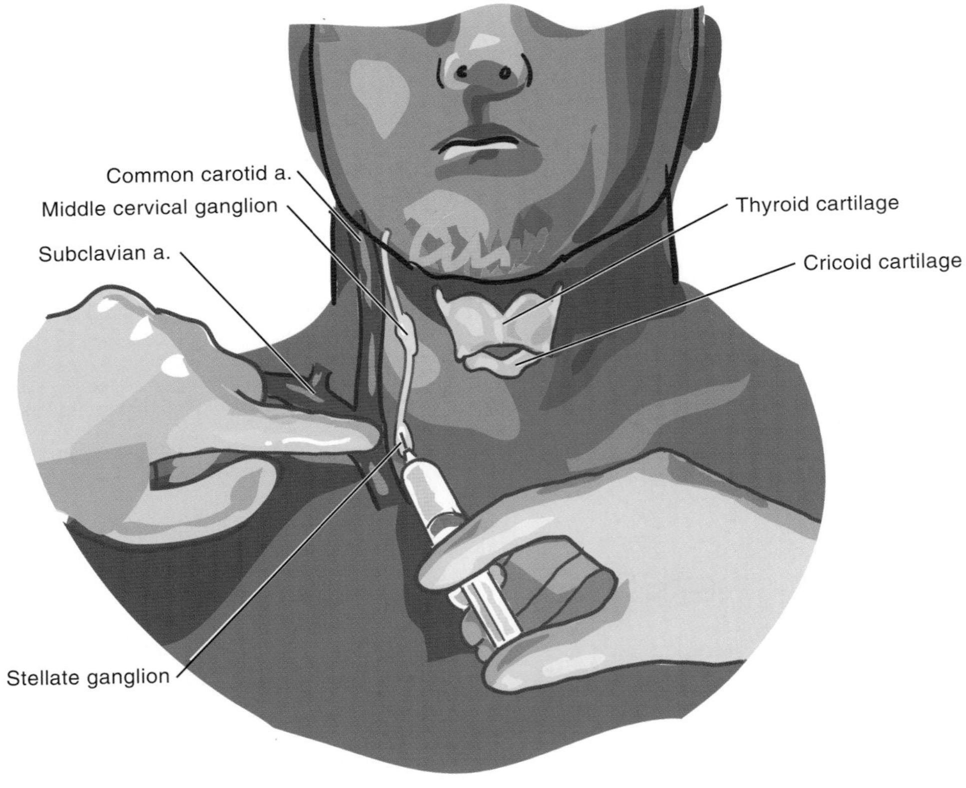

FIGURE 142–2 ■ Stellate ganglion block. C6 anterior tubercle is directly beneath the operator's index finger. The carotid artery is retracted laterally when necessary. The needle is perpendicular to all skin planes and is inserted directly posterior from the point of entry. *Inset,* Patient positioned for stellate ganglion block. A pillow or roll should be placed between the shoulders to extend the neck, bring the esophagus to the midline, and facilitate palpation of Chassaignac's tubercle.

differ, the tubercle itself being more anterior than the junction between body and tubercle. Regardless of the specific location encountered at C6, if the skin is being properly displaced posteriorly by the nondominant index finger, the depth is rarely more than 2 to 2.5 cm. The important difference between the medial and lateral location of bone at C6 relates to the presence of the longus colli muscle, which is located over the lateral aspect of the vertebral body and the medial aspect of the transverse process. It does not cover the C6 tubercle; only the prevertebral fascia that invests the longus colli muscle covers the C6 tubercle. If the needle contacts the medial aspect of the transverse process at a depth greater than expected, the operator should be prepared to withdraw the needle 0.5 cm to avoid injecting into the longus colli muscle. Injection into the muscle belly can prevent caudad diffusion of local anesthetic to the stellate ganglion. Location of the needle on the superficial tip of the C6 anterior tubercle requires withdrawal of the needle from the periosteum before injection.

The procedure is performed most easily if the syringe is attached before the needle is positioned. This prevents accidental dislodgement of the needle from the bone during syringe attachment after the needle is placed. When bone is encountered, the palpating finger maintains its pressure, the needle is withdrawn 2 to 5 mm, and the medication is injected. Alternatively, when bone is met, the operator's palpating hand can release and fix the needle by grasping its hub, leaving the dominant hand free to aspirate and inject. Although this technique can be performed blindly, more often fluoroscopy is used to confirm contrast spread (Fig. 142–3). With fluoroscopy, correct placement of the needle should be shown by anteroposterior and lateral views with spread of the contrast solution (Fig. 142–4).

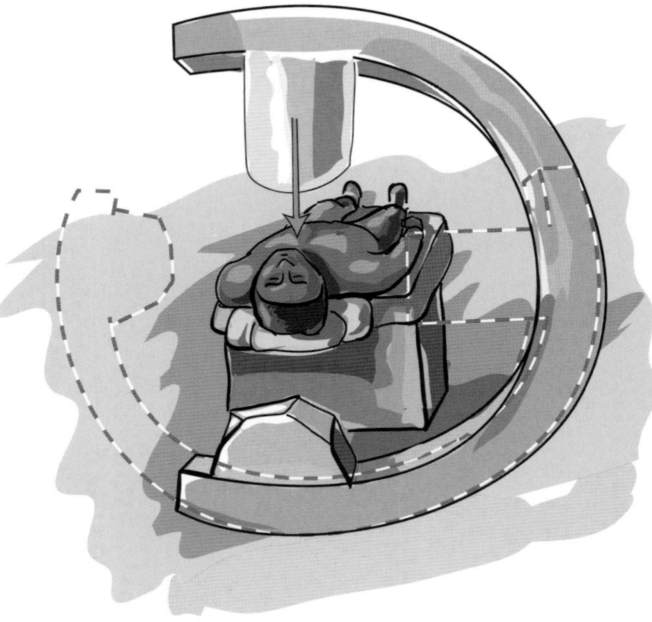

FIGURE 142–3 ■ The patient lies supine. If the fluoroscope is used, the C-arm should visualize the C6-7 vertebral region in anteroposterior and lateral views.

Final Injection

When proper needle placement is confirmed, injection of medication must be done in a routine and systematic fashion. A 50:50 mix of 2% lidocaine with 0.5% ropivacaine and 1 mL of 40 mg/mL of triamcinolone may be used. An initial test

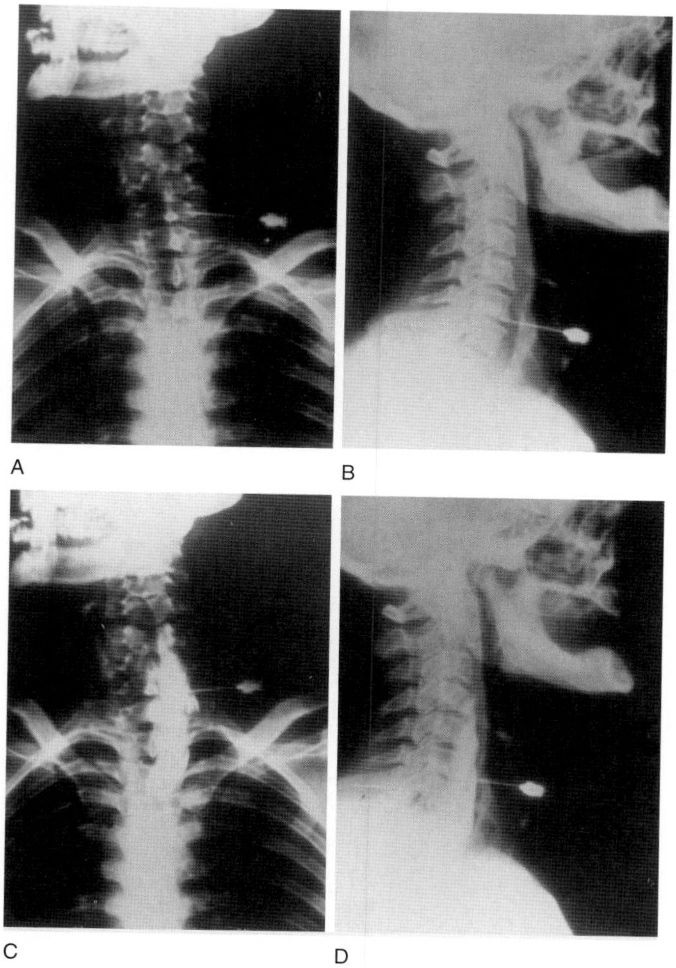

FIGURE 142–4 ■ **A-D,** Anteroposterior and lateral views of correct placement of the needle and the contrast medium spread after injection for stellate ganglion block. Anteroposterior (**A**) and lateral (**B**) views of needle placement and anteroposterior (**C**) and lateral (**D**) views of contrast medium spread. (From Waldman SD: Stellate ganglion block. Interventional Pain Management, 2nd ed. Philadelphia, WB Saunders, 2001, p 367.)

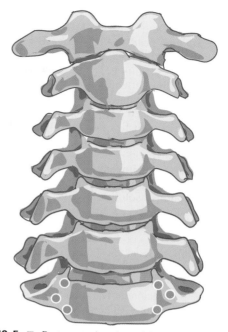

FIGURE 142–5 ■ Posteroanterior view of the cervical spine. Dots mark the target points for radiofrequency lesioning of the cervical sympathetic nerves. These are at the junction of the medial aspect of the transverse process and the lateral aspect of its respective vertebral body.

dose must be injected in all cases. Less than 1 mL of solution injected intravascularly has produced loss of consciousness and seizure activity. Before any injection, careful aspiration for blood and CSF must be performed. If the aspiration is negative, 0.5 to 1 mL of solution is administered, and the patient is asked to raise the thumb to indicate the absence of adverse symptoms. The patient should be informed beforehand and reminded during the blockade procedure that talking might cause movement of the neck musculature that could dislodge the needle from its proper location. To communicate during the block, the patient can be asked to point a thumb or finger upward in response to questions. After the initial test dose, the operator can inject the remainder of the solution, carefully aspirating after each 3 to 4 mL.

During injection or needle placement, paresthesia of the arm or hand may be elicited. It should always be interpreted to mean that the needle has been placed deeper to the anterior tubercle, adjacent to the C6 or C7 nerve root. Repositioning of the needle is necessary. Aspiration of blood or CSF also demands repositioning of the needle. Although the needle may be in the correct position, sometimes it is necessary to confirm that the injected solution is not flowing where it is not desired. The correct total volume of solution depends on what block is desired.[7] Properly placed, 5 mL of solution blocks the stellate ganglion.

■ C7 ANTERIOR APPROACH

The anterior approach to the stellate ganglion at C7 is similar to the approach described at C6. In contrast to C6, C7 has only a vestigial tubercle, so it is necessary to find Chassaignac's tubercle (C6). The palpating finger moves one fingerbreadth caudad from the inferior tip.

The advantage of blockade at C7 is manifested by the lower volume of local anesthetic needed to provide complete interruption of the upper extremity sympathetic innervation. Only 6 to 9 mL of solution suffices. The bothersome side effect of recurrent laryngeal nerve block is less common with this approach. The technique has two drawbacks: The less pronounced landmarks make needle positioning less reliable, and the risk of pneumothorax increases because the dome of the lung is close to the site of entry. The use of radiographic imaging during the approach helps to avoid the complications possible with the blind technique.

■ CHEMICAL NEUROLYSIS OF STELLATE GANGLION

The approach for chemical neurolysis is similar to that for stellate ganglion block performed at C7. The patient must be positioned with the neck and head in a neutral position (Fig. 142–5). Under direct anteroposterior fluoroscopy, the C7 vertebral body is identified. A skin wheal is raised over the ventrolateral aspect of the body of C7 with 1 mL of local anesthetic and a 25-gauge needle. A 22-gauge B-bevel needle is inserted through the skin wheal to contact the body of C7 in the ventrolateral aspect; this is at the junction of the transverse process with the vertebral body. Depth and direction should be confirmed with anteroposterior and lateral views. The needle tip is positioned deep to the anterior longitudinal ligament. The longus colli lies lateral to the needle tip. The needle should be stabilized with a long-handled Kelly clamp or hemostat. An intravenous extension should be attached to the needle and used for injection. Approximately 5 mL of water-soluble, nonirritating, nonionic, preservative-free, hypoallergenic contrast solution is injected after negative aspiration. Dye should spread around the vertebra, avoiding intravascular, epidural, intrathecal, thyroidal, or myoneural (longus colli) uptake. If good spread of the contrast medium is visualized, a mix of local anesthetic, phenol, and steroid is injected. The total volume of 5 mL should consist of 2.5 mL of 6% phenol in saline, 1 mL of 40 mg of triamcinolone, and 1.5 mL of 0.5% ropivacaine. (The total 5-mL dose contains a final mixture of 3% phenol.) The previously injected contrast material serves as a marker for the spread of the phenol. In the anteroposterior view, the contrast solution should spread caudad to the first thoracic sympathetic ganglion, cephalad to the inferior cervical ganglion, and cephalad to the superior cervical ganglion. In the lateral view, spread should be observed in the retropharyngeal space and in front of the longus colli and anterior scalene muscles. After injection, the patient remains supine with the head elevated slightly for approximately 30 minutes, to prevent spread of the phenol to other structures.[5]

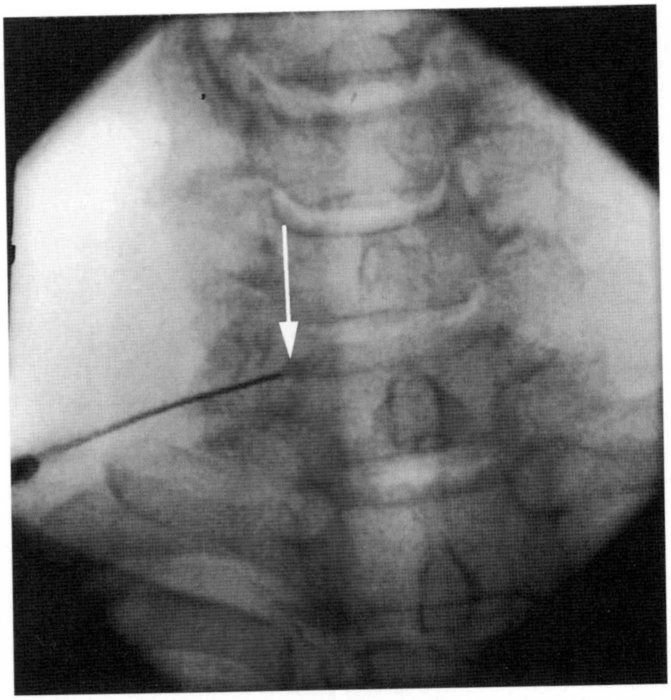

FIGURE 142–6 ■ Posteroanterior radiograph of the cervical spine. At the C7 level, the radiofrequency cannula rests at the junction of the lateral aspect of the vertebral body and the medial aspect of the transverse process *(arrow)*. This represents the correct cannula position for lesioning of the C7 sympathetic fibers. (From Raj PP, Lou L, Erdine S, et al: Stellate ganglion block. Radiographic Imaging for Regional Anesthesia and Pain Management. Philadelphia, Churchill Livingstone, 2003, p 78.)

RADIOFREQUENCY NEUROLYSIS

Radiofrequency neurolysis of the stellate ganglion may be accomplished under fluoroscopic guidance. After the target area is identified as for chemical neurolysis, a 16-gauge angiocatheter is inserted through the skin wheal instead of the B-bevel needle. A 20-gauge, curved, blunt-tipped cannula with a 5-mm active tip is guided through the extracath at the superolateral aspect. The tip should rest at the junction of the transverse process and the vertebral body. The depth and direction should be confirmed with anteroposterior and lateral views. Correct placement may be confirmed conclusively with the injection of contrast medium (Figs. 142–6, 142–7, and 142–8). A sensory (50 Hz, 0.9 V) and a motor (2Hz, 2 V) stimulation trial must be performed owing to the location of the phrenic nerve (lateral) and the recurrent laryngeal nerve (anterior and medial) relative to the proposed lesion. While motor stimulation is performed, the patient should say “ee” to ensure preservation of motor function. A small volume of local anesthetic (0.5 mL) should be injected before lesioning. The radiofrequency is applied for 60 seconds at 80°C. The cannula is redirected to the most medial aspect of the transverse process in the same plane. Placement is in the ventral aspect of the transverse process in the same plane. Placement in the ventral aspect must be confirmed with a lateral view. Before lesioning, the patient must be retested for sensory and motor stimulation. A repeat dose of the local anesthetic also should be given through the cannula. A third (and final) lesion

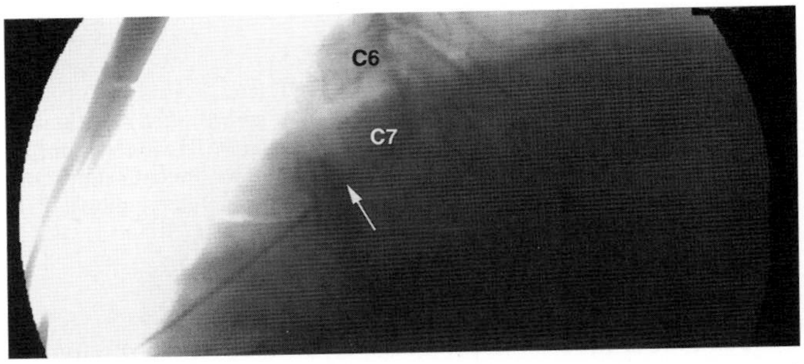

FIGURE 142–7 ■ Lateral view of correct placement of the needle *(arrow)* and the contrast spread after injection for stellate ganglion block. (From Raj PP, Lou L, Erdine S, et al: Stellate ganglion block. Radiographic Imaging for Regional Anesthesia and Pain Management. Philadelphia, Churchill Livingstone, 2003, p 79.)

should be directed at the upper portion of the junction of the transverse process and the body of C7. Potential complications include injury to the phrenic or the recurrent laryngeal nerve, neuritis, and vertebral artery injury.[6,7] Side effects of a stellate ganglion block should be distinguished from complications. Most unpleasant side effects result from the Horner syndrome—ptosis, miosis, and nasal congestion.

COMPLICATIONS

The two principal complications of stellate ganglion block are pneumothorax and intraspinal injection. A third risk

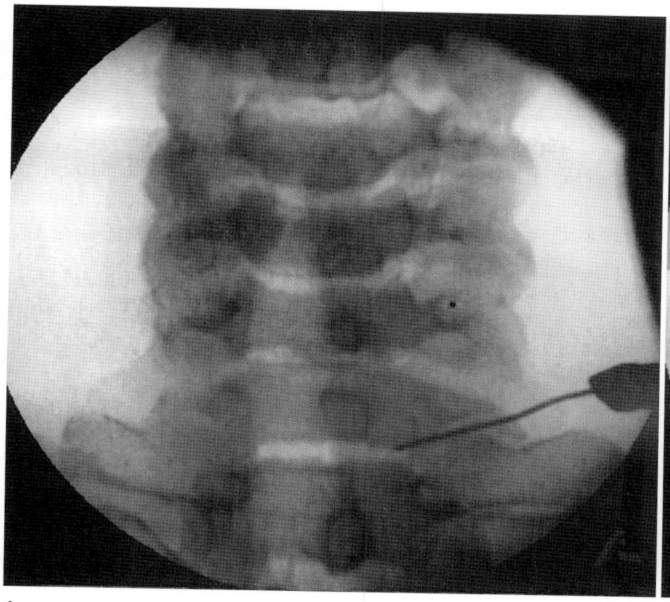

A

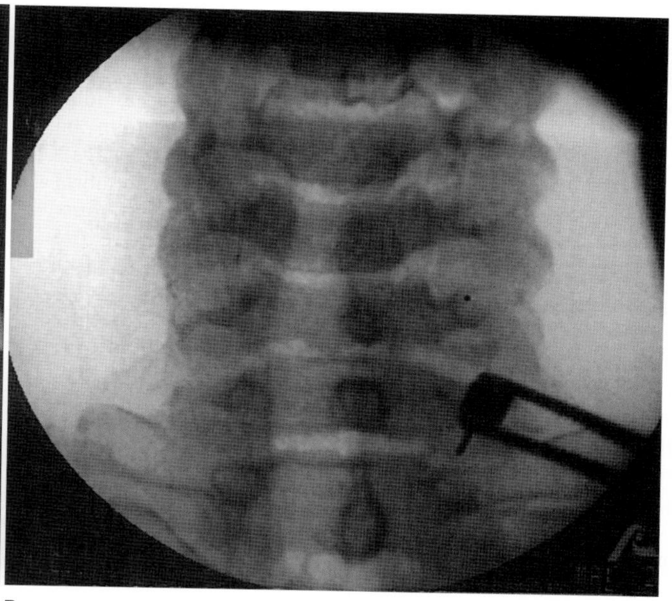

B

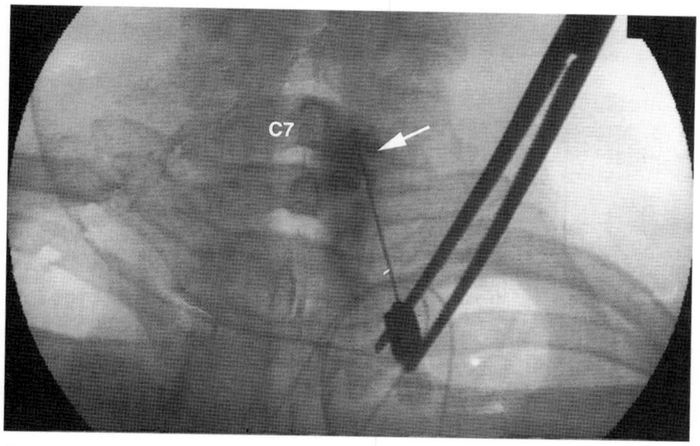

C

FIGURE 142–8 ■ **A-C,** The needle is in position for radiofrequency neurolysis at C7 (anteroposterior view). The *arrow* (**C**) shows the tip at the lateral border of vertebral body C7. (From Raj PP, Lou L, Erdine S, et al: Stellate ganglion block. Radiographic Imaging for Regional Anesthesia and Pain Management. Philadelphia, Churchill Livingstone, 2003, p 79.)

when neurolysis is performed is the possibility of persistent Horner syndrome. Pneumothorax can be avoided with careful placement of the needle, and if care is taken that the needle angulation is never lateral, and that the needle is advanced through the costotransverse ligaments (posterior and anterior) slowly and cautiously using the loss-of-resistance technique. Intraspinal injection most often occurs by diffusion through the intervertebral foramen and can be avoided by first injecting a water-soluble contrast dye and checking the needle position radiographically. The optimal method for checking needle position and solution spread is a CT scan.

To check for possible subsequent Horner syndrome, the clinician first can inject local anesthetic into the region and inspect the patient after 15 to 30 minutes. This practice does not always obviate Horner syndrome with neurolytic injection, however, and prior local anesthetic injection may not be considered optimal in all situations.

Common complications of a stellate ganglion block result from diffusion of local anesthetic onto nearby nerve structures. These include the recurrent laryngeal nerve with complaints of hoarseness, feeling of a lump in the throat, and sometimes a subjective shortness of breath. Bilateral stellate blocks are rarely advised because bilateral blocking of the recurrent laryngeal nerve can result in respiratory compromise and loss of laryngeal reflexes. Block of the phrenic nerve causes temporary paralysis of the diaphragm and can lead to respiratory embarrassment in patients whose respiratory reserve already is severely compromised. Partial brachial plexus block also can result secondary to spread along the prevertebral fascia[4] or positioning the needle too far posteriorly. The patient should be discharged with the arm in a sling and given careful instructions on how to care for a partially blocked arm, should this complication occur.

The two most feared complications of stellate ganglion block are intraspinal injection and seizures induced by intravascular injection. Respiratory embarrassment and the need for mechanical ventilation can result from injection into either the epidural space (if high concentrations of local anesthetic are used) or the intrathecal space. Should either occur, patients need continual reassurance that everything is being appropriately managed and that they will recover without sequelae. Some sedation is required while the local anesthetic wears off. No drugs are necessary for endotracheal cannulation because profound anesthesia of the larynx can be expected.

Intravascular injection most often involves the vertebral artery. Small amounts of local anesthetic cause unconsciousness, respiratory paralysis, seizures, and sometimes severe arterial hypotension. Increased intravenous fluids, vasopressors if indicated, oxygen, and endotracheal intubation may be necessary. If the amount of drug injected into the artery is less than 2 mL, the sequelae just listed are short-lived and self-limiting, with oxygen and increased fluid administration often being the only therapy needed. Care must be taken during a stellate ganglion block to ensure that no air is injected from the syringe. Cerebral air emboli have been reported from this procedure, and they are preventable.[2,8,9]

The risk of pneumothorax also attends the anterior approach. If the C7 tubercle is used and the needle is inserted caudally, the dome of the lung can be penetrated. This can cause pneumothorax. Approximately 10% to 15% of patients have postprocedure neuritis. This condition can last 3 to 6 weeks.[5,10]

CLINICAL PEARLS

Small amounts of local anesthetics (3 to 5 mL) do not reliably block all fibers to the upper extremities because contributions from T2 and T3 may be present. Injection of 10 mL of solution more reliably blocks all sympathetic innervation to the upper extremity, even in patients with the anomalous Kuntz nerves. If blockade is being performed for sympathetic-mediated pain of the thoracic viscera, including the heart, 15 to 20 mL of solution should be administered. Anomalous pathways, termed *Kuntz nerves*, can be reliably blocked only by a posterior approach,[3] although the posterior approach is technically more difficult than the anterior approach taught traditionally.

EFFICACY

Sympathetic interruption to the head, supplied by the stellate ganglion, can be documented easily by evidence of Horner syndrome: miosis (pinpoint pupil), ptosis (drooping of the upper eyelid), and enophthalmos (sinking of the eyeball). Associated findings include conjunctival injection, nasal congestion, and facial anhidrosis. These signs can be present without complete interruption of the sympathetic nerves to the upper extremity.

Evidence of sympathetic blockade to the upper extremity includes visible engorgement of the veins on the back of the hand and forearm, diminution of the psychogalvanic reflex, and plethysmographic and thermographic changes. Skin temperature also increases, provided that the preblock temperature did not exceed 33°C to 34°C.

References

1. Bonica JJ: The Management of Pain. Philadelphia, Lea & Febiger, 1953.
2. Moore DC: Stellate Ganglion Block. Springfield, IL, Charles C Thomas, 1954.
3. Bonica JJ: Sympathetic Nerve Blocks for Pain Diagnosis and Therapy. New York, Breon Laboratories, 1984.
4. Bridenbaugh PO, Cousins MJ: Neural Blockade in Clinical Anesthesia and Management of Pain. Philadelphia, JB Lippincott, 1988.
5. Racz G: Techniques of Neurolysis. Boston, Kluwer Academic, 1989.
6. Wenger C, Christopher C: Radiofrequency lesions for the treatment of spinal pain. Pain Digest 8:1, 1998.
7. Sluijter ME: Radiofrequency Lesions in the Treatment of Cervical Pain Syndromes. Burlington, MA, Radionics, 1990.
8. Moore DC: Regional Block, 4th ed. Springfield, IL, Charles C Thomas, 1975.
9. Adelman MH: Cerebral air embolism complicating stellate ganglion block. J Mt Sinai Hosp 15:28, 1948.
10. Skabelund C, Racz G: Indications and technique of thoracic neurolysis. Curr Rev Pain 3:400, 1999.

chapter 143

Cervical Facet Block

Laxmaiah Manchikanti, David M. Schultz, and Vijay Singh

HISTORICAL CONSIDERATIONS

Lifetime prevalence of spinal pain from the cervical spine has been reported as 65% to 80%.[1-14] Further, chronicity of neck pain has been demonstrated with chronic persistent pain resulting in 26% to 44% of patients after an initial episode of neck pain or whiplash.[12-16] Facet joints, ligaments, fascia, muscles, intervertebral disks, and nerve root dura have been identified as tissues capable of transmitting pain in the low back.[17] Facet joints are considered a common source of pain in the neck, head, and upper extremity.

Lumbar facet joints were identified as potential sources of back pain as early as 1911.[18] However, it was not until 1977 that Pawl[19] reported the reproduction of pain in patients with neck pain and headache after injections of hypertonic saline into the cervical facet joints. Bogduk and Marsland[20] studied the role of cervical facet joints in causation of idiopathic neck pain by using diagnostic cervical medial branch blocks and facet joint injections. Dwyer and colleagues[21] mapped out specific locations of referred neck pain by performing facet joint injections in normal volunteers. Aprill and associates[22] confirmed the accuracy of the pain chart developed by Dwyer and coworkers by anesthetizing the medial branches of the dorsal rami above and below the symptomatic joint. Fukui and coworkers[23] studied the referred pain distribution of cervical facet joints and cervical dorsal rami with similar results. Windsor and colleagues[24] also studied electrical stimulation-induced cervical medial branch referral patterns.

Sluijter and Koetsveld-Baart[25] described a technique for blocking the cervical dorsal rami near their origin and described a percutaneous radiofrequency technique to coagulate these nerves in 1980. Bogduk and Marsland[20] described cervical medial branch blocks distal to the target sites used by Sluijter and Koetsveld-Baart[25] in 1988. In 1981, Okada[26] introduced intra-articular cervical facet joint blocks using a lateral approach. Later, Dory[27] described a posterior approach based on a pillar view of the cervical facet joints. Subsequently, numerous others[28-31] have described intra-articular cervical facet joint blocks.

INDICATIONS

As with any synovial joint, degeneration, inflammation, and injury of facet joints can lead to pain on joint motion. Pain leads to restriction of motion, which eventually leads to overall physical deconditioning. Irritation of the facet joint innervation in itself also leads to secondary muscle spasm. It has been postulated that degeneration of the lumbar disk would lead to associated lumbar facet joint degeneration and subsequent spinal pain as the disk space loses height—resulting in excess stress on the posterior spinal elements. This process may also play a role in the cervical spine.

Cervical facet joints have been shown to be capable of being a source of pain in the neck and referred pain in the head and upper extremities.[19-24] Based on responses to controlled diagnostic blocks of cervical facet joints, in accordance with the criteria established by the International Association for the Study of Pain,[32] prevalence of cervical facet joint pain has been shown to be 54% to 67% in patients with chronic neck pain.[33-37]

Diagnostic Cervical Facet Blocks

Background

- Blocks of a cervical facet joint can be performed to test the hypothesis that the target joint is the source of the patient's pain.[38-40]
- The cervical facet joints can be anesthetized either with intra-articular injections of local anesthetic or by anesthetizing the medial branches of the dorsal rami that innervate the target joint.[38,39]
- If pain is relieved, the joint may be considered to be the source of pain.[38,39]
- True-positive responses are secured by performing controlled blocks, either in the form of placebo injections of normal saline or comparative local anesthetic blocks, in which on two separate occasions the same joint is anesthetized using local anesthetics with differing durations of action.[38,39]

Rationale

The rationale for using facet joint blocks for diagnosis is based on the following:

- The cervical facet joints are well innervated.
- The cervical facet joints have been shown to be capable of causing persistent neck pain and referred pain in the head and upper extremities.

- There is no reliable or valid indicator or clinical means to implicate cervical facet joints as the source of neck pain, headache, or upper extremity pain in a given patient.
- The referral patterns described for cervical facet joints are variable.
- A pattern of pain similar to that caused by cervical facet joints may be produced by other structures in the cervical spine, such as the disk, in the same segment.
- Many of the maneuvers used in physical examinations stress multiple structures simultaneously in the cervical spine in addition to facet joints and fail to provide useful diagnostic criteria.
- Numerous attempts by investigators to correlate neurophysiologic findings, radiologic findings, physical findings, and other signs and symptoms with the diagnosis of facet joint pain have been unsuccessful.[1]
- Strong evidence has been presented demonstrating the reliability of cervical facet joint nerve blocks in the diagnosis of neck pain, upper extremity pain, and headaches.[1,38-40]
- The face validity of intra-articular injections and medial branch blocks is demonstrated by determining the spread of contrast medium after injection of small volumes of local anesthetic under fluoroscopic visualization.[41]
- The construct validity of facet joint blocks has been demonstrated to rule out false-positive results.[42]
- The theory that evaluating a patient first with lidocaine and subsequently with bupivacaine provided a means of identifying placebo response has been tested and proven.[43-46]
- Significant false-positive rates with single facet joint blocks in the cervical spine have been documented (27% to 63%).[35-40,47]

Requirements

Tables 143–1 and 143–2 show indications and contraindications for diagnostic facet joint blocks. Cervical facet joint blocks are commonly performed in patients with the following:

- Neck pain, for which no cause is otherwise evident
- Pain patterns resembling that of pain evoked in normal volunteers on stimulation of the facet joints
- Lack of disk herniation or radiculopathy as the symptomatic lesion
- Lack of neurophysiologic abnormalities

Precautions

Caution must be exercised in patients receiving nonsteroidal anti-inflammatory medications. Raj and associates[48] provided a detailed description of the role of anticoagulants in interventional pain management. Nonetheless, there is lack of consensus as to the importance of discontinuation of nonsteroidal antiinflammatory drugs and aspirin before facet joint injection procedures. Patients on warfarin therapy should be checked for prothrombin time, which should be at acceptable levels. In stopping anticoagulant therapy, the interventional pain practitioner must take into consideration the risk-benefit ratio and also consult with the physician in charge of anticoagulant therapy to avoid unnecessary complications and consequent liability. Thus, it may be appropriate to advise the patient to contact the physician in charge of anticoagulant therapy to manage this aspect of care.

Table 143–1

Common Indications for Cervical Diagnostic Facet Joint Blocks

- Somatic or nonradicular neck and/or upper extremity pain
- Cervicogenic headache and upper back pain
- Lack of obvious evidence for diskogenic pain
- Lack of disk herniation or evidence of radiculitis
- Duration of pain of at least of 3 months
- Failure to respond to more conservative management, including physical therapy modalities with exercise, chiropractic management, and nonsteroidal antiinflammatory agents
- Average pain levels of greater than 5 on a scale of 0 to 10
- Intermittent or continuous pain causing functional disability
- No contraindications with understanding of consent, nature of the procedure, needle placement, or sedation
- No history of allergy to contrast administration, local anesthetic steroids, Sarapin, or other drugs potentially used
- No contraindications or inability to undergo physical therapy or chiropractic management
- Inability to tolerate nonsteroidal antiinflammatory drugs

Table 143–2

Common Contraindications for Cervical Facet Joint Blocks

- Infection
- Arnold-Chiari malformation
- Inability of the patient to understand consent, nature of the procedure, needle placement, or sedation
- Allergies to contrast, local anesthetic, steroids, Sarapin, or other drugs
- Needle phobia
- Psychogenic pain
- Suspected diskogenic pain or disk herniation
- Anticoagulant therapy
- Nonsteroidal antiinflammatory drug therapy (the authors disagree with this; no evidence that NSAIDs increase risk of serious bleeding)
- Non-aspirin antiplatelet therapy

Therapeutic Cervical Facet Blocks

A significant role has been described for therapeutic facet joint injections, either intra-articular or by medial branch block and medial branch neurotomy.[1] However, a single, randomized controlled trial has demonstrated lack of efficacy for intra-articular cervical facet joint steroid injections.[1] Manchikanti and coworkers,[1] in *Evidence-Based Practice Guidelines for Managing Spinal Pain*, reviewed the literature extensively. They concluded that, except for the one negative randomized trial for intra-articular injections, there were no other nonobservational trials qualifying to be included for evidence synthesis.

In addition to intra-articular blocks, medial branch blocks have been used for therapeutic purposes in the cervical spine.[49] However, evidence evaluating medial branch blocks for therapeutic purposes is limited.

Indications and contraindications for cervical facet joint blocks are described in Tables 143–1 and 143–2. Therapeutic facet joint blocks are performed only in patients with established facet joint pain by means of controlled diagnostic blocks.

CLINICALLY RELEVANT ANATOMY

- The cervical facet joints are paired, diarthrodial, synovial joints located between the superior and inferior articular pillars in the posterior cervical column (Fig. 143–1).[39]
  - Cervical facet joints extend from C2-C3 to C7-T1.
  - The atlanto-occipital and atlantoaxial synovial joints are also present in the cervical spine as two paired joints but are not considered to be facet joints because they are anterior rather than posterior spinal structures.
- The cervical facet joints are formed by the inferior articular process of the superior vertebral segment and superior articular process of the inferior vertebral segment.
- The superior aspect of the joint faces forward and downward at 45 degrees; whereas the inferior aspect of the joint faces backward and upward at 45 degrees.

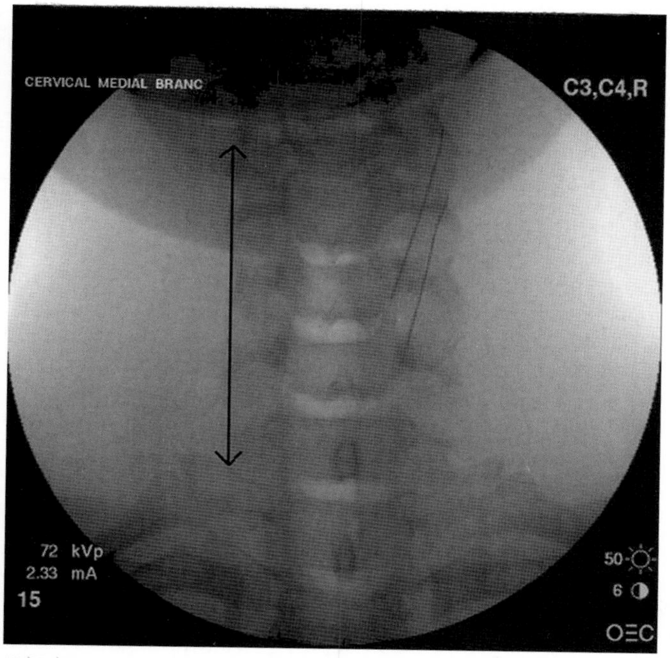

FIGURE 143–1 ■ Anteroposterior (AP) view of facet column.

- Cervical facet joints exhibit the features of typical synovial joints.
  - The articular facets are covered by articular cartilage and a synovial membrane bridges the margins of the articular cartilage of the two facets in each joint.
  - The cervical facet joints may contain a variety of intra-articular inclusions, with fibroadipose meniscoids being the most common inclusions.
- The capsular recesses exist at both superior and inferior aspects, with the superior recess adjacent to the neural foramina and the dorsal root ganglia. The average joint volume is less than 1 mL.[21]
- The articular surfaces of facet joints in the cervical spine are generally flat with only minimal concavity and convexity.[50] The obliquity of cervical facet joints averages about 45 degrees but is flatter at C2-C3 and steeper at C6-C7.[51] The C2-C3 joint is more oblique in its orientation than its adjacent counterpart. Thus, the inclination of lower joints is steeper.[52]
- The cervical facet joints are well innervated by the medial branches of the dorsal rami.[38-41,53-59] The cervical facet joints below C2-C3 are supplied by medial branches of the cervical dorsal rami above and below the joint, which also innervate the deep paramedian muscles. The C2-C3 joint is supplied by the third occipital nerve.[38,60] The innervation of the atlanto-occipital and atlantoaxial joints is derived from the C1 and C2 root, respectively.[38,60,61]
  - The fibrous joint capsule is richly innervated with mechanoreceptors, as well as nociceptors.[53-55]
- Each C3-C7 dorsal ramus crosses the transverse process of the same segment and divides into lateral and medial branches.
  - The medial branch curves around the waist of the articular pillar of the same-numbered vertebra.
  - The medial branches are bound by fascia, held against the articular pillar, and covered by the tendinous slips of the origin of the semispinalis capitis.[57]
  - Articular branches arise as the nerve approaches the posterior aspect of the articular pillar, with an ascending branch innervating the joint above and a descending branch innervating the joint below.
  - At C7, in contrast to C3-C6, the medial branch is located at a higher level owing to the transverse process. At C7, the base of the transverse process occupies most of the lateral aspect of the articular pillar pushing the medial branch higher.[35,61]
  - C4 to C7 medial branch nerves typically lack any cutaneous branches.
  - The course of the C4 and C5 medial branch nerves has been shown to be relatively constant, following the waist of their respective articular pillars in cadavers.[62]
  - The C3, C6, and C7 show more variation compared to C4 and C5.[62]
  - The C3 medial branch nerve with its more superior location at the upper third of the C3 articular pillar often overlaps the third occipital nerve, with the third occipital nerve being rostral to the C3 medial branch.[62] The C3 medial branch and the third occipital nerve have a common origin in the C3 dorsal ramus.
  - The C6 medial branch courses around the waist of the articular pillar or above it, between the waist and the superior articular process.

  - The majority (70%) of C7 medial branches are located high on the C7 articular pillar and cross the C6-C7 facet joint. However, a few may be lower on the C7 transverse process.
  - The distance between the nerves and bone varies from close proximity to separation by 2 mm to 3 mm.
- The C2-C3 facet joint is largely innervated from the third occipital nerve, which is the superficial medial branch of the C3 dorsal ramus.
  - The deep medial branch of the C3 dorsal ramus is referred to as the C3 medial branch.
  - Articular branches may also arise from a communicating loop that crosses the back of the joint between the third occipital nerve and the C2 dorsal ramus.[58,61]
  - The third occipital nerve continues around the lower lateral and dorsal surface of the C2-C3 joint embedded in the connective tissue that invests the joint capsule.[58,61] It also provides muscular branches to the semispinalis capitis and becomes cutaneous over the suboccipital region.
- The vertebral artery ascends through the cervical transverse foramina of C1 to C6, which are located anterolaterally.
  - The vertebral artery at C2-C7 is located anterior to the facet joints from both posterior and lateral injection approaches.
  - The vertebral artery passes directly superior in the neck until it reaches the transverse process of the axis where it courses upward and laterally to the transverse foramina of the atlas.[63]
  - The vertebral artery courses medially and superiorly from its lateral position at C1 to the medial foramen magnum. The course of the vertebral artery from the transverse foramen of the atlas to the foramen magnum may be tortuous and variable.

TECHNIQUE

Although the technique of cervical facet joint blockade has lagged behind that of lumbar facet joint block, multiple techniques have now been described. Cervical facet joint injections may be performed using either a posterior, lateral, or anterior approach. The posterior approach is the most commonly used method—followed by the lateral approach. Both approaches will be described subsequently.

Intra-articular Blocks

Posterior Approach

The posterior approach for cervical intra-articular facet joint block can be performed with the patient in a prone position, or if required, in a sitting position. It involves introducing a 22- or a 25-gauge needle into the target joint from behind, along an oblique trajectory that coincides with the plane of the joint.

- The patient is positioned in the prone position on a radiolucent fluoroscopy table with a cushion under the chest with the head and neck completely prone or with the neck rotated to the opposite side.
- Under aseptic conditions, the skin entry is carried out approximately two or more segments below the target joint. The skin entry point may be determined either by directing an imaginary line to the skin along the plane of the joint (as determined by a lateral view) or by direct visualization of the joint via a pillar view and making a skin mark along the plane of the x-ray beam into the center of the joint lucency.[64] The sagittal plane for skin entry is determined by identifying the sagittal plane of the lateral aspect of the facet joint column on prone fluoroscopic viewing
- The needle is passed with caution through the skin at approximately a 45-degree angle upward and ventrally through the posterior neck muscles until it makes contact with the posterior surface of the articular pillar below the target joint.
- Following this, the needle may be readjusted until it enters the joint cavity. However, this may require repeated posteroanterior and lateral fluoroscopic visualization to ensure the needle stays on course. **Caution:** Directing the needle medially toward the interlaminar space may result in epidural or intrathecal puncture and/or spinal cord trauma. The depth of the needle is evaluated by a lateral view; however, repeated posteroanterior and lateral screening is used to guide the insertion until the needle strikes the back of the target joint at its midpoint.[64]
- After satisfactory localization of the needle in the joint, water-soluble contrast medium is injected to obtain an arthrogram and verify accurate placement. Then, local anesthetic and/or corticosteroid is injected for diagnostic or therapeutic purpose. **Caution:** The capacity of the joint can be assessed from the volume of the injectate of the contrast, which is typically less than 1 mL. It is important to respect the capacity of the joint because the local anesthetic and steroid may leak into the recesses and block the dorsal root ganglion.
- The C7-T1 joint may be difficult to enter with a posterior approach and a lateral approach has been suggested. However, due to the risk of pneumothorax and the proximity of other neurovascular structures, the posterior approach is considered as preferred for the C7-T1 facet joint.[64] Figure 143–2 illustrates intra-articular needle placement with a posterior approach.

Overall, the posterior approach is considered safe because the needle penetrates only the skin and posterior neck muscles, with the deep cervical artery being the only structure at risk of inadvertent puncture. Further, posterior cervical arteries pose minimal risk of morbidity because they supply no major structures. However, if the needle is inserted too deeply or too aggressively, it could penetrate the anterior joint capsule moving into the neural foramen and the vicinity of the dorsal root ganglion, the cervical radicular artery and/or the vertebral artery. Leakage of local anesthetic and steroid to the dorsal root ganglion may negate any diagnostic information from this injection, whereas inadvertent contact with nerve root or anterior artery may have serious adverse consequences. In addition, there is potential for a misplaced needle to enter the epidural space or spinal cord.

Lateral Approach

Proponents of the lateral approach argue that it is technically less demanding, and may be performed with smaller-gauge needles.[26] They also argue that it is more comfortable for the

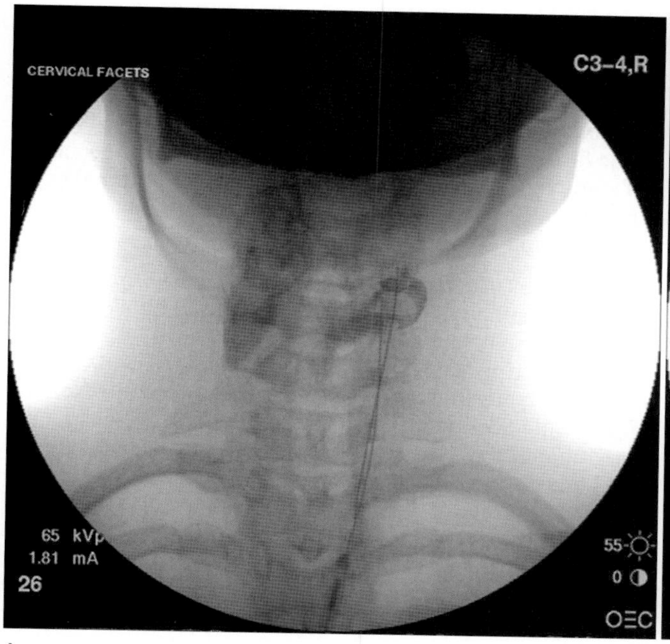

A

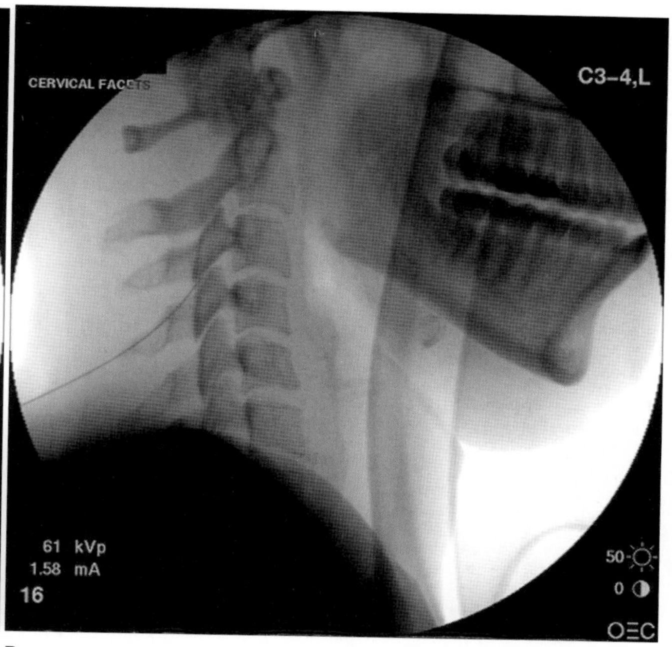

B

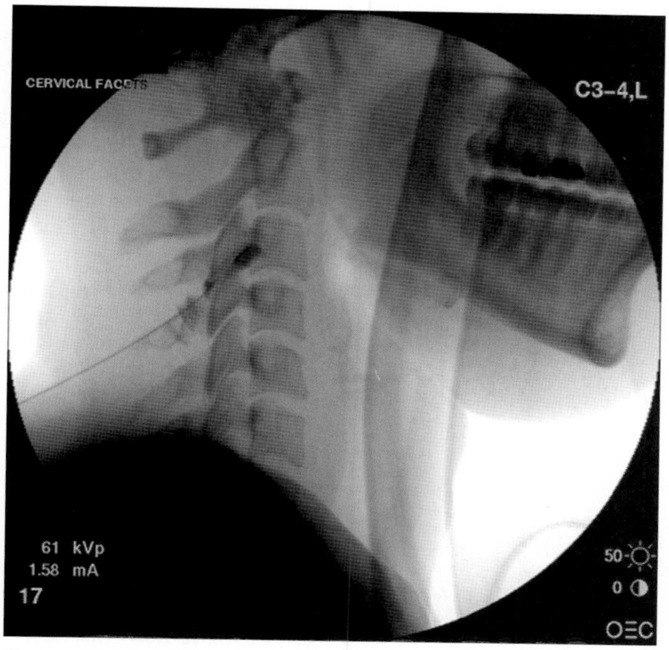

C

FIGURE 143–2 ■ Intra-articular needle placement with a posterior approach: **A,** ¾ PA view; **B,** ¾ needle placement lateral view; **C,** ¾ arthrogram lateral view.

patient because less soft tissue is traversed. Similar to the posterior approach during insertion, the risk of morbidity is minimal because only the skin and posterolateral neck muscles are penetrated with no other overlying structures being at risk of puncture. However, aggressive maneuvering or over-penetration may lead the needle into the epidural space or spinal cord. Many experts believe that the lateral technique is more technically demanding and requires more experience.

- The patient is positioned lying on the side with the target side up. The shoulders are pulled down to avoid obscuring the joints under fluoroscopy and rotated slightly posterior about 25 degrees into the plane of the upper torso and shoulders.[64]
- The target joint is identified on lateral imaging of the neck.
  - Lateral fluoroscopic imaging must appropriately identify both joints so that the uppermost target joint is differentiated from the down-side contralateral joint (Fig. 143–3).
  - The object is to identify the image of the target joint, which lies uppermost in the patient.
- The needle is introduced through the skin over the midpoint of the joint.
  - It is advanced deeply until it makes contact with the bone of either the superior or inferior articular process. *This*

technique promotes safety by providing the operator with a sense of accurate depth of insertion and prevents over-insertion.
  - Rotation of the intensifier may help to identify both joints. It is absolutely crucial that right and left joints be identified properly so that the uppermost joint is targeted.
- Once the correct joint is clearly identified, the needle is advanced until the superior articular process is contacted just above the joint line.
  - The needle is then directed and advanced through the joint capsule.
  - The needle may be felt to pierce the capsule and to enter the joint space. Only minimal penetration is required and the operator may also notice loss of resistance as the needle pierces the capsule.
- The appropriate position in the joint may be either confirmed by injection of a small dose of contrast medium to obtain an arthrogram or by multiple radiographic views. The facet joints in the cervical spine are more easily entered if one begins slightly superior to the joint and angles the needle inferiorly along the plane of the articular surfaces until the joint is entered.[64]

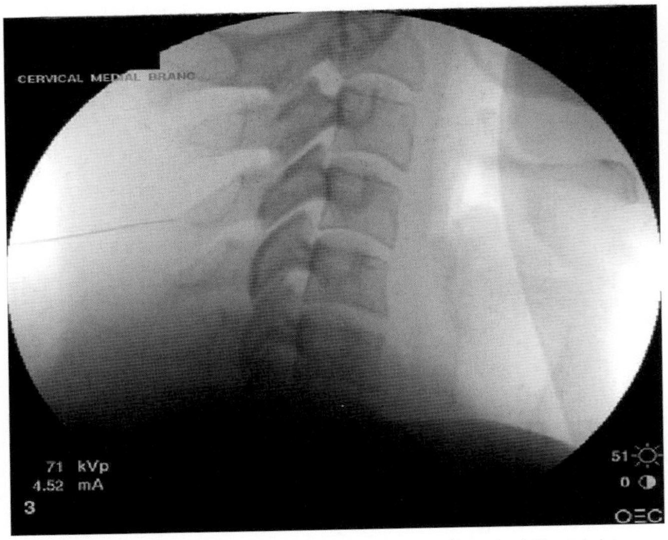

FIGURE 143–3 ■ Lateral fluoroscopic image of cervical facet joints.

With the lateral approach, the needle must remain posterior to the ventral ramus and the vertebral and radicular arteries to ensure safety. C3-C4, C4-C5, and C6-C7 joint injections are easily performed using the lateral approach with no disadvantages compared to the posterior approach. However, the C7-T1 joint injection may be more easily performed using the posterior approach. In patients with large neck and shoulders, C7-T1 may not be reached from a lateral approach and may require the posterior approach. C7-T1 may also require a much steeper superior to inferior approach than other mid-cervical levels to minimize the possibility of contacting more inferior neurovascular and pleural structures.

The C2-C3 joint may be technically more difficult to visualize and enter owing to its anatomic features. The C2-C3 joint is more angulated vertically and medially and is not clearly evident on lateral views. For C2-C3 the posterior approach may be modified by rotating the patient's head to bring the cavity of the C2-C3 joint into view as it moves forward on the long axis of the vertebral column. Other modifications with the fluoroscopic unit may also be made. Figure 143–4 illustrates intra-articular placement with a lateral approach.

It is of paramount importance that low volumes are injected into the cervical facet joints in a slow and incremental fashion. If volumes of more than 1 mL are injected or injection is carried out rapidly or forcefully, the joint capsule

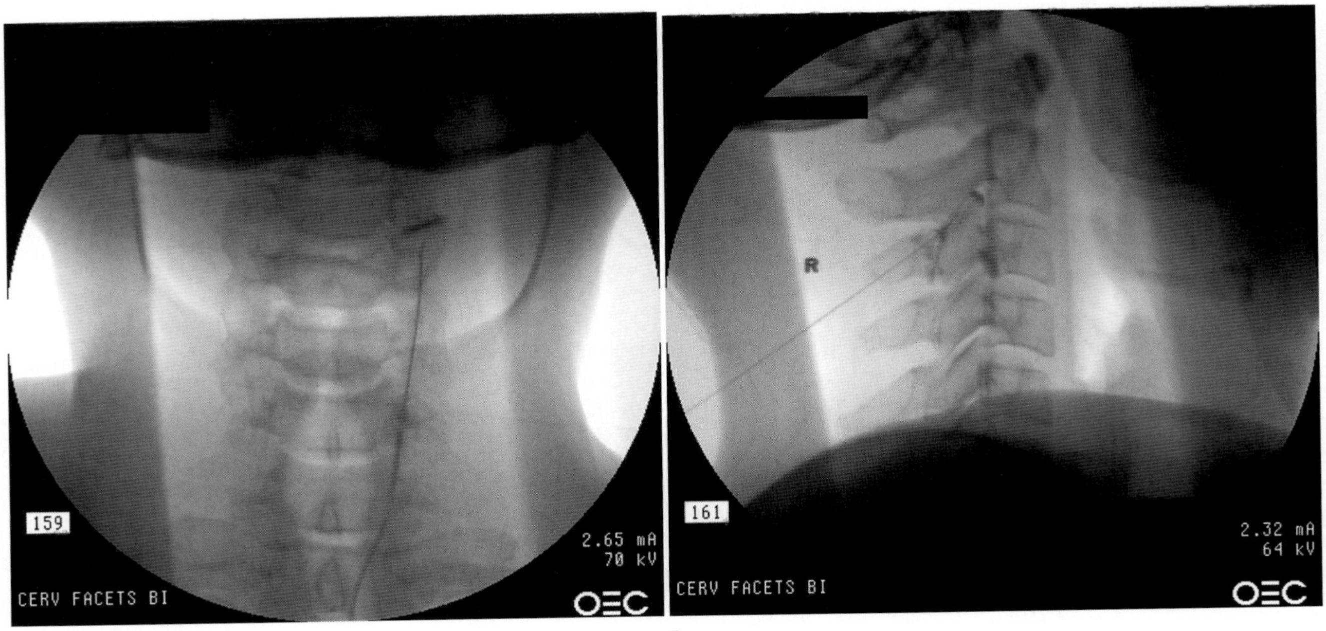

A B

FIGURE 143–4 ■ Intra-articular placement within C2-C3 with a lateral approach. **A,** Intra-articular placement of C2-C3 in PA view. **B,** Intra-articular placement of C2-C3 with a lateral approach.

may rupture and/or medication may spread onto nearby structures. Okada[26] showed that in a series of 142 arthrograms, a communicating pathway existed in 80% of subjects between the facet joint and the interlaminar space, the opposite facet joint, the extradural space, and/or the interspinous space when volumes in excess of 1 mL were injected (Fig. 143–5). Even with smaller volumes, extra-articular leaks have been observed in up to 7% of cases.[26,27,29] Extra-articular spread is extremely important, specifically when diagnostic blocks are performed, because this will compromise the specificity of the block.

Cervical Medial Branch Blocks

The cervical facet joints can be anesthetized by blocking the nerves that supply them, namely the medial branches of the cervical dorsal rami. To block the nerves supplying a cervical facet joint, two medial branches must be blocked owing to dual innervation of each facet joint. Table 143–3 illustrates the nerves to be blocked for each facet joint.

The target points for these nerves, other than the third occipital nerve, are the crossing points of the waists of the articular pillars—a point proximal to the origin of the articular branches and a point where the nerves have a constant relation to the bone.[38,64] These points may be reached by needles using either a posterior, lateral, or anterior approach. Posterior and lateral approaches are the commonly used techniques.

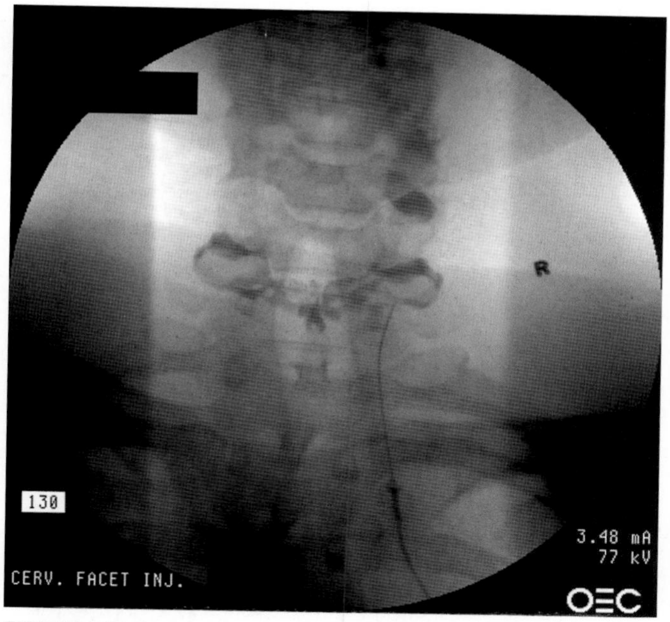

FIGURE 143–5 ■ Illustration of filling of a joint on the opposite side.

Posterior Approach

- The patient is placed in the prone position with a pillow under the chest. The head may be completely prone or turned to the opposite side.
- A posteroanterior view is obtained to identify the posterior aspect of the waists of the articular pillars from C3-C7.
  - In some patients, the articular pillars of the superior cervical spine (C3 and C4) may be difficult to identify, especially with the patient's head in neutral position. Turning the head to the opposite side may facilitate visualization of the target area.
  - An additional maneuver may be to ask the patient to open the mouth to remove the mandible from the radiologic field.
- After the identification of the waists of the articular pillars of the levels to be blocked, a 22- or 25-gauge, 2 to 3 inch spinal needle is inserted through the skin and posterior neck muscles aiming first for the dorsal aspect of the articular pillar medial to its lateral concavity.
- Once the needle has made contact with the bone, it is readjusted laterally to the deepest of this concavity where the C3 to C7 medial branches lie. **Caution:** Initially, directing the needle medially to bone ensures that the needle is not placed too deeply. The needle is then directed laterally until the tip reaches the lateral margin of the waist of the articular pillar. The needle should be felt to barely slip off the bone laterally in a ventral direction at the deepest point of concavity of the articular pillar.[64] Thus, it is prudent to obtain lateral images to ensure the needle tip rests at the centroid of the articular pillar. The centroid is found at the intersection of the two diagonals of the diamond-shaped pillar[64] (Fig.143–6).
- The C8 medial branch is blocked by placing the needle onto the transverse process of T1 and then directing it until it lies at the superolateral border of the transverse process. Figure 143–7 illustrates medial branch blocks with posterior approach.
- Lateral viewing of needle tip location may be difficult below C6. Moving the C-arm to an oblique projection may help to identify needle depth by moving the shoulders out of the line of the fluoroscopic beam.

Table 143–3

Facet Joint Nerves to Be Blocked for Each Facet Joint in Cervical Region

Facet Joint	*Facet Joint Nerves (Medial Branches) to Be Blocked*	*Level of Transverse Process*
C2-C3	Third occipital nerve or C2 and C3 medial branches	At C2-C3 joint
C3-C4	C3 and C4 medial branches	At C3 and C4 articular pillars
C4-C5	C4 and C5 medial branches	At C4 and C5 articular pillars
C5-C6	C5 and C6 medial branches	At C5 and C6 articular pillars
C6-C7	C6 and C7 medial branches	At C6 and C7 articular pillars
C7-T1	C7 and C8 medial branches	At C7 articular pillar At T1 transverse process for C8

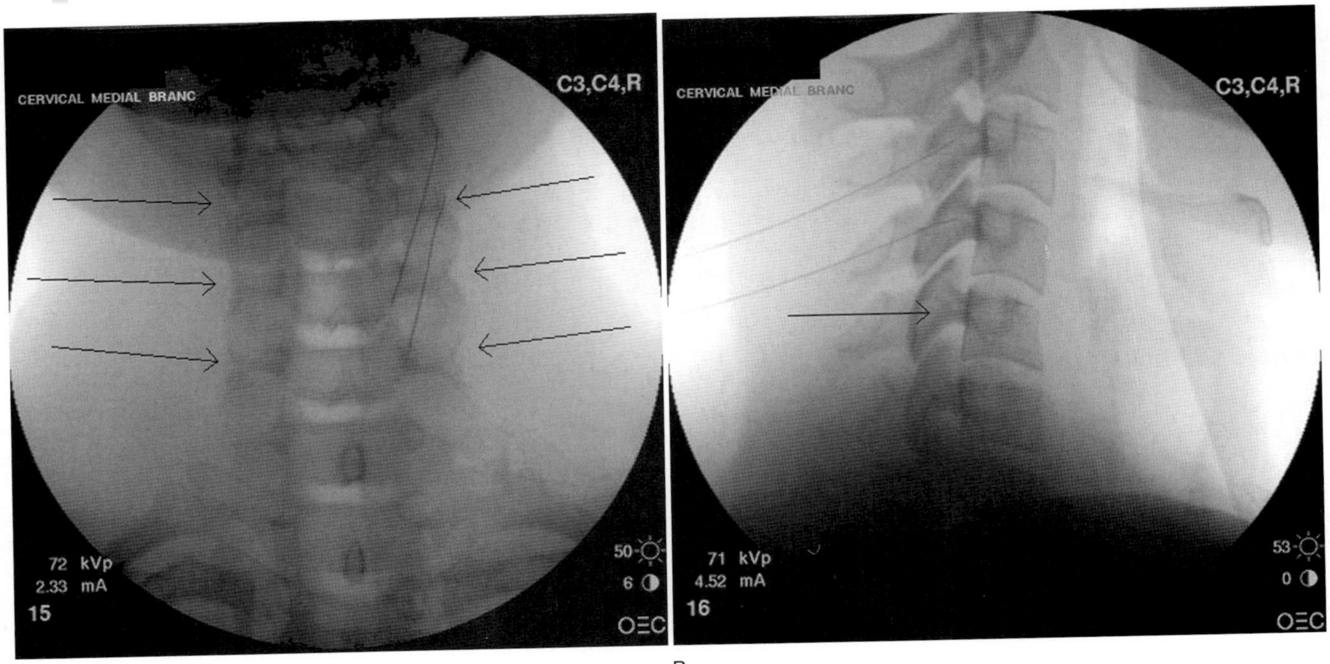

A B

FIGURE 143–6 ■ Illustration of center of centroid. **A,** Anteroposterior (AP)view; **B,** Lateral view.

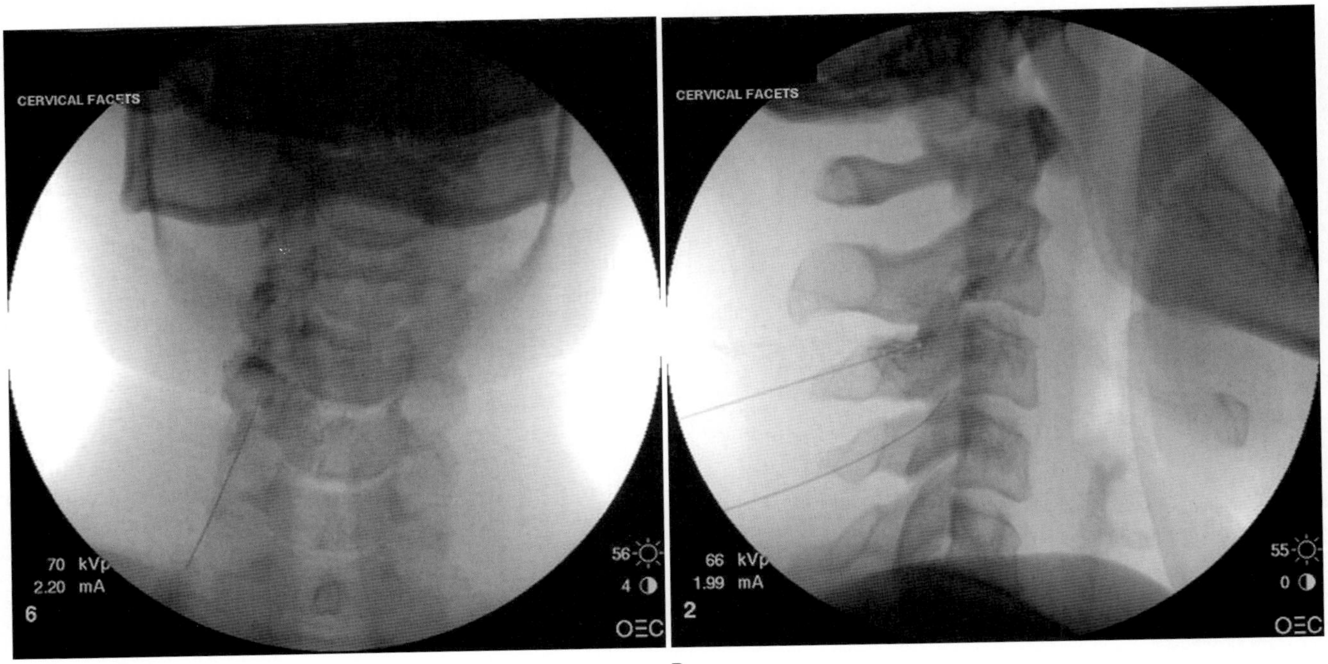

A B

FIGURE 143–7 ■ Medial branch blocks with posterior approach. **A,** Needle placement, anteroposterior (AP) view; **B,** Needle placement, lateral view.

Lateral Approach

- The patient is positioned in the lateral position with the target side up.
- Articular pillars are identified by lateral fluoroscopy.
  - The uppermost articular pillar can be distinguished from the opposite side by moving the fluoroscope. *The needle will be seen to travel with the uppermost articular pillar as the two articular pillars separate on the fluoroscopic image. This approach is well suited for C3 to C6 medial branches.*[64]
- The needle is directed through the skin and posterolateral neck muscles toward the centroid of the articular pillar as seen on a true lateral radiograph.[64]

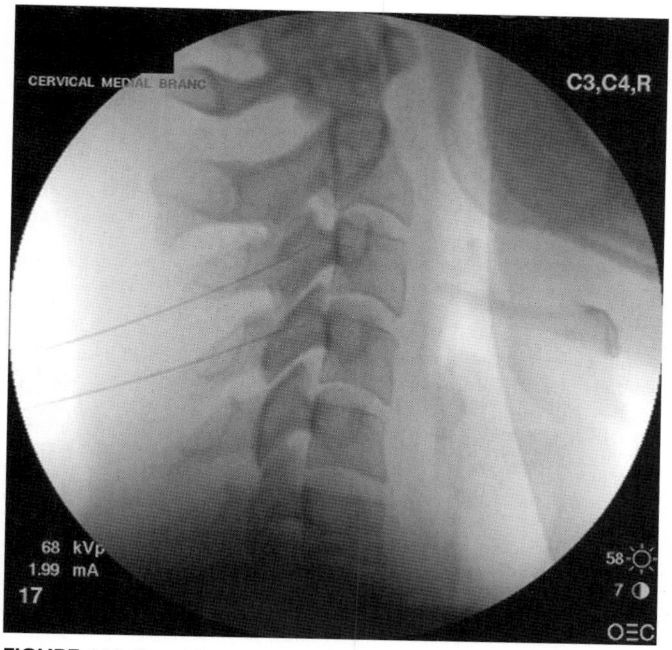

FIGURE 142–8 ■ C3-C4 medial branch blocks with a lateral approach.

- To block the C7 medial branch by the lateral approach, the needle is advanced so that it stays within the confines of the C7 superior articular process, which prevents excessive advancement into the C8 foramen and toward the vertebral artery.[64]
- Once the superior articular process is contacted, anteroposterior imaging should verify that the needle lies against the lateral aspect of the superior articular process.
- Figure 143–8 illustrates medial branch blocks with the lateral approach.

With posterior and lateral approaches, contrast in doses of 0.1 to 0.2 mL may be injected to confirm appropriate needle placement. However, contrast injection is not mandatory. After the confirmation of the needle position, local anesthetic with or without steroid is injected incrementally around the nerve.

Cervical medial branch blocks are extremely safe. Other than general risks associated with all cervical injections including fluoroscopic exposure, infection, and needle trauma, no specific complications have been reported. The relative safety of medial branch blocks lies in the fact that the blocks are performed on the external surface of the vertebral column—well away from any vital structures. Some state that the lateral approach is advantageous because target points are clearly visible and there is minimal tissue penetration. The posterior approach may require adjustment of the needle onto the lateral margin of the articular pillar using an additional step; however, with experience, this may be avoided.

Local anesthetic injection for intra-articular injections, as well as for medial branch blocks should be limited to 0.5 mL (0.3 mL to 0.6 mL) for a diagnostic block and approximately 1 mL for a therapeutic block. Numerous authors,[33,34,38,64] pioneering the concept of comparative local anesthetic blocks, have recommended potent local anesthetics such as 4% lidocaine and 0.75% bupivacaine, to minimize the risk of false-negative medial branch blockade, which may occur at a 10% rate with 2% lidocaine in the lumbar spine. Further, for diagnostic, as well as therapeutic blockade, the literature has been limited to using local anesthetic agents of different durations of action, namely, lidocaine and bupivacaine. Manchikanti and colleagues[35-37] in multiple investigations used concentrations of lidocaine 1% and bupivacaine 0.25% versus 4% lidocaine and 0.75% bupivacaine, as recommended by others, without compromising validity of diagnostic blocks and responsiveness to therapeutic blocks.

DRUGS

Local anesthetic injection should be limited to 0.4 to 0.6 mL for a diagnostic block and approximately 1 mL for a therapeutic block. Dreyfuss and associates[64] recommend potent local anesthetics (e.g., 4% lidocaine and 0.75% bupivacaine) to minimize the risk of false-negative medial branch blocks, which can occur at a 10% rate with 2% lidocaine. Kaplan and coworkers[65] described that failure to obtain relief with lumbar medial branch blocks in a case in which venous uptake of contrast is observed, despite needle redirection with avoidance of subsequent venous uptake, carries a 50% risk for false-negative results. Contrast injection of 0.1 to 0.3 mL also has been recommended for medial branch or dorsal ramus blocks to confirm selective flow along the path of the nerve and the absence of inadvertent venous uptake.[60]

For diagnostic, as well as therapeutic blocks, the literature has been limited to using local anesthetic agents of different durations of action, namely, lidocaine and bupivacaine. However, Manchikanti and colleagues[66] have shown that validity of diagnostic blocks is maintained with addition of adjuvant agents such as Sarapin and methylprednisolone, along with provision of a therapeutic benefit of much longer duration than with local anesthetic alone. In addition, in multiple investigations, Manchikanti and associates[35-37] demonstrated efficacy of 1% lidocaine and 0.25% bupivacaine for medial branch blocks versus 4% lidocaine and 0.75% bupivacaine as recommended by others.

SIDE EFFECTS AND COMPLICATIONS

Complications from intra-articular injections or medial branch blocks in the cervical spine are exceedingly rare.[1,25-31,33-48,56,57,64,66-77] However, disastrous complications may occur with cervical facet joint injections. These complications include those related to placement of the needle as well as complications related to the administration of various drugs. Proximity to the vertebral artery and spinal cord, along with nerve root ganglion, make intra-articular facet injections relatively high risk when compared to medial branch blocks. Complications may include dural puncture, spinal cord trauma, neural trauma, subdural injection, injection into the intervertebral foramen; intravascular injection into the veins, or more seriously into vertebral or radicular arteries, infectious complications including epidural abscess and bacterial meningitis, and side effects related to the administration of steroids, local anesthetics, and other drugs.

Other exceedingly rare but potential complications with cervical facet joint injections include vertebral artery and ventral ramus damage, embolus resulting in serious neurologic sequelae, spinal cord damage, and cerebral infarction. Other minor complications include light-headedness, flushing, sweating, nausea, hypotension, syncope, pain at the injection site, and headaches. Side effects related to the administration of steroids are generally attributed to the physiologic effects of the steroids.[77] These include suppression of pituitary-adrenal access, hypocorticism, Cushing syndrome, osteoporosis, avascular necrosis of the bone, steroid myopathy, epidural lipomatosis, weight gain, fluid retention, and hypoglycemia. However, Manchikanti and coworkers,[78] in evaluating the effect of neuraxial steroids and weight and bone mass density, showed no significant differences in patients undergoing various types of interventional techniques, with or without steroids.

CONCLUSION

Cervical facet joints are commonly identified as the cause of neck pain, upper extremity pain, and headaches. Cervical facet joint blocks can be performed to test the hypothesis that the target joint is the source of the patient's pain. The rationale for using facet joint blocks for diagnosis, as well as therapy, is based on the fact that cervical facet joints have been shown to be the source of neck pain and referred pain in the head and upper extremities. Although cervical facet joint pain may not be diagnosed based on referral patterns, physical examination, history, neurophysiologic testing, or radiologic evaluation, diagnostic cervical facet joint blocks have been shown to be highly valid and specific. Because degenerative processes of the cervical spine and the origins of cervical spine pain are extremely complex, the effectiveness of a large variety of therapeutic interventions in managing chronic pain arising from the cervical spine has not been demonstrated conclusively.

KEY POINTS

- Cervical facet joints have been shown to be capable of being a source of pain in the neck and referred pain in the head and upper extremities.
- Cervical facet joints are well innervated by the medial branches of the dorsal rami.
- Based on responses to controlled diagnostic blocks of cervical facet joints, in accordance with the criteria established by the International Association for the Study of Pain, prevalence of cervical facet joint pain has been determined to be 54% to 67%.
- To maintain validity of diagnostic blocks, either comparative local anesthetic blocks or placebo-controlled blocks must be performed because single blocks carry a false-positive rate of 27% to 63%.
- Multiple effective and therapeutic modalities are available in managing cervical facet joint pain.
- Adequate training and experience, proper technique, meticulous adherence to safety guidelines, and high-quality fluoroscopic imaging equipment are prerequisites for safe and effective injection of cervical structures.

References

1. Manchikanti L, Staats P, Singh V, et al: Evidence-based practice guidelines for interventional techniques in the management of chronic spinal pain. Pain Physician 6:3, 2003.
2. Bovim G, Schrader H, Sand T: Neck pain in the general population. Spine 19:1307, 1994.
3. Côté DC, Cassidy JD, Carroll L: The Saskatchewan Health and Back Pain Survey. The prevalence of neck pain and related disability in Saskatchewan adults. Spine 23:1689, 1998.
4. Côté DC, Cassidy JD, Carroll L: The factors associated with neck pain and its related disability in the Saskatchewan population. Spine 25:1109, 2000.
5. Lau EMC, Sham A, Wong KC: The prevalence of and risk factors for neck pain in Hong Kong Chinese. J Public Health Med 18:396, 1996.
6. Johnson G: Hyperextension soft tissue injuries of the cervical spine: A review. J Accid Emerg Med 13:3, 1996.
7. Ariëns GA, Borghouts JA, Koes BW: Neck pain. In Crombie IK, Croft PR, Linton SJ, et al (eds): Epidemiology of Pain. Seattle, IASP Press, 1999.
8. Frederiksson K, Alfredsson L, Koster M, et al: Risk factors for neck and upper limb disorders: Results from 24 years of follow-up. Occup Environ Med 56:59, 1999.
9. Leclerc A, Niedhammer I, Landre MF, et al: One-year predictive factors for various aspects of neck disorders. Spine 24:1455, 1999.
10. Marshall PD, O'Connor M, Hodgkinson JP: The perceived relationship between neck symptoms and precedent injury. Injury 26:17, 1995.
11. Linton SJ, Hellsing AL, Hallden K: A population based study of spinal pain among 35- to 45-year-old individuals. Spine 23:1457, 1998.
12. Miles K, Maimaris C, Finlay D, et al: The incidence and prognostic significance of radiological abnormalities in soft tissue injuries to the cervical spine. Skeletal Radiol 17:493, 1988.
13. Pennie B, Agambar I: Patterns of injury and recovery in whiplash. Injury 22:57, 1991.
14. Ylinen J, Ruuska J: Clinical use of neck isometric strength measurement in rehabilitation. Arch Phys Med Rehabil 75:465, 1994.
15. Hallgern RC, Greenman PE, Rechtien JJ: Atrophy of suboccipital muscles in patients with chronic pain: A pilot study. J Am Osteopath Assoc 12:1032, 1994.
16. Hildingsson C, Toolanen G: Outcome after soft-tissue injury of the cervical spine: A prospective study of 93 car accident victims. Acta Orthop Scand 61:357, 1990.
17. Kuslich SD, Ulstrom CL, Michael CJ: The tissue origin of low back pain and sciatica: A report of pain response to tissue stimulation during operation on the lumbar spine using local anesthesia. Orthop Clin North Am 22:181, 1991.
18. Goldthwait JE: The lumbosacral articulation: An explanation of many cases of lumbago, sciatica, and paraplegia. Boston Med Surg J 164:365, 1911.
19. Pawl RP: Headache, cervical spondylosis, and anterior cervical fusion. Surg Ann 9:391, 1977.
20. Bogduk N, Marsland A: The cervical zygapophyseal joints as a source of neck pain. Spine 13:610, 1988.
21. Dwyer A, Aprill C, Bogduk N: Cervical zygapophyseal joint pain patterns: A study in normal volunteers. Spine 6:453, 1990.
22. Aprill C, Dwyer A, Bogduk N: The prevalence of cervical zygapophyseal joint pain patterns II: A clinical evaluation. Spine 6:458, 1990.
23. Fukui S, Ohseto K, Shiotani M, et al: Referred pain distribution of the cervical zygapophyseal joints and cervical dorsal rami. Pain 68:79, 1996.
24. Windsor RE, Nagula D, Storm S, et al: Electrical stimulation induced cervical medial branch referral patterns. Pain Physician 6:411, 2003.
25. Sluijter ME, Koetsveld-Baart CC: Interruption of pain pathways in the treatment of the cervical syndrome. Anaesthesia 35:302, 1980.
26. Okada K: Studies on the cervical facet joints using arthrography of the cervical facet joint. J Jpn Orthop Assoc 55:563, 1981.
27. Dory MA: Arthrography of the cervical facet joints. Radiology 148:379, 1983.
28. Dussault RG, Nicolet VM: Cervical facet joint arthrography. J Can Assoc Radiol 36:79, 1985.
29. Wedel DJ, Wilson PR: Cervical facet arthrography. Reg Anesth 10:7, 1985.
30. Hove B, Glydensted C: Cervical analgesic facet joint arthrography. Neuroradiology 32:456, 1990.

31. Roy DF, Fleury J, Fontaine SB, et al: Clinical evaluation of cervical facet joint infiltration. J Can Assoc Radiol 39:118, 1988.
32. Merskey H, Bogduk N: Classification of Chronic Pain: Descriptions of Chronic Pain Syndromes and Definitions of Pain Terms, 2nd ed. Seattle, IASP Press, 1994, p 180.
33. Barnsley L, Lord SM, Wallis BJ, et al: The prevalence of chronic cervical zygapophyseal joint pain after whiplash. Spine 20:20, 1995.
34. Lord SM, Barnsley L, Wallis BJ, et al: Chronic cervical zygapophysial joint pain with whiplash: A placebo-controlled prevalence study. Spine 21:1737, 1996.
35. Manchikanti L, Singh V, Rivera J, et al: Prevalence of cervical facet joint pain in chronic neck pain. Pain Physician 5:243, 2002.
36. Manchikanti L, Singh V, Pampati S, et al: Is there correlation of facet joint pain in lumbar and cervical spine? Pain Physician 5:365, 2002.
37. Manchikanti L, Boswell MV, Singh V, et al: Prevalence of facet joint pain in chronic spinal pain of cervical, thoracic, and lumbar regions. BMC Musculoskelet Disord 5:15, 2004.
38. Bogduk N: International Spinal Injection Society guidelines for the performance of spinal injection procedures. Part 1: Zygapophyseal joint blocks. Clin J Pain 13:285, 1997.
39. Bogduk N, Lord S: Cervical zygapophysial joint pain. Neurosurgery 8:107, 1998.
40. Boswell MV, Singh V, Staats PS, et al: Accuracy of precision diagnostic blocks in the diagnosis of chronic spinal pain of facet or zygapophysial joint origin. Pain Physician 6:449, 2003.
41. Barnsley L, Bogduk N: Medial branch blocks are specific for the diagnosis of cervical zygapophyseal joint pain. Reg Anesth 18:343, 1993.
42. Lord SM, Barnsley L, Bogduk N: The utility of comparative local anesthetic blocks versus placebo-controlled blocks for the diagnosis of cervical zygapophysial joint pain. Clin J Pain 11:208, 1995.
43. Bonica JJ: Local anesthesia and regional blocks. In Wall PD, Melzack R (eds): Textbook of Pain, 2nd ed. Edinburgh, Churchill Livingstone, 1989, p 724.
44. Bonica JJ, Buckley FP: Regional analgesia with local anesthetics. In Bonica JJ (ed): The Management of Pain. Philadelphia, Lea & Febiger, 1990, p 1883.
45. Boas RA: Nerve blocks in the diagnosis of low back pain. Neurosurg Clin North Am 2:806, 1991.
46. Barnsley L, Lord S, Bogduk N: Comparative local anesthetic blocks in the diagnosis of cervical zygapophysial joints pain. Pain 55:99, 1993.
47. Barnsley L, Lord S, Wallis B, et al: False-positive rates of cervical zygapophysial joint blocks. Clin J Pain 9:124, 1993.
48. Raj PP, Shah RV, Kay AD, et al: Bleeding risk in interventional pain practice: Assessment, management, and review of the literature. Pain Physician 7:3, 2003.
49. Manchikanti L, Manchikanti KN, Damron K, et al: Effectiveness of cervical medial branch blocks in chronic neck pain: A prospective outcome study. Pain Physician 7:195, 2004.
50. Grieve GP: Applied anatomy—regional. In Grieve GP, Newman PH (eds): Common Vertebral Joint Problems, 2nd ed. London, Churchill Livingstone, 1988, p 7.
51. Nowitzke A, Westaway M, Bogduk N: Cervical zygapophyseal joints. Geometrical parameters and relationship to cervical kinematics. Clin Biomech 9:342, 1994.
52. Dvorak J, Dvorak V: Biomechanics and functional examination of the spine. In Manual Medicine-Diagnostics, 2nd ed. New York, Thieme, 1990, p 1.
53. McClain RF: Mechanoreceptor endings in human cervical facet joints. Spine 19:495, 1994.
54. Wyke B: Neurology of the cervical spinal joints. Physiotherapy 65:72, 1979.
55. Wyke B: Articular neurology: A review. Physiotherapy 58:563, 1981.
56. Bogduk N: Back pain: Zygapophyseal joint blocks and epidurals. In Cousins MJ, Bridenbaugh PO (eds): Neural Blockade in Clinical Anesthesia and Pain Management, 2nd ed. Philadelphia, JB Lippincott, 1990, p 935.
57. Lord SM, Barnsley L, Bogduk N: Cervical zygapophyseal joint pain in whiplash injuries. Spine State Art Rev 12:301, 1998.
58. Bogduk N: The clinical anatomy of the cervical dorsal rami. Spine 7:35, 1982.
59. Stilwell DL: The nerve supply of the vertebral column and its associated structures in the monkey. Anat Rec 125:139, 1956.
60. Dreyfuss P, Michaelsen M, Fletcher D: Atlanto-occipital and lateral atlanto-axial joint pain patterns. Spine 19:1125, 1994.
61. Lord SM, Barnsley L, Bogduk N: Percutaneous radiofrequency neurotomy in the treatment of cervical zygapophyseal joint pain: A caution. Neurosurgery 36:732, 1995.
62. Lord SM: Cervical Zygapophyseal Joint Pain after Whiplash Injury, Precision Diagnosis, Prevalence, and Evaluation of Treatment by Percutaneous Radiofrequency Neurotomy [doctoral thesis]. Newcastle, Australia, University of Newcastle, 1996.
63. Schultz D: Risk of transforaminal epidural injections. Pain Physician 6:390, 2003.
64. Dreyfuss P, Kaplan M, Dreyer SJ: Zygapophyseal joint injection techniques in the spinal axis. In Leonard (ed): Pain Procedures in Clinical Practice, 2nd ed. Philadelphia, Hanley & Belfus, 2000, p 276.
65. Kaplan M, Dreyfuss P, Halbrook B, et al: The ability of medial branch blocks to anesthetize the zygapopophyseal joint. Spine 23:1847, 1998.
66. Manchikanti L, Pampati VS, Fellows B, et al: The diagnostic validity and therapeutic value of medial branch blocks with or without adjuvants. Curr Rev Pain 4:337, 2000.
67. Windsor RE, Storm S, Sugar R: Prevention and management of complications resulting from common spinal injections. Pain Physician 6: 473, 2003.
68. Windsor RE, Pinzon EG, Gore HC: Complications of common selective spinal injections: Prevention and management. Am J Orthop 29:759, 2000.
69. Gladstone JC, Pennant JH: Spinal anaesthesia following facet joint injection. Anaesthesia 42:754, 1987.
70. Marks R, Semple AJ: Spinal anaesthesia after facet joint injection. Anaesthesia 43:65, 1988.
71. Cook NJ, Hanrahan P, Song S: Paraspinal abscess following facet joint injection. Clin Rheumatol 18:52, 1999.
72. Magee M, Kannangara S, Dennien B, et al: Paraspinal abscess complicating facet joint injection. Clin Nucl Med 25:71, 2000.
73. Manchikanti L, Cash K, Moss T, et al: Risk of whole body radiation exposure and protective measures in fluoroscopically guided interventional techniques: A prospective evaluation. BMC Anesthesiology 3:2, 2003.
74. Orpen NM, Birch NC. Delayed presentation of septic arthritis of a lumbar facet joint after diagnostic facet joint injection. J Spinal Disord Tech 16:285, 2003.
75. Manchikanti L, Cash K, Moss T, et al: Effectiveness of protective measures in reducing risk of radiation exposure in interventional pain management: A prospective evaluation. Pain Physician 6:301, 2003.
76. Berrigan T: Chemical meningism after lumbar facet joint block. Anesthesia 7:905, 1992.
77. Manchikanti L: Role of neuraxial steroids in interventional pain management. Pain Physician 5:182, 2002.
78. Manchikanti L, Pampati V, Beyer C, et al: The effect of neuraxial steroids on weight and bone mass density: A prospective evaluation. Pain Physician 3:357, 2000.

chapter 144

Cervical Epidural Nerve Block

Steven D. Waldman

Because cervical epidural nerve block has had a limited number of applications in surgical anesthesia, this procedure traditionally has been identified as an exotic technique of only passing historical interest. The more recent recognition of the clinical utility of cervical epidural nerve block in the management of head, face, neck, shoulder, and upper extremity pain has brought the technique into the mainstream of contemporary pain management. This chapter provides a practical overview of the indications for, technique of, and contraindications to cervical epidural nerve block.

HISTORICAL CONSIDERATIONS

Although the description by Pagés[1] of the paramidline approach to the lumbar epidural space in 1921 is considered the first clinically relevant report of the technique of lumbar epidural nerve block, it seems that Dogliotti[2] was the first to describe the technique of epidural block in the cervical region.[3]

Owing to the problems inherent in complete sensory blockade of the cervical nerve roots when cervical epidural nerve block is performed for surgical anesthesia, many anesthesiologists believed that cervical epidural nerve block was too risky, given the general anesthetic techniques available at the time. This fact led to two persistent beliefs that have colored contemporary thinking about the use of cervical epidural nerve block for pain management. The first belief is that cervical epidural nerve block is too risky for routine clinical use. The second belief is that it has a limited number of applications. The documented clinical utility of cervical epidural administration of steroids to manage cervical radiculopathy, tension-type headache, and other painful conditions, along with cervical epidural opioids to manage cancer-related pain, combined with the clinical experience of most contemporary pain specialists refute both of these beliefs.

INDICATIONS AND CONTRAINDICATIONS

Indications for cervical epidural nerve block are summarized in Table 144–1. In addition to a few applications for surgical anesthesia, cervical epidural nerve block with local anesthetics can be used as a diagnostic tool for differential neural blockade on an anatomic basis for the evaluation of head, neck, face, shoulder, and upper extremity pain.[4-8] If destruction of the cervical nerve roots is being considered, the technique is useful as a prognostic indicator of the extent of motor and sensory impairment that the patient may experience.

Cervical epidural nerve block with local anesthetics or opioids may be used to palliate acute pain emergencies during the wait for pharmacologic, surgical, or antiblastic methods to take effect.[9,10] The technique is useful in the management of postoperative pain and pain secondary to trauma involving the head, face, neck, and lower extremities. The pain of acute herpes zoster and cancer-related pain also are amenable to epidural administration of local anesthetics, steroids, or opioids.[11] Additionally, this technique is of value for acute vascular insufficiency of the upper extremities secondary to vasospastic and vaso-occlusive disease, including frostbite and ergotamine toxicity.[11] Evidence is increasing that the prophylactic or preemptive use of epidural nerve blocks in patients scheduled to undergo limb amputations for ischemia reduces the incidence of phantom limb pain.[12]

The administration of local anesthetics or steroids via the cervical approach to the epidural space is useful in the treatment of a variety of chronic benign pain syndromes, including cervical radiculopathy, cervicalgia, cervical spondylosis, cervical postlaminectomy syndrome, tension-type headache, phantom limb pain, vertebral compression fractures, diabetic polyneuropathy, chemotherapy-related peripheral neuropathy, postherpetic neuralgia, reflex sympathetic dystrophy, and neck and shoulder pain syndromes.[7,13-15]

The cervical epidural administration of local anesthetics in combination with steroids or opioids is useful in the palliation of cancer-related pain of the head, face, neck, shoulder, upper extremity, and upper trunk.[16] This technique has been especially successful in relieving pain secondary to metastatic disease of the spine. The long-term epidural administration of opioids has become a mainstay in the palliation of cancer-related pain.[17] The role of epidural opioids in the management of chronic benign pain syndromes is currently being evaluated.

Contraindications to the cervical epidural nerve block are listed in Table 144–2. Because of the potential for hematogenous spread via the epidural vasculature, local infection and sepsis represent absolute contraindications to using the cervical approach to the epidural space.[18] In contrast to the caudal approach to the epidural space, anticoagulation and coagulopathy are absolute contraindications to cervical epidural nerve block, owing to the risk of epidural hematoma.[19]

Table 144–1

Indications for Cervical Epidural Nerve Block

Surgical, Diagnostic, Prognostic	
Surgical anesthesia	
Differential neural blockade to evaluate head, neck, face, shoulder, and upper extremity pain	
Prognostic indicator before destruction of cervical nerves	
Acute Pain	
Palliation in acute pain emergencies	
Postoperative pain	
Head, face, neck, shoulder, and upper extremity pain secondary to trauma	
Pain of acute herpes zoster	
Acute vascular insufficiency of the upper extremities	
Prophylactic and Preemptive Pain	
Pain of tension-type headache	
Before amputation of ischemic limbs	
Chronic Benign Pain	
Cervical radiculopathy	
Cervical spondylosis	
Cervicalgia	
Vertebral compression fractures	
Diabetic polyneuropathy	
Postherpetic neuralgia	
Reflex sympathetic dystrophy	
Shoulder pain syndromes	
Upper extremity pain syndromes	
Phantom limb syndrome	
Peripheral neuropathy	
Postlaminectomy syndrome	
Pain of tension-type headache	
Cancer-Related Pain	
Pain secondary to head, face, neck, shoulder, and upper extremity malignancies	
Bony metastases to head, face, cervical spine, shoulder girdle, and upper extremity	
Chemotherapy-related peripheral neuropathy	

Table 144–2

Contraindications for Cervical Epidural Nerve Block

Absolute	*Relative*
Local infection	Hypovolemia
Sepsis	
Anticoagulant medication or coagulopathy	

Hypovolemia is a relative contraindication to cervical epidural nerve block with local anesthetics.[20]

CLINICALLY RELEVANT ANATOMY

Boundaries of the Cervical Epidural Space

The superior boundary of the cervical epidural space is the point at which the periosteal and spinal layers of dura fuse at the foramen magnum.[21] These structures allow drugs injected into the cervical epidural space to travel beyond their confines if the volume of injectate is large enough. This fact probably explains many of the early problems associated with the use of cervical epidural nerve block for surgical anesthesia, when large volumes of local anesthetics in vogue at the time were injected.

The epidural space continues inferiorly to the sacrococcygeal membrane.[22] The cervical epidural space is bounded anteriorly by the posterior longitudinal ligament and posteriorly by the vertebral laminae and the ligamentum flavum (Fig. 144–1). The ligamentum flavum is relatively thin in the cervical region and becomes thicker farther caudad, closer to the lumbar spine.[21] This fact has direct clinical implications, in that the loss of resistance felt during *cervical* epidural nerve block is more subtle than it is in the lumbar or lower thoracic region.

The vertebral pedicles and intervertebral foramina form the lateral limits of the epidural space (Fig. 144–2). The degenerative changes and narrowing of the intervertebral foramina associated with aging may be marked in the cervical region. Such changes reduce leakage of local anesthetic out of the foramina and account in part for the lower local anesthetic dose requirements of elderly patients undergoing cervical epidural nerve block. The distance between the ligamentum flavum and dura is greatest at the L2 interspace, measuring 5 to 6 mm in adults.[21] Because of the enlargement of the cervical spinal cord that corresponds to the neuromeres serving the upper extremities, this distance is only 1.5 to 2 mm at C7 (Fig. 144–3A).[21] Flexion of the neck moves this cervical enlargement more cephalad, resulting in widening of the epidural space to 3 to 4 mm at the C7-T1 interspace (Fig. 144–3B).[22] This fact has important clinical implications if cervical epidural block is performed with the patient in the lateral or prone position (see under Technique).

Contents of the Epidural Space

Fat

The epidural space is filled with fatty areolar tissue. The amount of epidural fat varies in direct proportion to the amount of fat stored elsewhere in the body.[21] The epidural fat is relatively vascular and seems to change to a denser consistency with aging. This change in consistency may account for the significant variations in required drug doses in adults, especially with the caudal approach to the epidural space. The epidural fat seems to perform two functions: (1) It serves as a shock absorber for the other contents of the epidural space and for the dura and the contents of the dural sac, and (2) it serves as a depot for drugs injected into the cervical epidural space. This second function has direct clinical implications for the choice of opioids for cervical epidural administration.

Epidural Veins

The epidural veins are concentrated principally in the anterolateral portion of the epidural space.[21] These veins are valveless and transmit intrathoracic and intra-abdominal pressures. As pressure in either of these body cavities increases, owing to Valsalva's maneuver or compression of the inferior vena cava by a gravid uterus or a tumor mass, the epidural veins

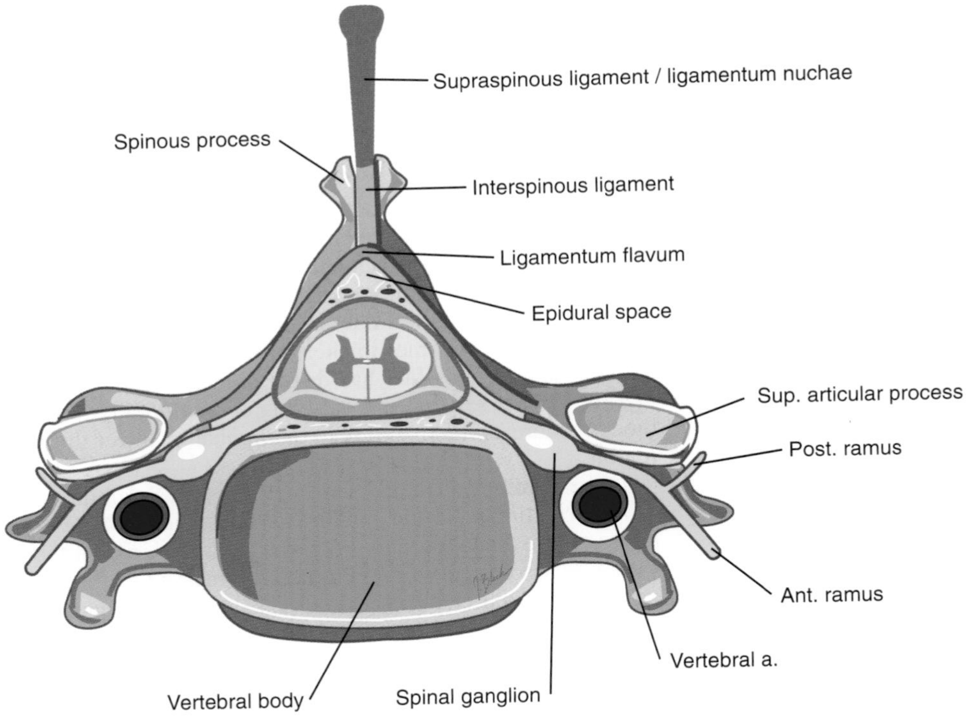

FIGURE 144–1 ■ Cross-sectional anatomy of the cervical epidural space.

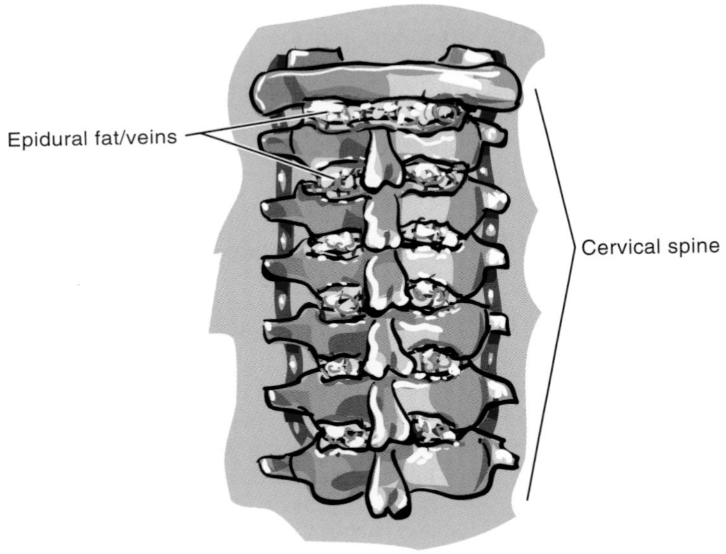

FIGURE 144–2 ■ Posterolateral view of cervical epidural space.

distend and reduce the volume of the epidural space. This decrease in volume can directly affect how much drug is needed to obtain a given level of neural blockade. Because this venous plexus serves the entire spinal column, it becomes a ready conduit for hematogenous infection.

Epidural Arteries

The arteries that supply the bony and ligamentous confines of the cervical epidural space and the cervical spinal cord enter the cervical epidural space via two routes—through the intervertebral foramina and through direct anastomoses from the intracranial portions of the vertebral arteries.[21,23] There are significant anastomoses between the epidural arteries, most of which lie in the lateral portions of the epidural space. Trauma to the epidural arteries can result in epidural hematoma formation and compromise the blood supply to the spinal cord itself.

Lymphatics

The lymphatics of the epidural space are concentrated in the region of the dural roots, where they remove foreign material from the subarachnoid and epidural spaces.

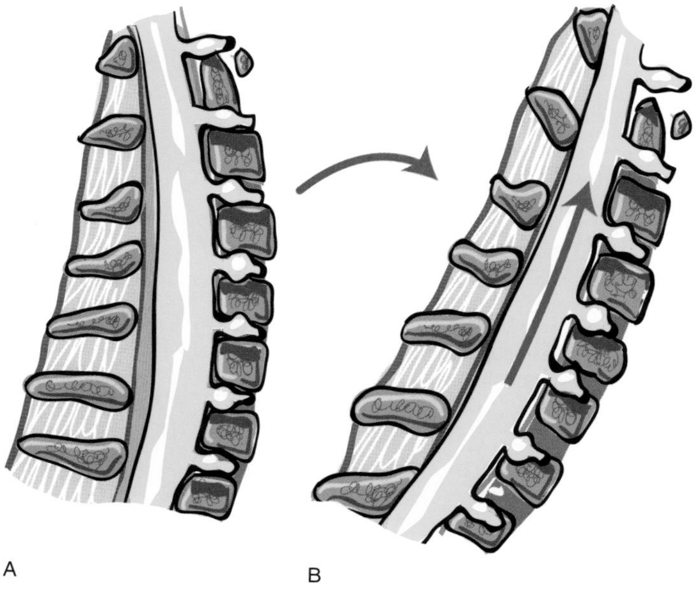

FIGURE 144–3 ■ **A,** Lateral view of cervical spine in neutral position. **B,** Lateral view of cervical spine flexed and moving the neuromeres cephalad.

Structures Encountered During Midline Insertion of a Needle into the Cervical Epidural Space

In the cervical region, after traversing the skin and subcutaneous tissues, the styletted epidural needle impinges on the ligamentum nuchae, which runs vertically between the apices of the cervical spinous processes.[24] The ligamentum nuchae offers some resistance to the advancing needle (Fig. 144–4A). This ligament is dense enough to hold a needle in position even when the needle is released.

The interspinous ligament, which runs obliquely between the spinous processes, is encountered next and offers additional resistance to needle advancement (Fig. 144–4B). Because the interspinous ligament is contiguous with the ligamentum flavum, the operator may perceive a "false" loss of resistance when the needle tip enters the space between the interspinous ligament and the ligamentum flavum. This phenomenon is more pronounced in the cervical region than in the lumbar region because the ligaments are less well defined.

A significant increase in resistance to needle advancement signals that the needle tip is impinging on the dense ligamentum flavum. Because the ligament is composed almost entirely of elastin fibers, resistance increases as the needle traverses the ligamentum flavum because of the drag of the ligament on the needle (Fig. 144–4C). A sudden loss of resistance occurs as the needle tip enters the epidural space (Fig. 144–4D). There should be essentially no resistance to injection of drug into the normal epidural space.

Pitfalls in Needle Placement

A comprehensive discussion of the pitfalls of needle placement for cervical epidural block is beyond the scope of this chapter. Close attention must be paid to the site of needle entry, the needle trajectory, and the final position of the needle tip; otherwise, the block may fail. Trauma to the nerves, arteries, veins, and dural sac and its contents also may occur, possibly with disastrous results.[25]

■ TECHNIQUE

All equipment—needles and supplies for nerve block, drugs, resuscitation equipment, oxygen supply, and suction—must be assembled and checked before the start of the cervical epidural nerve block. The patient's informed consent also must be obtained.

Positioning of the Patient

Cervical epidural nerve block may be done with the patient in the sitting, lateral, or prone position. Each position has advantages and disadvantages.

Sitting Position

The sitting position is easiest for the patient and the pain management specialist. Not only does it enhance the operator's ability to identify the midline, but also it ensures that the cervical spine is flexed, which widens the lower cervical epidural space. The sitting position avoids the rotation of the spine inherent in the lateral position, which makes identification of the epidural space difficult. The sitting position is not always an option, as with a patient with acute vertebral compression fractures. A history of vasovagal syncope with previous needle punctures precludes use of this position. In such situations, the lateral position is preferred, unless the patient is treated first with intravenous ephedrine.

Lateral Position

The lateral position is preferred for patients who cannot assume the sitting position or who are prone to vasovagal attacks. For the patient's comfort, the lateral position is more suitable for placement of tunneled epidural catheters or other implantable devices with an epidural terminus. If the lateral position is chosen, care must be taken to ensure that there is no rotation of the patient's spine, which would make epidural nerve block exceedingly difficult or impossible. Flexion of the

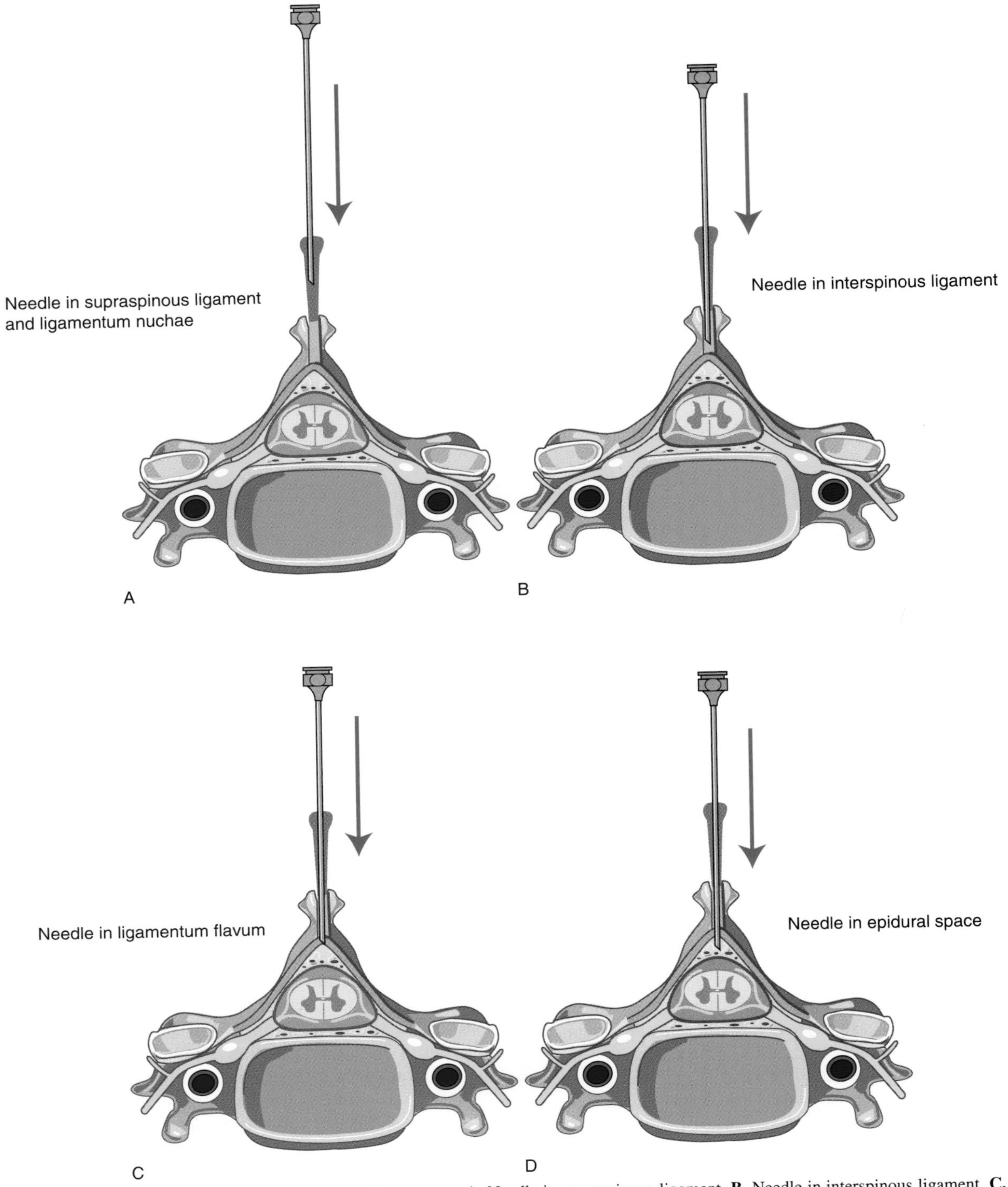

FIGURE 144–4 ■ Midline ligaments of the cervical epidural space. **A,** Needle in supraspinous ligament. **B,** Needle in interspinous ligament. **C,** Needle in ligamentum flavum. **D,** Needle through ligamentum flavum with "animated" loss of resistance.

cervical spine is mandatory to maximize the width of the epidural space.

Prone Position

The prone position is used principally for placement of tunneled epidural catheters and spinal stimulator electrodes. As with the other positions, care must be taken to flex the cervical spine to widen the epidural space. The prone position should be avoided if sedation is required because access to the airway is limited.

Preblock Preparation

After the patient is placed in the optimal position, the skin is prepared with an antiseptic solution, such as povidone-iodine, so that all of the surface landmarks can be palpated

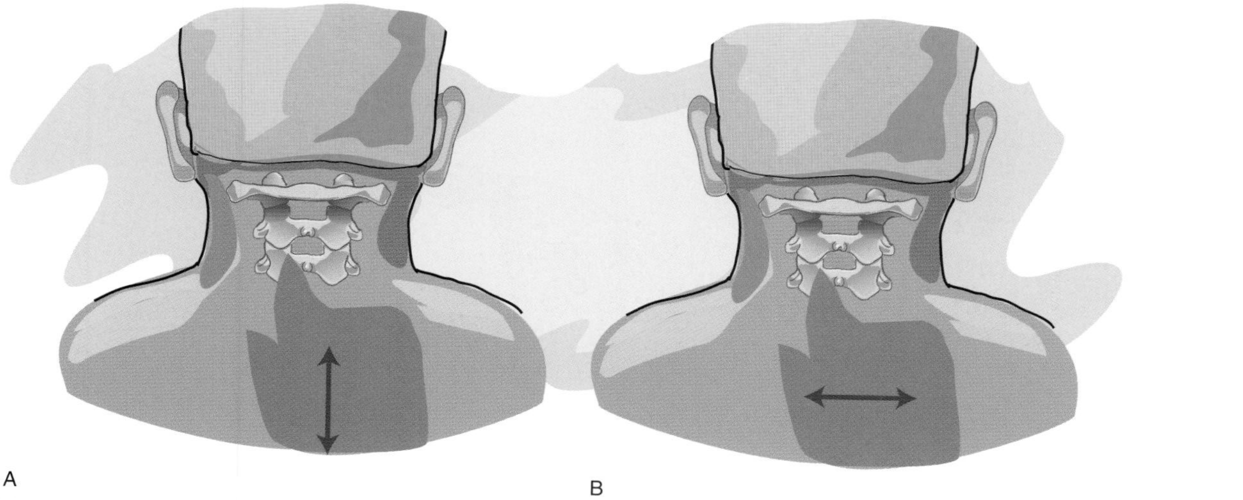

FIGURE 144–5 ■ **A,** Palpation of C6-7 intervertebral space with superoinferior rocking motion. **B,** Palpation of C6-7 midline with lateral rocking.

aseptically. A fenestrated sterile drape is placed to avoid contamination by the palpating fingers. The interspace suitable for the intended epidural block is identified. At the level of this interspace, the operator's middle and index fingers are placed on either side of the spinous processes (Fig. 144–5A). The position of the interspace is confirmed again with palpation, using a rocking motion in the superior and inferior planes. The midline of the selected interspace is identified by palpating the spinous processes above and below the interspace with a lateral rocking motion, to ensure that the needle entry site is exactly in the midline (Fig. 144–5B). Failure to identify the midline accurately is the most common cause of difficulty in performing cervical epidural nerve block.

Choice of Needle

For most adult patients, a 3½-inch 18-gauge Hustead or Tuohy needle is suitable for cervical epidural block; however, with the sharper Tuohy needle, the incidence of dural punctures may be higher.[26] Many centers now use smaller, sharper, and shorter needles with equally good results. These smaller, sharper, and shorter needles decrease the amount of procedure-related and postprocedure pain and decrease the cost of the procedure.

Identification of the Epidural Space

The choice of technique for identifying the epidural space usually is based on the pain specialist's training and personal experience, rather than on scientific data. Most experts agree that the loss-of-resistance technique has significant advantages over the hanging-drop technique.[27] Because the hanging-drop method is associated with a 2% failure rate as compared with less than 0.5% for the loss-of-resistance technique, the hanging-drop technique cannot be recommended.

Loss-of-Resistance Technique

After careful identification of the midline at the chosen interspace using the technique described earlier, 1 mL of local anesthetic is used to infiltrate the skin, the subcutaneous tissues, and the supraspinous and interspinous ligaments. Large amounts of local anesthetic should be avoided because they disrupt the ligamentous fibers and contribute to postprocedure pain.

The styletted needle is inserted exactly in the midline in the previously anesthetized area through the supraspinous ligament into the interspinous ligament.[27] The needle stylet is removed, and a well-lubricated 5-mL glass syringe filled with preservative-free sterile saline is attached. Because saline is not compressible, it provides better tactile feedback than air. Additionally, saline avoids the risk of air embolism via the cervical epidural veins.[27]

The following instructions are written for right-handed physicians and should be reversed for left-handed physicians. The operator holds the epidural needle firmly at the hub with the left thumb and index finger. The left hand is placed firmly against the patient's neck to ensure against uncontrolled needle movements should the patient move unexpectedly (Fig. 144–6A). The right hand holds the syringe with the thumb exerting *continuous* firm pressure on the plunger.[28] Bromage[21] admonished, "Never advance the needle without simultaneous pressure on the plunger to tell you where you are." Ballottement of the plunger, advocated by some clinicians, should not be used because it would increase the risk of inadvertent dural puncture.

As constant pressure is applied to the plunger of the syringe with the thumb of the physician's right hand, the needle and syringe are continuously advanced in a slow and deliberate manner with the left hand. As the needle bevel passes through the ligamentum flavum and enters the epidural space, there is a sudden loss of resistance, and the plunger slides effortlessly forward (Fig. 144–6B). This loss of resistance provides the operator with visual and tactile confirmation that the needle bevel has entered the epidural space. The syringe is gently removed from the needle.

An air or saline acceptance test is done by injecting 0.5 to 1 mL of air or sterile, preservative-free saline with a well-lubricated sterile glass syringe to help confirm that the needle lies within the epidural space. The force required for injection should not exceed that necessary to overcome the resistance

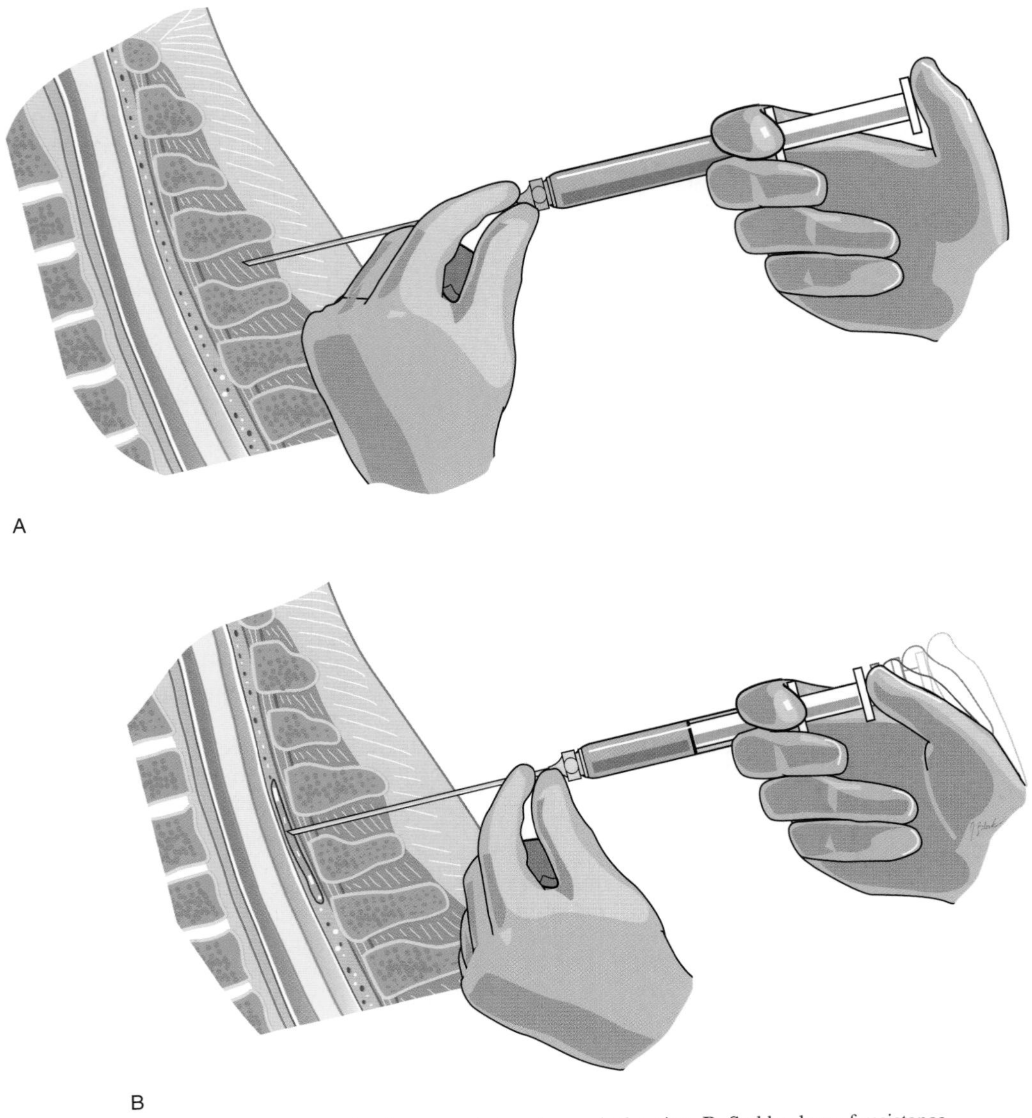

FIGURE 144–6 ■ **A,** Position of needle and hand for loss-of-resistance technique in cervical region. **B,** Sudden loss of resistance.

of the needle. Any significant pain or sudden increase in resistance during injection suggests incorrect needle placement. The injection should be stopped immediately, and the position of the needle should be reassessed. Some centers advocate the use of fluoroscopic guidance when performing cervical epidural nerve block in technically challenging situations (Fig. 144–7). Although not mandatory, fluoroscopic guidance can be a useful adjunct in selected patients.

Injection of Drugs

When satisfactory needle position is confirmed, a syringe containing the drugs to be injected is carefully attached to the needle. Gentle aspiration is carried out to identify CSF or blood.[28] Inadvertent dural puncture can occur in the best of hands, and careful observation for CSF is mandatory.[29] If CSF is aspirated, the epidural block may be attempted at a different interspace. In this situation, drug doses should be adjusted accordingly because subarachnoid migration of drugs through the dural rent can occur. Aspiration of blood can be due to damage to veins during insertion of the needle into the cervical epidural space or, less commonly, to intravenous placement of the needle.[28] If blood is aspirated, the needle should be rotated slightly, and the aspiration test should be repeated. If no blood is present, incremental doses of local anesthetic and other drugs may be administered while the patient is monitored closely for signs of local anesthetic toxicity or untoward reactions to the other drugs.

Choice of Local Anesthetic

The spread of drugs injected into the cervical epidural space depends on the volume and speed of injection; the anatomic variations of the epidural space; the extent of dilation of the epidural veins; and the position, age, and height of the patient.[30] Pregnant patients required significantly less drug to

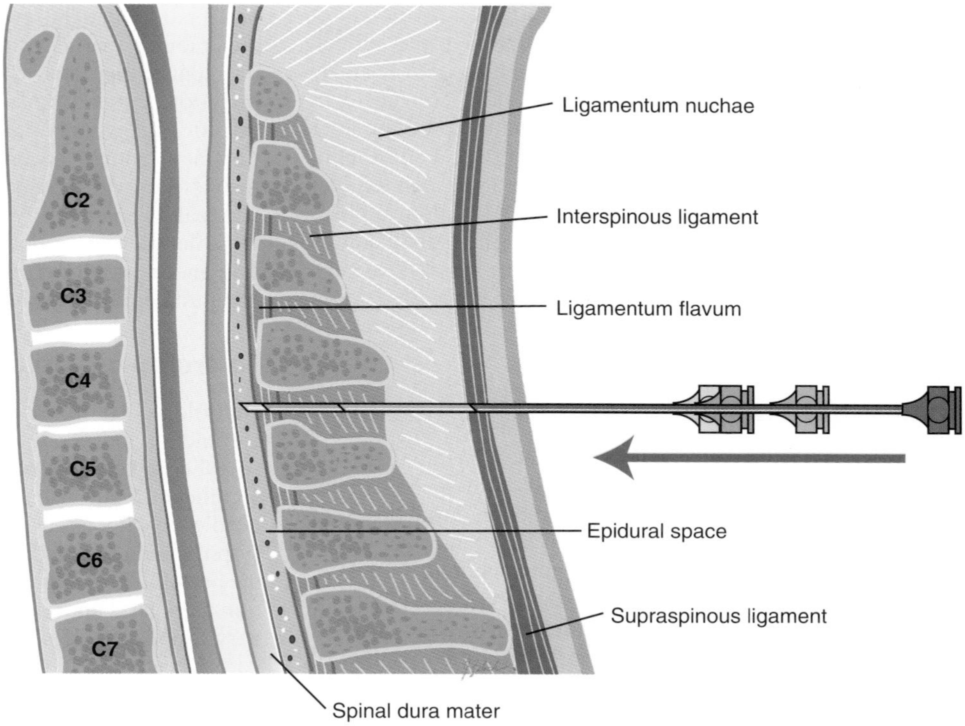

FIGURE 144–7 ■ Fluoroscopic spread of contrast solution within the cervical epidural space. (From Waldman SD: Cervical epidural nerve block. In: Atlas of Interventional Pain Management, 2nd ed. Philadelphia, WB Saunders, 2004, p 134.)

achieve a given level of blockade than did nongravid controls.[144]

Local anesthetics capable of producing adequate sensory block of the cervical nerve roots when administered via the cervical epidural route include 1% lidocaine, 0.25% bupivacaine, 2% chloroprocaine, and 1% mepivacaine. Increasing the concentration of drug increases the amount of motor block and speeds the onset of action. Adding epinephrine reduces systemic absorption and slightly prolongs the duration of action.[32] Generally, 5 to 7 mL of the previously listed agents is adequate for most pain management applications in adults.[7] Significant intrapatient variability exists, however, and additional incremental doses of local anesthetic may be needed to ensure adequate anesthesia in some adult patients. All local anesthetics administered via the cervical epidural route should be formulated for epidural use.[33]

For diagnostic and prognostic blocks, 0.5% or 1% preservative-free lidocaine is a suitable local anesthetic.[8] For therapeutic blocks, 0.5% preservative-free lidocaine or 0.25% preservative-free bupivacaine in combination with 80 mg of depot methylprednisolone (Depo-Medrol) is injected.[7,8] Subsequent nerve blocks are done in a similar manner, with 40 mg of methylprednisolone instead of the initial 80-mg dose. Daily cervical epidural nerve blocks with local anesthetic or steroid may be required to treat the acute painful conditions described earlier.[3] Chronic conditions, such as cervical radiculopathy, tension-type headache, and diabetic polyneuropathy, are treated daily, every other day, once a week, or as the clinical situation dictates.[3,4,7,13] Some centers choose to avoid the use of local anesthetic when performing therapeutic cervical epidural blocks and instead substitute preservative-free saline.

If the cervical epidural route is chosen for administration of opioids, 0.5 mg of morphine sulfate formulated for epidural use is a reasonable initial dose for opioid-tolerant patients. More lipid-soluble opioids, such as fentanyl, must be delivered by continuous infusion via a cervical epidural catheter. All opioids administered via the cervical epidural route should be formulated for epidural use.[33]

Cervical Epidural Catheters

An epidural catheter may be placed into the cervical epidural space through a Hustead or Tuohy needle. The catheter is advanced approximately 2 to 3 cm beyond the needle tip. The needle is carefully withdrawn over the catheter. Under no circumstance is the catheter withdrawn back through the needle, lest shearing of the catheter occur. After the injection hub is attached to the catheter, an aspiration test is carried out for blood or CSF.[34] A test dose of 1 to 2 mL of local anesthetic is given via the catheter. The patient is observed for signs of local anesthetic toxicity and inadvertent subarachnoid injection. If no side effects are noted, a continuous infusion or intermittent boluses of local anesthetics or opioids may be administered through the catheter. Because the risk of infection limits the long-term use of percutaneous cervical epidural catheters, tunneling of the catheter is strongly recommended if it is anticipated that it will be in place for more than 48 hours.[35]

■ SIDE EFFECTS AND COMPLICATIONS OF THE CERVICAL APPROACH

Inadvertent Dural Puncture

In the hands of an experienced pain specialist, the prevalence of inadvertent dural puncture during cervical epidural nerve block is less than 0.5%.[25,29] Although postdural puncture headache is upsetting to patient and pain specialist in and of itself, it should not result in permanent harm to the patient. Failure to recognize inadvertent dural puncture can result in permanent harm. If an epidural needle or catheter is accidentally placed in the subarachnoid space, and the problem goes unrecognized, injection of epidural doses of local anesthetics causes immediate total spinal anesthesia and associated loss of consciousness, hypotension, and apnea. If epidural doses of opioids are accidentally placed into the subarachnoid space, significant respiratory and central nervous system depression result. Should either of these problems occur, immediate supportive measures must be taken to restore homeostasis.

Inadvertent Subdural Puncture

It is possible to place a needle or catheter intended for the epidural space inadvertently into the subdural space. If subdural placement goes unrecognized, and epidural doses of local anesthetics are administered, the signs and symptoms are similar to those of massive subarachnoid injection, although the resulting motor and sensory block may be spotty.[36,37] The effect of inadvertent injection of large doses of opioids into the subdural space is probably similar to that of subarachnoid injection. Massive subdural injection of local anesthetics or opioids requires immediate supportive measures, as indicated, to restore homeostasis.

Inadvertent Intravenous Needle and Catheter Placement

The cervical epidural space is densely vascular. Intravenous placement of the epidural needle complicates approximately 0.5% to 1% of lumbar epidural anesthesia procedures.[21] The prevalence of inadvertent intravenous placement of the epidural needle in the cervical epidural space is assumed to be similar. This complication is more common in patients with distended epidural veins (e.g., parturients and patients with a large intra-abdominal tumor mass). If the misplacement is unrecognized, injection of local anesthetic directly into an epidural vein results in significant local anesthetic toxicity.[38] Careful aspiration before injection of drugs into the epidural space also is mandatory to identify this potentially serious problem. Observation of the patient during and after the injection process is mandatory.

Hematoma and Ecchymosis

The epidural space is densely vascular. Needle trauma to the epidural veins may cause self-limited bleeding and postprocedure pain. Uncontrolled bleeding into the epidural space may result in compression of the spinal cord with the rapid development of neurologic deficit. Although the incidence of significant neurologic deficit secondary to epidural hematoma after cervical epidural block is exceedingly rare, this devastating complication should be considered whenever rapidly developing neurologic deficit follows cervical epidural nerve block.[39]

Infection

Although uncommon, infection in the epidural space is an ever-present possibility, especially in immunocompromised patients and patients with cancer.[40] Because of the nature of the epidural venous system, hematogenous spread throughout the central nervous system is a possibility when epidural infection occurs.[25] Because the offending organism in epidural infections is usually *Staphylococcus aureus,* initial antibiotic treatment should be directed at this organism until culture results are available.[41] If epidural abscess occurs, emergent surgical drainage to avoid spinal cord compression and irreversible neurologic deficit is usually necessary. Early detection and treatment of infection is crucial to avoid potentially life-threatening sequelae.

Neurologic Complications

Neurologic complications of cervical nerve block are uncommon if proper technique is used. Direct trauma to the spinal cord or nerve roots usually is accompanied by pain. If significant pain occurs during placement of the epidural needle or catheter or during injection, the physician should stop immediately and ascertain the cause of the pain to avoid the possibility of additional neural trauma.[25] Intravenous sedation or general anesthesia before initiation of cervical epidural nerve block renders the patient unable to provide accurate verbal feedback if the needle is misplaced. Routine use of sedation or general anesthesia before cervical epidural nerve block is discouraged because it takes away this important safeguard.[28]

Urinary Retention and Incontinence

The administration of local anesthetics and opioids into the cervical epidural space may be associated with a greater incidence of urinary retention as compared with cervical epidural block performed with local anesthetic and steroid.[34] This side effect is more common in elderly men and multiparous women whose bladders are ptotic. Overflow incontinence may occur when such patients are unable to void or bladder catheterization is not used. All patients undergoing cervical epidural nerve block should be able to empty their bladder before discharge from the pain center.

SUMMARY

Cervical epidural nerve block is useful in the management of a variety of acute, chronic, and cancer-related pain syndromes. Clinical experience has shown that cervical epidural nerve block is safe as long as careful attention is paid to the technical aspects.

References

1. Pagés E: Anestesia metamerica. Rev Sanid Mil Madr 11:351, 1921.
2. Dogliotti AM: Segmental peridural anesthesia. Am J Surg 20:107, 1933.
3. Waldman SD: Cervical epidural nerve block. In: Atlas of Interventional Pain Management, 2nd ed. Philadelphia, WB Saunders, 2004, p 129.
4. Waldman SD: The role of neural blockade in the management of headaches and facial pain. Curr Rev Pain 1:346, 1997.
5. Waldman SD: Acute herpes zoster and postherpetic neuralgia. Intern Med 11:33, 1990.
6. Waldman SD: Reflex sympathetic dystrophy. Intern Med 11:62, 1990.
7. Cronen MC, Waldman SD: Cervical steroid epidural nerve blocks in the palliation of pain secondary to tension-type headaches. J Pain Symptom Manage 5:379, 1990.

8. Waldman SD: Acute and postoperative pain management. In Weiner RS (ed): Innovations in Pain Management. Orlando, PMD Press, 1993, p 12.
9. Waldman SD: The role of spinal opioids in the management of cancer pain. J Pain Symptom Manage 5:163, 1990.
10. Waldman SD, Feldstein GS, Waldman HJ: Cervical implantable narcotic delivery systems in the management of upper body pain of malignant origin. Anesth Analg 66:780, 1987.
11. Waldman SD: Cervical epidural block. In: Atlas of Interventional Pain Management Techniques. Philadelphia, WB Saunders, 1998, p 121.
12. Bonica JJ: Regional anesthesia with local anesthetics. In Bonica JJ (ed): The Management of Pain. Philadelphia, Lea & Febiger, 1990, p 1956.
13. Wilson WL, Waldman SD: Role of the epidural administration of steroids and local anesthetics in the palliation of pain secondary to vertebral compression fractures. Pain Digest 1:294, 1992.
14. Waldman SD, Waldman KA: Reflex sympathetic dystrophy of the face. Reg Anesth 12:15, 1987.
15. Cronen MC, Waldman SD: Cervical steroid epidural nerve block in the palliation of pain secondary to intractable muscle contraction headache. American Association for the Study of Headache 28:1444, 1988.
16. Waldman SD, Portenoy RK: Recent advances in the management of cancer pain. Pain Manage 4:19, 1991.
17. Waldman SD, Coombs DW: Selection of implantable narcotic delivery systems. Anesth Analg 68:377, 1989.
18. Cousins MJ, Bromage PR: Epidural neural blockade. In Cousins MJ, Bridenbaugh DO (eds): Neural Blockade, 2nd ed. Philadelphia, JB Lippincott, 1988, p 340.
19. Waldman SD, Feldstein GS, Waldman HJ: Caudal administration of morphine sulfate in anticoagulated and thrombocytopenic patients. Anesth Analg 66:267, 1987.
20. Bromage PR: Complications and contraindications. In: Epidural Analgesia. Philadelphia, WB Saunders, 1978, p 654.
21. Bromage PR: Anatomy. In: Epidural Analgesia. Philadelphia, WB Saunders, 1978, p 8.
22. Reynolds AF, Roberts PA, Pollay M, et al: Quantitative anatomy of the thoracolumbar epidural space. Neurosurgery 17:905, 1985.
23. Woollam DHM, Millen JW: An anatomical background to vascular disease of the spinal cord. Proc R Soc Med 51:540, 1958.
24. Katz J: Cervical approach-single injection technique. In: Atlas of Regional Anesthesia. Norwalk, CT, Appleton & Lange, 1994, p 204.
25. Waldman SD: Cervical steroid epidural nerve blocks—a prospective study of complications occurring during 790 consecutive blocks. Reg Anesth 11:149, 1989.
26. Bromage PR: Epidural needles. Anesthesiology 22:1018, 1961.
27. Bromage PR: Identification of the epidural space. In: Epidural Analgesia. Philadelphia, WB Saunders, 1978.
28. Cousins MJ, Bromage PR: Epidural neural blockade. In Cousins MJ, Bridenbaugh DO (eds): Neural Blockade. Philadelphia, JB Lippincott, 1988, p 333.
29. Waldman SD, Feldstein GS, Allen ML: Cervical epidural blood patch for treatment of cervical dural puncture headache. Anesth Rev 14: 23, 1987.
30. Burn JM, Guyer PB, Langdon L: The spread of solutions injected into the epidural space: A study using epidurograms in patients with the lumbosciatic syndrome. Br J Anaesth 45:338, 1973.
31. Bromage PR: Mechanism of action. In: Epidural Analgesia. Philadelphia, WB Saunders, 1978, p 141.
32. Mather LE, Tucker GT, Murphy TM, et al: The effects of adding adrenaline to etidocaine and lignocaine in extradural anaesthesia: II. Pharmacokinetics. Br J Anaesth 48:989, 1976.
33. Waldman SD: Issues in selection of local anesthetics. Hosp Formulary 26:590, 1991.
34. Armitage EN: Lumbar and thoracic epidural. In Wildsmith JAW, Armitage EN (eds): Principles and Practice of Regional Anesthesia. New York, Churchill Livingstone, 1987, p 109.
35. Waldman SD: Placement of subcutaneous tunnelled epidural catheters. J Pain Symptom Manage 2:163, 1987.
36. Waldman SD: Horner's syndrome following epidural nerve block. Reg Anesth 17:55, 1992.
37. Waldman SD: Subdural injection as a cause of unexplained neurological symptoms. Reg Anest 17:55, 1992.
38. Braid DP, Scott DB: The systemic absorption of local analgesic drugs. Br J Anaesth 37:394, 1965.
39. Cousins MJ: Hematoma following epidural block. Anesthesiology 37:263, 1972.
40. Donohoe CD, Waldman SD: Headache in the AIDS patient. Intern Med 14:68, 1993.
41. Waldman SD: Cervical epidural abscess following cervical steroid epidural nerve block. Anesth Analg 72:717, 1991.

chapter 145

Brachial Plexus Block

Steven D. Waldman

HISTORICAL CONSIDERATIONS

Brachial plexus block was first performed by two famous surgeons—Halsted in 1884, and Crile in 1887.[1] Both surgeons first surgically exposed the brachial plexus before applying cocaine to this neural structure under direct vision. The first percutaneous brachial plexus blocks were reported in 1911 by Hirschel and Hulenkampff.[2] Over the ensuing years, a variety of techniques, modifications, and advancements have made brachial plexus block one of the regional anesthetic techniques most frequently used in contemporary anesthesia practice. Recent work by Winnie has further elucidated the clinically relevant anatomy of the brachial plexus, which has led to further refinement of the technique and recognition of the role of brachial plexus block in the treatment of sympathetically maintained pain syndromes involving the upper extremity.[3]

CLINICALLY RELEVANT ANATOMY

A clear understanding of the clinically relevant anatomy of the brachial plexus is mandatory if the pain management specialist is to safely and successfully perform brachial plexus block, regardless of what technique is chosen. Failure to appreciate this fact will increase the incidence of failed blocks and complications. The brachial plexus is formed by the fusion of the anterior rami of the C5, C6, C7, C8, and T1 spinal nerves. There may also be a contribution of fibers from C4 and T2 spinal nerves. The nerves that make up the plexus exit the lateral aspect of the cervical spine and pass downward and laterally in conjunction with the subclavian artery. The nerves and artery run between the anterior scalene and the middle scalene muscle passing inferiorly behind the middle of the clavicle and above the top of the first rib to reach the axilla (Fig. 145–1). The scalene muscles are enclosed in an extension of prevertebral fascia that helps to contain drugs injected into this region.

Interscalene Block

Indications

The interscalene approach to the brachial plexus is the preferred technique for brachial plexus block when anesthesia or relaxation of the shoulder is desired.[4] In addition to applications for surgical anesthesia, interscalene brachial plexus nerve block with local anesthetics can be used as a diagnostic tool when performing differential neural blockade on an anatomic basis in the evaluation of shoulder and upper extremity pain. If destruction of the brachial plexus is being considered, this technique is useful as a prognostic indicator of the degree of motor and sensory impairment that the patient may experience. Interscalene brachial plexus nerve block with local anesthetic may be utilized to palliate acute pain emergencies including acute herpes zoster, brachial plexus neuritis, shoulder and upper extremity trauma, and cancer pain while waiting for pharmacologic, surgical, and antineoplastic methods to take effect.[5] Interscalene brachial plexus nerve block is also a useful alternative to stellate ganglion block when treating reflex sympathetic dystrophy of the shoulder and upper extremity.[4]

Destruction of the brachial plexus is indicated for the palliation of cancer pain, including invasive tumors of the brachial plexus and tumors of the soft tissue and bone of the shoulder and upper extremity.[6] Owing to the desperate nature of many patients' suffering from aggressively invasive tumors that have invaded the brachial plexus, blockade of the brachial plexus using the interscalene approach may be carried out in the presence of coagulopathy or anticoagulation by using a 25-gauge needle, albeit with increased risk of ecchymosis and hematoma formation.

Technique

The patient is placed in a supine position with the head turned away from the side to be blocked. A total of 20 to 30 mL of local anesthetic is drawn up in a 30-mL sterile syringe. When treating painful or inflammatory conditions that are mediated via the brachial plexus, a total of 80 mg of depot steroid is added to the local anesthetic with the first block and 40 mg of depot steroid with subsequent blocks.

The patient is then asked to raise his or her head against the resistance of the pain specialist's hand to help to identify the posterior border of the sternocleidomastoid muscle. In most patients, a groove can be palpated between the posterior border of the sternocleidomastoid muscle and the anterior scalene muscle. Identification of the intrascalene groove can be facilitated by having the patient inhale strongly against a closed glottis. The skin overlying this area is then prepared with antiseptic solution. At the level of the cricothyroid notch (C6) at the interscalene groove, a 25-gauge, 1½-

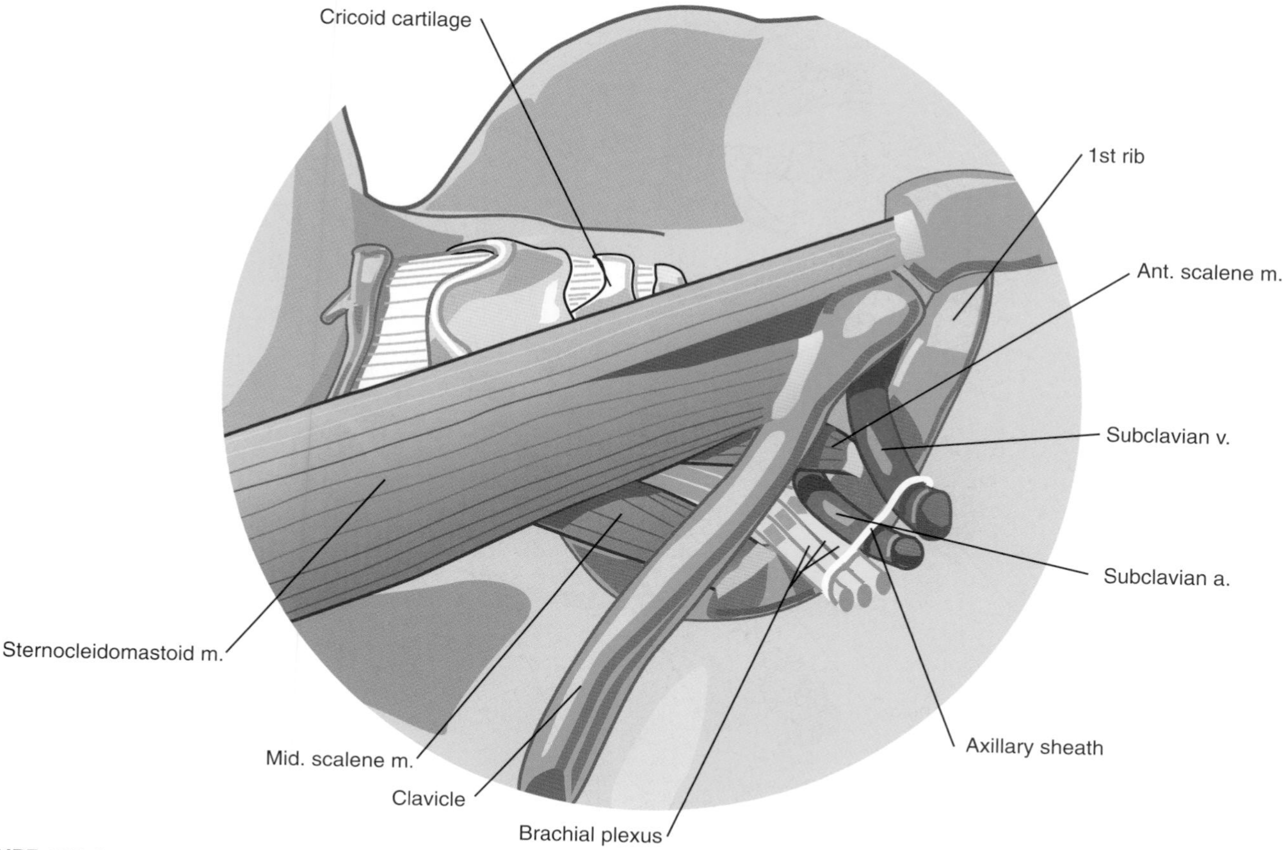

FIGURE 145–1 ■ Anatomy of the brachial plexus.

inch needle is inserted with a slightly caudad and inferior trajectory (Fig. 145–2). If the intrascalene groove cannot be identified, the needle is placed just slightly behind the posterior border of the sternocleidomastoid muscle. The needle should be advanced slowly because a paresthesia is almost always produced when the needle tip impinges on the brachial plexus as it traverses the interscalene space nearly at a right angle to the needle tip. The patient should be warned that at some point a paresthesia will occur and to say, "There!" as soon as it is felt. Paresthesia should be encountered at a depth of approximately ¾ to 1 inch. After paresthesia is elicited, gentle aspiration is carried out to identify blood or cerebrospinal fluid. If the aspiration test is negative and no paresthesia into the distribution of the brachial plexus persists, 20 to 30 mL of solution is slowly injected, as the patient is monitored closely for signs of local anesthetic toxicity or inadvertent subarachnoid injection. If surgical anesthesia is required for forearm or hand procedures, additional local anesthetic may have to be placed farther caudad along the brachial plexus to obtain adequate anesthesia of the lower portion of the plexus. Alternatively, specific nerves may be blocked farther distally if augmentation of the interscalene brachial plexus block is desired.[4]

Side Effects and Complications

The proximity of the brachial plexus to the subclavian artery and other large vessels suggests the potential for inadvertent intravascular injection or local anesthetic toxicity from intravascular absorption. Given the large doses of local anesthetic required for interscalene brachial plexus block, the pain specialist should carefully calculate the total milligram dose of local anesthetic that may safely be given. This vascularity also increases the incidence of post-block ecchymosis and hematoma formation. In spite of the vascularity of this anatomic region, this technique can safely be performed in the presence of anticoagulation by using a 25- or 27-gauge needle, albeit at increased risk of hematoma, if the clinical situation dictates a favorable risk-benefit ratio. Risk for these complications can be decreased if manual pressure is applied to the area of the block immediately after injection. Application of cold packs for 20-minute periods after the block also decreases the amount of post-procedure pain and bleeding.

In addition to the potential for complications involving the vasculature, the proximity of the brachial plexus to the central neuraxial structures and the phrenic nerve can result in side effects and complications. If the needle is placed too deep, inadvertent epidural, subdural, or subarachnoid injection is a possibility. If volume of local anesthetic used for this block is accidentally placed in any of these spaces, significant motor and sensory block will result. Unrecognized, these complications could be fatal. It should be assumed that the phrenic nerve will also be blocked during brachial plexus block using the interscalene approach. In the absence of significant pulmonary disease, unilateral phrenic nerve block should rarely create respiratory embarrassment. However, blockade of the recurrent laryngeal nerve with its attendant

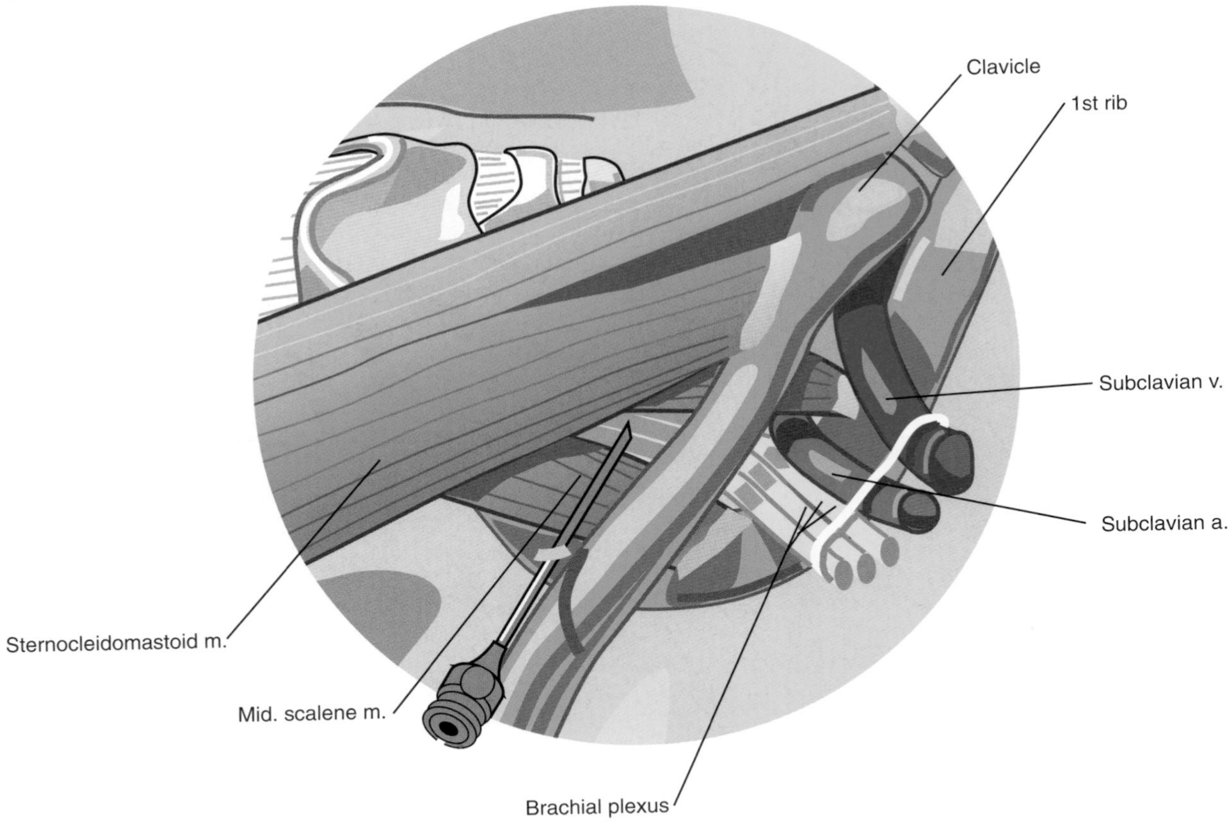

FIGURE 145–2 ■ Needle placement for interscalene brachial plexus block.

vocal cord paralysis, combined with paralysis of the diaphragm, may make clearing pulmonary and upper airway secretions difficult. Although less likely than with the supraclavicular approach to brachial plexus block, pneumothorax is a possibility.

Clinical Pearls

The key to the safe and successful interscalene brachial plexus block is a clear understanding of the anatomy and careful identification of the necessary anatomic landmarks. Poking around for a paresthesia without first identifying the interscalene groove is a recipe for disaster. The pain specialist should remember that the brachial plexus is quite close to the skin at the level where this block is performed. The needle should rarely be inserted deeper than 1 inch in any but the most obese patients. Supplementation of intrascalene brachial plexus block by more peripheral block of the ulnar nerve may be required because the C8 fibers are not always adequately anesthetized when using the interscalene approach. Careful neurologic examination for preexisting neurologic deficits that might later be attributed to the nerve block should be performed before beginning any brachial plexus block.

Supraclavicular Block

Indications

The supraclavicular approach to brachial plexus block is an excellent choice when dense surgical anesthesia of the distal upper extremity is required. This technique is less suitable for shoulder problems because it almost always requires supplementation with cervical plexus block to provide adequate cutaneous anesthesia of the shoulder.[7] In addition to applications for surgical anesthesia, supraclavicular brachial plexus nerve block with local anesthetics can be used as a diagnostic tool when performing differential neural blockade on an anatomic basis to evaluate upper extremity pain. If destruction of the brachial plexus is being considered, this technique is useful as a prognostic indicator of the degree of motor and sensory impairment that the patient may experience. Supraclavicular brachial plexus nerve block with local anesthetic may be used to palliate acute pain emergencies, including that of acute herpes zoster, brachial plexus neuritis, upper extremity trauma, and cancer while waiting for pharmacologic, surgical, and antineoplastic methods to take effect. Supraclavicular brachial plexus nerve block is also useful as an alternative to stellate ganglion block for treating reflex sympathetic dystrophy of the upper extremity.

Destruction of the supraclavicular brachial plexus is indicated for palliation of cancer pain, including invasive tumors of the brachial plexus, and tumors of the soft tissue and bone of the upper extremity.[6] Because of the potential for intrathoracic hemorrhage, the interscalene approach to brachial plexus block should be used in patients who are anticoagulated only if the clinical situation dictates a favorable risk-benefit ratio.

Technique

The patient is placed supine with the head turned away from the side to be blocked. A total of 10 mL of local anesthetic is drawn up in a 20-mL sterile syringe. When treating painful conditions that are mediated via the brachial plexus, a total of 80 mg of depot steroid is added to the local anesthetic with the first block and 40 mg of depot steroid is added with subsequent blocks.

The patient is then asked to raise his or her head against the resistance of the pain specialist's hand to aid in identifying the posterior border of the sternocleidomastoid muscle. The point at which the lateral border of the sternocleidomastoid attaches to the clavicle is then identified. At this point, just above the clavicle, after the skin is prepared with antiseptic solution, a 1.5-inch needle is inserted directly perpendicular to the table top (Fig. 145–3). The needle should be advanced slowly, as a paresthesia is almost always encountered at a depth of approximately $^3/_4$ to 1 inch. The patient should be warned that a paresthesia will occur and to say, "There" as soon as it is felt. If a paresthesia is not elicited after the needle has been slowly advanced to a depth of 1 inch, the needle should be withdrawn and advanced again with a slightly more cephalad trajectory. This maneuver should be repeated until a paresthesia is elicited. Conversely, if the first rib is encountered before a paresthesia is induced, the needle should be walked laterally along the first rib until a paresthesia is elicited (Fig. 145–4). To avoid pneumothorax, the needle should *never* be directed in a more medial trajectory.

After paresthesia is elicited, gentle aspiration is carried out to identify blood or cerebrospinal fluid. If the aspiration is negative and no persistent paresthesia into the distribution of the brachial plexus remains, 20 to 30 mL of solution is slowly injected as the patient is monitored closely for signs of local anesthetic toxicity or inadvertent neuraxial injection.

Side Effects and Complications

The proximity of the brachial plexus to the subclavian artery and other large vessels suggests the potential for inadvertent intravascular injection or local anesthetic toxicity from intravascular absorption. Given the large doses of local anesthetic required for supraclavicular brachial plexus block, the pain specialist should carefully calculate the total milligram dose of local anesthetic that may safely be given. This vascularity also increases the risk of post-block ecchymosis and hematoma formation. These complications can be minimized if manual pressure is applied to the area of the block immediately after injection. Applying cold packs for 20-minute periods after the block also reduces the amount of post-procedure pain and bleeding the patient may experience.

In addition to the potential for complications involving the vasculature, the proximity of the brachial plexus to the central neuraxial structures and the phrenic nerve can result in side effects and complications. Although these complications occur less frequently than with interscalene brachial plexus block, inadvertent epidural, subdural, or subarachnoid injection remains a possibility. If the volume of local anesthetic used for this block is accidentally placed in any of these spaces, significant motor and sensory block will result. Unrecognized, these complications could be fatal. It should be assumed that the phrenic nerve will also be blocked at least 30% of the time during brachial plexus block using the supraclavicular approach. In the absence of significant pulmonary disease, unilateral phrenic nerve block should rarely create

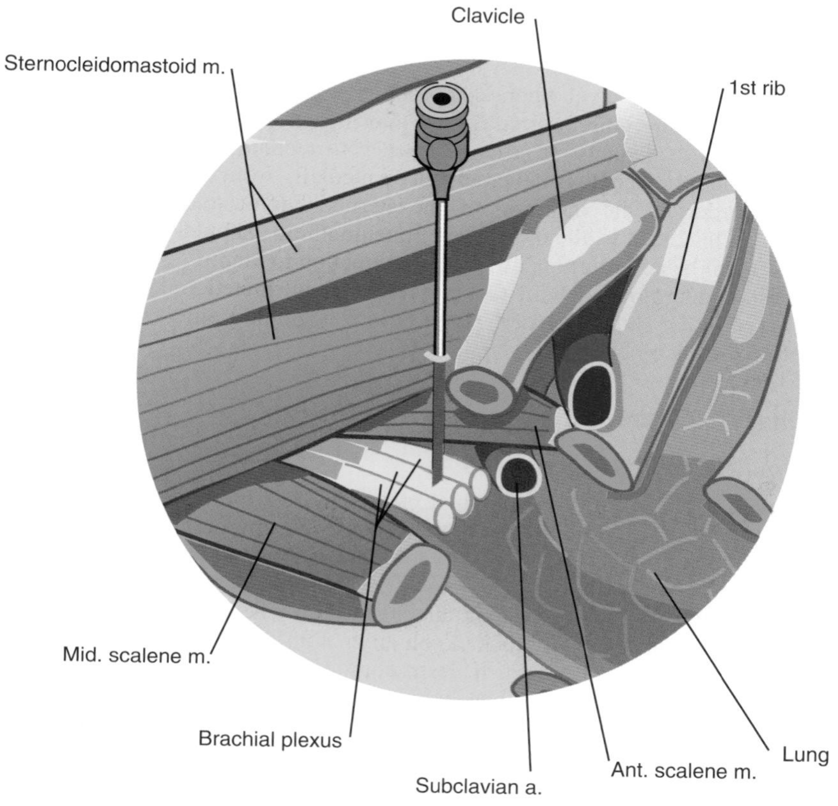

FIGURE 145–3 ■ Needle placement for supraclavicular brachial plexus block.

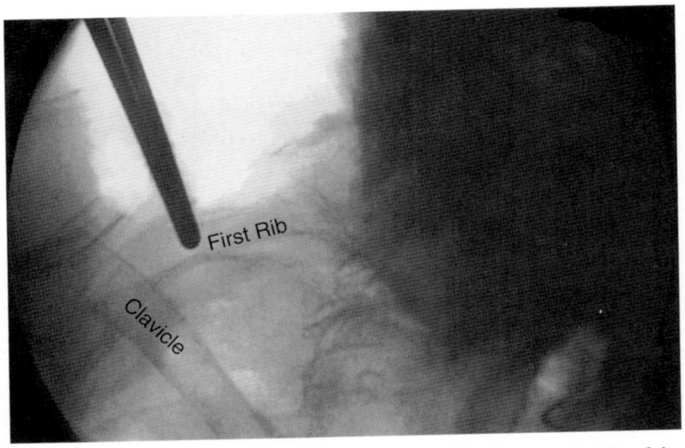

FIGURE 145–4 ■ Radiographic supraclavicular view of the middle of the first rib. (From Raj PP, Lou L, Erdine S, Staats PS, Waldman SD: Radiographic Imaging for Regional Anesthesia and Pain Management. Philadelphia, Churchill Livingstone, 2003, p 112, Figure 18–1, with permission).

respiratory embarrassment.[7] Blockade of the recurrent laryngeal nerve with its attendant vocal cord paralysis, combined with paralysis of the diaphragm, may make clearing pulmonary and upper airway secretions difficult. Owing to proximity of the apex of the lung, pneumothorax is a distinct possibility and the patient should be so informed.

Clinical Pearls

The key to performing safe and successful supraclavicular brachial plexus block is a clear understanding of the anatomy and careful identification of the necessary anatomic landmarks. Poking around for a paresthesia without first identifying the anatomic landmarks is a recipe for disaster. The pain specialist should remember that the brachial plexus is close to the surface at the level where this block is performed. The needle should rarely be inserted deeper than 1 inch in all but the most obese patients. If strict adherence to technique is observed and the needle is never advanced medially from the lateral border of the insertion of the sternocleidomastoid muscle on the clavicle, the incidence of pneumothorax should be less than 0.5%. Careful neurologic examination to identify preexisting neurologic deficits that might later be attributed to the nerve block should be performed before beginning any brachial plexus block.

Axillary Approach to the Brachial Plexus

Indications

The axillary approach to the brachial plexus is the preferred technique for brachial plexus block when dense anesthesia of the forearm and hand is required.[8] In addition to applications for surgical anesthesia, axillary brachial plexus block with local anesthetics can be used as a diagnostic tool when performing differential neural blockade on an anatomic basis to evaluate upper extremity pain. If destruction of the brachial plexus is being considered, this technique is useful as a prognostic indicator of the degree of motor and sensory impairment that the patient may experience. Axillary brachial plexus nerve block with local anesthetic may be used to palliate acute pain emergencies including that of acute herpes zoster, brachial plexus neuritis, shoulder and upper extremity trauma, and cancer pain while waiting for pharmacologic, surgical, and antineoplastic methods to take effect. Axillary brachial plexus nerve block is also useful as an alternative to stellate ganglion block when treating reflex sympathetic dystrophy of the upper extremity.[8]

Destruction of the brachial plexus is indicated for the palliation of cancer pain, including invasive tumors of the distal brachial plexus and tumors of the soft tissue and bone of the upper extremity. Because of the desperation of many patients suffering from aggressively invasive tumors that have invaded the brachial plexus, blockade using the axillary approach may be carried out even in the presence of coagulopathy or anticoagulation by using a 25-gauge needle, albeit with increased risk of ecchymosis and hematoma formation.

Clinically Relevant Anatomy

The brachial plexus is formed by the fusion of the anterior rami of the C5, C6, C7, C8, and T1 spinal nerves. There may also be a contribution of fibers from C4 and T2 spinal nerves. The nerves that make up the plexus exit the lateral aspect of the cervical spine and pass downward and laterally in conjunction with the subclavian artery. The nerves and artery run between the anterior scalene and the middle scalene muscle, passing inferiorly behind the middle of the clavicle and above the top of the first rib to reach the axilla. Because the sheath that encloses the axillary artery and nerves is less consistent than the sheath that encloses the brachial plexus at the level where interscalene and supraclavicular brachial plexus blocks are performed, a single-injection technique is less satisfactory. The median, radial, ulnar, and musculocutaneous nerves surround the artery within this imperfect sheath. David Brown has suggested that the position of these nerves relative to the axillary artery can best be visualized by placing them in the quadrants as represented on the face of a clock with the axillary artery at the center of the clock (Fig. 145–5).[9] The median nerve is found in the 12:00 to 3:00 o'clock quadrant, the ulnar nerve in the 3:00 to 6:00 o'clock quadrant, the radial nerve in the 6:00 to 9:00 o'clock quadrant, and the musculocutaneous nerve in the 9:00 to 12:00 o'clock quadrant. To ensure adequate block of these nerves, drugs must be injected into each quadrant to deposit it close to each of these nerves.

Technique

The patient is placed in a supine position with the arm abducted 85 to 90 degrees and the fingertips resting just behind the ear. A total of 30 to 40 mL of local anesthetic is drawn up in a 50-mL sterile syringe. When treating painful or inflammatory conditions that are thought to be mediated via the brachial plexus, a total of 80 mg of depot steroid is added to the local anesthetic with the first block and 40 mg of depot steroid with subsequent blocks.

The pain specialist then identifies the pulsations of the axillary artery with the middle and index fingers of the nondominant hand and traces the course of the artery distally by following the pulsations. After the skin has been prepared with antiseptic solution, a 1-inch, 25-gauge needle is inserted just below the arterial pulsations (Fig. 145–6). The needle should be advanced slowly because a paresthesia is almost always induced as the needle tip impinges on the radial or ulnar nerve. The patient should be warned that a paresthesia

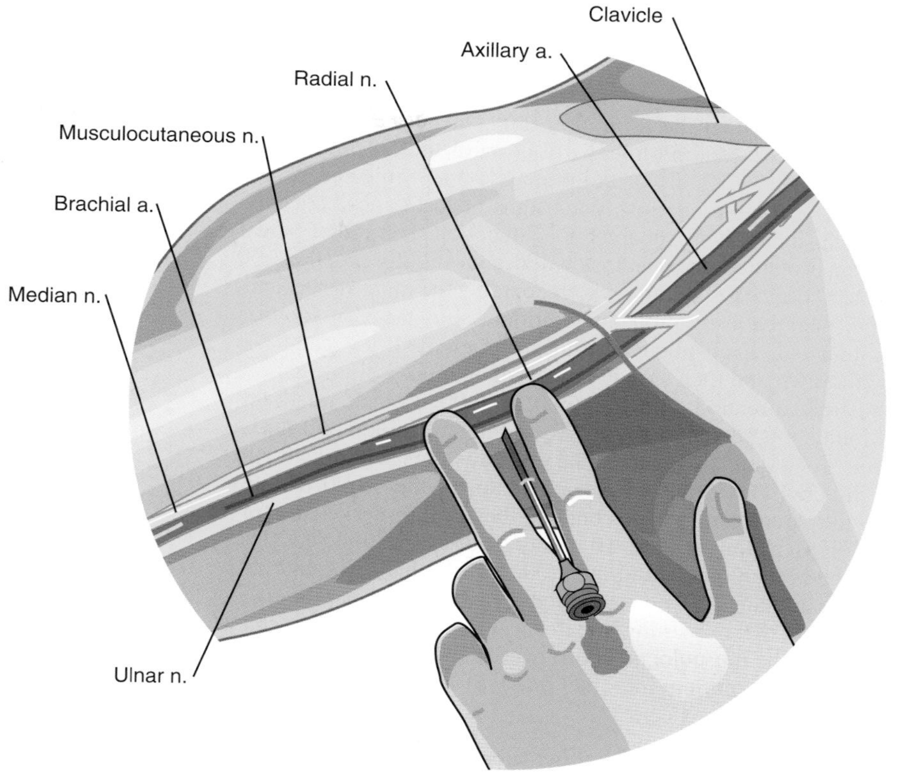

FIGURE 145–5 ■ Relative locations of the median, radial, and ulnar nerves.

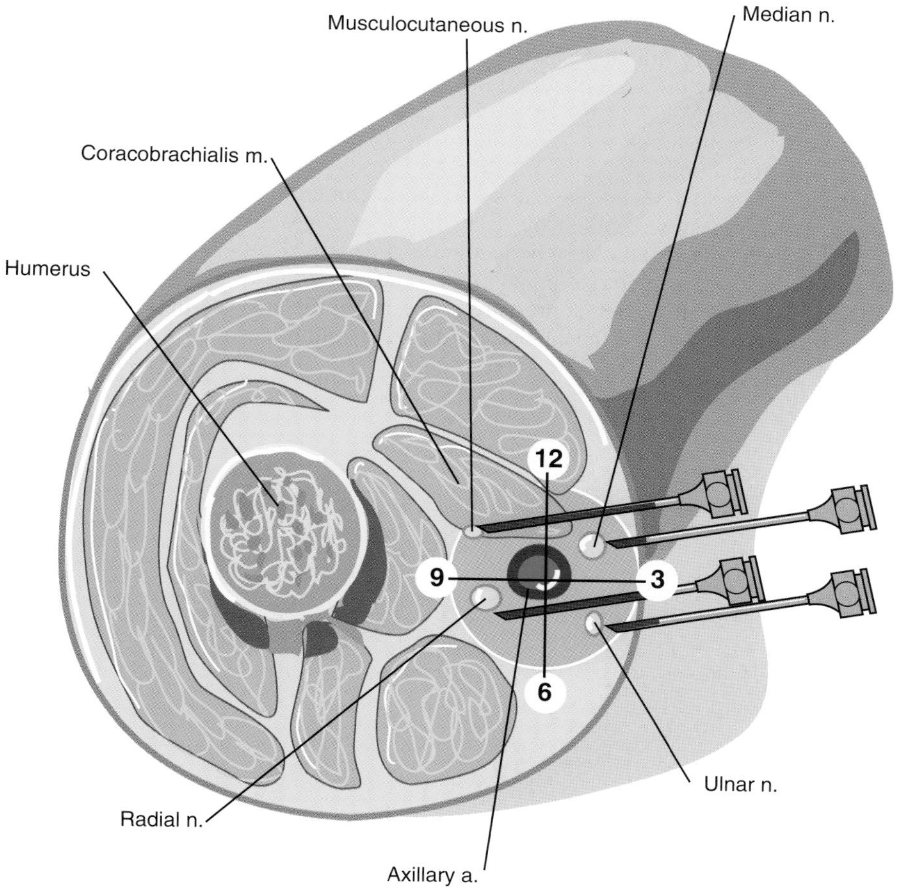

FIGURE 145–6 ■ Needle placement for axillary approach to brachial plexus block.

will occur and asked to say "There" as soon as it is felt. Paresthesia should be encountered at a depth of approximately ½ to ¾ inch. After paresthesia is elicited and its distribution is noted, gentle aspiration is carried out to identify blood or cerebrospinal fluid. If the aspiration test is negative and no persistent paresthesia into the distribution of the brachial plexus remains, 8 to 10 mL of solution is slowly injected as the patient is monitored closely for signs of local anesthetic toxicity or inadvertent subarachnoid injection. If a radial paresthesia is elicited, the needle is withdrawn slightly into the 3:00 to 6:00 o'clock quadrant, which contains the ulnar nerve, and, after negative aspiration, an additional 8 to 10 mL of solution is injected. If an ulnar paresthesia is elicited, the needle is withdrawn and then slowly advanced again in a slightly more superior direction into the 6:00 to 9:00 o'clock quadrant, which contains the radial nerve, and the aspiration and injection technique is repeated. The needle is then withdrawn and redirected above the arterial pulsation to the 12:00 to 3:00 o'clock quadrant, which contains the median nerve. If aspiration is negative, 8 to 10 mL of solution is injected. The needle is then directed to the 9:00 to 12:00 o'clock quadrant, which contains the musculocutaneous nerve. If aspiration is negative, the remaining local anesthetic is injected. Alternatively, the musculocutaneous nerve can be blocked by infiltrating the solution into the mass of the coracobrachialis muscle.

Side Effects and Complications

The proximity of the nerves to the axillary artery and other large vessels carries the risk for inadvertent intravascular injection or local anesthetic toxicity from intravascular absorption.[10] Given the large doses of local anesthetic required for axillary brachial plexus block, the pain specialist should carefully calculate the total milligram dose of local anesthetic that may safely be given. The dense vascularity also increases the risk of post-block ecchymosis and hematoma formation. In spite of the vascularity of this anatomic region, this technique can safely be attempted in a patient taking an anticoagulant by using a 25- or 27-gauge needle, albeit at increased risk of hematoma, if the clinical situation dictates a favorable risk-benefit ratio. These complications can be reduced if manual pressure is applied to the area of the block immediately after injection. Applying cold packs for 20-minute periods after the block also reduces the amount of post-procedure pain and bleeding.

The distance of the nerves to be blocked from the neuraxis and phrenic nerve makes the complications associated with injection of drugs onto these structures highly unlikely, which is an advantage of the axial approach as compared with the intrascalene and supraclavicular approaches to brachial plexus block. Because paresthesias are elicited, the potential for post-block persistent paresthesia is a possibility and the patient should be so advised.

Clinical Pearls

The axillary approach to brachial plexus block is a safe and simple way to anesthetize the distal upper extremity. For pain above the elbow, the interscalene or supraclavicular approach is probably a better choice. Careful neurologic examination for preexisting neurologic deficits that might later be attributed to the nerve block should be performed before any brachial plexus block.

References

1. Crile GW: Anesthesia of the nerve roots with cocaine. Cleve Med J 2:355, 1997.
2. Kulenkampff D: Anesthesia of the brachial plexus. Zentrabl Chir 38, 1337, 1911.
3. Winnie AP: Plexus Anesthesia: Perivascular Technique of Brachial Plexus Block, 2nd ed. Philadelphia, WB Saunders, 1990, p 56.
4. Waldman SD: Brachial plexus block: Interscalene approach. In Waldman SD (ed): Atlas of Interventional Pain Management Techniques. Philadelphia, WB Saunders, 1998, p 131.
5. Bonica JJ: Musculoskeletal disorders of the upper limb. In Bonica JJ (ed): The Management of Pain, 2nd ed. Philadelphia, Lea & Febiger, 1990, p 891.
6. Bonica JJ: Neurolytic blockade. In Bonica JJ (ed): The Management of Pain, 2nd ed. Philadelphia, Lea & Febiger, 1990, p 1996.
7. Waldman SD: Brachial plexus block: Supraclavicular approach. In Waldman SD (ed): Atlas of Interventional Pain Management Techniques. Philadelphia, WB Saunders, 1998, p 136.
8. Waldman SD: Brachial plexus block: Axiallary approach. In Waldman SD (ed): Atlas of Interventional Pain Management Techniques. Philadelphia, WB Saunders, 1998, p 140.
9. Brown DL: Axillary block. In Brown DL (ed): Atlas of Regional Anesthesia. Philadelphia, WB Saunders, 1999, p 49.
10. Katz J: Axillary block. In Katz J (ed): Atlas of Regional Anesthesia. Norwalk, Conn, Appleton-Century-Crofts, 1995, p 70.

chapter 146

Peripheral Nerve Blocks of the Upper Extremity

Robert H. Overbaugh

Distal blockade of the upper extremity nerves has often been seen as primarily a supplemental technique for inadequate brachial plexus anesthesia.[1] However, knowledge of the anatomy and blockade of the upper extremity nerves not only serves to enhance the armamentarium of the anesthetist, but also serves as an important diagnostic and therapeutic tool for the pain practitioner. Nerve entrapment syndromes of the upper extremity are not uncommon, and they are seen with greater frequency in patients with comorbidities such as diabetes mellitus, rheumatoid arthritis and alcoholism.[2] This chapter will focus on the blockade of the upper extremity nerves distal to the axilla (Fig. 146–1).

MEDIAN NERVE BLOCK

Indications

Blockade of the median nerve is essential to provide surgical anesthesia of the palmar surface of the hand. Median nerve block proximal to the wrist crease can be successfully used as a sole anesthetic technique for patients undergoing endoscopic carpal tunnel release.[3,4] When combined with ulnar nerve block, median nerve blockade at the wrist has proven efficacy for providing anesthesia for patients undergoing botulism type A therapy for palmar hyperhidrosis. This block not only provides anesthesia for this therapy, but may also increase its efficacy.[5] Median nerve blockade can be a useful tool to differentiate between chronic pain of a radicular (C6) etiology versus that which is caused by a peripheral nerve entrapment at either the elbow/forearm (pronator teres syndrome) or the wrist (carpal tunnel syndrome). Pronator teres syndrome is not uncommonly seen in mechanics and carpenters, and is secondary to compression of the median nerve in the cubital fossa by either the pronator teres muscle or the flexor digitorum superficialis.[2] When combined with steroids, blockade of the median nerve at the wrist has a direct therapeutic effect on pain secondary to nerve entrapment in the aforementioned locations. This block also has great utility in providing analgesia for patients who are undergoing painful occupational and physical therapy for flexion contractures of the index, ring, and middle fingers. Median nerve block may aid in the treatment of complex regional pain syndrome type I (CRPS I) by allowing these patients to better perform occupational and physical therapy.[6]

Blockade of the median nerve may also be useful in evaluating and guiding therapy of upper extremity contractures secondary to stroke, traumatic brain injury, and cerebral palsy.[7] When performed with neurolytic agents, median nerve block provides additional treatment for spasticity associated with these conditions.[8] Peripheral blockade of the median nerve using local anesthetics is recommended before any neural destructive therapy to elucidate the degree of sensory or motor deficit this procedure will produce.[9]

Clinically Relevant Anatomy

The median nerve forms from an amalgamation of the medial and lateral cords thereby encompassing contributions from the C5-T1 nerve roots. As the median nerve exits the axilla, it courses distally adjacent to the brachial artery. At the elbow, the median nerve enters the antecubital space adjacent to the insertion of the biceps tendon on the radius. At this location, the nerve is just medial to the brachial artery and lateral to the medial epicondyle of the humerus. The nerve then continues in the forearm giving off multiple small motor branches to the flexor muscles of the forearm and digits.[2] At this level, each of these small branches is subsequently susceptible to compression and entrapment by ligaments, trauma, and hypertrophied musculature. As the median nerve enters the wrist, it lies directly beneath the tendon of the palmaris longus. This tendon is found to be congenitally absent in approximately 15% of patients.[10] The nerve then continues in the carpal tunnel above the radius, lying beneath the flexor retinaculum and deep to the flexor carpi radialis and palmaris longus tendons. It is in the carpal tunnel that the median nerve is extremely sensitive to compression by the flexor tendons, leading to the possibility of carpal tunnel syndrome (Fig. 146–2). Just distal to the retinaculum, the median nerve sends a small recurrent branch to supply innervation to the opponens pollicis and flexor pollicis brevis muscles.[11] The median nerve gives off its terminal branches—the common and proper palmar digital nerves, which supply sensory innervation to the palmar surface of the thumb and index and middle

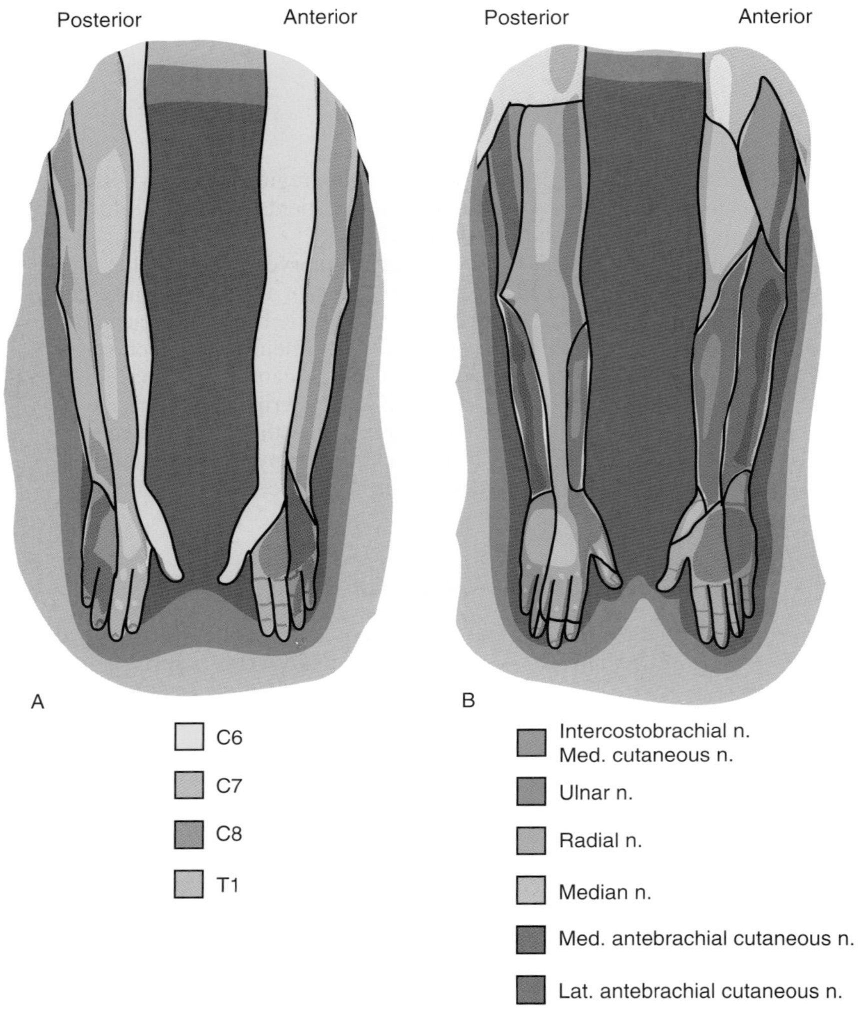

FIGURE 146–1 ■ **A,** Cutaneous distribution of the cervical roots. **B,** Cutaneous distribution of the peripheral nerves. (Adapted from Wedel DJ, Horlocker TT: Nerve blocks. In Miller RD [ed]: Miller's Anesthesia, 6th ed. Philadelphia, Churchill Livingstone, 2005, p 1687.)

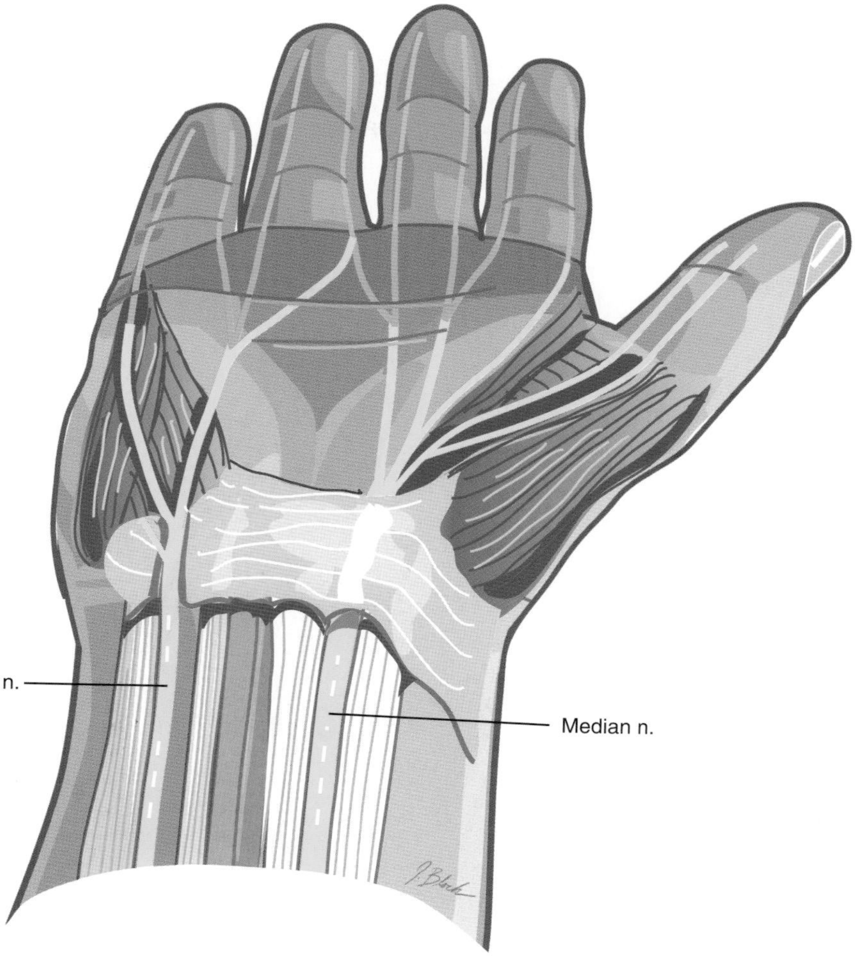

FIGURE 146–2 ■ Ulnar and median nerve anatomy at the wrist.

fingers and the medial half of the ring finger. The dorsal, distal aspects of these digits are also supplied by these branches.[10,11]

Blockade of the Median Nerve at the Elbow

Placing the patient in a supine position with the arm fully supinated, the skin overlying the antecubital region should be sterilely prepped and draped in the usual fashion. At the level of the anterior crease of the elbow, the brachial artery should be palpable just medial to the insertion of the biceps muscle. Active flexion of the biceps allows the operator to easily locate this landmark. Using a 1½-inch, 22-gauge B-bevel or 2-inch, 22-gauge stimulating needle, the skin is then entered at a slightly cephalad and medial angle medial to the brachial artery (Fig. 146–3). Blunt bevel needles are recommended for peripheral nerve blockade because there is evidence that they decrease the risk of nerve injury associated with these techniques.[12] The needle then is directed toward the medial epicondyle. The operator should slowly advance the needle until a paresthesia in a median nerve distribution or a motor-evoked response is elicited. Motor stimulation of the median nerve will be seen by either wrist/finger flexion or thumb opposition. Should the medial epicondyle be contacted before an appropriate motor response or paresthesia, the needle should be withdrawn approximately 0.5 cm and "walked" slightly medially. After appropriate paresthesia or motor response, (the author prefers accepting a distal motor twitch at or below 0.4 mA) and following negative aspiration for heme, 5 to 7 mL of local anesthetic is then injected. As with brachial plexus blockade, it is prudent to inject the first 1 mL of local anesthetic slowly before injecting the remaining volume. This technique will help identify intraneural needle placement.[13] If the needle tip is intraneural, low volumes of local anesthetic, 0.5 mL, will cause immediate lancinating pain. Should distal stimulation or paresthesia be unattainable, the medial epicondyle can be contacted and 5 to 7 mL of local anesthetic can be injected in a fan-like progression toward the brachial artery. One may also consider the addition of a depot steroid for the treatment of a nerve entrapment syndrome at this level.

Blockade of the Median Nerve at the Wrist

The median nerve can be easily blocked at the wrist. The patient's arm is first placed in a fully supinated position with a small towel beneath the dorsal aspect of the wrist to provide slight extension. The palmaris longus and flexor carpi ulnaris tendons should then be identified by having the patient flex his wrist against resistance. Should the palmaris longus be

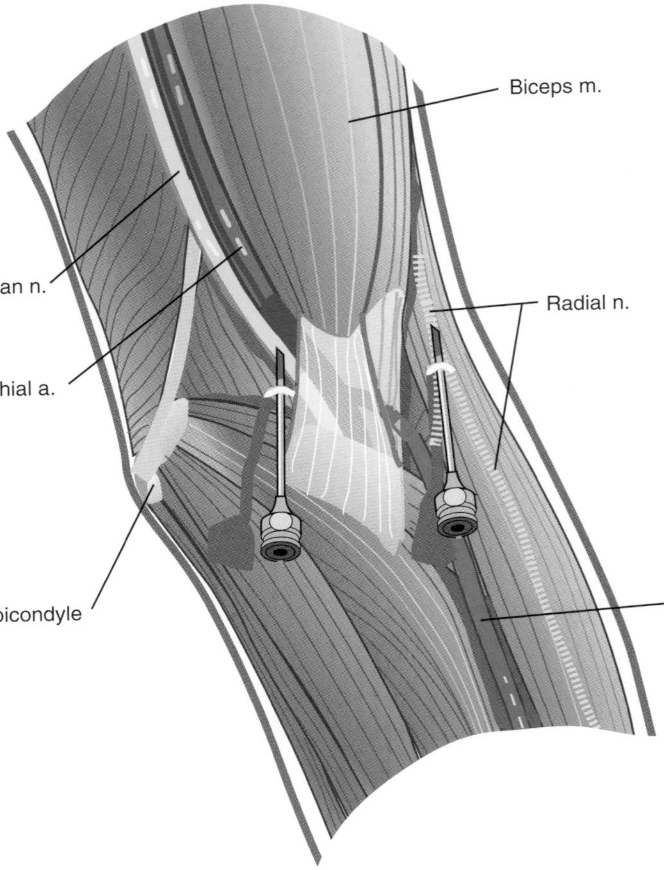

FIGURE 146–3 ■ Radial and median nerve blocks at the elbow. (Adapted from Wedel DJ, Horlocker TT: Nerve blocks. In Miller RD [ed]: Miller's Anesthesia, 6th ed. Philadelphia, Churchill Livingstone, 2005, p 1693.)

congenitally absent, the needle should be inserted just ulnar to the flexor carpi radialis tendon.[14,15] Using a 5/8-inch, 25-gauge B-bevel needle, the skin should be entered either perpendicularly or at a slight cephalad angle approximately at 1 to 1.5 cm proximal to the crease of the wrist. This location should lie just proximal to the flexor retinaculum.[13] The needle should then be advanced between the palmaris longus and flexor carpi ulnaris tendons (Fig. 146–4). The median nerve will usually be contacted and will elicit a paresthesia just deep to the palmaris longus tendon. If the carpal bones are contacted before paresthesia, the needle should be withdrawn approximately 2 to 3 mm and a total of 3 to 5 mL of local anesthetic should then be injected slowly. When performing a therapeutic blockade in patients with carpal tunnel syndrome, depot steroid can be added to the local anesthetic of choice.[9]

Side Effects and Complications

Blockade of the median nerve at both the elbow and wrist are generally safe techniques. As with all peripheral nerve blocks, nerve injury is possible secondary to direct needle trauma. Blockade of the median nerve at the wrist has the potential of exacerbating symptoms of carpal tunnel syndrome in certain patients because this is a relatively confined space. Bleeding and hematoma formation can occur secondary to direct puncture of the brachial artery at the elbow. This complication can usually be easily remedied by applying direct pressure to the area following the block. Inadvertent intravascular injection is also a possibility. Other relatively uncommon complications may include allergic reaction, localized infection, and systemic local anesthetic toxicity.

As mentioned earlier, blockade of the median nerve at the elbow and wrist is not only useful for providing anesthesia and analgesia of the palmar surface of the hand, but it also serves diagnostic and therapeutic functions. Median nerve blockade at the elbow can aid in the diagnosis of patients suffering from entrapment syndromes caused by accessory ligaments or muscular hypertrophy.[9] Although blockade of the median nerve at the wrist may provide relief of carpal tunnel symptoms, care should be taken to inject medication proximal to the flexor retinaculum so as not to further exacerbate median nerve compression as it courses through the carpal tunnel.

ULNAR NERVE BLOCK

Indications

Blockade of the ulnar nerve is essential to provide surgical anesthesia to the ulnar half of the middle and little fingers. Its anatomic location at the elbow makes this nerve susceptible not only to compression syndromes but also to direct trauma. In fact, the ulnar nerve is the most commonly injured peripheral nerve associated with positioning injuries during general

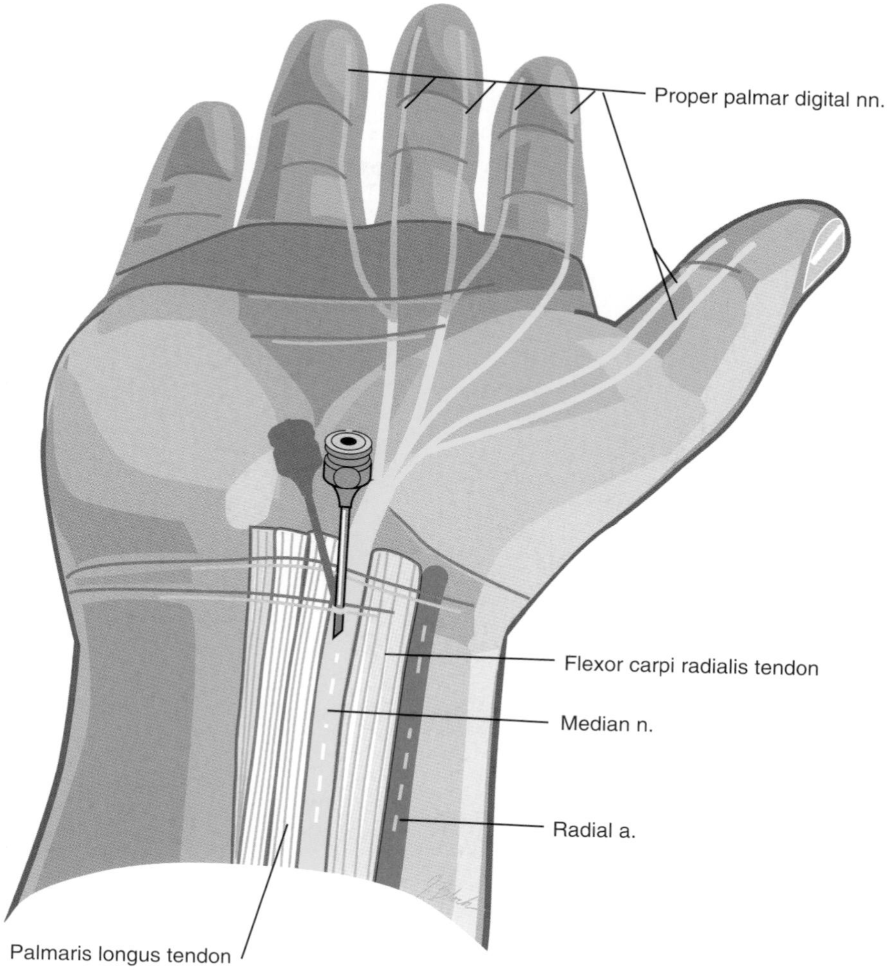

FIGURE 146–4 ■ Median nerve block at the wrist. (From Waldman SD: Atlas of Interventional Pain Management, 2nd ed. Philadelphia, Saunders, 2004, p 197.)

anesthesia.[16] Ulnar nerve blockade at the elbow can be combined with depot-steroid preparations to help manage the pain associated with cubital and ulnar tunnel syndromes. In ulnar tunnel syndrome, the ulnar nerve is compressed as it runs through the canal of Guyon (Fig. 146–5). Ulnar nerve compression at this site is often seen in professional bicyclists (a condition often referred to as cyclist's hand).[2,11] This syndrome occur when the hand is extended for prolonged periods against the handlebars of a bicycle, allowing the palmar branch of the ulnar nerve to become compressed by the hook of the hamate bone.[11] It may also occur as a result of compression secondary to ganglion cysts. Ulnar tunnel syndrome typically presents with pain and decreased sensation of the medial hand and occasionally weakness of the interossei and hypothenar musculature.[17] It is important to note that the cutaneous nerves to the fingers branch distally in the canal of Guyon. Consequently, compression of the ulnar nerve at this location typically spares sensation to the medial aspect of the hand but not the fingers.[2]

Ulnar nerve block may also be useful when combined with cervical MRI, EMG, and nerve conduction studies to elucidate the cause of neuropathic pain below the elbow. This is because C7 and C8 radiculopathies and compressive lesions of the brachial plexus (thoracic outlet syndrome, metastatic cancer, and apical lung tumors) may manifest with symptoms similar to those of ulnar neuropathy.[9] Blockade of the ulnar nerve may also be useful in evaluating and guiding therapy for upper extremity spasticity secondary to stroke, traumatic brain injury, and cerebral palsy.[7] When performed with neurolytic agents, this technique may provide additional treatment for the spasticity associated with these conditions.[8] Peripheral ulnar nerve block with local anesthetic is recommended before any neural destructive therapy to elucidate the degree of sensory and motor deficit following this procedure.

Clinically Relevant Anatomy

The ulnar nerve arises from the medial cord and thus primarily receives contributions from the C8 and T1 nerve roots. At the level of the axilla, the nerve runs just inferior and anterior to the axillary artery. After exiting the axilla, the ulnar nerve then traverses the upper arm medial to the brachial artery. At the middle portion of the upper arm, the nerve pierces the intramuscular septum entering the posterior compartment. It then travels between the medial humeral epicondyle and the olecranon process of the ulna. Running medial to the epicondylar groove, the ulnar nerve subsequently enters the cubital tunnel beneath the cubital retinaculum. It is at this

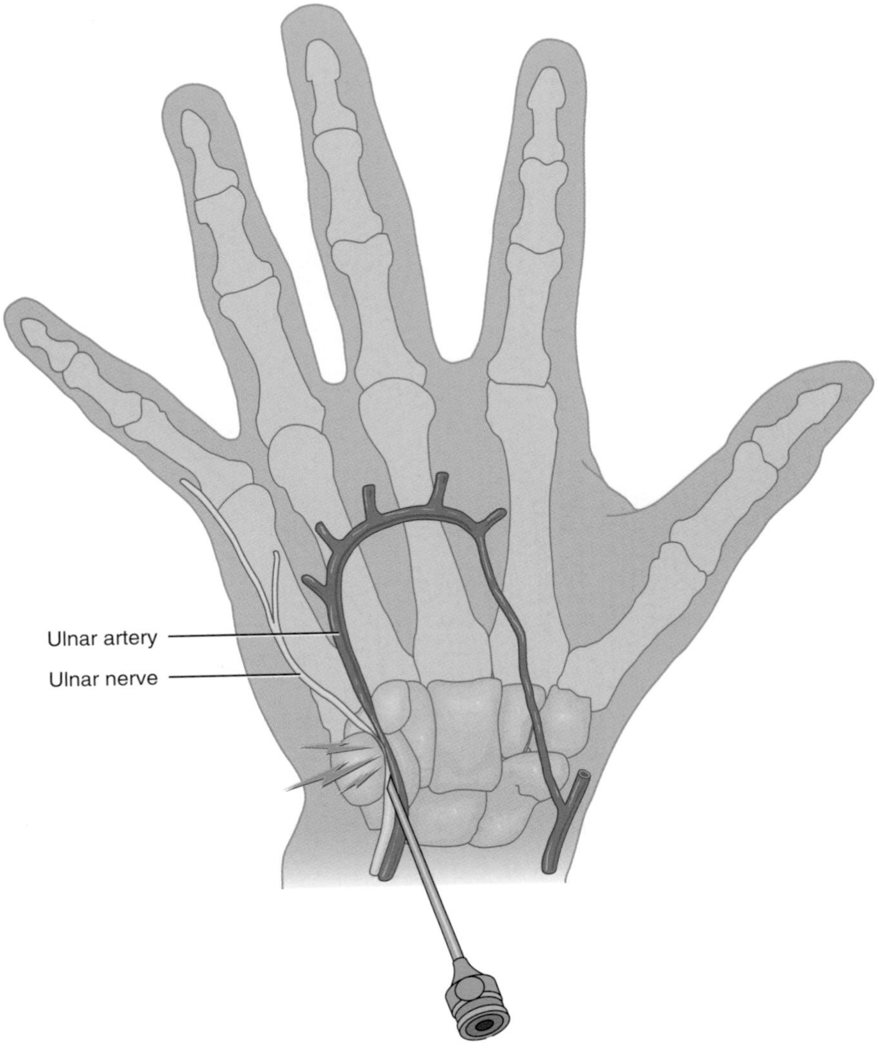

FIGURE 146–5 ■ Ulnar tunnel syndrome is caused by compression of the ulnar nerve as it passes through canal of Guyon at the wrist. (From Waldman SD: Atlas of Pain Management Injection Techniques. Philadelphia, Saunders, 2000, p 149.)

location that the nerve is susceptible to both compression and direct trauma. The ulnar nerve then travels with the ulnar artery between the heads of the flexor carpi ulnaris muscle in the anterior compartment of the forearm. It provides motor branches to both the flexor carpi ulnaris and the flexor digitorum profundus. The ulnar nerve branches into its palmar and dorsal branches at approximately 5 cm proximal to the volar skin crease of the wrist (see Fig. 146–2). The nerves that provide sensory innervation to the medial aspect of the hand, branch proximal to the canal of Guyon. The most distal branches must then travel through the canal of Guyon before providing sensory innervation to the little finger and the medial half of the ring finger.

Ulnar Nerve Block at the Distal Humerus

The ulnar nerve can be blocked at the elbow before entering the cubital tunnel. It is often preferred not to block this nerve directly in the ulnar groove because the nerve is more susceptible to compression at this location. The patient is first positioned in a supine position with the arm pronated and the elbow flexed at a 90-degree angle. The ulnar groove and medial epicondyle can then be easily palpated in most patients. Using a 25-gauge, 1½-inch B-bevel needle or a 22- or 24-gauge stimulating needle, the insertion site should be approximately 2 cm proximal to the midpoint of the ulnar groove.[18] The needle is then advanced in a perpendicular plane toward the humerus, until either an ulnar paresthesia or motor response of the ulnar nerve is elicited (ulnar deviation of the wrist, flexion of the wrist, finger adduction). Next, 5 to 7.5 mL of local anesthetic is injected after negative aspiration for heme (Fig. 146–6). In patients with chronic pain secondary to cubital tunnel syndrome, a depot steroid preparation can be added to the injectate. Should one choose to perform this block at the level of the ulnar groove, less than 5 mL of volume should be injected to prevent nerve injury from increased cubital tunnel pressure.

Ultrasound-guided block of the ulnar nerve in the forearm proximal to the wrist has been described by Gray.[19] In this technique, the nerve is located with the assistance of ultrasonography 15 cm proximal to the styloid process of the ulna.

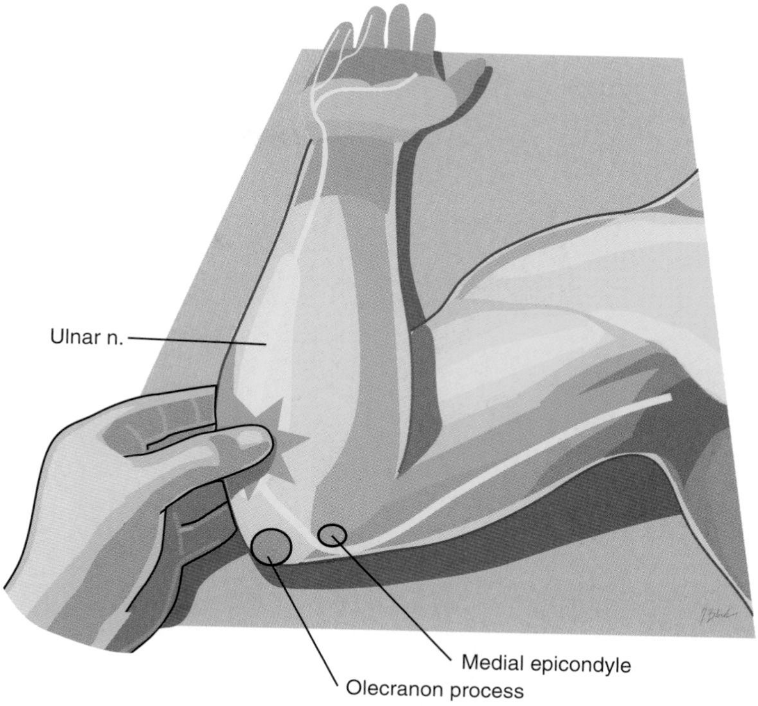

FIGURE 146–6 ■ Ulnar nerve block proximal to the elbow. (From Waldman SD: Atlas of Interventional Pain Management, 2nd ed. Philadelphia, Saunders, 2004, p 188.)

Ulnar Nerve Block at the Wrist

The ulnar nerve can be blocked safely and reliably at the wrist (Fig. 146–7). At the level of the styloid process of the ulna, the ulnar nerve is found just lateral to the flexor carpi ulnaris tendon and just medial to the ulnar artery. The patient's arm should be placed in a fully supinated position. Slight extension of the wrist is often helpful in identifying landmarks. Using a 25-gauge 5/8-inch, B-bevel needle the skin is entered at a perpendicular angle just ulnar to the flexor carpi ulnaris tendon and 2 cm proximal to the skin crease of the wrist. Paresthesia is usually elicited before bony contact. At this level, 3 to 5 mL of local anesthetic is usually sufficient to anesthetize the ulnar nerve (see Fig. 146–2).

Side Effects and Complications

As the cubital tunnel is a relatively confined space, the ulnar nerve is very susceptible to compression when it is blocked at the elbow. Therefore, careful neurologic evaluation should be performed before all blocks at this level. In fact, Stahl reports that even therapeutic blocks for medial epicondylitis may lead to ulnar nerve injury.[20] Intraneural injection and direct needle trauma can occur at both the elbow and the wrist. Intra-arterial injection and hematoma formation are also potential sequelae. Other relatively uncommon complications may include allergic reaction, localized infection, and systemic local anesthetic toxicity.

■ RADIAL NERVE BLOCK

Blockade of the radial nerve is essential to provide surgical anesthesia of the dorsal surface of the arm, forearm, and hand. Radial nerve block at the elbow can serve both diagnostic and therapeutic functions. Entrapment syndromes of the radial nerve (radial tunnel syndrome) may be misdiagnosed as tennis elbow (lateral epicondylitis).[2,21] Blockade of the radial nerve at the elbow completely relieves pain associated with this entrapment syndrome.[21] It will not appreciably decrease pain associated with lateral epicondylitis. By adding a depot steroid to radial blockade at this location, the chronic pain associated with the above entrapment syndromes can often be palliated. This modality can also be used for the management of cheiralgia paresthetica or Wartenberg syndrome. This syndrome, which occurs during forearm pronation, is secondary to compression of the sensory branches of the radial nerve by the brachioradialis distal to the musculospiral groove. It manifests with painful paresthesias and decreased sensation over the dorsum of the hand. Radial nerve blockade may also be useful in evaluating and guiding therapy for upper extremity spasticity secondary to stroke, traumatic brain injury, or cerebral palsy.[7] When performed with neurolytic agents, radial nerve blockade may provide additional treatment for the spasticity associated with these conditions.[8] Blockade of the posterior interosseous branch of the radial nerve has also been proposed as an important diagnostic and therapeutic modality in the treatment of chronic wrist pain.[22] Peripheral neural blockade of the radial nerve with local anesthetics is recommended before any neural destructive therapy to elucidate the degree of sensory and motor deficit this procedure will produce. As with other upper extremity pain syndromes, it is imperative that the pain practitioner rule out other etiologies of the patient's pain. Nerve blockade of the radial nerve is also useful when combined with cervical MRI, EMG, and nerve conduction studies to elucidate the cause of chronic pain radiating to the dorsal aspect of the arm, forearm, and the hand.

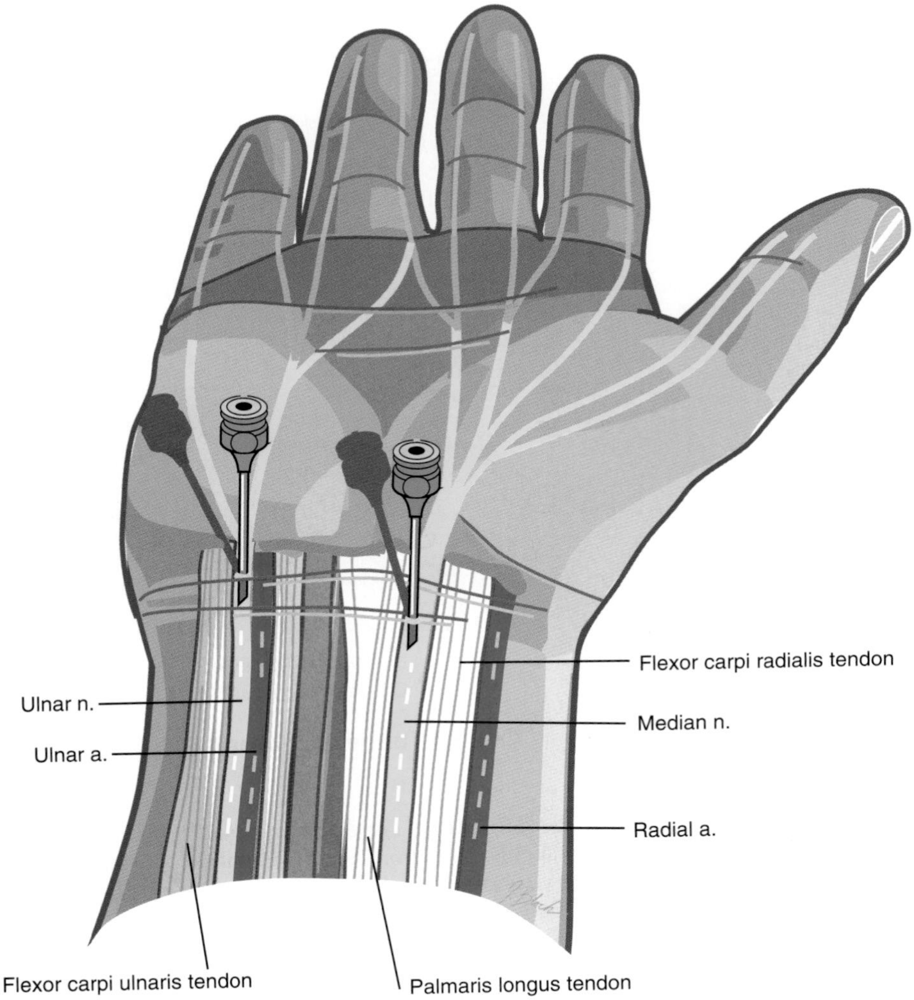

FIGURE 146–7 ■ Ulnar and median nerve blocks at the wrist. (Adapted from Wedel DJ, Horlocker TT: Nerve blocks. In Miller RD [ed]: Miller's Anesthesia, 6th ed. Philadelphia, Churchill Livingstone, 2005, p 1694.)

This is due to the fact that cervical radiculopathies and compressive lesions of the brachial plexus may manifest with symptoms similar to those of radial neuropathy.

Clinically Relevant Anatomy

The radial nerve is a direct continuation of the posterior cord of the brachial plexus and receives contributions from the C5-T1 cervical roots. In the axilla, the nerve resides just posterior to the axillary artery.[10] On leaving the axilla, the radial nerve then pierces between the long and middle heads of the triceps, providing motor branches to this muscle and giving off the posterior cutaneous nerve that innervates skin sensation overlying the posterior proximal arm. The nerve then runs along the posterior humeral groove and emerges between the musculospiral groove of the proximal arm before moving anterior and medial to the lateral epicondyle of the humerus. As the radial nerve leaves the cubital space, it enters the forearm under the brachioradialis muscle and subsequently divides into its deep and superficial branches. The deep branch ultimately becomes the posterior interosseous nerve, which provides motor innervation to the wrist flexors. The superficial branch then continues running distally between the brachioradialis and supinator muscles.[23] At the wrist, the superficial branch of the radial nerve lies in a lateral position in relation to the radial artery. This branch finally gives off dorsal digital branches that supply sensory innervation to the dorsal hand and the dorsal aspects of the thumb, index finger, and ring finger and radial half of the middle finger.

Radial Nerve Block at the Distal Humerus

The radial nerve can be blocked safely and with relative reliability proximal to the lateral epicondyle of the humerus (Fig. 146–8). The patient's arm should be flexed to approximately 90 degrees at the elbow with the patient's palm resting comfortably on the chest or abdomen. Using a 22-gauge, 2-inch stimulating needle, the skin is entered at a perpendicular angle 5 to 6 cm proximal to the lateral epicondyle of the humerus. This should roughly correspond to the most distal aspect of the musculospiral groove created by the lateral head of the triceps and the brachialis muscles. The needle should then be slowly advanced until either a radial paresthesia is elicited or distal motor stimulation of a radial nerve distribution is attained below 0.5 mA (wrist or finger extension, thumb abduction). If no paresthesia or motor stimulation occurs before contact with the humerus, the needle should be withdrawn slightly and "walked" in an anterior-posterior manner until an appropriate response is elicited. Following

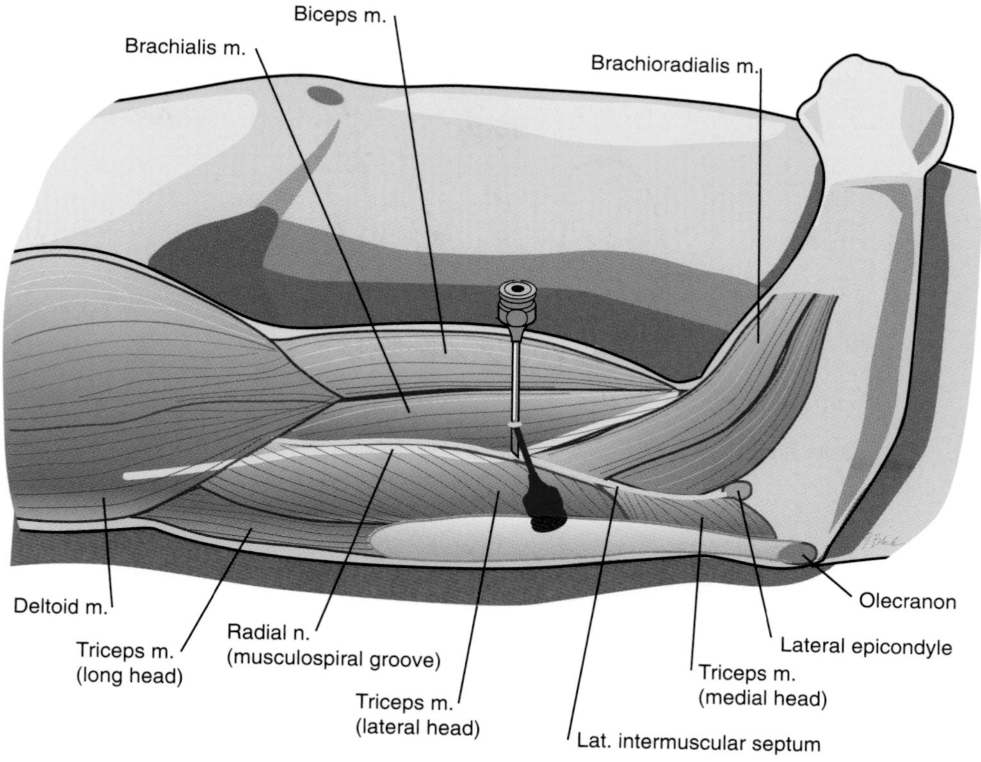

FIGURE 146–8 ■ Radial nerve block at the humerus. (From Waldman SD: Atlas of Interventional Pain Management, 2nd ed. Philadelphia, Saunders, 2004, p 169.)

appropriate stimulation and after negative aspiration for heme, 7 to 10 mL of local anesthetic is injected slowly. The provider may also consider the addition of a depot-steroid preparation when appropriate.

Radial Nerve Block at the Elbow

The patient's arm is first placed in a supinated and fully extended position. Using a 22-gauge, 2-inch stimulating needle, the skin is entered at the antecubital skin crease between the tendon of the biceps and the belly of the brachioradialis muscle. The needle is then advanced toward the lateral epicondyle with a slightly cephalad tilt (see Fig. 146–3). Proper placement is evidenced by either a radial paresthesia or distal motor stimulation of a radial nerve distribution below 0.5 mA. If paresthesia or motor stimulation do not occur before contact with the humerus, the needle should be withdrawn slightly and "walked in" a medial direction.[24] Following appropriate stimulation and after negative aspiration for heme, 7 to 10 mL of local anesthetic is injected slowly. The pain practitioner may also consider the addition of a depot-steroid preparation, when appropriate, for the treatment of pain secondary to inflammation or nerve entrapment.

Radial Nerve Block at the Wrist

The superficial radial nerve can be blocked at the wrist before giving off to the dorsal digital branches, which supply sensory innervation to the dorsum of the hand and dorsal aspects of the thumb, index finger, ring finger, and radial half of the middle finger.[2] To block the radial nerve at this level, the patient's forearm should be placed in a fully supinated position with a small towel resting beneath the dorsum of the wrist. A 25-gauge, 1½-inch B-bevel needle is first inserted at the styloid of the radius between the radial artery and the flexor carpi ulnaris tendon (Fig. 146–9). After paresthesia is elicited in the dorsal thumb, 4 to 5 mL of local anesthetic is injected after negative aspiration. To block the dorsal branches to the ring, index and middle fingers, the patient's hand is then placed in a fully pronated position. Using the same needle, 4 to 5 mL of local anesthetic is subcutaneously injected from the dorsal aspect of the radial styloid to the tendon of the extensor carpi radialis on the dorsum of the wrist.[24,25]

Side Effects and Complications

Blockade of the radial nerve at the distal humerus, elbow, and wrist are generally safe techniques. As with all peripheral nerve blocks, nerve injury is possible secondary to direct needle trauma. Bleeding and hematoma formation are also two relatively self-limiting complications. When the radial nerve is blocked at the wrist, inadvertent intra-arterial injection can occur due to the proximity of the radial nerve to the radial artery in the "anatomic snuff box." Should this occur, systemic toxicity may manifest with seizure or cardiac conduction block. Fortunately, the low volume used with this block makes this a rare occurrence.

■ MUSCULOCUTANEOUS NERVE BLOCK

Indications

Blockade of the musculocutaneous nerve is used primarily to provide surgical anesthesia of the arm and forearm and is usually performed in combination with brachial plexus blockade (axillary block). Because this nerve branches from the

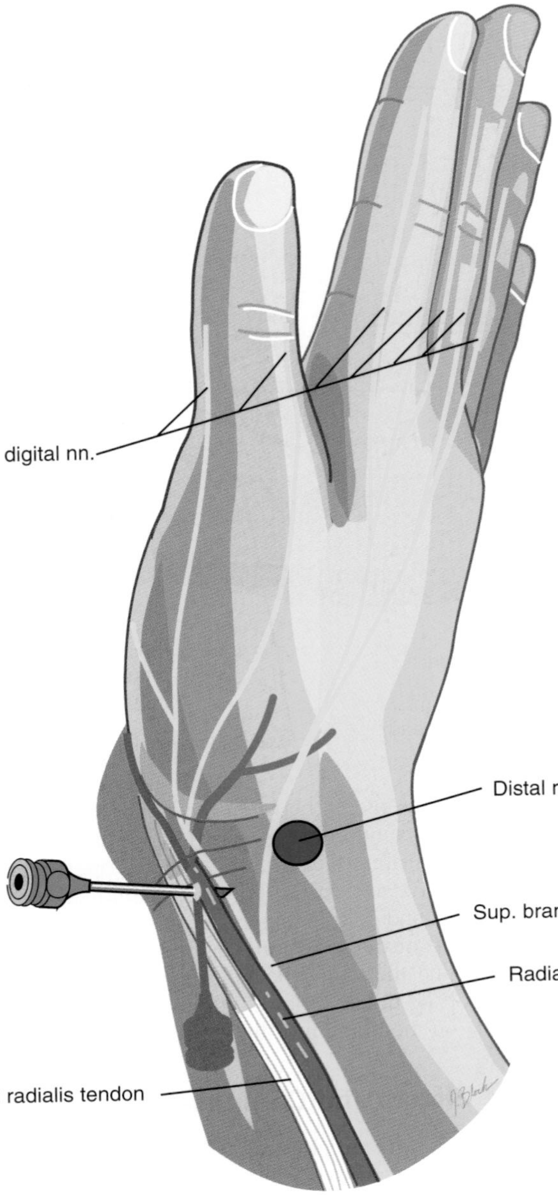

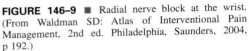

FIGURE 146–9 ■ Radial nerve block at the wrist. (From Waldman SD: Atlas of Interventional Pain Management, 2nd ed. Philadelphia, Saunders, 2004, p 192.)

lateral cord proximal to the axilla, it must be blocked separately at this level. The musculocutaneous nerve provides motor innervation to the coracobrachialis, brachialis, and biceps musculature. Blockade of the musculocutaneous nerve is useful in evaluating and guiding therapy for upper extremity spasticity secondary to stroke, traumatic brain injury, and cerebral palsy.[7] The musculocutaneous nerve continues below the elbow as the lateral antebrachial cutaneous nerve. This nerve provides sensory innervation to the dorsal-lateral forearm. Therefore, blockade of this nerve is helpful when combined with cervical MRI, EMG, and nerve conduction studies to elucidate the cause of neuropathic pain in the lateral forearm.[9]

Clinically Relevant Anatomy

The musculocutaneous nerve branches from the lateral cord of the brachial plexus and receives contributions from the C5-C7 nerve roots. This nerve branches from the lateral cord just distal to the pectoralis minor muscle.[10] The musculocutaneous nerve then travels between the bellies of the coracobrachialis muscle, running laterally as it approaches the elbow joint. At the elbow, the musculocutaneous nerve gives off a small branch to the elbow joint before continuing as the lateral antebrachial cutaneous nerve, which runs lateral to the cephalic vein in the forearm.[21]

Blockade of the Musculocutaneous Nerve in the Axilla

The patient should be first placed in a supine, recumbent position with the elbow flexed and the shoulder abducted and externally rotated. The coracobrachialis muscle should then be identified at a location just superior to the axillary artery. Using a 22-gauge, 2-inch insulated needle the skin is entered perpendicularly into the belly of the coracobrachialis muscle.

The needle should be moved in a fan-like manner through this muscle until motor stimulation produces a vigorous biceps contraction (elbow flexion). After obtaining a biceps twitch below 0.5 mA, 10 mL of local anesthetic can be injected after negative aspiration for blood. This block can also be performed without stimulation by inserting the needle as above and advancing the needle until the humerus is contacted. After contacting bone, the needle is withdrawn 0.5 cm and 10 mL of local anesthetic is injected into the belly of the coracobrachialis muscle in a fan-like manner.

Side Effects and Complications

Blockade of the musculocutaneous nerve at the proximal humerus is generally a safe technique. As with all peripheral nerve blocks, nerve injury is possible secondary to direct needle trauma. Bleeding and hematoma formation are also two relatively self-limiting complications. Inadvertent intra-arterial injection can occur owing to the proximity of the musculocutaneous nerve to the axillary artery. Should this occur, systemic toxicity may manifest with seizure or cardiac conduction block. Fortunately, the low volume used with this block makes this a rare occurrence.

MEDIAL BRACHIAL CUTANEOUS AND INTERCOSTOBRACHIAL NERVE BLOCKS

Blockade of the medial brachial cutaneous nerve and intercostobrachial nerve is used primarily in conjunction with brachial plexus block (axillary technique) to provide anesthesia to the proximal arm. The medial brachial cutaneous nerve arises from the cervical roots at C8-T1. The intercostobrachial nerve receives contributions from T1 and T2. These nerves provide sensory innervation to the medial aspect of the proximal arm and axilla. To block these nerves (Fig. 146–10), the patient's arm should be flexed at the elbow with the shoulder abducted 80 degrees. Because these nerves are both superficial, they are easily blocked by infiltrating 7 to 10 mL of local anesthetic in the subcutaneous tissue from the midpoint of the biceps muscle to the inferior axilla.[24]

Complications

Medial brachial cutaneous and intercostobrachial blocks are safe and simple blocks. Care should be taken to avoid inadvertent vascular injection by ensuring the needle remains in the subcutaneous tissue. Bleeding and hematoma formation are also potential complications of this injection.

CONCLUSION

Blockade of the peripheral nerves of the upper extremity are safe and relatively simple techniques. Unlike some proximal brachial plexus blocks, there is no risk of pneumothorax associated with peripheral blockade of the upper extremity nerves. These blocks can all be safely performed in the presence of systemic anticoagulation. Peripheral upper extremity blocks not only provide surgical anesthesia but also play important diagnostic and therapeutic roles. These blocks have been used for the diagnosis and treatment of neuropathic pain syndromes and entrapment neuropathies. Consequently, knowledge of

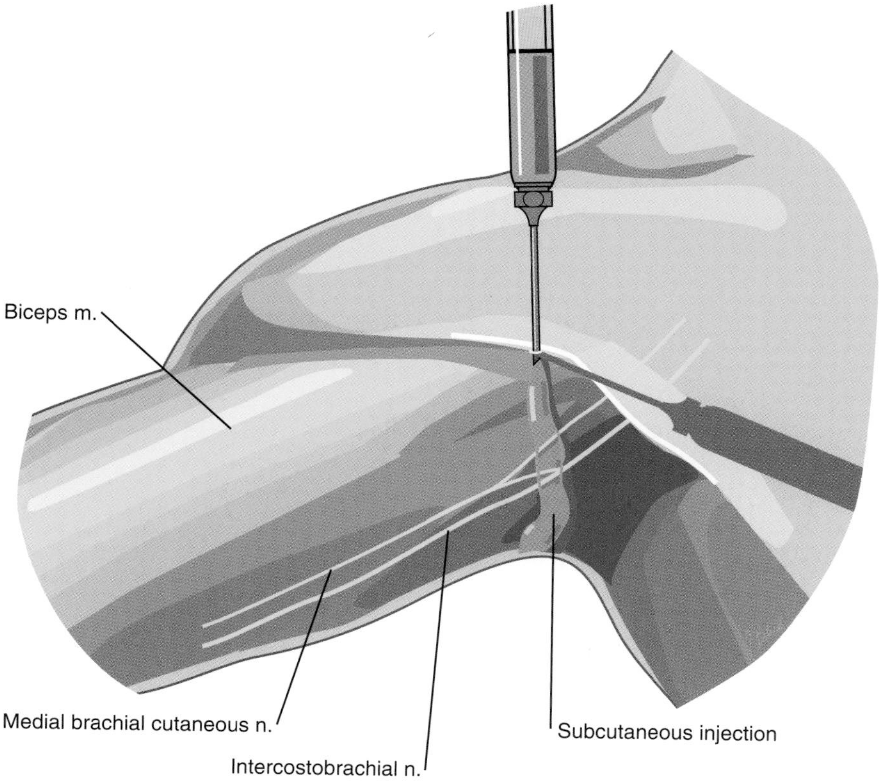

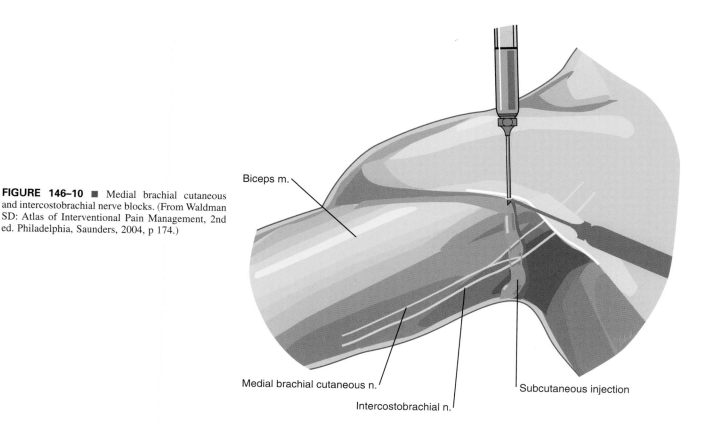

FIGURE 146–10 ■ Medial brachial cutaneous and intercostobrachial nerve blocks. (From Waldman SD: Atlas of Interventional Pain Management, 2nd ed. Philadelphia, Saunders, 2004, p 174.)

the anatomy and blockade of the upper extremity nerves can be a useful adjuvant in the armamentarium of the pain practitioner.

References

1. Urmey WF: Upper extremity blocks. In Brown DL (ed): Regional Anesthesia and Analgesia. Philadelphia, Saunders, 1995, p 254.
2. Goldstein B: Musculoseletal upper limb pain. In Loeser JD (ed): Bonica's Management of Pain, 3rd ed. Philadelphia, Lippincott-Raven, 2001, p 1032.
3. Delaunay L, Chelly JE: Blocks at the wrist provide effective anesthesia for carpal tunnel release. Can J Anaesth 48:656, 2001.
4. Wilson KM: Distal forearm regional block anesthesia for carpal tunnel release. J Hand Surg [Am] 18:438, 1993.
5. Campanati A, Lagalla G, Penna L, et al: Local neural block at the wrist for treatment of palmar hyperhidrosis with botulinum toxin: Technical improvements. J Am Acad Dermatol 51:345, 2004.
6. Phillips ME, Katz JA, Harden RN: The use of nerve blocks in conjunction with occupational therapy for complex regional pain syndrome type I. Am J Occup Ther 54:544, 2000.
7. Filipetti P, Decq P: Interest of anesthetic blocks for assessment of the spastic patient: A series of 815 motor blocks. Neurochirurgie 49:226, 2003.
8. Loubser PG: Neurolytic interventions for upper extremity spasticity associated with head injury. Reg Anesth 22:386, 1997.
9. Waldman SD: Atlas of Interventional Pain Management, 2nd ed. Philadelphia, Saunders, 2004, pp 166-201.
10. Agur A, Dalley A: Grant's Atlas of Anatomy. Philadelphia, Lippincott Williams & Wilkins, 2005, pp 500-505.
11. Mathers LH, Chase RA, Dolph J, et al: Clinical Anatomy Principles. St. Louis, CV Mosby, 1996, pp 365-377.
12. Selander D, Dhuner KG, Lundborg G: Peripheral nerve injury due to injection needles used for regional anesthesia. Acta Anaesth Scand 21:182, 1977.
13. Wedel DJ, Horlocker TT: Nerve blocks. In Miller RD (ed): Miller's Anesthesia, 6th ed. Philadelphia, Churchill Livingstone, 2005, p 1685.
14. Thompson WL, Malchow RJ: Peripheral blocks and anesthesia of the hand. Milit Med 167:478, 2002.
15. Kletzl Z, Krejca M, Simcik J: Role of sensory innervation variations for wrist block anesthesia. Arch Med Res 32:155, 2001.
16. Warner MA, Warner ME, Martin JT: Ulnar neuropathy: Incidence, outcome and risk factors in sedated or anesthetized patients. Anesthesiology 81:1332, 1994.
17. Berquist TH: Musculoskeletal Imaging Companion. Philadelphia, Lippincott Williams & Wilkins, 2002, p 506.
18. Brown DL, Bridenbaugh LD: The upper extremity somatic block. In Cousins MJ, Bridenbaugh PO (eds): Neural Blockade in Clinical Anesthesia and Management of Pain, 3rd ed. Philadelphia, Lippincott-Raven, 1998, p 345.
19. Gray AT, Schafhalter-Zoppoth I: Ultrasound guidance for ulnar nerve block in the forearm. Reg Anesth Pain Med 28:335, 2003.
20. Stahl S, Kaufman T: Ulnar nerve injury at the elbow after steroid injections for medial epicondylitis. J Hand Surg [Br] 22:69, 1997.
21. Grutter PW, Desilva GL, Meehan RE, Desilva SP: The accuracy of distal posterior interosseous and anterior interosseous nerve injection. J Hand Surg [Am] 29:865, 2004.
22. Abrams RA, Ziets RT, Lieber RL, Botte MJ: Anatomy of the radial nerve motor branches in the forearm. J Hand Surg [Am] 22:232, 1997.
23. Nishanian E, Gargarian M: Regional anesthesia. In Hurford WE, Bailin MT (eds): Clinical Anesthesia Procedures of the Massachusetts General Hospital, 5th ed. Philadelphia, Lippincott-Raven, 1998, p 264.
24. Howard RF: Hand and microsurgery. In Miller MD (ed): Review of Orthopaedics, 4th ed. Philadelphia, Saunders, 2004, p 358.
25. Porter JM, Inglefield CJ: An audit of peripheral nerve blocks for hand surgery. Ann R Coll Surg Engl 75:325, 1993.

chapter 147

Suprascapular Nerve Block

P. Prithvi Raj

HISTORICAL CONSIDERATIONS

Historically, suprascapular nerve block was used as a primary treatment for conditions that limited the range of motion of the shoulder, including adhesive capsulitis and calcific tendinitis and bursitis.[1] The advent of corticosteroids allowed earlier treatment of the maladies. Subsequently, the use of a suprascapular nerve block as a primary treatment modality for shoulder lesions declined. Recently, there has been renewed interest in suprascapular nerve block to allow early range of motion and rehabilitation after shoulder reconstruction or joint replacement.

INDICATIONS AND CONTRAINDICATIONS

Suprascapular nerve block with local anesthetics can be used as a diagnostic tool when performing differential neural blockade on an anatomic basis to evaluate shoulder girdle and shoulder joint pain.[2] If destruction of the suprascapular nerve is being considered, this technique is useful as a prognostic indicator of the degree of motor and sensory impairment that the patient might experience.[3] Suprascapular nerve block with local anesthetic may be used to palliate acute pain emergencies, including postoperative pain, pain secondary to trauma to the shoulder joint and girdle, and cancer pain while waiting for pharmacologic, surgical, or antiblastic treatment to become effective.[3] Suprascapular nerve block is also useful as adjunctive therapy for decreased range of motion of the shoulder secondary to reflex sympathetic dystrophy or adhesive capsulitis,[1,3] and it can be effective in allowing the patient to tolerate more aggressive physical therapy after shoulder reconstructive surgery.[3]

Destruction of the suprascapular nerve is indicated for palliation of cancer pain, including that of invasive tumors of the shoulder girdle.[3] It can be performed in patients who are taking anticoagulants, if the clinical situation dictates a favorable risk-benefit ratio. This procedure is contraindicated in patients with local infection, anatomic anomaly, or coagulopathies.

EQUIPMENT AND DRUGS

The required equipment includes 3- or 5-mL syringe for local infiltration; 5- or 10-mL syringe for local anesthetics/steroids; 25-gauge needle for local infiltration; 22-gauge spinal needle or 22-gauge, B-beveled needle for nerve block; and 10-cm curved, blunt radiofrequency needle with 10-mm active tip for pulsed radiofrequency.

For the block using local anesthetic, the drug preparations include: lidocaine 1% to 2%; bupivacaine 0.25% to 0.5%; ropivacaine 0.2% to 0.5%; and depot steroids 40 to 80 mg. For the neurolytic block the solution used is phenol 6%.

PREPARATION AND POSITIONING OF THE PATIENT

Physical examination should include (1) palpation of the area for needle entry; and (2) examination of the shoulder motion and documentation of the range of motion for evaluating success of the block. The patient is placed in the prone position with the arms at the side. A total of 10 mL of local anesthetic is drawn up in a 10-mL sterile syringe. When treating painful conditions that are mediated via the suprascapular nerve, a total of 80 mg of depot steroid is added to the local anesthetic with the first block and 40 mg of depot steroid with subsequent blocks. Medication protocol should be consistent with the American Society of Anesthesiologists conscious sedation guidelines.

CLINICALLY RELEVANT ANATOMY

The suprascapular nerve is formed from fibers originating from the C5 and C6 nerve roots of the brachial plexus and, in most patients, some fibers from the C4 root. The nerve passes inferiorly and posteriorly from the brachial plexus to pass underneath the coracoclavicular ligament through the suprascapular notch.[4] The suprascapular artery and vein accompany the nerve through the notch. The suprascapular nerve provides much of the sensory innervation to the shoulder joint and innervation to two of the muscles of the rotator cuff, the supraspinatus and infraspinatus (Fig. 147–1).

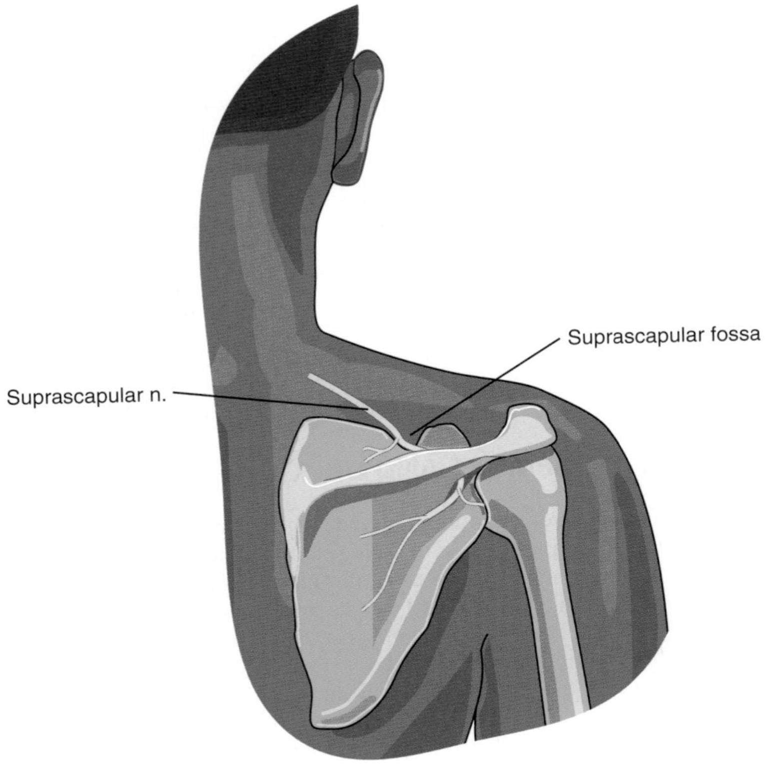

FIGURE 147–1 ■ Drawing of the anatomy of the suprascapular nerve. (From Raj PP, Lou L, Erdine S, et al: Radiographic Imaging for Regional Anesthesia and Pain Management. Philadelphia, Churchill Livingstone, 2003, p 128.)

TECHNIQUE FOR SUPRASCAPULAR NERVE BLOCK

Blind Technique

The operator identifies the spine of the scapula and then draws a line vertically through the midpoint of the spine and parallel to the vertebral column. The upper and outer quadrant so formed is bisected and a needle is inserted at a distance of 2 cm along this line. The needle is inserted at a right angle to the skin and advanced until the dorsal surface of the scapula is located. The needle is then "walked" along this dorsal surface until the suprascapular notch is identified. If a nerve stimulator is used, contractions of the supraspinatus and infraspinatus muscles will confirm placement. At this location, 5 mL of local anesthetics is injected. It is not always possible to ascertain any dermal analgesia as a result of this block. The success of block can be determined if motor-blocking concentrations of drug are used, when abduction of the arm will be compromised for the first 15 degrees before the deltoid muscle takes over (Fig. 147–2).

Radiographic Technique (Fig. 147–3)

The spine of the scapula is identified and the pain specialist then palpates along the length of the scapular spine laterally to identify the acromion (Fig. 147–4). At the point where the thicker acromion fuses with the thinner scapular spine, the skin is prepared with antiseptic solution. At this point, the skin and subcutaneous tissues are anesthetized using a $1\frac{1}{2}$-inch infiltration needle. After adequate anesthesia is obtained, a $3\frac{1}{2}$-inch, 25-gauge needle or a radiofrequency (RF) needle

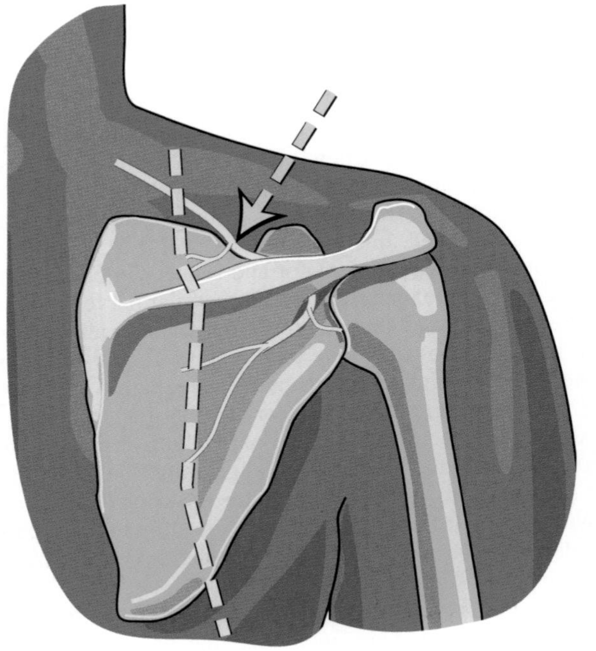

FIGURE 147–2 ■ Suprascapular nerve block. The nerve is blocked in the suprascapular fossa. The spine of the scapula is divided by a vertical line, and the upper and outer quadrant so formed is bisected and a needle is introduced 2 cm along this line and advanced to a depth of approximately 5 to 6 cm, at which point the dorsal surface of the scapula should be located. If this end point is not reached at this depth, the needle should be withdrawn and repositioned. When osseous contact is achieved, the needle is "walked" until the suprascapular notch is located, or, if an electrical stimulator is used, needle placement is confirmed by movements of the suprascapular and infrascapular muscles. At this point 5 mL of local anesthetic is injected.

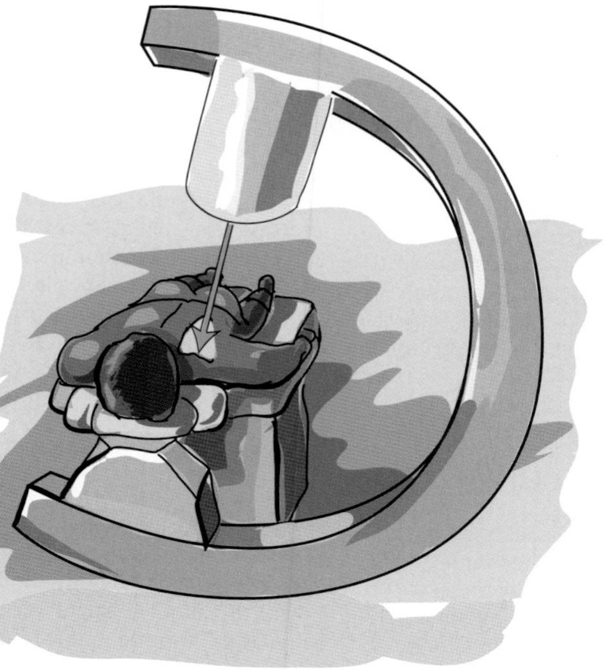

FIGURE 147–3 ■ Drawing of the patient in the prone position with the fluoroscope slightly lateral to midline at the T2-T3 level with a slight cephalocaudad tilt. (From Raj PP, Lou L, Erdine S, et al: Radiographic Imaging for Regional Anesthesia and Pain Management. Philadelphia, Churchill Livingstone, 2003, p 129.)

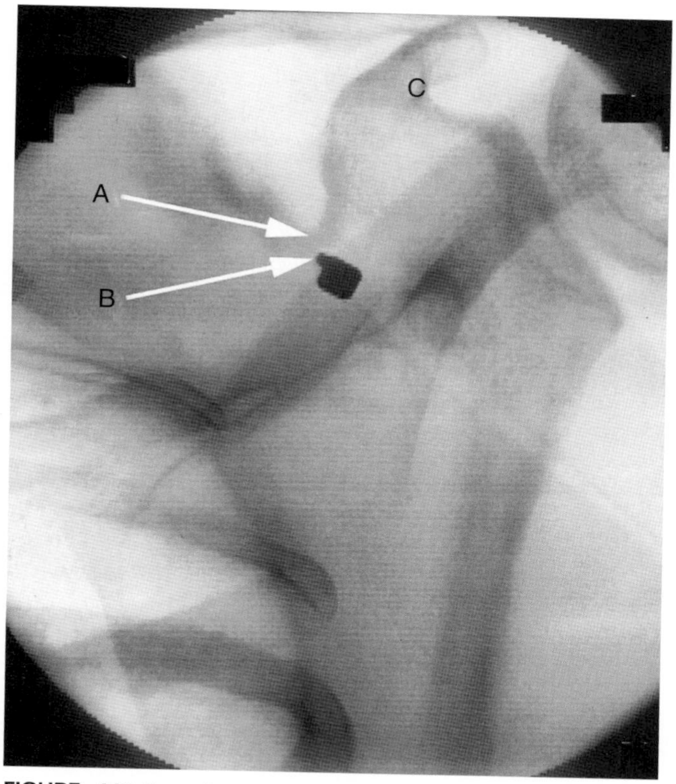

FIGURE 147–5 ■ Suprascapular nerve block with needle in place contacting bone just below the suprascapular nerve. *A,* suprascapular notch; *B,* curved blunt needle tip at the notch. (From Raj PP, Lou L, Erdine S, et al: Radiographic Imaging for Regional Anesthesia and Pain Management. Philadelphia, Churchill Livingstone, 2003, p 130.)

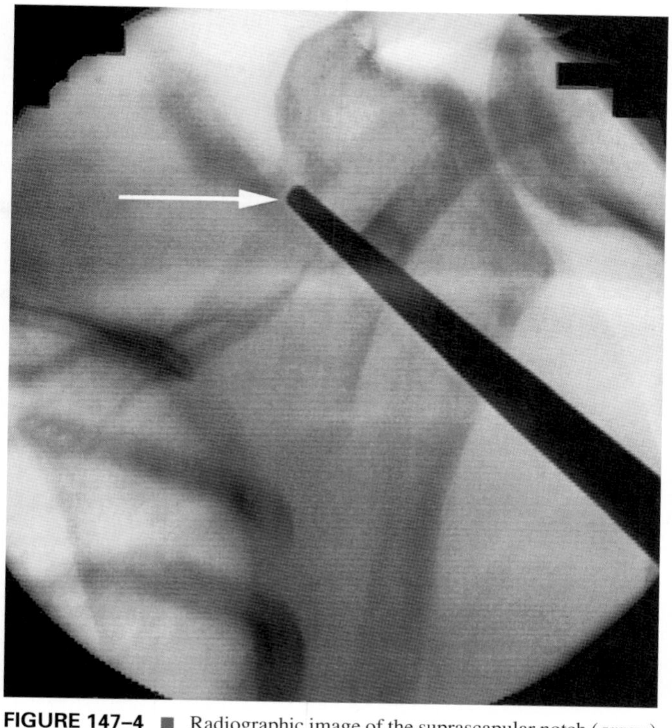

FIGURE 147–4 ■ Radiographic image of the suprascapular notch (*arrow*) emphasized by the oblique angulation of the fluoroscope. (From Raj PP, Lou L, Erdine S, et al: Radiographic Imaging for Regional Anesthesia and Pain Management. Philadelphia, Churchill Livingstone, 2003, p 130.)

with previously inserted catheter is inserted with an inferior trajectory toward the body of the scapula (Fig. 147–5). The needle should make contact with the body of the scapula at a depth of about 1 inch. The needle is then gently walked superiorly and medially until the tip walks off the scapular body into the suprascapular notch. If the notch is not identified, the same maneuver is repeated, directing the needle superiorly and laterally until the needle tip is positioned in the suprascapular notch. A paresthesia is often encountered as the needle tip enters the notch, and the patient should be warned. If a paresthesia is not elicited after the needle has entered the suprascapular notch, it is advanced an additional ½ inch, to place the tip beyond the substance of the coracoclavicular ligament. To avoid pneumothorax, the needle should *never* be advanced deeper.

After paresthesia is elicited or the needle has been advanced into the notch as described, gentle aspiration is carried out to identify blood or air. If the aspiration test is negative, 10 mL of solution is slowly injected as the patient is monitored closely for signs of local anesthetic toxicity (Fig. 147–6).

TECHNIQUE OF NEUROLYTIC BLOCK

After the needle is placed appropriately as described, 3 to 4 mL of Omnipaque (iohexol) is injected. An anteroposterior (AP) radiographic image is taken. The contrast solution

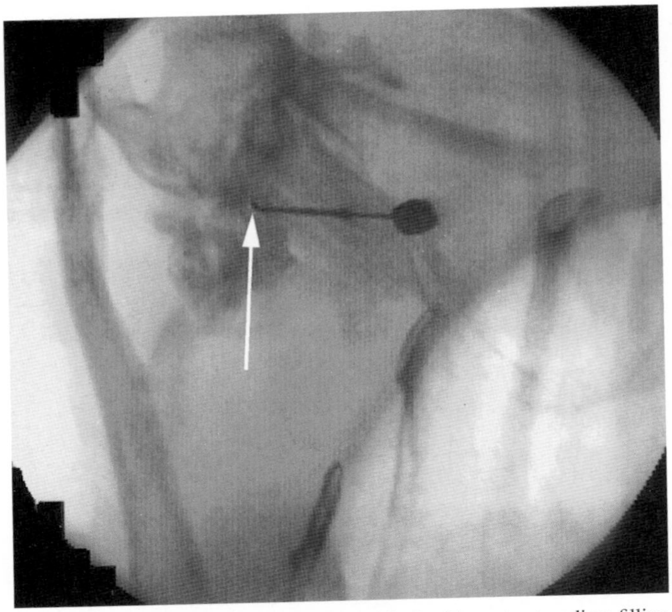

FIGURE 147–6 ■ Suprascapular nerve block with contrast medium filling the suprascapular fossa (*arrow*). (From Raj PP, Lou L, Erdine S, et al: Radiographic Imaging for Regional Anesthesia and Pain Management. Philadelphia, Churchill Livingstone, 2003, p 130.)

should fill the suprascapular notch and run toward the glenoid cavity. After the correct spread of the contrast medium is verified, 3 to 5 mL of local anesthetic is injected. If there are no side effects, then 3 to 5 mL of 6% phenol is injected.

PULSED ELECTROMAGNETIC FLOWMETER OF THE SUPRASCAPULAR NERVE

The landmarks and position are the same as described earlier. The needle chosen is a 10-cm blunt curved Racz-Finch Kit (RFK) needle with a (16-gauge introducer catheter). After the fluoroscopic view of the suprascapular notch is obtained the catheter is inserted. This is done with a "tunnel view." Following the catheter insertion, the Racz-Finch Kit (RFK) needle is introduced until it reaches the suprascapular notch. Contrast solution is then injected to confirm the position of the needle on the suprascapular nerve.

Ideally sensory stimulation at 50 Hz is positive at 0.3 to 0.6 volts to confirm proximity to the suprascapular nerve. Motor stimulation should not be more than two times sensory stimulation voltage and at 2 Hz. One proper placement is confirmed, the pulsating electromagnetic flowmeter lesion is created at 42°C for 120 seconds for two cycles. The needle is then removed. No local anesthetic is injected.

COMPLICATIONS

The proximity of the suprascapular nerve to the suprascapular artery and vein suggests the potential for inadvertent intravascular injection or local anesthetic toxicity from intravascular absorption. The pain specialist should carefully calculate the total (milligram) dose of local anesthetic that may safely be given for suprascapular nerve block. Because of the proximity of the lung, if the needle is advanced too deep through the suprascapular notch, pneumothorax is a possibility.

CLINICAL PEARLS

Suprascapular nerve block is a safe and simple regional anesthesia technique that has many pain management applications. It is probably underutilized as an adjunct to rehabilitation after shoulder reconstruction and for the shoulder-hand variant of reflex sympathetic dystrophy. It is important that the pain specialist be sure that the physical and occupational therapists caring for the patient understand that suprascapular nerve block renders not only the shoulder girdle but also the shoulder joint insensate. This means that deep heat modalities and range of motion exercises must be carefully monitored to avoid burns and damage to the shoulder.

EFFICACY

No reliable data for efficacy are available. Block success is dependent on patient response and pain relief.

Acknowledgment

Portions of this chapter have been excerpted from Raj PP, Lou L, Erdine S, Staats P, Waldman SD: Radiographic Imaging for Regional Anesthesia and Pain Management. Philadelphia, Churchill Livingstone, 2003, with permission.

References

1. Pitkin GP: Therapeutic nerve block. In Pitkin GP (ed): Conduction Anesthesia. Philadelphia, JB Lippincott, 1946, p 884.
2. Bonica JJ: Musculoskeletal disorders of the upper limb. In Bonica JJ (ed): The Management of Pain, 2nd ed. Philadelphia, Lea & Febiger, 1990, p 891.
3. Katz J: Suprascapular nerve block. In Katz J (ed): Atlas of Regional Anesthesia. Norwalk, CT, Appleton-Century-Crofts, 1995, p 72.
4. Waldman SD: Suprascapular nerve block. In Waldman SD: Atlas of Interventional Pain Management. Philadelphia, Saunders, 1998, p 144.

chapter 148

Thoracic Epidural Nerve Block

Somayaji Ramamurthy

The technique of thoracic epidural nerve block is being used with increasing frequency in the practice of pain management. The presence of the spinal cord at the thoracic levels demands that the clinician have significant technical proficiency in performing epidural techniques without complications. A thorough knowledge of anatomic and physiologic changes associated with a thoracic epidural block is essential to avoiding complications. This chapter outlines the anatomy, physiologic changes, indications, applications, and complications of thoracic epidural nerve block.

HISTORICAL CONSIDERATIONS

The development of thoracic epidural techniques followed developments in lumbar epidural techniques. Modification of the Tuohy needle with the Huber tip to facilitate insertion of the catheter further increased their utility and safety, as did the improvement in the catheter material and development of disposable, prepackaged sterile equipment. Advances in epidurally administered drugs, such as the opioids, and the ability to implant catheters for the management of cancer pain further advanced the clinical applications of thoracic epidural block. The addition of implantable epidural electrodes to stimulate the spinal cord in the thoracic region has made this technique extremely useful.

INDICATIONS

Surgical

Thoracic epidural catheters are increasingly used for providing intraoperative, and especially postoperative, analgesia for thoracic and upper abdominal surgical procedures. With the thoracic epidural, the physiologic stress of surgery is significantly reduced.[1-6] It has been used for thoracotomy and cardiac surgery[7-12] in conjunction with light general anesthesia.[13] The benefits and safety of thoracic epidural analgesia for breast surgery are well documented.[14-16]

Postoperative Analgesia

There has been much debate about whether thoracic epidural nerve block is indicated to provide postoperative analgesia. Many clinicians believe that a catheter placed in the lumbar epidural space, to deliver a narcotic, can provide significant analgesia in the thoracic area without risking the complications associated with the thoracic epidural technique.[17,18] Many studies show the superiority of the thoracic epidural technique.[19-24] With the thoracic epidural technique, the catheter can be placed close to the nerve roots innervating the painful area; this becomes especially important when using any local anesthetic. Small quantities of local anesthetics can be used to provide excellent analgesia with the thoracic approach.[20-22,25] The lumbar epidural technique requires large volumes of local anesthetic to provide analgesia in the thoracic dermatomes.[17] This may result in significant hypotension and significant blood levels of the local anesthetic, limiting its usefulness.

Even with opioids such as morphine, which ascend in the CSF, the thoracic epidural technique still has advantages because the onset of analgesia is faster.[20,22] Morphine placed in the lumbar epidural space takes quite a while to ascend to the thoracic area and provide analgesia. With highly lipid-soluble drugs, such as fentanyl and sufentanil, the doses required to maintain analgesia are such that either epidural technique may not offer any advantages over the intravenous route of administration.[18] Patient-controlled epidural analgesia has been used effectively and safely, even at thoracic levels.[26]

The thoracic epidural approach provides rapid onset of analgesia and minimizes the doses of local anesthetics and opioids needed to provide excellent analgesia. Small doses of bupivacaine with morphine do not prevent ambulation.[27] This is important because small quantities of local anesthetic play a significant role in reducing pain related to motion and episodic pain.[20,21,25,27] Thoracic epidural techniques also have been used in pediatric patients with good results. The analgesia obtained from the technique has been shown to be superior to that of interpleural or intravenous techniques.[28,29]

Herpes Zoster and Postherpetic Neuralgia

Herpes zoster infection is most common in the thoracic area. Pain from acute herpes zoster can be relieved by epidural administration of local anesthetic or steroids. For acute herpes zoster, the local anesthetic produces excellent pain relief and may prevent postherpetic neuralgia and limit eruption of more vesicles.[30] An epidural catheter placed close to the involved nerve root can provide excellent analgesia with 2 to 3 mL of 0.25% bupivacaine. Usually, the catheter is left in only 2 or 3 days. The drug is injected once or twice a day. Alternatively, single-shot epidural blocks can be performed on a daily to weekly basis using local anesthetic and steroid.

Epidural Steroids

Herniated disks are uncommon in the thoracic spine. The patient who has nerve root irritation secondary to a herniated intervertebral disk or inflammation of the nerve root secondary to cancer or radiation therapy responds extremely well to a series of epidural thoracic steroid nerve blocks. Methylprednisolone (Depo-Medrol), 80 mg, or triamcinolone (Aristocort), 25 to 50 mg, is given, alone or mixed with saline or local anesthetic on a daily to weekly basis as the clinical situation dictates.

Acute Pain Secondary to Trauma

Patients with multiple fractured ribs and fractured vertebra get excellent analgesia with a properly positioned epidural catheter. Local anesthetic, such as 0.125% to 0.25% bupivacaine, or an opioid or a steroid, or both, can be used. Even with short-term administration of local anesthetic by the epidural route, the patient may experience prolonged pain relief after the muscle spasm and other secondary phenomena are relieved.

Angina

Angina secondary to myocardial ischemia has been treated via the thoracic epidural technique.[1,31,32] It provides excellent analgesia and decreases myocardial oxygen consumption, anxiety associated with pain, and catecholamine levels. Thoracic epidural techniques also have been used for long-term home self-treatment.[33] Spinal cord stimulation with the electrode placed in the epidural space has been used to control angina,[34,35] and such stimulation does not mask the pain of acute myocardial infarction.[36]

Cancer Pain

Catheters placed in the thoracic epidural space can be used to provide long-term analgesia using opioids such as morphine or local anesthetic. Through a tunneled epidural catheter, excellent long-term analgesia can be provided. Catheters also can be completely buried under the skin using a reservoir that is accessed through the skin for injection. Epidural phenol[37] or alcohol[38] also has been used for analgesia in cancer patients. The catheter is placed in the area of the involved nerve roots. Alcohol is injected through the catheter in 0.5-mL increments to a maximum of 5 mL. Previous injection of local anesthetic and sedation help to reduce the pain associated with injection of the alcohol. The injection has to be repeated daily for at least 3 days. More than 79% of patients report significant pain relief (50%). Phenol also has been used epidurally. The technique is similar to that of epidural alcohol: 5% phenol in dextrose or in 0.9% saline is injected slowly and repeated daily for 3 days. Both techniques have been reported to provide excellent analgesia without producing significant sensory or motor deficit. Epidural clonidine can be a useful advancement for various types of cancer pain or benign neuropathic pain that has failed to respond to more traditional measures.

Spinal Cord Stimulation

Electrodes for spinal cord stimulation are commonly placed through the lumbar or thoracic area. The technique is similar to that of thoracic epidural catheter insertion except that the needle is beveled so that the catheter can be gently withdrawn and redirected. The procedure uses an image intensifier. Stimulation of the cervical spinal cord usually is approached through a thoracic epidurally placed electrode, which is advanced into the cervical area. The catheter is tunneled subcutaneously and connected to a pulse generator. Thoracic epidural administration of local anesthetic and steroid administered via a single-shot injection can be extremely useful in the palliation of pain secondary to bony metastatic disease.

Management of Acute Pancreatitis

Patients with severe pain secondary to acute pancreatitis benefit from an epidural catheter placed in the lower thoracic area to deliver local anesthetics, such as bupivacaine, or an opioid such as morphine with or without the addition of steroids.[6] The severe pain is controlled until the pancreatitis is under control. Alternatively, daily single-shot thoracic epidural blocks with local anesthetic, opioids, or steroids may be used.

CONTRAINDICATIONS

Contraindications are the same as the contraindications for any other epidural approach:

- Patient refusal
- Infection in the area or septicemia
- Bleeding or clotting disorders, such as thrombocytopenia, or current anticoagulant therapy
- Uncorrected hypovolemia

ANATOMY

The thoracic epidural space extends from the lower margin of the C7 vertebra to the upper margin of L1.[1-5] The vertebral column in the thoracic area normally has a kyphotic curvature with its apex at approximately T6. Slight scoliosis to the right can occur, even in normal individuals. Significant scoliosis is associated with the rotation of the vertebral column, which can produce significant technical difficulty in performing this block. The inclination of the spinous processes is different at different levels of the thoracic vertebral column (Fig. 148–1). The spines from T1-4 have little inclination, whereas the spines of T5-8 tilt significantly downward, making a midline approach to the epidural space practically impossible. The T9-12 spines point dorsally without significant inclination, so the midline approach is possible. The ligamentum flavum is not as thick as it is in the lumbar spine, and occasionally the epidural space can be entered without encountering much resistance. The attachment of the ligamentum flavum to the lower margin of the lamina on its inner aspect

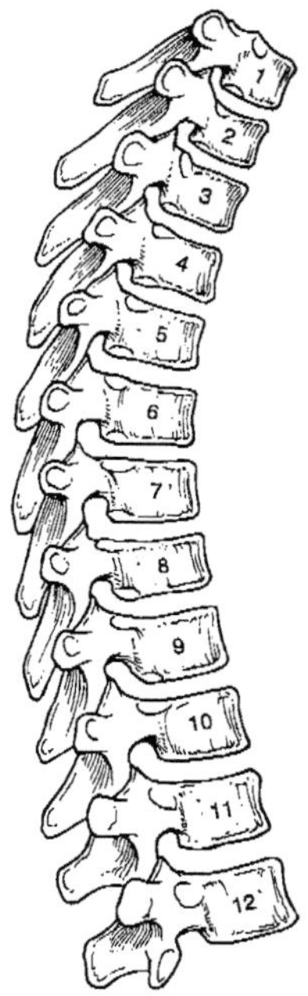

FIGURE 148–1 ■ The inclination of the spinous processes from T1-12. (Adapted from Waldman SD: Thoracic epidural nerve block. In: Interventional Pain Management, 2nd ed. Philadelphia, WB Saunders, 2001, p 392.)

reduces the size of the epidural space, whereas the space is wider at the upper margin of the lamina because the ligamentum flavum is attached to the outer aspect of the upper margin of the lower lamina. The epidural space is 3 to 4 mm wide in the thoracic area. The thoracic epidural space, similar to the rest of the epidural space, contains loose areolar tissue, fat, and vertebral venous plexus.

Nerve Roots

The T1 nerve root is fairly large and participates in the formation of the brachial plexus. The nerve roots at T2 and below gradually increase in size, but are still smaller than any of the lumbar or cervical roots. The epidural space communicates through the intervertebral foramina into the paravertebral space. The spinal cord has a lumbar enlargement at T9-12. Although the nerve roots in the subarachnoid space travel caudad for significantly increasing distances below T2 before they exit the intervertebral foramina, their course in the epidural space is horizontal. The dorsal and ventral roots unite just proximal to the intervertebral foramina.

Epidural Pressure

The pressure in the thoracic epidural space is approximately −15 cm H_2O, which is very close to the pressure of the intrapleural pressure.[6] It is more pronounced in the sitting position. The negative pressure in the thoracic epidural space also is considered to be secondary to the tenting of the dura by a blunt epidural needle.[39] In 12% of patients, the pressure is not negative.

The insignificant amount of fat in the epidural space of children younger than 5 or 6 years old makes it possible to thread a caudally introduced epidural catheter straight up into the thoracic epidural space.[40] Blanco and coworkers[41] reported, however, that lumbar epidural catheters were successfully advanced to T12 level only in 22% of the 199 patients.

Physiologic Changes

Cardiovascular

The cardiovascular effects of a thoracic epidural nerve block depend on its level.[4,6] The preganglionic sympathetic fibers are present in all of the thoracic anterior nerve roots. Levels of block to T10 produce minimal cardiovascular changes. The degree of hypotension secondary to this level of block depends on the blood volume and the position of the patient. The cardiovascular effects could be minimal because of the compensatory vasoconstriction in the upper extremities. If the local anesthetic block extends to T6, the cardiovascular effects are mainly due to peripheral vasodilation, venous pooling, decreased right heart filling, and hypotension. Blocking of the fibers to the abdominal viscera, including the fibers to the adrenal medulla, can reduce the response to stress for lower abdominal and pelvic surgical procedures.

If the block extends to T1, the sympathetic fibers innervating the heart also are affected. The block of the cardioaccelerator fibers can produce bradycardia and hypotension owing to the unopposed action of the parasympathetic fibers derived from the vagus nerve, sometimes resulting in cardiac standstill.[42] Studies also have shown decreased myocardial contractility.[43] The hypotension can be significant. It may respond to treatment with ephedrine initially, but may require aggressive treatment with epinephrine or dopamine or both.

The myocardial oxygen consumption is reduced with a thoracic epidural. Blomberg and colleagues[31,32] showed that thoracic epidural analgesia can relieve the pain of angina, decrease stenosis, and reduce the oxygen requirement, facilitating oxygenation of the myocardium. Pulmonary hypertension[44] is decreased with thoracic epidural analgesia, and the ST-T segment changes can be reversed.

Pulmonary

Weakening of the intercostal muscles can affect respiratory parameters. When a block affects all the intercostals, normal ventilation and $Paco_2$ still can be maintained by the activity of the diaphragm because the phrenic nerve is not affected. Improved diaphragmatic shortening and tidal volume have been reported secondary to intercostal paralysis.[45] The inspiratory reserve volume and functional reserve capacity are significantly decreased, as is vital capacity. Thoracic or abdominal pain can produce shallow breathing and decreased oxygen saturation. Oxygenation can improve after pain relief because of the thoracic epidural block.[46]

Horner Syndrome

Thoracic epidural block of T1 nerve roots can result in unilateral or bilateral Horner syndrome.[47]

■ CLINICAL PEARLS

Placement of the thoracic epidural catheter can be done with the patient sitting or in the lateral decubitus position. The sitting position provides better alignment of the skin midline to the spine and facilitates identification of landmarks. A patient who is anxious may have a vasovagal reaction in the sitting position with hypotension and nausea. The procedure also can be done with the patient prone. Because there is no significant flexion and extension, flexion of the patient contributes little to expanding the interlaminar space in the thoracic spine. Thousands of postoperative thoracic epidural procedures have been performed without complication and without radiographic guidance. Fluoroscopy or an image intensifier is required only for spinal cord stimulator placement or in patients in whom technical considerations dictate. Verification of the position of the catheter using a nonionic contrast medium may be advisable before performing a neurolytic block.

Midline Approach

The midline approach (Fig. 148–2) is applicable in the upper part of the thoracic spine between C7 and T5 and in the lower part, including T9-L1, because the spinous processes project directly posteriorly and are horizontal. The level of the spinous process corresponds to the level of the vertebra. The epidural technique is similar to that used in the lumbar areas, with a 90-degree approach, but I prefer starting at the lower part of the interspace, just above the lower spine, so that the needle is angled cephalad, which facilitates insertion and advancement of the catheter.

After infiltration of a local anesthetic, such as lidocaine, intradermally with a short, 25-gauge or 27-gauge needle, injection of a local anesthetic with a slightly longer needle, such as a 1½-inch 22-gauge needle, into the paraspinal

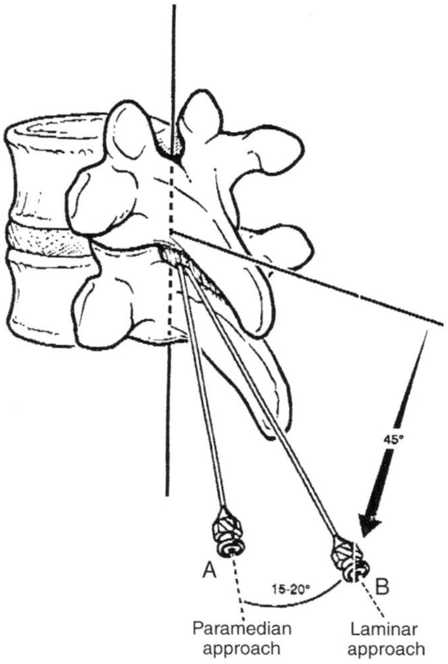

FIGURE 148–2 ■ **A,** Paramedian approach. Needle is inserted 1 cm lateral to the midline with a 45-degree cephalad angle and a 15- to 20-degree angle in the coronal plane to enter the ligamentum flavum in the midline. **B,** Laminar approach. Needle is inserted right next to the cephalad edge of the spine and is advanced straight forward without any deviation toward the midline. (Adapted from Waldman SD: Thoracic epidural nerve block. In: Interventional Pain Management, 2nd ed. Philadelphia, WB Saunders, 2001, p 393.)

muscles on either side of the spine provides significant analgesia for the procedure by blocking the nerve fibers as they come from lateral areas toward the midline. I prefer to use a 3½ inch 16-gauge to 18-gauge Touhy needle, although many pain management specialists use shorter, sharper needles. The Touhy needle is advanced with the bevel cephalad so that the smooth part of the curvature bounces off the lamina. The needle is advanced through the skin, subcutaneous tissue, supraspinous ligament, intraspinous ligament, and ligamentum flavum. If ligament resistance is encountered, and the lamina is contacted after that, the needle is at the upper margin of the lower lamina. Redirection farther cephalad facilitates entry into the epidural space, which entry is recognized by one of the many techniques described earlier.

The most common technique is the loss-of-resistance technique using air or a fluid-filled syringe containing a small bubble of air to allow compression (because a liquid is not compressible). If a liquid is used, I prefer 0.9% saline without preservatives. Hanging-drop technique has been used, especially in the thoracic area, because of the significant negative pressure. Despite a low incidence of dural puncture, the drop is sucked in only 88% of the time. Because both hands are used to advance the needle slowly, entry into the epidural space is recognized even when the drop is not sucked in.

Some authors take the ability to advance the significant length of the catheters without difficulty as an indication of entry into the epidural space. If the needle is off course and enters the paraspinal muscles or a defect in the interspinous ligament, there could be misleading loss of resistance. This error can be identified by the paraspinal compression technique,[48] in which the index and middle fingers of the nondominant hand compress the paraspinal tissues on either side of the needle. If the resistance that was lost reappears, the tip of the needle is superficial to the ligamentum flavum. If the external pressure does not affect pressure in the syringe, the needle is deep to the ligamentum flavum.

A catheter is advanced 3 to 4 cm. As in any epidural technique, the catheter should not be withdrawn after it passes the tip of the needle because the catheter may be sheared off. Needles used for electrode placement in the epidural space are specially designed to allow for gentle withdrawal. Inserting the catheter too far may result in migration through the intervertebral foramen or epidural vein or true knot formation. Tunneling the catheter for 5 cm using another epidural needle reduces the risk of catheter migration.[49]

I prefer to use the technique described by Raj[50] (Fig. 148–3) for taping the catheter, using Steri-Strips (sterile stips), Mastisol (liquid adhesive), and Tegaderm (transparent dressing). This technique reduces the possibility of catheter dislodgment and facilitates maintaining the catheter for a longer time. The catheter is connected to an adapter, a filter, and an injection site and taped over the infraclavicular area to afford easy access for reinjection. An externalized catheter can be well protected over the long-term with a colostomy bag.[51]

Epidural Drugs

Medication similar to that used in the lumbar area is chosen, although smaller volumes of local anesthetics are needed. Positioning the catheter in the middle of the desired area of analgesia minimizes the necessary volume. The necessary doses depend on individual factors, such as age, height,

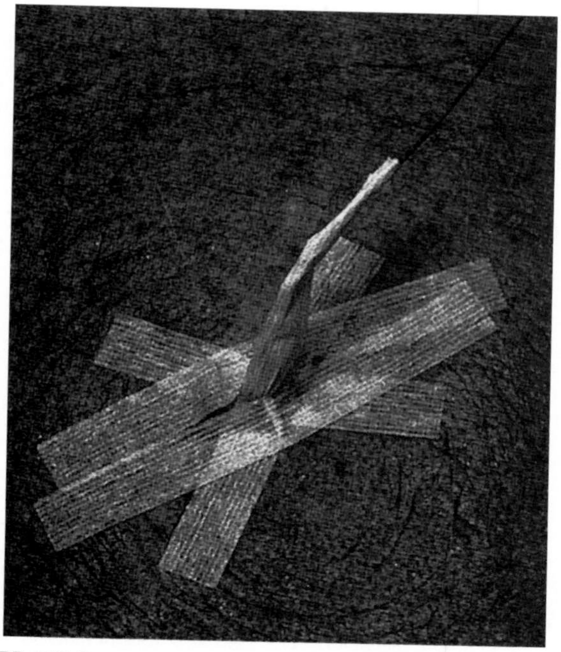

FIGURE 148–3 ■ Technique of anchoring the epidural catheter for prolonged use. (Adapted from Waldman SD: Thoracic epidural nerve block. In: Interventional Pain Management, 2nd ed. Philadelphia, WB Saunders, 2001, p 394.)

weight, intercurrent disease (e.g., diabetes), and extent of desired analgesia. Short-acting and long-acting local anesthetics and opioids have been used for single administration or infusion. Concentrations are similar to those for lumbar epidural analgesia.

Paramedian Lateral Approach

The paramedian lateral approach can be used at any level of the thoracic spine. Usually, the starting point is 1 to 2 cm lateral to the superior margin of the spinous process. In most patients, a 1½-inch 22-gauge needle can contact the lamina, and 1 mL of short-acting local anesthetic can be injected to decrease the pain related to "walking" on the lamina. The epidural needle is advanced at a 45- to 55-degree angle cephalad and a 15- to 30-degree angle toward the midline. Extreme angles can result in nerve root contact on the opposite side of the spine or the needle passing between the spinous processes into the paraspinal muscle without contacting the ligamentum flavum. I prefer starting right next to the lateral margin of the cephalad edge of the spine, minimizing the angle required to make the puncture in the ligamentum flavum, close to the midline. Contacting the lamina with the epidural needle significantly increases the safety of the technique because the epidural space can be entered by walking off the superior margin of the lamina. The steep angle required to enter the epidural space in the midthoracic area also facilitates the insertion of the catheter.

Laminar Approach

For a laminar approach, the starting point is the same as that for the paramedian approach, but the needle is not angled toward the midline. Only the lateral portion of the epidural space is entered. The disadvantages of the technique are that the epidural space is narrower, and veins are more numerous in the lateral portion of the epidural space. Also, if the starting point is too far lateral, or even with the slight lateral angle, the needle contacts the articular processes. Walking it more cephalad would not achieve entry into the epidural space. I prefer starting right next to the cephalad margin of the spinous process and minimizing the angle, which increases the chance of entering the epidural space. The laminar approach is more useful when attempting to get a predominantly unilateral block, especially while using epidural steroids. A small volume of injectate has a tendency to stay on one side for two to three segments.

■ PITFALLS

1. Because the spinal cord is present in the thoracic vertebral level, a thoracic epidural technique should be attempted only by an operator who has extensive experience doing lumbar epidurals. Bromage[4] recommended that an individual who performs a thoracic epidural should have done at least 50 consecutive lumbar epidurals without a dural puncture or a complication.
2. Because of the inclination of the spine in the midthoracic area, the technique could be technically difficult, although it can be mastered with some practice.
3. Because the nerve roots contain the sympathetic nerves to the heart, a block of these fibers can produce significant bradycardia and hypotension.

Intercostal muscle weakness resulting from thoracic epidural block can produce significant difficulty, especially in obese patients and patients with respiratory impairment. In a patient with impaired function of the diaphragm, chronic obstructive lung disease, or obesity, intercostal paralysis can contribute significantly to the respiratory impairment.

■ COMPLICATIONS

The complications of the thoracic epidural technique are similar to the complications of the lumbar epidural and include infection, epidural hematoma, injury to the nerve roots, intravascular injection, respiratory depression, and subdural and subarachnoid injection.[52] The presence of the spinal cord in the thoracic vertebral canal brings in the possibility of spinal cord damage. The incidence of spinal cord damage owing to attempted thoracic epidural analgesia is unknown. There are few reports of this complication. In one series of 1071 postoperative patients, no long-term serious complications were reported. In a study of 4185 patients, absence of serious neurologic complications was documented.[53] Many studies documented safety and absence of infection.[54,55]

Infection

Epidural abscess[17,56,57] secondary to a thoracic epidural catheter left in place is a possibility, especially with the increasing use of long-term catheter placement for the management of cancer pain. There is some evidence that the incidence of infection is higher in the thoracic area than in other areas.[17]

Pleural Puncture

Accidental pleural puncture and placement of the catheter was recognized during surgery. Although uncommon, this complication can be life-threatening if not recognized.[58]

CONCLUSION

Thoracic epidural nerve block has become a mainstay of contemporary pain management. Careful attention to the functional anatomy of the thoracic spine increases the clinician's success rate and decreases complications.

References

1. Scott D: Central neural blockade. In: Techniques of Regional Anaesthesia. Norwalk, CT, Appleton & Lange, 1989, p 178.
2. Katz J, Renck H: Lumbar epidural block. In: Handbook of Thoracoabdominal Nerve Block. Orlando, Grune & Stratton, 1987, p 111.
3. Anderson JE: The back. In: Grant's Atlas of Anatomy, 7th ed. Baltimore, 1978.
4. Bromage PR: Surgical applications. In: Epidural Analgesia. Philadelphia, WB Saunders, 1978, p 490.
5. Cousins MJ, Bridenbaugh PO (eds): Neural Blockade in Clinical Anesthesia and Management of Pain, 2nd ed. Philadelphia, JB Lippincott, 1988.
6. Lema MJ, Sinha I: Thoracic epidural anesthesia and analgesia. Pain Digest 4:3, 1994.
7. Liem TH, Booij LHDJ, Hasenbos MAWM: Coronary artery bypass grafting using two different anesthetic techniques: Part 1. Hemodynamic results. J Cardiothorac Vasc Anesth 6:148, 1992.
8. Liem TH, Hasenbos MAWM, Booij LHDJ: Coronary artery bypass grafting using two different anesthetic techniques: Part 2. Postoperative outcome. J Cardiothorac Vasc Anesth 6:156, 1992.
9. Mallick A, Bhaskaran NC: Thoracic epidural analgesia and coronary artery bypass graft surgery. Anaesthesia 53:511, 1998.
10. Turfrey DJ, Scott NB: Thoracic epidural analgesia started after cardiopulmonary bypass (letter). Anaesthesia 52:914, 1997.
11. Turfrey DJ, Ray DA, Sutcliffe NP, et al: Thoracic epidural anaesthesia for coronary artery bypass graft surgery: Effects on postoperative complications. Anaesthesia 52:1090, 1997.
12. Riedel BJ, Wright IG: Epidural anesthesia in coronary artery bypass grafting surgery. Curr Opin Cardiol 12:515, 1997.
13. Stenseth R, Berg EM, Bjella L, et al: The influence of thoracic epidural analgesia alone and in combination with general anesthesia on cardiovascular function and myocardial metabolism in patients receiving β-adrenergic blockers. Anesth Analg 77:463, 1993.
14. Lai CS, Yip WH, Lin SD, et al: Continuous thoracic epidural anesthesia for breast augmentation. Ann Plast Surg 36:113, 1996.
15. Lynch EP, Welch KJ, Carabuena JM, et al: Thoracic epidural anesthesia improves outcome after breast surgery. Ann Surg 222:663, 1995.
16. Nesmith RL, Herring SH, Marks MW, et al: Early experience with high thoracic epidural anesthesia in output submuscular breast augmentation. Ann Plast Surg 24:299, 1990.
17. Redekop GJ, Del Maestro RF: Diagnosis and management of spinal epidural abscess. Can J Neurol Sci 19:180, 1992.
18. Guinard JP, Mavrocordatos P, Chiolero R, et al: A randomized comparison of intravenous versus lumbar and thoracic epidural fentanyl for analgesia after thoracotomy. Anesthesiology 77:1108, 1992.
19. Salomaki TE, Laitinen JO, Nuutiene LS: A randomized double-blind comparison of epidural versus intravenous fentanyl infusion for analgesia after thoracotomy. Anesthesiology 75:790, 1991.
20. Sawchuck WT, Ong B, Unruh HW, et al: Thoracic versus lumbar epidural fentanyl for postthoracotomy pain. Ann Thorac Surg 55:1472, 1993.
21. George KA, Chisakuta AM, Gamble JAS, et al: Thoracic epidural infusion for postoperative pain relief following abdominal aortic surgery: Bupivacaine, fentanyl or a mixture of both? Anaesthesia 47:388, 1992.
22. George KA, Wright PMC, Chisakuta A: Continuous thoracic epidural fentanyl for post-thoracotomy pain relief: With or without bupivacaine? Anaesthesia 46:732, 1991.
23. Scott NB, James K, Murphy M, et al: Continuous thoracic epidural analgesia versus combined spinal/thoracic epidural analgesia on pain, pulmonary function and the metabolic response following colonic resection. Acta Anaesthesiol Scand 40:691, 1996.
24. Pelton JJ, Fish DJ, Keller SM: Epidural narcotic analgesia after thoracotomy. South Med J 86:1106, 1993.
25. Mourisse J, Hasenbos M, Gielen MJM, et al: Epidural bupivacaine, sufentanil or the combination for post-thoracotomy pain. Acta Anaesthesiol Scand 36:70, 1992.
26. Liu SS, Allen HW, Olsson GL: Patient-controlled epidural analgesia with bupivacaine and fentanyl on hospital wards: Prospective experience with 1,030 surgical patients. Anesthesiology 88:688, 1998.
27. Moiniche S, Hjortso N-C, Blemmer T, et al: Blood pressure and heart rate during orthostatic stress and walking with continuous postoperative thoracic epidural bupivacaine/morphine. Acta Anaesthesiol Scand 37:65, 1993.
28. Tobias JD, Lowe S, O'Dell N, et al: Anaesthetic techniques: Thoracic epidural anaesthesia in infants and children. Can J Anaesth 40:879, 1993.
29. Tobias JD: Analgesia after thoracotomy in children: A comparison of interpleural, epidural, and intravenous analgesia. South Med J 84:158, 1991.
30. Winnie AP, Hartwell PW: Relationship between time of treatment of acute herpes zoster with sympathetic blockade and prevention of post-herpetic neuralgia: Clinical support for a new theory of the mechanism by which sympathetic blockade provides therapeutic benefit. Reg Anesth 18:277, 1993.
31. Blomberg S, Emanuelsson H, Kvist H, et al: Effects of thoracic epidural anesthesia on coronary arteries and arterioles in patients with coronary artery disease. Anesthesiology 73:840, 1990.
32. Blomberg S, Emanuelsson H, Ricksten SE: Thoracic epidural anesthesia and central hemodynamics in patients with unstable angina pectoris. Anesth Analg 69:558, 1989.
33. Blomberg SG: Long-term home self-treatment with high thoracic epidural anesthesia in patients with severe coronary artery disease. Anesth Analg 79:413, 1994.
34. Mannheimer C, Eliasson T, Augustinsson LE, et al: Electrical stimulation versus coronary artery bypass surgery in severe angina pectoris: The ESBY study. Circulation 97:1157, 1998.
35. Hautvast RW, Blanksma PK, DeJongste MJ, et al: Effect of spinal cord stimulation on myocardial blood flow assessed by positron emission tomography in patients with refractory angina pectoris. Am J Cardiol 77:462, 1996.
36. Andersen C, Hole P, Oxhoj H: Does pain relief with spinal cord stimulation for angina conceal myocardial infarction? Br Heart J 71:419, 1994.
37. Racz GB, Heavner J, Haynsworth P: Repeat epidural phenol injections in chronic pain and spasticity. In Lipton S (ed): Persistent Pain: Modern Methods of Treatment. New York, Grune & Stratton, 1985, p 157.
38. Korevaar WC: Transcatheter thoracic epidural neurolysis using ethyl alcohol. Anesthesiology 69:989, 1988.
39. Okutomi T, Watanabe S, Goto F: Time course in thoracic epidural pressure measurement. Can J Anaesth 40:1044, 1993.
40. Gunter JB, Eng C: Thoracic epidural anesthesia via the caudal approach in children. Anesthesiology 76:935, 1992.
41. Blanco D, Llamazares J, Rincon R, et al: Thoracic epidural anesthesia via the lumbar approach in infants and children. Anesthesiology 84:1312, 1996.
42. Ng KP: Complete heart block during laparotomy under combined thoracic epidural and general anaesthesia. Anaesth Intensive Care 24:257, 1996.
43. Goertz AW, Seeling W, Heinrich H, et al: Influence of high thoracic epidural anesthesia on left ventricular contractility assessed using the end-systolic pressure-length relationship. Acta Anaesthesiol Scand 37:38, 1993.
44. Armstrong P: Thoracic epidural anaesthesia and primary pulmonary hypertension. Anaesthesia 47:496, 1992.
45. Polaner DM, Kimball WR, Fratacci MD, et al: Thoracic epidural anesthesia increases diaphragmatic shortening after thoracotomy in the awake lamb. Anesthesiology 79:808, 1993.
46. Cicala RS, Voeller GR, Fox T, et al: Epidural analgesia in thoracic trauma: Effects of lumbar morphine and thoracic bupivacaine on pulmonary function. Crit Care Med 18:229, 1990.
47. Liu M, Kim PS, Chen CK, et al: Delayed Horner's syndrome as a complication of continuous thoracic epidural analgesia. J Cardiothorac Vasc Anesth 12:195-196, 1998.

48. Wilson MA, Swartzman S, Ramamurthy S: A simple test to confirm correct identification of the epidural space. Reg Anesth 8:158, 1983.
49. Bougher RJ, Corbett AR, Ramage DT: The effect of tunnelling on epidural catheter migration. Anaesthesia 51:191, 1996.
50. Raj P: Postoperative pain. In: Handbook of Regional Anesthesia. New York, Churchill Livingstone, 1985, p 106.
51. Kenworthy KL, Hoffman J, Rogers JN: A new dressing technique for temporary percutaneous catheters used for pain management (letter to the editor). Anesthesiology 76:482, 1992.
52. Tanaka K, Watanabe R, Harada T, et al: Extensive application of epidural anesthesia and analgesia in a university hospital: Incidence of complications related to technique. Reg Anesth 18:148, 1993.
53. Giebler RM, Scherer RU, Peters J: Incidence of neurologic complications related to thoracic epidural catheterization. Anesthesiology 86:55, 1997.
54. Strafford MA, Wilder RT, Berde CB: The risk of infection from epidural analgesia in children: A review of 1620 cases. Anesth Analg 80:2148, 1995.
55. Scherer R, Schmutzler M, Giebler R, et al: Complications related to thoracic epidural analgesia: A prospective study in 1071 surgical patients. Acta Anaesthesiol Scand 37:370, 1993.
56. Blomberg S, Curelaru I, Emanuelsson H, et al: Thoracic epidural anaesthesia in patients with unstable angina pectoris. Eur Heart J 10:437, 1989.
57. Yuste M, Canet J, Garcia M, et al: An epidural abscess due to resistant *Staphylococcus aureus* following epidural catheterization. Anaesthesia 52:163, 1997.
58. Zaugg M, Stoehr S, Weder W, et al: Accidental pleural puncture by a thoracic epidural catheter. Anaesthesia 53:69, 1998.

chapter 149

Intercostal Nerve Block

Dan J. Kopacz and Gale E. Thompson

In the future, acute pain management will tend to emphasize the application of analgesic drugs directly to the surgical wound edges or to smaller peripheral nerve branches. In this way, the many side effects (hypotension, itching, nausea, vomiting, urinary retention) that often accompany central neuraxis blockade will be avoided. At some point, intercostal nerve block will finally and fully achieve a major role in pain management. It will likely become the most often used peripheral nerve block. As we show later, there must be one major development in local anesthetic drugs before this advance can be realized.

HISTORICAL CONSIDERATIONS

On reviewing the early writings of Schleich,[1] Braun,[2] Pauchet and coworkers,[3] and Labat,[4] one is struck with the idea that the technique of intercostal nerve block developed through a series of evolutionary steps. At the turn of the 20th century, surgeons were fascinated by infiltration anesthesia. Elaborate descriptions and recipes defined how surgery of the chest and abdomen could be accomplished using large volumes (100 to 150 mL) of dilute solutions of local anesthetic drugs, procaine being the mainstay after it was synthesized in 1904. Over time, many of the descriptions and illustrations began to define the reality of blocking the intercostal nerve trunk, in preference to the more elaborate process of infiltration or "field block" of the more peripheral twigs and branches. In addition, paravertebral injections began to be used as an alternative to spinal injections.[5] These lumbar and thoracic blocks became popular because of increasing doubt and concern about possible neurotoxicity from the injection of cocaine and its synthetic allies directly into the spinal canal. Techniques were defined whereby major nerve trunks could be blocked after they exited the vertebral canal. Proximal and more distal sites for blocking intercostal nerves were gradually defined. By 1922, Labat's textbook[4] contained an elaborate description of intercostal nerve block that is quite similar to present-day conceptions.

INDICATIONS

No method of pain relief is more specific and effective for fractured ribs than intercostal nerve block.[6] The pain from chest wall contusion, pleurisy, and flail chest also is relieved quickly.[7,8] Often unappreciated is the fact that the pain from median sternotomy, pericardial window, or fractured sternum can be controlled successfully by blocks in the parasternal region (Fig. 149–1).[4] This point might well be applied to many cardiac and pulmonary surgery cases of today.[9,10] Blockade of two or more nerves is a simple way to prepare for insertion of thoracostomy tubes and can be used to provide analgesia for percutaneous biliary drainage or liver biopsy. Perhaps the most important but least exploited use of this block is for control of postoperative pain of the chest or abdomen.[11] A simple study by Bunting and McGeachie[12] vividly showed this point. They performed lateral intercostal blocks of right T10, T11, and T12 at the conclusion of appendectomy. With this investment of a few milliliters of local anesthetic drug, the study patients required only one third as much postoperative narcotic as the patients who did not receive intercostal blocks.

Intercostal blocks (CPT code 64420 [single], 64421 [multiple, regional block]) also are useful in several chronic pain scenarios. When combined or alternated with celiac plexus block, they can help resolve a common diagnostic dilemma and distinguish abdominal wall pain from visceral pain. A unilateral paravertebral T12 and L1 nerve block (CPT code 64440 [single], 64441 [multiple, regional block]) can help unravel the question of nerve entrapment syndromes after inguinal hernia repair. Numerous references have been made to the diagnostic and therapeutic benefits of this block in patients with acute and chronic pain from herpes zoster.[13] A few neurolytic intercostal blocks (CPT code 64620) have limited applications in some patients with terminal cancer.

ANATOMY

The intercostal nerves are composed of the ventral rami of the first through the twelfth thoracic nerves. The first, second, and twelfth nerves differ from the other nine in several respects. T1 gives off a small contribution to the brachial plexus. T2-3 sends cutaneous branches to the arm as the intercostobrachial nerve. T12 is not strictly an intercostal nerve, but rather is more appropriately called a subcostal nerve. It runs its course in the abdominal wall below the twelfth rib and sends fibers to join L1.

Evidence from cadaver studies indicates that the classic medical school teaching that the intercostal vein, artery, and

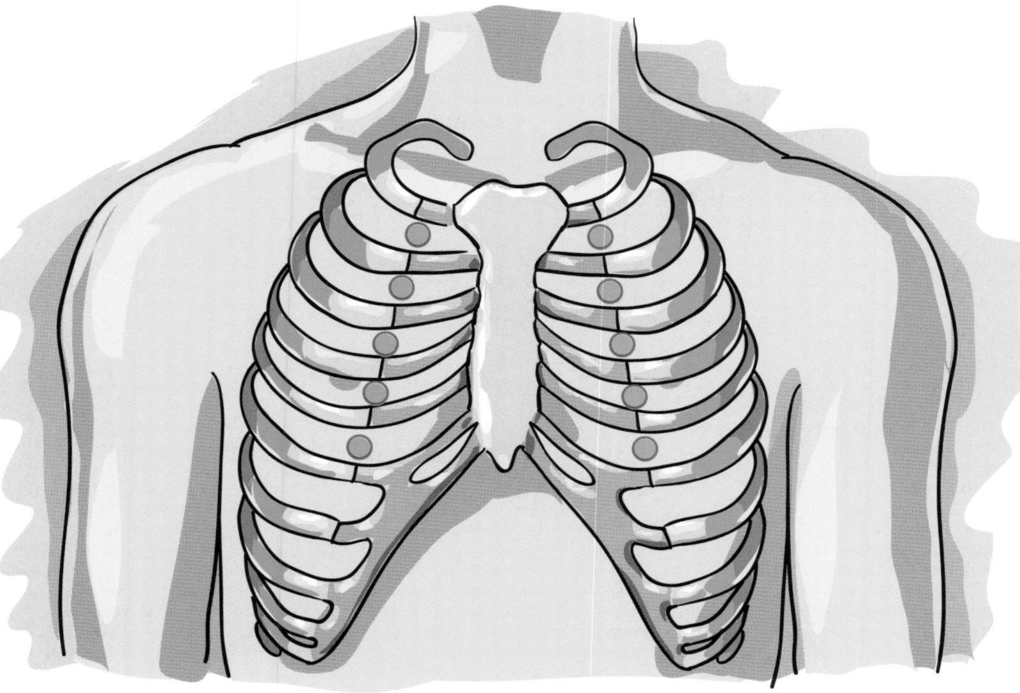

FIGURE 149–1 ■ Circles indicate approximate sites for parasternal block of the upper anterior intercostal nerves. This is an effective way to relieve pain from median sternotomy or a fractured sternum.

nerve are located in precise order and comfortably tucked into the subcostal groove is unrealistic. The nerve may vary from a subcostal to midcostal to supracostal location. In his cadaver study, Hardy[14] found the following frequencies of these variations: classic subcostal, 17%; midzone, 73%; and supracostal, 10%.

Another anatomic subtlety for the anesthesiologist's appreciation is intercostal nerve branching, of which there are two types. First, the nerve may split into separate bundles that have no common enclosing fascial sheath. These may rejoin or subdivide further as the nerve continues its lateral course; there is not a single, well-defined nerve at every site in the intercostal space. Second, each intercostal nerve gives off four well-defined branches as it proceeds on its circuitous route anteriorly (Fig. 149–2). The *first* is the gray rami communicantes, which goes to the appropriate sympathetic ganglion. The *second* branch arises as the posterior cutaneous branch and supplies skin and muscles in the paravertebral region and possibly as far lateral as the posterior axillary line. The *third* branch, the lateral cutaneous division, arises just anterior to the midaxillary line. The clinical importance of the takeoff of this branch historically has been emphasized and perhaps exaggerated. This is a concern during blocking of intercostal nerves for pain relief because the third branch sends subcutaneous fibers coursing posteriorly and anteriorly, and a lateral injection conceivably could be directed too far anterior and miss the point of takeoff. The *terminal* or final branch is the anterior cutaneous branch, which provides cutaneous innervation to the midline of the chest and abdomen. In contrast to the situation at the vertebral spines, there seems to be some slight overlap of sensory fibers across the anterior midline of the chest and abdomen.

The paravertebral space warrants separate discussion. The dura mater and the arachnoid membrane fuse with the epineurium as the nerve exits the vertebral foramen (Fig. 149–3). This has two important implications. Local anesthetics (or other drugs) injected directly intraneurally to the peripheral nerve may spread centrally, to the nerve roots or spinal cord. It also is possible to produce epidural or spinal anesthesia if a large volume of local anesthetic is injected into the paravertebral region and flows centrally around the nerve in the vertebral foramen. Conacher[15] showed that even quick-setting resin can be propelled into the vertebral epidural space. He also showed that correctly placed paravertebral intercostal injections can spread over several intercostal spaces and can dissect the pleura laterally from the vertebral bodies. In transverse section, the paravertebral space is wedge-shaped. The posterior wall is the costotransverse ligament, anterolaterally is the parietal pleura, and medially lie the vertebral body and vertebral foramen. From the paravertebral space to the posterior angle of the rib, there is no structure between the intercostal nerve and the pleura. At the angle of the rib, the internal intercostal muscle arises and lies internal to the nerve, all the way around to the costosternal cartilages.

In the paravertebral region, the intercostal artery and vein are usually single structures. Laterally, they show multiple branches. This has implications for intercostal block because vessel puncture can lead to hematoma formation or rapid uptake of local anesthetic drug. Flank hematomas can become extensive in a patient taking anticoagulants.[16] Other high-risk scenarios involve patients with neurofibromatosis, Marfan syndrome, and arterial dilation or stretching, as in coarctation of the aorta or severe scoliosis.[17]

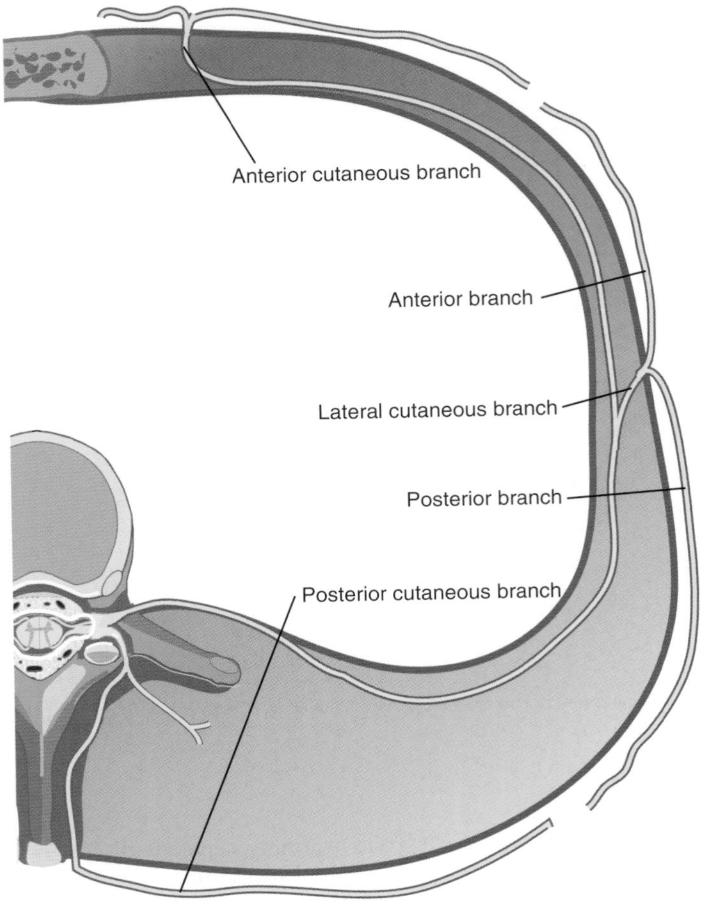

FIGURE 149–2 ■ The four branches of a typical intercostal nerve.

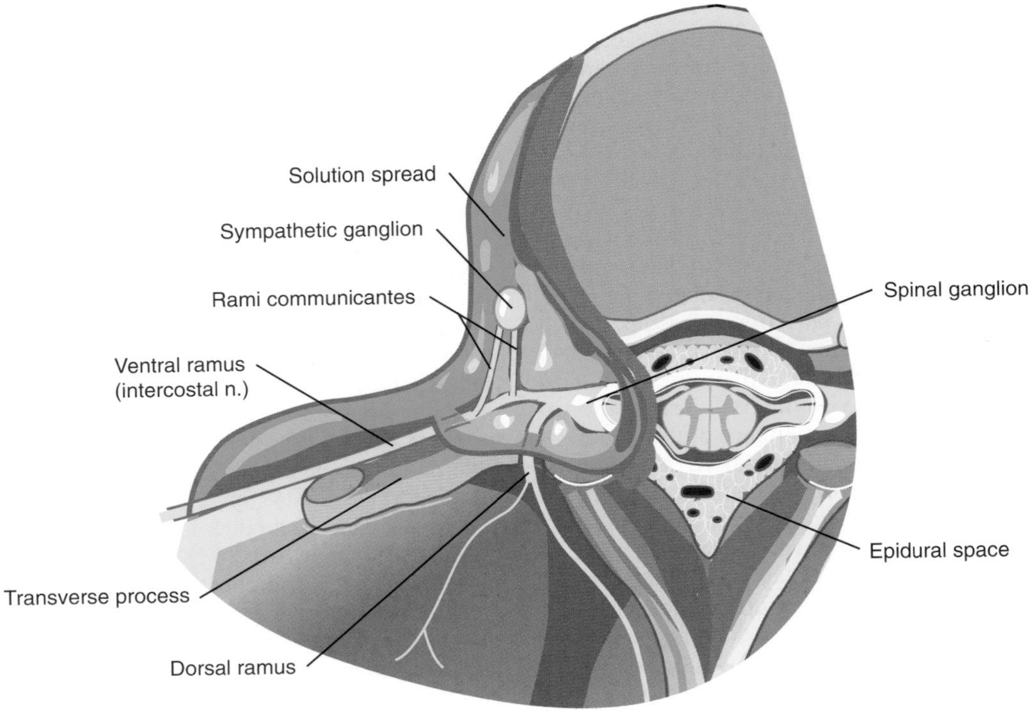

FIGURE 149–3 ■ Possible central neuraxial spread of solutions injected into the paravertebral space or intercostal nerve.

TECHNIQUE: PEARLS AND PRINCIPLES

Classic Approach

In the classic approach, intercostal nerve block is performed posteriorly at the angle of the ribs and just lateral to the sacrospinalis group of muscles.[18] At this point, the thickness of the rib is about 8 mm. If the needle is advanced 3 mm into the triangular fat-filled space where the nerve runs, there is a 5-mm margin of safety before it penetrates the pleura. In most instances, the blocks are easiest to learn and perform with the patient in a prone position with a pillow under the midabdomen. This position is optimal for rib identification by posterior palpation of the intercostal spaces. The patient's arms are kept hanging over the sides of the cart or operating table to rotate the scapulae laterally and make it easier to block the nerves under the upper ribs. After the patient is positioned, it is helpful to use a skin-marking pen to identify the inferior edge of each rib. This constitutes a map to illustrate and review anatomic detail and ultimately makes the process of blocking smoother and quicker. First, a vertical line is drawn connecting the posterior thoracic vertebral spines. Then, by palpation, the lateral edge of the sacrospinalis group of muscles is identified and marked as another vertical line on each side. This lateral line is usually 7 to 8 cm from the posterior midline and should angle medially at the upper levels to avoid the scapulae. The inferior border of each rib is marked along these two lateral vertical lines.

When these markings and local anesthetic mixing preparations have been completed, the initial step is to raise skin wheals (30-gauge needle) at each of the previously marked intersections of vertical and horizontal lines. A 2- to 3-cm, 22-gauge or 23-gauge needle is used to inject each intercostal nerve. If a disposable long-beveled needle is used, the operator must remember that the tip may be bent easily with the repeated bone contacts necessary to do this block. The needle can become barbed and possibly cause bleeding or nerve damage.

The practitioner's hand and finger position is of utmost importance to performing this block properly. Beginning at the lowest rib, a right-handed operator uses the index finger of the left hand to pull the skin up and over at the lower edge of the rib (FIg. 149–4). The needle is introduced to the rib as the palpating left index finger defines it. Care should be taken to prevent the needle's penetrating beyond this palpated depth because it could enter the interpleural or intra-alveolar space. The practitioner should think of the palpating finger as having sonar capabilities. When the needle reaches the rib, the right hand pushes to maintain firm contact between needle and rib. The left hand is shifted to gain control of the needle by holding the hub and shaft with the thumb and index and middle fingers. In addition, firm placement of the left hand's hypothenar eminence against the patient's back is crucial; this allows precise and constant control of needle depth as the left hand now "walks" the needle off the lower edge of the rib (Fig. 149–5). While the needle is being advanced, a slight loss of resistance is often felt as the tip enters the correct space. At each interspace, 3 to 5 mL of local anesthetic solution is injected. The left hand walks the needle back onto the rib and finally releases control to the right hand and to the left index finger for palpation of the next higher rib. Keeping the needle in firm contact with the previously injected rib until the next space is identified serves to avoid missing a rib or doing a second block of the same rib.

This process is repeated for each of the nerves to be blocked. An experienced operator can block 12 to 14 ribs safely and successfully in 3 to 5 minutes. Intercostal blocks may be repeated as needed.

Midaxillary Approach

It is reasonable to perform intercostal nerve blocks in the midaxillary line. Some authors have advised against this approach, out of concern that it might be more likely to cause pneumothorax and to miss anesthetizing the lateral cutaneous branch of the nerve, which takes off near the midaxillary line and becomes superficial to innervate the skin of the anterolateral chest wall. Two realities make intercostal block effective, however, when done at a midaxillary site (Fig. 149–6).[19] First, the solution always spreads longitudinally in the intercostal groove for a distance of several centimeters from the site of injection. Second, the final milliliter of solution can be injected as the needle is being moved away from the rib toward the skin, to anesthetize the lateral cutaneous branch in its subcutaneous site.

The midaxillary approach makes intercostal block much more feasible in patients who cannot be turned to a supine or lateral position, such as postoperative or trauma patients who experience severe pain with any motion. This block also can be used to complement a general anesthetic after induction and intubation of a supine patient. The anesthesiologist can reach down and quickly do a series of unilateral or bilateral midaxillary line blocks without ever leaving the position at the head of the operating table. If the patient is being ventilated during this time, it is advisable to synchronize the block with the ventilator (i.e., to avoid walking the needle off the rib at the point of maximum inspiration) to help avoid pneumothorax as a complication.

The upper intercostal nerves can be blocked by raising the patient's arm and palpating the ribs high in the axilla. Good analgesia also can be produced by blocking the intercostal nerve even farther anterior than the midaxillary line. Parasternal blocks can provide good pain relief after median sternotomy. Rectus sheath block is yet another variation.[20]

Paravertebral Approach

Intercostal blocks can be performed posteriorly at any site medial to the posterior angle of the ribs. There is some point medially at which every intercostal block is best characterized as a paravertebral block. In some sense, the distinction is moot, but there are two interesting clinical concerns or observations. One is that central neuraxis spread of solution becomes more worrisome farther medially. The other is that subpleural spread of anesthetic from one intercostal space to another becomes more likely as injections are placed closer to the spine. Although some physicians believe that paravertebral somatic block is now of more interest to historians than to practicing anesthesiologists, there are still reasons to explore the technique. A catheter can be inserted here for a variation on the theme of interpleural anesthesia or "continuous" intercostal nerve block. Such a catheter would lie in the extrapleural space.[21,22]

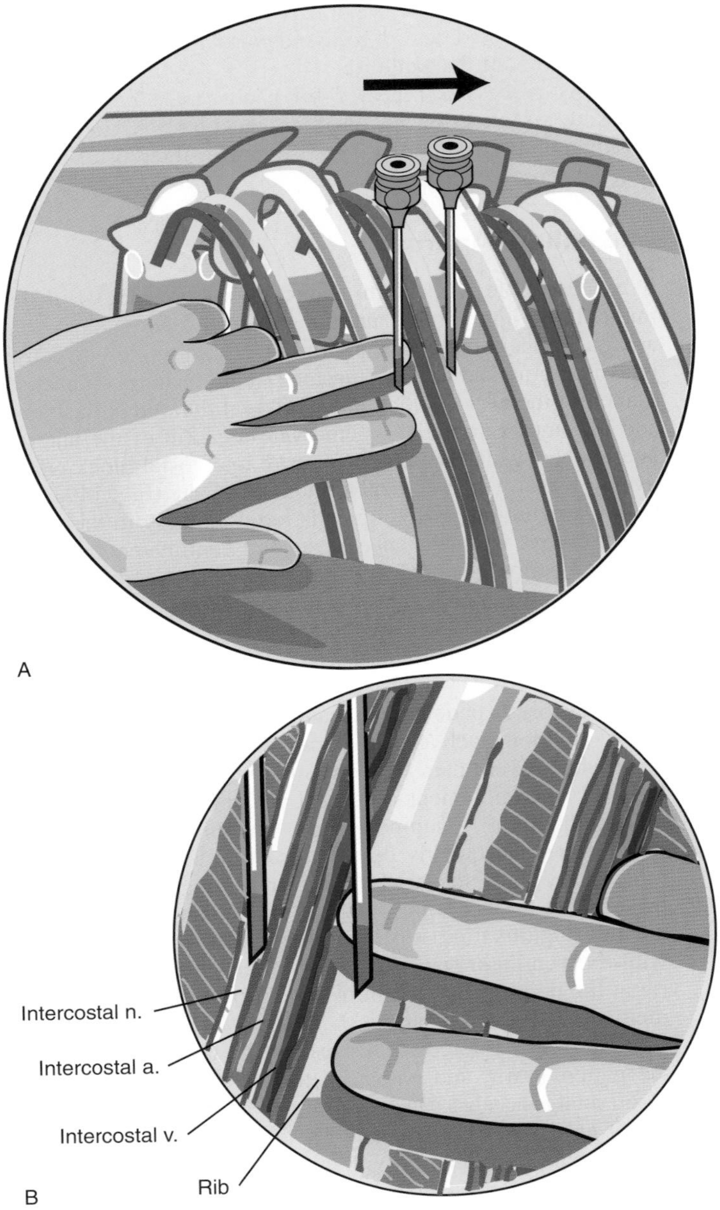

FIGURE 149–4 ■ Overview of anatomy and technique for performing the classic posterior approach to intercostal block. The left index finger palpates to identify the rib. The skin and subcutaneous tissues are retracted cephalad. The needle is advanced until contact is made with the rib and then is withdrawn into the subcutaneous tissue. The needle is "walked" off the inferior border of the rib.

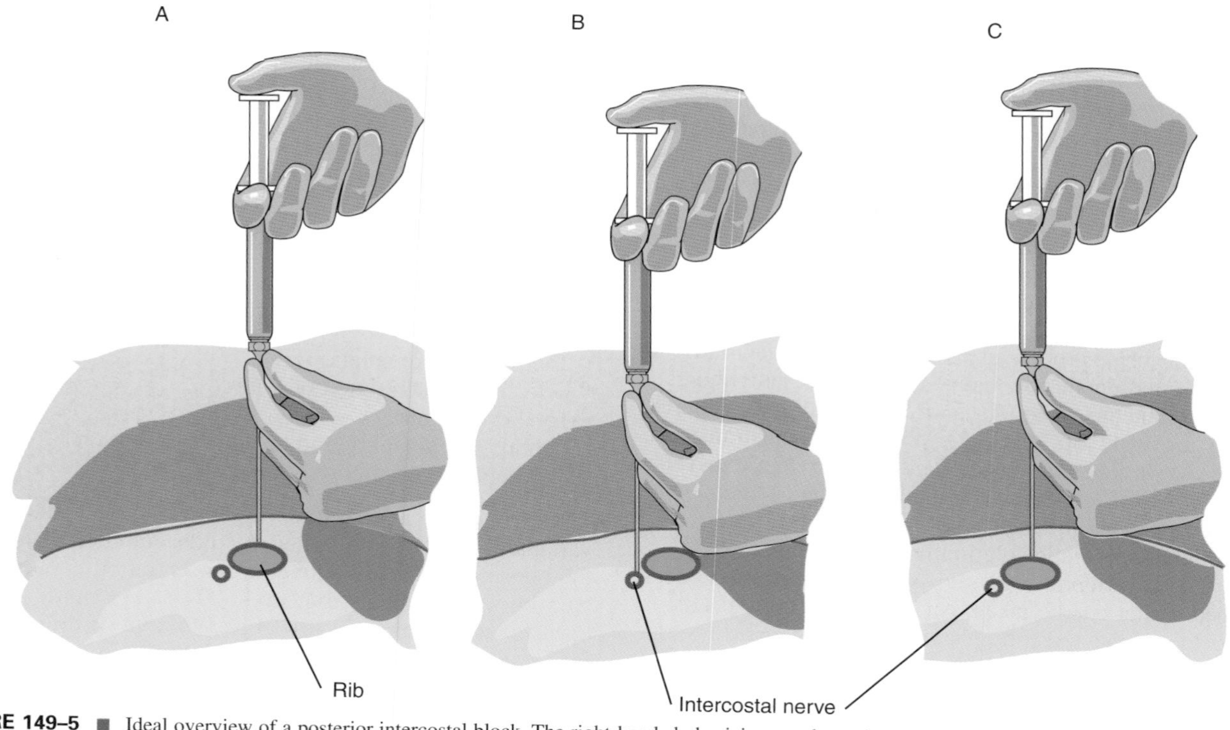

FIGURE 149–5 ■ Ideal overview of a posterior intercostal block. The right-handed physician stands on the left side of the prone patient, whose arms hang down to retract the scapulae laterally. The palpating left index finger identifies the rib to determine depth and direction for the advancing needle. The depth of the needle is firmly controlled by the anesthesiologist's left hand, which is constantly in contact (hypothenar eminence) with the patient's back. Now the right hand is shifted to inject 3 to 5 mL of solution. The depth of the needle is controlled by the left hand. The left hand again controls return of the needle to the "safety" of osseous contact. The previous steps are repeated at the next higher rib level.

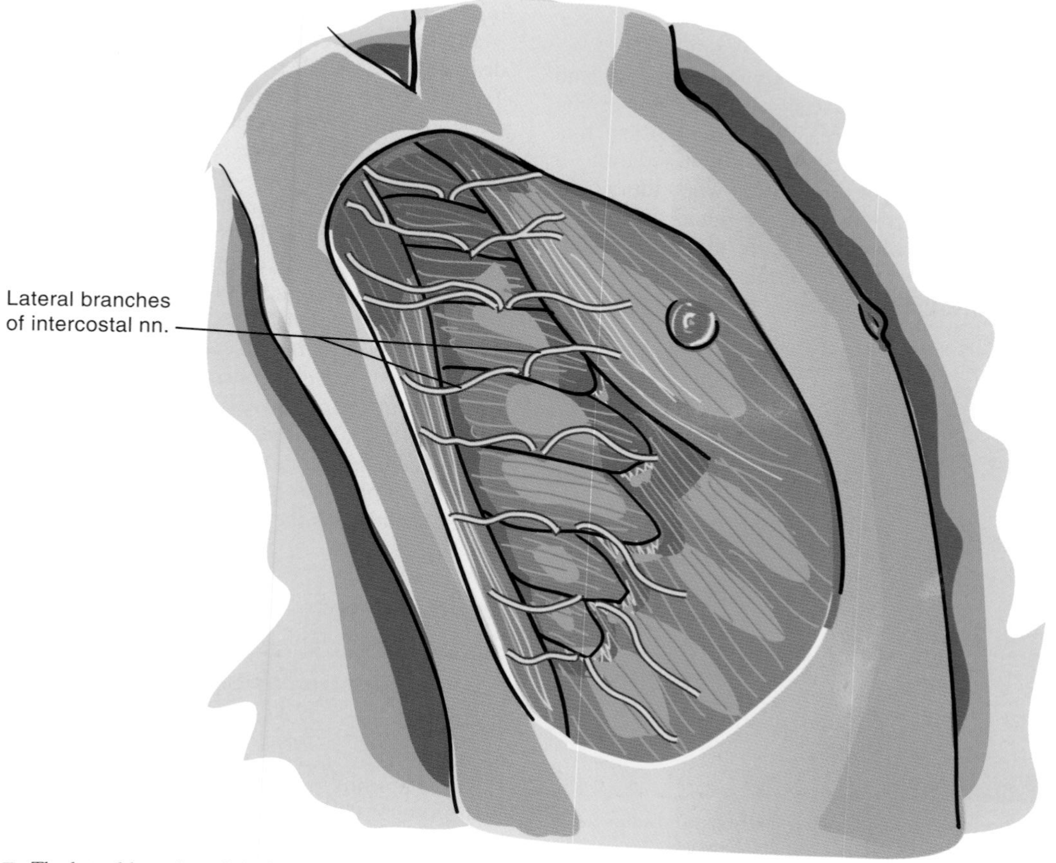

FIGURE 149–6 ■ The lateral branches of the intercostal nerves near the midaxillary line. Blocks made at or near these sites are effective and can be done easily on the supine patient.

To perform a paravertebral block, a skin wheal is raised 2.5 to 3 cm from the posterior midline at the superior edge of the vertebral spinous process of the nerve to be blocked. It is possible to palpate the ribs at this point because they are tilted steeply inward toward their attachments to the vertebral bodies and are covered by the thick paraspinous muscles. If palpation is begun laterally at the angle of the rib, however, it is usually possible to project a mental image of its attachment to the spine. A 10-cm 22-gauge needle is inserted perpendicular to the skin at the site of the skin wheal. Contact with the transverse process usually is made at a depth of 2 to 4 cm. With that depth now defined, the needle is withdrawn to a subcutaneous position and angled slightly inferior (caudal) to "walk off" the inferior edge of the transverse process. As it passes 1 to 1.5 cm deep to the transverse process, a loss of resistance may be felt as the needle pierces the costotransverse ligament. After negative aspiration, 3 to 6 mL of local anesthetic solution is injected (Fig. 141-7).

If a paravertebral catheter is to be used, the steps described earlier can be taken. An 18-gauge Tuohy needle is used to locate the loose areolar tissue of the paravertebral space. A catheter should be advanced only 1 to 2 cm beyond the tip of the needle; otherwise it could enter the epidural space. A 3-mL test dose of local anesthetic drug should be used to rule out intravascular and central neuraxis injection. Eason and Wyatt[23] reported that one 15-mL injection can be expected to cover four intercostal spaces.

PITFALLS

Use of Sedative Drugs

Intercostal nerve block may cause significant skin and periosteal stimulation that can be easily relieved by giving light sedation before the procedure. This is not to say that these nerve blocks cannot be performed without sedation. It may be mandatory to use little or no sedation when the blocks are performed on seriously ill patients or when a block is being used to help solve a diagnostic pain dilemma. Drugs commonly used to supplement these blocks include midazolam, fentanyl, ketamine, thiopental, and propofol.[24] The clinical situation should dictate which agent should be used. Is there need for hypnosis, analgesia, tranquilization, or some combination of these effects? It is important to titrate all sedative drugs in small intravenous doses while observing closely for the desired action.

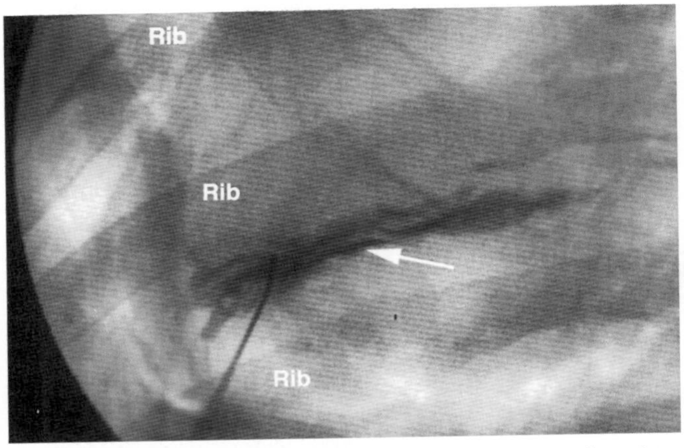

FIGURE 149–7 ■ Spread of local anesthetic and contrast medium along the intercostal groove. (From Raj PP, Lou L, Erdine S, Staats PS, Waldman S: Radiographic Imaging for Regional Anesthesia and Pain Management. Philadelphia, Churchill Livingstone, 2003.)

Local Anesthetic Drugs

In preparing a solution of local anesthetic for bilateral intercostal nerve block, the following calculations are made:

- Total volume of solution
- Effective concentration of drug
- Total dose of drug
- Volume of epinephrine to be added
- Total dose of epinephrine

There are safe or ideal limits for each of these interrelated variables. Volume multiplied by concentration determines total dose. Excessive volume or concentration may be tolerated by some patients, but toxic effects are more likely to occur. Small volumes or low concentrations of drug produce ineffective anesthesia. Any block might be termed ineffective were it inadequate in area, duration, or extent of motor or sensory fiber blockade. The drug should be tailored to the block, and doing so requires more than just a vague knowledge of local anesthetic drug doses and effective concentrations (Table 141-1).

For each local anesthetic, recommendations for maximum total dose are approved. These recommendations may vary from country to country or region to region, according to the prevailing bias, custom, or regulatory agencies. Many regional techniques (e.g., subarachnoid block) require drug doses far smaller than the maximum recommended dose. To perform multiple bilateral intercostal blocks, however, the anesthesiologist often needs to approach the maximum recommended dose to achieve a successful result. Blood levels of local anesthetic drug are higher after multiple intercostal nerve blocks than after any other commonly used regional anesthetic procedure. Tucker and colleagues[25] measured arterial plasma levels after epidural, caudal, intercostal, brachial plexus, and sciatic–femoral nerve block with a single injection of 500 mg of mepivacaine. The blocks were performed using 1% and 2% mepivacaine, with and without epinephrine. The highest plasma concentrations (5 to 10 mg/mL) were observed after intercostal nerve blocks without epinephrine. When a 1:200,000 concentration of epinephrine was added to the injected solution, plasma levels decreased to the range of 2 to 5 mg/mL. These lower blood levels were similar to the levels found with the other regional block procedures.

Table 149–1

Drugs for Intercostal Nerve Block for Pain Relief

Drug	*Duration (hr)*	*Concentration*	*Dose (mg/kg)*
Bupivacaine	8-12	0.25-0.5	2-3
Ropivacaine	8-12	0.25-0.5	2-3
Mepivacaine	4-8	0.5-1.5	7
Lidocaine	4-7	0.5-1.5	7

Respiratory Effects

Intercostal blockade produces effective analgesia with little central respiratory depression and minimal interference with pulmonary function. With the exception of peak expiratory flow, indices of respiratory function are essentially unaltered in healthy volunteers.[26] After thoracotomy, lung function is better in patients with intercostal blocks than in nonblocked controls.[27] Good information or comparative studies of patients with underlying pulmonary disease are not available.

COMPLICATIONS

Pneumothorax

The most feared complication of intercostal nerve block is pneumothorax. Many physicians avoid this block because they believe the risk of pneumothorax is too high. With proper attention to technique, however, the risk should be extremely low. Moore and Bridenbaugh[28] reported an incidence of pneumothorax of only 0.082% in an analysis of 17,000 patients. Most of the blocks reported in their study were done by residents in training. Other authors have reported incidences of pneumothorax closer to 1% or 2%.[29] In these series, the lesions were generally silent and asymptomatic and were discovered only on follow-up chest radiographs.

An asymptomatic pneumothorax is of little clinical consequence and usually requires no treatment beyond close observation. If further treatment is required, needle aspiration usually suffices. Reabsorption of a small pneumothorax also can be aided by administration of oxygen. A thoracostomy tube should be placed only if there is continued ventilatory embarrassment or a steady increase in the size of the pneumothorax.[30,31]

To produce a pneumothorax from an intercostal injection, the needle must puncture not only the parietal pleura, but also the visceral pleura, to allow air to leak from the lung into the pleural cavity. With coughing, over time, this condition can progress to tension pneumothorax. The most common technical error that results in pneumothorax is improper positioning of the hands during the performance of the block and failure to control needle depth.

Systemic Toxicity

A second type of complication from intercostal block is the toxic effects of absorbed local anesthetic drugs. This problem is most likely to occur when large amounts of concentrated drug are injected. Systemic toxic reactions are less likely with blocks for diagnosis or postoperative pain relief because ordinarily smaller volumes of more dilute local anesthetic solution are used.

Hypotension and Respiratory Failure

A third complication of intercostal block is hypotension.[32] Usually, hypotension has occurred when intrathoracic intercostal blocks were performed under direct vision by the surgeon. It seems that in each case a high epidural or total spinal block resulted from central spread of solution and subsequent to a rapid and profound drop in blood pressure. Hypotension develops occasionally, when intercostal blocks are performed to provide postoperative pain relief for patients in the intensive care unit. Although the cause is unclear, hypotension seems to occur in patients who are hypovolemic and vasoconstricted because of severe pain. When analgesia is produced by the intercostal blocks, the compensatory vasoconstriction eases, and the patient becomes hypotensive. In a similar manner, intercostal nerve block can lead to respiratory failure when pain relief from the block unmasks the ventilatory depression of previously administered, but ineffective, parenteral narcotics.[33]

FUTURE CONSIDERATIONS

The success rate of intercostal nerve block should approach 100%. The problem is not in the doing, but in the duration of this block. Currently available local anesthetic drugs provide analgesia for only 8 to 12 hours. Cryoanalgesia has been advocated as a method of obtaining blocks of long duration by freezing the nerves. This technique is, however, unreliable, cumbersome, and declining in use.[34,35]

Another future consideration is that techniques might be developed that do not require needle injections. There are reports of using the jet injection system originally designed and used for mass inoculations, which also has been adapted to intercostal and other superficial peripheral nerve blocks. The injector jet is applied directly to the skin, but does not penetrate it. The injectate is forced through the skin and is subsequently absorbed into the bloodstream. Advantages purportedly include little or no risk of pneumothorax and capability for performing multiple blocks easily and rapidly. The procedure is not totally painless; transdermal spread of local anesthetic drug is unpredictable, and the jet gun has some major deficits. One is that only 1 mL of solution can be ejected per "shot." Although this limitation conceivably could be overcome by design modifications, a larger volume likely would be more painful when injected. Seddon[36] reported using 1 mL of 1.5% bupivacaine, which was specially prepared for his study, as this concentration is not available commercially.[36] This drug concentration did not seem to be neurotoxic, and the results compared favorably with postcholecystectomy pain relief from intramuscular narcotics. Katz and associates[37] compared two separate 1-mL injections of 0.75% bupivacaine with more traditional intercostal nerve blocks (3 mL) by needle injection. Neither patient group seemed to receive effective analgesia in that study.

New drug formulations currently are being developed that may prolong the duration of intercostal blockade from hours to days or weeks. The incorporation of bupivacaine into liposomes and polymer microspheres has been shown to extend its duration of action greatly.[38,39] The duration of sensory anesthesia after intercostal block in sheep is increased from 4 to 13 days after the injection of bupivacaine in microspheres (8 to 80 mg/kg). Despite this extremely large load of bupivacaine within the microspheres, plasma concentrations (<0.25 mg/mL) are only a fraction of what is detected after injection of aqueous bupivacaine.[40] When these new formulations become available, the slight pain and time involved in performing intercostal block will be more than offset by the benefits and duration of pain relief.

References

1. Schleich DS: Schmerzlöse Operationen. Berlin, J Springer, 1894.
2. Braun H: Local Anesthesia: Its Scientific Basis and Practical Use. Philadelphia, Lea & Febiger, 1914.
3. Pauchet V, Sourdat P, Labat G: L'Anesthesie Regionale, 3rd ed. Paris, Librairie Octave Doin, 1921.
4. Labat G: Regional Anesthesia: Its Technic and Clinical Application. Philadelphia, WB Saunders, 1922.
5. Mandl F: Paravertebral Block. New York, Grune & Stratton, 1947.
6. Moore DC, Bridenbaugh LD: Intercostal nerve block in 4333 patients: Indications, technique, and complications. Anesth Analg 41:1, 1962.
7. Moore DC: Intercostal nerve block for postoperative somatic pain following surgery of thorax and upper abdomen. Br J Anaesth 47:284, 1975.
8. Mozell EJ, Sabanathan S, Mearns AJ, et al: Continuous extrapleural intercostal nerve block after pleurecotomy. Thorax 46:21, 1991.
9. Conacher I, Kokri M: Postoperative paravertebral blocks for thoracic surgery. Br J Anaesth 59:155, 1987.
10. Baxter AD, Jennings FO, Harris RS, et al: Continuous intercostal blockade after cardiac surgery. Br J Anaesth 59:162, 1987.
11. Nunn JF, Slavin C: Posterior intercostal nerve block for pain relief after cholecystectomy. Br J Anaesth 52:253, 1980.
12. Bunting P, McGeachie JF: Intercostal nerve blockade producing analgesia after appendicectomy. Br J Anaesth 61:169, 1988.
13. Sihota MK, Holmblad BR: Horner's syndrome after interpleural anesthesia with bupivacaine for post-herpetic neuralgia. Acta Anesth Scand 32:593, 1988.
14. Hardy PAJ: Anatomical variation in the position of the proximal intercostal nerve. Br J Anaesth 61:338, 1988.
15. Conacher ID: Resin injection of thoracic paravertebral spaces. Br J Anaesth 61:657, 1988.
16. Baxter AD, Flynn JF, Jennings FO: Continuous intercostal nerve blockade. Br J Anaesth 56:665, 1984.
17. Butchart EG, Grott GJ, Barnsley WC: Spontaneous rupture of an intercostal artery in a patient with neurofibromatosis and scoliosis. J Thorac Cardiovasc Surg 69:919, 1975.
18. Thompson GE, Brown DL: The common nerve blocks. In Nunn FF, Utting JE, Brown BR (eds): General Anaesthesia, 5th ed. London, Butterworth, 1989, p 1070.
19. Moore D, Bush W, Scurlock J: Intercostal nerve block: A roentgenographic anatomic study of technique and absorption in humans. Anesth Analg 59:815, 1980.
20. Smith BE, Suchak M, Siggins D, Challands J: Rectus sheath block for diagnostic laparoscopy. Anaesthesia 43:947, 1988.
21. Kvalheim L, Reistad F: Interpleural catheter in the management of postoperative pain. Anesthesiology 61:A231, 1984.
22. Murphy DF: Continuous intercostal nerve blockade: An anatomical study to elucidate its mode of action. Br J Anaesth 56:627, 1984.
23. Eason MJ, Wyatt R: Paravertebral thoracic block—a reappraisal. Anaesthesia 34:638, 1979.
24. Thompson GE, Moore DC: Ketamine, diazepam and Innovar: a computerized comparative study. Anesth Analg (Cleve) 50:458, 1971.
25. Tucker GT, Moore DC, Bridenbaugh PO, et al: Systemic absorption of mepivacaine in commonly used regional block procedures. Anesthesiology 141:276, 1972.
26. Jakobson S, Fridiksson H, Hedenstrom H, Ivarsson I: Effects of intercostal nerve blocks on pulmonary mechanics in healthy men. Acta Anaesthesiol Scand 24:482, 1980.
27. Hecker BR, Fjurstrom R, Schoene RB: Effect of intercostal nerve blockade on respiratory mechanics and CO_2 chemosensitivity at rest and exercise. Anesthesiology 70:13, 1989.
28. Moore DC, Bridenbaugh LD: Pneumothorax: Its incidence following intercostal nerve block. JAMA 174:842, 1960.
29. Bridenbaugh PO, DuPen SL, Moore DC, et al: Postoperative intercostal nerve block analgesia versus narcotic analgesia. Anesth Analg (Cleve) 52:81, 1973.
30. Jones JS: A place for aspiration in the treatment of spontaneous pneumothorax. Thorax 40:66, 1985.
31. Vallee P: Sequential treatment of a simple pneumothorax. Ann Emerg Med 17:936, 1988.
32. Skretting P: Hypotension after intercostal nerve block during thoracotomy under general anesthesia. Br J Anaesth 53:527, 1981.
33. Cory PC, Mulroy MF: Postoperative respiratory failure following intercostal block. Anesthesiology 54:418, 1981.
34. Lloyd JW, Barnard JDW, Glynn CJ: Cryoanalgesia, a new approach to pain relief. Lancet 2:932, 1976.
35. Maiwand O, Makey AR: Cryoanalgesia for relief of pain after thoracotomy. BMJ 282:1749, 1981.
36. Seddon SJ: Intercostal nerve block by jet injection. Anaesthesia 39:484, 1984.
37. Katz J, Knarr D, Juneja M: Intercostal nerve block by jet injection. Anaesthesia 75:A726, 1991.
38. Curley J, Castillo J, Hotz J, et al: Prolonged regional nerve blockade. Anesthesiology 84:1401, 1996.
39. Mowat JJ, Mok MJ, MacLeod BA, Madden TD: Liposomal bupivacaine. Anesthesiology 85:635, 1996.
40. Drager C, Benziger D, Gao F, Berde CB: Prologed intercostal nerve blockade in sheep using controlled-release of bupivacaine and dexamethasone from polymer microspheres. Anesthesiology 89:969, 1998.

chapter 150

Interpleural Catheters: Indications and Techniques

Kathleen A. O'Leary, Anthony T. Yarussi, and David P. Myers

The concept of interpleural anesthesia (IPA) was originally described by Mandl[1] in 1947, who used 6% phenol injected into the interpleural space of experimental animals and produced no signs of pleural irritation or necrosis. IPA resurfaced in 1986, when it was used as an investigational tool for postoperative pain relief after breast surgery, kidney surgery, and cholecystectomy by Reiestad and Stromskag.[2] In their study, a single 20-mL dose of bupivacaine, 0.5%, with epinephrine was administered after surgery. Of the 81 enrolled patients, 78 required no additional analgesic measure during the first 24 hours postoperatively. Duration of analgesia ranged from 6 to 27 hours.

Most recently, interest in IPA for chronic pain management has increased. Durrani and colleagues[3] alleviated pancreatic carcinoma pain using interpleural bupivacaine. Fineman[4] used IPA for metastatic bronchogenic carcinoma pain in the pleura and chest wall.

MECHANISMS OF ACTION

Three theories of the mechanism of action of IPA have been advanced. First is diffusion of local anesthetic from the pleural space through the parietal pleural and the innermost intercostal muscles, producing multiple unilateral intercostal nerve blocks. Second, a unilateral block of the thoracic sympathetic chain and the splanchnic nerves is produced by drug traversing the parietal pleura paraspinally. Third, diffusion of the anesthetic to the ipsilateral brachial plexus produces analgesia to the arm.

Riegler and Vadeboncouer[5] used evoked potential monitoring in dogs to demonstrate that IPA produces multiple sensory nerve blocks. Clinical studies by Durrani and colleagues,[3] Reiestad and Kvalheim,[6] and Alhburg and coworkers,[7] in which sympathetically mediated pain syndromes were treated with IPA, imply that autonomic blockade can also occur. Ramajoli and DeAmici[8] proposed that bilateral block of the sympathetic and splanchnic nerves occurs after unilateral IPA. In their patients with diffuse visceral pain, they noted marked reduction in pain scores bilaterally and bilateral increases in cutaneous temperatures as compared with controls after injection of 20 mL of 0.25% or 0.5% bupivacaine via an interpleural catheter. They hypothesized that the anesthetic agent diffused through the pleura at the costovertebral margin to the mediastinum to reach the ipsilateral and contralateral sympathetic chains. The force of aspiration is caused by the greater negative pressure in the mediastinum (−25 to −30 cm H_2O) as compared with the pleura (−5 to −10 cm H_2O).[9]

Diffusion of local anesthetic into the brachial plexus and stellate ganglion has produced relief for head and neck and upper extremity pain syndromes. Horner syndrome is commonly seen if the drug is allowed to diffuse cephalad to block the stellate ganglion.

INDICATIONS

Interpleural analgesia is commonly used for unilateral subcostal postoperative pain relief. It also provides anesthesia for minor surgical procedures and chronic pain. Table 150–1 lists procedures in which IPA has been effective for either analgesia or anesthesia. It is important to remember that IPA is considered a unilateral block and is not currently recommended for pain extending across the midline. Because bilateral pneumothoraces can occur, bilateral interpleural analgesia should never be attempted unless catheters can be placed under direct surgical vision.

Interpleural analgesia has been used effectively to treat chronic pain in terminally ill patients with pancreatic, renal cell, and breast cancers and lymphomas.[10] For patients in whom traditional methods of analgesic therapy have failed and whose expected survival is short, IPA can produce immediate pain relief. For patients with advanced cancer who may survive >3 months, interpleural phenol injections have been used with good results. Phenol injections into the pleural cavity of one cancer patient produced no microscopic or macroscopic changes in lung, pleura, or nerve tissue despite excellent analgesia over a 3-month period until his death.[11] Tunneled interpleural catheters have also been useful in the palliation of chronic cancer-related pain. The interpleural catheter is tunneled in the same manner as an epidural catheter. IPA has also been used for symptomatic management of acute herpes zoster,[12] postherpetic neuralgia,[13-15] reflex sympathetic dystrophy,[16] upper limb ischemia,[17] and cystic fibrosis.[18]

CONTRAINDICATIONS

Relative contraindications to the use of IPA include pleuritis, pulmonary fibrosis, pleural adhesions, emphysema, hemothorax, pleural effusions, empyema, bronchopleural fistula, and surgical or chemical pleurodesis. These processes either increase the risk of pneumothorax or cause erratic distribution and absorption of local anesthetic as well as difficulty in identifying the interpleural space. If a patient is being ventilated with positive end-expiratory pressure (PEEP) at the time of catheter insertion, the risk of pneumothorax is greatly increased. Absolute contraindications to IPA include allergy to local anesthetic, extensive infection around the catheter insertion site, and bleeding diatheses.

Table 150–1

Indications for Use of Intrapleural Anesthesia

- Postoperative analgesia
  - Cholecystectomy
  - Breast surgery
  - Renal surgery
  - Other subcostal incisions
  - Multiple rib fractures
  - Thoracotomy
  - Cardiac surgery
- Surgical anesthesia
  - Breast biopsy and lumpectomy
  - Percutaneous hepatic and renal drainage procedures
- Lithotripsy
- Chronic pain management
  - Chronic pancreatitis
  - Postherpetic neuralgia
  - Reflex sympathetic dystrophies of the arm/face
  - Frozen shoulder
  - Upper abdominal cancer pain
  - Chest wall and thoracic visceral pain
  - Pain of pancreatic cancer and other abdominal cancer
  - Upper limb ischemia
  - Cystic fibrosis

PATIENT POSITIONING

Proper patient positioning is exceeded only by correct catheter placement and successful injection into the pleural space as critical determinants of the extent of the resulting block. Table 150–2 describes the three best positions for IPA. In all blocks except multiple intercostal rib blocks sparing the thoracic sympathetic chain, the patient must be positioned with the *affected side up.* Because the block sets up by mass action, delivery of local anesthetic agent along the paravertebral gutter by gravitational flow is essential to have the bulk of solution bathe the affected nerves (Fig. 150–1). The position of the patient after injection of local anesthetic into the pleural space also determines, in large part, the nature, intensity, and extent of the resulting blockade. The preferred approach for unilateral blockade of cervical or superior thoracic segments is to place the patient in a lateral decubitus position with the head tilted down 20 degrees for 20 to 30 minutes after the injection.

Patients who are suffering from somatic or visceral pain, such as that from pancreatic carcinoma, may also benefit from interpleural analgesia.[3] For those who are unable to lie prone or in lateral decubitus position owing to pain, celiac plexus blockade is not an option. IPA can be provided by putting the patient in either the sitting or reverse Trendelenburg position, depending on the patient's tolerance.

INSERTION OF CATHETERS

In a 70-kg man, the pleural space is 10 to 20 μm wide and occupies a surface area of 2000 cm^2. This cavity is created between the visceral pleura lining the heart and lungs and the parietal pleura covering the thoracic cage and diaphragm.

Table 150–2

Patient Positioning for Intrapleural Anesthesia

Purpose of Block	*Recommended Position and Comments*
Unilateral blockade of cervical and superior thoracic segments of sympathetic chain	Lateral decubitus position with affected side up and head down about 20 degrees for 20-30 min after injection of local anesthetic Partial blockade of ipsilateral brachial plexus is also achieved by this position, as demonstrated by hypesthesia in C3-T1 dermatomes and motor weakness of shoulder, arm, and forearm
Surgical anesthesia for unilateral breast tumor resection	Lateral decubitus position with affected side down and head down about 20 degrees for 20-30 min after injection of local anesthesia Produces unilateral blockade of intercostal nerves from T1-T9 with complete skin anesthesia
Postoperative pain management, including chest trauma	Side-lying position at angle of about 20 degrees with the affected side up during injection and injection time of 5-6 min for 30 mL of local anesthetic: after injection, patient is turned supine. Produces blockade of both sympathetic chain and intercostal nerves of affected side

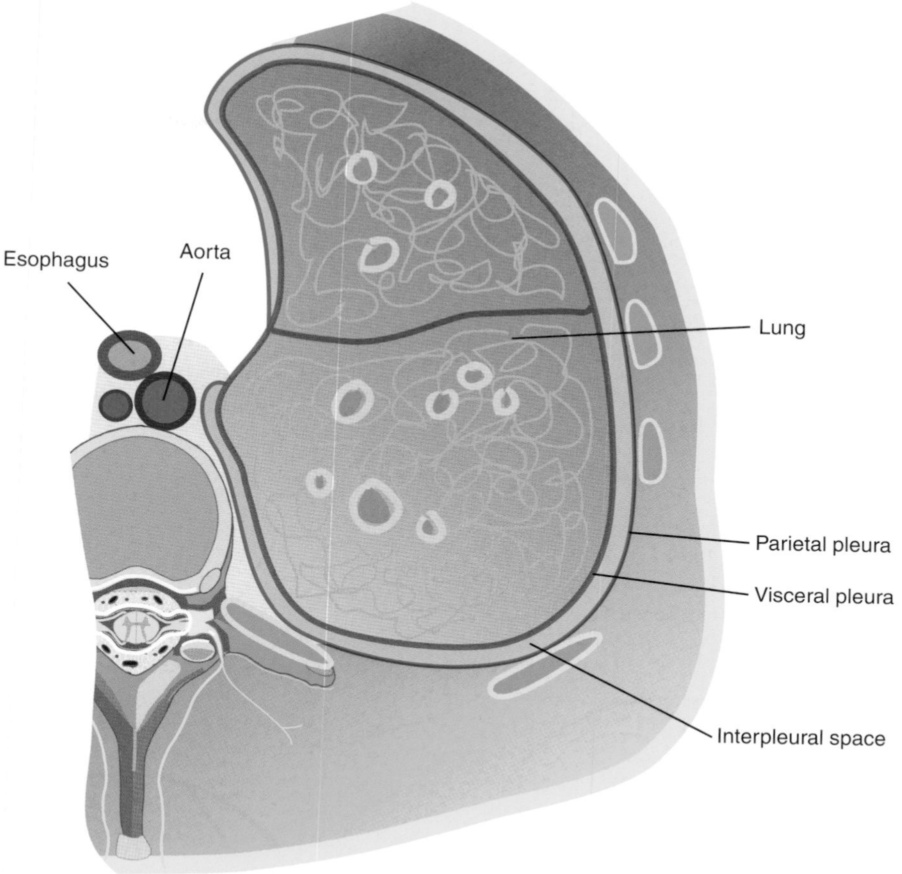

FIGURE 150–1 ■ Cross-sectional view of thorax shows paravertebral gutter between visceral and parietal pleura.

Pleural pressure varies from −12 cm H_2O in the apical portion of the lungs to less negative values (−5 cm H_2O) at the bases. This negative interpleural pressure is the key to proper identification of the pleural space and is a function of the elastic recoil of the chest outward and the tendency of the lungs to collapse.

Blood pressure, heart rate, and respiration should be monitored during and immediately after placement of the interpleural catheter. The patient lies in the lateral decubitus position with the affected side up. An interpleural kit (Arrow) is ideal, but a continuous epidural tray will suffice. The major advantages of the interpleural kit are its blunter needle and softer-tipped catheter (Flexitip), which reduce the chance of pneumothorax.

With sterile technique, an area is identified for insertion, most commonly the T7-T8 intercostal space. The site of puncture is 8 to 10 cm from the posterior midline (Fig. 150–2A). After local anesthetic injection (see Fig. 150–2B), the blunt-tipped needle is introduced in a medial direction with the cutting edge uppermost until it reaches the lower rib of the selected interspace (see Fig. 150–2C). When the parietal pleura is penetrated, which is perceived as a clicking sensation (see Fig. 150–2D), the negative pleural pressure and the plunger weight itself cause the air to escape into the thorax (see Fig. 150–2E). The syringe is then removed, and the catheter is introduced 6 to 8 cm into the pleural space (see Fig. 150–2F). The needle is removed next and the catheter is left in place (see Fig. 150–2G). After aspiration for blood and air, the catheter is taped in place.

A test dose of local anesthetic with epinephrine can then be administered. If there are no adverse reactions, a bolus dose can be given. On return of pain, additional bolus doses may be given, again with the patient in the lateral decubitus position and the affected side up.

Although this has been the standard technique for interpleural catheter placement, the introduction of air into the interpleural space is difficult to avoid as the Touhy needle is open to air to allow passage of the catheter. As much as 20 mL of air can be entrained into the pleural space during insertion, and the resulting air pockets can be responsible for patchy blocks that may sometimes be encountered with interpleural anesthesia. Modified techniques have been developed to create a closed system and reduce the chance of air entering the interpleural space.[19,20]

Gomar and associates used an electronic device (Episensor [Palex, Spain]) that detects negative pressure under −1.8 cm H_2O to identify the interpleural space.[21] This technique was used in 25 patients postoperatively and catheter positions were confirmed radiographically. None of the patients developed pneumothorax. Electronic devices may prove to be useful adjuncts to interpleural catheter placement, especially in obese patients or those with pleural disease.

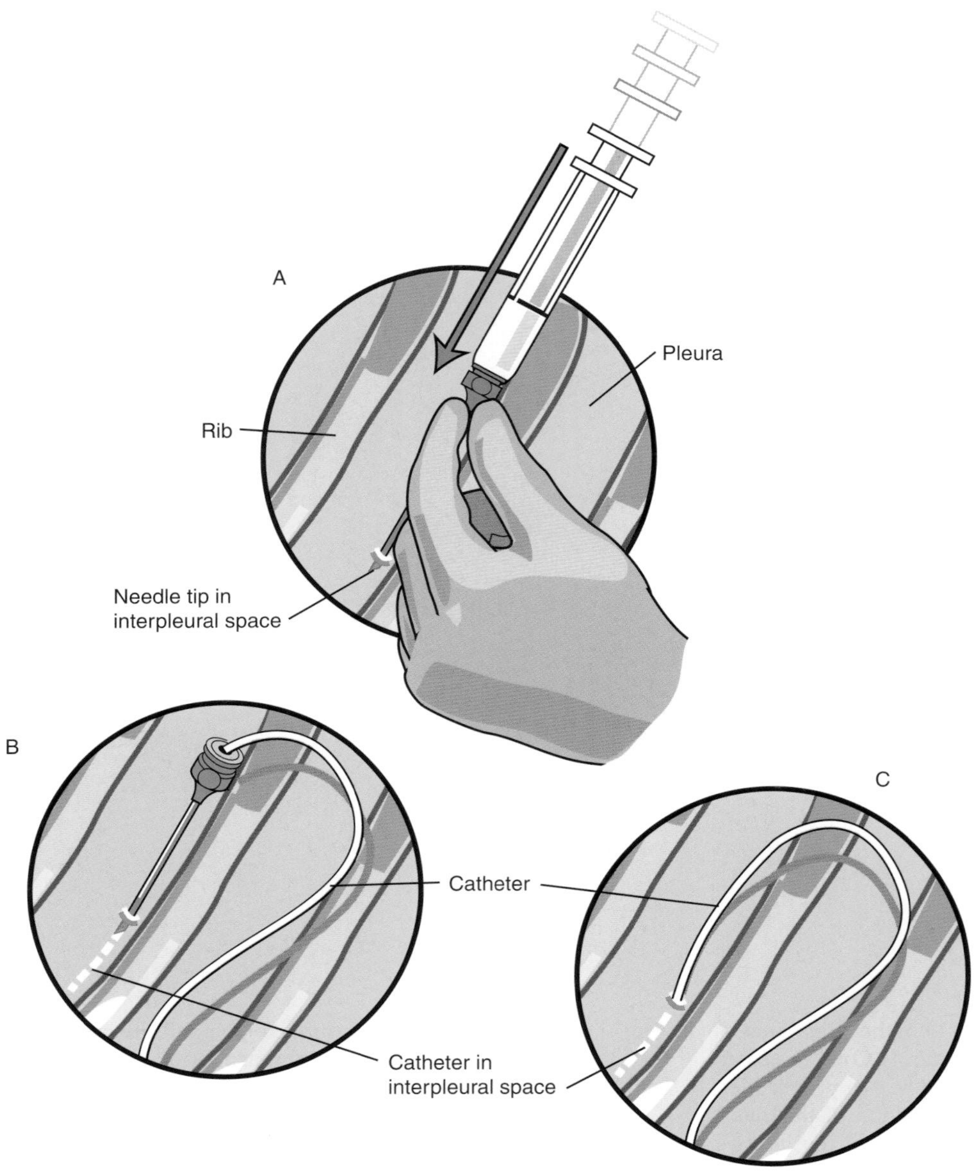

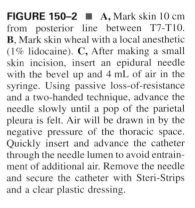

FIGURE 150–2 ■ **A,** Mark skin 10 cm from posterior line between T7-T10. **B**, Mark skin wheal with a local anesthetic (1% lidocaine). **C,** After making a small skin incision, insert an epidural needle with the bevel up and 4 mL of air in the syringe. Using passive loss-of-resistance and a two-handed technique, advance the needle slowly until a pop of the parietal pleura is felt. Air will be drawn in by the negative pressure of the thoracic space. Quickly insert and advance the catheter through the needle lumen to avoid entrainment of additional air. Remove the needle and secure the catheter with Steri-Strips and a clear plastic dressing.

DOSAGE

Various dosing regimens have been advocated for IPA, but controversy about the optimal dosage, volume, and concentration of local anesthetic persists. The need for adequate analgesia must be balanced with the risk of possible toxicity, because the margin of safety with IPA is small.

Perhaps the most common method of delivering IPA is the intermittent bolus method. Typically, a bolus dose is given at the end of the surgical procedure, before the conclusion of the general anesthetic. This initial dose is followed up with doses given either at established intervals (usually every 6 hours) or as needed when the patient experiences pain.

Bolus doses using 20 mL of both 0.25% and 0.5% bupivacaine with epinephrine 1:200,000 have proved efficacious for postoperative analgesia.[2,22] Stromskag and colleagues[23] compared the analgesic effects of 40 mL of 0.25% bupivacaine with epinephrine and 20 mL of 0.5% bupivacaine with epinephrine in postcholecystectomy patients. They found no difference between the two groups—concluding that, as long as the amount of drug administered is adequate, the volume of bupivacaine with epinephrine has little effect within the range of 20 to 40 mL.

Continuous infusion of bupivacaine has also been used. Laurito and associates[24] compared continuous infusions of 0.25% bupivacaine (plain) at a rate of 0.125 mL/kg/hour with bolus doses of 0.5% bupivacaine with epinephrine 1:200,000 at 0.4 mL/kg every 6 hours in postcholecystectomy patients. They found that the continuous infusion produces better analgesia and lower plasma bupivacaine levels than bolus dosing. Van Kleef and coworkers[25] compared continuous infusions of 0.25% and 0.5% bupivacaine with epinephrine 1:200,000 at 5 mL/hour in postoperative patients who had either flank or subcostal incisions. They found comparable clinical effects but lower plasma concentrations in the group who received 0.25% bupivacaine.

Continuous infusions of 0.25% bupivacaine with epinephrine are safe, effective, and less labor intensive than intermittent bolus doses. When continuous infusions are not possible, intermittent bolus doses of 20 to 30 mL of 0.25% bupivacaine with epinephrine can safely be administered. In either situation, the patients should be monitored for evidence of systemic toxicity during the course of treatment.

Clinical studies have also evaluated the effect of interpleural opioids on postoperative pain control.[26,27] Welte and colleagues found that interpleural morphine had no beneficial effect in reducing postoperative pain scores or improving pulmonary function after thoracotomy, as compared with the intravenous route.[27] Morphine via the interpleural route does not appear to activate peripheral opioid receptors at primary afferent neurons, thus giving it no greater effect than when administered intravenously.

COMPLICATIONS

Although the IPA technique has been safe in clinical use, there has been some disagreement about its safety. Gomez and colleagues[28] demonstrated a high malposition rate with intraoperative placement of 18 catheters. They concluded that the procedure was unsafe, but several factors contributed to the high failure rate. They inserted catheters to 30 cm and used sharp-tipped needles and stiffer epidural catheters. The patients also received positive-pressure ventilation during insertion of the interpleural catheter.

The risks of inserting an interpleural catheter (Table 150–3) are low if one takes the time to slowly advance a catheter with a soft, flexible tip to a distance of 6 to 8 cm. The use of a blunt epidural-style needle and a heavier-barreled 10-mL glass syringe allows for easier confirmation of positioning in the interpleural space. Despite meticulous technique, however, complications can occur.

Clinically significant pneumothorax is the most common complication (reported incidence <5%). Thus, a chest radiograph is mandatory after placement of an interpleural catheter. In such cases, a small pocket of air may be seen over the apex of the lung. This finding represents injected air that entered the pleural space during positioning of the interpleural catheter, not air leaking from a perforated lung. This air is rapidly absorbed and presents no clinical problem. One tension pneumothorax[29] has been reported. It resulted from use of the loss-of-resistance technique to identify the interpleural space.

Table 150–3

Complications of Interpleural Anesthesia
Pneumothorax
Pleural effusion
Horner syndrome
Catheter displacement
Catheter loss
Systemic reaction
Empyema
Bronchopleural fistula
Laceration of intercostal neurovascular bundle

The reported prevalence of systemic toxicity from local anesthetics is 1.3%.[29] The clinical manifestations are neurologic, ranging from somnolence and disorientation to seizure activity. It is likely that absorption of local anesthetic is increased in patients with inflamed pleura, and they are the ones most at risk for systemic toxicity.

Pleural effusion after IPA is rare (incidence 0.4%).[30] Causes include damage to intercostal vessels, minor trauma from needle insertion, failure of local anesthetic absorption, and diaphragmatic tracking of inflammatory fluid after abdominal surgery. Other reported complications include catheter displacement, Horner syndrome, empyema, and formation of a bronchopleural fistula.[30]

SUMMARY

The correct technique for placement of interpleural catheters is relatively easy as compared with other anesthetic procedures, such as thoracic epidural catheter insertion. Another advantage of IPA is the development of a unilateral sympathetic block, versus the bilateral sympathetic and somatic block produced by thoracic epidural analgesia. Unilateral sympathetic blockade avoids bradycardia and hypotension, because the contralateral sympathetic chain is intact.

In spite of the advantages of this technique, IPA has not gained momentum in anesthesiology. To many, the risk of inserting a needle into the thoracic cavity for routine postoperative analgesia far outweighs the benefits. Its success in relieving subdiaphragmatic chronic organ pain, however, makes it an intriguing alternative to the more complex plexus blocks for pain management.

At present, IPA appears to be most clinically useful for analgesia for subdiaphragmatic incisions, chronic benign pain, and neurolytic cancer pain in terminally ill persons. Further clinical studies will continue to elucidate the place of IPA in the armamentarium of the regional anesthesiologist.

References

1. Mandl F: Paravertebral Block. New York, Grune & Stratton, 1947, p 34.
2. Reiestad F, Stromskag K: Interpleural catheter in the management of postoperative pain. Reg Anesth 11:89, 1986.
3. Durrani Z, Winnie A, Ikuta P: Interpleural catheter analgesia for pancreatic pain. Anesth Analg 67:479, 1988.
4. Fineman S: Long-term postthoracotomy cancer pain management with interpleural bupivacaine. Anesth Analg 68:694, 1989.
5. Riegler F, Vadeboncouer T: Interpleural anesthetics in the dog: Differential somatic neural blockade. Anesthesiology 71:744, 1989.
6. Reiestad F, Kvalheim L: Continuous intercostal blocks for postoperative pain relief. Norweg Med Assoc J 104:485, 1984.
7. Ahlburg P, Noreng M, Molgaard J, Egebo K: Treatment of pancreatic pain with interpleural bupivacaine: An open trial. Acta Anesthesiol Scand 34:156, 1990.
8. Ramajoli F, DeAmici D: Is there a bilateral block of the thoracic sympathetic chain after unilateral intrapleural analgesia? Anesth Analg 87:360, 1998.
9. Miserocchi GM, Pistoleis M, Miriati M, et al: Pleural liquid pressure gradients and intrapleural distribution of injected bolus. J Appl Physiol 56:526, 1984.
10. Myers DP, Lema MJ, de Leon-Casasola OA, Bacon DR: Interpleural analgesia for the treatment of severe cancer pain in terminally ill patients. J Pain Symptom Manage 8:505, 1993.
11. Lema MJ, Myers DP, de Leon-Casasola OA, Penetrante R: Pleural phenol therapy for treatment of chronic esophageal pain. Reg Anesth 17:166, 1992.

12. Johnson LR, Racco AG, Fellonte FM: Continuous subpleural paravertebral block in acute thoracic herpes zoster. Anesth Analg 67:1105, 1988.
13. Reiestad F, McIlvaine WB, Barnes M, et al: Interpleural analgesia in the treatment of severe thoracic post herpetic neuralgia. Reg Anesth 15:113, 1990.
14. Reiestad F, Stokke T, Barnes M: Interpleural analgesia in chronic pain. Acta Anaesth Scand 33:A101, 1989.
15. Sihuta MK, Holmblad BR: Horner's syndrome after intrapleural anesthesia with bupivacaine for postherpetic neuralgia. Acta Anaesth Scand 32:593, 1988.
16. Reiestad F, McIlvaine WB, Kvalheim L, et al: Interpleural analgesia in the treatment of upper extremity reflex sympathetic dystrophy. Anesth Analg 69:671, 1989.
17. Perkins G: Interpleural anesthesia in the management of upper limb ischemia. A report of three cases. Anaesth Intensive Care 19:575, 1991.
18. Bruce DL, Gerken MV, Lyon GD: Post cholecystectomy pain relief by intrapleural bupivacaine in patients with cystic fibrosis. Anesth Analg 66:1187, 1987.
19. Marsh B, McDonald P: A modified technique for the insertion of an interpleural catheter. Anaesthesia 46(10):889, 1991.
20. Ho A, Cortardi L: A simple technique to facilitate interpleural catheter placement. Anesth Analg 79:614, 1994.
21. Gomar C, Cabres L, DeAndres T, et al: An electronic device (Episensor) for detection of the interpleural space. Reg Anesth 16:112, 1991.
22. Stromskag KE, Reiestad F, Holmquist ELO: Intrapleural administration of 0.25%, 0.37%, and 0.5% bupivacaine with epinephrine after cholecystectomy. Anesth Analg 67:430, 1988.
23. Stromskag KE, Minor BG, Lindeberg A: Comparison of 40 milliliters of 0.25% intrapleural bupivacaine with epinephrine with 20 milliliters of 0.5% intrapleural bupivacaine with epinephrine after cholecystectomy. Anesth Analg 73:397, 1991.
24. Laurito CE, Kirz LI, Vadeboncouer TR, et al: Continuous infusion of interpleural bupivacaine maintains effective analgesia after cholecystectomy. Anesth Analg 72:516, 1991.
25. Van Kleef JW, Logeman A, Burns AGL, et al: Continuous interpleural infusion of bupivacaine for postoperative analgesia after surgery with flank incisions: A double-blind comparison of 0.25% and 0.5% solutions. Anesth Analg 75:268, 1992.
26. Schulte-Steinberg H, Weringer G, Jokisch O, et al: Intraperitoneal versus interpleural morphine or bupivacaine for pain after laparoscopic cholecystectomy. Anesthesiology 82:634, 1995.
27. Welte M, Haimerl E, Groh J, et al: Effect of interpleural morphine on postoperative pain and pulmonary function after thoracotomy. Br J Anaesth 69:637, 1992.
28. Gomez MN, Symreng T, Rossi NP, Chiang CK: Interpleural bupivacaine for intraoperative analgesia: A dangerous technique? Anesth Analg 67:578, 1988.
29. Stromskag KE, Minor B, Steen PA: Side effects and complications related to interpleural analgesia: An update. Acta Anaesth Scand 34:473, 1990.
30. Harrison P, Kent E, Lema M: Interpleural analgesia: Its use and complication in a quadriplegic patient with chronic pain. J Pain Symptom Manage 8:2150, 1993.

chapter 151

Splanchnic and Celiac Plexus Nerve Block

Steven D. Waldman and Richard B. Patt

HISTORICAL CONSIDERATIONS

In 1914, Kappis[1] introduced a percutaneous technique for blockade of the splanchnic nerves and celiac plexus with local anesthetic.[*] He described a posterior approach intended primarily for surgical anesthesia that used two needles, the tips of which were placed into the retroperitoneum via a retrocrural approach. He rapidly gained experience with this technique and reported on it in a series of 200 patients in 1918.[2]

The same year, Wendling[3] described a method of blocking the celiac plexus and splanchnic nerves using a single needle placed anteriorly through the liver. Judged to be riskier than Kappis' posterior approach, it rapidly fell into disfavor.

Labat, Farr, and others introduced further modifications of the Kappis technique over the ensuing 30 years.[4-6] Because of the technical demands and variable results of celiac plexus and splanchnic nerve block as a surgical anesthetic, over time, this technique was supplanted by spinal anesthesia and segmental blockade of the somatic paravertebral nerves.[7]

In the classic textbook *Conduction Anesthesia,* published in 1946, Pitkin,[8] surveying the status of the use of splanchnic nerve block for surgical anesthesia, wrote, "Posterior splanchnic block gained some popularity with a limited number of anesthetists, but because of unsatisfactory results, it was never continued beyond the experimental stage." There is no doubt that, as with many other regional anesthesia techniques, the introduction of neuromuscular blocking agents into the clinical practice of anesthesia led to the final demise of celiac plexus and splanchnic nerve block for surgical anesthesia, except at a limited number of institutions.

As celiac plexus and splanchnic nerve blocks were falling into disuse for surgical anesthesia, the clinical utility of these techniques was becoming apparent in the new specialty of pain management. In 1947, Gage and Floyd[9] described the use of celiac plexus and splanchnic nerve block in the management of pain secondary to pancreatitis. Esnaurrizar[10] and others recommended it to palliate abdominal pain secondary to a variety of causes. Recognizing the difficulty in distinguishing the somatic and visceral components of abdominal pain, Popper[11] recommended the use of splanchnic nerve block with local anesthetic as a diagnostic tool.

Alcohol neurolysis of the splanchnic nerves and celiac plexus for long-lasting relief of abdominal pain was first described by Jones[12] in 1957. Bridenbaugh and colleagues[13] reported on the role of neurolytic celiac plexus block to treat the pain of upper abdominal malignancy. In 1965, Moore[14] further modified original technique of Kappis and brought celiac plexus block into the mainstream of pain management practice.

In spite of these modifications over the last 80 years, the Kappis classic posterior approach to blockade of the celiac plexus and splanchnic nerves continues to serve as the basis for contemporary techniques. Interestingly, there is renewed interest in the anterior approach to celiac plexus block, using computed tomography or ultrasound to allow more accurate needle placement.[15,16]

INDICATIONS

Indications for celiac plexus block are several. Celiac plexus block with local anesthetic is indicated as a diagnostic tool to determine whether flank, retroperitoneal, or upper abdominal pain is sympathetically mediated via the celiac plexus.[17] Daily celiac plexus blocks with local anesthetic are also useful in the palliation of pain secondary to acute pancreatitis.[18,19] Clinical reports suggest that early implementation of celiac plexus block with local anesthetic and/or steroid markedly reduces the morbidity and mortality associated with acute pancreatitis.[20,21] Celiac plexus block is also used successfully to palliate the acute pain of arterial embolization of the liver for cancer therapy and to reduce the pain of abdominal "angina" associated with visceral arterial insufficiency.[22] Celiac plexus block with local anesthetic may be used for prognosis before performing celiac plexus neurolysis.[23]

*Note: There is significant confusion about the nomenclature for the neural structures that innervate the abdominal viscera. Different investigators have used a variety of terms, including splanchnic plexus, splanchnic nerve, solar plexus, and abdominal brain of Bichat, to describe all or some of the same structures. In this chapter, we have tried to use all neuroanatomic nomenclature in an "anatomically correct" manner whenever possible.

Neurolysis of the celiac plexus with alcohol or phenol is indicated to treat pain secondary to malignancies of the retroperitoneum and upper abdomen.[24,25] Neurolytic celiac plexus block may also be useful in some chronic benign abdominal pain syndromes, including chronic pancreatitis, in carefully selected patients.[26,27] Most investigators report a lower success rate when using celiac plexus and splanchnic nerve block to treat patients suffering from chronic nonmalignant abdominal pain as compared with the rate for abdominal pain of neoplastic origin.[23]

CONTRAINDICATIONS

Owing to the proximity to vascular structures, celiac plexus block is contraindicated in patients who are on anticoagulant therapy or who suffer from coagulopathy secondary to congenital abnormality, antiblastic cancer therapies, or liver abnormalities associated with ethanol abuse.[23,25] Local or intra-abdominal infection and sepsis represent absolute contraindications to celiac plexus block.

Because blockade of the celiac plexus results in greater bowel motility, the technique should be avoided in patients with bowel obstruction.[20] Neurolytic celiac plexus block should probably be deferred in patients who suffer from chronic abdominal pain, who are chemically dependent, or who exhibit drug-seeking behavior until these relative contraindications have been adequately addressed.[18] The use of alcohol as a neurolytic agent should be avoided in patients on disulfiram therapy for alcohol abuse.

CLINICALLY RELEVANT ANATOMY

To perform celiac plexus and splanchnic nerve block safely and effectively, it is necessary to understand the anatomy of the autonomic nervous system and the relationships of the anatomic structures surrounding the celiac plexus. Computed tomography (CT) has enhanced our understanding of the functional anatomy of the region and better documents where injected drugs are ultimately to be deposited. This information has been used to improve the efficacy and safety of celiac plexus and splanchnic nerve block.

The Autonomic Nervous System

The sympathetic innervation of the abdominal viscera originates in the anterolateral horn of the spinal cord (Fig. 151–1).[28] Preganglionic fibers from T5 through T12 exit the spinal cord in conjunction with the ventral roots to join the white communicating rami on their way to the sympathetic chain. Instead of synapsing with the sympathetic chain, these

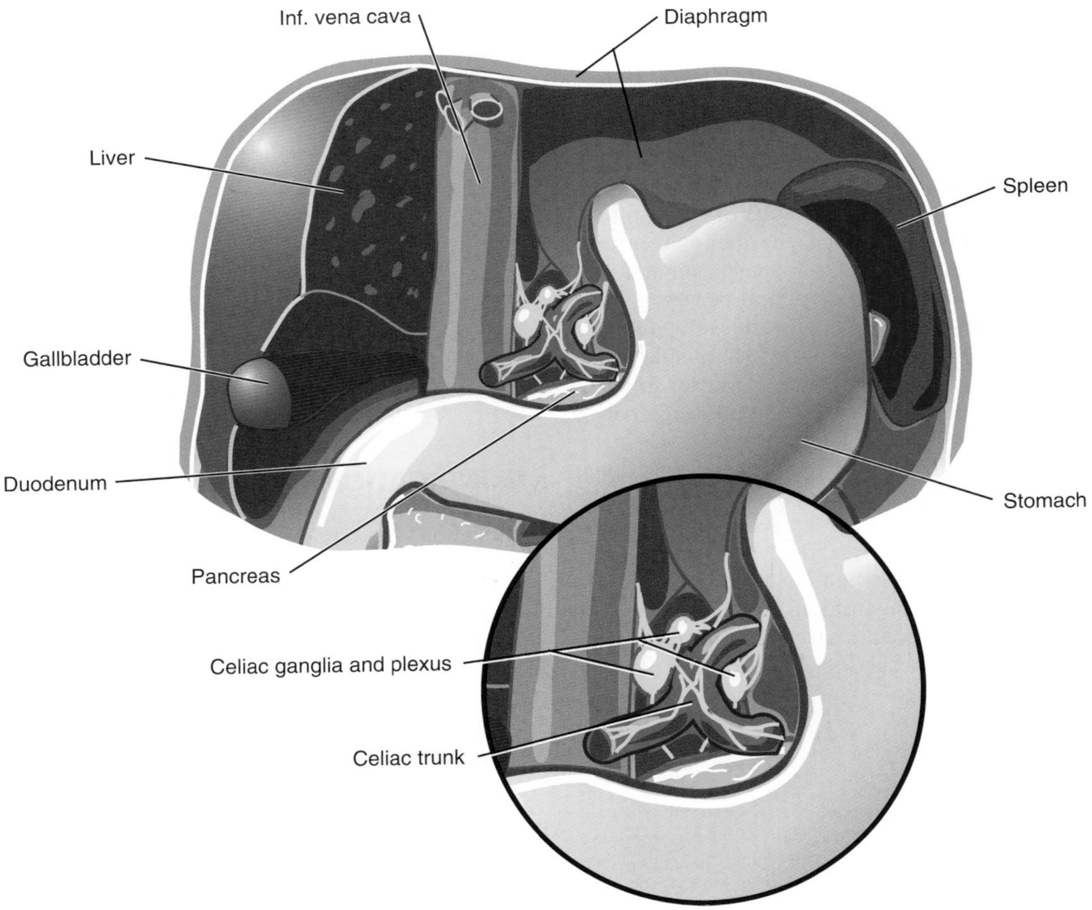

FIGURE 151–1 ■ The sympathetic innervation of the abdominal viscera.

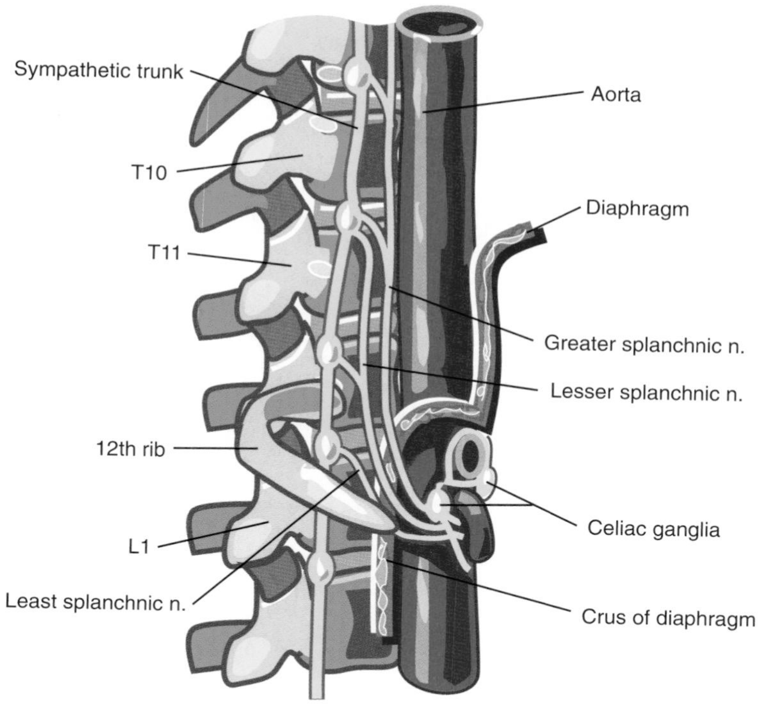

FIGURE 151–2 ■ The splanchnic nerves.

preganglionic fibers pass through it, ultimately to synapse on the celiac ganglia.[29]

The Splanchnic Nerves

The greater, lesser, and least splanchnic nerves provide the major preganglionic contribution to the celiac plexus (Fig. 151–2).[30] The greater splanchnic nerve has its origin from the T5-T10 spinal roots. The nerve travels along the thoracic paravertebral border, through the crus of the diaphragm, and into the abdominal cavity, ending on the ipsilateral celiac ganglion. The lesser splanchnic nerve arises from the T10-T11 roots and passes with the greater nerve to end at the celiac ganglion. The least splanchnic nerve arises from the T11-T12 spinal roots and passes through the diaphragm to the celiac ganglion. It is important to note that the greater, lesser, and least splanchnic nerves are *preganglionic* structures that synapse at the celiac ganglia.[20] Blockade limited solely to these nerves is properly termed *splanchnic nerve block* (see later).

The Celiac Ganglia

The three splanchnic nerves synapse at the celiac ganglia (see Fig. 151–2). Despite significant variability among patients of the anatomy of the celiac ganglia, the following generalizations can be drawn from anatomic studies.[31] The number of ganglia ranges from one to five and their diameters from 0.5 to 4.5 cm. The ganglia lie anterior and anterolateral to the aorta. The ganglia located on the left are uniformly farther inferior than their right-sided counterparts by as much as a vertebral level, but both groups of ganglia lie below the level of the celiac artery. In most instances, the ganglia lie approximately at the level of L1.

Postganglionic fibers radiate from the celiac ganglia along the course of the blood vessels and innervate the abdominal viscera, which are derived from the embryonic foregut[25] (i.e., much of the distal esophagus, stomach, duodenum, small intestine, ascending and proximal transverse colon, adrenal glands, pancreas, spleen, liver, and biliary system).

The Celiac Plexus

Ganglia and *plexus* are often used interchangeably, but, in point of fact, the ganglia and their respective dense network of preganglionic and postganglionic fibers constitute the celiac plexus. Anatomically, the celiac plexus arises from the preganglionic splanchnic nerves, vagal preganglionic parasympathetic fibers, sensory fibers from the phrenic nerve, and postganglionic sympathetic fibers.[28]

The celiac plexus is anterior to the diaphragmatic crura.[32] It extends in front of and around the aorta, the greatest concentration of fibers being anterior to the aorta (see Fig. 151–2). Blockade of these neural structures, which include the afferent fibers carrying nociceptive information, is properly termed *celiac plexus block.* It should be noted that the phrenic nerve also transmits nociceptive information from the upper abdominal viscera,[28] which may be perceived as poorly localized pain referred to the supraclavicular region.

Structures Surrounding the Celiac Plexus

The relation of the celiac plexus to the surrounding structures is depicted in Figure 151–3. The normal configuration of these structures may be dramatically distorted owing to organomegaly or tumor. The aorta lies anterior and slightly to

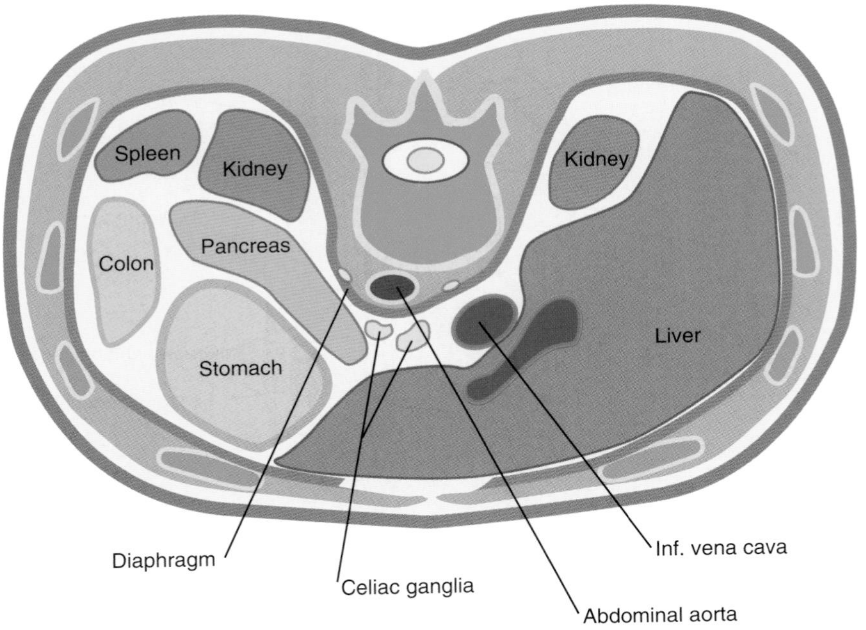

FIGURE 151–3 ■ The structures surrounding the celiac plexus.

the left of the anterior margin of the vertebral body. The inferior vena cava lies to the right of the midline, and the kidneys are posterolateral to the great vessels. The pancreas lies anterior to the celiac plexus. All of these structures lie within the retroperitoneal space.

TECHNIQUE OF CELIAC PLEXUS AND SPLANCHNIC NERVE BLOCK

The Classic Retrocrural Technique

The technique of celiac plexus block that is traditionally taught and, thus, most commonly used by anesthesiologists for blocking the celiac plexus, is the retrocrural technique first described by Kappis[2] and subsequently refined and popularized by Moore.[14]

As with other techniques for celiac plexus and splanchnic nerve block, preparation includes administration of intravenous fluids to attenuate the hypotension associated with neural blockade of these structures. Evaluation for coagulopathy is especially indicated in those patients who have undergone antiblastic therapy or who have a history of significant alcohol abuse.[23] If radiographic contrast is to be used, evaluation of the patient's renal function is indicated as well.

The patient is placed in the prone position with a pillow beneath the abdomen to reverse the thoracolumbar lordosis. This position increases the distance between the costal margins and the iliac crests and between the transverse processes of adjacent vertebral bodies. For comfort, the patient's head is turned to the side, and the arms are permitted to hang freely off the sides of the table. The operative field is prepared and draped in standard aseptic manner.

Some clinicians find it beneficial to delineate the pertinent landmarks on the skin with a sterile marker. The landmarks include the iliac crests, 12th ribs, dorsal midline, vertebral bodies (T12-L2), and lateral borders of the paraspinal (sacrospinalis) muscles (Fig. 151–4). Moore[14] recommends that the intersection of the 12th rib and the lateral border of the paraspinal muscles on each side (which corresponds to L2) be marked and connected with lines to each other and to the cephalic portion of the L1 spine, forming an isosceles triangle, the sides of which serve as an additional guide to needle positioning.

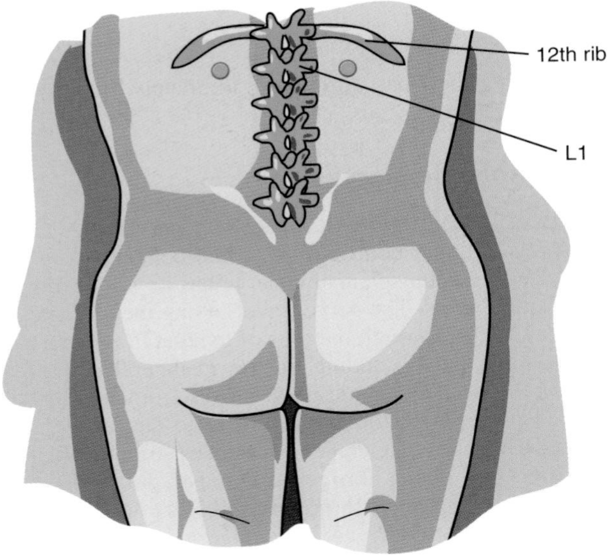

FIGURE 151–4 ■ Topographic landmarks for celiac plexus block.

The skin and underlying subcutaneous tissues and musculature are infiltrated with 1.0% lidocaine at the points of needle entry, which is about four fingerbreadths (7.5 cm) lateral to the midline, just beneath the 12th ribs. Either 20- or 22-gauge, 13-cm stylet needles are inserted bilaterally

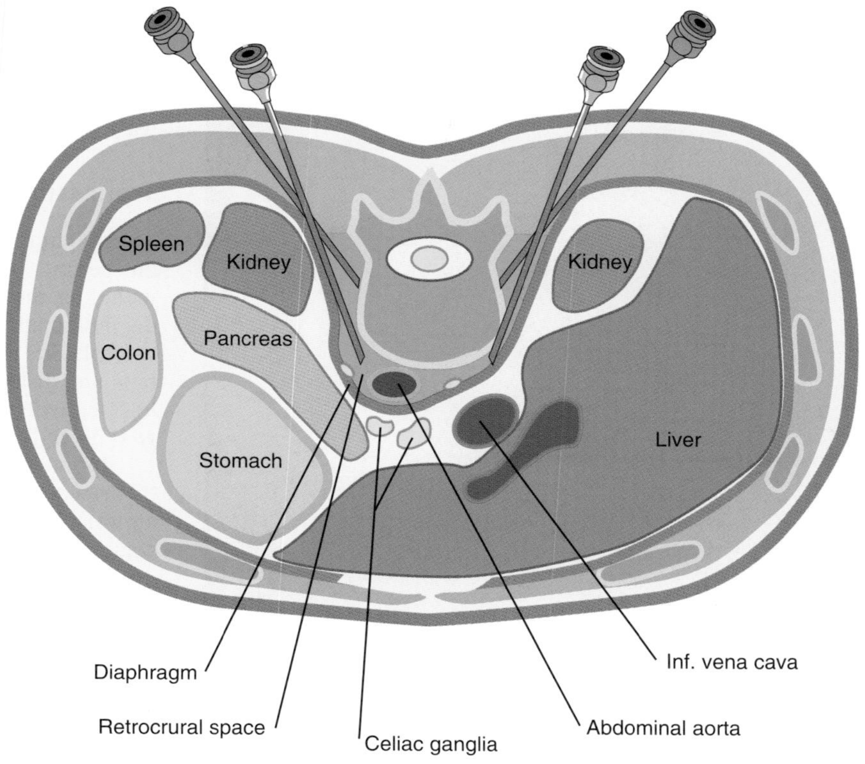

FIGURE 151–5 ■ Needle placement for "classic" celiac plexus block.

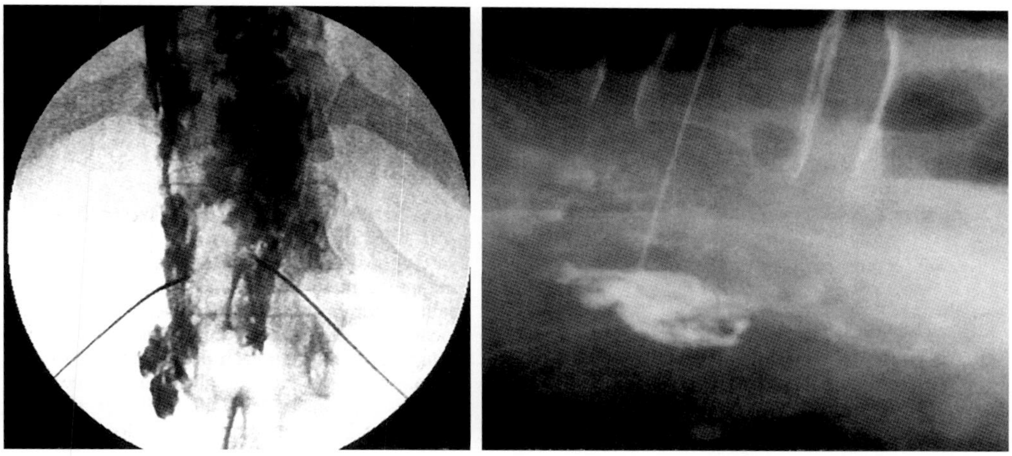

FIGURE 151–6 ■ Anteroposterior fluoroscopic view of the midline placement of contrast agent at L1.

through the previously anesthetized areas. The needles are initially oriented 45 degrees toward the midline and about 15 degrees cephalad, to ensure contact with the L1 vertebral body (Fig. 151–5). Once contact with the vertebral body has been verified, the depth at which bone contact occurred is noted. (Some clinicians find it useful to actually mark this measurement on the shaft of the needle with a sterile gentian violet marker after the needle is withdrawn.)

After bone contact is made and the depth is noted, the needles are withdrawn to the level of the subcutaneous tissue and redirected slightly less mesiad (about 60 degrees from the midline) so as to "walk off" the lateral surface of the L1 vertebral body. The needles are reinserted to the depth at which contact with the vertebral body was first noted. At this point, if no contact with bone is made, the left-sided needle is gradually advanced 1.5 to 2 cm or until the pulsations emanating from the aorta and transmitted to the advancing needle are felt.[33,34] The right-sided needle is then advanced slightly farther (i.e., 3 to 4 cm past contact with the vertebral body). Ultimately, the tips of the needles should be just posterior to the aorta on the left and to the anterolateral aspect of the aorta on the right (see Fig. 151–5).

The stylets are removed, and the needle hubs are inspected for blood, cerebrospinal fluid, and urine. If radiographic guidance is being used, a small volume of contrast material is injected bilaterally and its spread is observed radiographically.

Ideally, on the fluoroscopic anteroposterior view, contrast material is confined to the midline and concentrated near the L1 vertebral body (Fig. 151–6). A smooth posterior contour

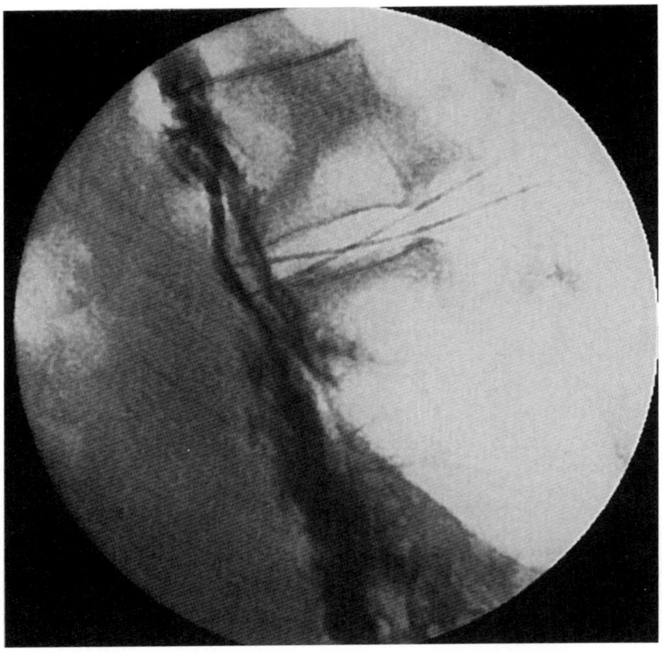

FIGURE 151–7 ■ Lateral fluoroscopic view of contrast agent bounded by psoas fascia.

can be observed that corresponds to the psoas fascia on the lateral view (Fig. 151–7).

Alternatively, if CT guidance is used, contrast material should appear lateral to and behind the aorta. If contrast material is confined entirely to the retrocrural space, the needles should be advanced to the precrural space to minimize the risk of posterior spread of local anesthetic or neurolytic agent to the somatic nerve roots (see later).[35]

If radiographic guidance is not used, a local anesthetic with rapid onset and in sufficient concentration to produce motor block (such as 1.5% lidocaine or 3.0% 2-chloroprocaine) is given before administration of neurolytic agents. If the patient experiences no motor or sensory block after an adequate waiting time, it is likely that additional drugs injected through the needles will not reach the somatic nerve roots if given in similar volumes.

For diagnostic and prognostic block using the retrocrural technique, 12 to 15 mL of 1.0% lidocaine or 3.0% 2-chloroprocaine is administered through each needle.[18] For therapeutic local anesthetic block, 10 to 12 mL of 0.5% bupivacaine is administered through each needle. Owing to the potential for local anesthetic toxicity, all local anesthetics should be administered in incremental doses.[24] For treatment of the pain of acute pancreatitis, an 80-mg dose of depot methylprednisolone is advocated for the initial celiac plexus block, and 40 mg for subsequent blocks.[36]

Most investigators suggest that 10 to 12 mL of 50% ethyl alcohol or 6.0% aqueous phenol be injected through each needle for retrocrural neurolytic block. Thomson and colleagues,[34] however, strongly recommend that 25 mL of 50% ethyl alcohol be injected via each needle.

After the neurolytic solution has been injected, each needle should be flushed with sterile saline solution. (There have been anecdotal reports of neurolytic solution being tracked posteriorly along with the needles as they are withdrawn.) Radiographic guidance, in particular CT guidance, offers the pain specialist an added margin of safety when performing neurolytic celiac plexus block and thus should be used whenever possible.

Transcrural Techniques

The diaphragm separates the thoracic and abdominal cavities but permits the passage of the thoracoabdominal structures, including the aorta, vena cava, and splanchnic nerves. The diaphragmatic crura are bilateral structures that arise from the anterolateral surfaces of the upper two or three lumbar vertebrae and disks. The crura of the diaphragm serve as a barrier to effectively separate the splanchnic nerves from the celiac ganglia and plexus below.[28]

In the modified Kappis approach to celiac plexus block, described previously, the needles are behind the crura in almost all instances. That is to say, the needles and injected solution are placed posterior and cephalad to the crura of the diaphragm. On the basis of CT and cadaver studies, it has been suggested that the classic method of retrocrural block is more likely to produce splanchnic nerve block rather than blockade of the celiac plexus. Instead of depositing injected material around and anterior to the aorta and directly onto the celiac plexus at the level of the L1 vertebral body, as was previously thought, the injectate appears to (1) concentrate posterior to the aorta and in front of and along the side of the L1 vertebral body, where it may anesthetize retroaortic celiac fibers; (2) diffuse cephalad to anesthetize the splanchnic nerve at a site rostrad to the origin of the plexus; and (3) finally encircle the aorta at the site of the celiac plexus only when a sufficient volume of drug is injected to transgress the diaphragm by diffusing caudad through the aortic hiatus.[33,37]

Although the retrocrural approach has been shown to be generally effective and safe, advocates of the transcrural approaches believe that simple modifications maximize the spread of injected solutions anterior to the aorta, where the celiac plexus is most concentrated, and minimize the risk of somatic nerve root blocks. The term *transcrural* reflects placement of needle tips and drug anterior and caudal to the diaphragmatic crura.

Singler[37] and Boas[62] recommend a transcrural approach using, respectively, CT scan and fluoroscopic guidance as important modifications of the traditional retrocrural technique. Transcrural block is carried out in a manner essentially the same as that for retrocrural block, except that needles are advanced farther anteriorly. Slightly smaller volumes of local anesthetic and neurolytic agents are used for the bilateral transcrural approach. Efficacy equal to or slightly greater than that of the classic retrocrural approach is reported by most investigators.[38]

Transaortic Techniques

In 1983, Ischia and colleagues[39] introduced a new approach to transcrural celiac plexus block that involved placing a single needle on the left side and posteriorly through the aorta, to ensure that the injected drugs are placed in the precrural space directly onto the celiac plexus. This method is, in some respects, analogous to the transaxillary approach to brachial plexus block. The safety of the transaortic approach is suggested by previous experience with both axillary block and translumbar aortograms.[40]

Despite concerns about the potential for aortic trauma and subsequent occult retroperitoneal hemorrhage with the transaortic approach to celiac plexus block, it may, in fact, be safer than the classic two-needle posterior approach.[41,42] The lower incidence of complications is thought to be due in part to the use of a single fine needle rather than two larger ones. The fact that the aorta is relatively well-supported in this region by the diaphragmatic crura and prevertebral fascia also contributes to the technique's apparent relative safety.[41]

The transaortic approach to celiac plexus block has three additional advantages over the classic two-needle approach. First, it avoids the risks of neurologic complications related to posterior retrocrural spread of drugs. Second, the aorta provides a definitive landmark for needle placement when radiographic guidance is not available. Third, much smaller volumes of local anesthetic and neurolytic solutions are required to achieve efficacy equal to or greater than that of the classic retrocrural approach.[42]

Fluoroscopically Guided Transaortic Celiac Plexus Block

The fluoroscopically guided transaortic approach uses the usual landmarks for the posterior placement of a left-sided, 22-gauge, 13-cm stylet needle. Some investigators use a needle entry point 1.0 to 1.5 cm closer to the midline than that for the classic retrocrural approach, combined with a needle trajectory closer to the perpendicular, to reduce the incidence of renal trauma.

The needle is advanced with the goal of passing just lateral to the anterolateral aspect of the L1 vertebral body. If that vertebral body is encountered, the needle is withdrawn into the subcutaneous tissues and redirected in a manner analogous to that for the classic retrocrural approach. The stylet needle is gradually advanced until its tip rests in the posterior periaortic space. As the needle impinges on the posterior aortic wall, the operator feels transmitted aortic pulsations via the needle and greater resistance to its passage.

Passing the needle through the wall of the aorta has been likened to passing a needle through a large rubber band. Presence of the needle within the aortic lumen is evidenced by free flow of arterial blood when the stylet is removed. The stylet is replaced, and the needle is advanced until it impinges on the intraluminal anterior wall of the aorta. At this point, the operator again feels increased resistance to needle advancement. A pop is felt as the needle tip passes through the anterior aortic wall, indicating that it probably lies within the preaortic fatty connective tissue and the substance of the celiac plexus. A saline loss-of-resistance technique, as described earlier, may help in identification of the preaortic space.

Because the needle is sometimes inadvertently advanced beyond the retroperitoneal space into the peritoneal cavity, confirmatory fluoroscopic views of injected contrast medium are advised, especially when neurolytic blockade is to be done. On anteroposterior views, the contrast medium should be confined to the midline, with a tendency toward greater concentration around the lateral margins of the aorta. Lateral views should demonstrate a predominantly preaortic orientation extending from around T12 through L2, sometimes accompanied by pulsations.[25] Incomplete penetration of the anterior wall is indicated by a narrow longitudinal "line image."

Failure of the contrast medium to completely surround the anterior aorta may occur in the presence of extensive infiltration of the preaortic region by tumor or in patients who have undergone previous pancreatic surgery or radiation therapy. It is our experience that the chance of success is smaller when poor or irregular preaortic spread of contrast is observed. In this setting, selective alcohol neurolysis of the splanchnic nerves may provide better pain relief.

For diagnostic and prognostic block using the fluoroscopically guided transaortic technique, 10 to 12 mL of 1.5% lidocaine or 3.0% 2-chloroprocaine is administered through the needle. For therapeutic block, 10 to 12 mL of 0.5% bupivacaine is administered. Owing to the potential for local anesthetic toxicity, all local anesthetics should be administered in incremental doses. For treatment of the pain of acute pancreatitis, the same dosages of depot methylprednisolone mentioned previously for the retrocrural and transcrural techniques are indicated. Absolute alcohol or 6.0% aqueous phenol, 12 to 15 mL, is used for neurolytic block.

CT-Guided Transaortic Celiac Plexus Block

The CT-guided transaortic celiac plexus block is probably the safest way to achieve neurolysis of the celiac plexus. CT allows the pain management physician to clearly identify the clinically relevant anatomy, including the crura of the diaphragm, aorta, vena cava, and kidneys, to ensure accurate precrural needle placement. Observation of the spread of contrast medium, as described here, enables the physician to know exactly where the injectate is deposited, and provides an added margin of patient safety in comparison with fluoroscopic or blind techniques.

The patient is prepared for CT-guided transaortic celiac plexus block just as for the techniques described earlier. After proper positioning on the CT scanning table, a scout film is obtained to identify the T12-L1 interspace (Fig. 151–8). A CT image is then taken through the interspace. The scan is reviewed for the position of the aorta relative to the vertebral body, the position of intra-abdominal and retroperitoneal organs, and any distortions of normal anatomy by tumor, previous surgery, or adenopathy (Fig. 151–9). The aorta at this level is evaluated for significant aortic aneurysm, mural thrombus, or calcifications; any of these would recommend against use of a transaortic approach.[23]

The level at which the scan was taken is identified on the patient's skin and marked with a gentian violet marker. The skin is prepared with antiseptic solution. The skin, subcutaneous tissues, and muscle at a point approximately 2.5 inches from the left of the midline is anesthetized with 1.0% lidocaine. A 13-cm, 22-gauge stylet needle is placed through the anesthetized area and is advanced until the posterior wall of the aorta is encountered, as evidenced by transmission of arterial pulsations and greater resistance to needle advancement. The needle is advanced into the lumen of the aorta. The stylet is removed, and the needle hub is observed for free flow of arterial blood (Fig. 151–10).

A well-lubricated 5-mL glass syringe filled with preservative-free saline is attached to the needle hub. The needle and syringe are then advanced through the anterior wall of the aorta using a loss-of-resistance technique in the same way that it is used to identify the epidural space.[43] The glass syringe is

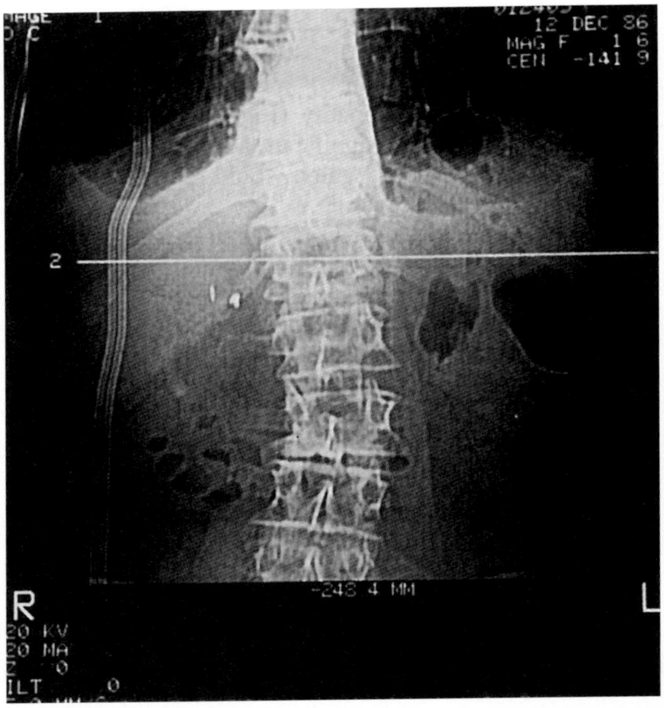

FIGURE 151–8 ■ Identification of the T12-L1 interspace for CT-guided transaortic celiac plexus block.

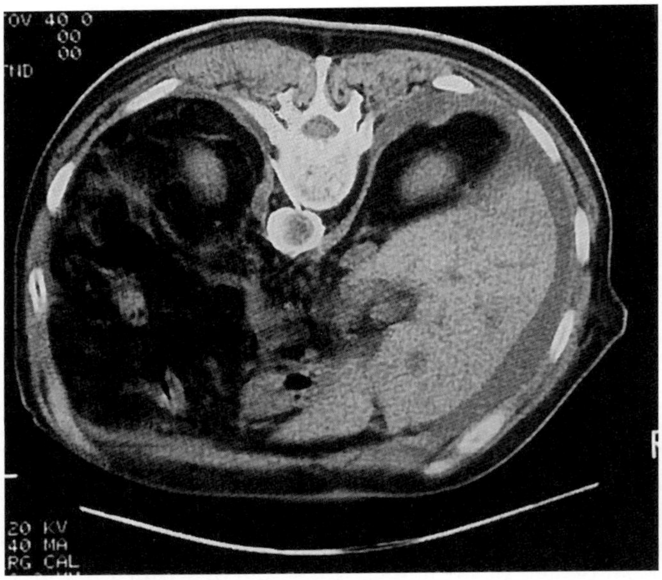

FIGURE 151–9 ■ CT scan through the T12-L1 interspace.

removed, and 3.0 mL of 1.5% lidocaine in solution with an equal amount of water-soluble contrast medium is injected through the needle.

A CT scan at the level of the needle's tip is taken. The scan is reviewed for the placement of the needle and, most importantly, for the spread of contrast medium,[23] which should be seen in the preaortic area and surrounding the aorta (Fig. 151–11). No contrast medium should be observed in the retrocrural space (Fig. 151–12). After proper needle

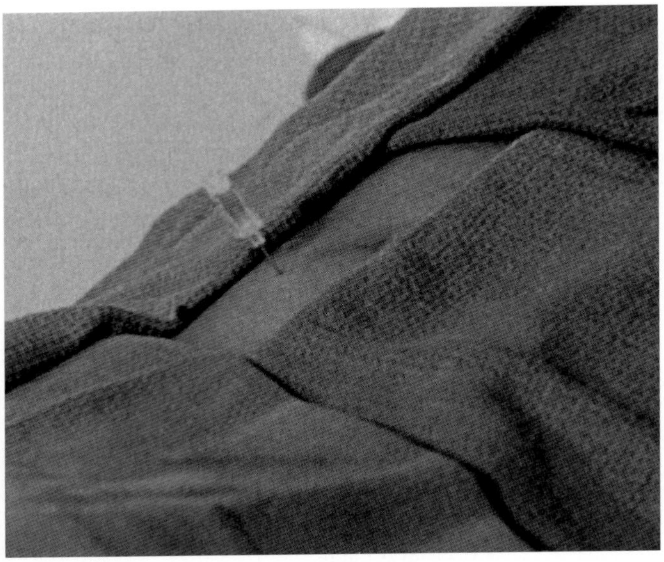

FIGURE 151–10 ■ Needle in position with tip in lumen of aorta.

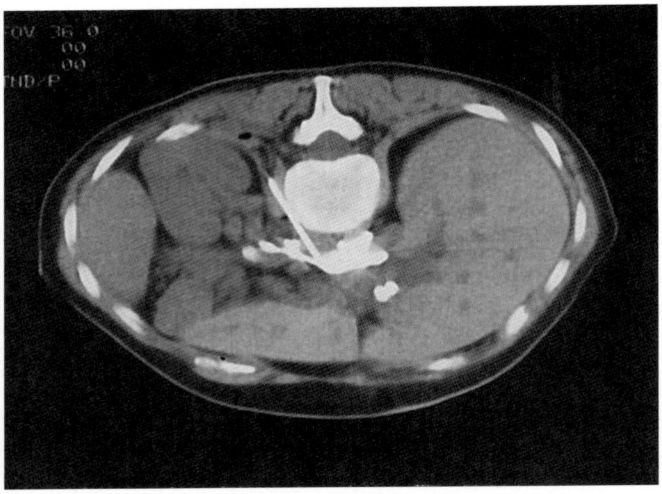

FIGURE 151–11 ■ Preaortic spread of contrast agent.

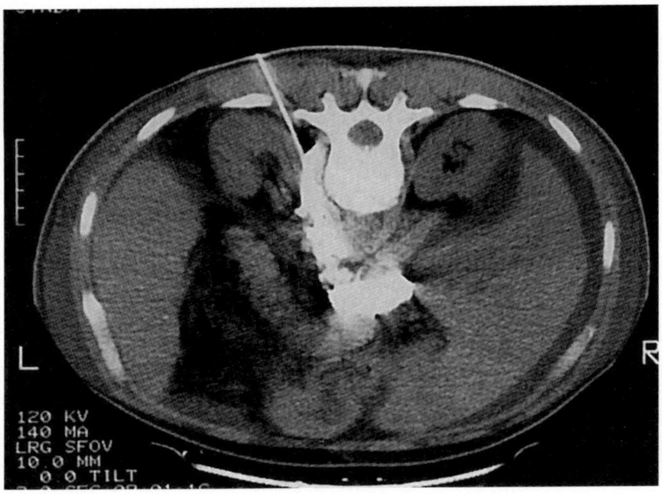

FIGURE 151–12 ■ Retrocrural spread of contrast agent.

placement and spread of contrast medium is confirmed, 12 to 15 mL of absolute alcohol or 6% aqueous phenol is injected through the needle.[42] The needle is flushed with a small amount of sterile saline and then removed. The patient is observed carefully for hemodynamic changes, including hypotension and tachycardia secondary to the resulting profound sympathetic blockade.

Lieberman and Waldman[43] reported on the success and efficacy of transaortic celiac plexus block using the loss-of-resistance technique in a large series of patients suffering from cancer pain.[43] In this study, 91% of patients reported marked immediate pain relief after CT-guided transaortic celiac plexus block using the loss-of-resistance technique. At 6 weeks, 39% of surviving patients were pain free and did not require opioid analgesics. An additional 50% of patients reported great improvement but required adjunctive treatment with opioids. No unusual complications or side effects were encountered in this large series of patients.

Anterior Approaches to Celiac Plexus Block

Percutaneous Gangliolysis

A percutaneous anterior approach to the celiac plexus was advocated early in this century, only to be abandoned because of the high incidence of complications.[3,44] The advent of fine needles, improvements in radiologic guidance technology, and the maturation of the specialty of interventional radiology have since led to renewed interest in the anterior approach to blockade of the celiac plexus.

Extensive experience with transabdominal fine-needle aspiration biopsy has confirmed the relative safety of this approach and provides the rationale and method for the modification of this radiologic technique for anterior celiac plexus block. The anterior approach to the celiac plexus necessarily involves the passage of a fine needle through the liver, stomach, intestine, vessels, and pancreas. Surprisingly, it is associated with very low rates of complications.[45-48]

Advantages of the anterior approach to blocking the celiac plexus include its relative ease, speed, and reduced periprocedural discomfort as compared with posterior techniques.[16,25] Perhaps the greatest advantage of the anterior approach is the fact that patients are spared having to remain prone for long periods, which can be a significant problem for patients suffering from intra-abdominal pain. The supine position is also advantageous for patients with iliostomies and colostomies.

The anterior approach is probably associated with less discomfort because only one needle is used. The needle does not impinge on either periosteum or nerve roots or pass through the bulky paraspinous musculature. Because needle placement is precrural, there is less risk of accidental neurologic injury related to retrocrural spread of drug to somatic nerve roots or epidural and subarachnoid spaces.

Potential disadvantages of the anterior approach to celiac plexus block include the risks of infection, abscess, hemorrhage, and fistula formation.[46] Although preliminary findings indicate that these complications are exceedingly rare, further experience is needed to draw a definitive conclusion. By the same token, although preliminary data suggest the efficacy of the anterior approach, further experience is needed to permit adequate comparisons with better-established techniques.

The anterior technique can be carried out under CT or ultrasound guidance. Patient preparation is similar to that for posterior approaches to celiac block. The patient is placed in the supine position on the CT or ultrasound table. The skin of the upper abdomen is prepared with antiseptic solution. The needle entry site is identified 1.5 cm below and 1.5 cm to the left of the xyphoid process (Fig. 151–13).[45] At that point, the skin, subcutaneous tissues, and musculature are anesthetized with 1.0% lidocaine. A 22-gauge, 15-cm needle is introduced through the anesthetized area perpendicular to the skin and advanced to the depth of the anterior wall of the aorta, as calculated using CT or ultrasound guidance (Figs. 151–14 and 151–15).

If CT guidance is being used, 4 mL of water-soluble contrast in solution with an equal volume of 1.0% lidocaine is injected to confirm needle placement (Fig. 151–16). If ultrasound guidance is being used, 10 to 12 mL of sterile saline can be injected to help confirm needle position (Fig. 151–17).[16] After satisfactory needle placement is confirmed, diagnostic and prognostic block is carried out using 15 mL of 1.5% lidocaine or 3.0% 2-chloroprocaine. Therapeutic block is performed with an equal volume of 0.5% bupivacaine. Owing to the potential for local anesthetic toxicity, all local anesthetics should be administered in incremental doses.

Matamala and associates[16] recommend 35 to 40 mL of 50% ethyl alcohol for neurolytic blocks of the celiac plexus via the anterior approach. Other investigators have had equally good results using 15 to 20 mL of absolute alcohol.

An alternative technique uses fluoroscopy to guide the passage of a single needle just to the right of the center of the L1 vertebral body, after which it is withdrawn 1 to 3 cm.[45] Important precautions for the anterior approach to celiac plexus block include the administration of prophylactic antibiotics and the use of needles no larger than 22 gauge to minimize the risks of infection and trauma to the vasculature and viscera.

Intraoperative Gangliolysis

The intraoperative anterior approach to the blockade of the celiac plexus and splanchnic nerves was first advocated by Braun[4] in 1921 as a means to provide intraoperative visceral anesthesia. This technique was used in combination with field block of the abdominal wall. Braun's approach involved gentle retraction of the stomach and placement of a digit between the aorta and vena cava to serve as a guide to the injection of an anesthetic over the ventral surface of the L1 vertebral body. This technique enjoyed only limited acceptance for surgical anesthesia for abdominal operations.

In 1978, Kraft and associates described a similar approach to block the splanchnic nerves and celiac plexus for pain management.[49,50] They identified the origin of the celiac artery and advanced a 20-gauge spinal needle over the exploring finger. Then, 15 to 20 mL of 6% aqueous phenol was injected intraoperatively.

The main advantage of intraoperative celiac block is the elimination of a separate procedure for pain control. In addition, intraoperative celiac block provides an opportunity to prophylactically treat the patient with only mild or no pain who is known to have an intra-abdominal malignancy that in all likelihood will produce pain as it progresses.

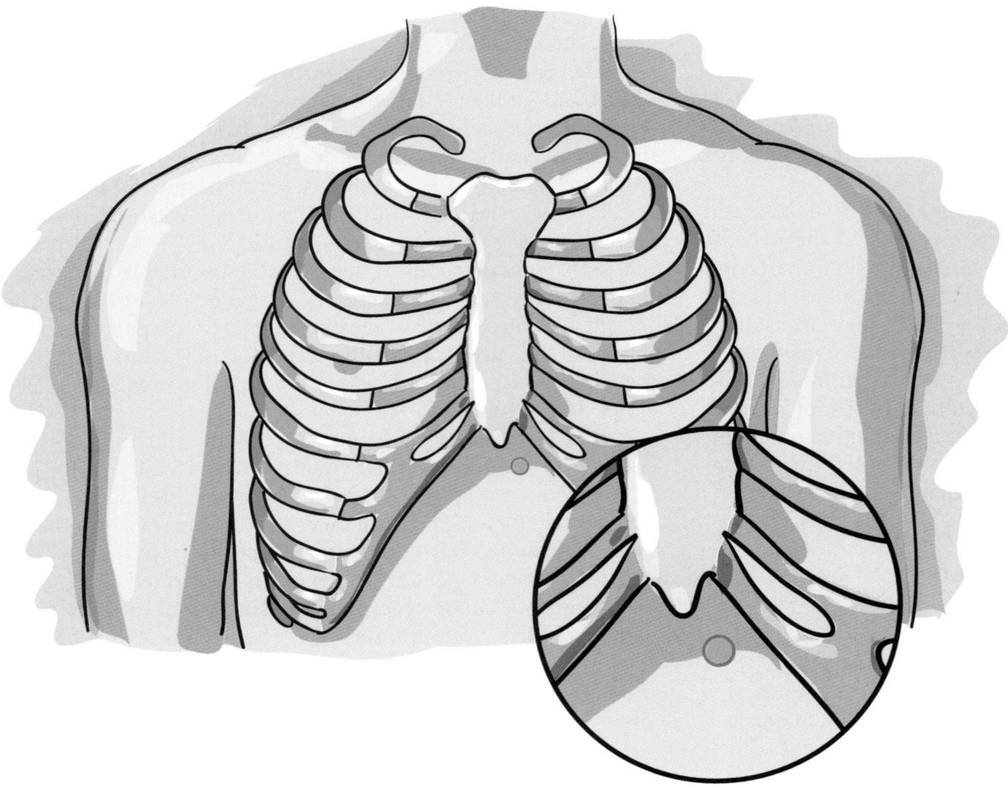

FIGURE 151–13 ■ Needle entry site for anterior celiac plexus block. Inset, The site is located 1.5 cm below and 1.5 cm to the left of the xyphoid process.

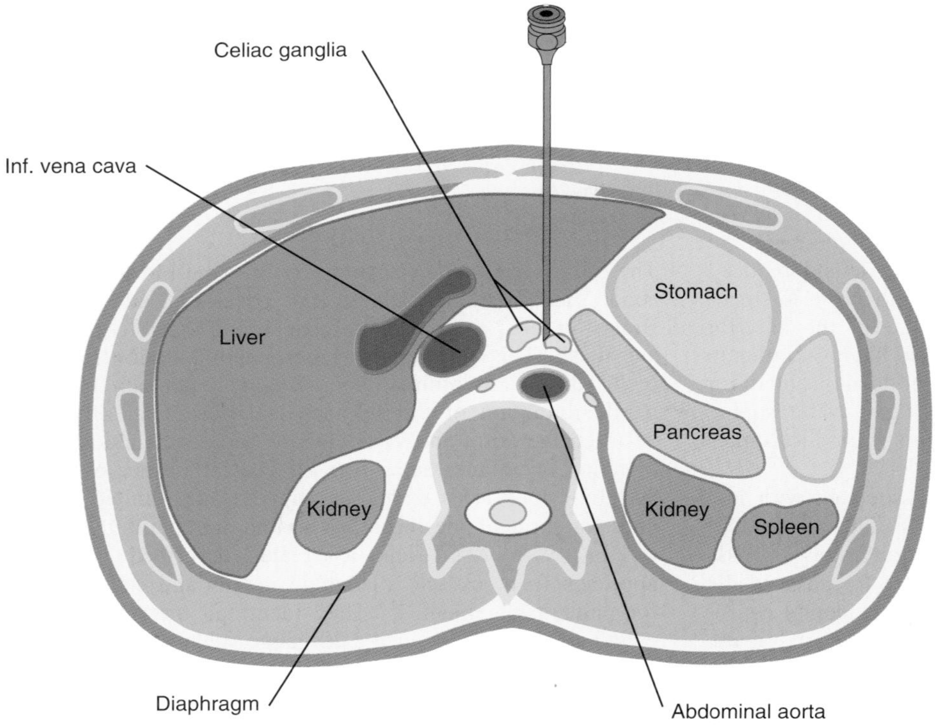

FIGURE 151–14 ■ Needle placement for anterior celiac plexus block.

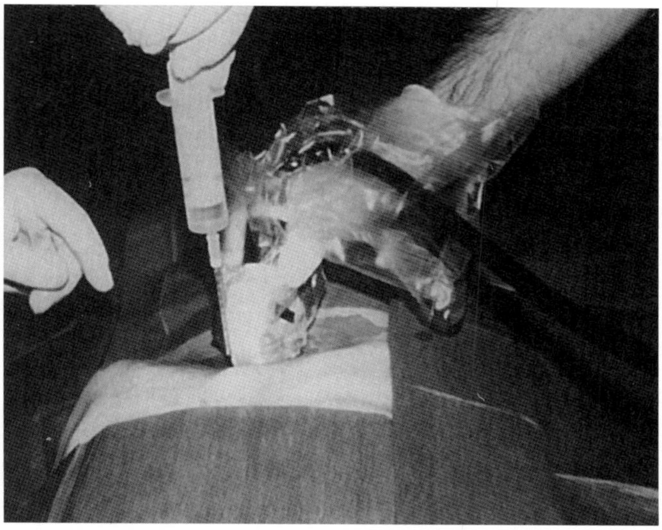

FIGURE 151–15 ■ Anterior celiac plexus block.

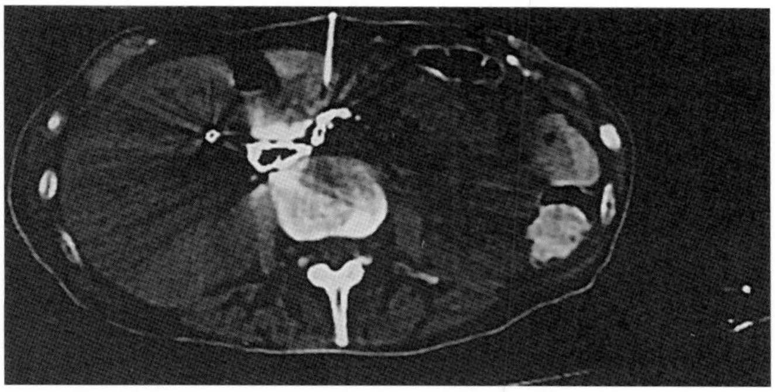

FIGURE 151–16 ■ CT scan confirms proper needle placement for anterior celiac plexus block.

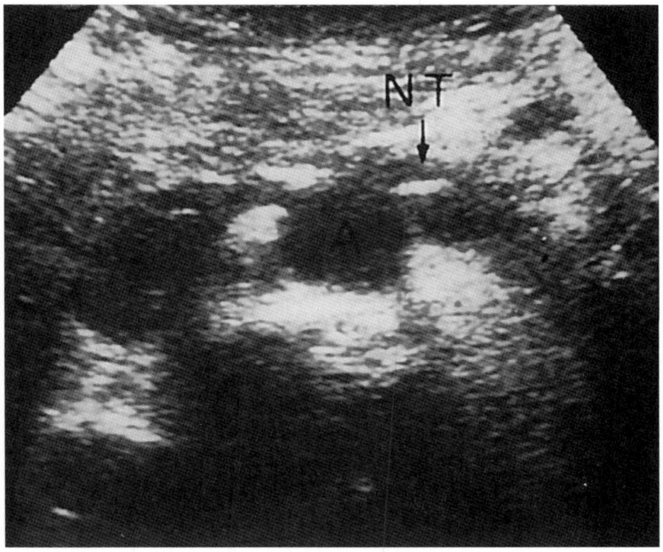

FIGURE 151–17 ■ Ultrasonogram confirms proper needle placement for anterior celiac plexus block.

Disadvantages of intraoperative anterior celiac plexus neurolysis include the unfamiliarity of most surgeons with (1) the functional regional anatomy, (2) injection techniques, and (3) the use of neurolytic agents required for the block.[25] Furthermore, safe access to the specified injection site may be prohibited by bulky intra-abdominal disease and phlegmon. Because intraoperative dissection may result in leakage of the injected solution out of the intended injection site, the risk of neurologic injury is increased and the overall efficacy is decreased.[25] Concurrent general anesthesia renders a test dosing with local anesthetic invalid and further raises the patient's risk, because of the patient's inability to report untoward reactions to the local anesthetic.

Given the current availability of effective percutaneous methods of achieving celiac block, intraoperative celiac plexus block cannot be recommended except when laparotomy is already planned for exploration or bypass of the gastrointestinal or biliary tract.[49] Even in these cases, the efficacy and relative safety of the technique are controversial. A valuable alternative in such cases is placement of surgical clips in the vicinity of the celiac axis to facilitate postoperative neural blockade.[51]

Catheter Techniques

Anecdotal reports documenting the efficacy and safety of temporary periaortic catheters to facilitate daily celiac nerve blocks have been presented.[52,53] A percutaneous polytetrafluoroethylene periaortic catheter was in place for 14 days in a patient with pancreatitis, during which time serial injections of local anesthetic were administered before a definitive neurolytic block was performed.[54] Fluoroscopy and CT performed 13 days after placement revealed no catheter migration and no perivascular erosion or pleural reaction. A second report, documenting a single case of intraoperative placement of a percutaneously tunneled epidural catheter that was used after surgery to produce neurolysis suggests another potential treatment option.[55] In a third report, after a temporary periaortic catheter was placed percutaneously, the patient had persistent hematuria, and evidence of transrenal catheter placement was obtained. That case suggests that CT guidance may be advisable during placement of percutaneous catheters for celiac plexus block.[28]

At present, indications for periaortic catheterization are ill-defined. If shown to be safe and efficacious, this approach may ultimately prove beneficial in patients with chronic nonmalignant conditions.

Splanchnic Nerve Block

The recognition that splanchnic nerve block may provide relief of pain in a subset of patients who fail to obtain relief from celiac plexus block has renewed interest in this technique.[25,56] The splanchnic nerves transmit the majority of nociceptive information from the viscera.[28] These nerves are contained in a narrow compartment made up by the vertebral body and the pleura laterally, the posterior mediastinum ventrally, and the pleural attachment to the vertebra dorsally. This compartment is bounded caudally by the crura of the diaphragm. Abram and Boas[56] have determined that the volume of this compartment is approximately 10 mL on each side.

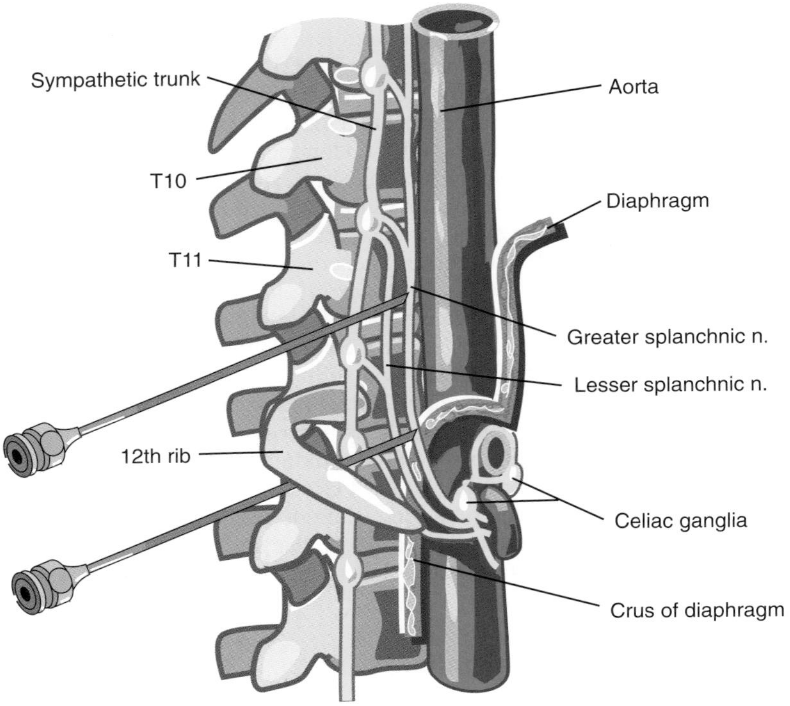

FIGURE 151–18 ■ Splanchnic nerve block.

The technique for splanchnic nerve block differs little from the classic retrocrural approach to the celiac plexus, except that the needles are aimed more cephalad so as to rest ultimately at the anterolateral margin of the T12 vertebral body (Fig. 151–18). It is imperative that both needles be placed medially against the vertebral body to reduce the incidence of pneumothorax.

An alternative approach to splanchnic nerve block uses 22-gauge, 3.5-inch spinal needles.[57] The needles are placed 3 to 4 cm lateral to the midline, just below the 12th ribs. Their trajectory is slightly mesiad, so that the tips come to rest at the anterolateral margin of the T12 body.

Abram and Boas[56] have described a simplified technique for splanchnic nerve block that uses a paravertebral transthoracic approach. Standard 22-gauge, 3.5-inch spinal needles are introduced bilaterally 6 cm from the midline through the 11th intercostal space (see Fig. 151–18). The needle is advanced to rest against the anterolateral aspect of the T11 vertebral body. Precautions include attendance to a medial entry point and observation of the lower limit of the lung, which during quiet breathing is generally observed to lie one segment higher in the costophrenic angle. These precautions allow the needles to safely traverse the transpleural spaces. If experience eventually demonstrates that this simplified technique is comparable in safety and efficacy to the more difficult classic technique, it will clearly become the procedure of choice for splanchnic nerve block.

For diagnostic and prognostic splanchnic nerve block, 7 to 10 mL of 1.5% lidocaine or 3.0% 2-chloroprocaine is administered through the needle; for therapeutic block, 7 to 10 mL of 0.5% bupivacaine. Owing to the potential for local anesthetic toxicity, all local anesthetics should be administered in divided doses. A 10-mL volume of absolute alcohol or 6.0% aqueous phenol is used for neurolytic block.

The risks of splanchnic nerve block are similar to those of celiac plexus block. Additionally, the rates of pneumothorax, thoracic duct injury, and inadvertent spread of injected drugs to the somatic nerve roots are higher than those for transcrural approaches to celiac plexus block.[56] Because of the need for accurate needle placement, it is advisable to perform splanchnic nerve block under fluoroscopic or CT guidance.

CHOICE OF AGENT, VOLUME, NEEDLE, RADIOGRAPHIC GUIDANCE, AND TECHNIQUE

Choice of Agent

Investigators tend to disagree about the ideal volume, concentration, or drug for celiac plexus and splanchnic nerve blocks. Diagnostic and prognostic celiac plexus and splanchnic nerve blocks should be performed with a local anesthetic that has rapid onset and is sufficiently concentrated to produce sensory and motor block. For the classic two-needle retrocrural approach, a total volume of 20 to 25 mL of 1.0% lidocaine or 3.0% 2-chloroprocaine is appropriate. A volume of 12 to 15 mL is adequate for a single-needle transcrural approach to the celiac plexus block. Splanchnic nerve block is performed with 7 to 10 mL of 1.5% lidocaine or 3.0% 2-chloroprocaine. Similar volumes (as specified for each technique) of longer-acting local anesthetics such as 0.5% bupivacaine are used for therapeutic nerve block. Owing to the potential for local anesthetic toxicity, all local anesthetics should be administered in incremental doses. For the pain of inflammatory conditions such as pancreatitis, depot preparations of methylprednisolone may be administered in an initial dose of 80 mg and subsequent doses of 40 mg.

Neurolytic blockade of the celiac plexus and splanchnic nerves may be carried out with either ethyl alcohol or aqueous phenol. Because of limitations associated with the classic retrocrural technique, some authors have advocated 50 mL of 50% ethyl alcohol. Others have used concentrations of alcohol (25% to 100%) in volumes ranging from 20 to 80 mL without apparent differences in efficacy or side effects.[27,58,59] Smaller volumes (12 to 15 mL) of absolute alcohol are recommended for single-needle transcrural techniques.

Many investigators believe that as a neurolytic agent, alcohol is superior to phenol in duration of neural blockade; however, alcohol has the disadvantage of producing transient severe pain on injection. Furthermore, alcohol is not miscible with contrast medium. Unless alcohol is accidentally injected into a vessel, actual alcohol intoxication should not occur. Susceptible patients undergoing alcohol neurolysis may be subject to acetaldehyde syndrome, a relatively innocuous side effect (see discussion of complications).[34,60,61] Alcohol should be avoided in patients on disulfiram therapy for alcohol abuse.

Several workers have recommended 6% to 10% phenol for celiac plexus and splanchnic nerve block.[25,49,50] An advantage of phenol over alcohol is that it can be combined with contrast medium. The combination allows radiographic documentation of the distribution of neurolytic solution during and after injection, instead of relying on verification of needle placement before injection of neurolytic solution, as is necessary for alcohol injection. Mixtures of 10% phenol and iodinated contrast medium (Conray 420 or Renografin 76) remain stable up to 3 months.[62] The fact that phenol is not commercially available and must be prepared for each patient by a pharmacist is a practical disadvantage of this agent. The apparently greater affinity of phenol for vascular, rather than neurologic, tissue also represents a theoretical disadvantage, in view of the vascularity of the region surrounding the celiac plexus and splanchnic nerves.[63] Some investigators believe that phenol produces a block of shorter duration than that produced by alcohol, making it a less desirable agent for the intractable and progressive pain of cancer. It is important to note that controlled comparisons between alcohol and phenol for this application have not been conducted but they appear to be equally safe and efficacious.

Choice of Needles

Both 20- and 22-gauge needles have been advocated for celiac plexus and splanchnic nerve block. Thompson and Moore[58] note that the resistance to injection provided by a long 22-gauge needle interferes with the appreciation of differences in tissue compliance, which can provide much useful information about needle position.[58] In addition, owing to the greater flexibility of 22-gauge needles, it is more difficult to maintain a straight trajectory during placement.[28] If 22-gauge needles are used, it is advisable to rely on radiologic guidance to confirm needle placement. A 22-gauge needle is preferred for anterior and transaortic approaches.[64]

Choice of Radiographic Guidance

The use of radiologic guidance for celiac plexus and splanchnic nerve block was once very controversial. Today, it is in favor. Provided that proper precautions are observed, celiac plexus and splanchnic nerve block with local anesthetic can safely be accomplished by experienced practitioners relying on topographic guidance alone.[34] In our opinion, and that of others, radiologic guidance is virtually mandatory for neurolytic celiac plexus and splanchnic nerve block.[23,35] Interestingly, when large series of cases are compared, it is not clear that the use of fluoroscopy actually reduces the incidence of complications.[64] It does appear, however, that CT guidance may add a margin of safety as compared with fluoroscopy, although a small number of serious complications have been reported when CT has been used for celiac plexus block.[43,64] It is our strong belief that the use of radiographic guidance must still be encouraged on practical, empirical, and medicolegal grounds.

It is clear that even sophisticated radiologic guidance by itself does not ensure against complications. Routine application of simple precautionary measures, including careful serial aspiration and incremental injections of local anesthetic, is essential to minimize the likelihood of an adverse outcome. CT permits visualization of, not only bony structures, but also vascular and soft tissue elements (including diaphragmatic crura and tumor spread). It is particularly useful when anterior and transcrural approaches are planned. The disadvantages of CT include limited availability in some areas, the need for specialized support personnel, and the slightly higher cost relative to fluoroscopy.[28]

Choice of Technique

Numerous techniques have been advocated to achieve celiac plexus and splanchnic nerve block. Most of the experience is with the classic retrocrural technique, which, as a result, is regarded as the standard against which other techniques are compared. It is anticipated that the newer techniques for celiac plexus and splanchnic nerve block will gain greater acceptance as experience accrues because they appear safe and efficacious and offer certain practical and theoretical advantages. The transaortic approach is particularly attractive, because it requires only a single needle—the position of which is easily verifiable—ensuring anterior deposition of the drug.[43] The anterior approach, although it requires CT or ultrasound guidance, is quick and relatively painless. It is an excellent option for patients who cannot assume the prone position.[16] The transcrural approach, with or without CT, is theoretically more desirable than retrocrural techniques, because injectate spreads reliably around the aorta, thereby avoiding the somatic nerves.[28] Ultimately, the choice of technique should be individualized to the facility, the patient's physical status, the extent of tumor spread, and the clinician's experience and preparation.

COMPLICATIONS

In the hands of the skilled clinician, serious complications should rarely occur from celiac plexus and splanchnic nerve block. Because of the proximity of other vital structures, coupled with the use of large volumes of neurolytic drugs, the following side effects and complications may be seen:

- Hypotension
- Paresthesia of lumbar somatic nerve
- Intravascular injection (venous or arterial)
- Deficit of lumbar somatic nerve

- Subarachnoid or epidural injection
- Diarrhea
- Renal injury
- Paraplegia
- Pneumothorax
- Chylothorax
- Vascular thrombosis or embolism
- Vascular trauma
- Perforation of cysts or tumors
- Injection of the psoas muscle
- Intradiskal injection
- Abscess
- Peritonitis
- Retroperitoneal hematoma
- Urinary tract abnormalities
- Failure of ejaculation
- Pain during and after procedure
- Failure to relieve pain

Hypotension, Altered Gastrointestinal Motility, and Pain

Hypotension[65] and increased gastrointestinal motility occur to some extent in most patients following celiac plexus and splanchnic nerve block. The high frequency of these side effects dictates that they should be anticipated with either prophylactic treatment or a well-conceived management plan. Hypotension occurs as a result of regional vasodilation and pooling of blood within the splanchnic vessels. This side effect is more likely to occur in patients who are elderly, debilitated, and chronically or acutely dehydrated. Without prophylaxis, clinically significant hypotension can be expected in 30% to 60% of patients but may be prevented by administration of 500 to 1000 mL of balanced salt solution intravenously before the procedure.[58] Small increments of intravenous ephedrine are occasionally required, in addition to intravenous fluids, to maintain an adequate blood pressure. Careful monitoring of blood pressure during the procedure and the recovery period is mandatory. A gradual return to a sitting position is indicated to allow early identification and treatment of unrecognized orthostatic hypotension.

Gastrointestinal hypermotility may occur as a result of unopposed parasympathetic activity. It occasionally manifests as diarrhea, except in cancer patients, who tend to be chronically constipated from high doses of opioids. For them, the hypermotility improves bowel habits. Self-limited diarrhea lasting 36 to 48 hours has been reported in as many as 60% of patients after alcohol celiac block.[39] Unrecognized, this side effect can be life threatening.[66]

Although not a complication per se, pain can occur during and after celiac plexus and splanchnic nerve block. The interval to maximal pain relief after the procedure is variable. In the majority of patients, relief is immediate and complete; in others, it develops over a few days.[59] It is not uncommon for a patient to experience transient self-limited back or pleuritic pain after the procedure.[55]

Neurologic and Vascular Complications

Among 3000 cases of celiac plexus and splanchnic nerve block, Moore[58] reported 18 episodes of dural puncture (0.006%). In all but one case, it was manifested as the appearance of clear fluid in the needle hub.[58] In the majority of these cases, radiographic guidance was not used. The results of a more contemporary series suggest that this complication can be avoided by consistent use of radiographic guidance, as can epidural puncture. One case of unilateral paraplegia was reported in a patient who, because of obesity and ascites, was positioned laterally.[34] No form of radiologic guidance was used in that case. It is probable that paraplegia was the result of unrecognized injection of the psoas muscle that accidentally produced neurolysis of lumbar somatic nerve roots.

With the classic retrocrural technique, the anesthetic may track posteriorly (even when "correct" needle placement has been confirmed) and be deposited near somatic nerve roots. The consequent neurologic injury may manifest as numbness over the anterior thigh and lower abdominal wall and quadriceps weakness.[26] This complication is less likely when transcrural techniques are used.[37,43]

Another potential mechanism of neurologic injury is disruption of or accidental injection into the small nutrient vessels of the spinal cord (i.e., the artery of Adamkiewicz).[28] This mechanism was postulated to be responsible for the rapid development of persistent paraplegia after celiac plexus block with 6 mL of 6% aqueous phenol in a patient with carcinoma of the pancreas.[67] Neither test doses of local anesthetic nor radiologic guidance was used in this case. To avoid this serious complication, pre-neurolysis test doses of local anesthetic and either fluoroscopy to detect "vascular runoff" or CT guidance should be used to confirm exact needle placement.[68] It is not uncommon for larger vessels to be entered, either by accident or by intention.[43,64] An obvious and essential precaution, intermittent aspiration is not entirely reliable for detecting intravascular placement. Giving test doses of local anesthetics and using radiographic guidance decrease the incidence of this potentially lethal complication. Clinically significant bleeding and hematoma formation have not been reported in the literature, even after transaortic blocks. It is essential that each patient's coagulation status be investigated, and if necessary, optimized before the procedure.

Visceral Injury

The advent of CT guidance for celiac plexus and splanchnic nerve block revealed that perforation of adjacent viscera, including the kidney, occurred more often than we had appreciated. Renal puncture is characteristically a self-limited complication suggested by the appearance of transient hematuria. Accidental injection of an appreciable volume of neurolytic drug into the renal parenchyma, however, may produce serious injury and renal infarction. Moore[58] believes that renal puncture is more likely when (1) needles are inserted farther than 7.5 cm from the midline; (2) the needle tip comes to rest too far lateral to the vertebral body; and (3) a relatively higher vertebral body (T11) is targeted.

Careful attention to technique reduces the incidence of perforation of the viscera. The risk can be further reduced by using CT guidance. An obvious advantage of CT is the ability to visualize the anatomic relationships of visceral structures before and during needle placement.[36] This practice is particularly useful in patients whose normal anatomy is distorted because of a bulky tumor or a previous surgical insult.

Pneumothorax and Pleural Effusion

Pneumothorax may occur as a result of celiac plexus and splanchnic nerve block, even when the operator has radiologic guidance. This complication may or may not require tube thoracostomy. Pleural effusion after celiac plexus neurolysis has also been reported.[69] The proposed mechanism of pleural effusion is diaphragmatic irritation resulting from overflow of alcohol into the subdiaphragmatic space. Other suggested mechanisms include acute pancreatitis and hemorrhage. Chylothorax, an occasional complication of translumbar aortography, has been reported to have occurred on one occasion after phenol celiac plexus block.[70,71] Ejaculatory failure has also been reported after celiac plexus neurolysis.[72]

Metabolic Complications

Although accidental intravascular injection of alcohol could conceivably produce intoxication, several investigators have measured serum ethanol levels after celiac block and have determined that circulating levels are insufficient to produce systemic effects.[61,68,73] After 50 mL of 50% alcohol administered via the classic retrocrural approach, peak serum ethanol levels ranged from 21 to 39 mg/dL. These levels are well below the legally defined levels for intoxication.

Accumulation of high levels of acetaldehyde has been observed in persons with an atypical phenotype for the enzyme aldehyde dehydrogenase. This genetic defect, which is more common in Asians, has been implicated in facial flushing, palpitations, and hypotension in susceptible persons.[60] Such patients report a history of facial flushing after ingesting small amounts of alcoholic beverages, which represents potentially useful data. The use of alcohol as a neurolytic agent should also be avoided in patients undergoing disulfiram therapy for alcoholism.

The finding that amylase levels measured before and after celiac plexus block remained normal in a series of 20 patients suggests that pancreatic injury does not typically occur with this procedure.[73] Alterations in creatine phosphokinase (CPK) levels were minimal in most of the patients studied, suggesting absence of significant skeletal muscle injury. Interestingly, the only two patients with significantly elevated CPK levels (4242 and 1640 IU/L) also experienced side effects consistent with damage to nearby muscle tissue (bilateral L1 neuritis and back pain). A single case of a generalized seizure and transient loss of consciousness has been reported after apparent accidental intravascular injection of phenol.[74]

FUTURE DIRECTIONS

Further technologic advances in radiology should produce continued improvements in the efficacy and safety of celiac plexus and splanchnic nerve blocks. Faster image acquisition and higher resolution will continue to make CT guidance a more attractive option for celiac plexus and splanchnic nerve block. Three-dimensional image reconstruction may also provide the pain specialist a better understanding of the functional clinical anatomy and allow further refinement of these neurolysis techniques. As more experience is gained with ultrasound, it will play a role in the evolution of the anterior approach. The development of safer and longer-acting local anesthetics and neurolytic agents would be a welcome advance for the pain management specialist who performs celiac plexus and splanchnic nerve block.

References

1. Kappis M: Erfahrungen mit Lokalansthesie bei Bauchoperationen. Verh Dtsch Ges Circ 43:87, 1914.
2. Kappis M: Die Ansthesierung des Nervus splanchnicus. Zentralbl 45:709, 1918.
3. Wendling H: Ausschaltung der Nervi splanchnici durch Leitungsanesthesie bei Magenoperationen und anderen Eingriffen in der oberen Bauchule. Beitr Klin Chir 110:517, 1918.
4. Braun H: Ein Hilfsinstrument zur Ausfuhrung der Splanchnicusanesthesie. Zentralbl Chir 48:15151, 1921.
5. Labat G: L'anesthésie splanchnique dans les interventions chirurgicales et dans les affections douloureuses de la cavité abdominale. Gaz d'Hôp 93:662, 1920.
6. Roussiel M: Anesthésie des nerfs splanchniques et des plexus mésenteriques supérieur et inferieurs en chirurgie abdominale. Presse Med 31:4, 1923.
7. De Takats G: Splanchnic anesthesia: A critical review of the theory and practice of this method. Surg Gynecol Obstet 151:501, 1927.
8. Pitkin GP: Segmental block for visceral surgery. In Southworth JL, Hingson RA (eds): Conduction Anesthesia. Philadelphia, JB Lippincott, 1946, p 517.
9. Gage M, Floyd JB: The treatment of acute pancreatitis: With discussion of mechanism of production, clinical manifestations and diagnosis and report of four cases. Treatment Symp South Aust 59:415, 1947.
10. Esnaurrizar M: The surgical relief of abdominal pain by splanchnic block. Ann R Coll Surg Engl 4:192, 1949.
11. Popper HL: Acute pancreatitis: An evaluation of the classification, symptomatology, diagnosis and therapy. Am J Digest Dis 15:1, 1948.
12. Jones RR: A technique of injection of the splanchnic nerves with alcohol. Anesth Analg 36:75, 1957.
13. Bridenbaugh LD, Moore DC, Campbell DD: Management of upper abdominal cancer pain: Treatment with celiac plexus block with alcohol. JAMA 190:877, 1964.
14. Moore DC: Regional Block, ed 4. Springfield, Ill. Charles C Thomas, 1965, p 137.
15. Matamala AM, Lopez FV, Martinez LI: Percutaneous approach to the celiac plexus using CT guidance. Pain 34:285, 1988.
16. Matamala AM, Sanchez JL, Lopez FV: Percutaneous anterior and posterior approach to the celiac plexus: A comparative study using four different techniques. Pain Clinic 5:21, 1992.
17. Portenoy RK, Waldman SD: Managing cancer pain. Contemp Oncol 13:33, 1993.
18. Waldman SD: Management of acute pain. Postgrad Med 87:15, 1992.
19. Waldman SD: Celiac plexus block. In Waldman SD: Atlas of Interventional Pain Management Techniques. Philadelphia, WB Saunders, 1998, p 269.
20. Raj PP: Chronic pain. In Raj PP (ed): Handbook of Regional Anesthesia. New York, Churchill Livingstone, 1985, p 113.
21. Kune GA, Cole R, Bell S: Observations on the relief of pancreatic pain. Med J Aust 2:789, 1975.
22. Loper KA, Coldwell DM, Leck J, et al: Celiac plexus block for hepatic arterial embolization: A comparison with intravenous morphine. Anesth Analg 69:398, 1989.
23. Waldman SD: Celiac plexus block. In Weiner RS (ed): Innovations in Pain Management. Orlando, Fla., PMD Press, 1990, p 10.
24. Waldman SD, Portenoy RK: Recent advances in the management of cancer pain. Part II. Pain Manage 4:19, 1991.
25. Patt RB: Neurolytic blocks of the sympathetic axis. In Patt RB (ed): Cancer Pain. Philadelphia, JB Lippincott, 1993, p 393.
26. Bell SN, Cole R, Roberts-Thomson IC: Coeliac plexus block for control of pain in chronic pancreatitis. Br Med J 281:1604, 1980.
27. Hegedus V: Relief of pancreatic pain by radiography-guided block. AJR 133:1101, 1979.
28. Bonica JJ: Autonomic innervation of the viscera in relation to nerve block. Anesthesiology 29:793, 1968.
29. Lobstrom JB, Cousins MJ: Sympathetic neural blockade. In Cousins MJ, Bridenbaugh PO (eds): Neural Blockade, 2nd ed. Philadelphia, JB Lippincott, 1988, p 479.

30. Brown DL: Celiac plexus nerve block. In Brown DL (ed): Atlas of Regional Anesthesia. Philadelphia, WB Saunders, 1999, p 281.
31. Ward EM, Rorie DK, Nauss LA, et al: The celiac ganglion in man: Normal and anatomic variations. Anesth Analg 58:461, 1979.
32. Woodburne RT, Burkel WE: Essentials of Human Anatomy. New York, Oxford University Press, 1988, p 552.
33. Moore DC, Bush WH, Burnett LL: Celiac plexus block: A roentgenographic, anatomic study of technique and spread of solution in patients and corpses. Anesth Analg 60:369, 1981.
34. Thomson GE, Moore DC, Bridenbaugh PO, et al: Abdominal pain and celiac plexus nerve block. Anesth Analg 56:1, 1987.
35. Jain S: The role of celiac plexus block in intractable upper abdominal pain. In Racz GB (ed): Techniques of Neurolysis. Boston, Kluwer Academic, 1989, p 161.
36. Waldman SD: Acute and postoperative pain management. In RS Weiner (ed): Innovations in Pain Management. Orlando, Fla., PMD Press, 1993, p 28.
37. Singler RC: An improved technique for alcohol neurolysis of the celiac plexus. Anesthesiology 56:137, 1982.
38. Brown D, Moore DC: The use of neurolytic celiac plexus block for pancreatic cancer: Anatomy and technique. Pain Sympt Manage 3:206, 1988.
39. Ischia S, Luzzani A, Ischia A, et al: A new approach to the neurolytic block of the celiac plexus: The transaortic technique. Pain 16:333, 1983.
40. Hessel SJ, Adams DF, Abrams HL: Complications of angiography. Radiology 138:273, 1981.
41. Ostheimer GW: Pain and its treatment. In Miller RD, Kirby RR, Ostheimer GW, et al (eds): Year Book of Anesthesia. Chicago, Year Book, 1984, p 364.
42. Feldstein GS, Waldman SD: Loss of resistance technique for transaortic celiac plexus block. Anesth Analg 65:1089, 1986.
43. Lieberman RP, Waldman SD: Celiac plexus neurolysis with the modified transaortic approach. Radiology 175:274, 1990.
44. Labat G: Splanchnic analgesia. In Labat G (ed): Regional Anesthesia: Its Technique and Clinical Application, ed 2. Philadelphia, WB Saunders, 1928, p 398.
45. Lieberman RP, Nance PN, Cuka DJ: Anterior approach to the celiac plexus during interventional biliary procedures. Radiology 167:562, 1988.
46. Mueller PR, van Sonnenberg E, Casola G: Radiographically guided alcohol block of the celiac ganglion. Semin Intervent Radiol 4:195, 1987.
47. Lieberman RP, Crummy AB, Matallana RH: Invasive procedures in pancreatic disease. Semin Ultrasound CT MR 1:192, 1980.
48. Wajsman Z, Gamarra M, Park JJ, et al: Transabdominal fine needle aspiration of retroperitoneal lymph nodes in staging of genitourinary tract cancer. J Urol 128:1238, 1982.
49. Flanigan DP, Kraft RO: Continuing experience with palliative chemical splanchnicectomy. Arch Surg 113:5089, 1978.
50. Copping J, Willix R, Kraft RO: Palliative chemical splanchnicectomy. Arch Surg 98:418, 1969.
51. Charlton JE: Relief of the pain of unresectable carcinoma of the pancreas by chemical splanchnicectomy during laparotomy. Ann R Coll Surg Engl 67:136, 1985.
52. Corbitz C, Leavens M: Alcohol block of the celiac plexus for control of upper abdominal pain caused by cancer and pancreatitis. J Neurosurg 34:575, 1971.
53. Balamoutsos NG: Infiltration block of the celiac plexus using plastic catheter. Reg Anesth 5:64, 1982.
54. Humbles FH, Mahaffey JE: Teflon epidural catheter placement for intermittent celiac plexus blockade and celiac plexus neurolytic blockade. Reg Anesth 15:103, 1990.
55. Illuminati M, Kizelshteyn G, Ackert M, et al: Neurolytic celiac plexus block: Intraoperative catheter technique. Reg Anesth 14(Suppl):90, 1989.
56. Abram SE, Boas RA: Sympathetic and visceral nerve blocks. In Benumof JL (ed): Clinical Procedures in Anesthesia and Intensive Care. Philadelphia, JB Lippincott, 1992, p 787.
57. Parkinson SK, Mueller JB, Little WL: A new and simple technique for splanchnic nerve block using a paramedian approach and 3½ inch needles. Reg Anesth 14(Suppl):41, 1989.
58. Moore DC: Celiac (splanchnic) plexus block with alcohol for cancer pain of the upper intra-abdominal viscera. In Bonica JJ, Ventafridda V (eds): Advances in Pain Research and Therapy, vol 2. New York, Raven, 1979, p 357.
59. Jones J, Gough D: Coeliac plexus block with alcohol for relief of upper abdominal pain due to cancer. Ann R Coll Surg Engl 59:46, 1977.
60. Noda J, Umeda S, Mori K, et al: Acetaldehyde syndrome after celiac plexus block. Anesth Analg 65:1300, 1986.
61. Jain S, Hirsh R, Shah N, et al: Blood ethanol levels following celiac plexus block with 50% ethanol. Anesth Analg 68(Suppl):S135, 1989.
62. Boas RA, Hatangdi VS, Richards EG: Lumbar sympathectomy: A percutaneous chemical technique. In Bonica JJ, Albe-Fessard D (eds): Advances in Pain Research and Therapy, vol 1. New York, Raven, 1976, p 685.
63. Nour-Eldin F: Preliminary report: Uptake of phenol by vascular and brain tissue. Microvasc Res 2:224, 1970.
64. Lieberman RP, Lieberman SL, Cuka DJ, et al: Celiac plexus block and splanchnic nerve block: A review. Semin Intervent Radiol 5:213, 1988.
65. Myhre J, Hilsted J, Tronier B, et al: Monitoring of celiac plexus block in chronic pancreatitis. Pain 38:269, 1989.
66. Matson JA, Ghia JN, Levy JH: A case report of a potentially fatal complication associated with Ischia's transaortic method of celiac plexus block. Reg Anesth 10:193, 1985.
67. Galizia EJ, Lahiri SK: Paraplegia following coeliac plexus block with phenol. Br J Anaesth 46:539, 1974.
68. Waldman SD: Avoiding complications when performing celiac plexus block. Pain Clinic 6:62-63, 1993.
69. Fujita Y, Takori M: Pleural effusion after CT-guided alcohol celiac plexus block. Anesth Analg 66:911, 1987.
70. Cook FE, Jr, Flaherty RA, Willmarth CL, et al: Chylothorax: A complication of translumbar aortography. Radiology 75:251, 1960.
71. Fine PG, Bubela C: Chylothorax following celiac plexus block. Anesthesiology 63:454, 1985.
72. Black A, Dwyer B: Coeliac plexus block. Anaesth Intensive Care 1:315, 1973.
73. Lebenow TR, Ivankovich AD: Serum alcohol, CPK and amylase levels following celiac plexus block with alcohol. Reg Anesth 13(Suppl):64, 1988.
74. Benzon HT: Convulsions secondary to intravascular phenol: A hazard of celiac plexus block. Anesth Analg 58:150, 1979.

chapter 152

Lumbar Epidural Nerve Block

Laxmaiah Manchikanti and Sairam Atluri

HISTORICAL CONSIDERATIONS

Epidural administration of corticosteroids is one of the commonly used interventions in managing chronic low back pain.[1] Several approaches available to access the lumbar epidural space include caudal, interlaminar, and transforaminal routes. Reports of the effectiveness of epidural corticosteroids have varied from 18% to 90%.[1] Numerous publications over the years have described in detail the administration of lumbar epidural steroid injections by various routes.[1-15]

Sicard,[16] a radiologist, was the first to describe injection of dilute solutions of cocaine through the sacral hiatus (the caudal route) into the epidural space in 1901, to treat patients suffering from severe, intractable sciatic pain or lumbago. One week later, but independently, in 1901, Cathelin,[17] a urologist, described caudal administration of local anesthetic for surgical procedures and also injection of cocaine for relief of pain due to inoperable carcinoma of the rectum. Pasquier and Leri,[18] also in 1901, independently reported the use of caudal epidural injection for the relief of sciatic pain. The extension of this technique to the treatment of sciatica is attributed to Caussade and Queste[19] in 1909, Viner[20] in 1925, Evans[21] in 1930, Ombregt[22] and Cyriax[23] from 1937 to the 1970s, and Brown[24] in 1960.

However, some consider that the first to use epidural anesthesia was Corning, a neurologist whose intentions were to treat some neurologic disorders by using cocaine spinally (Fig. 152–1).[25,26] In the October 1885 issue of the *New York Medical Journal*, a case report by Corning[26] was based on two subjects: one a dog and the other a patient who suffered from spinal weakness and seminal incontinence.

The description of the para-midline approach to the lumbar epidural space was proposed by Pagés[27] in 1921. This is considered the first clinically relevant report of the technique of lumbar epidural injection. Multiple modifications were suggested to the technique described by Pagés.[28] In 1933, Dogliotti[29] introduced the loss of resistance technique into the clinical practice. Gutierrez,[30] also in 1933, suggested that the negative pressure of the epidural space might be used to identify the epidural space and described the hanging-drop technique. In 1936, Rovenstein[31] established a nerve block service. By the 1950s, many nerve block clinics were in operation.[32,33]

The clinical introduction of cortisone, a purified glucocorticoid preparation, introduced in 1949, revolutionized medical care of patients with a host of diseases and provided life-sustaining physiologic replacement in patients with acute or chronic adrenal insufficiency.[34,35] Soon after that, the first use of steroids in epidural injections was reported by Robecchi and Capra[36]; however, the first report of the use of epidural steroid injections has been attributed by various authorities to Lievre and coworkers[37] in 1953. The initial American reports of epidural steroid injections by Goebert and colleagues appeared in 1961.[38]

INDICATIONS

Tissues in the lower back capable of transmitting pain include the disk, nerve root dura, muscle, ligament, fascia, and facet joint.[39] Pain from lumbar disk herniation can arise from nerve root compression and stimulation of nociceptors in the annulus or posterior longitudinal ligament. Mixter and Barr,[40] in 1934, described intervertebral disk herniation, which led many practitioners to assume that intervertebral disk herniation is the most common cause of back problems. However, modern evidence implicates intervertebral disk herniation in only a small percentage of back complaints.[1,41-43] Thus, a simple compression or mass effect cannot be the mechanism of pain due to disk disease. In fact, several studies evaluating the progress of disk herniation have shown that, even though the resolution of symptoms tends to be associated diminution of the size of the disk herniations, it is not always the case because compression may continue in spite of resolution of the symptomatology.[43-46] In addition, it is also well known that disk herniations that are evident on computerized tomographic (CT) axial scan or magnetic resonance imaging (MRI) scan can be asymptomatic.[47,48] Various proposed mechanisms for radicular pain include partial axonal damage, neuroma formation, and focal demyelination[49]; intraneural edema[50-53]; and impaired microcirculation.[52,53] The other explanation surrounds the theory of chemical irritation and inflammation around the disks and nerve roots, which is considered a pain generator in conjunction with or without mechanical factors.[54]

RATIONALE

The philosophy of epidural steroid injections is based on the premise that the corticosteroid delivered into the epidural

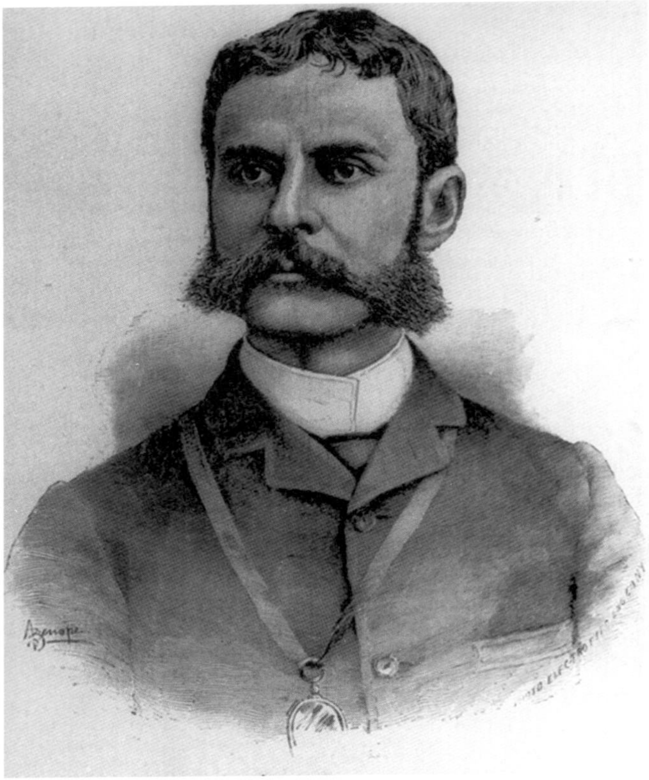

FIGURE 152–1 ■ New York neurologist James Leonard Corning (1855-1923). (Figure courtesy of the National Library of Medicine.)

Table 152–1

Disadvantages of Caudal, Lumbar, Interlaminar, and Transforaminal Epidural Injections

Transforaminal	
Intraneural injection	
Neural trauma	
Technical difficulty in presence of fusion and/or hardware	
Intravascular injection	
Spinal cord trauma	
Caudal	
Requirement of substantial volume of fluid	
Dilution of the injectate	
Extra-epidural placement of the needle	
Intravascular placement of the needle	
Atypical anatomy	
Dural puncture	
Interlaminar	
Dilution of the injectate	
Extra-epidural placement of the needle	
Intravascular placement of the needle	
Preferential cranial flow of the solution	
Preferential posterior flow of the solution	
Difficult placement in postsurgical patients	
Difficult placement below L4/L5 interspace	
Deviation of needle to nondependent side	
Dural puncture	
Trauma to spinal cord	

From Manchikanti L, Singh V, Kloth D, et al: Interventional techniques in the management of chronic pain: Part 2.0. Pain Physician 4:24, 2001.

space attains higher local concentrations over an inflamed nerve root and will be more effective than a steroid administered either orally or by intramuscular injection.[1,2,5]

Target site concentration of steroids depends on multiple injection variables, including the route of administration. Steroids may be prevented from migrating from the posterior epidural space to the anterior or ventral epidural space by the presence of epidural ligaments or scar tissue, either with caudal or interlaminar administration. Interlaminar lumbar epidural injections are alleged to be superior to caudal epidural injections by some because of the requirement of the apparently lesser volume. Interlaminar epidural injections are also considered more target specific than caudal epidural injections. However, among the many disadvantages of interlaminar epidural injections, the extradural placement of the needle, which may go unrecognized without fluoroscopic guidance, is crucial.[1,5,55-57] Other disadvantages of the interlaminar approach include erroneous placement of the needle, which may miss the targeted interspace without fluoroscopic guidance[56,57]; preferential cranial flow of the solution in the epidural space[58,59]; deviation of the needle to the nondependent side[60]; difficulty entering the epidural space and delivery of injectate below L5 for S1 nerve root involvement[1,2,56]; potential risk of dural puncture and post-lumbar puncture headache[5]; and the rare, but serious, risk of spinal cord trauma.[61] Disadvantages of various types of epidural administration of drugs are listed in Table 152–1.[2]

Similar to interlaminar epidural injections, transforaminal epidural injections also have some disadvantages, which include intravascular penetration of the needle, neural penetration, spinal cord trauma, and paraplegia.[55,62] In addition to lumbar radiculitis or chronic low back pain, lumbar epidural injections with local anesthetics, opioids, or steroids may be used in multiple other chronic painful conditions, as well as acute painful conditions.

The present clinical rationale for steroid usage in epidurals is primarily based on the benefits, which include pain relief outlasting by hours, days, and sometimes weeks, the pharmacologic action of steroids and local anesthetics.[63] However, appropriate explanations for such benefits continue to lack scientific validity. Additional explanations include alteration or interruption of nociceptive input, reflex mechanism of the afferent limb, self-sustaining activity of the neuronal pools in the neuraxis, and the pattern of central neural activities by neural blockade, including caudal epidural steroids.[64] The basis for these explanations is twofold. First, it is postulated that corticosteroids reduce inflammation either by inhibiting the synthesis or release of a number of proinflammatory substances or by causing a reversible local anesthetic effect.[63-76] Second, administration of epidural solutions clears or dilutes the chemical irritants. Corticosteroids are postulated to exert their effect by multiple modes, including membrane stabilization, inhibition of neural peptide synthesis or action, blockade of phospholipase A_2 activity, prolonged suppression of ongoing neuronal discharge, and suppression of sensitization of dorsal horn neurons.[63]

Interlaminar epidural steroid injections are indicated in patients with chronic low back pain who have failed to respond to conservative modalities of treatments. Patients should present with a strong radicular component or diskogenic pain—or at the least—they must not have facet joint pain or sacroiliac joint pain. Patients with combined pain generators with diskogenic pain as well as facet joint pain may also receive interlaminar epidural steroid injections.

In the past, a multitude of investigators have attempted to identify predictors of outcome of epidural injections, as well as facet joint injections. However, these have been proven to be futile; hence, no such recommendations are made in this review. Various contraindications include the patient's inability to be in the prone position, contraindications for fluoroscopy, local or systemic infection, abnormalities of the sacrum, and allergy to any of the drugs used. Multiple indications for interlaminar epidural injections are illustrated in Table 152–2. These indications are related to other than surgical or obstetric anesthesia.

CLINICALLY RELEVANT ANATOMY

The epidural space extends from the base of the skull to the end of dural sac at S2. It is a cylindrical structure enveloping the dura. The epidural space exists between the dura and ligamentum flavum.[77] The actual size of epidural space varies greatly. The distance from the skin to the epidural space in normal adults usually ranges from 3 to 5 cm. In the midlumbar region, the depth of the posterior epidural space is about 5 to 6 mm, and it gradually decreases to 2 mm at the S1 level. The epidural space is widest in the midline below the junction of the lamina and it narrows laterally. Laterally the ligamentum flavum joins with the facet joint capsule. The posterior epidural space is divided by the plica mediana dorsalis and additional transverse connective tissue planes, providing a compartmentalized nature. The ligamentum flavum is also 5 to 6 mm in the lumbar region.

The epidural space contains fat, veins, spinal arteries, and lymphatics. The epidural veins are a part of the large internal vertebral venous plexus, which communicates with the occipital, sigmoid and basilar sinuses superiorly in the cranium. If needle placement in the epidural veins is not recognized, it may result in the injectate's reaching the cranial sinuses. The spinal arteries enter the epidural space through the intervertebral foramen laterally. During the performance of the interlaminar lumbar epidural steroid injection, it is important to make sure that the needle is not too lateral in the epidural space because of the possibility of injury to the spinal artery, which is entering the epidural space laterally through the intervertebral foramen. The largest of the spinal arteries is the artery of Adamkiewicz. This artery provides major arterial supply to the lumbar spine. It enters the spinal canal through a single intervertebral foramen anywhere between T8 and L3 and is located on the left side 78% of the time.

The spinal cord ends in most people at the L1 or L2 level. Epidurals done above this level can result in cord trauma if the needle is inadvertently advanced too far. The dural sac terminates at S2.

Table 152–2

Nonsurgical Indications for Lumbar Epidural Block
Acute pain
Herpes zoster and postherpetic neuralgia
Ischemic pain syndromes
Renal colic
Preemptive analgesia prior to amputation
Complex regional pain syndrome I and II
Lumbar radiculopathy
Lumbar disk herniation
Lumbar spinal stenosis
Post-lumbar laminectomy syndrome
Lumbar degenerative disk disease
Chronic low back pain
Vertebral compression fractures
Diabetic polyneuropathy
Pelvic pain syndromes
Phantom limb syndrome
Peripheral neuropathy
Metastatic pain

TECHNIQUE

Lumbar epidural injection is performed either with fluoroscopy or blindly without fluoroscopy. For all chronic pain settings, specifically for low back pain, fluoroscopic epidural is recommended.

Fluoroscopic Technique

All necessary protection against radiation should be used to avoid complications.[78,79]

Positioning

The patient should be placed in the prone position with a pillow under the abdomen. Sterile preparation should be carried out extensively. The desired interlaminar space must be identified, which should be in the middle of the viewing monitor in the anteroposterior (AP) view. The C-arm may be rotated toward the patient's right side or left side until the spinous process is exactly equidistant from the right and the left pedicle (Fig. 152–2). The cranial (C-arm is angled toward the patient's head) or caudal (C-arm is angled toward the patient's feet) angulation is done until the desired interlaminar space is maximally opened. Sometimes no cranial or caudal angulation is necessary, especially if the L5-S1 space is chosen. Typically the L5-S1 space is the widest, and the interspaces get smaller as one goes superior to L4-L5 and L3-L4. T12-L1 and L1-L2 are again easily accessible.

Procedure

If the patient is having unilateral pain, the needle entry point should be on that side of the interlaminar space (Fig. 152–3). If the patient is having bilateral pain, the needle entry should be in the midline of the interlaminar space. The epidural

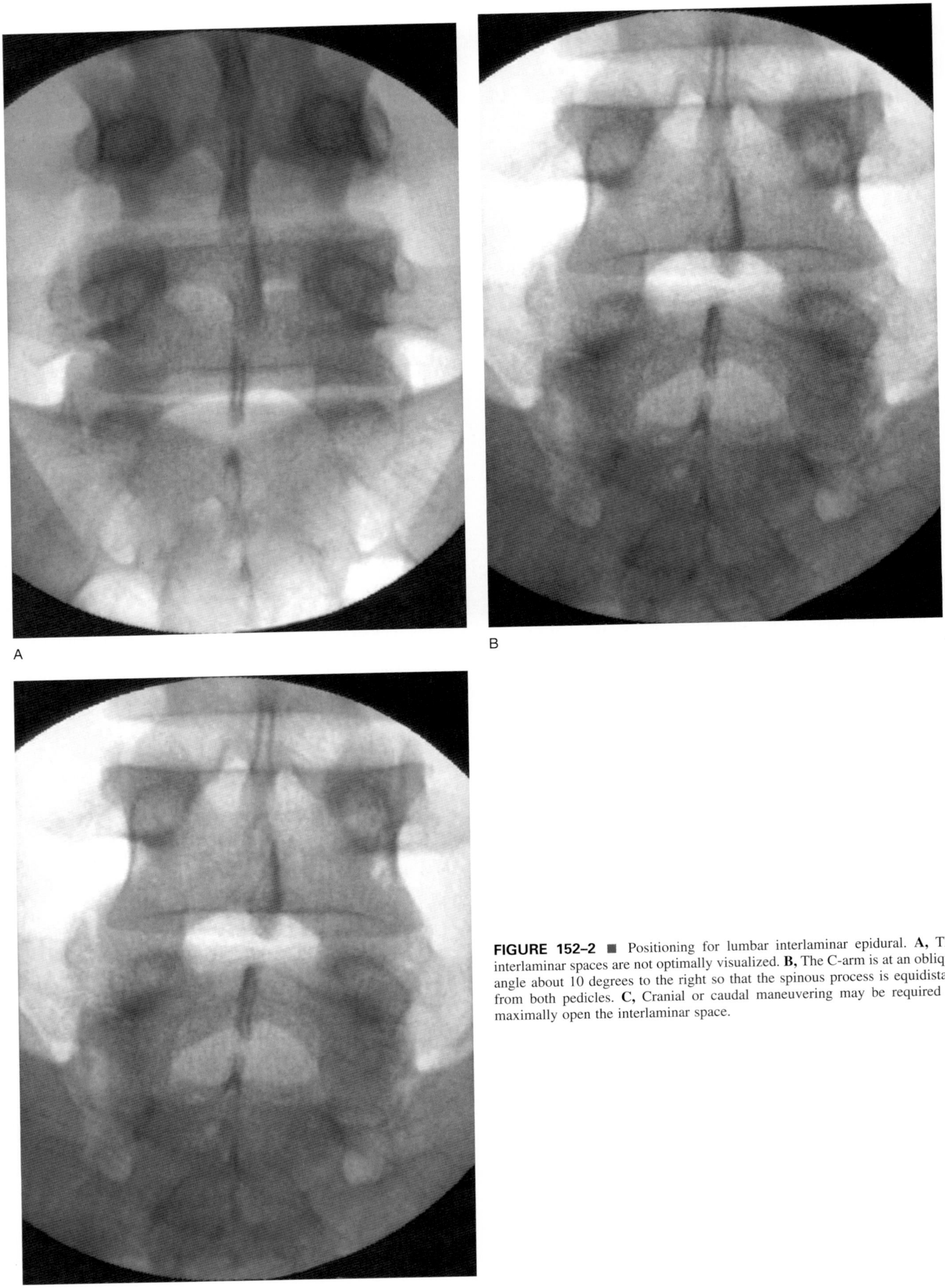

A

B

C

FIGURE 152–2 ■ Positioning for lumbar interlaminar epidural. **A,** The interlaminar spaces are not optimally visualized. **B,** The C-arm is at an oblique angle about 10 degrees to the right so that the spinous process is equidistant from both pedicles. **C,** Cranial or caudal maneuvering may be required to maximally open the interlaminar space.

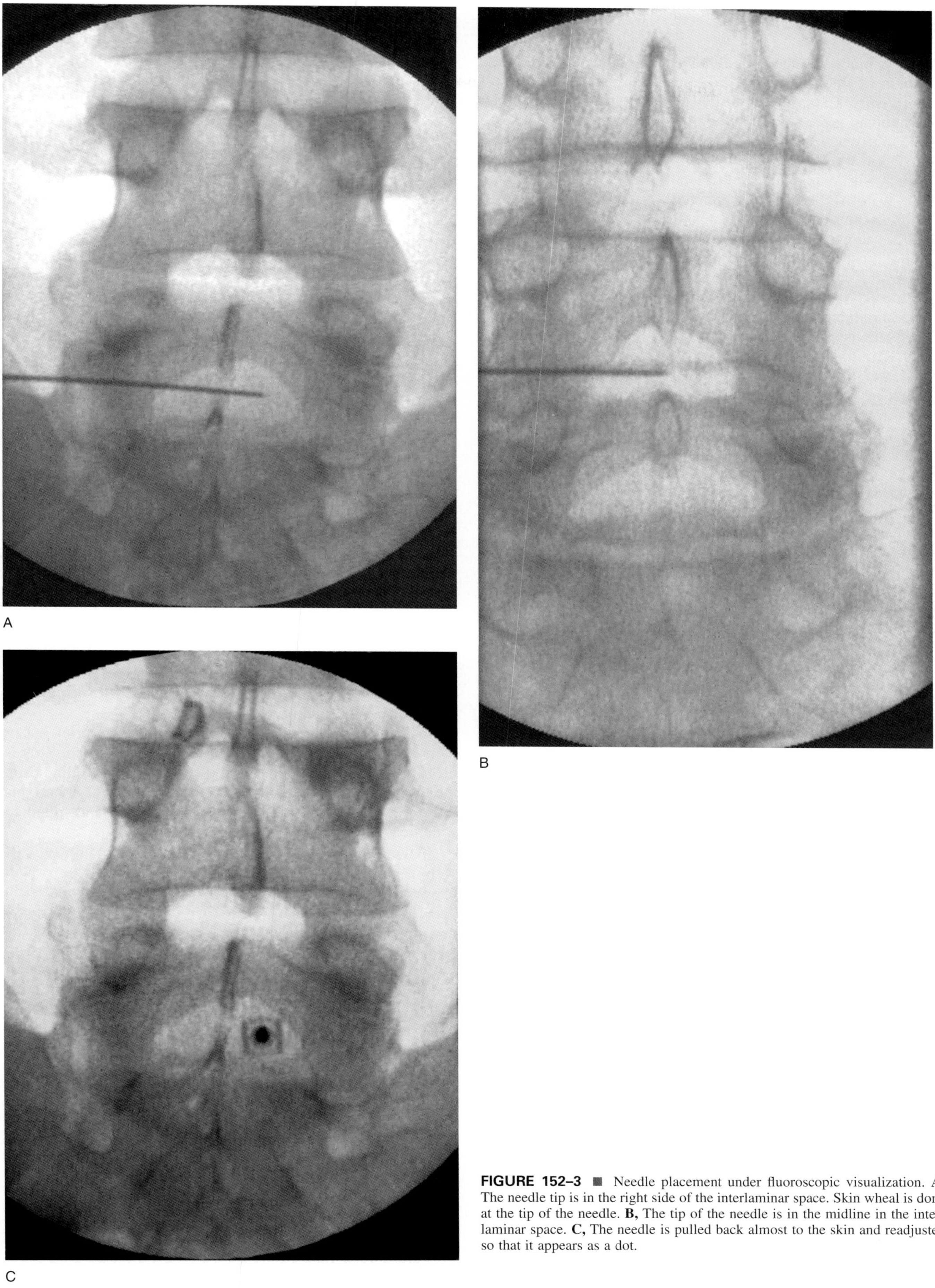

FIGURE 152–3 ■ Needle placement under fluoroscopic visualization. **A,** The needle tip is in the right side of the interlaminar space. Skin wheal is done at the tip of the needle. **B,** The tip of the needle is in the midline in the interlaminar space. **C,** The needle is pulled back almost to the skin and readjusted so that it appears as a dot.

needle is placed on the patient horizontally and adjusted with the help of fluoroscopy until the needle tip is at the site of needle entry. Extreme lateral placement of the needle in the interlaminar space should be avoided to minimize the risk of nerve injury and to stay away from vascular structures.

A skin wheal is raised, preferably with a 25- to 30-gauge needle, with 1% lidocaine at the needle entry site. This is done at the tip of the needle. Deeper infiltration with local anesthetic can be done. Again, using fluoroscopic guidance, the needle is adjusted so that it is seen as a "dot" (see Fig. 152–3). The dot must be in the interlaminar space and on the intended right or left side if the patient is having right or left radiculopathy, and it must be midline if the patient is suffering from bilateral radiculopathy. In this case, it was placed on the right side, as the patient was having right-sided radiculopathy. The stylet is removed. The loss-of-resistance syringe (plastic or glass) is attached to the Touhy needle. The needle is advanced straight in, inline with the x-ray beam. For the right-handed operator, the needle hub is held with the left thumb and index finger; and this hand should rest on the patient's back to provide stability. Continuous pressure is applied on the syringe plunger with the other hand, and the needle is advanced. There is increased bounce or pressure in the syringe, especially when the needle enters the ligamentum flavum. As the needle passes through the ligament and enters the epidural space, this pressure or bounce is suddenly lost. This is the loss-of-resistance or bounce technique. Live fluoroscopy is not necessary during advancement, but occasional spot pictures may be helpful to make sure that the needle is not off course. It is important to realize that because the Touhy needle has a curved tip, the principle of bevel control comes into play. It is possible to use this feature to advantage. Turning the bevel to the side of the intended direction results in the needle's going in that direction as it is advanced. This is analogous to the curved-needle technique that is commonly used in other spinal procedures. Getting false loss of resistance is not uncommon even in experienced hands. It cannot be emphasized enough that, if one is not sure where the needle is, the immediate course of action should be to check the lateral view. Inadvertent advancement without the knowledge of needle position can result in unnecessary dural puncture and even possibly spinal cord damage if lumbar epidural steroid injection is performed at the L1 or L2 level or higher.

Once one is convinced that the epidural space is found with loss of resistance, make sure that aspiration is negative for CSF or blood. Inject nonionic contrast (Omnipaque or Isovue) and look for the typical contrast spread to confirm. Epidural contrast spread can have one or all of the following patterns, which can help confirm correct needle placement:

1. Contrast has a smooth, continuous flow during injection. The contrast quickly moves away (runs off) from the tip of the needle as it is injected. Usually this flow is superior to the needle tip, but inferior spreads are also seen. If one gets a false loss of resistance and is posterior to the epidural space, a "blob" or "cotton ball" appearance is commonly seen. At this time it will be useful to use live fluoroscopy to visualize the contrast flow and spread. By using a small extension tubing during contrast injection, the physician's hand can be spared from radiation.
2. Areolar appearance (small bubbles within the contrast spread) is often seen (Fig. 152–4A).
3. Sometimes contrast can be seen surrounding the nerves, giving the typical appearance of the radiculogram (see Fig. 152–4B).

On the lateral view, the needle must be clearly in the spinal column and posterior to the neural foramen. In the lateral view, the contrast should be in the confines of the spinal canal. The contrast should not be posterior to the spine (see Fig. 152–4C). If the needle tip is posterior to the spine, it is posterior to the epidural space. If the needle tip is at the neural foramen or anterior to the foramen, then it may be in the intrathecal space. Contrast spread can be checked in both the AP view and lateral view: but as more experience is obtained, watching the contrast spread in the AP view will suffice.

Because the spine is a cylindrical structure, if needle entry is in the midline of the interlaminar space in the AP view, the needle tip will be barely in the spine. But if the needle entry is on the right or left side of the interlaminar space in the AP view, the needle tip will be clearly within the spine in the lateral view, and it will be posterior to the intervertebral foramen. If one is using the midline technique and in the lateral view, or if one is not sure if the needle is in the epidural space because the needle tip is barely at the posterior edge of the spine, the only way to confirm this is by injecting contrast and watching its spread. In the lateral view, it should be within the spine and not posterior to the spine (see Fig. 152–4C). In the AP view, the typical epidural contrast spread should be seen.

The compliance of the epidural space is very low; therefore, after the contrast is injected, it is common to see the contrast flowing back subtly (dripping back) through the needle (but with negative aspiration). This can be an additional assurance that the needle is in the correct place. Obvious flow-back of the fluid, especially with aspiration, indicates dural puncture.

It is not uncommon for the patient to feel a brief jolt or pain when the needle first enters the epidural space. This is probably from the sudden decompression of air or saline from the loss-of-resistance syringe into the epidural space, and this decompression irritates the already sensitized and inflamed spinal canal structures.

There should be no resistance during the injection. If there is resistance to injection, a simple turn of the bevel will resolve the problem. Many patients may feel radicular pain during injection; and if this pain is concordant to their pain, it is an additional confirmation that the steroid is reaching the desired inflamed nerve root. Severe and excruciating pain should alert the practitioner of the possibility of intraneural injection, which can cause nerve damage and obviously must be avoided. In such situations, the injection should be stopped immediately and the needle position reexamined (is it too lateral in the interlaminar space?).

Getting false loss of resistance is not uncommon, even in experienced hands. False loss of resistance is obtained commonly with the following:

1. The needle is posterior to the epidural space (not deep enough). This problem cannot be identified in the AP view. A lateral view must be checked. It is not uncommon to have a false loss of resistance. If one is not sure or if one is a beginner, the only way to confirm one is in the epidural space is to check the lateral view. When contrast is injected, it will be posterior to the spine. If the needle

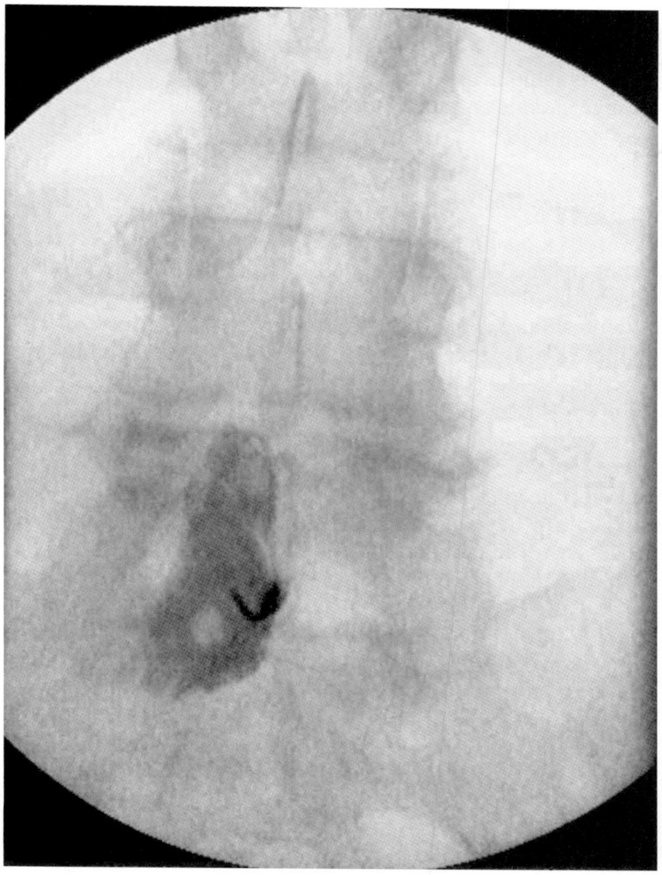

A

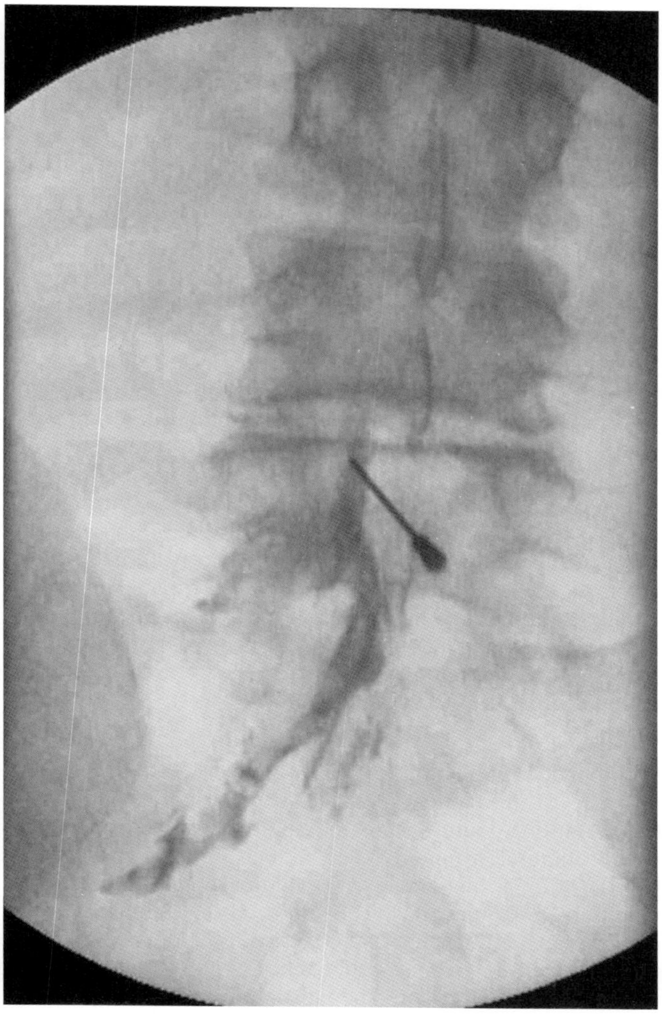

B

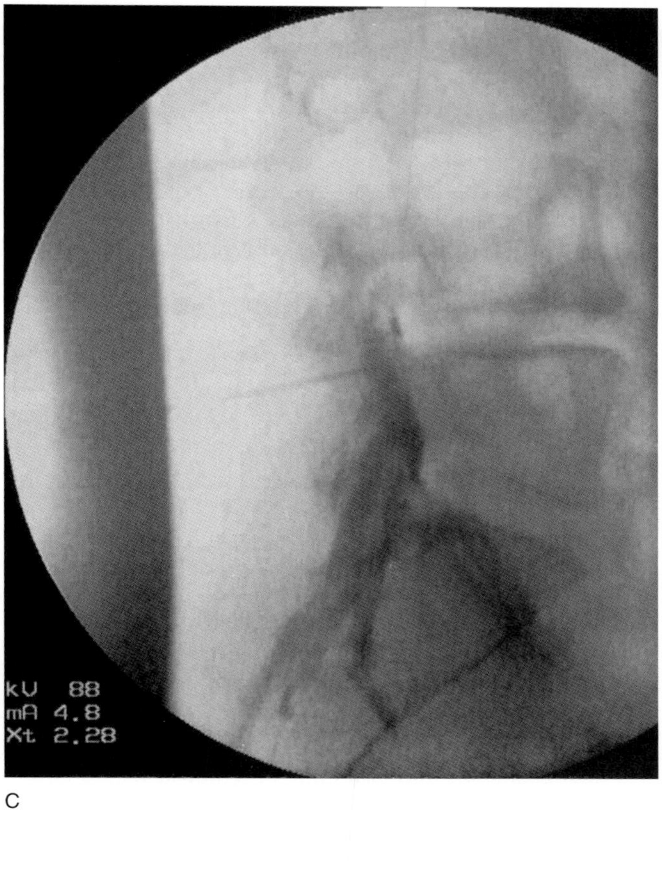

C

FIGURE 152–4 ■ Contrast injection under fluoroscopy. **A,** The areolar appearance of the contrast is noted on the left side of the epidural space. **B,** The contrast is seen surrounding the L5 and S1 nerves. **C,** The contrast is in the confines of the spine and not posterior to the spine.

and/or contrast is posterior to the epidural space, reattach the syringe to the needle and resume the loss of resistance until the needle position and contrast spread are appropriate as described (see Fig. 152–4C).

2. One is in the epidural space. When one injects the contrast, the typical spread in the AP view can be seen. In the lateral view, the needle is in the spine (not posterior to the spine) and the contrast is in the spinal canal (not posterior to the spine). Aspiration is negative for CSF or heme. No vascular spread of the contrast is seen. Frequently, it may be difficult to visualize the needle tip in the lateral view, especially in obese patients. This problem can be offset by using epidural needles with a metal stylet.
3. One is in the intrathecal space (the needle is in too deep). Clear fluid (CSF) is obtained on aspiration. It is impossible to tell on the AP view if the needle is in the epidural space or the intrathecal space and also difficult to see in the lateral view. Injecting contrast into the intrathecal space will show a myelogram pattern that is clearly distinct from the epidurogram. If one is not sure about this spread, the radiology department in the hospital should be able to furnish myelogram films for review. If one thinks the needle is deep enough and there is no loss of resistance or if one is not sure where the needle is, check the lateral view before further needle advancement to avoid dural puncture.

Figures 152–5 and 152–6 also indicate the interlaminar approach to the epidural space under fluoroscopy with epidural filling pattern showing multiple nerve roots and ventral epidural filling. Botwin and associates[80] described epidural filling patterns with fluoroscopic interlaminar epidural steroid injections. They showed that among the 25 epidurograms, all of them had contrast in the dorsal epidural space. Further, 36% of the patients had contrast visualized in the ventral epidural space. They also noted that contrast patterns showed unilateral flow in 84% of the patients, whereas bilateral contrast pattern was seen in only 16%. The mean caudad spread of contrast from the injection site was recorded and found to be a mean of 0.88 levels, in contrast to cephalad spread of 1.28 levels (Fig. 152–7). They also noted higher levels of cephalad flow in herniated disk patients with a lower level of caudad flow with means of 1.12 and 0.96 levels, respectively. Cephalad flow was also noticed to be higher in stenosis patients (Table 152–3).

Blind Technique

Blind technique may be performed with the patient in the sitting, lateral, or prone position with a midline or paramedian approach.

Sitting Position

The sitting position is preferred for obese patients because it facilitates the identification of the midline. In obese patients, other bony landmarks may not be palpable. Preferably, the patient should bend forward, with the knees close to the abdomen, or rest the legs on a stool, to abolish the lumbar lordosis and widen the posterior interspinous space. Following the appropriate sterile preparation and a skin wheal, an 18- or 20-gauge epidural needle is inserted and the posterior part of the spinous process may be identified. Following this, the epidural needle is slightly withdrawn and directed more cephalad in the sagittal plane and "walked off" the spinous process with identification of a clear pathway. At this point, or immediately after identification of the interspinous process, the stylet from the needle may be removed and a syringe with air or saline solution is attached to the hub of the needle. The epidural needle is advanced slowly with a two-handed technique stabilizing it so that unwanted movements and subdural puncture are prevented. Once the ligamentum flavum is reached, the operator will feel the resistance followed by sudden loss of resistance to air or saline. Once the epidural space is identified, aspiration should be carried out, which should be negative not only for CSF, but also for blood.

The paramedian approach for the sitting position is carried out in the same fashion by preparing the overlying skin. By introducing the needle approximately 1 inch lateral to the spinous process below the space to be entered, infiltration may be carried out copiously into the skin, as well as the deeper tissues along the intended pathway. An 18- or 20-gauge epidural needle is inserted cephalad and medially so that it makes a 15-degree angle to the sagittal plane. After the needle is advanced 3 to 4 cm, the stylet should be removed and a syringe containing air or saline solution should be attached to the hub of the needle. At this time, the needle is advanced slowly with the same steps as in the sitting position until the loss of resistance to air or saline solution is felt and epidural space is identified. Once again, negative aspiration should be confirmed.

Table 152–3

Mean Levels of Contrast Flow from Injection Site in 25 Injections

	HNP Injection (n = 13)	*LSS Injection (n = 12)*	*Total (n = 25)*	*P Value*
Caudad	0.96 ± 0.43 (0.5-2.0)	0.79 ± 0.26 (0.5-1.0)	0.88 ± 0.36 (0.5-2.0)	0.249
Cephalad	1.12 ± 0.46 (0.5-2.0)	1.46 ± 0.58 (0.5-2.0)	1.28 ± 0.54 (0.5-2.0)	0.120
P value	0.390	0.002	0.004	

HNP, herniated nucleus pulposus; LSS, lumbosacral spine.
Values in parentheses indicate range.
One level is defined as being from the middle of the intervertebral disk from where the injection was performed to the vertebral disk cephalad or caudad.
From Botwin KP, Natalicchio J, Hanna A: Fluoroscopic guided lumbar interlaminar epidural injections: A prospective evaluation of epidurography contrast patterns and anatomical review of the epidural space. Pain Physician 7:77, 2004.

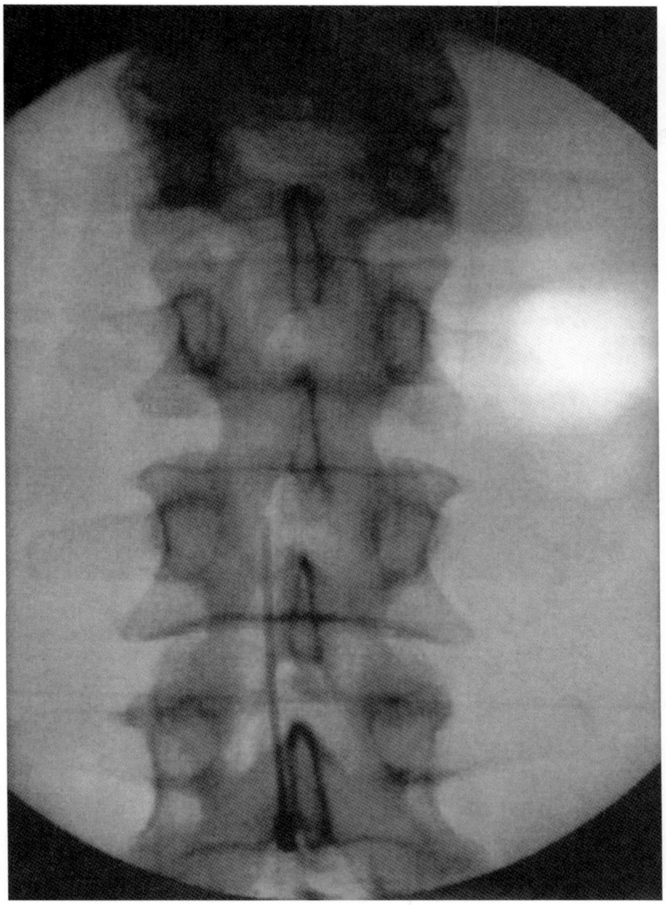

A

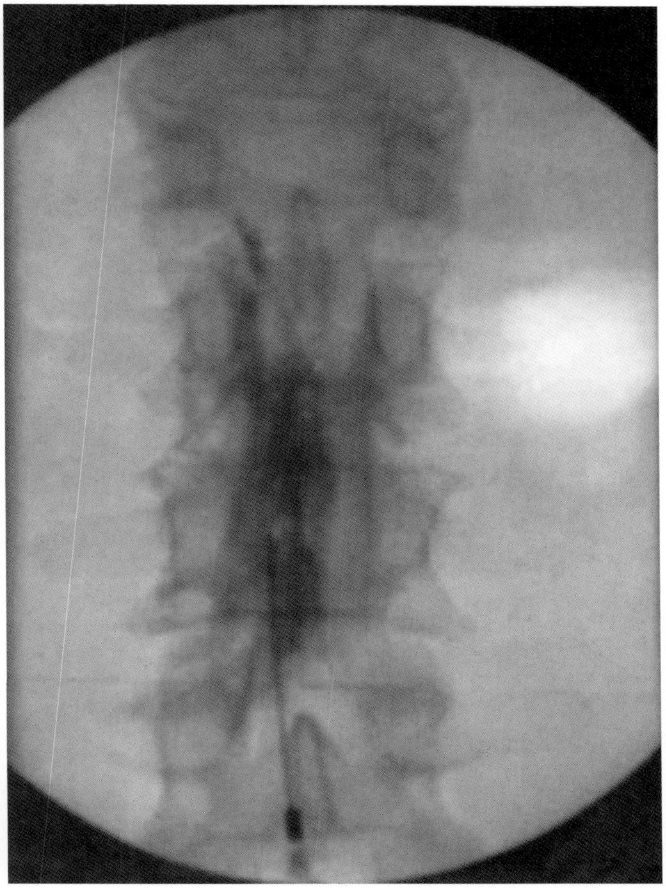

B

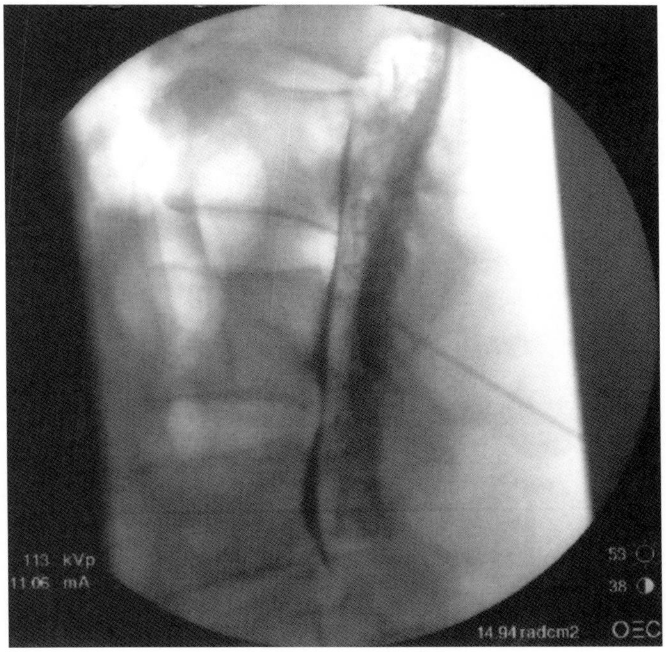

C

FIGURE 152–5 ■ Left-sided interlaminar approach to the epidural space under fluoroscopy with epidural filling pattern. **A,** Posteroanterior view with needle placement. **B,** Posteroanterior view with contrast injection. **C,** Lateral view with excellent ventral filling of epidural space.

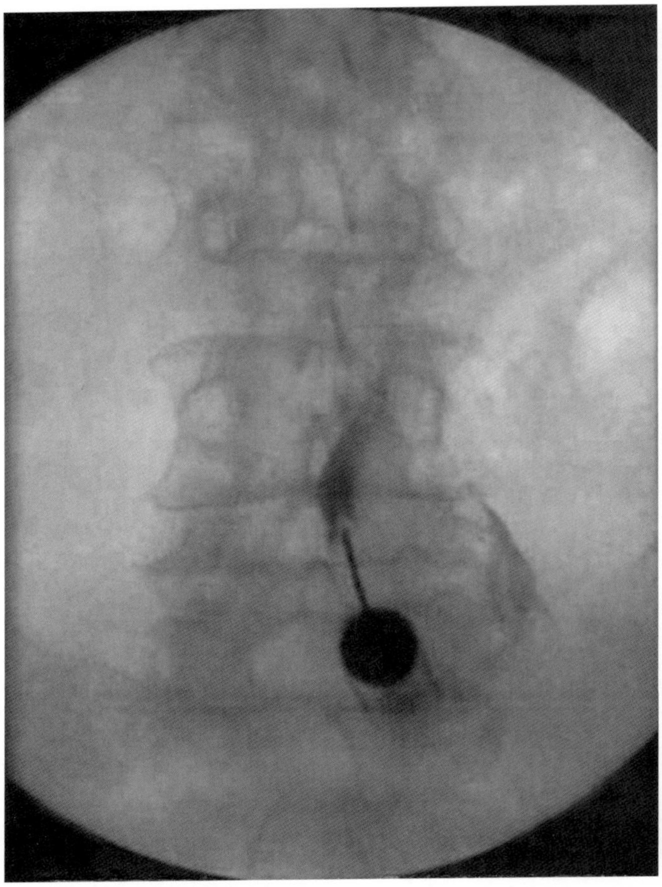

A

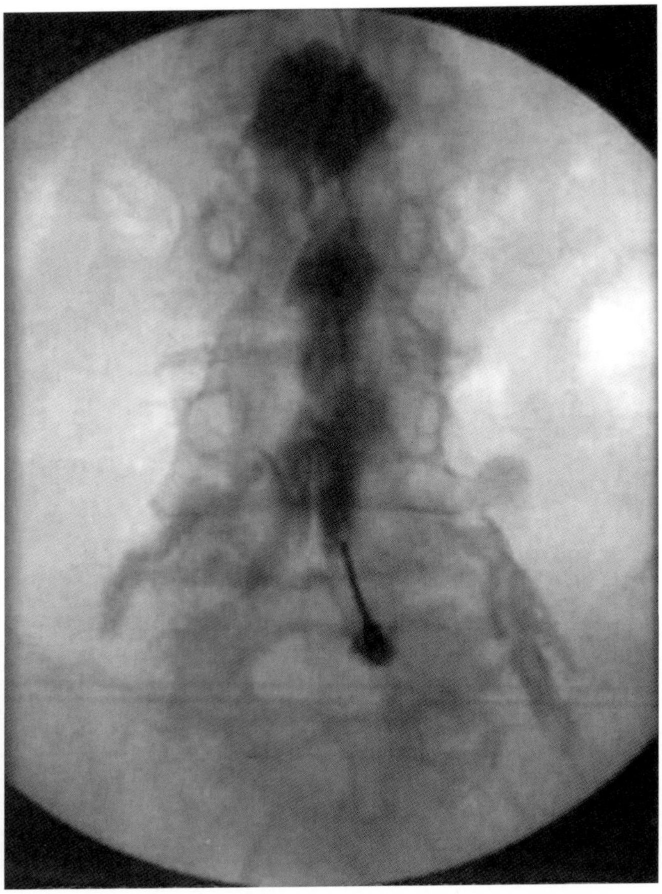

B

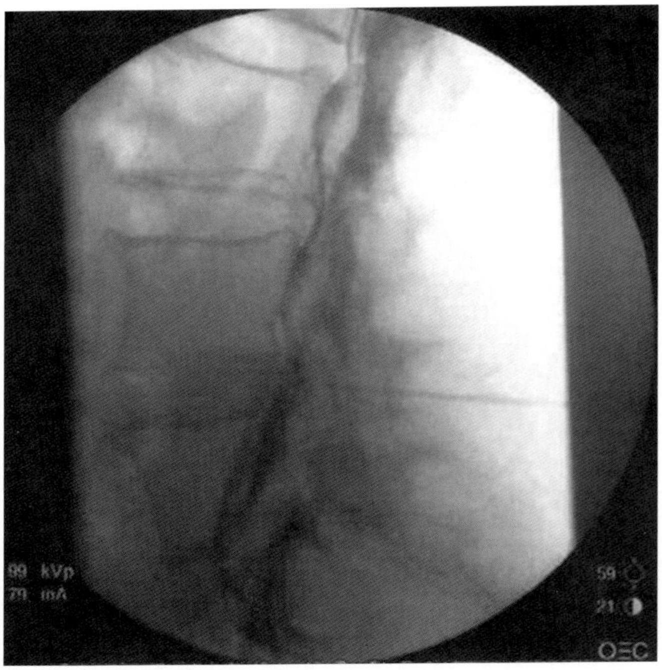

C

FIGURE 152–6 ■ Right-sided interlaminar approach to the epidural space. **A,** Posteroanterior view with needle placement. **B,** Posteroanterior with contrast injection. **C,** Lateral view with excellent ventral filling of epidural space.

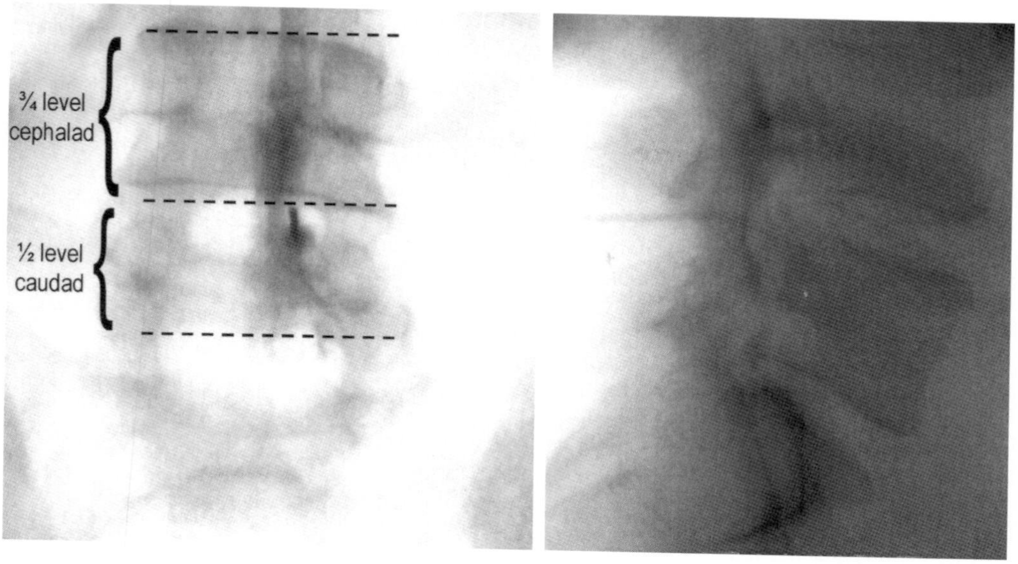

FIGURE 152–7 ■ Anteroposterior radiograph *(left)* of interlaminar injection at L4-L5. Note contrast flow cephalad of ¾ levels and caudad contrast flow of ½ levels. Lateral radiograph *(right)* reveals contrast flow in dorsal epidural space. (From Botwin KP, Natalicchio J, Hanna A: Fluoroscopic guided lumbar interlaminar epidural injections: A prospective evaluation of epidurography contrast patterns and anatomical review of the epidural space. Pain Physician 7:77, 2004.)

Lateral Position

The procedure is similar to the sitting position along with preparation, and so on, for both midline and paramedian approach. The advantage of the lateral approach is the avoidance of hypotension. As a cautionary note, it is ideal in pain management to perform these procedures under fluoroscopic visualization for managing chronic low back pain or other related conditions.

■ SIDE EFFECTS AND COMPLICATIONS

Corticosteroid-Related Side Effects

Most of the side effects reported are minor and transient.[63] They are related to systemic absorption and include insomnia, erythema, nausea, rash, and pruritus. Depression of plasma cortisol levels and the pituitary-hypothalamic axis can occur for about 2 weeks, but it normalizes by 3 weeks. Patients can develop Cushing's syndrome, but it is extremely rare. Diabetic patients can commonly have temporary elevations in blood-sugar levels for up to 3 to 7 days. In rare cases, fluid retention can occur, which can precipitate congestive heart failure in the susceptible. Weight gain is rare.

Local Anesthetic-Related Side Effects

Unrecognized intrathecal injection of the local anesthetic will result in spinal anesthesia. Venous injection of local anesthetic may or may not produce any symptoms, and this once again depends on the dose of the local anesthetic. The symptoms can range from minor transient manifestations such as dizziness, disorientation, tinnitus, metallic taste in the mouth, circumoral numbness, and muscle twitching to life-threatening seizures, unconsciousness, coma, and cardiovascular collapse. Arrhythmias resulting from local anesthetic overdose are usually refractory to the advanced cardiac life support (ACLS) protocol and are extremely difficult to treat. Central nervous system symptoms precede cardiovascular collapse. If the patient is having muscle twitching, benzodiazepines (Versed or Valium) should be used immediately. If seizures occur, intravenous thiopental sodium must be given along with the necessary ventilatory support. Fortunately, these complications are rare during lumbar epidural steroid injection because high doses of local anesthetics are rarely needed. If aspiration for blood is negative and there is no vascular runoff during contrast injection, venous injection is extremely rare. Higher concentrations of local anesthetics can lead to hypotension secondary to sympathetic blockade. This condition can be easily resolved with intravenous fluids and vasopressors such as ephedrine or phenylephrine hydrochloride (Neo-Synephrine).

Procedure-Related Side Effects

Some of the reported complications include vasovagal reactions, spinal headache, and spinal block. Subdural injection can result if the needle is between the dural membrane and the arachnoid membrane. The block resembles that of a spinal block, but it is patchy. Management is similar to spinal block. Fortunately, subdural needle placement is extremely rare. Nerve damage can occur, and any severe pain during placement of the needle or injection should alert the operator of potential neural injury. The procedure must be stopped immediately, and the needle position reevaluated. The patient must be able to report severe radicular pain in the case of intraneural injection—for this reason, the patient should *never* be oversedated.

Spinal cord injury can occur by two mechanisms: first, by direct injury to the cord with the epidural needle; second, by a rare mechanism, either by traumatizing the artery of Adamkiewicz with the needle or by injecting particulate steroid-like methylprednisolone acetate into it. This artery provides major arterial supply to the lumbar spinal cord. It enters the spinal canal through a single intervertebral foramen anywhere between T8 and L3 and is located on the left side 78% of the time. Injury to this artery or any spinal artery can be avoided by making sure that the needle is not too lateral in the interlaminar space in the AP view.

Epidural abscess is a serious event, but if meticulous attention is paid to sterility, this complication will not be a problem, especially if the patient is not having any systemic or local infection. The most common offending agent is *Staphylococcus aureus*. The incubation period is 7 to 10 days before signs or symptoms are noted. Patients complain of severe back pain, fevers with chills, and localized tenderness; they have leukocytosis with elevated erythrocyte sedimentation rate (ESR) and C-reactive protein. If not diagnosed early and treated, they may develop neurologic deficits. Treatment can range from intravenous antibiotics to urgent laminectomy and débridement. Because the epidural veins communicate directly with the cranial sinuses, this infection can spread to the CNS. Meningitis has also been reported, possibly from the aforementioned mechanism.

Epidural hematoma is a rare event in patients with normal clotting mechanisms. It can lead to rapidly progressing neurologic deficits secondary to compression of the spinal cord, and it is very important to recognize it early because deficits can be reversed if the hematoma is evacuated soon enough. If not, the consequences can be disastrous. Some patients have increased pain after lumbar epidural steroid injection; but in a majority of the cases, it is transient.

CONCLUSION

Lumbar epidural steroid injections are the most commonly used interventional modality for management of low back pain; however, the differentiation between caudal and lumbar is not available statistically. Although the rationale for lumbar epidural steroid injections is the logical presumption that delivery of the steroids as close as possible to the inflamed nerve root results in high concentration of the steroid, the results of randomized trials showing the effectiveness of interlaminar epidural steroids is disappointing.

References

1. Manchikanti L, Staats P, Singh V, et al: Evidence-based practice guidelines for interventional techniques in the management of chronic spinal pain. Pain Physician 6:3, 2003.
2. Manchikanti L, Singh V, Kloth D, et al: Interventional techniques in the management of chronic pain: Part 2.0. Pain Physician 4:24, 2001.
3. Kepes ER, Duncalf D: Treatment of backache with spinal injections of local anesthetics, spinal and systemic steroids. Pain 22:33, 1985.
4. Benzon HT: Epidural steroid injections for low back pain and lumbosacral radiculography. Pain 24:277, 1986.
5. Bogduk N, Christophidis N, Cherry D, et al: Epidural use of steroids in the management of back pain. Report of working party on epidural use of steroids in the management of back pain. National Health and Medical Research Council. Canberra, Commonwealth of Australia, 1994, p 1.
6. Koes BW, Scholten RJPM, Mens JMA, et al: Efficacy of epidural steroid injections for low back pain and sciatica: A systematic review of randomized clinical trials. Pain 63:279, 1995.
7. Bogduk N: Epidural steroids for low back pain and sciatica. Pain Digest 9:226, 1999.
8. Koes BW, Scholten R, Mens JMA, et al: Epidural steroid injections for low back pain and sciatica. An updated systematic review of randomized clinical trials. Pain Digest 9:241, 1999.
9. Benzon HT: Epidural steroid injections. Pain Digest 1:271, 1992.
10. Benzon HT, Molly RE: Outcomes, efficacy, and compliances from management of low back pain. In Raj PP, Abrams BM, Benzon HT et al (eds): Practical Management of Pain, 3rd ed. Philadelphia, Mosby, 2000, p 891.
11. Watts RW, Silagy CA: A meta-analysis on the efficacy of epidural corticosteroids in the treatment of sciatica. Anaesth Intens Care 23:564, 1995.
12. McQuay HJ, Moore RA: Epidural Corticosteroids for Sciatica. An Evidence-Based Resource for Pain Relief. New York, Oxford University Press, 1998, p 216.
13. Nelemans PJ, deBie RA, deVet HCW: Injection therapy for subacute and chronic benign low back pain. Spine 26:501, 2001.
14. van Tulder MWV, Koes BW, Bouter LM: Conservative treatment of acute and chronic nonspecific low back pain. A systematic review of randomized controlled trials of the most common interventions. Spine 22:2128, 1997.
15. Boswell MV: Epidural steroids in the management of chronic spinal pain and radiculopathy. Pain Physician 6:319, 2003.
16. Sicard JA: Les injections medicamenteuse extradurales per voie saracoccygiene. Comptes Renues des Senances de la Societe de Biolgie et de ses Filliales 53:396, 1901.
17. Cathelin F: Mode d'action de a cocaine injete dans l'escapte epidural par le procede du canal sacre. Comptes Rendies des Senaces de la Societe de Biologic et de ses Filliales 53:452, 1901.
18. Pasquier NM, Leri D: Injection intra-et extradurales de cocaine a dose minime daus le traitment de la sciatique. Bull Gen Ther 142:196, 1901.
19. Caussade G, Queste P: Traitement de la neuralgie sciatique par la mèthode de Sicard. Résultats favorables même dans les cas chroniues par la cocaine à doses élevées et répétées à intervalles raproches. Bull Soc Med Hosp Paris 28:865, 1909.
20. Viner N: Intractable sciatica—the sacral epidural injection—an effective method of giving pain relief. Can Med Asso J 15:630, 1925.
21. Evans W: Intrasacral epidural injection in the treatment of sciatica. Lancet 2:1225, 1930.
22. Ombregt L, Ter Veer HJ: Treatment of the lumbar spine. In Ombregt L, Bisschop P, Ter Veer HJ, et al (eds): A System of Orthopaedic Medicine. London, WB Saunders, 1995, p 633.
23. Cyriax JH: Epidural anesthesia and bedrest in sciatica. Br Med J 1:20, 1961.
24. Brown JH: Pressure caudal anesthesia and back manipulation. Northwest Med 59: 905-909, 1960.
25. Kafiluddi R, Hahn MB: Epidural neural blockade. In Raj PP (ed): Practical Management of Pain, 3rd ed. St. Louis, Mosby, 2000, p 637.
26. Corning JL: Spinal anesthesia and local medication of the cord with cocaine. NY Med J 42:483, 1885.
27. Pagés E: Anestesia metamerica. Rev Sanid Mil Madr 11:351, 1921
28. Bromage PR: Identification of the epidural space. In Bromage PR (ed): Epidural Analgesia. Philadelphia, WB Saunders, 1978, p 178.
29. Dogliotti AM: Segmental peridural anesthesia. Am J Surg 20:107, 1033.
30. Gutierrez A: Valor de la aspiracion liquada en al espacio peridural en la anestesia peridural. Rev Circ 12:225, 1933.
31. Rovenstein EA, Wertheim HM: Therapeutic nerve block. JAMA 117:1599, 1941.
32. Jacobsen L, Mariano A, Chabal C, et al: Beyond the needle. Expanding the role of anesthesiologist in the management of chronic non-malignant pain. Anesthesiology 87:1210, 1997.
33. Ruben JE: Experience with a pain clinic. Anesthesiology 5:574, 1951.
34. Hench PS, Slocum CH, Polley HF, et al: Effect of cortisone and pituitary adrenocorticotrophic hormone (ACTH) on rheumatic diseases. JAMA 144:1327, 1950.
35. Orth DN, Kovacs WJ: The adrenal gland. In Wilson JD, Foster DW, Kronenberg HM, Larsen PR (eds): Williams Textbook of Endocrinology, 9th ed. Philadelphia, WB Saunders, 1998, p 517.
36. Robecchi A, Capra R: L'idrocortisone (composto F). Prime esperienze cliniche in campo reumatologico. Minerva Med 98:1259, 1952.
37. Lievre JA, Bloch-Michel H, Pean G, et al: L'hydrocortisone en injection locale. Rev Rheum 20:310, 1953.
38. Goebert HW, Jallo SJ, Gardner WJ, et al: Painful radiculopathy treated with epidural injections of procaine and hydrocortisone acetate results in 113 patients. Anesth Analg 140:130, 1961.
39. Kuslich SD, Ulstrom CL, Michael CJ: The tissue origin of low back pain and sciatica: A report of pain response to tissue stimulation during operation on the lumbar spine using local anesthesia. Orthop Clin North Am 22:181, 1991.
40. Mixter WJ, Barr JS: Rupture of the intervertebral disc involvement of the spinal canal. N Engl J Med 211:210, 1934.
41. Carette S, Lecaire R, Marcoux S, et al: Epidural corticosteroid injections for sciatica due to herniated nucleus pulposus. N Engl J Med 336:1634, 1997.

42. Frymoyer JW: Lumbar disk disease: Epidemiology. Instr Course Lect 41:217, 1992.
43. Saal JA, Saal JS, Herzog RJ: The natural history of lumbar intervertebral disc extrusions treated nonoperatively. Spine 15:683, 1990.
44. Bush K, Cowan N, Katz DE, et al: The natural history of sciatica associated with disc pathology: A prospective study with clinical and independent radiologic follow-up. Spine 17:1205, 1992.
45. Maigne JY, Rime B, Delinge B: Computed tomographic follow-up study of forty-eight cases of nonoperatively treated lumbar intervertebral disc herniation. Spine 17:1071, 1992.
46. Delauche-Cavallier MC, Budet C, Laredo JD, et al: Lumbar disc herniation: Computed tomography scan changes after conservative treatment of nerve root compression. Spine 17:927, 1992.
47. Jensen MC, Bran-Zawadzki MN, Obucjowski N, et al: Magnetic resonance imaging of the lumbar spine in people without back pain. N Engl J Med 331:69, 1994.
48. Wiesel SW: A study of computer-assisted tomography. 1. The incidence of positive CAT scans in an asymptomatic group of patients. Spine 9:549, 1986.
49. Devor M: Pain arising from the nerve root and the dorsal root ganglia and chronically injured axons: A physiological basis for the radicular pain of nerve root compression. Pain 3:25, 1977.
50. Olmarker K, Rydevik B, Holm S: Edema formation in spinal nerve roots induced by experimental, graded compression: An experimental study on the pig cauda equina with special reference to differences in effects between rapid and slow onset of compression. Spine 14:569, 1989.
51. Yoshizawa H, Nakai S, Koboyashi S, et al: Intraradicular edema formation as a basic factor in lumbar radiculopathy. In Weinstein JN, Gordon SL (eds): Low Back Pain: A Scientific and Clinical Overview. Rosemont, Ill, American Academy of Orthopaedic Surgeons, 1996, p 235.
52. Olmarker K, Rydevik B, Holm B, et al: Effects of experimental graded compression on blood flow in spinal nerve roots: A vital microscopic study on the porcine cauda equina. J Orthop Res 7:817, 1989.
53. Homma Y, Brull SJ, Zhang J: A comparison of chronic pain behavior following local application of tumor necrosis factor a to the normal and mechanically compressed lumbar ganglia in the rat. Pain 95:239, 2002.
54. Chen C, Cavanaugh JM, Song Z, et al: Effects of nucleus pulposus on nerve root neural activity, mechanosensitivity, axonal morphology, and sodium channel expression. Spine 29:17, 2003.
55. Manchikanti L: Transforaminal lumbar epidural steroid injections. Pain Physician 3:374, 2000.
56. Fredman B, Nun MB, Zohar E, et al: Epidural steroids for treating "failed back surgery syndrome": Is fluoroscopy really necessary? Anesth Analg 88:367, 1999.
57. Mehta M, Salmon N: Extradural block. Confirmation of the injection site by x-ray monitoring. Anaesthesia 40:1009, 1985.
58. Burn JM, Guyer PB, Langdon L: The spread of solutions injected into the epidural space: A study using epidurograms in patients with lumbosciatic syndrome. Br J Anaesth 45:338, 1973.
59. Nishimura N, Khahara T, Kusakabe T: The spread of lidocaine and I-131 solution in the epidural space. Anesthesiology 20:785, 1959.
60. Hodgson PSA, Mack B, Kopacz D, et al: Needle placement during lumbar epidural anesthesia deviates toward the non-dependent side [abstract]. Reg Anesth 21:26, 1996.
61. Bromage PR, Benumof JL: Paraplegia following intracord injection during attempted epidural anesthesia under general anesthesia. Reg Anesth Pain Med 23:104, 1998.
62. Houten JK, Errico TJ: Paraplegia after lumbosacral nerve root block: Report of three cases. Spine J 2:70, 2002.
63. Manchikanti L: Role of neuraxial steroids in interventional pain management. Pain Physician 5:182, 2002.
64. Fox AJ, Melzack R: Transcutaneous electrical stimulation to acupuncture. Comparison of treatment of low back pain. Pain 2:141, 1976.
65. Fowler RJ, Blackwell GJ: Anti-inflammatory steroid induced biosynthesis of a phospholipase A_2 inhibitor which prevents prostaglandin generation. Nature 278:456, 1979.
66. Devor M, Govrin-Lippmann R, Raber P: Corticosteroids suppress ectopic neural discharges originating in experimental neuromas. Pain 22:127, 1985.
67. Hua SY, Chen YZ: Membrane receptor-mediated electrophysiological effects of glucocorticoid on mammalian neurons. Endocrinology 24; 687, 1989.
68. Johansson A, Hao J, Sjolund B: Local corticosteroid application blocks transmission in normal nociceptor C-fibers. Acta Anaesthesiol Scand 34:335, 1990.
69. Hayashi N, Weinstein JN, Meller ST, et al: The effect of epidural injection of betamethasone or bupivacaine in a rat model of lumbar radiculopathy. Spine 23:877, 1998.
70. Olmarker K, Byrod G, Cornefijord M, et al: Effects of methylprednisolone on nucleus pulposus-induced nerve root injury. Spine 19:1803, 1994.
71. Lee HM, Weinstein JN, Meller ST, et al: The role of steroids and their effects on phospholipase A_2. An animal model of radiculopathy. Spine 23:1191, 1998.
72. Minamide A, Tamaki T, Hashizume H, et al: Effects of steroids and lipopolysaccharide on spontaneous resorption of herniated intervertebral discs. An experience study in the rabbit. Spine 23:870, 1998.
73. Johansson A, Bennett GJ: Effect of local methylprednisolone on pain in a nerve injury model. A pilot study. Reg Anesth 22:59, 1997.
74. Kingery WS, Castellote JM, Maze M: Methylprednisolone prevents the development of autotomy and neuropathic edema in rats, but has no effect on nociceptive thresholds. Pain 80:555, 1999.
75. Kantrowitz F, Robinson DR, McGuire MB, et al: Corticosteroids inhibit prostaglandin production by rheumatoid synovia. Nature 258:737, 1975.
76. Byrod G, Otani K, Brisby H, et al: Methylprednisolone reduces the early vascular permeability increase in spinal nerve roots induced by epidural nucleus pulposus application. J Orthop Res 18:983, 2000.
77. Blomberg RG, Olsson SS: The lumbar epidural space in patients examined with epiduroscopy. Anesth Analg 68:157, 1989.
78. Manchikanti L, Cash K, Moss T, et al: Effectiveness of protective measures in reducing risk of radiation exposure in interventional pain management: A prospective evaluation. Pain Physician 6:301, 2003.
79. Manchikanti L, Cash K, Moss T, et al: Risk of whole body radiation exposure and protective measures in fluoroscopically guided interventional techniques: A prospective evaluation. BMC Anesthesiology 3:2, 2003.
80. Botwin KP, Natalicchio J, Hanna A: Fluoroscopic guided lumbar interlaminar epidural injections: A prospective evaluation of epidurography contrast patterns and anatomical review of the epidural space. Pain Physician 7:77, 2004.

chapter 153

Subarachnoid Neurolytic Blocks

Alon P. Winnie and Kenneth D. Candido

Dogliotti[1] first described the technique of subarachnoid chemical neurolysis using alcohol for the treatment of sciatic pain more than 70 years ago. In the same year, Suvansa[2] described intrathecal carbolic acid for the treatment of tetanus. A quarter of a century later, Maher,[3,4] in two landmark articles, described his experience with hyperbaric phenol and silver nitrate for subarachnoid neurolysis, stating, "It is easier to lay a carpet than to paper a ceiling." Over the ensuing years, however, lack of experience with either technique and fear of the anticipated complications resulted in underuse of this valuable modality. Better understanding and increased use of neuraxial opiates for cancer pain since the 1980s have decreased the use of subarachnoid chemical neurolysis even further. Nonetheless, because of the physical separation of the sensory and motor roots of spinal nerves within the spinal canal, intrathecal dorsal rhizotomy (more appropriately called *rhizolysis*) is the only neurolytic procedure that allows sensory block without concomitant motor block. Because of this and because of the relative precision with which the affected nerve roots can be blocked, the technique is particularly useful for treating cancer pain in an extremity, where preservation of motor function is so important. In short, the physical separation of motor and sensory fibers in the subarachnoid space preserves forever a small but unique role for subarachnoid neurolysis in the management of cancer pain in carefully selected patients.

SELECTION CRITERIA

Because the duration of action of neurolytic agents in the subarachnoid space is finite but unpredictable, great care must be exercised in choosing appropriate candidates for the procedure. Neurolytic blockade by this route is especially suited to patients in whom conventional treatment regimens have failed and who have a short life expectancy, usually less than 1 year. As with all neurolytic procedures, patients must be completely apprised of the possibility of debilitating side effects and other serious associated complications that can follow even a successful block, most notably, motor weakness and incontinence. The selection criteria for subarachnoid neurolysis include the following:

- The diagnosis is well established.[5]
- The patient's life expectancy is short, usually 6 to 12 months.
- The patient's pain is unresponsive to antineoplastic therapy (chemotherapy, radiation).
- The patient's pain has failed to respond to adequate trials of analgesic agents and adjunctive drugs.
- The pain is localized to two or three dermatomes.
- The pain is predominantly somatic in origin.
- The pain is unilateral (neurolytic blocks for bilateral pain should be staggered).[6]

INFORMED CONSENT

It is crucial that not only the patient, but also the patient's family fully understand the anticipated procedure, its potential risks, the alternative forms of therapy available, and, most importantly, the possibility of serious complications. It is important that the patient and family understand that the procedure does not simply "take away pain," but rather substitutes numbness (loss of sensation) for the pain. So important is this concept that, with rare exceptions, before the decision is made to proceed with a subarachnoid neurolytic block, a prognostic subarachnoid block should be carried out using a local anesthetic so that the patient can experience the pain relief that may be anticipated after a neurolytic block and the accompanying sensory block. Although an occasional patient may decide that he or she cannot tolerate the numbness, most patients prefer this lack of sensation to the pain and choose to proceed with the neurolytic procedure.

TECHNIQUE

Because unfamiliarity with the details of this technique has been a major obstacle to its use, and because proper execution of the technique determines its success and safety, the focus of the present discussion is on the technical aspects of subarachnoid neurolysis. First, because of the "permanence" of the complications of this technique, subarachnoid neurolysis should be attempted only after careful review of a dermatome chart to determine precisely which nerve or nerves are subserving the patient's pain (Fig. 153–1). If the patient's pain is due to one or more metastases to bone, it may be useful to refer to a sclerotome chart because the innervation of some parts of the skeleton differs from that of the overlying soft tissues (Fig. 153–2).

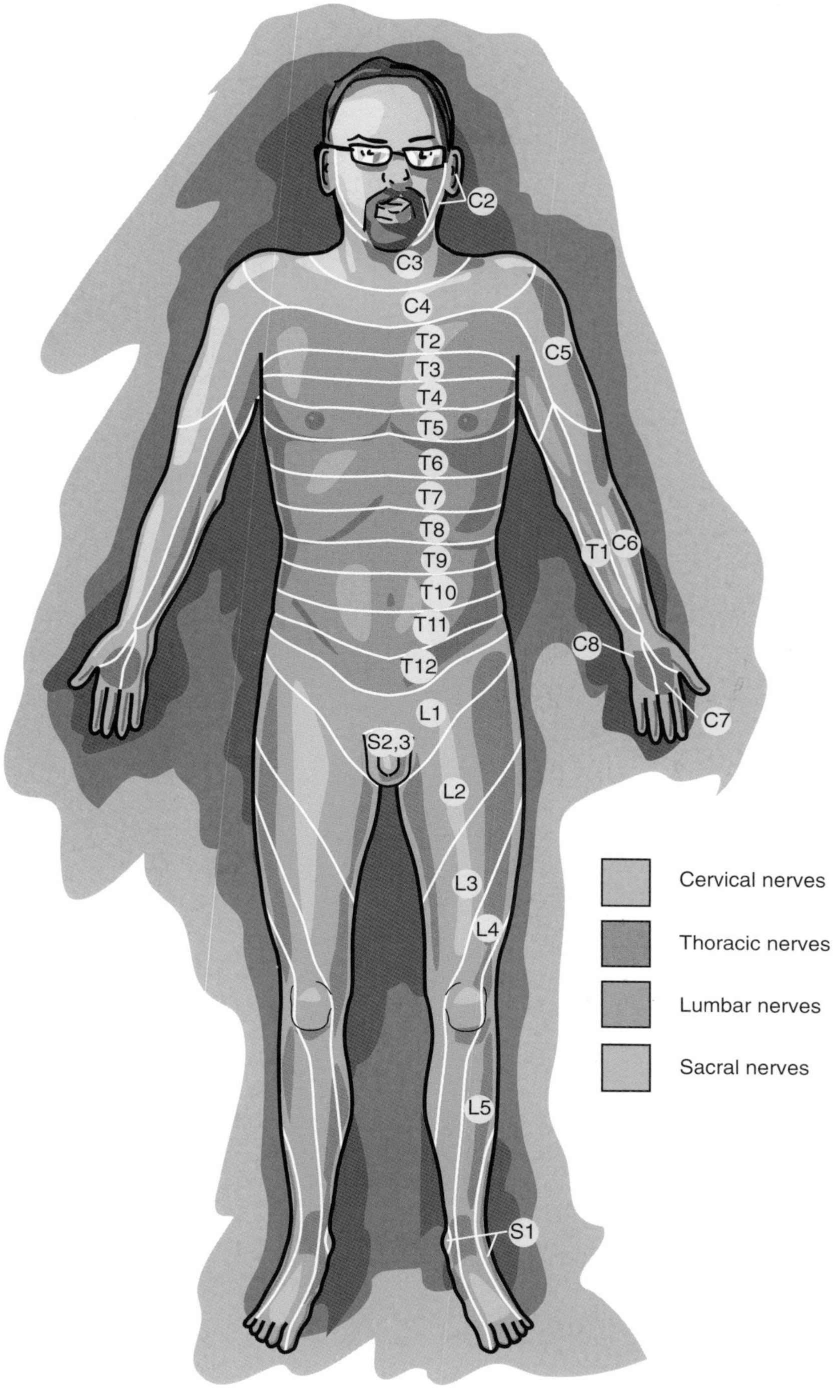

FIGURE 153–1 ■ View of the dermatomes. (Foerster, I. The dermatomes of man. Brain, 1993; 56:1-39)

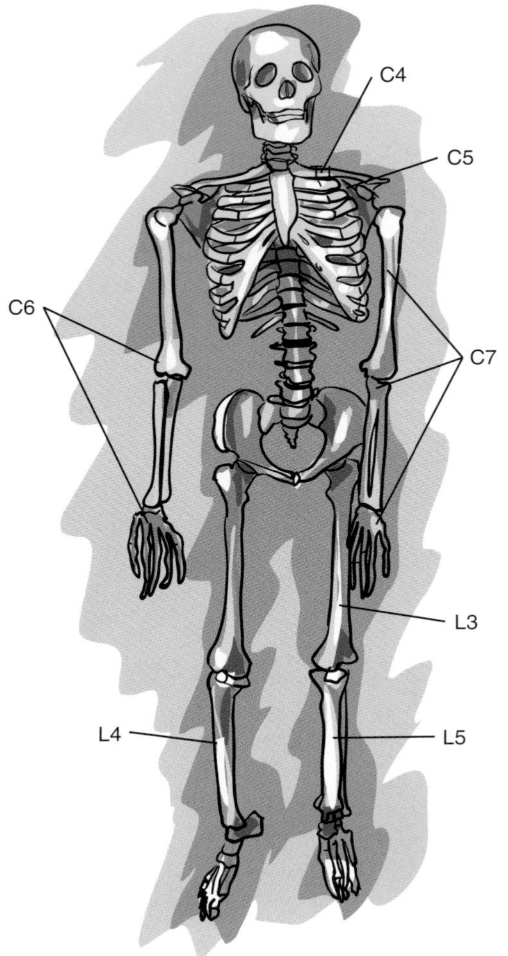

FIGURE 153–2 ■ Innervation of the skeleton by spinal segments from the anterior aspect. The various scelerotomes are indicated by the different styles of shading. (Modified from Déjerine J: Séminologie du Systéme Nerveux. Paris, Masson, 1914.)

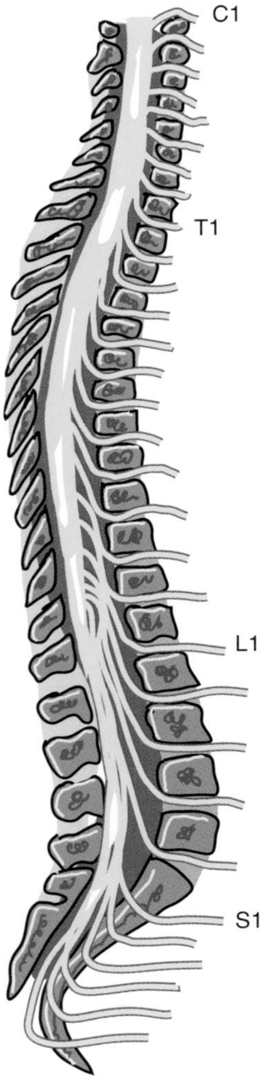

FIGURE 153–3 ■ The alignment of spinal segments with vertebrae. The bodies and spinous processes of the vertebrae are shown, and the spinal segments and their respective nerves are indicated by Arabic numbers. The cervical nerves exit through intervertebral foramina above their respective vertebral bodies, and the other nerves issue below those bodies.

Second, because a neurolytic subarachnoid block must be carried out at the level where the dorsal root to be blocked leaves the spinal cord (to spare motor function), it is essential to determine which interlaminar foramen affords access to that root. Although the cervical nerves exit at a level higher than their respective vertebral bodies, all of the other nerves exit at a level below their respective vertebral bodies because of the differential growth of the spinal cord and vertebral column in utero and for the first few years of life (Fig. 153–3).[7] Finally, a choice must be made before the procedure is undertaken to determine whether a hyperbaric (phenol in glycerin) or hypobaric (absolute alcohol) technique is more appropriate. No controlled studies have compared the outcomes with subarachnoid alcohol and phenol, but in our experience hypobaric alcohol has been the technique of choice in most cases because most patients with severe, intractable pain cannot lie on the painful side, a requirement when using hyperbaric phenol. Although at one time clinicians believed that phenol might exert a preferential effect on the small fibers subserving pain, it has been determined that neither alcohol nor phenol is a selective neurolytic agent, eliminating this as a rationale for choosing phenol over alcohol.[8-10]

SUBARACHNOID NEUROLYSIS WITH ALCOHOL

Because absolute alcohol is extremely hypobaric, when this agent is used, the patient is first placed in the lateral decubitus position with the painful site uppermost and is then rolled anteriorly approximately 45 degrees to place the dorsal (sensory) root uppermost (Fig. 153–4).[11] The patient is stabilized with straps and made as comfortable as possible with pillows because he or she needs to remain in this position throughout the procedure. An assistant is mandatory to stabilize the patient and to allay anxiety. After the patient has been positioned properly, and the patient's role in the procedure has been reviewed, a 22-gauge spinal needle is inserted and advanced through the interlaminar space at the level of the dorsal root to be blocked. If the procedure is being carried out at a thoracic level, because of the long, caudally sloping spinous processes, a paravertebral approach is usually easier

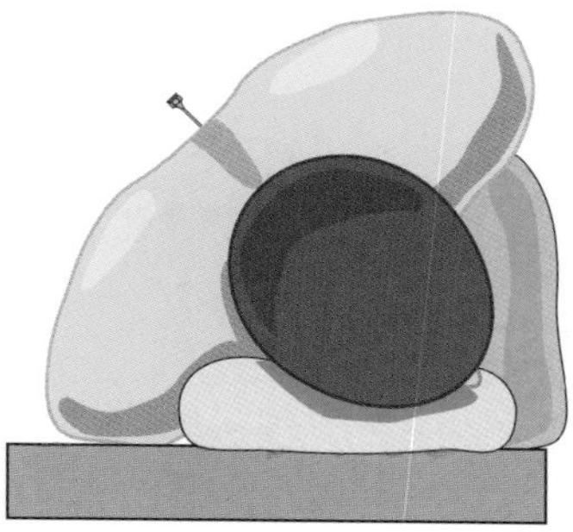

FIGURE 153–4 ■ **A** and **B,** Proper positioning of the patient with left-sided pain for intrathecal injection of alcohol. Note the 45-degree anterior tilt, intended to bathe the posterior (sensory) nerve roots with hypobaric alcohol, while sparing the anterior (motor) roots. (From Waldman SD: Atlas of Interventional Pain Management, 2nd ed. Philadelphia, WB Saunders, 2004, Chapter 114, Lumbar Subarachnoid Neurolytic Block, pp 529-530.)

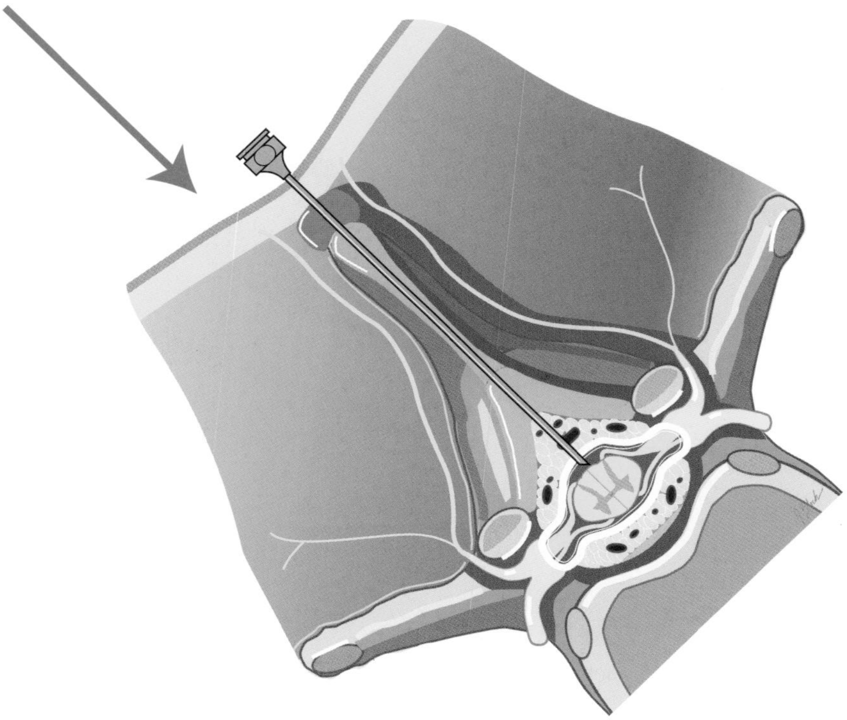

A

(Figure continues on page 1298)

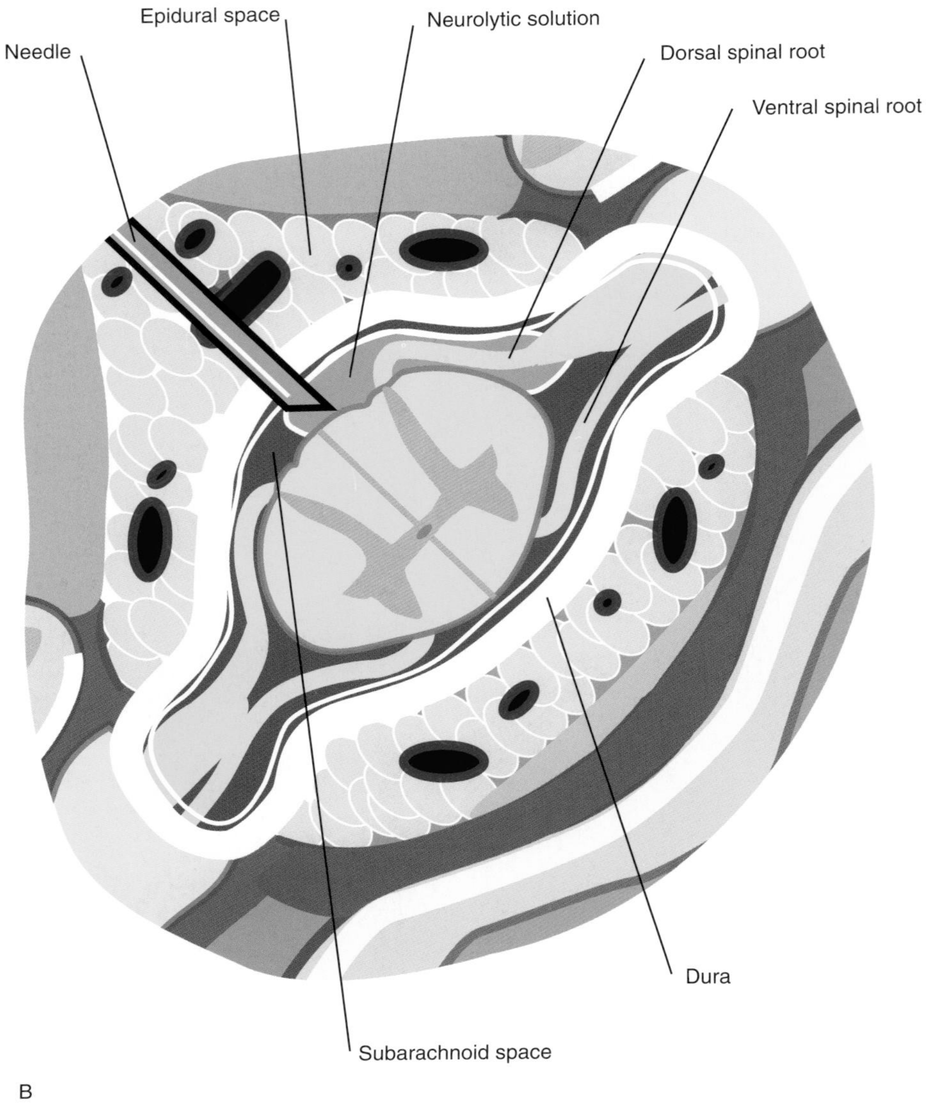

FIGURE 153–4—Cont'd

than a midline approach; whatever the approach, the needle tip should penetrate the dura in the midline. Needles smaller than 22-gauge should not be selected for this technique because the free flow of CSF is essential, and because post-dural puncture headache is extremely rare after subarachnoid alcohol neurolysis. A prognostic block with local anesthetic should already have been carried out to determine whether the pain can be relieved by the technique, and, equally important, whether the patient can tolerate the numbness.

Contrary to the recommendation in many texts, a test dose of local anesthetic should *not* be given when the needle is in place for a neurolytic block. The reason is that none of the available local anesthetics can be made as hypobaric as absolute alcohol, so a hypobaric local anesthetic "test dose" would not find its way to and block the same nerve root as the much more hypobaric alcohol, resulting in misinformation as to the placement of the neurolytic solution. Also contrary to the recommendation in most textbooks, a local anesthetic should not be administered before the injection of the alcohol because the pain produced by the injection of the alcohol is an essential indicator that enhances the accuracy and effectiveness of the procedure. Instead of preventing the burning pain caused by the alcohol, the physician must tell the patient *to expect* severe, localized, burning pain, *but only for a fraction of a second* after each injection, and to *focus attention* on whether that burning occurs *at, above,* or *below* the level of the pain. The patient also is instructed to report any other sensations, such as tingling, warmth, or numbness.

Subarachnoid alcohol neurolysis is a precise procedure, and to ensure efficacy and safety, the alcohol should be injected in 0.1-mL aliquots using a tuberculin syringe. The syringe containing the alcohol should not be attached to the needle until the free flow of CSF indicates that the needle is definitely in the subarachnoid space. When the syringe has been attached to the needle, aspiration should *not* be carried out to verify proper needle placement because alcohol causes the CSF to form a white coagulum within the syringe. When the syringe has been attached to the needle, the subjective experience of each injection and the importance of the brief burning sensation to the success of the technique are reiterated one more time, after which sequential injection of 0.1-mL increments of alcohol begins. The operator asks the patient the same questions about the presence and location of the burning after each aliquot. The first one or two increments of alcohol usually do not produce the expected burning pain simply because this volume is just enough to fill the hub and shaft of the spinal needle. The third or fourth 0.1-mL increment invariably produces the expected burning, however, and it reassures the patient as to how short-lived it is.

More important, the level at which the burning is perceived in relation to the location of the pain serves as an indicator as to whether the needle has been placed at the proper level. If the burning occurs at precisely the level of the patient's pain, a total volume of absolute alcohol not greater than 0.7 mL is injected in 0.1-mL increments; after about the fifth or sixth increment, there should be little or no additional burning. If the burning produced by the third or fourth increment of alcohol occurs *above* the site of the patient's pain, injections through that needle are discontinued, although the needle is left in place as a marker. A second needle (and if necessary even a third) must be inserted through progressively lower interspaces until the burning produced by the incremental injection of alcohol corresponds *exactly* to the distribution of the patient's pain. Likewise, if the initial injection of alcohol produces burning pain *below* the level of the patient's pain, a second needle (and if necessary a third) must be inserted through progressively higher interspaces until the injection of the 0.1-mL increments of alcohol produces burning in the precise distribution of the pain. At this point, the entire 0.7 mL is injected in 0.1-mL increments to produce the desired neurolysis. When the total volume of alcohol has been injected through each needle, the stylet is replaced, and the needle is left in place until the entire procedure has been completed.

When a nerve subserving a patient's pain has been identified and blocked by this process, and a total of 0.7 mL of alcohol has been injected, the process is repeated above or below (or above *and* below) the level of the initial full injection to abolish the pain completely. No more than three or four nerves should ever be blocked at one session, but as indicated in the selection criteria, this procedure is best reserved for patients with pain limited to two or three dermatomes. In contrast to subarachnoid injections of local anesthetics for surgical anesthesia, the injection of alcohol for subarachnoid neurolysis must be made through a separate needle to block each nerve root. The reason that alcohol cannot be "floated" to a higher or lower level through a single needle, as is done when performing a hypobaric spinal for surgery, is that alcohol "fixes" too quickly and would not float far enough to block the adjacent dermatomes. Matsuki and coworkers[12] showed that the CSF concentration of alcohol is rapidly reduced after intrathecal injection, a finding that implies rapid uptake by nerve tissue. In short, for best results, a separate needle *must* be placed at the level of each nerve root to be blocked. When the injections through the appropriate three or four needles are completed, and before each needle is withdrawn (including needles placed at inappropriate levels), 0.2 to 0.3 mL of air should be injected to clear the shaft and hub of alcohol to minimize the possibility that alcohol trickling from the needle as it is withdrawn from dura to skin will form a fistula. Experience indicates that the 0.1 to 0.2 mL of alcohol injected at levels that turned out to be inappropriate does not cause any demonstrable neurologic damage.

SUBARACHNOID NEUROLYSIS WITH PHENOL

Intrathecal phenol in glycerin may be used as an alternative to alcohol for subarachnoid neurolysis. The technique is similar to that described earlier except that the patient must be positioned with the painful side down because phenol in glycerin is a *hyperbaric* solution. Because most patients with pain of malignant origin have difficulty lying on the painful side, in our experience alcohol remains the neurolytic of choice in most patients. If phenol neurolysis is appropriate for a particular patient, however, the technique is similar to that used for alcohol neurolysis except that the patient is positioned with the dorsal root lowermost and with the head of the bed slightly elevated (Fig. 153–5).[11]

The patient must be tilted posteriorly with the back as close to the edge of the bed as possible, using bolsters, straps, or pillows to maintain the patient securely in position. The presence of an assistant to hold the patient securely and to provide emotional and physical reassurance is mandatory. For this technique, a 22-gauge (or even better, a 20-gauge) spinal needle should be used because of the viscosity of the phenol-glycerin mixture. In a manner essentially opposite to the technique of subarachnoid alcohol neurolysis, the bevel of the spinal needle should be directed inferiorly (laterally toward the table). Because of the viscosity of phenol in glycerin, it takes significant pressure applied to the plunger of the syringe to force the phenol into the subarachnoid space, so the injection must be done slowly and carefully to prevent the escape of phenol from the syringe and onto the skin of the patient or the practitioner. Warming the phenol lessens its viscosity and makes it easier to inject. Because phenol has local anesthetic properties, its injection into the subarachnoid space is not accompanied by the burning pain produced by alcohol, although the patient may feel warmth, tingling, or even mild dysesthesia in the distribution of the nerve being injected. Similar to alcohol, the concentration of phenol in the CSF declines rapidly after the initial injection, implying rapid absorption by neural tissues.[13] This has important implications as to how long *after* the neurolytic agent has been injected patients must remain as originally positioned. Traditionally, they have been kept in these (obviously uncomfortable) positions for at least 30 minutes after the neurolytic injection, but probably patients can be allowed to assume a more comfortable posture after 15 to 20 minutes, keeping in mind the relative position of the dorsal roots in the spinal canal when doing so. As with alcohol, after the subarachnoid injection of phenol in glycerin, 0.1 to 0.3 mL of air is injected to flush the lytic solution from each needle before it is removed.

SUCCESS AND COMPLICATION RATES

Careful patient selection and equally careful technique are essential for successful subarachnoid neurolysis and for the prevention of complications. Although subarachnoid neurolysis may be attempted at cervical, thoracic, or lumbosacral

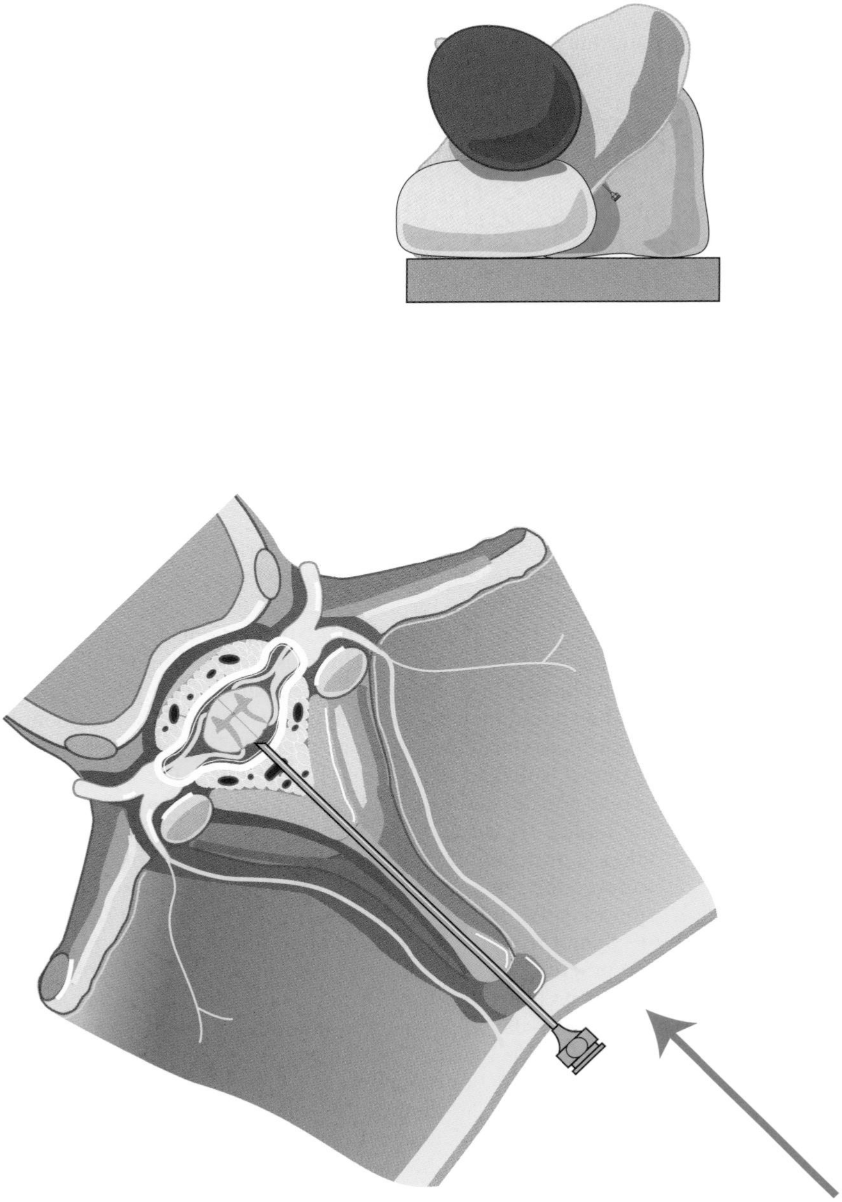

A

FIGURE 153–5 ■ **A** and **B,** Proper positioning of the patient with left-sided pain for intrathecal injection of phenol in glycerin. Note the 45-degree posterior tilt, intended to bathe the posterior (sensory) nerve roots with hyperbaric phenol, while sparing the anterior (motor) roots. (From Waldman SD: Atlas of Interventional Pain Management, 2nd ed. Philadelphia, WB Saunders, 2004. Lumbar Subarachnoid Neurolytic Block, pp 531-532.)

(Figure continues on page 1301)

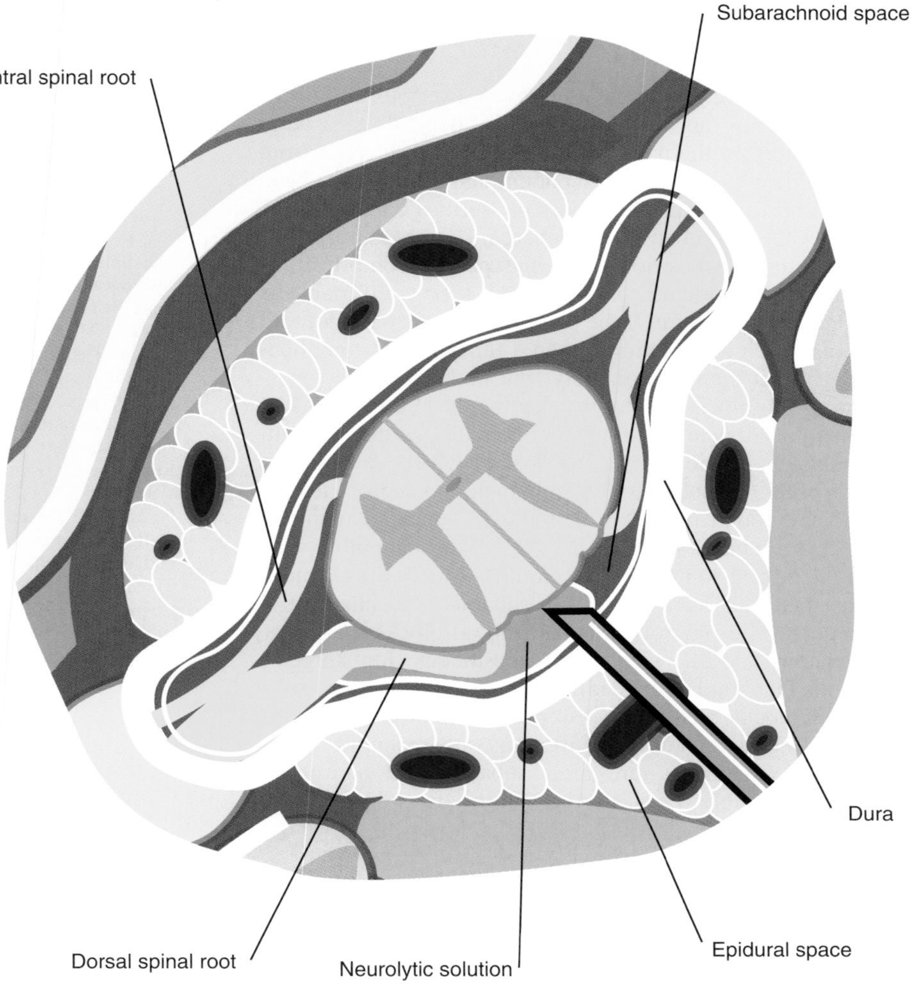

FIGURE 153–4—Cont'd

levels, the success rates and the incidence of complications vary, depending on the level of injection, primarily because of the anatomic differences at different levels. The distance between the origins of nerve roots decreases progressively in the lumbosacral area so that the lower an injection is made, the more difficult it becomes to block a single nerve root without involving adjacent roots. Yet cervical subarachnoid neurolytic blocks seem to be less successful than similar blocks carried out at thoracic or even lumbosacral levels.[14] Penetration of the spinal cord by the needle is a concern whenever these techniques are undertaken, especially at cervical or thoracic levels. This is a rare occurrence, but when it does occur, Perese[15] reported that no permanent injury results, only transient pain, which warns the clinician of the position of the needle and prevents subsequent injection into the cord.

From the point of view of complications, neurolytic subarachnoid blocks may be safest when undertaken in the midthoracic region because this region is relatively distant from the fibers that subserve limb, bowel, and bladder function,[16] so any motor loss would be of little consequence. Conversely, in the lumbosacral region, owing to the proximity of sensory and motor fibers to each other (because of the decreasing size of the conus medullaris, the dorsal and ventral roots are very close together) and to the proximity of both to the autonomic fibers subserving bowel and bladder function, lumbar subarachnoid neurolysis usually is reserved strictly for select individuals in whom the risk-to-benefit ratio has been clearly delineated. For patients who already have compromised sphincter function, lumbosacral subarachnoid phenol neurolysis has been advocated for rectal and pelvic malignancies because of the tendency of phenol to spare motor function.[17]

It is difficult to compare the success rates achieved with subarachnoid neurolysis by various investigators because of the different methods used to quantify pain and pain relief, but it would seem that one should expect a "beneficial effect" in about 75% of the patients, "excellent results" in 50%, and "fair results" in another 25%.[16] A review of the literature seems to indicate that the success rate is slightly greater with alcohol than with phenol, whereas the complication rate is slightly greater with phenol than with alcohol.[3,4,17-31] In assessing the success of a subarachnoid neurolytic procedure, even if a block produces only moderate pain relief, it may be sufficient to allow analgesic agents that could not control the pain previously to render the patient pain-free, or at least to make the patient comfortable. One should not consider a neurolytic block to be successful *only* if the patient is rendered pain-free without any supplemental analgesics, although such success is very rewarding.

The impact of a complication, even a serious complication, on a patient and his or her family depends to a large extent on whether the patient has significant pain relief from the neurolytic procedure. If the patient and family have been properly apprised of all of the possible serious complications that can follow a subarachnoid neurolytic procedure, many find even the most serious and unexpected complications acceptable *if* the patient is pain-free or at least comfortable as a result of the procedure. If the patient and family are not told of the possible complications, even a fairly minor complication may upset them inordinately (but understandably), particularly if the block fails to produce the desired relief. Most complications of neurolytic subarachnoid blocks are transient. Gerbershagen[32] reviewed reports that provided data on the duration of 303 complications of subarachnoid neurolytic procedures and found that 51% of them disappeared within 1 week, 21% within 1 month, and 9% within 4 months, with only 18% lasting longer than 4 months. Although postdural puncture headache can follow any subarachnoid block, it is less frequent after neurolytic subarachnoid blocks than after subarachnoid blocks with local anesthetics for surgery, despite the fact that larger needles are used for neurolytic subarachnoid blocks.[33] Similarly, aseptic meningitis (and even septic meningitis) can develop after any subarachnoid block; it also is exceedingly rare after subarachnoid neurolytic blocks, presumably because the neurolytic solutions are self-sterilizing.

CONCLUSION

Because of the physical separation of the sensory and motor nerve roots in the spinal canal, intrathecal chemical dorsal rhizotomy is the only neurolytic procedure that allows sensory block without concomitant motor block. For this reason subarachnoid neurolysis is a unique, effective modality for the management of cancer pain in certain patients. If the patients are carefully selected, and the technique is carefully carried out, pain relief can be provided in most cases without an excessive rate of complications.

References

1. Dogliotti AM: Traitement des syndromes doloreaux de la peripherie par l'alcoholisation subarachnoidienne des racines posterieures a leur émergence de la moelle epineri. Presse Med 39:1249, 1931.
2. Suvansa S: Treatment of tetanus by intrathecal injection of carbolic acid. Lancet 1:1075, 1931.
3. Maher RM: Relief of pain in incurable cancer. Lancet 1:18, 1955.
4. Maher RM: Neurone selection in relief of pain: Further experiences with intrathecal injections. Lancet 1:16, 1957.
5. Katz J: Current role of neurolytic agents. Adv Neurol 4:471, 1974.
6. Hollis PH, Malis LI, Zappulla RA: Neurological deterioration after lumbar puncture below complete spinal subarachnoid block. J Neurosurg 64:253, 1986.
7. Haymaker W, Woodhall B: Peripheral Nerve Injuries. Philadelphia, WB Saunders, 1945.
8. Nathan PW, Sears TA: Effects of phenol on nervous tissue. J Physiol 150:565, 1960.
9. Nathan PW, Sears TA, Smith MC: Effects of phenol solutions on the nerve roots of the cat: An electrophysiological and histological study. J Neurol Sci 2:7, 1965.
10. Patt R, Jain S: Management of a patient with osteoradionecrosis of the mandible with nerve blocks. J Pain Symptom Manage 5:59, 1990.
11. Swerdlow M: Neurolytic blocks. In Patt RB (ed): Cancer Pain. Philadelphia, JB Lippincott, 1993, pp 427-442.
12. Matsuki M, Kato Y, Ichiyanagi K: Progressive changes in the concentration of ethyl alcohol in the human and canine subarachnoid spaces. Anesthesiology 36:617, 1972.
13. Ichiyanagi K, Matsuki M, Kinefuchi S, Kato Y: Progressive changes in the concentrations of phenol and glycerine in the human subarachnoid space. Anesthesiology 42:622, 1975.
14. Swerdlow M: Spinal and peripheral neurolysis for managing Pancoast syndrome. Adv Pain Res Ther 4:135, 1982.
15. Perese DM: Subarachnoid alcohol block in the management of pain of malignant disease. Arch Surg 76:347, 1958.
16. Patt RB, Cousins MJ: Techniques for neurolytic neural blockade. In Cousins MJ, Bridenbaugh PO (eds): Neural Blockade. Philadelphia, JB Lippincott, 1998, p 1007.
17. Lifshitz S, Debacker LJ, Buchsbaum HJ: Subarachnoid phenol block for pain relief in gynecologic malignancy. Obstet Gynecol 48:316, 1976.
18. Stovner J, Endresen R: Intrathecal phenol for cancer pain. Acta Anaesth Scand 16:17, 1972.
19. Papo I, Visca A: Intrathecal phenol in the treatment of pain and spasticity. Proc Neurol Surg 7:56, 1976.
20. Papo I, Visca A: Phenol subarachnoid rhizotomy for the treatment of cancer pain: A personal account of 290 cases. Adv Pain Res Ther 2:339, 1979.
21. Ischia S, Luzzani A, Ischia A, et al: Subarachnoid neurolytic block (L_5-S_1) and unilateral percutaneous cervical cordotomy in the treatment of pain secondary to pelvic malignant disease. Pain 20:139, 1984.
22. Mark VH, White JC, Zervas NT, et al: Intrathecal use of phenol for the relief of chronic severe pain. N Engl J Med 267:589, 1962.
23. Hay RC: Subarachnoid alcohol block in the control of intractable pain: Report of results in 2153 patients. Anesth Analg 41:12, 1962.
24. Bruno G: Intrathecal alcohol block—experiences on 41 cases. Paraplegia 12:305, 1975.
25. Tank TM, Dohn DF, Gardner WJ: Intrathecal injections of alcohol or phenol for relief of intractable pain. Cleve Clin Q 30:111, 1963.
26. Superville-Sovak P, Rasminsky M, Finlayson MH: Complications of phenol neurolysis. Arch Neurol 32:226, 1975.
27. Holland AJC, Youssef M: A complication of subarachnoid phenol blockade. Anaesthesia 34:260, 1978.
28. Totoki T, Kato T, Nomoto Y, et al: Anterior spinal artery syndrome—a complication of cervical intrathecal phenol injection. Pain 6:99, 1979.
29. Evans RJ, Mackay IM: Subarachnoid phenol nerve blocks for relief of pain in advanced malignancy. Can J Surg 15:50, 1972.
30. Derrick W: Subarachnoid alcohol block for the control of intractable pain. Acta Anesth Scand 24(Suppl):167, 1966.
31. Stern EL: Dangers of intraspinal (subarachnoid) injection of alcohol: Their avoidance and contraindications. Am J Surg 35:99, 1937.
32. Gerbershagen HU: Neurolysis: Subarachnoid neurolytic blockade. Acta Anaesth Belg 1:45, 1981.
33. Patt RB, Wu CL, Reddy S, et al: Incidence of postdural puncture headache following intrathecal neurolysis with large caliber needles. Reg Anesth 19:86, 1994.

chapter 154

Lumbar Facet Block

Laxmaiah Manchikanti, David M. Schultz, and Vijay Singh

HISTORICAL CONSIDERATIONS

In 1911, Goldthwait[1] recognized lumbar facet joints as potential sources of back pain and explained facet joints as a cause of many cases of lumbago, sciatica, and paraplegia. Some twenty years later in 1933, Ghormley[2] coined the term *facet syndrome*, and defined it as lumbosacral pain with or without sciatic pain, particularly occurring suddenly after a twisting or rotatory strain of the lumbosacral region. In 1941, Badgley[3] suggested that facet joints themselves could be a primary source of pain separate from spinal nerve compression pain and made a plea for continuing focus on facet joints in order to explain the large numbers of patients with low back pain whose symptoms were not due to a ruptured disk. Hirsch and colleagues[4] demonstrated that low back pain distributed along the sacroiliac and gluteal areas with radiation to the greater trochanter could be induced by injecting hypertonic saline into the region of the facet joints.

Mooney and Robertson[5] and McCall[6] used fluoroscopic technique to inject hypertonic saline into the facet joints of asymptomatic volunteers and demonstrated causation of back and lower extremity pain. Marks[7] and Fukui and colleagues[8] also described the pattern of pain caused by facet joint stimulation and confirmed the findings of previous researchers. Windsor and colleagues[9] also confirmed that lumbar facet joints can be a source of pain in the low back. Mooney and Robertson[5] and McCall and coworkers[6] showed that stimulation of the facet joints produced back pain and somatic-referred pain identical to that commonly seen in patients; Kaplan and coworkers[10] and Dreyfuss and colleagues[11] showed that this pain can be relieved by anesthetizing the facet joints responsible for low back pain.

INDICATIONS

The prevalence of persistent low back pain secondary to the involvement of lumbosacral facet joints has been described in controlled studies as varying from 15% to 45% based on types of population and settings studied.[12-28]

Blocks of facet or zygapophysial joints can be performed for therapeutic purpose or to test the hypothesis that the target joint is the source of the patient's pain. Facet joints can be anesthetized by intra-articular injection of local anesthetic or by blocking the medial branches of the dorsal rami that innervate the target joint.

Lumbar facet joint blocks are useful in the diagnosis, as well as the therapeutic management of chronic low back pain.[26-28] Indications for diagnostic facet joint blocks include low back pain for which no cause is otherwise evident and for which pain patterns resemble that evoked in normal volunteers on stimulation of the facet joints. Imaging studies provide anatomic information, but cannot determine independently if a particular structure is painful.

DIAGNOSTIC FACET BLOCKS

Background

Lumbosacral facet joints can be anesthetized either with intra-articular injection of local anesthetic or by anesthetizing the medial branches of the dorsal rami that innervate the target joint.[27] The joint may be considered to be the source of pain if the pain is relieved by joint blockade. Steps need to be taken to ensure that the observed response is not false positive. True-positive responses are secured by performing controlled blocks, either in the form of placebo injections of normal saline or by using comparative local anesthetic blocks (blocks of the same joint performed on two separate occasions, using local anesthetics with different durations of action).

Rationale

The rationale for using lumbosacral facet joint blocks for diagnosis is based on the following:

- The lumbar facet joints have abundant innervation.[29-37]
- The lumbar facet joints have been shown to be capable of being a source of low back pain and referred pain in the lower limb in normal volunteers.[5-9]
- There are no historical or clinical features that are either indicative or diagnostic of facet joint pain.[12,26-28,38-43]
- Referral patterns described for various joints are variable.[5-9]
- A pattern of pain similar to that of facet joint pain is produced by many other structures in the lumbosacral spine.
- Most maneuvers used in physical examination are likely to simultaneously stress several structures, including disks, muscles, and facet joints.

- The diagnosis of facet joint pain lacks correlation with demographic features, pain characteristics, physical findings, and specific signs or symptoms.[12,15,16,26-28,38-43]
- Imaging technologies have not provided valid or reliable means of identifying symptomatic lesions.[40-42]
- The use of controlled local anesthetic facet joint blocks for the diagnosis of chronic low back pain has been reviewed and validated.[27,28,44]

Thus, placebo-controlled blocks or, more commonly in the United States, comparative local anesthetic blocks using two different local anesthetics, are the only means of confirming the diagnosis of facet joint pain.

Validity

The face validity of intra-articular facet injections and medial branch blocks has been established by injecting small volumes of local anesthetic into the joint or onto the sensory nerves of the joint.[11] The construct validity of facet joint blocks has been established.[27] The placebo effect of facet joint injections may be controlled by using strict criteria for determining positive response to blockade.[27] The theory that testing a patient first with lidocaine and subsequently with bupivacaine will identify placebo responders has been tested and proven.[45-49] The specificity of controlled diagnostic blocks has been demonstrated in multiple controlled trials. Pain provocation response of facet joint injections has been shown to be unreliable.[43] The false-negative rate for diagnostic facet joint blocks has been shown to be approximately 8% due to unrecognized intravascular injection of local anesthetic.[11] Confounding psychological factors were shown to lack influence on the validity of comparative, controlled diagnostic local anesthetic blocks of facet joints in the lumbar spine.[50] False-positive rates for facet joint blockade have been evaluated in multiple investigations and are reported to be 22% to 47% in the lumbar spine.[14-22,25,51] The indications and contraindications for diagnostic facet joint blocks are described in Tables 154–1 and 154–2.[52]

Precautions

Relative contraindications to facet injection have been described in patients receiving treatment with nonsteroidal antiinflammatory medications (especially aspirin), because of concerns that these agents may compromise coagulation.[53] Raj and colleagues have provided a detailed description of the role of anticoagulants in interventional pain management. There is a lack of consensus as to the importance of discontinuation of nonsteroidal antiinflammatory drugs and aspirin before lumbar facet joint injection procedures. Patients on warfarin therapy should have prothrombin time (PT) checked and documented to be at acceptable levels before spinal injection. In stopping anticoagulant therapy, one should take into consideration the risk-benefit ratio of the procedure and also consult with the physician in charge of anticoagulant therapy before a decision to proceed. It is prudent to advise the patient to contact the physician in charge of anticoagulant therapy and let him or her make the decision as to the date to stop and for how long.

Table 154–1

Indications for Lumbar Diagnostic Facet Joint Blocks

Somatic or nonradicular low back and/or lower extremity pain
Lack of evidence, either for diskogenic or sacroiliac joint pain
Lack of disk herniation or evidence of radiculitis
Duration of pain of at least of 3 months
Failure to respond to more conservative management, including physical therapy modalities with exercises, chiropractic management, and nonsteroidal antiinflammatory drugs
Average pain levels of greater than 5 on a scale of 0 to 10
Intermittent or continuous pain causing functional disability
No contraindications with understanding of consent, nature of the procedure, needle placement, or sedation
No history of allergy to contrast administration, local anesthetic steroids, Sarapin, or other drugs that may be used
Negative provocative diskography and sacroiliac joint blocks
Contraindications or inability to undergo physical therapy, chiropractic management, or inability to tolerate nonsteroidal antiinflammatory drugs

Table 154–2

Contraindications for Lumbosacral Facet Joint Blocks

Infection
Inability of the patient to understand consent, nature of the procedure, needle placement, or sedation
Allergies to contrast, local anesthetic, steroids, Sarapin, or other drugs
Needle phobia
Psychogenic pain
Suspected diskogenic, sacroiliac joint, or myofascial pain
Anticoagulant therapy
Nonsteroidal antiinflammatory drug therapy
Non-aspirin antiplatelet therapy

THERAPEUTIC FACET BLOCKS

There is a paucity of literature on the role of therapeutic facet joint injections. However, it is well accepted that facet joint pain may be successfully managed by intra-articular injections of steroid, medial branch blockade, and/or neurolysis of medial branch nerves.

Therapeutic benefit has been reported with the injection of corticosteroids, local anesthetics, or normal saline into the facet joints. The literature describing the effectiveness of these interventions is abundant.[54,55] Manchikanti and coworkers[54] in developing evidence-based practice guidelines for interventional techniques in managing chronic spinal pain reviewed the available literature. This literature included four randomized clinical trials,[56-59] multiple nonrandomized trials, and observational reports.[60-63] Based on a definition of short-term relief as relief of less than 3 months' duration and long-term relief as relief for 3 months or longer, a single, randomized trial[56] meeting the inclusion criteria showed positive results at 6 months. The authors (Carette and coworkers[56]) of this study, however, described it as negative. Among the nonrandomized trials, positive results were noted for short-term relief in all of the studies; whereas, long-term relief was noted in only three of the five studies. Thus, Manchikanti and colleagues[54] concluded that the data from randomized and nonrandomized trials (prospective and retrospective evaluations), regarding efficacy of therapeutic intra-articular facet joint injections provided moderate evidence of short-term relief and limited evidence of long-term relief of chronic low back pain.

Medial branch blocks have been extensively used for diagnostic and prognostic purposes with limited use for therapeutic purposes. The therapeutic role of medial branch blockade was evaluated in three randomized clinical trials,[57,58,64] and one nonrandomized clinical trial.[15] Based on the earlier definition (short-term <3 months and long-term ≥3 months) data on medial branch blockade provide strong evidence for short-term relief and moderate evidence for long-term relief from pain of lumbar facet joint origin.

Indications and contraindications for therapeutic lumbar facet joint injection are the same as for diagnostic blockade except that a negative response to diagnostic facet joint block is a contraindication for therapeutic facet joint injection.

Clinically Relevant Anatomy

The lumbar facet joints are formed by the articulation of the inferior articular process of one lumbar vertebra with the superior articular process of the next vertebra. The lumbar joints exhibit the features typical of synovial joints: (1) the articular facets are covered by articular cartilage, and a synovial membrane bridges the margins of the articular cartilages of the two facets in each joint;[29] and (2) surrounding the synovial membrane is a joint capsule that attaches to the articular processes a short distance beyond the margin of the articular cartilage.

The lumbar facet joints are well innervated. The capsules of the lumbar facet joints are richly innervated with encapsulated and unencapsulated free nerve endings.[29-32] The lumbar facet joints are appropriately equipped with sensory apparatus to transmit nociceptive and proprioceptive information. Nerve fibers and nerve endings also occur in the subchondral bone of the facet joints.[30] Nerve fibers and nerve endings are present in erosion channels extending from the subchondral bone to the articular cartilage.[33] These fibers may provide a pathway for nociception from these joints other than from the capsules.[30] Nerve fibers are distributed to the intra-articular inclusions of the facet joints.[34-36] Even though these fibers are known to contain substance P,[33] it is unclear whether these nerves are nociceptive[35] or predominantly vasoregulatory.[37] Interspinous ligaments are also richly innervated with nociceptive fibers and contain free nerve endings.[65-68] Each lumbar facet joint has dual innervation, being supplied by two medial branch nerves. Multiple variations have been described in the number and nature of branches of the lumbar dorsal rami that innervate the lumbar facet joints. The occasional origin of an articular branch from the dorsal ramus proper as well as atypical innervation of the ventral aspect of the adjacent joint have been described.[69] Various other descriptions of innervation also exist, but none has been confirmed.[30]

The L1-L4 dorsal rami are short nerves that arise at nearly right angles from the lumbar spinal nerves.[70] Each nerve measures approximately 5 mm in length[71] with the dorsal ramus directed backward to the upper border of the subjacent transverse process.[30] The L5 dorsal ramus differs from the other lumbar dorsal rami in that it is longer and travels over the top of the ala of the sacrum.[71] The L1-L4 dorsal rami divide into two or three branches as they approach their transverse processes. A medial branch and a lateral branch are always represented at every level. A variable third branch termed *intermediate branch*, although always represented, frequently arises from the lateral branch instead of the dorsal ramus itself.[71] The L5 dorsal ramus forms only a medial branch and a branch that is equivalent to the intermediate branches of the other lumbar dorsal rami.

The medial branches are of paramount clinical importance and relevance because they provide sensory innervation to the facet joints. The medial branches of the L1-L4 dorsal rami run across the top of their respective transverse processes and pierce the dorsal leaf of the intertransverse ligament at the base of the transverse process.[30] Subsequently, each nerve runs along bone at the junction of the root of the transverse process with the root of the superior articular process hooking medially around the base of the superior articular process, covered by the mamilloaccessory ligament. Finally, the medial branch crosses the vertebral lamina, where it divides into multiple branches that supply the multifidus muscle, the interspinous muscle and ligament, and two facet joints.

Each medial branch supplies the facet joints above and below its course.[10,11,30,31,69-73] The medial branch of the L5 dorsal ramus has a different course and distribution than those of the L1-L4 dorsal rami in that, instead of crossing a transverse process, it crosses the ala of the sacrum. The medial branch of the L5 dorsal ramus runs in the groove formed by the junction of the ala and the root of the superior articular process of the sacrum before hooking medially around the base of the lumbosacral facet joint.[30] It sends an articular branch to the facet joint before ramifying within the multifidus muscle.

The muscular distribution of the medial branches of the lumbar dorsal rami is very specific—each medial branch supplies only those muscles that arise from the lamina and spinous process of the vertebra with the same segmental number as the nerve.[71,74] This relationship indicates that the principal muscles that move a particular segment are innervated by the nerve of that segment.[30]

The lateral branches of the lumbar dorsal rami are principally distributed to the iliocostalis lumborum muscle, but those from the L1, L2, and L3 levels can emerge from the dorsal lateral border of this muscle to become cutaneous. The intermediate branches of the lumbar dorsal rami have only a musculature distribution—to the lumbar fibers of the longissimus muscle—and within this muscle they form an intersegmental plexus. The intermediate branch of the L5 dorsal ramus supplies the most caudal fibers of the longissimus, which arise from the L5 transverse process and attach to the medial aspect of the iliac crest.[30]

TECHNIQUE

Lumbar Facet Joint Intra-articular Injections

The patient is placed in the prone position on the fluoroscopy table. A towel roll or pillow can be placed under the abdomen, for easier entry into the joint. As with any lumbar intervention, a baseline anteroposterior (AP) fluoroscopic view of the lumbar spine is obtained and the fluoroscope is oriented. Facet joints may or may not be visible on AP fluoroscopy depending on the specific anatomy of the patient (Fig. 154–1).

Fluoroscopic views of the target joint are obtained. The fluoroscopy beam is rotated from the AP view toward the oblique view until the target facet joint is visible. The upper lumbar facet joints are typically aligned toward the sagittal plane and may be visible on AP imaging, whereas the lower joints are typically oriented increasingly toward the coronal plane so that oblique imaging is necessary to identify joint lines.[75] The target joint is then visualized under fluoroscopic guidance and the skin is marked.

A 22- to 25-gauge, 3½ inch spinal needle is then inserted through the anesthetized area. The needle is directed downward and obliquely (from lateral to medial) toward the selected joint under direct fluoroscopic visualization. Contact is made with the inferior articular processes. The needle is then withdrawn slightly and redirected to enter the target facet joint. As the needle is felt to penetrate the joint, advancement is stopped to prevent any potential damage to the articular cartilage.

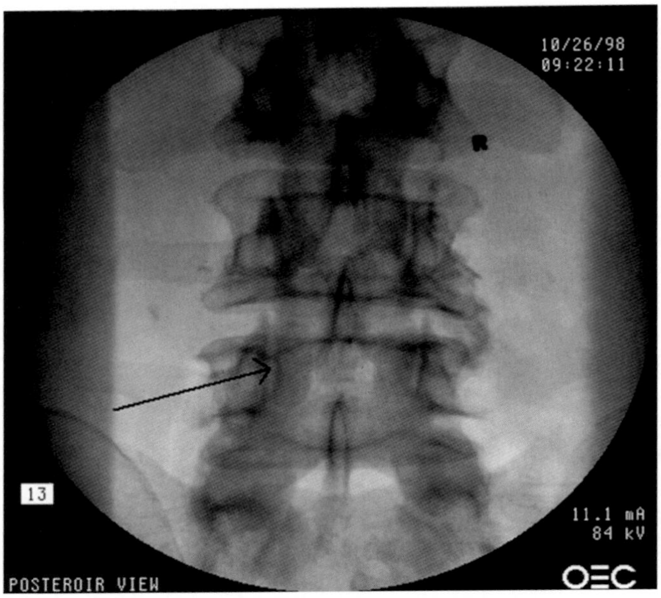

FIGURE 154–1 ■ Facet joints may or may not be visible on anteroposterior (AP) fluoroscopy depending on the specific anatomy of the patient.

If there is difficulty in obtaining capsular penetration, then one may try to access the articular recesses by redirection of the needle just off the margins of the inferior articular processes. Another method of gaining intracapsular entry is to redirect the needle slightly medial or lateral to the posterior joint line so that the needle gains access via its medial placement to the insertion of the capsule on the articular process.[60,76]

When the needle is in an appropriate position, 0.2 to 0.5 mL of contrast is then injected into the joint to confirm proper placement. An arthrographic image should then be visualized.[77] During contrast injection outline of the oval-shaped joint capsule should be visualized with lack of vascular uptake and/or epidural spread. After contrast confirmation of intra-articular needle tip placement, the joint is injected with anesthetic agent to complete a diagnostic block or in combination with a steroid for therapeutic injection.[60,76] Figure 154–2 illustrates intra-articular placement of needles and injection of contrast.

Medial Branch Blocks

To block the sensory innervation to a lumbar facet joint, it is necessary to block the two medial branch nerves that supply the joint. Table 154–3 illustrates the nerves to be blocked for each facet joint in the lumbar region. It is simple to remember which nerves need to be blocked to anesthetize a particular joint:

- Block the medial branch at the transverse process at the same level as the joint
- Block the medial branch at the level below the joint.

Thus, to anesthetize the L3-L4 facet joint, block the L2 medial branch at the transverse process of L3 and the L3 medial branch at the transverse process of L4. Similarly, to anesthetize the L5-S1 facet joint, block the L4 medial branch at the L5 transverse process and the L5 dorsal ramus at the sacral ala. For the L5-S1 facet joint, it has been suggested that additional innervation may be supplied by the communicating branch from the dorsal ramus of S1, which may be blocked just above the exit from the S1 posterior foramen.[75] However, it is has been demonstrated that blockade of the L4 medial branch and the L5 dorsal ramus alone adequately anesthetizes the L5-S1 facet joint from an experimental stimulus without the need for blockade of a potential ascending branch from S1.[10]

L1-L4 Medial Branch Blocks

Dreyfuss and coworkers[11,78] described that the nerves should be blocked proximal to the mamilloaccessory ligament and notch for the L1-L4 medial branches. They described that the target location for the L1-L4 medial branches is at the junction of the superior articular process and the transverse process where the nerve crosses, midway between the superior border of the transverse process and the location of the mamillo-accessory notch. In their opinion, L1-L4 medial

FIGURE 154–2 ■ Intra-articular placement of needles and injection of contrast for lumbar facet joint intra-articular injections. **A,** AP image of lumbar spine with coronally oriented facet joints. **B,** Oblique view with joint lines visible, L4-5, L5-S1. **C,** Oblique view with joint lines visible at L3-4, L4-5, and L5-S1. **D,** With "down the beam" needle placement the skin insertion point is directly over the target. **E,** A 25-gauge spiral needle curving into L5-S1 facet joint. **F,** L4-5 arthrogram.

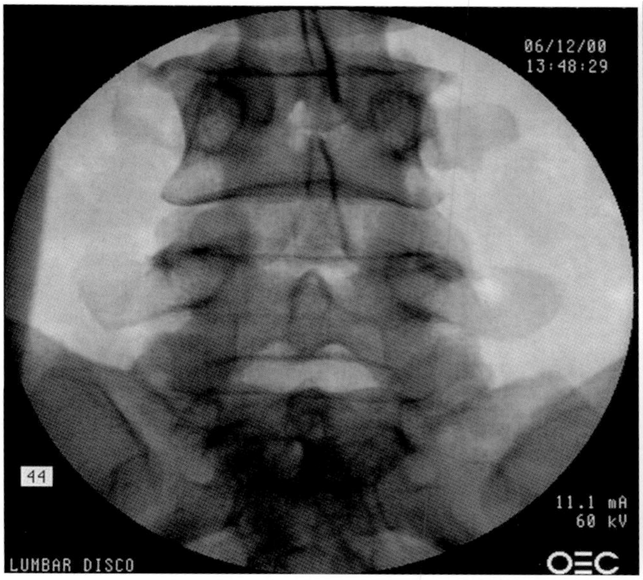
06/12/00
13:48:29
44
11.1 mA
60 kV
LUMBAR DISCO
A

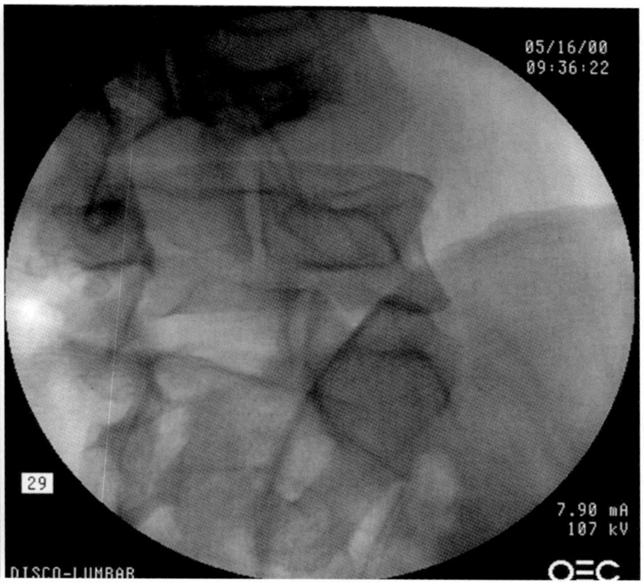
05/16/00
09:36:22
29
7.90 mA
107 kV
DISCO-LUMBAR
B

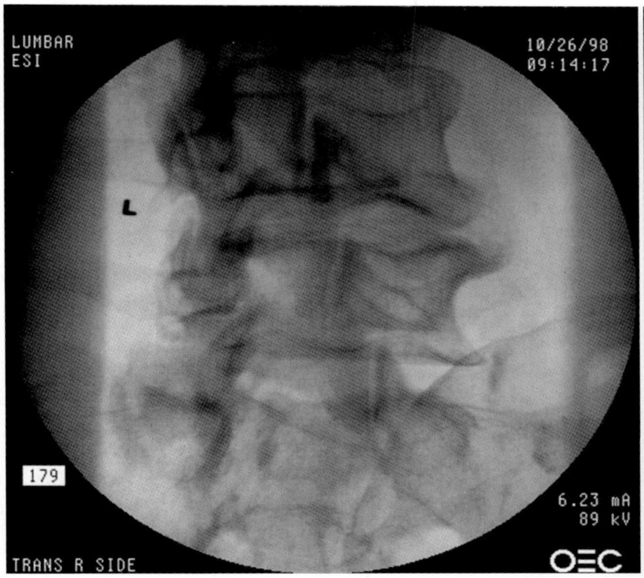
LUMBAR
ESI
10/26/98
09:14:17
L
179
6.23 mA
89 kV
TRANS R SIDE
C

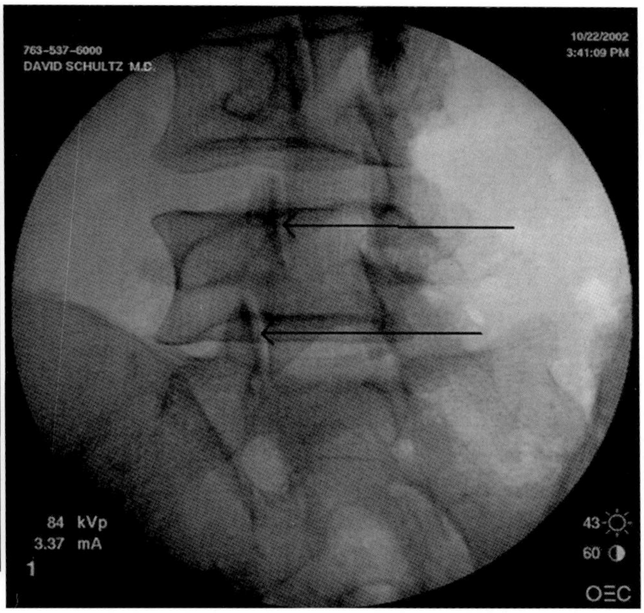
763-537-6000
DAVID SCHULTZ M.D.
10/22/2002
3:41:09 PM
84 kVp
3.37 mA
1
43
60
D

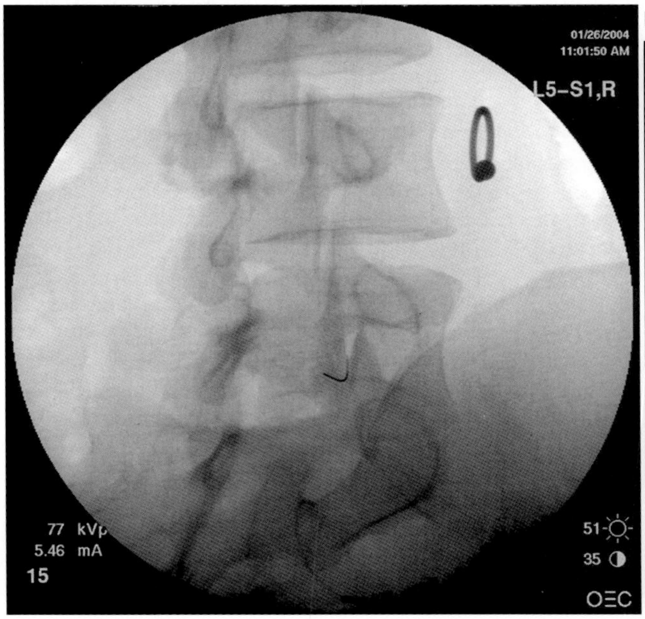
01/26/2004
11:01:50 AM
L5-S1,R
77 kVp
5.46 mA
15
51
35
E

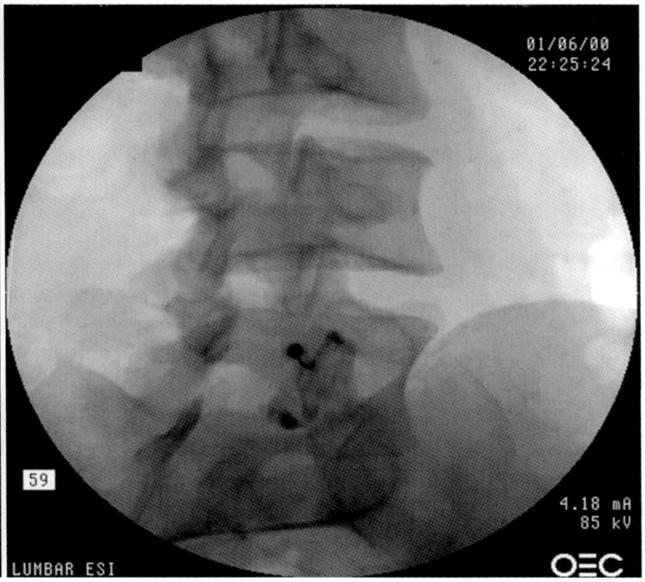
01/06/00
22:25:24
59
4.18 mA
85 kV
LUMBAR ESI
F

Table 154–3

Facet Joint Nerves Required to be Blocked for Each Facet Joint in Lumbar Region

Facet Joint	Facet Joint Nerves to be Blocked (Medial Branches or L5 Dorsal Ramus)	Level of Transverse Process or Sacral Ala
L1-L2	T12 and L1 medial branches	At L1 transverse process for T12 At L2 transverse process for L1
L2-L3	L1 and L2 medial branches	At L2 transverse process for L1 At L3 transverse process for L2
L3-L4	L2 and L3 medial branches	At L3 transverse process for L2 At L4 transverse process for L3
L4-L5	L3 and L4 medial branches	At L4 transverse process for L3 At L5 transverse process for L4
L5-S1	L4 medial branch L5 dorsal ramus	At L5 transverse process for L4 medial branch at sacral groove for L5 dorsal ramus

branch blocks at this location were not associated with inadvertent spread of injectate into the intervertebral foramen or epidural space. They also described that on oblique views, the target point lies high on the "eye" of the "Scottie dog" (Fig. 154–3). Placement more superior at the most superior junction of the superior articular process and transverse process as previously recommended apparently leads to an unacceptable incidence of spread into the neuroforamen. Dreyfuss and coworkers[11] validated a slightly superior-to-inferior and lateral-to-medial needle approach to medial branch blocks. However, if an inferior-to-superior needle approach is used, the injected anesthetic theoretically may spread toward the spinal nerve root or the sinuvertebral nerve, thereby substantially decreasing the specificity of the block. For all medial branch blocks a 22- or 25-gauge spinal needle may be used.

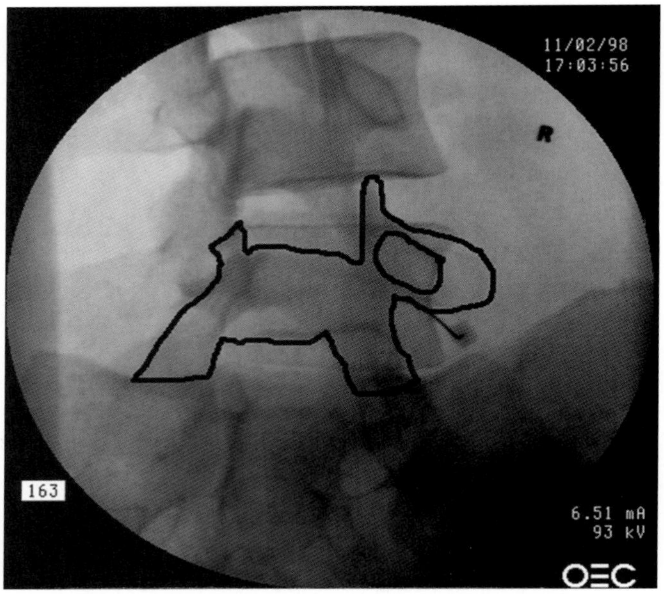

FIGURE 154–3 ■ "Scottie dog" appearance of the target location for the L1-L4 medial branches.

Prone Position—Oblique: L1-L4 Medial Branch Blocks

The patient is positioned in the prone position with a pillow under the abdomen. Fluoroscopic imaging is obtained. The C-arm must be adjusted to an oblique position. To maximally visualize the landmarks of the "Scottie dog," an approximate 25- to 30-degree angle is necessary depending on the specific level from L1-L4 medial branches. The needle is advanced toward the dorsal aspect of the root of the transverse process to ensure safe needle depth away from the ventral ramus. Using an oblique view with the "Scottie dog" identified, the needle is advanced "down the beam" toward the target using a slightly superior starting position to the final target.

The needle will be directed anterior, medial, and caudad to reach the target location, using a "Scottie dog" view (see Fig. 154–3). Needles are typically placed down to contact with the bony end point using oblique fluoroscopic imaging. Before injection, however, final needle tip position must be confirmed using both AP and lateral imaging to ensure that the needle tip is neither too deep nor too medial. On AP imaging, the tip of the needle should be at least in line with the lateral margin of the silhouette of the superior articular process and, if possible, medial to this margin.[78] On lateral imaging, the needle tip should be within the confines of the shadow of the dorsal elements and not protruding into the foramen. The superior articular process frequently bulges laterally, overlapping the target point dorsally. If the needle appears lateral to this point, it has contacted a thick transverse process instead of the superior articular process. In this case, the needle usually needs to be adjusted dorsally until correct position is obtained on both AP and oblique or lateral views.

Before injection, the bevel opening should be medial and slightly inferior to reduce lateral and superior flow to the intervertebral foramen, especially if the needle is placed inadvertently higher than the target position. Figure 154–4 illustrates medial branch blocks with oblique approach.

Prone Position—Posteroanterior: L1-L4 Medial Branch Blocks

The patient is positioned in the prone position with a pillow under the abdomen and fluoroscopic imaging is obtained. The C-arm must be adjusted straight anteroposterior from the skin

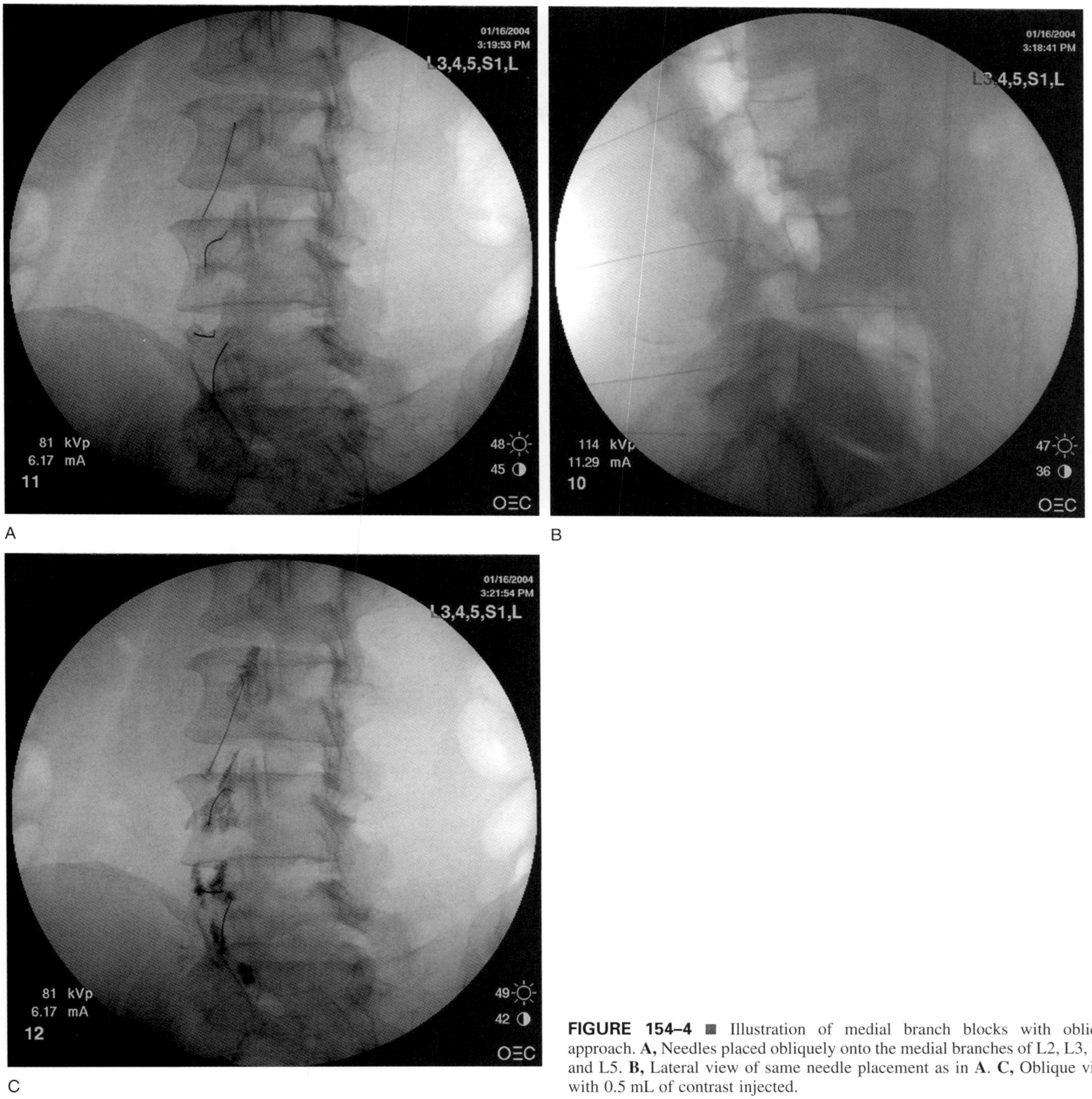

FIGURE 154–4 ■ Illustration of medial branch blocks with oblique approach. **A,** Needles placed obliquely onto the medial branches of L2, L3, L4, and L5. **B,** Lateral view of same needle placement as in **A**. **C,** Oblique view with 0.5 mL of contrast injected.

entry point laterally using AP imaging which is usually just above the tip of the target transverse process. The needle is advanced toward the back of the root of the transverse process to ensure safe needle depth away from the ventral ramus. The needle will be directed anterior, medial, and caudad to reach the target location. On AP imaging, the tip of the needle should be at least in line with the lateral margin of the silhouette of the superior articular process and, if possible, medial to this margin.[78]

The superior articular process frequently bulges laterally, overlapping the target point dorsally. If the needle appears lateral to this point, it has contacted a thick transverse process instead of the superior articular process. In this case, the needle usually needs to be adjusted dorsally until correct position is obtained. Before injection, the bevel opening should be medial and slightly inferior to reduce lateral and superior flow to the intervertebral foramen, especially if the needle is placed inadvertently higher than the target position.

L5 Dorsal Ramus Blocks

Position the patient in prone position with a pillow under the abdomen. Begin with an AP view of the L5-S1 segment.

Rotate the fluoroscope approximately 10 to 15 degrees oblique toward the side to be blocked to view the junction of the sacral ala and the superior articular process of S1. Further obliquity usually places the medial iliac crest in front of the trajectory to the target position. If the ilium obscures the view of the target point as the C-arm is rotated obliquely, cephalad tilt of the C-arm will usually bring the target into clear view by moving the ilium caudad within the fluoroscopic image. An angled needle tip will allow for adequate steering of the needle to the target despite a cephalad to caudad needle trajectory.

When a clear path to the target point for the L5 dorsal ramus is identified, a skin insertion point is chosen. The target point is recognized as a notch between the sacral ala and the superior articulating process of S1. The target point lies opposite the middle of the base of the superior articular process and is slightly below the silhouette at the top of the sacral ala. Higher placement is associated with spread into the L5-S1 epidural space and lower placement with spread to the S1 posterior sacral foramen. The needle is advanced directly "down the beam" to the target position. AP imaging is then obtained to verify that the needle is placed at, or preferably medial to, the lateral silhouette of the S1 superior articular process. Lateral imaging should confirm that the needle tip lies within the shadow of the posterior spinal elements and does not protrude into the L5-S1 neuroforamen. After the needle tip is confirmed to be in the proper location, the bevel opening should be rotated medial. This has been shown to reduce inadvertent spread to the S1 posterior foramen or the L5 vertebral foramen.[11,78] Figure 154–5 illustrates medial branch blocks with prone posteroanterior approach.

DRUGS

Local anesthetic injection should be limited to 0.4 to 0.6 mL for a diagnostic block and approximately 1 mL for a therapeutic block. Dreyfuss and colleagues[11,78] recommend potent local anesthetics, e.g., 4% lidocaine and 0.75% bupivacaine, to minimize the risk of false-negative medial branch blocks, which can occur at a 10% rate with 2% lidocaine. Kaplan and coworkers[10] described that failure to obtain relief with lumbar medial branch blocks in a case in which venous uptake of contrast is observed, despite needle redirection with avoidance of subsequent venous uptake, carries a 50% risk for false-negative results. Contrast injection of 0.1 to 0.3 mL also has been recommended for medial branch or dorsal ramus blocks to confirm selective flow along the path of the nerve and the absence of inadvertent venous uptake.[78]

For diagnostic and therapeutic blocks, the literature has been limited to using local anesthetic agents of different durations of action, namely, lidocaine and bupivacaine. However, Manchikanti and coworkers[16] have shown that validity of diagnostic blocks is maintained with addition of adjuvant agents such as Sarapin and methylprednisolone, along with provision of a therapeutic benefit of much longer duration than with local anesthetic alone. In addition, in multiple investigations, Manchikanti and colleagues[14-22,25] demonstrated efficacy of 1% lidocaine and 0.25% bupivacaine for medial branch blocks rather than 4% lidocaine and 0.75% bupivacaine as recommended by others.

SIDE EFFECTS AND COMPLICATIONS

Complications from facet joint nerve blocks or intra-articular injections in the lumbar spine are exceedingly rare.[78-80] The most common complications of this technique are twofold.[78-91] These include complications related to the placement of the needle, and complications related to the administration of various drugs. Most problems such as local swelling, pain at the site of the needle insertion, and pain in the low back are short-lived and self-limited. More serious complications may include dural puncture, spinal cord trauma, subdural injection, neural trauma, injection into the intervertebral foramen and hematoma formation; infectious complications including epidural abscess and bacterial meningitis; and side effects related to the administration of steroids, local anesthetics, and other drugs.[79-91] Thomson and coworkers[89] reported instances of chemical meningitis after two-level facet joint injections and a one-level medial branch block from penetration of the dural cuff leading to subarachnoid placement of medication. However, large volumes of injectate were used and the descriptions of the needle placement and contrast flow under fluoroscopic imaging before injection were not discussed. Berrigan[90] also reported chemical meningeal irritation. With the use of fluoroscopy with or without contrast, damage to a spinal nerve root or needle placement into the epidural or subarachnoid spaces should be exceedingly rare. Spinal anesthesia following lumbar facet joint injections also has been reported.[81,82] Infection associated with facet joint injections has been reported.[83,84,86]

Other minor complications may include light-headedness, flushing, sweating, nausea, hypotension, syncope, and nonpostural headaches. Some of these side effects may be related to the systemic uptake of injected steroids.[91] The major theoretical complications of corticosteroid administration include suppression of pituitary-adrenal axis, hypocorticism, Cushing syndrome, osteoporosis, avascular necrosis of bone, steroid myopathy, epidural lipomatosis, weight gain, fluid retention, and hypoglycemia. However, Manchikanti and coworkers,[92] in evaluating the effect of neuraxial steroids on weight and bone mass density, showed no significant differences in patients undergoing various types of interventional techniques with or without steroids.

CONCLUSION

Lumbar facet joints are sources of local and referred pain in patients with low back and lower extremity pain in approximately 40% of cases. The definitive diagnosis of facet joint pain relies on properly performed, controlled, comparative local anesthetic or placebo-controlled blocks. These techniques provide an important diagnostic and potentially therapeutic role in the management of low back pain. They should not be used in isolation but rather in the context of other diagnostic and therapeutic methodology. The role of therapeutic facet joint nerve blocks is emerging; however, many questions remain regarding their clinical utility and role in the daily practice of interventional pain management. Further research is required to better define the role of diagnostic and therapeutic facet joint nerve blocks as well as other interventional techniques in the management of chronic low back pain.

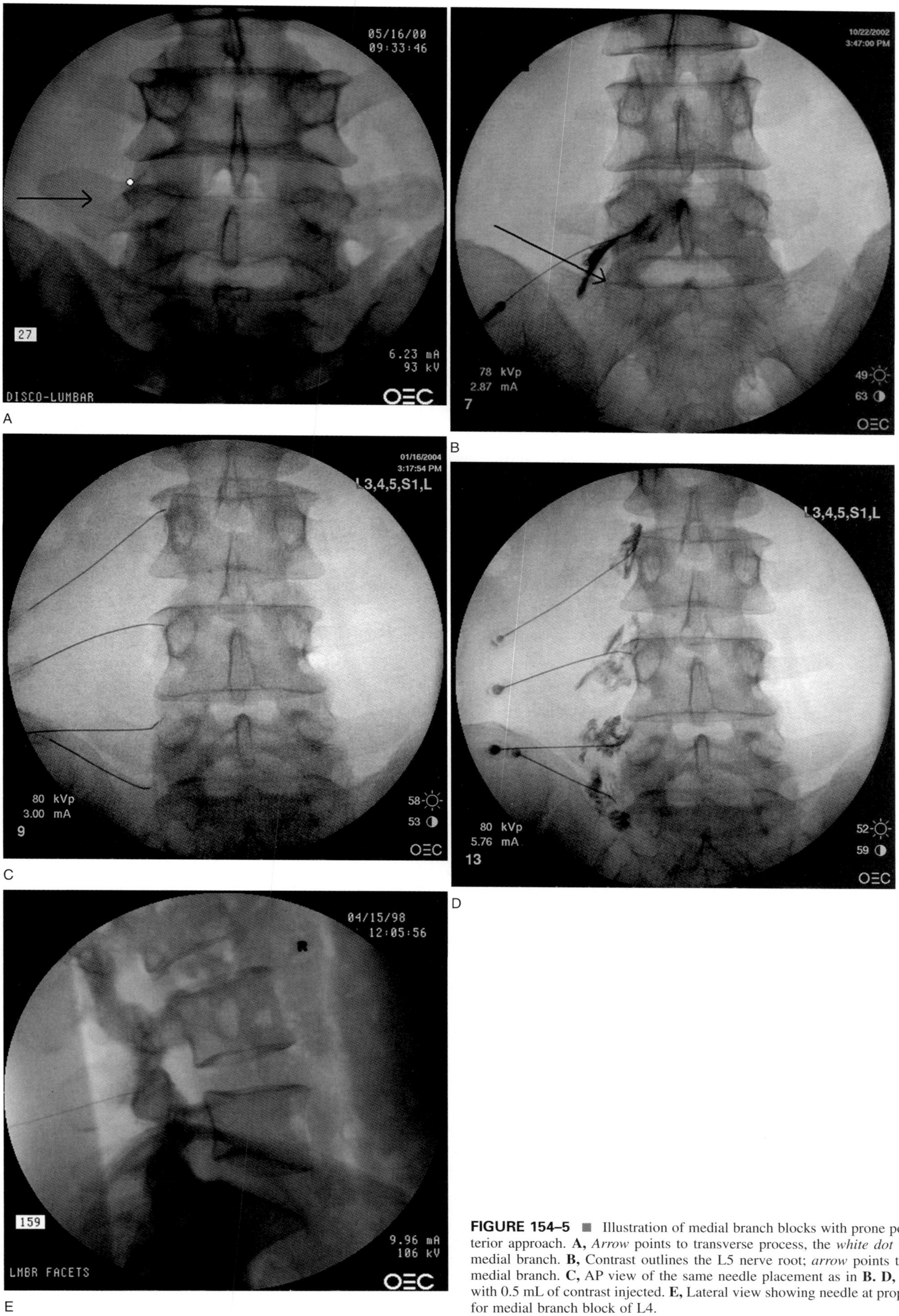

FIGURE 154–5 ■ Illustration of medial branch blocks with prone posteroanterior approach. **A,** *Arrow* points to transverse process, the *white dot* is on the medial branch. **B,** Contrast outlines the L5 nerve root; *arrow* points to the L5 medial branch. **C,** AP view of the same needle placement as in **B. D,** AP view with 0.5 mL of contrast injected. **E,** Lateral view showing needle at proper depth for medial branch block of L4.

References

1. Goldthwait JE: The lumbosacral articulation: An explanation of many cases of lumbago, sciatica, and paraplegia. Boston Med and Surg J 164:365, 1911.
2. Ghormley RK: Low back pain. With special reference to the articular facets, with presentation of an operative procedure. JAMA 101:1773, 1933.
3. Badgley CE: The articular facets in relation to low back pain and sciatic radiation. J Bone Joint Surg 23:481, 1941.
4. Hirsch D, Inglemark B, Miller M: The anatomical basis for low back pain. Acta Orthop Scand 33:1, 1963.
5. Mooney V, Robertson J: The facet syndrome. Clin Orthop 115:149, 1976.
6. McCall IW, Park WM, O'Brien JP: Induced pain referral from posterior elements in normal subjects. Spine 4:441, 1979.
7. Marks R: Distribution of pain provoked from lumbar facet joints and related structures during diagnostic spinal infiltration. Pain 39:37, 1989.
8. Fukui S, Ohseto K, Shiotani M, et al: Distribution of referral pain from the lumbar zygapophyseal joints and dorsal rami. Clin J Pain 13:303, 1997.
9. Windsor RE, King FJ, Roman SJ, et al: Electrical stimulation induced lumbar medial branch referral patterns. Pain Physician 5:347, 2002.
10. Kaplan M, Dreyfuss P, Halbrook B, et al: The ability of lumbar medial branch blocks to anesthetize the zygapophysial joint. Spine 23:1847, 1998.
11. Dreyfuss P, Schwarzer AC, Laup, et al: Specificity of lumbar medial branch and L5 dorsal ramus blocks: A computed tomography study. Spine 22:895, 1997.
12. Schwarzer AC, Aprill CN, Derby R, et al: Clinical features of patients with pain stemming from the lumbar zygapophysial joints. Is the lumbar facet syndrome a clinical entity? Spine 19:1132, 1994.
13. Schwarzer AC, Wang S, Bogduk N, et al.: Prevalence and clinical features of lumbar zygapophysial joint pain. A study in an Australian population with chronic low back pain. Am Rheum Dis 54:100, 1995.
14. Manchikanti L, Pampati VS, Pakanati RR, et al: Prevalence of facet joint pain in chronic low back pain. Pain Physician 2:59, 1999.
15. Manchikanti L, Pampati RR, Fellows B, et al: The diagnostic validity and therapeutic value of medial branch blocks with or without adjuvants. Curr Rev Pain 4:337, 2000.
16. Manchikanti L, Pampati VS, Fellows B, et al: The inability of the clinical picture to characterize pain from facet joints. Pain Physician 3:158, 2000.
17. Manchikanti L, Singh V, Pampati V, et al: Evaluation of the relative contributions of various structures in chronic low back pain. Pain Physician 4:308, 2001.
18. Manchikanti L, Pampati V, Singh V, et al: Evaluation of the role of facet joints in persistent low back pain in obesity: A controlled, prospective, comparative evaluation. Pain Physician 4:266, 2001.
19. Manchikanti L, Pampati VS, Baha A, et al: Contribution of facet joints to chronic low back pain in postlumbar laminectomy syndrome: A controlled comparative prevalence evaluation. Pain Physician 4:175, 2001.
20. Manchikanti L, Pampati V, Rivera J, et al: Role of facet joints in chronic low back pain in the elderly: A controlled comparative prevalence study. Pain Practice 1:332, 2001.
21. Manchikanti L, Singh V, Pampati V, et al: Evaluation of influence of gender, occupational injury, and smoking on chronic low back pain of facet joint origin. Pain Physician 5:30, 2002.
22. Manchikanti L, Hirsch JA, Pampati V: Chronic low back pain of facet (zygapophysial) joint origin: Is there a difference based on involvement of single or multiple spinal regions? Pain Physician 6:399, 2003.
23. Pang WW, Mok MS, Lin ML, et al: Application of spinal pain mapping in the diagnosis of low back pain—analysis of 104 cases. Acta Anaesthesiol Sin 36:71, 1998.
24. Schwarzer AC, Aprill CN, Derby R, et al: The relative contributions of the disc and zygapophyseal joint in chronic low back pain. Spine 19:801, 1994.
25. Manchikanti L, Singh V, Pampati V, et al: Is there correlation of facet joint pain in lumbar and cervical spine? An evaluation of prevalence in combined chronic low back and neck pain. Pain Physician 5:365, 2002.
26. Manchikanti L, Singh V: Review of chronic low back pain of facet joint origin. Pain Physician 5:83, 2002.
27. Bogduk N: International spinal injection society guidelines for the performance of spinal injection procedures. Part 1. Zygapophysial joint blocks. Clin J Pain 13:285, 1997.
28. Boswell MV, Singh V, Staats PS, et al: Accuracy of precision diagnostic blocks in the diagnosis of chronic spinal pain of facet or zygapophysial joint origin. Pain Physician 6:449, 2003.
29. Bogduk N: The zygapophysial joints. In Clinical Anatomy of the Lumbar Spine and Sacrum. New York, Churchill Livingstone, 1997, p 33.
30. Bogduk N: Nerves of the lumbar spine. In Clinical Anatomy of the Lumbar Spine and Sacrum. New York, Churchill Livingstone, 1997, p 127.
31. Bogduk N: The innervation of the lumbar spine. Spine 8:286, 1983.
32. Jackson HC, Winkelmann RK, Bickel WH: Nerve endings in the human lumbar spinal column and related structures. J Bone Joint Surg 48A: 1272, 1966.
33. Beaman DN, Graziano GP, Glover RA, et al: Substance P innervation of lumbar spine facet joints. Spine 18:1044, 1993.
34. Giles LG: Human lumbar zygapophyseal joint inferior recess synovial folds: A light microscope examination. Anat Rec 220:117, 1988.
35. Giles LG, Harvey AR: Immunohistochemical demonstration of nociceptors in the capsule and synovial folds of human zygapophysial joints. Brit J Rheumatol 26:362, 1987.
36. Giles LG, Taylor JR: Innervation of lumbar zygapophyseal joint synovial folds. Acta Orthop Scand 58:43, 1987.
37. Gronblad M, Korkala O, Konttinen Y, et al: Silver impregnation and immunohistochemical study of nerves in lumbar facet joint plical tissue. Spine 16:34, 1991.
38. Revel M, Poiraudeau S, Auleley GR, et al: Capacity of the clinical picture to characterize low back pain relieved by facet joint anesthesia. Proposed criteria to identify patients with painful facet joints. Spine 23:1972, 1998.
39. Schwarzer AC, Derby R, Aprill CN, et al: Pain from the lumbar zygapophysial joints: A test of two models. J Spinal Disord 7:331, 1994.
40. Schwarzer AC, Scott AM, Wang SC, et al: The role of bone scintigraphy in chronic low back pain: A comparison of SPECT and planar images and zygapophysial joint injection. Aust NZJ Med 22:185, 1992.
41. Schwarzer AC, Wang SC, O'Driscoll D, et al: The ability of computed tomography to identify a painful zygapophysial joint in patients with chronic low back pain. Spine 20:907, 1995.
42. Magora A, Bigos SJ, Stolov WC, et al: The significance of medical imaging findings in low back pain. Pain Clinic 7:99, 1994.
43. Schwarzer AC, Derby R, Aprill CN, et al: The value of the provocation response in lumbar zygapophysial joint injections. Clin J Pain 10:309, 1994.
44. Manchikanti L, Singh V, Pampati V: Are diagnostic lumbar medial branch blocks valid? Results of 2-year follow up. Pain Physician 6:147, 2003.
45. Bonica JJ: Local anesthesia and regional blocks. In Wall PD, Melzack R (eds): Textbook of Pain, 2nd ed. Edinburgh, Churchill Livingstone, 1989, p 724.
46. Bonica JJ, Buckley FP: Regional analgesia with local anesthetics. In Bonica JJ (ed): The Management of Pain. Philadelphia, Lea & Febiger, 1990, p 1883.
47. Boas RA: Nerve blocks in the diagnosis of low back pain. Neurosurg Clin North Am 2:806, 1991.
48. Barnsley L, Lord S, Bogduk N: Comparative local anesthetic blocks in the diagnosis of cervical zygapophysial joints pain. Pain 55:99, 1993.
49. Lord SM, Barnsley L, Bogduk N: The utility of comparative local anesthetic blocks versus placebo-controlled blocks for the diagnosis of cervical zygapophysial joint pain. Clin J Pain 11:208, 1995.
50. Manchikanti L, Pampati V, Fellows B, et al: Influence of psychological factors on the ability to diagnose chronic low back pain of facet joint origin. Pain Physician 4:349, 2001.
51. Schwarzer AC, Aprill CN, Derby R, et al: The false-positive rate of uncontrolled diagnostic blocks of the lumbar zygapophysial joints. Pain 58:195, 1994.
52. Manchikanti L, Singh V: Diagnostic lumbar facet joint injections. In Manchikanti L, Slipman CW, Fellows B (eds): Interventional Pain Management: Low Back Pain—Diagnosis and Treatment. Paducah, KY, ASIPP Publishing, 2002, p 239.
53. Raj PP, Shah RV, Kaye AD, et al: Bleeding risk in interventional pain practice: Assessment, management, and review of the literature. Pain Physician 7:3, 2004.
54. Manchikanti L, Staats P, Singh V, et al: Evidence-based practice guidelines for interventional techniques in the management of chronic spinal pain. Pain Physician 6:3, 2003.
55. Manchikanti L: Facet joint pain and the role of neural blockade in its management. Cur Rev Pain 3:348, 1999.

56. Carette S, Marcoux S, Truchon R, et al: A controlled trial of corticosteroid injections into facet joints for chronic low back pain. N Engl J Med 325:1002, 1991.
57. Marks RC, Houston T, Thulbourne T: Facet joint injection and facet nerve block. A randomized comparison in 86 patients with chronic low back pain. Pain 49:325, 1992.
58. Nash TP: Facet joints. Intra-articular steroids or nerve blocks? Pain Clinic 3:77, 1990.
59. Lilius G, Laasonen EM, Myllynen P, et al: Lumbar facet joint syndrome. A randomized clinical trial. J Bone Joint Surg (Br) 71:681, 1989.
60. Destouet JM, Gilula LA, Murphy WA, et al: Lumbar facet joint injection: Indication, technique, clinical correlation, and preliminary results. Radiology 145:321, 1982.
61. Lynch MC, Taylor JF: Facet joint injection for low back pain. A clinical study. J Bone Joint Surg (Br) 68:138, 1986.
62. Lippitt AB: The facet joint and its role in spine pain. Management with facet joint injections. Spine 9:746, 1984.
63. Lau LS, Littlejohn GO, Miller MH: Clinical evaluation of intra-articular injections for lumbar facet joint pain. Med J Aust 143:563, 1985.
64. Manchikanti L, Pampati V, Bakhit CE, et al: Effectiveness of lumbar facet joint nerve blocks in chronic low back pain: A randomized clinical trial. Pain Physician 4: 101, 2001.
65. Jiang H, Russell G, Raso J, et al: The nature and distribution of the innervation of human supraspinal and interspinal ligaments. Spine 20:869, 1995.
66. Rhalmi S, Yahia L, Newman N, et al: Immunohistochemical study of nerves in lumbar spine ligaments. Spine 18:264, 1993.
67. Yahia LH, Newman NA: A light and electron microscopic study of spinal ligament innervation. Z Mikroskop Anat Forsch Leipzig 103:664, 1989.
68. Yahia LH, Newman N, Rivard CH: Neurohistology of lumbar spine ligaments. Acta Orthop Scandi 59:508, 1988.
69. Lazorthes G, Juskiewenski S: Etude comparative des branches posterieures des nerfs dorsaux et lmbaires et leurs rapports avec les articulations interapophysaires vertebrales. Bulletin de l'Association des Anatomistes. 1025, 49e Reunion.
70. Bradley KC: The anatomy of backache. Aust NZ J Surg 44:227, 1974.
71. Bogduk N, Wilson AS, Tynan W: The human lumbar dorsal rami. J Anat 134:383, 1982.
72. Lewin T, Moffet B, Viidik A: The morphology of the lumbar synovial intervertebral joints. Acta Morphol Neerlando-Scandinav 4:299, 1962.
73. Pedersen HE, Blunck CFJ, Gardner E: The anatomy of lumbosacral posterior rami and meningeal branches of spinal nerves (sinu-vertebral nerves): With an experimental study of their function. J Bone Joint Surg 38A:377, 1956.
74. Macintosh JE, Valencia F, Bogduk N, et al: The morphology of the lumbar multifidus muscles. Clin Biomech 1:196, 1986.
75. Derby R, Bogduk N, Schwarzer A: Precision percutaneous blocking procedures for localizing spinal pain. Part 1: The posterior lumbar compartment. Pain Digest 3:89, 1993.
76. Destouet JM: Lumbar facet block: Indications and technique. Orthop Rev 14:57, 1985.
77. Dory MA: Arthrography of the lumbar facet joints. Radiology 140:23, 1981.
78. Dreyfuss P, Kaplan M, Dreyer SJ: Zygapophyseal joint injection techniques in the spinal axis. In Leonard (ed): Pain Procedures in Clinical Practice, 2nd ed. Philadelphia, Hanley & Belfus, 2000, p 276.
79. Windsor RE, Storm S, Sugar R: Prevention and management of complications resulting from common spinal injections. Pain Physician 6:473, 2003.
80. Windsor RE, Pinzon EG, Gore HC: Complications of common selective spinal injections: Prevention and management. Am J Orthop 29:759, 2000.
81. Gladstone JC, Pennant JH: Spinal anaesthesia following facet joint injection. Anaesthesia 42:754, 1987.
82. Marks R, Semple AJ: Spinal anaesthesia after facet joint injection. Anaesthesia 43:65, 1988.
83. Cook NJ, Hanrahan P, Song S: Paraspinal abscess following facet joint injection. Clin Rheumatol 18:52, 1999.
84. Magee M, Kannangara S, Dennien B, et al: Paraspinal abscess complicating facet joint injection. Clin Nucl Med 25:71, 2000.
85. Manchikanti L, Cash KA, Moss TL, et al: Radiation exposure to the physician in interventional pain management. Pain Physician 5:385, 2002.
86. Orpen NM, Birch NC: Delayed presentation of septic arthritis of a lumbar facet joint after diagnostic facet joint injection. J Spinal Disord Tech 16:285, 2003.
87. Manchikanti L, Cash K, Moss T, et al: Effectiveness of protective measures in reducing risk of radiation exposure in interventional pain management: A prospective evaluation. Pain Physician 6:301, 2003.
88. Manchikanti L, Cash K, Moss T, et al: Risk of whole body radiation exposure and protective measures in fluoroscopically guided interventional techniques: A prospective evaluation. BMC Anesthesiology 3:2, 2003.
89. Thomson SJ, Lomax DM, Collett BJ: Chemical meningism after lumbar facet joint nerve block with local anesthetic and steroids. Anesthesia 46:563, 1993.
90. Berrigan T: Chemical meningism after lumbar facet joint block. Anesthesia 47:905, 1992.
91. Manchikanti L: Role of neuraxial steroids in interventional pain management. Pain Physician 5:182, 2002.
92. Manchikanti L, Pampati V, Beyer C, et al: The effect of neuraxial steroids on weight and bone mass density: A prospective evaluation. Pain Physician 3:357, 2000.

chapter 155

Lumbar Sympathetic Nerve Block and Neurolysis

Michael Stanton-Hicks

Lumbar sympathetic ganglion block is useful in the evaluation and management of sympathetically mediated pain of the kidneys, ureters, genitalia, and lower extremities. Included in this category are phantom limb pain, reflex sympathetic dystrophy, causalgia, and a variety of peripheral neuropathies. Lumbar sympathetic ganglion block also is useful in the palliation of pain secondary to vascular insufficiency of the lower extremity, including pain secondary to frostbite, atherosclerosis, Buerger disease, and arteritis secondary to collagen vascular disease, and to maximize blood flow after vascular procedures on the lower extremities. Lumbar sympathetic ganglion block with local anesthetic can be used as a diagnostic tool when performing differential neural blockade on an anatomic basis in the evaluation of flank, pelvic, and lower extremity pain. If destruction of the lumbar sympathetic chain is being considered, this technique is useful as a prognostic indicator of the degree of pain relief that the patient may experience. Lumbar sympathetic ganglion block with local anesthetic also is useful in the treatment of acute herpes zoster and postherpetic neuralgia involving the lumbar and sacral dermatomes. Destruction of the lumbar sympathetic chain is indicated for the palliation of pain syndromes that have responded to lumbar sympathetic blockade with local anesthetic.

HISTORICAL CONSIDERATIONS

The first report of lumbar sympathetic block was by Brunn and Mandl,[1] who in a 1924 article described Selheim's technique of injecting the lumbar sympathetic nerves as a component of his paravertebral approach to blocking the mixed spinal outflow in the lumbar region. Eighteen years after Novocain was released in 1905, Kappis[2] described the technique of lumbar sympathetic block and surgical resection of the lumbar sympathetic nerves. Other authors associated with the technique of lumbar sympathetic block are von Gaza,[3] Mandl,[4] and Läwen[5] in Germany; Jonnesco[6] and Lériche and Fountain[7] in France; and White[8] in the United States. During the 1950s, Bonica,[9] Moore,[10] and Arnulf[11] described in detail the importance of lumbar sympathetic blockade, particularly its relationship to the treatment of causalgia and posttraumatic reflex dystrophies in servicemen after World War II. Although the technique described by Mandl[4] in 1926 remains one of the most popular approaches to the lumbar sympathetic trunk, Reid and colleagues,[12] in a large series published in 1970, described a more lateral approach that avoids contact with the transverse process. Two techniques are described in this chapter: the "classic" technique first described by Kappis[2] and Mandl[4] and the lateral technique first described by Mandl[4] and refined by Reid and colleagues.[12]

INDICATIONS

The indications for lumbar sympathetic block may be divided into three broad categories: (1) circulatory insufficiency in the leg, including arteriosclerotic vascular disease, diabetic gangrene, Buerger disease, Raynaud phenomenon and disease, and reconstructive vascular surgery after arterial embolic occlusion; (2) pain from renal colic, reflex sympathetic dystrophy, or causalgia (chronic regional pain syndrome types I and II), intractable urogenital pain, amputation stump pain, phantom pain, and frostbite; and (3) other conditions, such as hyperhidrosis, phlegmasia alba dolens, erythromelalgia, acrocyanosis, and trench foot.

The rationale for sympathetic blocks, particularly in the treatment of pain, is based on the observation that pain under certain conditions is potentiated or mediated by sympathetic activity. Laboratory evidence has shown that the sympathetic postganglionic neuron may act not only at its effector terminal, but also on the primary afferent neuron in certain pathologic conditions; it may communicate with the primary afferent neuron at other sites (direct and indirect coupling).[13] Although the mechanism is unclear, blocks of the sympathetic nervous system may have two actions: (1) Interruption of preganglionic and postganglionic sympathetic efferents may influence function of the primary afferent neuron,[14,15] or (2) visceral afferents from deep visceral structures in the leg that travel with the sympathetic nerves may be blocked.[16] As a diagnostic and prognostic tool, sympathetic blocks are helpful in determining the nature of the pain (i.e., whether it is sympathetically maintained or whether it is independent of sympathetic function). Such procedures are always used to test the effects of destructive (neurolytic, chemical) sympatholysis or surgical sympathectomy.

CONTRAINDICATIONS

Contraindications to sympathetic blocks are a bleeding diathesis, local infection, and certain anatomic anomalies, which may be considered relative contraindications if they are likely to render the procedure difficult or hazardous.

FUNCTIONAL ANATOMY

The general anatomy of the sympathetic nervous system consists of central and peripheral components. The central components are the hypothalamus, midbrain, pons, medulla, and lateral columns of the spinal cord extending from T1 to L2. Peripherally, the sympathetic nervous system consists of preganglionic and postganglionic efferent fibers that innervate deep somatic structures, skin, and viscera. The two paravertebral sympathetic trunks are connected segmentally by preganglionic neurons, whose cell bodies are situated in the lateral horn, intermediate nucleus, and paracentral nuclei of the thoracolumbar cord. The cell bodies responsible for vasoconstriction in the lower limbs are in the lower three thoracic and first three lumbar segments. The preganglionic fibers pass by way of their corresponding nerves as white rami communicantes, which communicate with considerable convergence in the paravertebral ganglia with postganglionic efferents and in the prevertebral ganglia by postganglionic efferents to the pelvic viscera. A small percentage of postganglionic fibers pass directly to ganglia in the aortic plexus and the superior and inferior hypogastric plexus. The postganglionic fibers leave the sympathetic trunk as gray rami communicantes, some passing to the L1 nerve to contribute to the iliohypogastric and genitofemoral nerve territories, some to the L2-5 nerves, and some to the upper three sacral nerves, where they pass on to their respective destinations in the lumbosacral plexus.

Intermediate ganglia found in the psoas and iliacus muscles also communicate with postganglionic fibers that pass through the segmental lumbar and sacral nerves. The S1 and S2 nerves contain the largest numbers of postganglionic fibers. Most of these represent gray rami communicantes that subserve vasomotor, pilomotor, and sudomotor functions. It has been determined that, although each root of the lumbosacral plexus receives one group of gray rami communicantes, the S1-3 nerves contain several (i.e., a large convergence)[17] because they innervate the blood vessels in the lower extremity. Each lumbar sympathetic chain enters the retroperitoneal space under the right and left crura, continuing inferiorly in the interval between the anterolateral aspect of the vertebral bodies and the origin of the psoas muscle to enter the pelvis at the L5-S1 disk. Posteriorly, the periosteum overlies the vertebral bodies and the fibroaponeurotic origin of the psoas muscles and their fascial coverings. Anterior is the parietal reflection of the peritoneum, the aorta lying anteromedial to the left trunk and the vena cava anterior to the right trunk. The white and gray rami communicantes pass to their respective ganglia beneath the fibrous arcades of psoas attachments to each vertebral body. Also, they tend to pass alongside the middle of the vertebral body, an observation that is important to positioning of the blocking needle.

The sympathetic ganglia of the lumbar sympathetic chains vary in number and position. Rarely are five ganglia found on each side in the same individual.[18] In most cases, only four are found. There tends to be fusion of L1 and L2 ganglia in most patients, and ganglia are aggregated at the L2-3 and L4-5 disks. Also, there is considerable variability in the size of the ganglia, some being fusiform and 10 to 15 mm long and others being round and approximately 5 mm long.[19] Because of this aggregation and the fact that the right crus extends to L3 and the left to L2, sympathetic blockade is more efficacious when performed at the L3, L4, or L5 level, rather than at the L2 vertebral body, as is most common. Although most postganglionic sympathetic efferents join spinal nerves that form the lumbar plexus and pass distally as components of the femoral, sciatic, and obturator nerves, their branches distribute segmentally to their respective vessels in the lower limb. Block of L2-3 ganglia should interrupt most of the efferent sympathetic supply to the lower limb. In patients whose sympathetic pathways bypass the sympathetic chain and make synapses with their respective postganglionic efferents in somatic spinal nerves, complete sympathetic interruption is not achieved after surgical sympathectomy.[20] Important branches of the lumbar sympathetic trunk contain postganglionic efferents, visceral afferents, and lumbar somatic afferents that supply the axial skeleton and musculoskeletal structures in the hip and the lower limbs. With this understanding, there can be no "pure" sympathetic block. Some component of somatosensory block, if only a small one, always is present with every sympathetic blocking procedure.

TECHNIQUE

Although the "classic" or paramedian technique describes the insertion of three needles from L2 to L4, this method has been modified to one using only two needles at L2 and L4[21] and, more recently, a single-needle technique[22] at either L2 or L3. When a neurolytic procedure is to be undertaken, it is important to use at least two needles, if not three, to prevent too much local pressure developing at the injection sites. Although not mandatory for diagnostic or therapeutic blocks with local anesthetics, for neurolytic blockade, an image intensifier (fluoroscopy) or CT should be mandatory. Because of the expense and frequently the inconvenience of scheduling, CT is used in only a small percentage of cases. The prone position is most convenient for lumbar sympathetic blockade, but pain or anatomic deformity may make it necessary to place the patient in the left or right lateral decubitus position.

Classic or Traditional Technique

After sterile preparation of the skin and draping of the area, wheals are made 5 to 6 cm lateral to the spinous processes and on lines that are drawn through the upper margins of the second, third, or fourth lumbar spinous processes.[23] This placement can be verified by anteroposterior fluoroscopy (Fig. 155–1). With an 8-cm 22-gauge needle, a local anesthetic solution is infiltrated down to the respective transverse processes, forming tracts through which the 15-cm 20-gauge sympathectomy needle and stylet can be introduced. Each sympathectomy needle is introduced at an angle of 5 to 10 degrees from the parasagittal plane and is advanced so as to contact the transverse process (Fig. 155–2). At this point, a lateral view with the image intensifier is taken to observe the alignment, and any small adjustments necessary are made to set up the proper angle so that the needle reaches the anterolateral aspect of the vertebral body (Fig. 155–3). The latter view is obtained by "looking down the needle" with the image intensifier. The needle is introduced by following the axis of the image intensifier camera, and an imaginary line is subtended to reach the anterolateral aspect of the vertebral body of interest. The needle depth can be determined by taking a lateral view (Fig. 155–4). Care should be taken when the needle is passed below the transverse process because it may contact the posterior or anterior primary rami at that level. Should the needle contact the vertebral body, medial pressure on the paraspinous muscle usually induces sufficient bend in the needle to deflect it from the side of the vertebral body and allow it to pass forward through the psoas muscle and its investing fascia to reach the retroperitoneal space (Fig. 155–5).[24]

With a loss-of-resistance syringe and light percussion with the tip of a finger, the retroperitoneal space may be identified (Fig. 155–6).[25] The position of the needle tip can

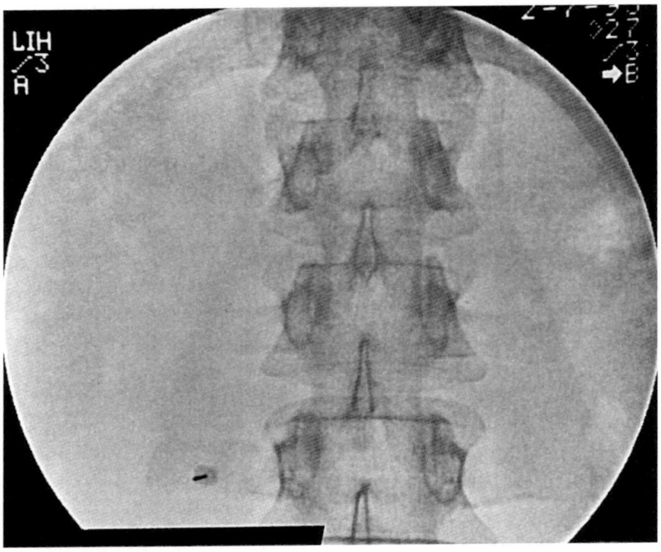

FIGURE 155–1 ■ Anteroposterior view of the needle seen end-on after being introduced to the transverse process of L3. (From Waldman SD: Interventional Pain Management, 2nd ed. Philadelphia, WB Saunders, 2001, Chapter 43, p 487.)

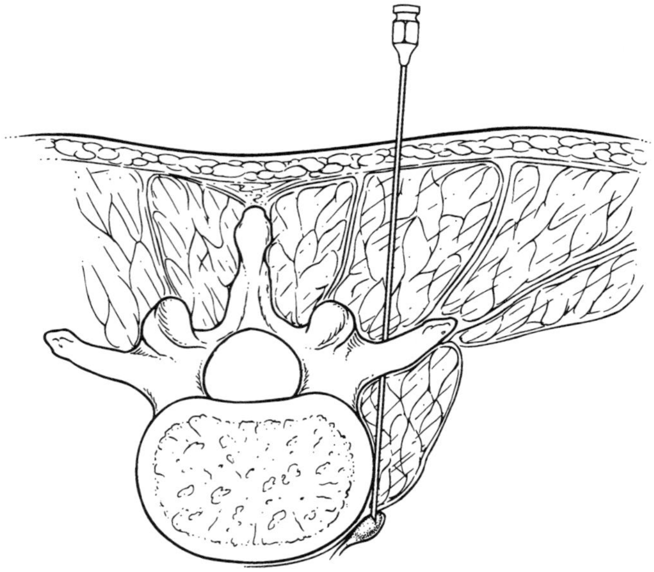

FIGURE 155–3 ■ Needle tip in correct portion for lumbar sympathetic block.

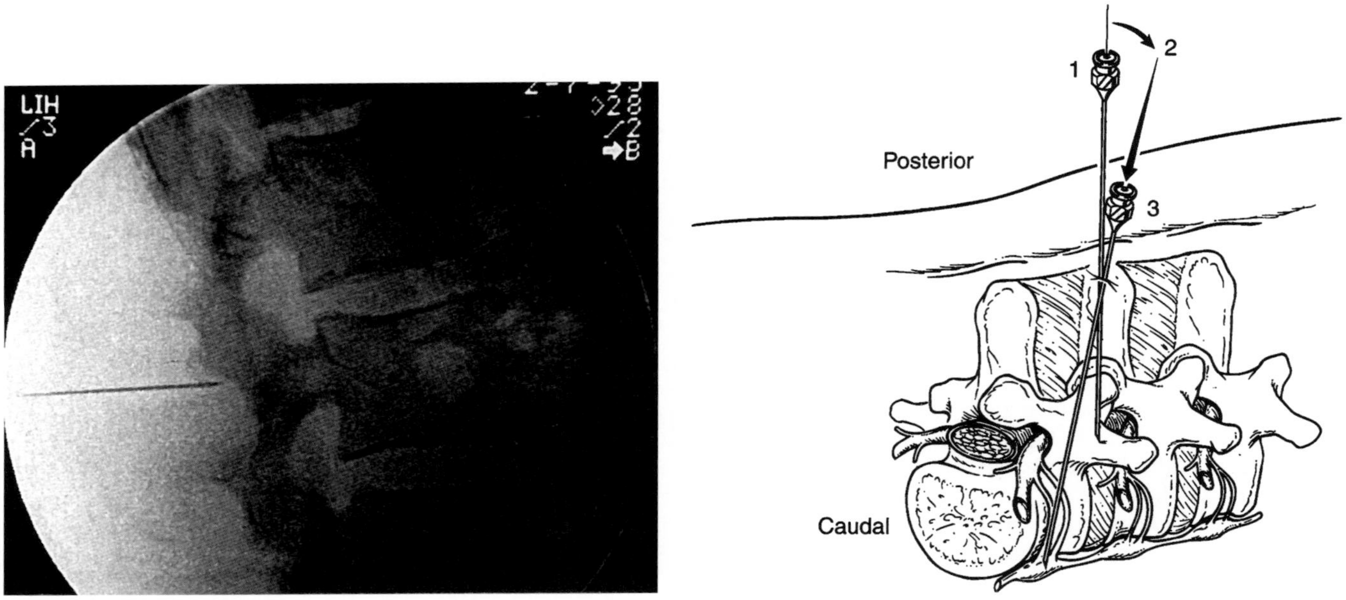

A B

FIGURE 155–2 ■ **A,** Lateral radiograph shows proper needle position. **B,** Lateral view shows the needle tip and alignment on the inferior aspect of the transverse process of L3. (From Waldman SD: Interventional Pain Management, 2nd ed. Philadelphia, WB Saunders, 2001, p 487.)

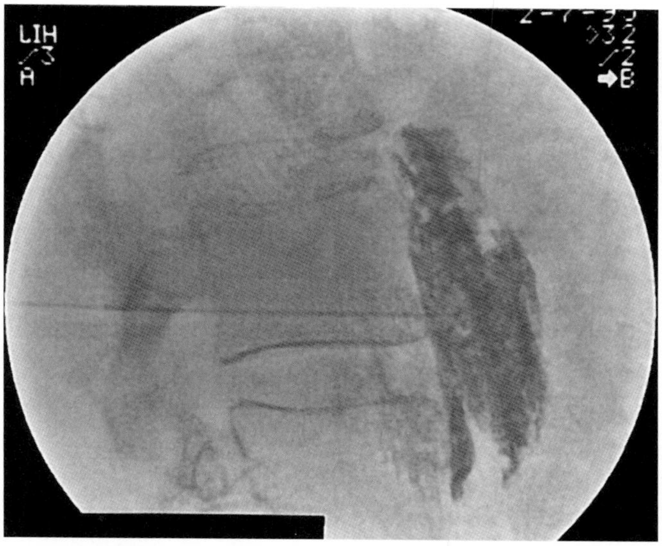

FIGURE 155–4 ■ Lateral image shows the needle at the anterolateral aspect of the vertebral body with the retroperitoneal space identified by longitudinal spread of contrast material. (From Waldman SD: Interventional Pain Management, 2nd ed. Philadelphia, WB Saunders, 2001, p 488.)

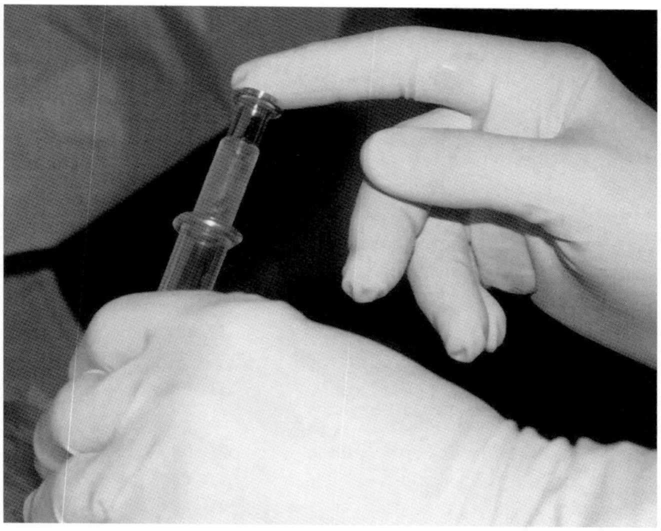

FIGURE 155–6 ■ The retroperitoneal space is identified using a loss-of-resistance syringe and light percussion with the tip of the finger. (From Waldman SD: Interventional Pain Management, 2nd ed. Philadelphia, WB Saunders, 2001, p 488.)

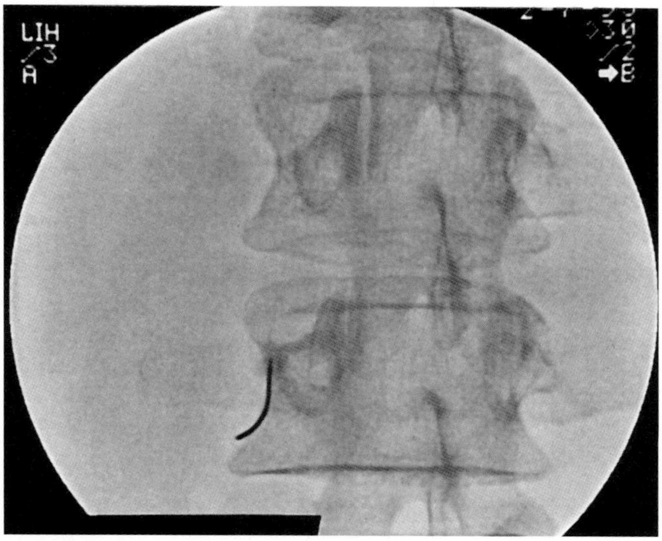

FIGURE 155–5 ■ Oblique (and slightly inclined) view of the spine shows deflection of the needle produced by lateral pressure on the trunk and slight curving of the needle to allow it to pass alongside the vertebral body. (From Waldman SD: Interventional Pain Management, 2nd ed. Philadelphia, WB Saunders, 2001, p 488.)

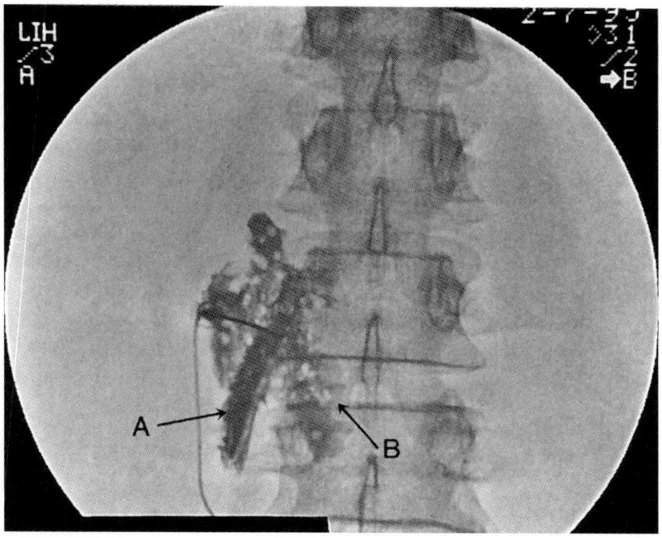

FIGURE 155–7 ■ Compound figure shows the correct position of the needle, and contrast is depicted in two tissue planes. **A,** The striated linear spread is within the psoas fascia and is incorrect. **B,** The "vacuolated" appearance is retroperitoneal. and the spread of contrast material is in the correct plane. (From Waldman SD: Interventional Pain Management, 2nd ed. Philadelphia, WB Saunders, 2001, p 488.)

be verified by injection of a small amount of air to produce an "airogram" or nonionizable, water-soluble contrast material.[26,27]

The technique just described is repeated at each additional level. If the needles have been placed in the correct space (retroperitoneal), the injected contrast material should be confluent at each vertebral level (Fig. 155–7B; see Fig. 155–4). If the contrast material has been placed within the substance of the psoas or just beneath its fascia, the appearance is as shown in Figure 155–7A. This position produces incomplete sympatholysis.

Lateral Technique

The lateral technique is favored over the paramedian technique because it causes less discomfort for the patient, does not require contact with the transverse process, is unlikely to encounter a segmental nerve, and provides a direct path and optimal position to contact the lumbar sympathetic trunk and its ganglia.[12] This technique requires only two needles, and, with experience, a single-needle technique can be used successfully in almost 80% of cases.[28]

It is unnecessary to measure the point of needle insertion; rather, this point is determined by using the fluoroscope's C-arm as a sighting device (Figs. 155–8 and 155–9). Distance from the midline, depending on the girth of the patient, is 8 to 12 cm. After a skin wheal is raised, a tract of local anesthetic can be infiltrated using a 22-gauge spinal needle. The 15-cm 20-gauge sympathetic block needle is introduced at an angle that allows it to arrive at the anterolateral aspect of the vertebral body margin. The axis of the C-arm camera, when positioned to look down the needle (Fig. 155–10), should facilitate insertion of the needle into the retroperitoneal space (Fig. 155–11). Using a lateral view to check its depth (Figs. 155–12 and 155–13), the final few millimeters of the needle's travel can be undertaken by the loss-of-resistance syringe until the retroperitoneal space is reached. If the needle should

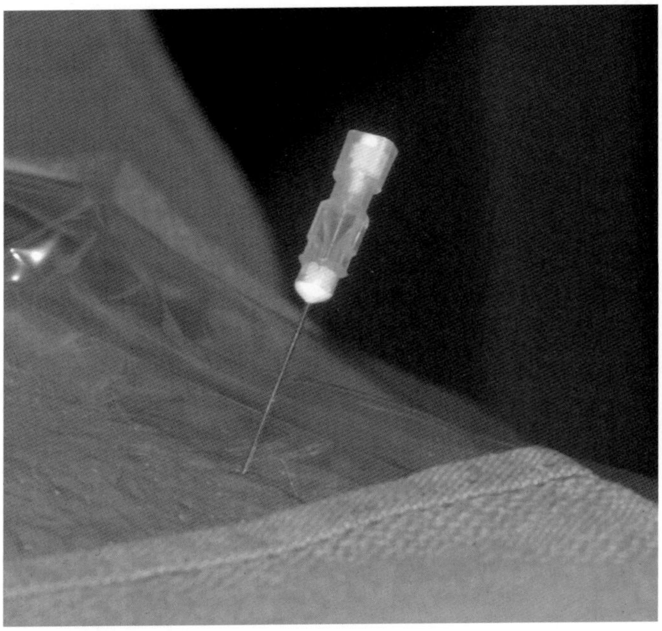

FIGURE 155–8 ■ View of the needle entry site for the Reid or lateral approach. (From Waldman SD: Interventional Pain Management, 2nd ed. Philadelphia, WB Saunders, 2001, p 489.)

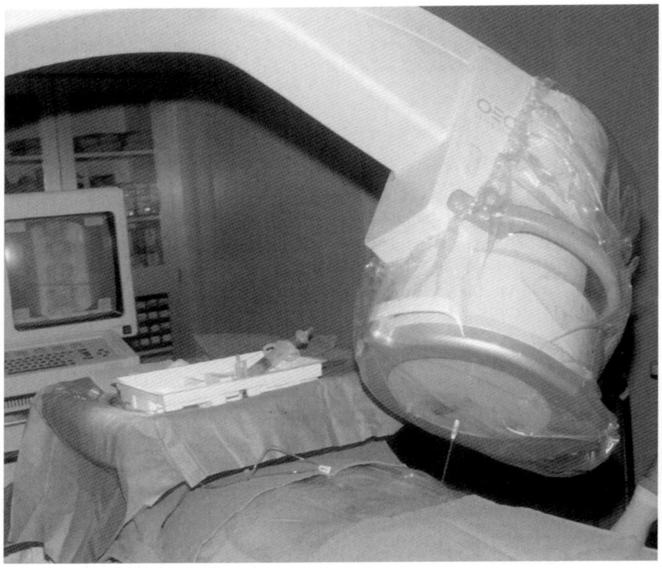

FIGURE 155–9 ■ View of the image intensifier positioned to "look down" the needle during the Reid or lateral approach. (From Waldman SD: Interventional Pain Management, 2nd ed. Philadelphia, WB Saunders, 2001, p 489.)

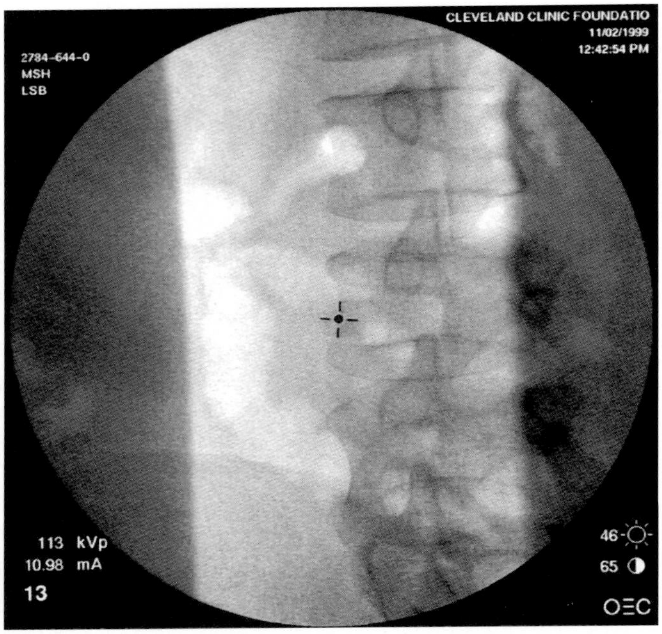

FIGURE 155–10 ■ Oblique view shows the needle end-on ("looking down the needle") as it is introduced into the retroperitoneal space. The image intensifier also has been rotated caudad to allow a clear path for the needle to reach the lower third of the vertebral body without contacting the transverse process. (From Waldman SD: Interventional Pain Management, 2nd ed. Philadelphia, WB Saunders, 2001, p 489.)

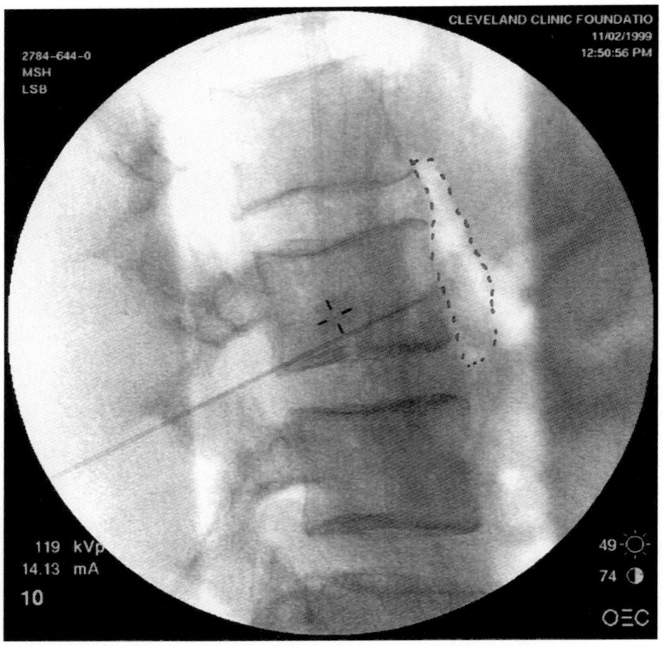

FIGURE 155–11 ■ Transverse view shows position of the needle tip at the sympathetic trunk using the Reid or lateral approach. (From Waldman SD: Interventional Pain Management, 2nd ed. Philadelphia, WB Saunders, 2001, p 490.)

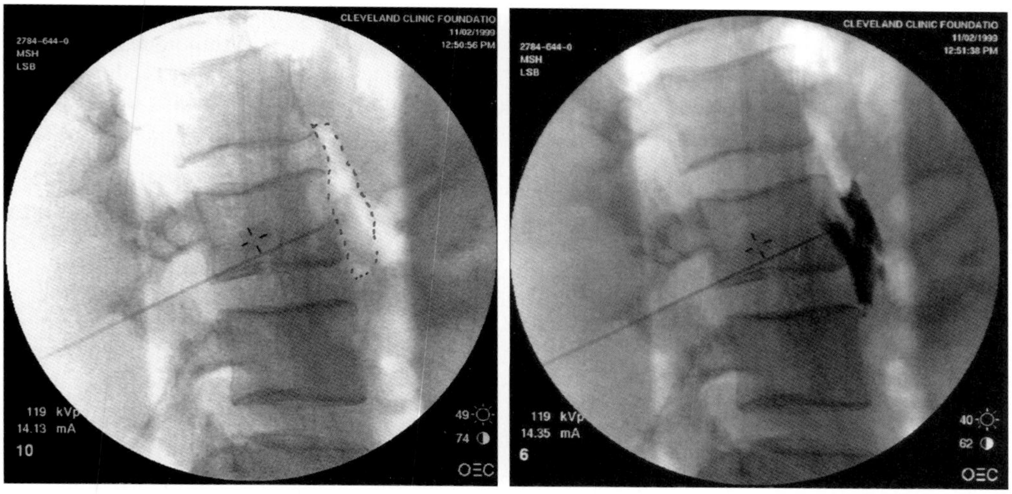

FIGURE 155–12 ■ **A,** Lateral image of needle in position with "airogram" obtained after injection of 2 mL of air. **B,** Lateral image of needle in the same patient after the injection of 2 mL of radiopaque contrast material. (From Waldman SD: Interventional Pain Management, 2nd ed. Philadelphia, WB Saunders, 2001, p 490.)

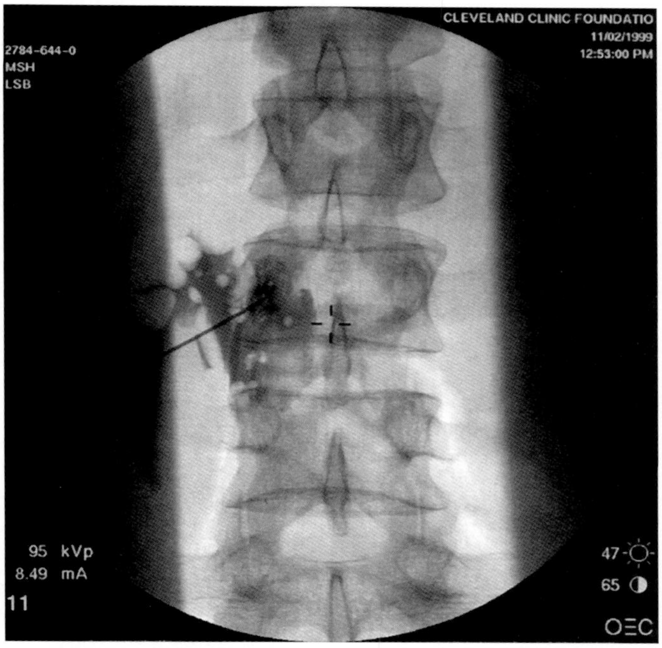

FIGURE 155–13 ■ Anteroposterior projection of contrast spread in patient shown in Figure 155–12. (From Waldman SD: Interventional Pain Management, 2nd ed. Philadelphia, WB Saunders, 2001, p 490.)

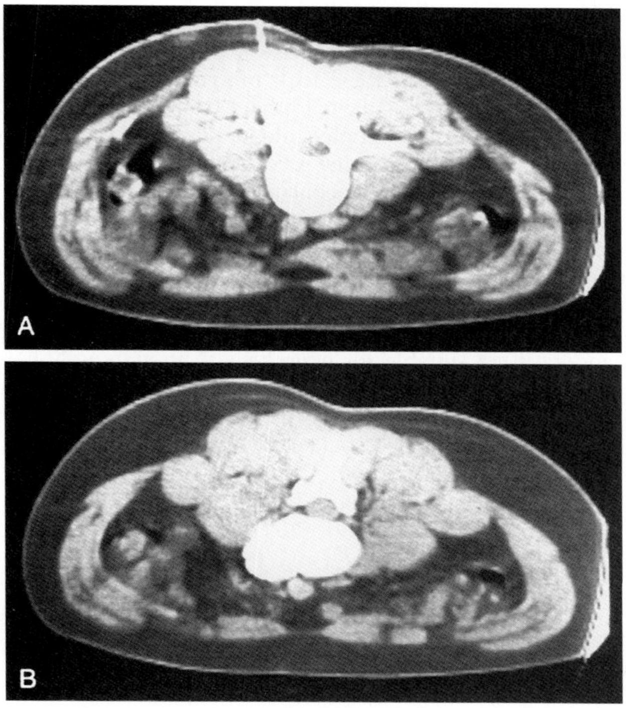

FIGURE 155–14 ■ **A,** CT-guided needle placement for lumbar sympathetic block. **B,** Proper spread of contrast medium outlining the sympathetic chain. (From Waldman SD: Interventional Pain Management, 2nd ed. Philadelphia, WB Saunders, 2001, p 491.)

contact the side of the vertebral body, the needle may be deflected from this position by first being withdrawn 2 to 3 cm and then being passed alongside the vertebral body by medial pressure on the paraspinous musculature (see Fig. 155–5). Correct alignment of the needle and its position in the retroperitoneal space can be determined by injecting either a small amount of air to produce an airogram (see Fig. 155–12A) or nonionizable, water-soluble contrast medium (see Fig. 155–12B). Use of CT as an aid to needle placement is shown in Figure 155–14.

Comment

When determining loss of resistance, it is necessary to ballotte the plunger of the syringe gently with a finger because the thumb is too insensitive in most cases to feel the small change in pressure as the needle tip enters the retroperitoneal space. Sometimes, as a result of previous retroperitoneal surgery, peritoneal inflammatory disease, or neurolytic sympatholysis, the retroperitoneal space is obliterated, and no loss of resistance is recognizable. Under such circumstances, it may be necessary to place the needle tip anatomically in relation to the vertebral body, taking advantage of biplanar views, and to dissect the space by injection of saline and contrast material. I have used this technique successfully in most instances.

Injection of any therapeutic or diagnostic solutions should be monitored by continuous imaging. Movement of the contrast tracer confirms its correct dispersion and alerts the observer to any anomalous spread. Injected solutions may enter a lymphatic, vein, or artery and may spread in an unwanted tissue plane, such as alongside the rami communicantes to the lateral foramen. Imaging time should be kept to a minimum, but the progress of injection always should be monitored throughout. Bonica[9] suggested that, in the presence of an unexpectedly poor sympatholysis, it may be necessary to undertake prognostic blocks of the lower thoracic sympathetic ganglia in addition to the lumbar ganglia, in case postganglionic fibers have taken routes other than the lumbar trunk to reach the lower extremities.

MEDICATIONS EMPLOYED FOR SYMPATHOLYSIS

Although short-acting local anesthetics commonly are used for prognostic and therapeutic sympathetic blocks, I believe that a long-acting agent, such as bupivacaine, is advantageous for therapy and prognosis because it provides the patient a longer time to evaluate the effects of sympatholysis and any effect this might have on the pain, apart from any greater duration that may accrue with physiologic adaptation. A concentration of 0.375% bupivacaine gives optimal duration without the need for an added vasoconstrictor. The disadvantage of bupivacaine is its relatively long latency (5 to 8 minutes). It may be shortened by mixing 2% chloroprocaine and 0.75% bupivacaine in equal proportions, or using a small 5- to 6-mL injection of 2% chloroprocaine as a test solution.

A solution of 10% to 16% phenol in diatrizoate sodium (Renografin) is suitable for neurolysis. Although an "older" ionized contrast material, it is the only solution that has undergone stability testing, and it has a long shelf life.[29] This combination has not been associated with any hypersensitivity response in my experience.

COMPLICATIONS

Similar to all regional anesthetic blocks, sympatholysis may result in intravascular injection; however, the chance of intravenous injection should be negligible if fluoroscopic guidance is used throughout the injection.[30,31] The most common complication associated with lumbar sympatholysis is neuralgia of the genitofemoral nerve, particularly for the lateral approach.[32] The incidence of genitofemoral neuralgia has been reported to be 15%, but it may be only 4% with a single-needle technique. Most cases are transient and resolve with nonprescription analgesics, but the condition may last 6 weeks. A repeat local anesthetic sympathetic block commonly produces immediate remission. Similarly, intravenous lidocaine may be used in a dose of 1 to 2 mL/kg, or transcutaneous nerve stimulation may be employed over the thigh for genitofemoral neuralgia.

Other complications are necrosis of the psoas muscle and sloughing of the ureter (D. Reed, personal communication, 1985). Bleeding may occur in a patient with a clotting deficiency, which, in any case, would be a contraindication to sympathetic block. Otherwise, any bleeding from needle puncture should be self-limiting. Patients should be warned that they may have some hypotension immediately after sympatholysis, and men should be apprised that they may experience impotence or failure of ejaculation, particularly if a neurolytic procedure is undertaken. No incidence has been established for this latter complication.

INTERPRETATION OF AND RESPONSES TO LUMBAR SYMPATHETIC BLOCK

It is important to understand the patient's personality when interpreting the subsequent effects of sympatholysis. Although evidence of sympatholysis—vasodilation, increased temperature, and reduction of edema—is important, the qualitative effect on the preexisting symptoms, which may be manifested as continuous pain, hyperalgesia, or touch-evoked pain such as allodynia, requires careful assessment after sympatholysis. Technical failure may be the cause of therapeutic failure, even on repeated occasions. A placebo response is normal and may merely be the response of a grateful patient to the fact that something fundamental has been done to unravel a particular medical condition. The amount of local anesthetic used for sympatholysis, as the result of its own uptake, may have an effect on multisynaptic pathways in the central nervous system, producing central inhibition of nociception, an effect that erroneously may be attributed to sympatholysis.[33] Lumbar sympatholysis is associated with few complications and is normally a reproducible technique when carried out with proper imaging guidance. Appropriate knowledge of anatomy and good technique are required to minimize the risk of harm to the patient, and the procedure is valuable in the management of a comparatively small but treatment-refractory group of painful conditions. Finally, Treede and coworkers[35] questioned the efficacy and reproducibility of sympathetic block (as did Bonica[9]), particularly in relation to pain relief, as a response. Nevertheless, carefully performed, sympathetic block is a useful and important therapeutic diagnostic procedure.

References

1. Brunn F, Mandl F: Die paravertebrale Injektion zur Bekämpfung visceraler Schmerzen. Wien Klin Wochenschr 37:511, 1924.
2. Kappis M: Weitere Erfahrungen mit der Sympathektomie. Klin Wochenschr 2:1441, 1923.
3. von Gaza W: Die Resektion der paravertebralen Nerven und die isolierte Durchschneidung des Ramus communicans. Arch Klin Chir 133:479, 1924.
4. Mandl F: Die Paravertebrale Injektion. Vienna, J Springer, 1926.
5. Läwen A: Über segmentare Schmerzaufhegungen durch paravertebrale Novokaininjektion zur differential Diagnose intraabdominaler Erkrankungen. München Med Wochenschr 69:1423, 1922.
6. Jonnesco R: Angine de poitrien guérié par le résection du sympathique cervico-thoracique. Bull Acad Med 84:93, 1920.
7. Lériche R, Fountain R: L'Anesthésie isolée du ganglion étoile: Sa technique, ses indications, ses résultats. Presse Med 42:849, 1934.
8. White JC: Diagnostic novocaine block of the sensory and sympathetic nerves. Am J Surg 9:264, 1930.
9. Bonica JJ: The Management of Pain. Philadelphia, Lea & Febiger, 1953.
10. Moore DC: Stellate Ganglion Block. Springfield, IL, Charles C Thomas, 1954.
11. Arnulf G: Practique des Infiltrations Sympathetiques. Lyon, Camugli, 1954.
12. Reid W, Watt JK, Gray RG: Phenol injection of the sympathetic chain. Br J Surg 57:45, 1970.

13. Devor M, Wall PD, Jänig W: Cross-excitation of dorsal root ganglion neurons in nerve injured rats by neighboring afferents and by postganglionic sympathetic efferents. Soc Neurosci 17:1559, 1991.
14. Procacci P, Francini F, Zoppi M, Maresca M: Cutaneous pain threshold changes after sympathetic block in reflex dystrophies. Pain 1:167, 1975.
15. Price D, Bennett GJ, Raffi A: Psychophysical observations on patients with neuropathic pain relieved by sympathetic block. Pain 36:273, 1989.
16. Mense G: Slowly conducting afferent fibers from deep tissues: Neurological properties and central nervous actions. Prog Sensory Physiol 6:139, 1986.
17. Gabella G: Structure of the Autonomic Nervous System. London, Chapman & Hall, 1976.
18. Hovelacque A: Anatomie des Nerfs Craniens et Rachidens et du Systeme Grand Sympathique chez 1 'Homme. Paris, G Doin, 1927.
19. Rocco AG, Palomgi D, Raeke D: Anatomy of the lumbar sympathetic chain. Reg Anesth 20:13, 1995.
20. Bonica JJ, Buckley FP. Regional analgesia with local anesthetics. In Bonica JJ (ed): The Management of Pain, 2nd ed. Philadelphia, Lea & Febiger, 1990, p 883.
21. Boas RA, Hatangdi VS: Chemical sympathectomy techniques and responses. In Yokua T, Dubner R (eds): Current Topics in Pain Research and Therapy—Proceedings of the International Symposium on Pain, Kyoto, December 19, 1982. Amsterdam, Excerpta Medica, 1983.
22. Hatangdi VS, Boas RA: Lumbar sympathectomy: A single needle technique. Br J Anaesth 57:285, 1985.
23. Bergan JJ, Conn JJR: Sympathectomy for pain relief. Med Clin North Am 52:147, 1968.
24. Eriksson E: Illustrated Handbook of Local Anaesthesia. Copenhagen, Munksgaard, 1980.
25. Stanton-Hicks MDA: Blocks of the sympathetic nervous system. In Stanton-Hicks MDA (ed): Pain and the Sympathetic Nervous System. Boston, Kluwer Academic, 1990, p 155.
26. Boas RA, Hatangdi VS, Richards EG: Lumbar sympathectomy—a percutaneous technique. Adv Pain Res Ther 1:685, 1976.
27. Eaton AC, Wright M, Cullum KG: The use of the image intensifier in phenol lumbar sympathetic block. Radiography 46:298, 1980.
28. Loh L, Nathan PW: Painful peripheral states and sympathetic blocks. J Neurol Neurosurg Psychiatry 41:664, 1978.
29. Gregg RV, Constantini TH, Ford DJ, Raj PP: Electrophysiologic investigation of phenol in diatrizoate sodium as a neurolytic agent. Reg Anesth 10:46, 1985.
30. Walsh JA, Glynn CJ, Cousins MJ, Basedow RW: Blood flow, sympathetic activity and pain relief following lumbar sympathetic blockade or surgical sympathectomy. Anaesth Intensive Care 13:18, 1984.
31. Cousins MJ, Reeve TS, Glynn CJ, et al: Neurolytic lumbar sympathetic blockade: Duration of denervation and relief of rest pain. Anaesth Intensive Care 7:121, 1979.
32. Dam WH: Therapeutic blockade. Acta Chir Scand Suppl 3155:89, 1965.
33. Woolf CJ, Wiesenfeld-Hallin Z: The systemic administration of local anaesthetics produces a selective depression of C-afferent fibre evoked activity in the spinal cord. Pain 23:361, 1985.
34. Rowbotham MC, Fields HL: Topical lidocaine reduces pain in postherpetic neuralgia. Pain 38:297, 1989.
35. Treede RD, David KD, Campbell JN, Rajc SN: The plasticity of cutaneous hyperalgesia during sympathetic ganglionic blockade in patients with neuropathic pain. Brain 115:607, 1992.

chapter 156

Ilioinguinal-Iliohypogastric Nerve Block

Son Truong Nguyen, Vimal Akhouri, and Carol Warfield

HISTORICAL CONSIDERATIONS

Ponka was one of the first to describe a technique of ilioinguinal, iliohypogastric, and 12th intercostal nerve block.[1] Several modifications of this technique have been created, which vary mainly in the choice of the local anesthetics and the injection sites. In 1978, a major article in the surgical literature propounded its broad use in adult herniorrhaphy.[2] In 1987, its value gained further importance for the diagnosis of ilioinguinal and genitofemoral entrapment neuralgia when Starling described a series of patients for whom an ilioinguinal block was essential in differentiating post-herniorrhaphy neuralgia.[3] In the last 30 years, the anesthetic and analgesic efficacies of the block have been studied in combination or in comparison with other regional techniques, including spinal anesthesia, instillation, and infiltration techniques.[4-6,10] Various approaches have also examined its efficacy when combined with sedation or general anesthesia. This block seems now to have gained wide acceptance by anesthesiologists and surgeons especially for ambulatory groin surgery. In particular, a recent article by Song and colleagues showed the cost-effectiveness of this anesthetic technique when combined with monitored anesthesia care with respect to speed of recovery, patient comfort, and associated incremental cost.[7]

INDICATIONS

Diagnostic Use

Neuropathic groin, testicular, or medial thigh pain in the distribution of the ilioinguinal and iliohypogastric nerves is caused by chronic inflammation or entrapment of the nerve following surgical, blunt abdominal trauma, or other pathological processes.[3,8] The ilioinguinal-iliohypogastric (INIH) nerve* block with local anesthetics is used diagnostically in differentiating localized entrapment against other lumbosacral etiology for neuropathic pain.[2,3] Owing to the overlap of the INIH nerve sensory distribution with that of a lumbar radiculopathy, ineffective ilioinguinal block suggests that other causes of neuropathy may exist. A differential list may include involvement of the genitofemoral nerve, L1 lumbar radiculopathy, lumbar plexus lesions, infection, malignancy invading the lumbar plexus or epidural or vertebral metastatic disease at T12-L1, referred pain, myofascial pain, and central causes.[3,8] Lumbosacral spine pathology must be suspected especially in patients whose groin pain occurs without a history of hernia or previous herniorrhaphy.[9] Electromyography and magnetic resonance imaging of the lumbar plexus are indicated in this patient population. If neurolysis or destruction of the nerve is to be performed, the ilioinguinal nerve block may be useful as a prognostic indicator of the degree of motor and sensory impairment.

Analgesic Use

Whether a diagnosis is made clinically or by differential blockade, a palliative ilioinguinal-iliohypogastric nerve block can be used as an adjunct to pharmacologic methods. In the acute setting, the INIH nerve block has been used with variable success after inguinal herniorrhaphy, cesarean section, abdominal hysterectomy, appendectomy, varicocelectomy, and hydrocelectomy.[4,15,16] Following a cesarean section, a postoperative ilioinguinal nerve block may prolong the time to administration of morphine following a cesarean section.[10] Another randomized controlled trial showed similar results with an intraoperative block.[4] There is no evidence that combining INIH nerve block with neuraxial anesthesia provides any benefits. For example, in one randomized study, no additional benefits 6 hours postoperatively were found in patients receiving both ilioinguinal-iliohypogastric block and spinal anesthesia for herniorrhaphy.[11] In contrast, an alternative approach to postoperative analgesia involving local wound instillation or infiltration[6,12,13] following inguinal herniorrhaphy has been shown to be effective in children and may especially be useful in uncooperative children afraid of needles.[6,14] However, except for post-herniorrhaphy pain, one systematic review of wound infiltration for different abdominal operations showed no conclusive benefits.[15,16]

*Because of considerable overlap in their anatomic locations and courses, the ilioinguinal and iliohypogastric nerves are frequently referred to as the *ilioinguinal-iliohypogastric nerve*.

Persistent or chronic pain in the groin and testicular areas is a difficult problem. The frequency of chronic pain after inguinal herniorrhaphy may be as high as 54%.[17] Yet, there are no reliable, standardized treatments for persistent or chronic groin pain and orchialgia. Persistent or chronic pain may be caused by inflammation, entrapment, or deafferentation from infection or trauma. Once the neuralgia has been specifically attributed to either ilioinguinal or iliohypogastric, or both, nerves a solution of local anesthetic with steroid is usually injected directly onto the nerve.[18] The use of an indwelling catheter for repeated ilioinguinal-iliohypogastric blocks into an inter-abdominis plane has been described[19] and may promote further research into devices for continuous infusion. Radiofrequency lesioning of the ilioinguinal nerve for post-herniorrhaphy pain and orchialgia has been successful in a small anecdotal series of three patients in whom relief was 100% at 6-month follow-up.[20] This technique is particularly promising for having the longest duration of analgesia, but more definitive randomized trials are needed to evaluate its efficacy and safety. Randomized studies on cryoanalgesic ablation of the ilioinguinal nerve do not show any benefits.[21,22]

Anesthesia

For surgical anesthesia, the ilioinguinal-iliohypogastric nerve block may be used separately or in combination with a genitofemoral nerve block, depending on the extent of the operation. The most accepted use of this anesthetic block in the United States is for groin surgery. However, reports exist in the literature on common uses in lower abdominal surgery, pelvic surgery with Pfannenstiel incision (cesarean section, hysterectomy, myomectomy, Burch), varicocelectomy, hydrocelectomy, and orchidopexy.[23-25] Based on the preferences of the patient, the anesthesiologist, or the surgeon, this block can be used as part of a regional technique with or without sedation, or as a supplement to general anesthesia. Many studies have attempted to evaluate the efficacy of the block at various perioperative stages. Currently, there is no conclusive evidence correlating efficacy of analgesia favoring either preoperative, intraoperative, or postoperative INIH blockade.[26,27] INIH nerve block is commonly used in pediatric outpatient surgery because of quicker recovery and decreased postoperative analgesic requirements.[28] Contraindications are common to any regional blockade and include patient refusal, local anesthetic allergy, severe coagulation disorders, and local infection.

CLINICALLY RELEVANT ANATOMY

The ilioinguinal nerve (Fig. 156–1) branches from the L1 nerve root, with some contribution from T12. The nerve runs obliquely across the quadratus lumborum muscle and the iliacus posterior to the kidney. It continues anteriorly at the level of the anterior superior iliac spine to perforate the transversus abdominis muscle. The nerve may interconnect with the iliohypogastric nerve where it continues inferiorly and medially along the spermatic cord, through the superficial inguinal ring, and into the inguinal canal. Its lateral branch pierces the muscle of the lateral abdominal wall to supply the skin over the lateral gluteal region. In general, the sensory distribution includes the superomedial thigh, the root of the penis and upper scrotum in the male, or the mons pubis and lateral labium majus in the female (Fig. 156–2). Overlap can exist with the sensory distribution of the iliohypogastric nerve, which may interconnect with the ilioinguinal nerve.

The iliohypogastric nerve branches from the L1 nerve root, with some contribution from T12 (see Fig. 156–1). The nerve runs obliquely across the quadratus lumborum and iliacus and perforates the transversus abdominis muscle to lie between it and the oblique muscle. An anterior branch pierces the external oblique muscle to provide cutaneous sensory innervation to the abdominal skin above the pubis (Fig. 156–3). A lateral branch provides cutaneous sensory innervation to the posterolateral gluteal region.

TECHNIQUES

Anesthetic Technique

The patient is placed in the supine position with a pillow under the knees. A line is drawn between the anterior superior iliac spine (ASIS) and the umbilicus and an injection site is located approximately 2 inches superomedial to the ASIS (Fig. 156–4). Another line is drawn between the ASIS and the pubic symphysis; the injection site is approximately 2 inches inferomedial to the ASIS.

After sterile preparation, a 25-gauge, short-bevel needle is inserted at a 45-degree angle to the skin, in a caudal direction toward the pubic symphysis (see Fig. 156–4). The bevel is kept parallel to the plane. After passing through the skin and subcutaneous tissue, the needle meets the firm resistance of the external oblique sheath. The needle is pushed to penetrate this sheath with a definite snap. From 5 to 7 mL of local anesthetic solution is injected in a fan-like manner into the plane deep to the external oblique aponeurosis. Attention should be given when piercing the fascia of the external oblique muscle to avoid entering the peritoneal cavity. For additional anesthesia of the distal portion of the INIH nerve, another 5 mL of anesthetic solution is injected into the subcutaneous region at the pubic spine. Supplemental infiltrations of the spermatic cord may also be performed. Separate blockade of the iliohypogastric nerve is difficult due to its close approximation to the ilioinguinal nerve, but it may be possible by choosing an injection site 1 inch medial and inferior to the ASIS.[18] After the block, pressure may be applied to the injection site to prevent ecchymosis and hematoma formation.[18] For longer blocks up to 12 hours, ropivacaine 0.5% may be used.[29] Injections of 0.25 mL/kg ropivacaine result in safe plasma concentrations of ropivacaine that peak at 30 to 45 minutes.[30,31] In pediatric regional anesthesia, ropivacaine and levobupivacaine may be favored because of their safer pharmacokinetic properties of longer absorption times and lower peak plasma concentrations.[30-32]

Analgesic or Diagnostic Technique

The analgesic technique is much simpler. A single injection site is located 2 cm medially and inferiorly from the anterior superior iliac spine. At a 45-degree angle, staying parallel to the plane of the aponeurosis, again a 25-gauge, short-bevel needle is advanced inferiomedially toward the symphysis pubis while aspirating for blood, until a snap marks the pierc-

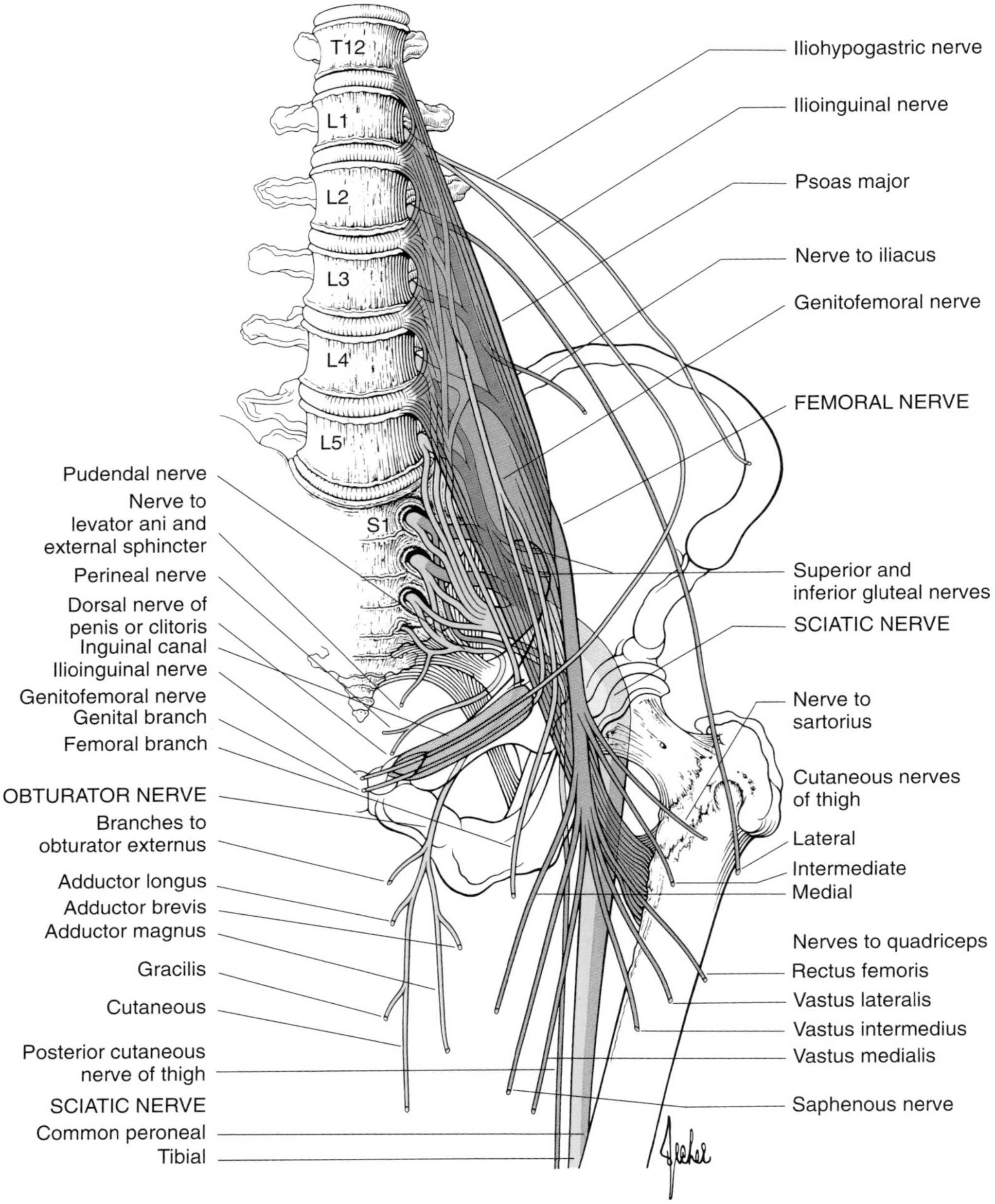

FIGURE 156–1 ■ Anatomic location and course of the ilioinguinal and iliohypogastric nerves.

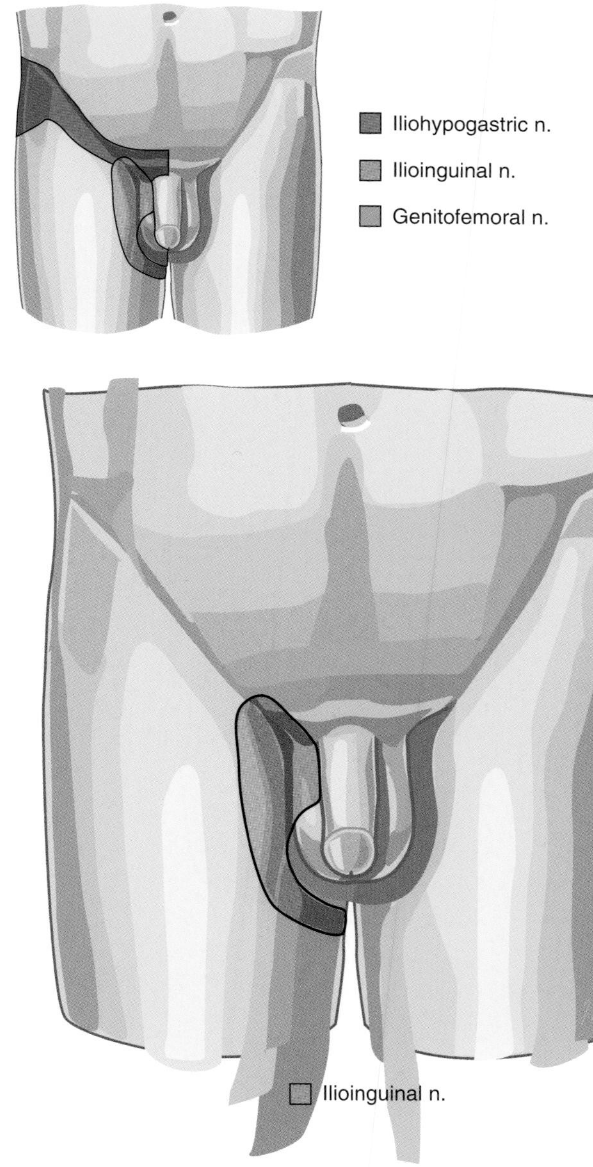

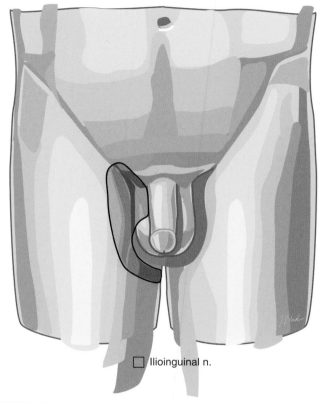

FIGURE 156–2 ■ Sensory distribution of the ilioinguinal nerve.

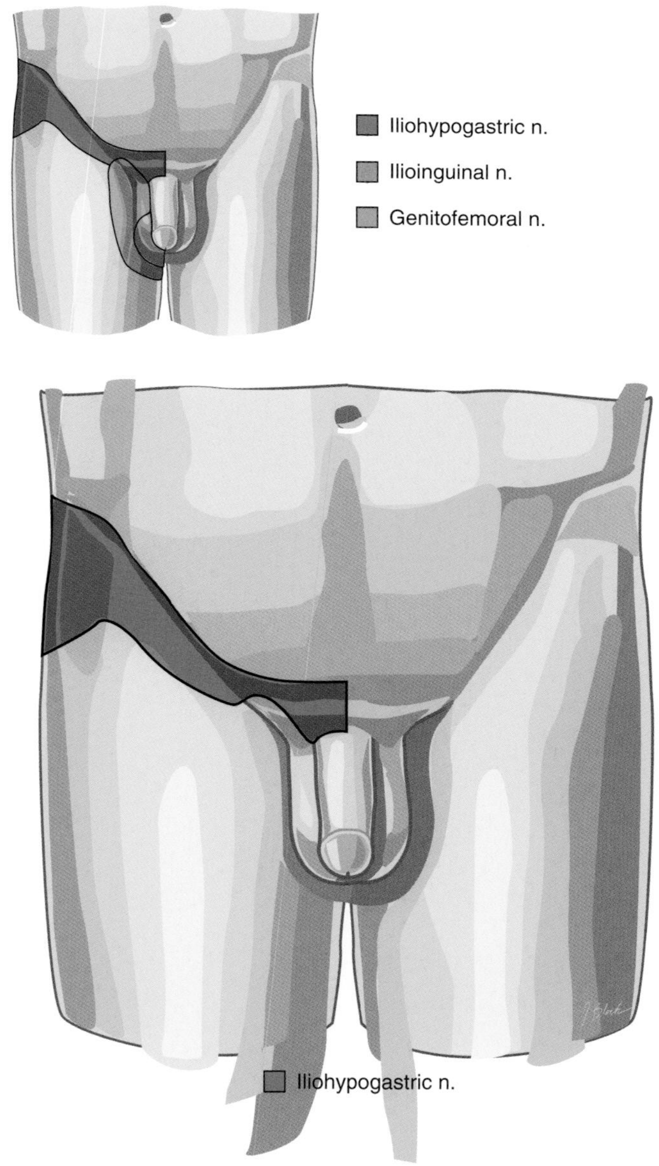

FIGURE 156–3 ■ Sensory distribution of the iliohypogastric nerve.

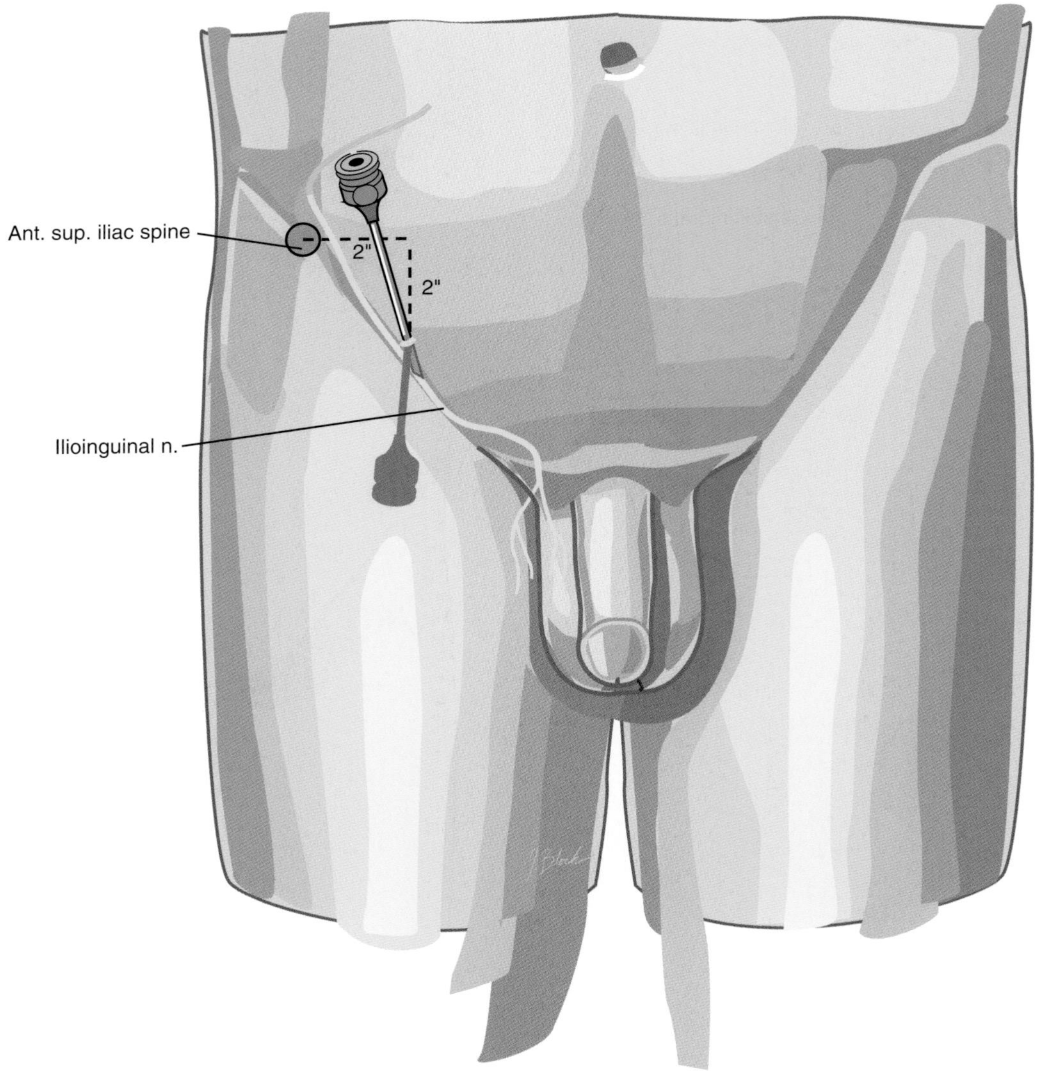

FIGURE 156–4 ■ Injection technique for ilioinguinal-iliohypogastric nerve block.

ing of the external oblique aponeurosis. At this time, after standard testing against intravascular injection, 5 to 15 mL of local anesthetic with or without steroids is injected in a fan-like manner in the layer between the internal and external oblique muscles.

■ SIDE EFFECTS AND COMPLICATIONS

Complications from ilioinguinal-iliohypogastric nerve blockade are rare, but can be devastating. Precautions that are common to regional anesthesia techniques should be taken throughout the procedure. Intravascular injection of bupivacaine can be catastrophic, and particular care should be taken to aspirate before any volume is injected. The safety of the local anesthetic again may depend on the agent used. In particular, avoidance of toxicity may be observed in both adults and pediatric patients by using ropivacaine or levobupivacaine instead of bupivacaine.[19-23,29-33] Higher plasma concentrations of bupivacaine occur in smaller children after ilioinguinal block.[39] Similarly, hematoma and ecchymosis can be prevented by constant aspiration of the needle on entry into the inter-abdominis area.

Penetration of the peritoneum and perforation of viscera are rare, but potentially disastrous, often requiring surgical repair. A few cases have been reported mainly involving children.[33-35] Using a short, blunt-bevel needle may reduce the risk of accidental visceral puncture, although caution regarding the depth of needle penetration should still be kept because one report occurred with this type of needle.[35] Femoral nerve palsy is a benign complication, which is self-resolving[33-35] but may delay recovery and day-surgery discharge.[35,36] The mechanism for this palsy is well described by Rosario[36] and suggests that femoral nerve palsy may occur more commonly than has been reported. The local anesthetic may diffuse in the plane connecting the transversalis fascia and the iliacus fascia, which contains the femoral nerve.

Studies may be needed to evaluate the incidence of palsy with different volumes of injectate. Conversely, failed blockade may occur if the needle position is too superficial. When a block fails in the awake patient, a supplemental dose of local anesthetic may be injected or infiltrated into the surgical site, such as the hernia orifice and spermatic cord. Overall, ilioinguinal nerve blockade is a safe procedure. As with any regional technique, the operator should pay careful attention to technique, anatomy, proper equipment, and appropriate testing against intravascular injection.

CONCLUSION

The ilioinguinal-iliohypogastric nerve block is a simple regional block with minimal adverse effects. The block is easily performed, effective, and safe in both adults and children requiring anesthesia or analgesia. Used as an individual regional technique or with monitored anesthesia care, this block improves day surgery efficiency with minimal risks. In eliciting a temporary neurotomy, it serves as a minimally invasive method for differential diagnosis of chronic groin and testicular pain and may save patients from unnecessary groin re-exploration after herniorrhaphy and from potentially worsening neurectomy.[20] Improvements are needed in extending the duration of its therapeutic use for chronic pain. Current modalities for neurolysis hold future promise but require further investigation.

References

1. Ponka JL. Seven steps to local anesthesia for inguino-femoral hernia repair. Surg Gynecol Obstet 117:115, 1963.
2. Bowen JR, Thompson WR, Dorman BA, et al: Change in the management of adult groin hernia. Am J Surg 135: 564, 1978.
3. Starling JR, Harms BA, Schroeder ME, Eichman PL: Diagnosis and treatment of genitofemoral and ilioinguinal entrapment neuralgia. Surgery 102:581, 1987.
4. Bunting P, McConachie I: Ilioinguinal nerve blockade for analgesia after caesarian section. Br J Anaesth 61: 773, 1988.
5. Casey WF, Rice LJ, Hannallah RS, et al: A comparison between bupivacaine instillation versus ilioinguinal/iliohypogastric nerve block for postoperative analgesia following inguinal herniorrhaphy in children. Anesthesiology 72(4):637, 1990.
6. Suraseranivongse S, Chowranayotin S, Pirayavarpom S, et al: Effect of bupivacaine with epinephrine wound instillation for pain relief after pediatric inguinal herniorrhaphy and hydrocelectomy. Reg Anesth Pain Med 28 (1):24, 2003.
7. Song D, Greilich NB, White PF, et al: Recovery profiles and costs of anesthesia for outpatient unilateral inguinal herniorrhaphy. Anesth Analg 91 (4):876, 2000.
8. Geis K, Dietl J: Ilioinguinal nerve entrapment after tension-free vaginal tape procedure. Int Urogynecol J Pevic Floor Dysfunct 13(2):136, 2002.
9. Deysine M, Deysine WP, Reed WP Jr, et al: Groin pain in the absence of hernia: A new syndrome. Hernia 6(2):64-7, 2002.
10. Bell EA, Jones BP, Olufolabi AJ, et al: Iliohypogastric-ilioinguinal peripheral nerve block for post-cesarean delivery analgesia decreases morphine use but not opioid-related side effect. Can J Anaesth 49(7):694, 2002.
11. Toivonen J, Permi J, Rosenberg PH, et al: Effect of preincisional ilioinguinal and iliohypogastric nerve bloc on postoperative analgesic requirement in day-surgery patients undergoing herniorrhaphy under spinal anesthesia. Acta Anaesthesiol Scand 45(5):603, 2001.
12. Casey WF, Rice LJ, Hannallah RS, et al: A comparison between bupvacaine instillation versus ilioinguinal/iliohypogastric nerve block for postoperative analgesia following inguinal herniorrhaphy in children. Anesthesiology 72(4):637, 1990.
13. Reid MF, Harris R, Phillips PD, et al: Day-case herniotomy in children. A comparison of ilio-inguinal nerve block and wound infiltration for postoperative analgesia. Anaesthesia 42(6):658, 1987.
14. Casey WF, Rice LJ, Hannallah RS, et al: A comparison between bupvacaine instillation versus ilioinguinal/iliohypogastric nerve block for postoperative analgesia following inguinal herniorrhaphy in children. Anesthesiology 72(4):637, 1990.
15. Ganta R, Samra SK, Maddineni VR, et al: Comparison of the effectiveness of bilateral ilioinguinal nerve block and wound infiltration for postoperative analgesia after cesarean section. Br J Anaesth 72 (2):229, 1994.
16. Moiniche S, Mikkelsen S, Welterslev J, Dahl JB, et al: A qualitative systematic review of incisional local anaesthesia for postoperative pain relief after abdominal operations. Br J Anaesth 81(3):377, 1998.
17. Poobalan AS, Bruce J, Smith BJ, et al: A review of chronic pain after inguinal herniorrhaphy. Clin J Pain 19(1):48, 2003.
18. Waldman SD: Atlas of Interventional Pain Management, 2nd ed, Philadelphia, WB Saunders, 2004.
19. Ghia JN, Blank JW, McAdams CG, et al: A new inter-abdominis approach to inguinal region block for the management of chronic pain. Reg Anesth 16(2):72, 1991.
20. Cohen SP, Foster A. Pulsed radiofrequency as a treatment for groin pain and orchialgia. Urology 61(3):645, 2003.
21. Khiroya RC, Davenport HT, Jones JG, et al: Cryoanalgesia for pain after herniorrhaphy. Anaesthesia 41(1):73, 1986.
22. Callesen T, Bech K, Thorup J, et al: Cryoanalgesia: Effect on post-herniorrhaphy pain. Anesth Analg 87(4):896, 1998.
23. Lipp A: Ilioinguinal nerve block for orchidopexy. Anaesthesia 53(5):515, 1998.
24. Kelly MC, Beers HT, Huss BK, et al: Bilateral ilioinguinal nerve blocks for analgesia after total abdominal hysterectomy. Anaesthesia 51(4):406, 1996.
25. Yazigi A, Jabbour K, Jebara SM, et al: [Bilateral ilioinguinal nerve block for ambulatory varicocele surgery] Ann Fr Anesth Reanim 21(9):710, 2002.
26. Huffnagle HJ, Norris MC, Leighton BL, et al: Ilioinguinal iliohypogastric nerve blocks—before or after cesarean delivery under spinal anesthesia? Anesth Analg 82:8, 1996.
27. Ding Y, White PF: Post-herniorrhaphy pain in outpatients after pre-incision ilioinguinal-hypogastric nerve block during monitored anaesthesia care. Can J Anaesth 42 12, 1995.
28. Shandling B, Steward DJ: Regional analgesia for postoperative pain in pediatric outpatient surgery. J Pediatr Surg 15(4):477, 1980.
29. Wulf H, Worthmann F, Behnke H, et al: Pharmacokinetics and pharmacodynamics of ropivacaine 2 mg/mL, 5 mg/mL, or 7.5 mg/mL after ilioinguinal blockade for inguinal hernia repair in adults. Anesth Analg 89(6):1471, 1999.
30. Gunter JB, Gregg T, Varughese AM, et al: Levobupivacaine for ilioinguinal/iliohypogastric nerve block in children. Anesth Analg 89(3):647, 1999.
31. Ala-Kokko TI, Karinen J, Raiha E, et al: Pharmacokinetics of 0.75% ropivacaine and 0.5% bupivacaine after ilioinguinal-iliohypogastric nerve block in children. Br J Anaesth 89(3):438, 2002.
32. Dalens B, Ecoffey C, Joly A, et al: Pharmacokinetics and analgesic effect of ropivacaine following ilioinguinal/iliohypogastric nerve block in children. Paediatr Anaesth 11(4):415, 2001.
33. Amory C, Mariscal A, Guyot E, et al: Is ilioinguinal/iliohypogastric nerve block always totally safe in children? Paediatr Anaesth 13(2):164, 2003.
34. Ghani KR, McMillan R, Patterson-Brown S, et al: Transient femoral nerve palsy following ilio-inguinal nerve blockade for day case inguinal hernia repair. J R Coll Surg Edinb 47(4):626, 2002.
35. Johr M, Sossai R: Colonic puncture during ilioinguinal nerve block in a child. Anesth Analg 88(5):1051, 1999.
36. Rosario DJ, Jacob S, Luntley J, et al: Mechanism of femoral nerve palsy complicating percutaneous ilioinguinal field block. Br J Anaesth 78(3): 314, 1997.
37. Leng SA: Transient femoral nerve palsy after ilioinguinal nerve block. Anaesth Intensive Care 25(1):92, 1997.
38. Ghani KR, McMillan R, Patterson-Brown S, et al: Transient femoral nerve palsy following ilio-inguinal nerve blockade for day surgery case inguinal hernia repair. J R Coll Surg Edinb 47(4):626, 2002.
39. Smith T, Moratin P, Wulf H, et al: Smaller children have greater bupivacaine plasma concentrations after ilioinguinal block. Br J Anaesth 76(3):452, 1996.

chapter 157

Lateral Femoral Cutaneous Nerve Block

David P. Bankston

HISTORICAL CONSIDERATIONS

Lateral femoral cutaneous neuropathy is one of the earliest entrapment neuropathies, having been reported in Germany in 1895 by W. K. Roth and M. Bernhardt. Bernhardt coined the phrase "meralgia tica," meaning thigh pain. Five years later, Harvey Cushing reported operating on a patient with meralgia paresthetica who transiently improved but ultimately became worse than preoperatively. Sigmund Freud had meralgia paresthetica. Freud initially believed it to be psychogenic, although he subsequently altered his thoughts.

INDICATIONS

1. The procedure may be used to block sensation to skin graft donor sites on the thigh.
2. It may be used in combination with sciatic and femoral blocks for surgical procedures performed on the lower extremities.
3. Perhaps the most common application of the lateral femoral cutaneous block is to treat meralgia paresthetica, a compressive disorder of the nerve (Table 157–1).
4. If a neurolytic block is contemplated, the block may be used for prognostic value to determine the degree of impairment that may be present after destruction of the lateral femoral cutaneous nerve.

CLINICALLY RELEVANT ANATOMY

The lateral femoral cutaneous nerve originates from the posterior divisions at L2 and L3 nerve roots. The nerve pierces the psoas muscle, traveling inferior-lateral until it runs inferior or occasionally invades the ilioinguinal ligament[1,2] just medial to the anterior superior iliac spine. It then divides into anterior and posterior branches under the fascia lata. The anterior branch supplies sensation to the anterior lateral thigh, whereas the posterior branch supplies the lateral thigh from above the greater trochanter to the knee.

TECHNIQUE

Place the patient supine and identify the anterior superior iliac spine. A point 2 to 3 cm medial and 2 to 3 cm inferior, depending on the patient's size, to the spine is then marked. A 25-gauge $1\frac{1}{2}$-inch needle is passed perpendicular to the skin until a fascial pop is felt or paresthesia is obtained (Fig. 152–1). An injection of 10 to 15 mL of local anesthetic together with 80 mg Depo Medrol or Kenalog should be made in a fan-like manner. If the iliac crest is contacted, injection can continue more medially. Care should be taken not to advance the needle too far, especially in a thin patient, to avoid the peritoneal cavity and possible visceral perforation, as illustrated in these MR images (Fig. 152–2). After injection, pressure may be applied to the injection site to decrease the possibility of bleeding or ecchymosis, which is more likely to occur in anticoagulated patients.

ASSESSING THE ADEQUACY OF THE BLOCK

The lateral femoral cutaneous nerve is purely sensory with no motor fibers. These sensory nerves innervate the lateral thigh and buttock. The block can be considered successful if the patient is unable to feel a pinch high on the lateral thigh (Fig. 152–3).[3]

SIDE EFFECTS AND COMPLICATIONS

Complications include nerve damage, bleeding, infection, and local anesthetic toxicity. In addition, the proximity of the peritoneal cavity makes contact with visceral structure (i.e., the intestine), a possibility if the needle is inserted too deeply.

CONCLUSION

The lateral femoral cutaneous nerve block is a simple, easily performed peripheral nerve block, which is not commonly associated with complications. It is most frequently used to treat entrapment neuropathy meralgia paresthetica. Lateral femoral cutaneous nerve block may be used for diagnostic

Table 157–1

Causes and Differential Diagnosis of Meralgia Paresthetica

Causes	***Differential Diagnosis***
Abdominal or pelvic tumors (may cause compression)	Abdominal pathology
Anterior pelvic surgery	Trochanteric bursitis
Backpacks	Diabetes mellitis
Cardiac catheterization	Lumbar radialopathy (including disk pathology)
Hip extension	Peripheral neuropathy
Iliac crest bone harvest	Retroperitoneal tumors
Intramuscular injection	
Jogging	
Obesity	
Pregnancy	
Self-retaining retractors (surgical)	
Spine surgery	
Tight garments	
Tool belts	
Trauma (the nerve is superficial)	

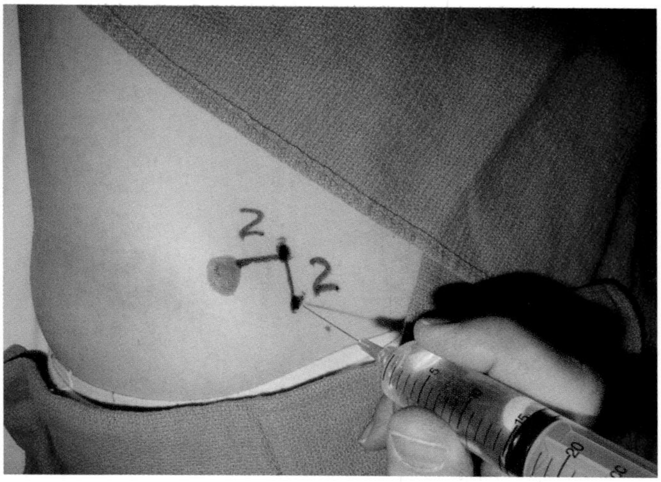

FIGURE 157–1 ■ Injection technique for lateral femoral cutaneous nerve block.

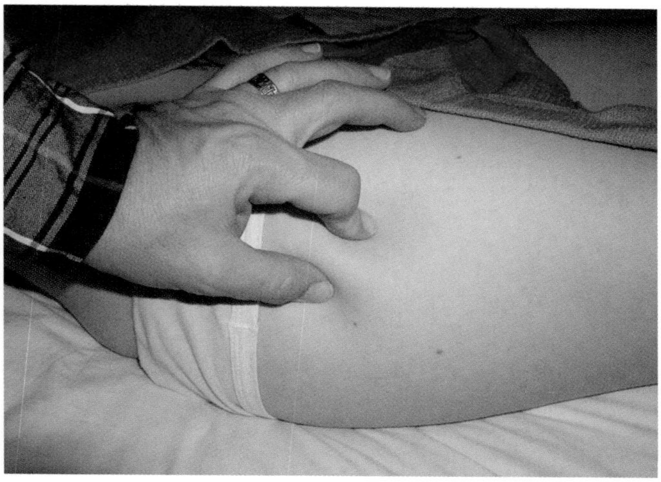

FIGURE 157–3 ■ Assessing the adequacy of lateral femoral cutaneous nerve block.

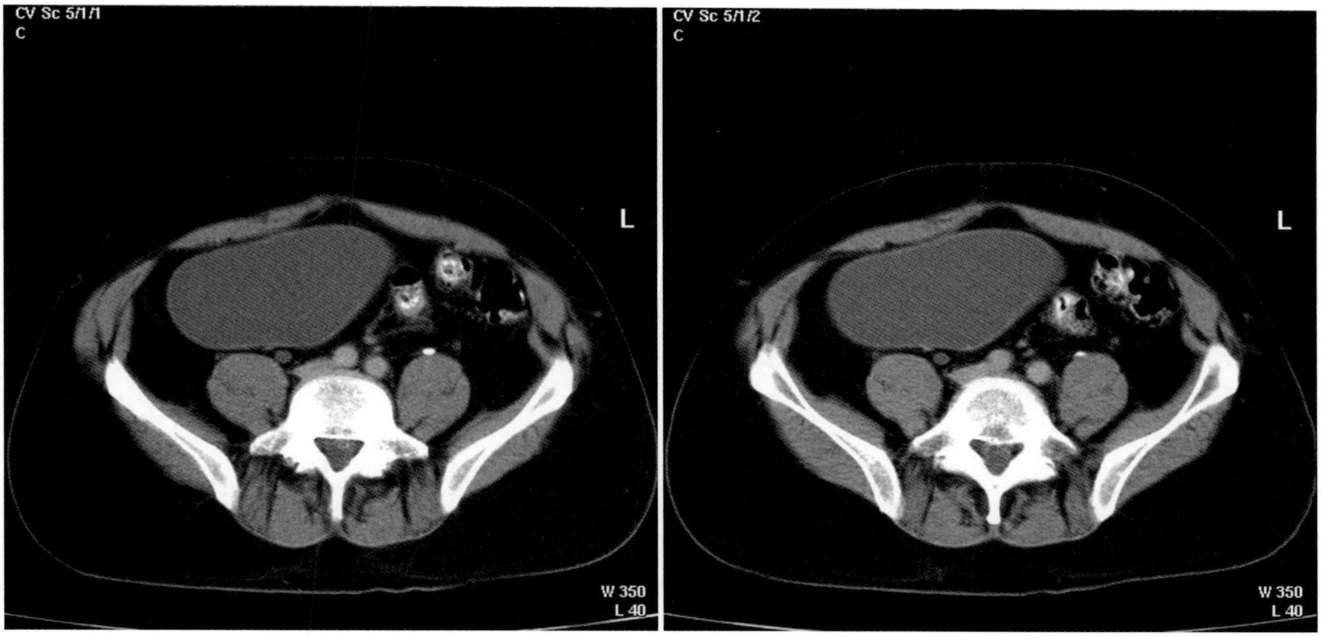

A B

FIGURE 157–2 ■ These MR images depict structures underlying the injection site for lateral femoral cutaneous nerve block that may be at risk if the needle is inserted too deeply. **A,** axial view at the level of the anterior superior iliac spine. **B,** view 2 cm inferior to panel **A**.

purposes and also may offer extended relief when several blocks are administered in short intervals.[4] Lateral femoral cutaneous nerve block is also a valuable tool for skin grafting procedures or may be combined with other lower extremity nerve blocks (i.e., sciatic, obturator, femoral) for surgical anesthesia.

References

1. Dawson DM: Lateral femoral cutaneous nerve entrapment. In Dawson DM (ed): Entrapment Neuropathies, 2nd ed. Boston, Little, Brown, 1990, p 301.
2. Loeser JD: Pain of neurologic origin in the hips and lower extremities. In Loeser JD, Butler SH, Chapman CR, Turk DC (eds): Bonica's Management of Pain, 3rd ed. Philadelphia, Lippincott Williams & Wilkins, 2001, p 1565.
3. Neal JM: Assessment of lower extremity nerve block: Reprise of the four P acronym. Reg Anesth Pain Med 27:618, 2002.
4. Warfield CA: Peripheral neuropathies. In Warfield CA, Fausett HJ (eds): Manual of Pain Management, 2nd ed. Philadelphia, Lippincott Williams & Wilkins, 2002, p 206.

chapter 158

Obturator Nerve Block

Somayaji Ramamurthy

Blockade of the obturator nerve is a clinically useful technique in the management of hip and lower extremity pain and spasticity. The increased use of nerve stimulators to aid in correct needle placement has significantly improved the success of the obturator nerve block and has made it less uncomfortable for the patient.[2] Results of blind paresthesia techniques used before the days of the nerve stimulator or the multiple reinsertion and the infiltration technique were extremely unpredictable and could be very painful for the patient.

Clinically Relevant Anatomy

The obturator nerve originates from anterior primary rami of L2-L3 and L4 lumbar nerve roots. The contribution of L3 is the most predominant; contributions from L2 and L4 are small. The nerve passes through the psoas major muscle, emerging at its lateral border. It travels posterior to the iliac vessels and reaches the undersurface of the superior ramus of the pubis.[1] It passes through the obturator internus and externus muscles to emerge from the obturator foramen.(Fig. 158–1) Shortly thereafter, it divides into anterior and posterior branches. The anterior branch innervates the anterior adductor muscles and gives a branch to innervate the hip joint. The posterior branch innervates mainly the adductor magnus muscle. It travels inferiorly and communicates with the saphenous branch of the femoral nerve. It travels along the femoral vessels to the popliteal fossa and gives a branch to innervate the knee joint. The innervation of both the hip joint and the knee joint by the obturator nerve can explain why a patient with a lesion in the hip joint sometimes complains of pain in the knee and vice versa. The obturator nerve is almost entirely a motor nerve. Sensory contribution to dermatomal distribution to the lower medial aspect of the thigh is variable and could be nonexistent in some patients.

■ INDICATIONS

Surgical Anesthesia

The obturator nerve has to be blocked for any procedure above the knee or when a pneumatic tourniquet is placed over the thigh. It is blocked along with the femoral, lateral femoral cutaneous, and sciatic nerves for this purpose.[3] One of the most important surgical indications is due to the anatomic relationship of the obturator nerve as it runs close to the neck of the bladder and the prostate.[4-7] Because of the proximity of the nerve to the prostate, this nerve can be electrically stimulated during the transurethral resection. This stimulation can produce significant contraction of the adductors, which can interfere with the surgical procedure, and on occasion can even result in the perforation of the bladder. This can occur even with adequate spinal analgesia that blocks the nerve roots proximal to the site of stimulation. Local anesthetic block of the obturator nerve has been well documented to abolish the spasms and facilitate the prostatic surgery.

Acute Pain

Blockade of the obturator nerve with local anesthetics such as bupivacaine is useful in the management of acute hip and lower medial thigh pain following pelvic trauma, total hip replacement surgery, and other acute pain emergencies. Because compromise or irritation of the obturator nerve may produce significant spasm in addition to pain, this technique can be extremely useful in providing symptomatic relief to allow the patient to comfortably undergo radiographic studies, magnetic resonance, or computerized tomographic scanning of the hip or pelvic bones.

Chronic Pain

Because the hip joint derives significant innervation from the obturator nerve, blockade of this nerve was one of the main indications in patients who had degenerative hip disease.[8] Since the advent of total joint replacement, however, the number of patients who require this type of block has significantly decreased. It still can be of use as a diagnostic block for a complex pain problem.[9,10] Even under these circumstances, a direct hip joint injection provides more valuable diagnostic information than blockade of the obturator nerve.[11] Obturator nerve entrapment has been described in athletes[12] and after pelvic surgery.[13,14] The obturator nerve has been surgically released with good success. A diagnostic nerve block may help to make the diagnosis.

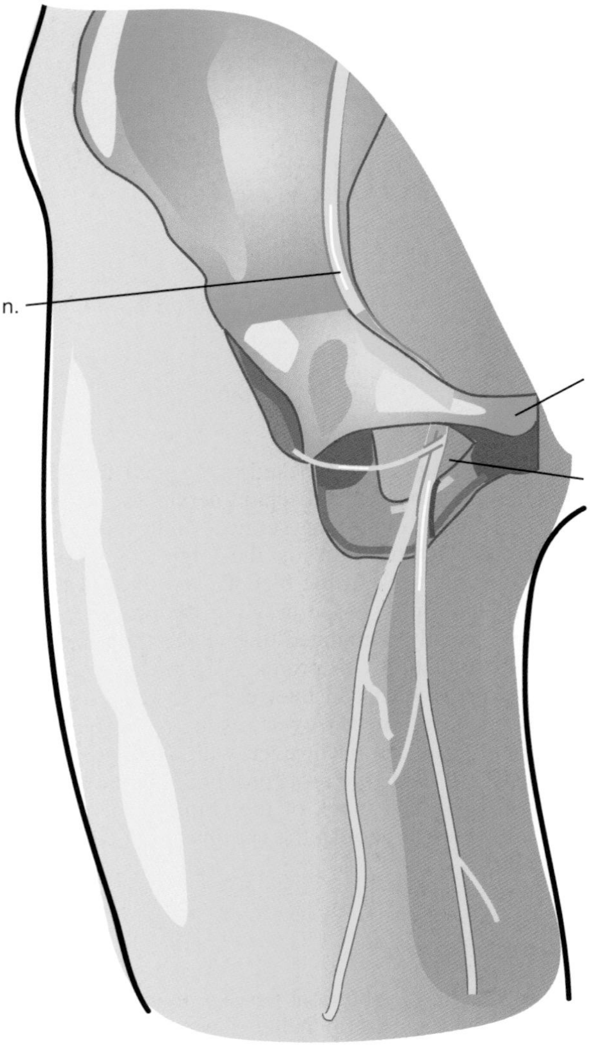

FIGURE 158–1 ■ Anatomy of obturator nerve, showing bony landmarks used in nerve block technique.

Spasticity

One of the most important nonsurgical indications was for adductor muscle spasticity. Obturator nerve block was used extensively to relieve adductor spasm to improve the personal hygiene of patients with spasticity. Oral and intrathecal dosing with baclofen has very significantly reduced the use of neurolytic obturator nerve block for this purpose but it remains a useful technique for those patients in whom pharmacologic methods are not tolerated or do not produce the desired results.

■ TECHNIQUE

Direct Approach

The direct approach (Fig. 158–2) blocks the nerve as it exits the obturator foramen underneath the superior ramus of the pubis. The patient is placed in the supine position. The thigh is slightly abducted. The pubic area is sterilized with a nonirritating antiseptic such as Betadine. The pubic tubercle, the most important landmark, is identified. The entry point is 1.5 cm lateral and inferior to the pubic tubercle. The skin is anesthetized with a 25- or 27-gauge, short needle and a fast-acting local anesthetic such as 1% lidocaine. A 22-gauge (8-cm) spinal needle is advanced vertically downward. The needle usually contacts the bone of the upper one third of the pubis. The negative electrode from a stimulator is attached to the needle, and the positive electrode is placed on the patient in an area where no paresthesia from the obturator nerve is expected. Over the bone 0.5 mL of 1% lidocaine is infiltrated to reduce the pain of "walking" the needle on the bone. The needle is redirected laterally and superiorly to induce contraction of the adductor muscles. When strong contractions are elicited, the nerve stimulator is adjusted until good contractions are produced with current less than 1 mA with an uninsulated needle or less than 0.5 mA with an insulated needle. A 2-mL test dose of local anesthetic should abolish the contraction, confirming proximity of the needle tip to the obturator nerve. At this point, 7 to 12 mL of local anesthetic is injected. During the lateral and superior redirection, if the pubic ramus is encountered, the needle must be walked slightly inferiorly to enter the obturator foramen. The needle should not be advanced more than 2 to 3 cm into

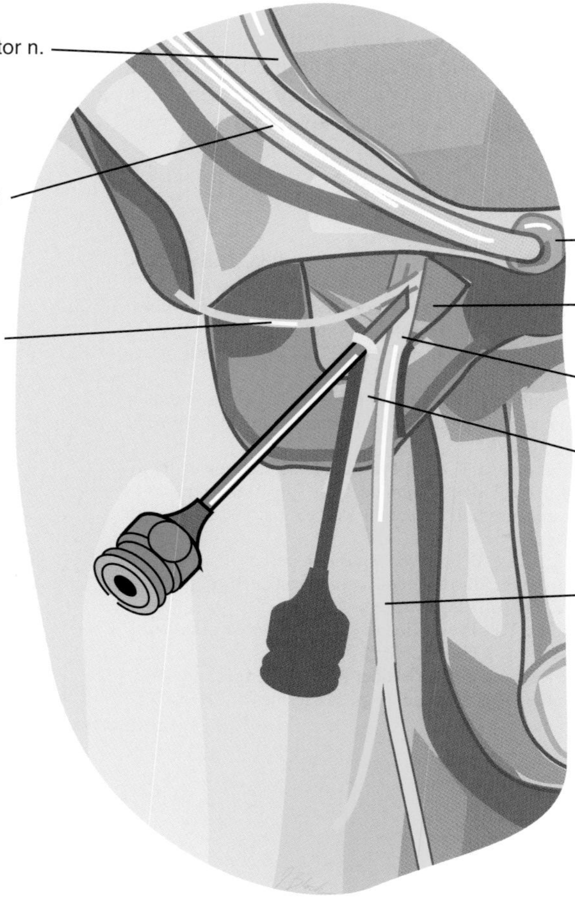

FIGURE 158–2 ■ The direct technique of obturator nerve block. (From Waldman SD [ed]: Atlas of Interventional Pain Management, 2nd ed. Philadelphia, Saunders, 2003; page 462, Figure 100-3.)

the obturator foramen lest it enter the pelvis and damage the bladder.

An alternative approach consists of identifying the adductor longus muscle and advancing the needle underneath the proximal end of the adductor longus muscle in a medial to lateral direction and looking for contraction of the other adductor muscles with nerve stimulation.[15] A successful block can be identified when the patient is asked to adduct the thigh against resistance. The accompanying dermatomal analgesia is quite variable and can be nonexistent.

Neurolytic Block

The direct approach is the most suitable for neurolytic block of the obturator nerve. The author uses an insulated needle with a stimulator to ensure proximity of the needle tip to the nerve. Most clinicians use a 6% or higher concentration of phenol to block the nerve. Radiofrequency coagulation can also be utilized.

INDIRECT TECHNIQUE

Winnie and coworkers described a three-in-one block. During this technique, the femoral nerve is identified and a volume of local anesthetic greater than 20 mL is injected, which is expected to spread to the lumbar plexus and block the obturator and the lateral femoral cutaneous nerves, in addition to the femoral nerve. This could be a significant advantage because the obturator nerve can be blocked easily without the pain of multiple injections. Whether the obturator nerve is consistently blocked is a matter of debate. The results of the three-in-one block were originally assessed by checking for cutaneous analgesia over the thigh. It was believed that analgesia over the anterior and lateral aspect of the thigh in the distribution of all three nerves indicated that the obturator nerve was also blocked. This may not be so when the obturator innervation of the skin is minimal or nonexistent. There have been cadaver studies[16] in which injection of methylene blue indicated that the dye does not spread to the lumbar plexus or to the obturator nerve. Studies compared three-in-one block with direct block of the obturator nerve with a nerve stimulator and assessed the results with motor evoked potentials.[17-20] It was clear that the three-in-one block did not produce consistent block of the obturator nerve.[17-20] Thus, if an obturator nerve block is needed to prevent abductor spasm during transurethral surgery or for neurolysis, the direct approach is preferred.

COMPLICATIONS

Nerve block with a local anesthetic using the landmarks and techniques described here usually does not result in serious complications. The usual complications are infection, bleeding, and pain at the site of the injection, but usually they are not serious. If the needle is advanced more than 3 cm into the pelvis, it can damage pelvic organs including the bladder. Neurolytic blockade in a patient who has normal sensation can result in neuritis, which can produce severe burning pain along the inside of the thigh.

References

1. Warwick R, Williams PL (eds): Gray's Anatomy, ed 35. Philadelphia, WB Saunders, 1973, p 1052.
2. Magora F, Rozin R, Ben-Menachem Y, Magora A: Obturator nerve block: An evaluation of technique. Br J Anaesth 41(8):695, 1969.
3. Lim W, Kennedy N: Hemi-arthroplasty of the hip under triple nerve block. Anaesth Intensive Care 22(6):722, 1994.
4. Deliveliotis C, Alexopoulou K, Picramenos D, et al: The contribution of the obturator nerve block in the transurethral resection of bladder tumors. Acta Urol Belg 63(3):51, 1995.
5. Fujita Y, Kimura K, Furukawa Y, et al: Plasma concentrations of lignocaine after obturator nerve block combined with spinal anaesthesia in patients undergoing transurethral resection procedures. Br J Anaesth 68(6):569, 1992.
6. Moulaert P, Verbaeys A, De Brock M: Obturator nerve block in preventing bladder perforation during endoscopic transurethral bladder surgery. Acta Urol Belg 56(4):523, 1988.
7. Augspurger RR, Donohue RE: Prevention of obturator nerve stimulation during transurethral surgery. J Urol 123(2):170, 1980.
8. James CD, Little TF: Regional hip blockade. A simplified technique for the relief on intractable osteoarthritic pain. Anaesthesia 31(8):1060, 1976.
9. Hong Y, O'Grady T, Lopresti D, et al: Diagnostic obturator nerve block for inguinal and back pain: A recovered opinion. Pain 67:507, 1996.
10. Trainer N, Bowser BL, Dahm L: Obturator nerve block for painful hip in adult cerebral palsy. Arch Phys Med Rehabil 67(11):829, 1986.
11. Edmonds-Seal J, Turner A, Khodadadeh S, et al: Regional hip blockade in osteoarthrosis. Effects on pain perception. Anaesthesia 37(2):1158, 1982.
12. Bradshaw C, McCrory P: Obturator nerve entrapment. Clin J Sports Med 7(3):217, 1997.
13. Crews DA, Dohlman LE: Obturator neuropathy after multiple genitourinary procedures. Urology 29(5):504, 1987.
14. Warfield CA: Obturator neuropathy after forceps delivery. Obstet Gynecol 64(3):158S, 1984.
15. Wassef MR: Interadductor approach to obturator nerve blockade for spastic conditions of adductor thigh muscles. Reg Anesth 18(1):13, 1993.
16. Ritter JW: Femoral nerve "sheath" for inguinal paravascular lumbar plexus block is not found in human cadavers. J Clin Anesth 7(6):1580, 1995.
17. Atanassoff PG, Weiss BM, Brull SJ, et al: Compound motor action potential recording distinguishes differential onset of motor block of the obturator nerve in response to etidocaine or bupivacaine. Anesth Analg 82(2):317, 1996.
18. Lang SA: Electromyographic comparison of obturator nerve block to 3-in-1-block (Letter). Anesth Analg 83(2):436, 1996.
19. Atanassoff PG, Weiss BN, Brull SJ, et al: Electromyographic comparison of obturator nerve block to three-in-one block. Anesth Analg 81(3):529, 1995.
20. Lang SA, Yip RW, Chang PC, et al: The femoral 3-in-1 block revisited. J Clin Anesth 5(4):292, 1993.

chapter 159

Caudal Epidural Nerve Block

Steven D. Waldman

Although it once seemed destined for extinction, the use of the caudal approach to the epidural space has enjoyed a remarkable resurgence in the care of the patient in pain. This resurgence has been fueled by several disparate factors: (1) an improved understanding of the functional anatomy of the sacral hiatus, sacrococcygeal ligament, and sacral canal from information gleaned from imaging (MRI and CT) of the region, which dispelled the commonly held belief that anatomic variations of this anatomic region made caudal block too technically challenging; (2) the increased use of sharper, shorter needles when performing other epidural blocks; and (3) the constant pressure on pain management specialists to provide pain management techniques in the most cost-effective manner possible, which placed performance of the caudal approach to the epidural space in a favorable light relative to lumbar epidural block, which required the use of more expensive Hustead or Touhy epidural needles. This renewed interest in caudal epidural block has been fueled further by studies indicating that the caudal approach to the epidural space may be more efficacious than the lumbar approach for many pain management applications. This chapter provides an overview of the current status of caudal epidural block in contemporary pain management.

HISTORICAL CONSIDERATIONS

Although the discovery of a practical way to administer drugs via the caudal approach to the epidural space preceded that for the lumbar approach by almost 20 years, the popularity of the caudal epidural nerve block has waxed and waned relative to the lumbar approach to the epidural space. In 1901, Cathelin[1] published the first accurate description of the caudal approach to the epidural space. Despite the initial enthusiasm for the caudal approach after Cathelin's report, worldwide acceptance of the technique was inconsistent, at best. The reasons included lack of understanding of the clinical anatomy, overemphasis on the importance of the anatomic variations of the sacrum, and, perhaps most important, misapplication of the caudal approach for indications for which it was anatomically unsuited (i.e., to deliver drugs to the upper thoracic dermatomes). A tendency to compare the caudal epidural approach with the spinal and lumbar epidural approaches also contributed to misunderstanding of the appropriate role of this technique in surgical (and later in obstetric) anesthesia.

The description of the midline approach to the lumbar epidural space proposed by Pagés[2] in 1921 and refined by Dogliotti[3] and Gutierrez[4] in 1933 led to a further decline in use of the caudal approach. Just when it seemed that caudal nerve block was destined for extinction, in 1943, Hingson and Edwards[5] repopularized it for pain relief in childbirth. Anesthesiologists, obstetricians, and patients rapidly embraced the technique. This resurgence of interest was short-lived, however, owing in part to several widely publicized reports of fetal demise secondary to injection of local anesthetic into the fetus during caudal block and in part to the introduction of neuromuscular blocking agents in 1946. Persistent ignorance of the detailed anatomy and technique of the caudal approach to the epidural space led to reported failure rates of 5% to 7%,[6] rates that did not compare favorably with the much lower ones of spinal and general anesthesia reported at the time.

Throughout the 1950s and 1960s, the caudal approach to the epidural space was left in the hands of a few enthusiasts, who, in the words of Bromage,[7] "somewhat inexplicably, made it their hobby." The second repopularization of the caudal approach to the epidural space occurred during the 1970s and 1980s, in tandem with the increasing interest in the role of neural blockade in pain management. The growing use of the caudal approach in the pediatric population and as a route for administration of opioids in anticoagulated patients has increased use of this valuable technique further.

INDICATIONS AND CONTRAINDICATIONS

Indications for caudal epidural nerve block are summarized in Table 159–1. In addition to applications for surgical and obstetric anesthesia, caudal epidural nerve block with local anesthetics can be used as a diagnostic tool when differential neural blockade is performed on an anatomic basis to evaluate pelvic, bladder, perineal, genital, rectal, anal, and lower extremity pain.[8,9] If destruction of the sacral nerves is being considered, caudal epidural nerve block is useful as a prognostic indicator of the extent of motor and sensory impairment that the patient may experience.[9]

Caudal epidural nerve block with local anesthetics may be used to palliate acute pain emergencies in adults and children—postoperative pain, acute low back pain, acute radiculopathy, pain secondary to pelvic and lower extremity trauma,

Table 159–1

Indications for the Caudal Approach to the Epidural Space

Surgical, Obstetric, Diagnostic, and Prognostic	
Surgical anesthesia	
Obstetric anesthesia	
Differential neural blockade to evaluate pelvic, bladder, perineal, genital, rectal, anal, and lower extremity pain	
Prognostic indicator before destruction of sacral nerves	
Acute Pain	
Acute low back pain	
Acute lumbar radiculopathy	
Palliation in acute pain emergencies	
Postoperative pain	
Pelvic and lower extremity pain secondary to trauma	
Pain of acute herpes zoster	
Acute vascular insufficiency of the lower extremities	
Hidradenitis suppurativa	
Chronic Benign Pain	
Lumbar radiculopathy	
Spinal stenosis	
Low back syndrome	
Vertebral compression fractures	
Diabetic polyneuropathy	
Postherpetic neuralgia	
Reflex sympathetic dystrophy	
Orchialgia	
Proctalgia	
Pelvic pain syndromes	
Cancer Pain	
Pain secondary to pelvic, perineal, genital, or rectal malignancy	
Bony metastases to pelvis	
Chemotherapy-related peripheral neuropathy	
Special Situations	
Patients with previous lumbar spine surgery	
Patients who are "anticoagulated" or have coagulopathy	

pain of acute herpes zoster, and cancer-related pain—during the wait for pharmacologic, surgical, or antiblastic treatment to take effect.[10,11] The technique also is valuable in patients with acute vascular insufficiency of the lower extremities secondary to vasospastic or vaso-occlusive disease, including frostbite and ergotamine toxicity.[12] Caudal nerve block also is recommended to palliate the pain of hidradenitis suppurativa of the groin.[13]

Administration of local anesthetics or steroids via the caudal approach to the epidural space is useful in the treatment of a variety of chronic benign pain syndromes, including lumbar radiculopathy, low back syndrome, spinal stenosis, postlaminectomy syndrome, vertebral compression fractures, diabetic polyneuropathy, postherpetic neuralgia, reflex sympathetic dystrophy, phantom limb pain, orchalgia, proctalgia, and pelvic pain syndromes.[14-18] Because of the simplicity, safety, and patient comfort associated with the caudal approach to the epidural space, this technique is replacing the lumbar epidural approach for these indications in some pain centers.[15]

The caudal approach to the epidural space is especially useful in patients who have previously undergone low back surgery, which may make the lumbar approach to the epidural space less efficacious.[19] The caudal approach to the epidural space can be used in the presence of anticoagulation or coagulopathy, so local anesthetics, opioids, and steroids can be administered via this route, even when other regional anesthetic techniques, including the spinal and lumbar epidural approaches, are contraindicated.[20] This fact is advantageous for patients with vascular insufficiency who are fully anticoagulated and for cancer patients who have developed coagulopathy secondary to radiation or chemotherapy.

The caudal epidural administration of local anesthetics in combination with steroids or opioids is useful in the palliation of cancer-related pelvic, perineal, and rectal pain.[21] This technique has been especially successful in the relief of pain secondary to the bony metastases of prostate cancer and the palliation of chemotherapy-related peripheral neuropathy. Another benefit is that it can be used to administer local anesthetics, opioids, or steroids despite anticoagulation or coagulopathy.

Contraindications to the caudal approach to the epidural space are the following:

- Local infection
- Sepsis
- Pilonidal cyst
- Congenital abnormalities of the dural sac and its contents

Because of the potential for hematogenous spread via Batson's plexus, local infection and sepsis are absolute contraindications to the caudal approach to the epidural space. Pilonidal cyst and congenital anomalies of the dural sac and its contents are relative contraindications.

CLINICALLY RELEVANT ANATOMY

Sacrum

The triangular sacrum consists of the five fused sacral vertebrae, which are dorsally convex (Fig. 159–1).[22] The sacrum inserts in a wedgelike manner between the two iliac bones, articulating superiorly with the L5 vertebra and caudally with the coccyx. On the anterior concave surface are four pairs of unsealed anterior sacral foramina that allow passage of the anterior rami of the upper four sacral nerves. The unsealed nature of the anterior sacral foramina allows the escape of drugs injected into the sacral canal.[23]

The convex dorsal surface of the sacrum has an irregular surface because the elements of the sacral vertebrae all fuse there. Dorsally, there is a midline crest called the *median sacral crest.* The posterior sacral foramina are smaller than their anterior counterparts. The sacrospinal and multifidus muscles effectively prevent leakage of drugs injected into the sacral canal. The vestigial remnants of the inferior articular processes project downward on each side of the sacral hiatus. These bony projections, called the *sacral cornua,* represent important clinical landmarks for caudal epidural nerve block (see Fig. 159–1).[24] Although there are gender-determined and race-determined differences in the shape of the sacrum, they

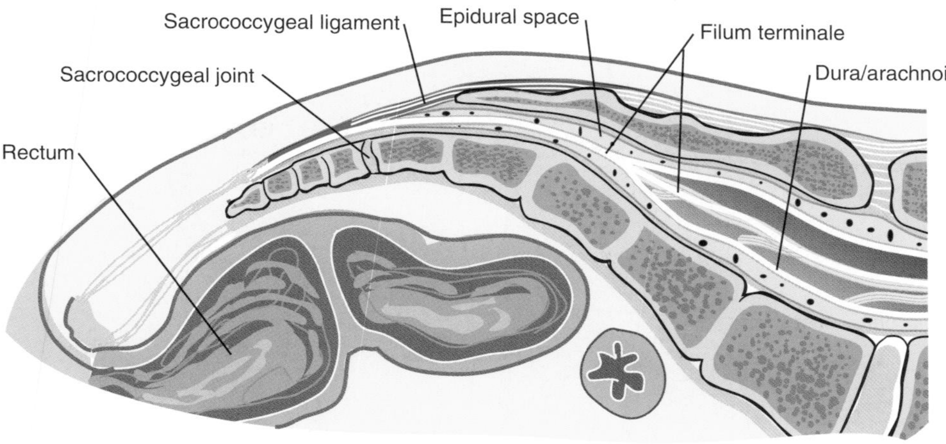

FIGURE 159–1 ■ Anatomy of the sacrum and coccyx.

are of little importance relative to the ultimate ability to perform caudal epidural nerve block successfully on a given patient.[14]

Coccyx

The triangular coccyx is composed of three to five rudimentary vertebrae (see Fig. 159–1). Its superior surface articulates with the inferior articular surface of the sacrum. Two prominent coccygeal cornua adjoin their sacral counterparts. The ventral surface of the coccyx is angulated anteriorly and superiorly. The tip of the coccyx is an important landmark for caudal epidural nerve block.[19]

Sacral Hiatus

The sacral hiatus is the result of incomplete midline fusion of the posterior elements of the lower portion of the S4 and the entire S5 vertebrae. This U-shaped space is covered posteriorly by the sacrococcygeal ligament, which is also an important clinical landmark for caudal epidural nerve block (see Fig. 159–1). Penetration of the sacrococcygeal ligament provides direct access to the epidural space of the sacral canal.[22]

Sacral Canal

A continuation of the lumbar spinal canal, the sacral canal continues inferiorly to terminate at the sacral hiatus (Fig. 159–2). The canal communicates with the anterior and posterior sacral foramina. The volume of the sacral canal, with all of its contents removed, averages approximately 34 mL in dried bone specimens.[14]

Contents of the Sacral Canal

The sacral canal contains the inferior termination of the dural sac, which ends between S1 and S3 (Fig. 159–3).[23] The five sacral nerve roots and the coccygeal nerve all traverse the canal, as does the terminal filament of the spinal cord, the filum terminale. The anterior and posterior rami of the S1-4 nerve roots exit from their respective anterior and posterior sacral foramina. The S5 roots and coccygeal nerves leave the sacral canal via the sacral hiatus. These nerves provide sensory and motor innervation to their respective dermatomes and myotomes. They also supply partial innervation to several pelvic structures, including the uterus, fallopian tubes, bladder, and prostate.[19]

The sacral canal also contains the epidural venous plexus, which generally ends at S4, but may continue caudad (see Fig. 159–3). Most of these vessels are concentrated in the anterior portion of the canal.[23] The dural sac and the epidural vessels are susceptible to trauma during cephalad advancement of needles or catheters into the sacral canal.[24] The remainder of the sacral canal is filled with fat, which is subject to age-related increase in density. Some investigators believe that this change is responsible for the higher incidence of "spotty" caudal epidural nerve blocks in adults.[6]

■ TECHNIQUE

All equipment, including the needles and supplies for nerve block, drugs, resuscitation equipment, oxygen supply, and suction, must be assembled and checked before beginning a caudal epidural nerve block.

Positioning the Patient

Caudal epidural nerve block is done with the patient in the prone or the lateral position. Each position has advantages and disadvantages. The prone position is easier for the pain management physician, but it may not be an option if the patient (1) cannot rest comfortably on the abdomen or (2) wears an ostomy appliance, such as a colostomy or ileostomy bag. The prone position limits easy access to the airway, which might be needed if problems occur during the procedure. The lateral position affords better access to the airway, but makes the approach technically more demanding.

Prone Position

The patient is placed in the prone position with the head on a pillow and turned away from the operator. Another pillow is placed under the hips, to tilt the pelvis and make the sacral hiatus more prominent. The legs and heels are abducted to prevent tightening of the gluteal muscles, which could make identification of the sacral hiatus more difficult (Fig. 159–4).[8]

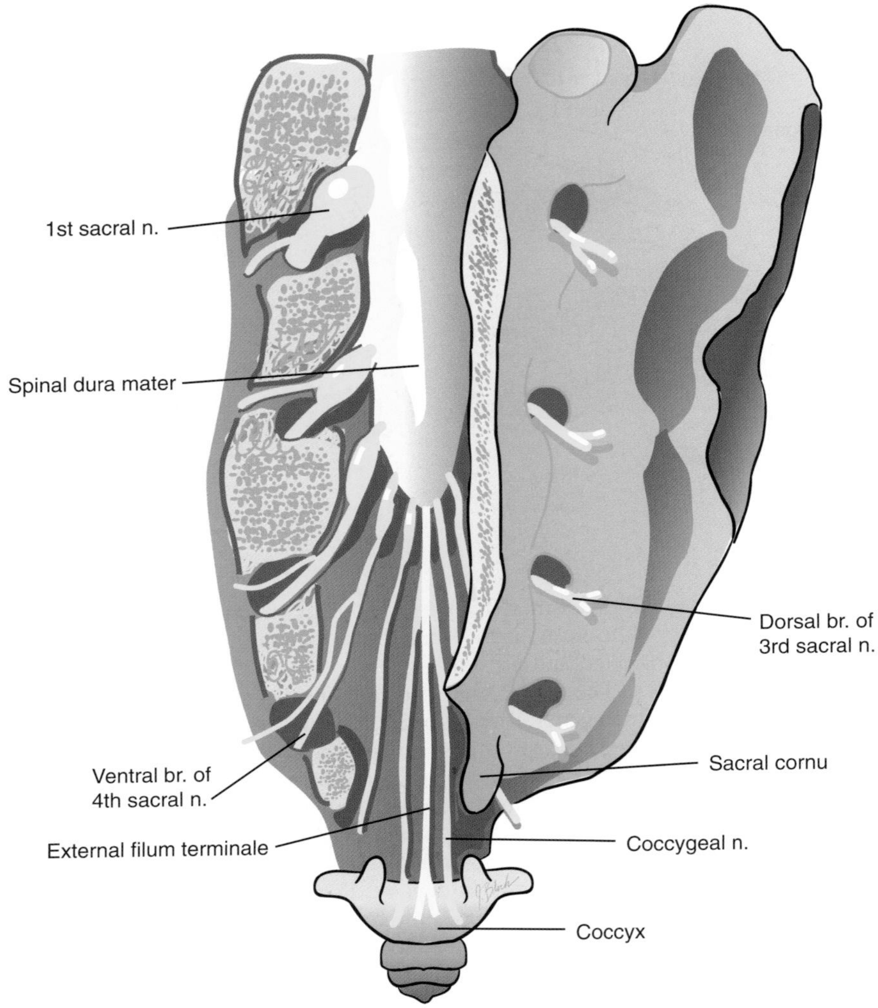

FIGURE 159–2 ■ Lateral view of the sacral canal.

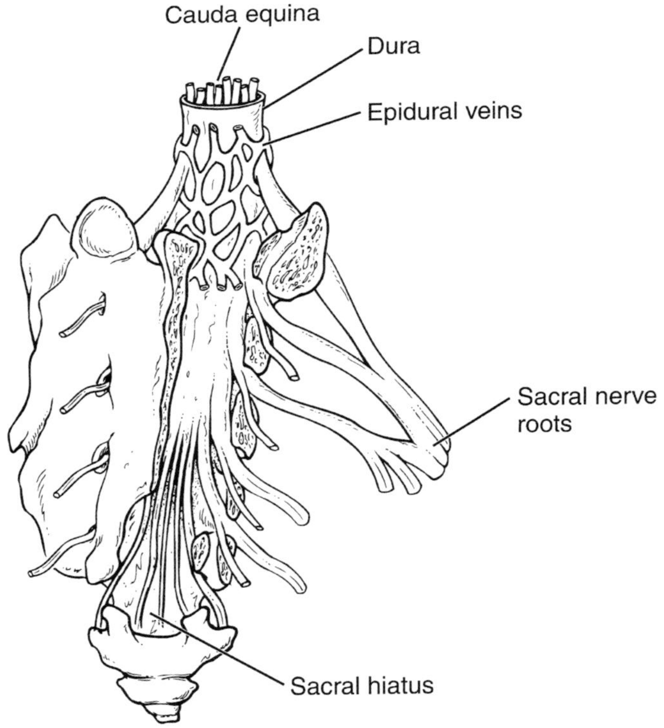

FIGURE 159–3 ■ Sacral canal and its contents.

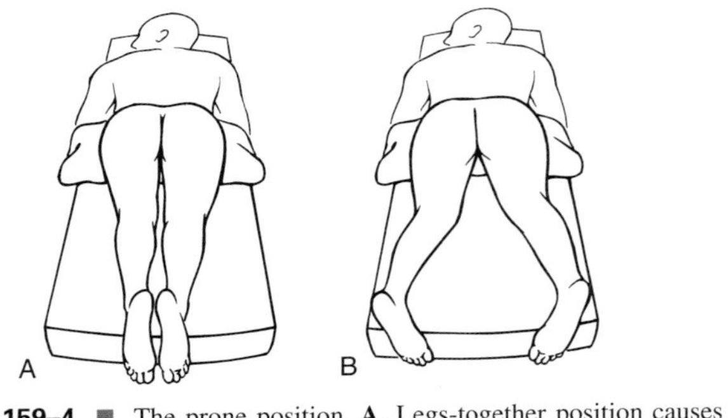

FIGURE 159–4 ■ The prone position. **A,** Legs-together position causes contraction of the gluteus medius muscles. **B,** Legs-apart position with heels rotated externally allows relaxation of the gluteus medius muscles.

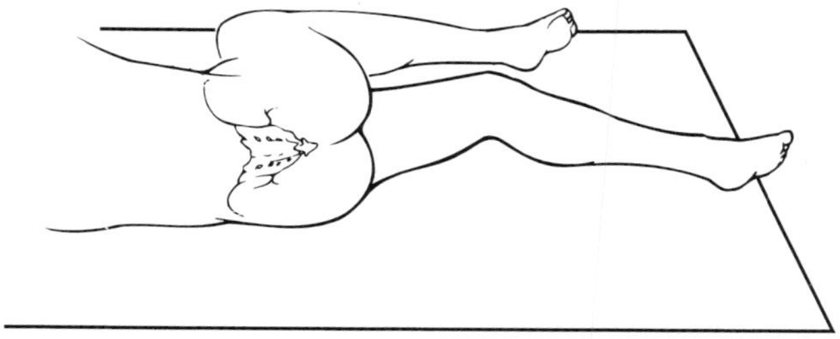

FIGURE 159–5 ■ The lateral position.

Lateral Position

The patient is placed in the lateral position with the left side down for a right-handed pain management physician (Fig. 159–5). The dependent leg is slightly flexed at the hip and knee for the patient's comfort. The upper leg is flexed so that it lies over and above the lower leg and also in contact with the bed. This modified Sims position separates the buttocks, making identification of the sacral hiatus easier. Because the buttocks sag in the lateral position, the gluteal fold is usually inferior to the level of the sacral hiatus and is a misleading landmark for needle placement (see Fig. 159–5).[6]

Choice of Needle

A 1½-inch 22-gauge needle is suitable for most adult patients. A ⅝-inch 25-gauge needle is indicated for pediatric applications. A 1½-inch 25-gauge needle is used when caudal epidural nerve block is performed in the presence of coagulopathy or anticoagulation.[20] The use of longer needles, as advocated by some earlier investigators, increases the incidence of complications, including intravascular injection and inadvertent dural puncture. The use of longer needles contributes nothing to the overall success of this technique.

Location of the Sacral Hiatus

A wide area of skin is prepared with an antiseptic solution such as povidone-iodine so that all landmarks can be palpated aseptically. A fenestrated sterile drape is placed to avoid contamination of the palpating finger. The middle finger of the physician's nondominant hand is placed over the sterile drape into the natal cleft with the fingertip at the tip of the coccyx (Fig. 159–6). This maneuver allows easy confirmation of the sacral midline and is especially important when the patient is in the lateral position.

After careful identification of the midline, the area under the physician's proximal interphalangeal joint is located (Fig. 159–7). The middle finger is moved cephalad from the area that was previously located under the proximal interphalangeal joint (Fig. 159–8). This spot is palpated using a lateral rocking motion to identify the sacral cornua. If the operator's glove size is 7.5 or 8, the sacral hiatus is found at this level. If the operator's glove size is smaller, the sacral hiatus is located just superior to the area below the proximal interphalangeal joint when the fingertip is at the tip of the coccyx. If the operator's glove size is larger, the sacral hiatus is located just inferior to the area below the proximal interphalangeal joint when the fingertip is at the tip of the coccyx (Fig. 159–9).

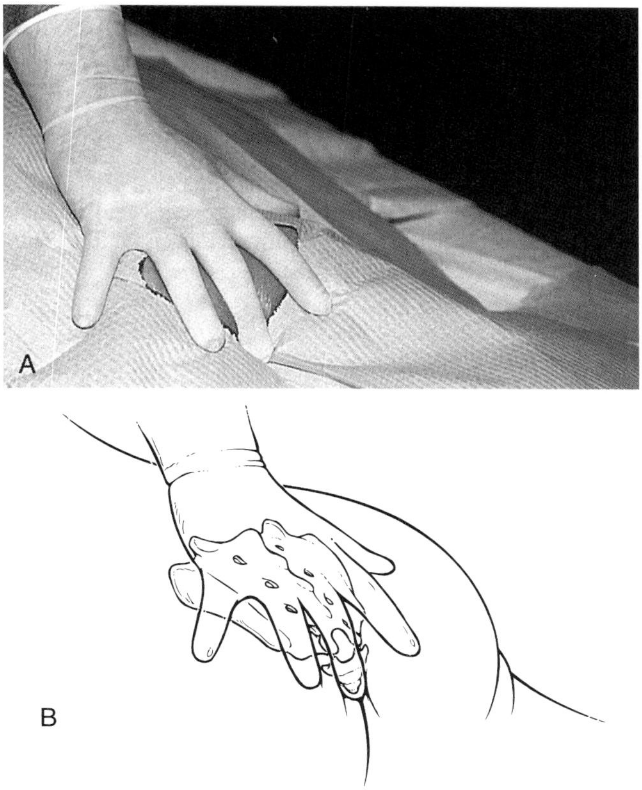

FIGURE 159–6 ■ The operator's finger identifies the tip of the coccyx. **A,** photograph. **B,** line drawing.

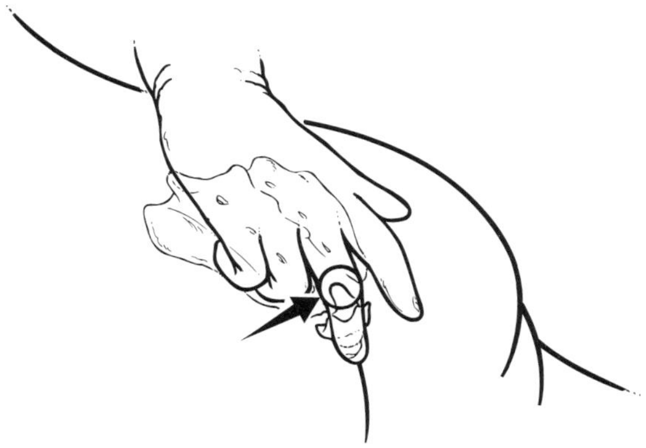

FIGURE 159–7 ■ Identification of the area under the operator's proximal interphalangeal joint *(arrow)*.

Although significant anatomic variation of the sacrum and sacral hiatus is normal, the spatial relationship between the tip of the coccyx and the location of the sacral hiatus remains amazingly constant. When the approximate position of the sacral hiatus is located by palpating the tip of the coccyx, identifying the midline and locating the area under the proximal interphalangeal joint as just described, inability to identify and enter the sacral hiatus should occur in less than 0.5% of cases.

After the sacral hiatus is located, 1 mL of local anesthetic is used to infiltrate the skin, subcutaneous tissues, and sacrococcygeal ligament (Fig. 159–10). Large amounts of anes-

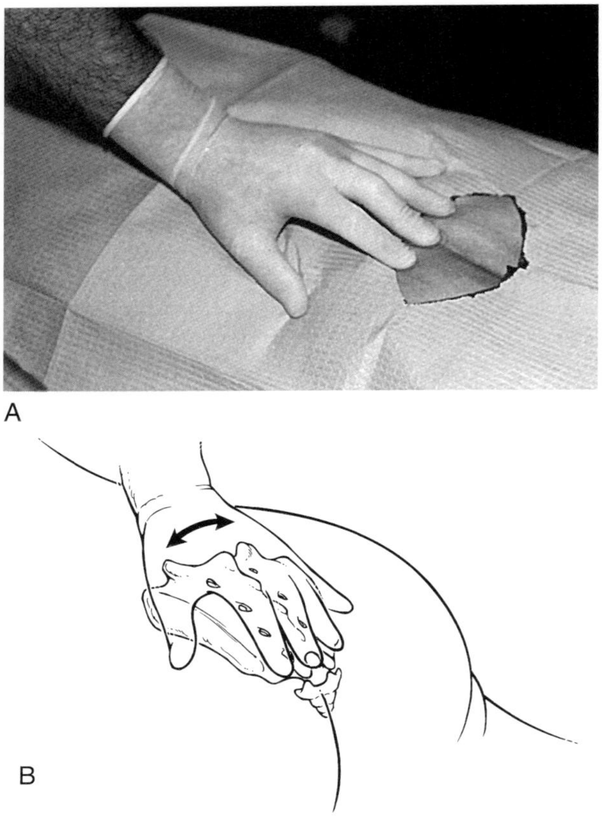

FIGURE 159–8 ■ Palpation of the sacral hiatus. **A,** photograph. **B,** line drawing.

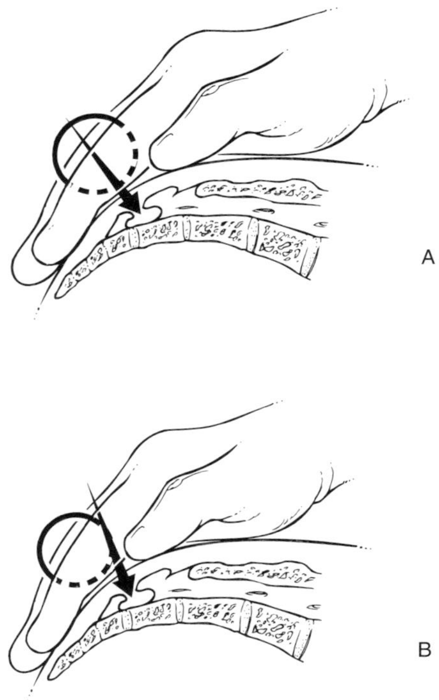

FIGURE 159–9 ■ Location of the sacral hiatus relative to glove size. **A,** Location of the sacral hiatus below the proximal interphalangeal joint for an operator with a size 8 glove. **B,** Location of the sacral hiatus above the proximal interphalangeal joint for an operator with a size 7 glove.

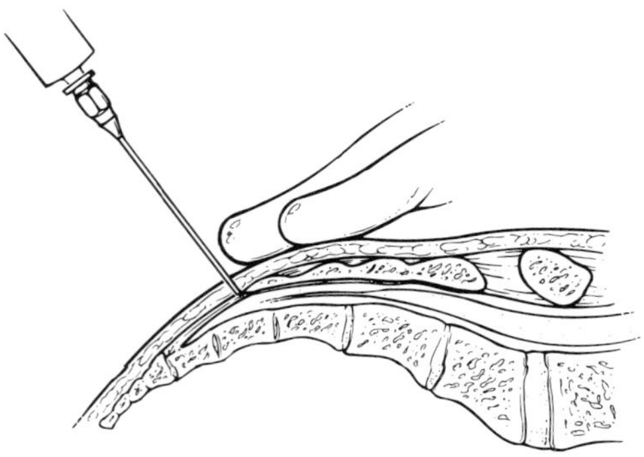

FIGURE 159–10 ■ Infiltration of the skin, subcutaneous tissues, and sacrococcygeal ligament.

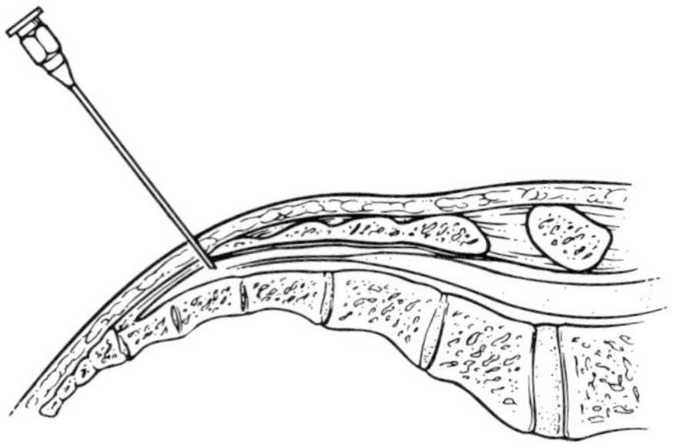

FIGURE 159–11 ■ Needle through the sacrococcygeal ligament at a 45-degree angle.

thetic should be avoided because the bony landmarks necessary for successful completion of this technique may be obscured. Many pain management specialists omit this technique because the pain from infiltration of local anesthetic is often greater than simply placing a 22-gauge or 25-gauge needle directly through the unanesthetized skin and subcutaneous tissues directly into the sacral canal.

The needle is inserted through the anesthetized area at a 45-degree angle into the sacrococcygeal ligament (Fig. 159–11). As the ligament is penetrated, the operator should feel a "pop" or "giving way." If contact with the interior bony wall of the sacral canal occurs, the needle should be withdrawn slightly, to disengage the needle tip from the periosteum. The needle is advanced approximately 0.5 cm into the canal, to ensure that the entire needle bevel is beyond the sacrococcygeal ligament, to avoid injection into the ligament.

At this point, the needle should be held firmly in place by the bone ligament and subcutaneous tissues and should not sag if released by the pain management physician (Fig. 159–12). If there is any question as to whether the needle is correctly placed into the sacral canal, an air-acceptance test may performed by injecting 1 mL of air through the needle. There should be no bulging or crepitus of the tissues overlying the sacrum. The injection of air and the subsequent injection of drugs should feel to the operator like any other injection into the epidural space. The force required for injection should not exceed what was necessary to overcome the resistance of the needle. If there is initial resistance to injection, the needle should be rotated 180 degrees because it might be correctly placed in the canal while the bevel is occluded by the internal wall of the sacral canal (Fig. 159–13). Any significant pain or sudden increase in resistance during injection suggests incorrect needle placement; the physician should stop injecting immediately and reassess the position of the needle. If the physician encounters difficulty in placing the needle properly, fluoroscopic guidance may be used. A lateral fluoroscopic view can help ensure that the needle is within the sacral canal (Fig. 159–14).

Injection of Drugs

When the needle is satisfactorily positioned, a syringe containing the drugs to be injected is attached to the needle. Gentle aspiration is carried out to identify cerebrospinal fluid or blood (Fig. 159–15). Although rare, inadvertent dural puncture can occur, and careful observation for CSF must be carried out. Aspiration of blood occurs more commonly. It can be due to damage to veins during insertion of the needle into the caudal canal or, less often, to intravenous placement of the needle.

If the aspiration test is positive for either CSF or blood, the needle is repositioned, and the aspiration test is repeated. If the repeat test is negative, subsequent injection of 0.5-mL increments of local anesthetic is done. Careful observation for

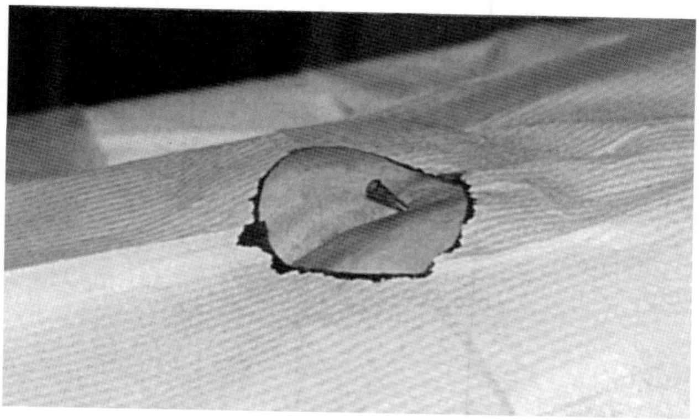

FIGURE 159–12 ■ Needle in place.

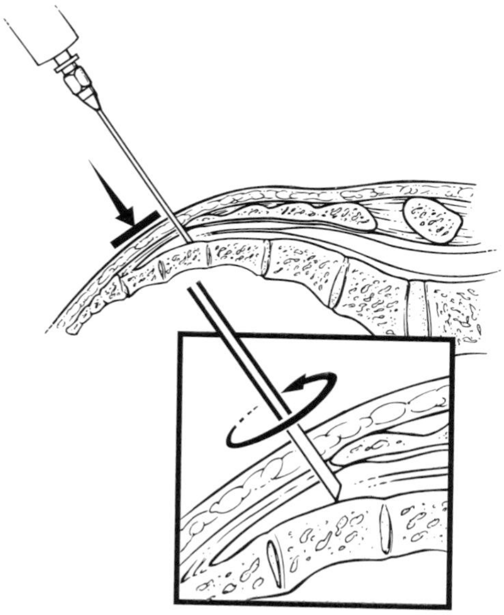

FIGURE 159–13 ■ Rotation of the needle 180 degrees away from the canal wall.

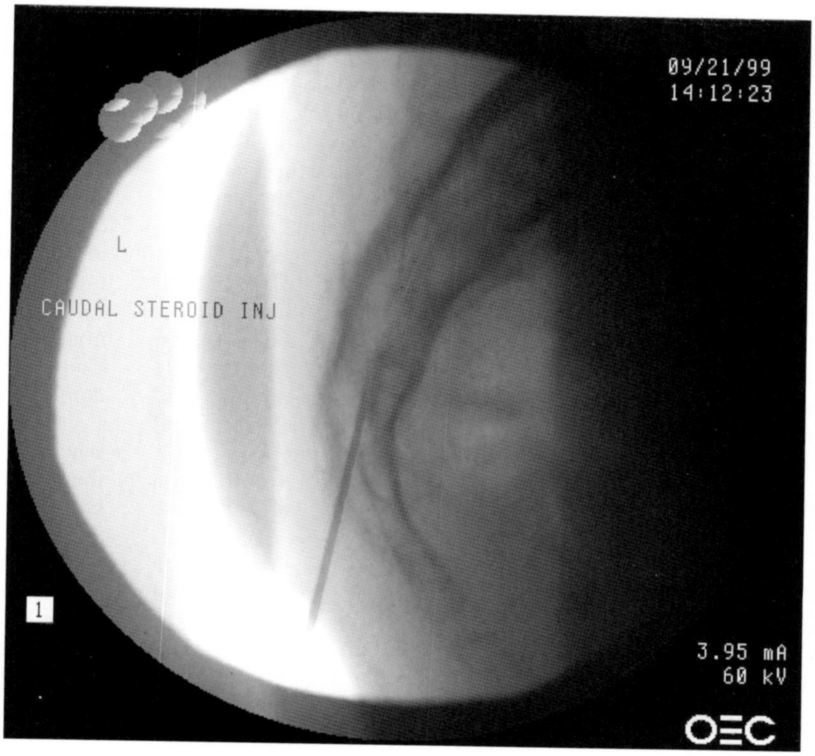

FIGURE 159–14 ■ Lateral fluoroscopic view of needle within sacral canal. (From Waldman SD: Caudal epidural nerve block prone position. In Waldman SD: Atlas of Interventional Pain Management, 2nd ed. Philadelphia, WB Saunders, 2003, p 389.)

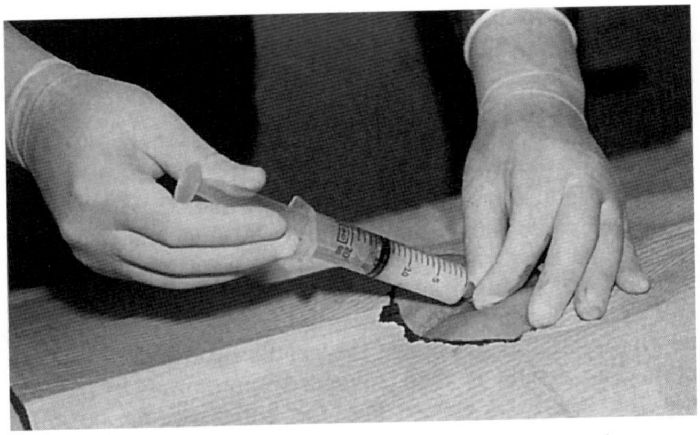

FIGURE 159–15 ■ Gentle aspiration to identify CSF or blood.

signs of local anesthetic toxicity and subarachnoid spread of local anesthetic during the injection and after the procedure is indicated.

Choice of Local Anesthetic

The spread of drugs injected into the sacral canal depends on the volume and speed of injection, the anatomic variations of the bony canal, and the age and height of the patient.[14] Pregnant patients require a significantly smaller volume to achieve the same level of blockade than do nongravid controls.[6] As the injection proceeds, the drugs spread upward in the epidural space. There is a variable amount of leakage through the anterior sacral foramina, which can alter the upward spread of the injected drugs substantially. The onset of action is generally slower than with the lumbar approach to the epidural space.[14]

Local anesthetics capable of producing adequate sensory block of the sacral and lower lumbar nerve roots when administered via the caudal route include 1% lidocaine, 0.25% bupivacaine, 2% chloroprocaine, and 1% mepivacaine.[14] The addition of epinephrine decreases the amount of systemic absorption and lengthens the duration of action slightly. Increasing the concentration of drug increases the depth of motor block and speeds onset of action. A 20-mL volume of the drugs mentioned earlier, given in incremental doses, generally provides adequate sensory blockade of the sacral and lower lumbar dermatomes to allow surgical interventions in most adults.[14] Significant intrapatient variability exists, however, and additional incremental doses of local anesthetic may have to be administered to ensure adequate anesthesia in adults. All local anesthetics administered via the caudal epidural route should be formulated for epidural use.[25]

In pediatric patients, there is a much greater correlation between the dose of local anesthetic and body weight. A dose of 1 mL/kg of 0.25% bupivacaine seems to be safe in children.[14] The established maximum for the total doses of each local anesthetic always must be observed, regardless of patient age, to avoid local anesthetic toxicity. For diagnostic and prognostic blocks, 1% preservative-free lidocaine is a suitable local anesthetic.[9] For therapeutic blocks, 3 to 5 mL of 0.25% preservative-free bupivacaine or 0.5% preservative-free lidocaine in combination with 80 mg of depot methylprednisolone (Depo-Medrol), is injected.[10] Subsequent nerve blocks are done in a similar manner, but using only 40 mg of methylprednisolone. Daily caudal epidural nerve blocks with local anesthetic or steroid may be required to treat acute painful conditions.[10] Chronic conditions, such as lumbar radiculopathy and diabetic polyneuropathy, are treated daily to once a week, as the situation dictates.[9] Increasing clinical experience has indicated that higher volumes of local anesthetics increase side effects and complications, but add little, if anything, to the overall efficacy of caudal steroid epidural blocks if there is not a significant sympathetic component to the pain. For selective neurolytic block of an individual sacral nerve, incremental 0.1-mL injections of 6.5% phenol in glycerin or alcohol to a total volume of 1 mL may be used after the level of pain relief and potential side effects have been confirmed with local anesthetic blocks.[13]

If the caudal epidural route is chosen for administration of opioids, 4 to 5 mg of morphine sulfate formulated for epidural use is a reasonable initial dose.[20] More lipid-soluble opioids, such as fentanyl, must be delivered by continuous infusion via a caudal catheter.

Pitfalls in Needle Placement

It is possible to insert the needle incorrectly during performance of caudal epidural nerve block. The needle may be placed outside the sacral canal, resulting in the injection of air or drugs into the subcutaneous tissues (Fig. 159–16A). Palpation of crepitus and bulging of tissues overlying the sacrum during injection indicate needle malposition.[8] Greater resistance to injection accompanied by pain also is noted.

A second possible needle misplacement is into the periosteum of the sacral canal (Fig. 159–16B). This needle misplacement is suggested by considerable pain on injection, very high resistance to injection, and the inability to inject more than a few milliliters of drug.[22] A third possibility for needle malposition is partial placement of the needle bevel in the sacrococcygeal ligament (Fig. 159–16C). There is significant resistance to injection and significant pain as the drugs are injected into the ligament.

A fourth possible needle malposition is to force the point of the needle into the marrow cavity of the sacral vertebra, which results in very high blood levels of local anesthetic (Fig. 159–16D).[6] It can occur in elderly patients with significant osteoporosis. Such needle malposition is detected as initial easy acceptance of a few milliliters of local anesthetic followed by a rapid increase in resistance to injection, as the noncompliant bony cavity fills with local anesthetic. Significant local anesthetic toxicity can occur as a result of this complication.

The fifth and most serious needle malposition occurs when the needle is inserted through the sacrum or lateral to the coccyx into the pelvic cavity beyond (Fig. 159–16E),[23] where it could enter the rectum or the birth canal, resulting in contamination of the needle. Repositioning of a contaminated needle into the sacral canal carries with it the danger of infection. Although in competent hands this complication is exceedingly rare, some investigators believe that caudal analgesia for obstetric applications is inadvisable when the infant's head has entered the pelvis because inadvertent injection of local anesthetic into the head would cause fetal demise.

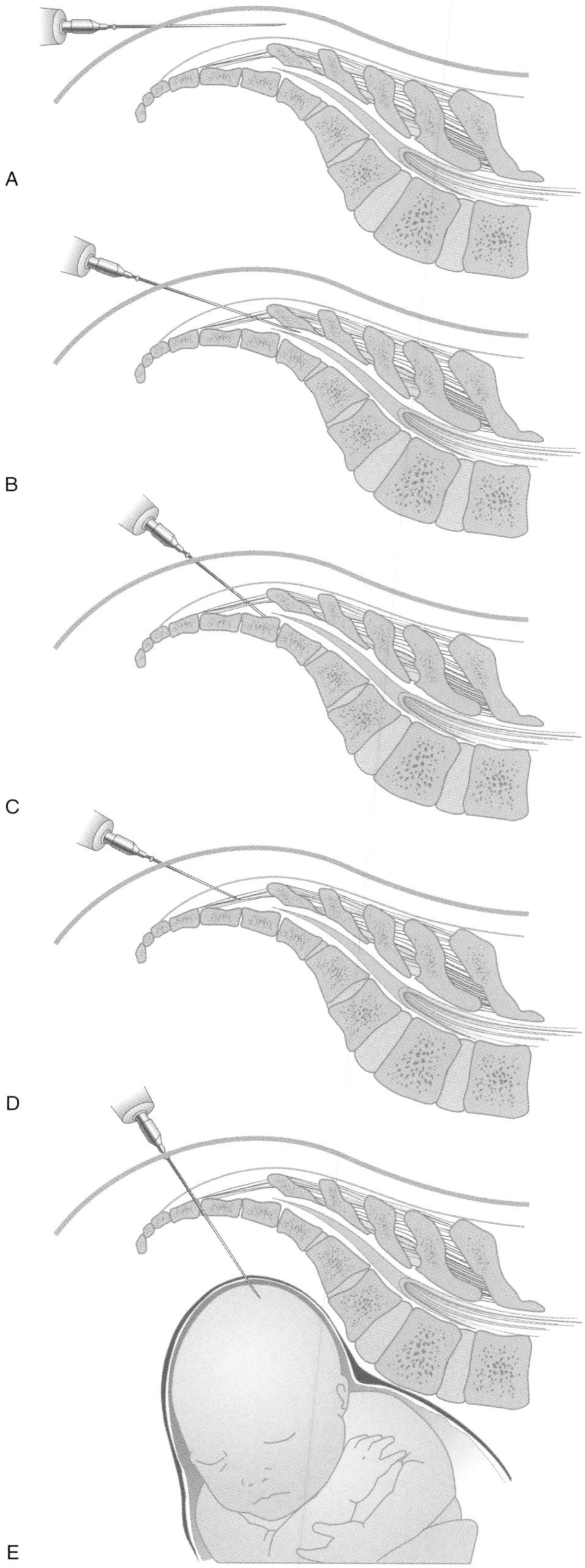

FIGURE 159–16 ■ Possible misplacements of needle. **A,** Outside sacral canal. **B,** Subperiosteal. **C,** In sacrococcygeal ligament. **D,** Into marrow cavity. **E,** Through sacrum into fetal cranium.

Caudal Epidural Catheters

An epidural catheter may be placed into the caudal canal through a Crawford needle, in a manner analogous to that for continuous lumbar epidural anesthesia.[6] The catheter is advanced approximately 2 to 3 cm beyond the needle tip.[26] The needle is carefully withdrawn over the catheter. To avoid shearing of the catheter, under no circumstances is the catheter withdrawn back through the needle. After the injection hub is attached to the catheter, an aspiration test is done to identify the presence of blood or CSF. A test dose of 3 to 4 mL of local anesthetic is given via the catheter. The patient is observed for signs of local anesthetic toxicity or inadvertent subarachnoid injection. If no side effects are noted, a continuous infusion or intermittent boluses of local anesthetics or opioids may be administered through the catheter. Because of proximity to the anus, the risk of infection limits the long-term use of caudal epidural catheters.[14]

SIDE EFFECTS AND COMPLICATIONS OF THE CAUDAL APPROACH TO THE EPIDURAL SPACE

Local Anesthetic Toxicity

The caudal epidural space is highly vascular; the possibility of intravascular uptake of local anesthetic is significant with this technique.[14] Careful aspiration and incremental dosing with local anesthetic are important to allow early detection of toxicity. Careful observation of the patient during and after the procedure is mandatory.[9]

Hematoma and Ecchymosis

The epidural venous plexus generally ends at S4, but it may extend the entire length of the canal in some patients. Needle trauma to this plexus can result in bleeding and cause post-procedure pain. Subperiosteal injection of drugs, which also may result in bleeding, is associated with significant pain during and after injection. The chances of these two complications and the incidence of injection site eccyhmosis can be reduced by using short, small-diameter needles. Significant neurologic deficit secondary to epidural hematoma after caudal block is exceedingly rare.[14]

Infection

Although uncommon, infection remains an ever-present possibility, especially in immunocompromised cancer patients.[23] Studies comparing cultures of the skin puncture sites of patients in whom lumbar and caudal epidural catheters were placed simultaneously for obstetric anesthesia have shown consistently that the caudal sites produced a significantly larger number of positive results.[27] Early detection of infection is crucial to avoiding potentially life-threatening sequelae.

Neurologic Complications

Neurologic complications after caudal nerve block are exceedingly rare. Usually, they are associated with a preexisting neurologic lesion or with surgical or obstetric trauma, rather than with the caudal block itself.[14]

Urinary Retention and Incontinence

The application of local anesthetics and opioids to the sacral nerve roots results in a higher incidence of urinary retention.[14] This side effect of caudal epidural nerve block is seen more commonly in elderly men and multiparous women and after inguinal and perineal surgery. Overflow incontinence may occur in such patients if they are unable to void or if bladder catheterization is not used. It is advisable that all patients undergoing caudal epidural nerve block show the ability to void before discharge from the pain center.

SUMMARY

Caudal epidural nerve block is a simple, safe, and effective technique for a variety of surgical anesthetic applications. It is especially useful for outpatient surgery and in pediatric patients. The ability to perform caudal epidural nerve block in the presence of anticoagulation or coagulopathy is unique among the major neuraxial regional anesthesia techniques. The utility of caudal epidural analgesia in the management of a variety of acute, chronic, and cancer-related pain syndromes makes the technique an excellent addition to the armamentarium of pain management specialists.

References

1. Cathelin MF: Une nouvelle voie d'injection rachidienne: Méthode des injections épidurales par le procedé du canal sacre. C R Soc Biol Paris 53:452, 1901.
2. Pagés E: Anestesia metamerica. Rev Sanid Mil Madr 11:351, 1921.
3. Dogliotti AM: Segmental peridural anesthesia. Am J Surg 20:107, 1933.
4. Gutierrez A: Valor de la aspiracion liquada en al espacio peridural en la anestesia peridural. Rev Circ 12:225, 1933.
5. Hingson RA, Edwards WB: An analysis of the first ten thousand confinements managed with continuous caudal analgesia with a report of the authors' first one thousand cases. JAMA 125:538, 1943.
6. Bromage PR: Caudal anesthesia. In Bromage PR: Epidural Analgesia. Philadelphia, WB Saunders, 1978, p 489.
7. Bromage PR: Introduction. In Bromage PR: Epidural Analgesia. Philadelphia, WB Saunders, 1978, p 2.
8. Moore DC: Single-dose caudal anesthesia. In Moore DC (ed): Regional Block, 4th ed. Springfield, IL, Charles C Thomas, 1965, p 439.
9. Waldman SD: The current status of caudal epidural nerve block in contemporary practice. Pain Dig 7:187, 1997.
10. Waldman SD: Management of acute pain. Postgrad Med 87:15, 1992.
11. Portenoy RK, Waldman SD: Alleviating cancer pain: A guide for urologists. Contemp Urol 6:40, 1994.
12. Waldman SD: Acute and postoperative pain management. In Weiner RS (ed): Innovations in Pain Management. Orlando, FL, PMD Press, 1993, p 12.
13. Gee WF, Ansell JS: Pelvic and perineal pain of urological origin. In Bonica JJ (ed): The Management of Pain. Philadelphia, Lea & Febiger, 1990, p 1392.
14. Willis RJ: Caudal epidural blockade. In Cousins MJ, Bridenbaugh DO (eds): Neural Blockade. Philadelphia, JB Lippincott, 1988, p 376.
15. Waldman SD, Greek CR, Greenfield, MA: The caudal administration of steroids in combination with local anesthetics in the palliation of pain secondary to radiographically documented lumbar herniated disc—a prospective outcome study with six-month follow-up. Pain Clin 11:43, 1998.
16. Waldman SD: Reflex sympathetic dystrophy. Intern Med 11:62, 1990.
17. Waldman SD: Acute herpes zoster and postherpetic neuralgia. Intern Med 11:33, 1990.
18. Wilson WL, Waldman SD: Role of the epidural administration of steroids and local anesthetics in the palliation of pain secondary to vertebral compression fractures. Pain Dig 1:294-295, 1992.
19. Katz J: Caudal approach-single injection technique. In Katz J: Atlas of Regional Anesthesia. Norwalk, CT, Appleton & Lange, 1994, p 129.
20. Waldman SD, Feldstein GS, Waldman HJ: Caudal administration of morphine sulfate in anticoagulated and thrombocytopenic patients. Anesth Analg 66:267, 1987.
21. Portenoy RK, Waldman SD: Managing cancer pain. Contemp Oncol 13:33, 1993.
22. Brown DL: Caudal block. In Brown DL (ed): Atlas of Regional Anesthesia. Philadelphia, WB Saunders, 1999, p 347.
23. Martin LV: Sacral epidural (caudal) block. In Wildsmith JAW, Armitage EN (eds): Principles and Practice of Regional Anesthesia. New York, Churchill Livingstone, 1987, p 102.
24. Lofstrom B: Caudal anesthesia. In Eriksson E (ed): Illustrated Handbook of Local Anesthesia. Copenhagen, Sorensen & Co, 1969, p 129.
25. Waldman SD: Issues in selection of local anesthetics. Hosp Form 26:590, 1991.
26. Katz J: Caudal approach-continuous technique. In Katz J: Atlas of Regional Anesthesia. Norwalk, CT, Appleton & Lange, 1994, p 132.
27. Abouleish E, Orig T, Amortegui AJ: Bacteriologic comparison between epidural and caudal techniques. Anesthesiology 53:511, 1980.

chapter 160

Lysis of Epidural Adhesions: The Racz Technique

Miles Day and Gabor Racz

Chances are, each of us will experience low back pain at some point in our lives. The usual course is rapid improvement, but 5% to 10% of patients develop persistent symptoms.[1] In 1997, the total impact of low back pain on industry in the United States was estimated at $171 billion.[2] The medical treatment of low back pain in 1990 amounted to 13 billion dollars.[3] Treatment varies from conservative therapy with medication and physical therapy to minimally and highly invasive pain management interventions. Surgery is sometimes required in those patients who have progressive neurologic deficits or those who have failed other therapies. Surgery is successful in the majority of patients, but an unlucky few continue to have pain and neurologic symptoms. A quandary arises as to whether a repeat surgery should be attempted or an alternative intervention should be sought. *This is the exact quandary that the epidural adhesiolysis procedure was designed to address.* It was developed to break down scar formation, deliver site-specific corticosteroids and local anesthetic drugs directly to the target, and reduce edema with hypertonic saline. Epidural adhesiolysis has afforded patients reduction in pain and neurologic symptoms without the expense and sometimes long recovery period associated with repeat surgery and often prevents the need for surgical intervention.

RADIOLOGICAL DIAGNOSIS OF EPIDURAL FIBROSIS

Magnetic resonance imaging and computerized tomography (CT) scanning are diagnostic tools; sensitivity and specificity are 50% to 70%, respectively.[4] CT myelography may also be helpful, although none of the aforementioned modalities can identify epidural fibrosis with 100% reliability. In contrast, epidurography is a technique used with considerable success and it is believed that epidural fibrosis is best diagnosed by performing an epidurogram.[5-8] It can detect filling defects in good correlation with a patient's symptoms in real time.[8] A combination of several of these techniques will undoubtedly increase the ability to identify epidural fibrosis.

INDICATIONS FOR EPIDURAL ADHESIOLYSIS

Although originally designed to treat radiculopathy secondary to epidural fibrosis following surgery, the use of epidural adhesiolysis has been expanded to treat a multitude of pain etiologies. These include the following:[9]

1. Post-laminectomy syndrome of the neck and back after surgery
2. Disk disruption
3. Metastatic carcinoma of the spine leading to compression fractures
4. Multilevel degenerative arthritis
5. Facet pain
6. Spinal stenosis
7. Pain unresponsive to spinal cord stimulation and spinal opioids

CONTRAINDICATIONS

The following are absolute contraindications for performing epidural adhesiolysis:

1. Sepsis
2. Chronic infection
3. Coagulopathy
4. Local infection at the site of the procedure
5. Patient refusal

A relative contraindication is the presence of arachnoiditis. With arachnoiditis, the tissue planes may be adherent to one another increasing the chance of loculation of contrast or medication. It may also increase the chance of spread of the medications to the subdural or subarachnoid space, which can increase the chance of complications. Practitioners with limited experience with epidural adhesiolysis should consider referring these patients to a clinician with more experience.

PATIENT PREPARATION

When epidural adhesiolysis has been deemed an appropriate treatment modality, the risks and benefits of the procedure should be discussed with the patient and an informed consent signed. The benefits are pain relief, improved physical function, and possible reversal of neurologic symptoms. Risks include bruising, bleeding, infection, reaction to medications used (hyaluronidase, local anesthetic, corticosteroids, hypertonic saline), damage to nerves or blood vessels, no or little pain relief, bowel/bladder incontinence, worsening of pain, and paralysis. Patients with a history of urinary incontinence should have an evaluation by a urologist prior to performing the procedure to document the preexisting urodynamic etiology and pathology.

ANTICOAGULANT MEDICATION

Medications that prolong bleeding parameters should be withheld prior to performing epidural adhesiolysis. The length of time varies depending on the medication taken. A consultation with the patient's primary physician should be obtained before stopping any of these medications. Nonsteroidal anti-inflammatory drugs (NSAIDs) and aspirin, respectively, should be withheld 4 days and 7 to 10 days before the procedure. Although there is much debate regarding these medications and neuraxial procedures, we tend to be on the conservative side. Clopidogrel (Plavix) should be stopped 7 days before, whereas ticlopidine (Ticlid) is withheld 10 to 14 days before the adhesiolysis.[10] Warfarin (Coumadin) stoppage is variable, but 5 days is usually adequate.[10] Patients on subcutaneous heparin should have it withheld at a minimum of 12 hours before the procedure, whereas those on low-molecular-weight heparin require a minimum of 24 hours.[10] Over-the-counter homeopathic medications that prolong bleeding parameters should also be withheld. These include vitamin E, gingko biloba, garlic, ginseng, and St. John's wort.[11,12] Adequate coagulation status can be confirmed by the prothrombin time, partial thromboplastin time, and a platelet function assay or bleeding time. The tests should be performed as close to the day of the procedure as possible. Tests performed only a few days after stopping the anticoagulant medication may come back elevated because not enough time has elapsed to allow the anticoagulant effects of the medication to resolve. The benefits of the procedure must be weighed against the potential sequelae of stopping the anticoagulant medication and this should be discussed thoroughly with the patient.

PREOPERATIVE LABORATORY

Before the procedure a complete blood count and a clean-catch urinalysis are obtained to check for any undiagnosed infection. An elevated white count and/or a positive urinalysis should prompt the physician to postpone the procedure and refer the patient to the primary care physician for further work-up and treatment. In addition, a prothrombin time, a partial thromboplastin time, and a platelet function assay or a bleeding time are obtained to check for coagulation abnormalities. Any elevated value warrants further investigation and postponement of the procedure until those studies are complete.

TECHNIQUE

This procedure can be performed in the cervical, thoracic, lumbar, and caudal regions of the spine. The caudal and transforaminal placement of catheters will be described in detail, whereas highlights and slight changes in protocol will be provided for cervical and thoracic catheters. Our policy is to perform this procedure under strict sterile conditions in the operating room. Prophylactic antibiotics with broad neuraxial coverage are given preprocedure. Patients will receive either ceftriaxone 1 g intravenously, or Levaquin 500 mg orally in those allergic to penicillin. The same dose is also given on day 2. An anesthesiologist or nurse anesthetist provides monitored anesthesia care.

Caudal Approach

The patient is placed in the prone position with a pillow placed under the abdomen to correct the lumbar lordosis and a pillow under the ankles for patient comfort. The patient is asked to put his/her toes together and heels apart. This relaxes the gluteal muscles and facilitates identification of the sacral hiatus. After sterile preparation and draping, the sacral hiatus is identified via palpation just caudal to the sacral cornu or with fluoroscopic guidance. A skin wheal is raised with local anesthetic 1 inch lateral and 2 inches caudal to the sacral hiatus on the side opposite the documented radiculopathy. The skin is nicked with an 18-gauge cutting needle, and a 15- or 16-gauge RX Coudé (Epimed International) epidural needle is inserted through the nick at a 45-degree angle and guided fluoroscopically or by palpation toward the sacral hiatus. When the needle is through the hiatus, the angle of the needle is dropped to approximately 30 degrees and advanced. The advantages of the RX Coudé over other needles are the angled tip, which enables easier direction of the catheter, and the tip of the needle is less sharp. The back edge of the distal opening of the needle is designed to be a noncutting surface that allows manipulation of the catheter in and out of the needle. A Touhy needle should never be used for this procedure because the back edge of the distal opening is a cutting surface and can easily shear a catheter. A properly placed needle will be inside the caudal canal below the level of the S_3 foramen on anteroposterior (AP) and lateral fluoroscopic images. A needle placed above the level of the S_3 foramen could potentially punctured a low-lying dura. The needle tip should cross the midline of the sacrum toward the side of the radiculopathy.

An epidurogram is performed using 10 mL of a nonionic, water-soluble contrast agent. Confirm a negative aspiration for blood or cerebrospinal fluid (CSF) before any injection of contrast or medication. Omnipaque and Isovue are the two agents most frequently used and are suitable for myelography.[13,14] Do not use ionic, water-insoluble contrast agents such as Hypaque or Renografin or ionic, water-soluble agents such as Conray.[15,16] These agents are not indicated for myelography. Accidental subarachnoid injections can lead to serious untoward events such as seizure and possible death. Slowly inject the contrast agent and observe for filling defects (Fig. 160–1). A normal epidurogram will have a "Christmas tree" pattern with the central canal being the trunk and the outline of the nerve roots making up the branches. An abnormal epidurogram will have areas where the contrast does not fill. These are the areas of presumed scarring and typically correspond to the patient's radicular complaints. If vascular uptake is observed, the needle needs to be redirected.

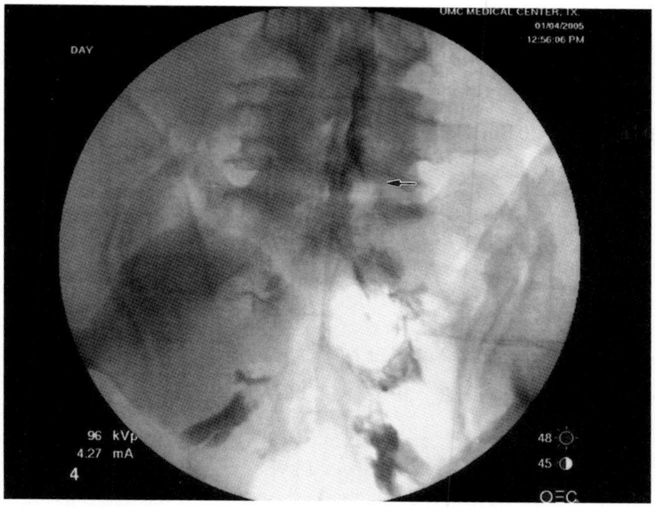

FIGURE 160–1 ■ Initial epidurogram. There are several filling defects, but note the partial filling defect at the right L_5 nerve root (*arrow*).

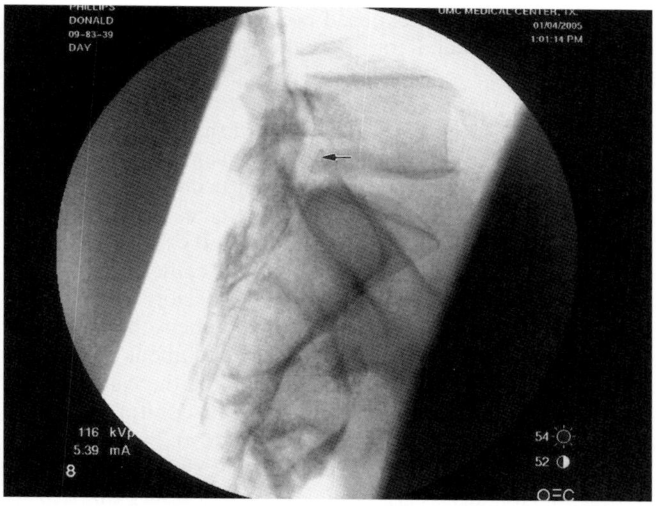

FIGURE 160–2 ■ Lateral view of the epidural catheter in the ventral-lateral aspect of the right L_5 foramen (*arrow*).

After turning the distal opening of the needle ventral-lateral, insert a TunL Kath or TunL-XL (stiffer) catheter (Epimed International) with a bend on the distal tip through the needle. The bend should be 2.5 cm from the tip of the catheter and at a 30-degree angle. The bend will enable the catheter to be steered to the target level. Under continuous AP fluoroscopic guidance, advance the tip of the catheter toward the ventral-lateral epidural space of the desired level. The catheter can be steered by gently twisting the catheter in a clockwise or counterclockwise direction. Avoid "propellering" the tip (i.e., twisting the tip in circles) because this makes it more difficult to direct the catheter. Do not advance the catheter up the middle of the sacrum because this makes guiding the catheter to the ventral-lateral epidural space more difficult. Ideal location of the tip of the catheter in the AP projection is in the foramen just below the midportion of the pedicle shadow (Fig. 160–2). Check a lateral projection to confirm that the catheter tip is in the ventral epidural space (Fig. 160–3).

Under real-time fluoroscopy, inject 2 to 3 mL of additional contrast through the catheter in an attempt to outline the "scarred in" nerve root. If vascular uptake is noted, reposition the catheter and reinject contrast. Preferably there should not be vascular runoff, but infrequently—secondary to venous congestion—an epidural pattern is seen with a small amount of vascular spread. This is acceptable as long as the vascular uptake is venous in nature and not arterial. Extra caution should be taken when injecting the local anesthetic to prevent local anesthetic toxicity. Any arterial spread of contrast always warrants repositioning of the catheter. We have never observed intra-arterial catheter placement in 25 years of placing soft, spring-tipped catheters.

Inject 1500 U of hyaluronidase dissolved in 10 mL of preservative-free normal saline. This may cause some discomfort, so a slow injection is preferable. Observe for "opening up,"(i.e., visualization) of the "scarred in" nerve root. A 3-mL test-dose of a 10-mL local anesthetic/steroid (LA/S) solution is then given. Our institution uses 4 mg of dexamethasone mixed with 9 mL of 0.2% ropivacaine.

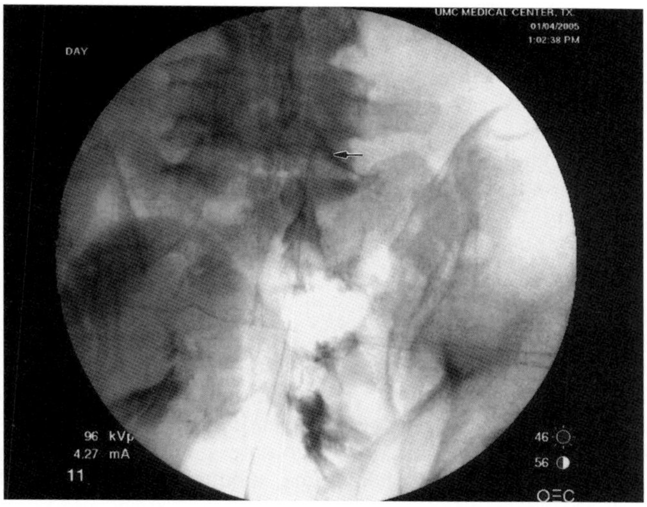

FIGURE 160–3 ■ Repeat epidurogram after placement of the epidural catheter in the ventral-lateral aspect of the right L5 foramen and injection of 1500 U hyaluronidase. Note filling of contrast around the L_5 nerve root (*arrow*) that was not seen on the initial epidurogram.

Ropivacaine is used instead of bupivacaine for two reasons: the former produces a preferential sensory versus a motor block, and it is less cardiotoxic than racemic bupivacaine. Doses for other corticosteroids commonly used are 40 to 80 mg methylprednisolone (Depo-Medrol), 25 to 50 mg triamcinolone diacetate (Aristocort), 40 to 80 mg triamcinolone acetonide (Kenalog), and 6 to 12 mg betamethasone (Celestone Solu span).[17] If, after 5 minutes, there is no evidence of intrathecal or intravascular injection of medication, inject the remaining 7 mL of the LA/S solution.

Remove the needle under continuous fluoroscopic guidance to ensure the catheter remains at the target level. Secure the catheter to the skin using nonabsorbable suture and coat the skin puncture site with antimicrobial ointment. Apply a sterile dressing and attach a 20-µ filter to the end of the catheter. Affix the exposed portion of the catheter to the patient with tape and transport the patient to the recovery area.

A 20-minute period should elapse between the last injection of the LA/S solution and the start of the hypertonic (10%) saline infusion. This is necessary to ensure that a subdural injection of the LA/S solution has not occurred. A subdural block mimics a subarachnoid block but takes longer to establish. If the patient develops a subarachnoid or subdural block at any point during the procedure, the catheter should be removed and the remainder of the adhesiolysis canceled. The patient needs to be observed to document the resolution of the motor and sensory block and to document that 10 mL of hypertonic saline is then infused through the catheter over 30 minutes. If the patient complains of discomfort, the infusion is stopped and an additional 2 mL of 0.2% ropivacaine is injected and the infusion is restarted. Alternatively, 50 to 100 μg of fentanyl can be injected epidurally in lieu of the local anesthetic. After completion of the hypertonic saline infusion, the catheter is slowly flushed with 2 mL of preservative-free normal saline and the catheter is capped.

Our policy is to admit the patient for a 23-hour observation status and do a second and a third hypertonic saline infusion the following day. On post-catheter insertion day 2, the catheter is twice injected (separated by 4 hours) with 10 mL of 0.2% ropivacaine without steroid and infused with 10 mL hypertonic saline (10%) using the same technique and precautions as the day 1 infusion. At the end of the third infusion, the catheter is removed and a sterile dressing applied. The patient is discharged home with 5 days of oral cephalexin at 500 mg twice a day or oral Levaquin at 500 mg once a day for penicillin-allergic patients. Clinic follow-up is in 30 days.

COMPLICATIONS

As with any invasive procedure, complications are possible. These include bleeding, infection, headache, damage to nerves or blood vessels, catheter shearing, bowel/bladder dysfunction, paralysis, spinal cord compression from loculation of the injected fluids or hematoma, subdural or subarachnoid injection of local anesthetic or hypertonic saline, and reactions to the medications used. We also include on the permit that the patient may experience an increase in pain or no pain relief at all.

OUTCOMES

Racz and Holubec first reported on epidural adhesiolysis in 1989.[18] There were slight variations in the protocol compared to today's protocol, namely the dose of local anesthetic and the fact that hyaluronidase was not used. Catheter placement was lesion-specific (i.e., the tip of the catheter was placed in the foramen corresponding to the vertebral level and side of the suspected adhesions). This retrospective analysis conducted 6 to 12 months post-procedure reported initial pain relief in 72.2% of patients ($N = 72$) at time of discharge. Relief was sustained in 37.5% and 30.5% of patients at 1 and 3 months, respectively. Forty-three percent decreased their frequency and dosage of medication use and 16.7% discontinued their medications altogether. In total, 30.6% of patients returned to work or returned to daily functions.

At a presentation at the 7th World Congress on pain, Arthur and colleagues reported on epidural adhesiolysis in 100 patients, of whom 50 received hyaluronidase as part of the procedure.[19] In the hyaluronidase group, 81.6% of the participants had initial pain relief with 12.3% having persistent relief; 68% of the no hyaluronidase group had relief of pain, with 14% having persistent relief.

In 1994, Stolker and colleagues added hyaluronidase to the procedure, but omitted the hypertonic saline. In a study of 28 patients, they reported greater than 50% pain reduction in 64% of patients at 1 year.[20] They stressed the importance of patient selection and felt that the effectiveness of adhesiolysis was based on the effect of the hyaluronidase on the adhesions and the action of the local anesthetic and steroids on the sinuvertebral nerve.

Devulder and colleagues published a study of 34 patients with failed back surgery syndrome in whom epidural fibrosis was suspected or proved with MRI.[21] An epidural catheter was inserted via the sacral hiatus to a distance of 10 cm into the caudal canal. Injections of contrast dye, local anesthetic, corticosteroid, and hypertonic saline (10%) were carried out daily for 3 days. No hyaluronidase was used. Filling defects were noted in 30 of 34 patients, but significant pain relief was noted in only 7 patients at 1 month; 2 patients at 3 months; and no patients at 12 months. They concluded that epidurography may confirm epidural filling defects for contrast dye in patients with filling defects, but a better contrast dye spread, assuming scar lysis, does not guarantee sustained pain relief. This study was criticized for lack of lesion-specific catheter placement resulting in nonspecific drug delivery.[22]

Heavner and colleagues performed a prospective randomized trial of lesion -specific epidural adhesiolysis on 59 patients with chronic intractable low back pain.[23] The patients were assigned to one of four epidural adhesiolysis treatment groups: (1) hypertonic (10%) saline plus hyaluronidase, (2) hypertonic saline, (3) isotonic (0.9%) saline, or (4) isotonic saline plus hyaluronidase. All treatment groups received corticosteroid and local anesthetic. Overall, across all four treatment groups, 83% of patients had significant pain relief at 1 month compared to 49% at 3 months, 43% at 6 months, and 49% at 12 months.

Manchikanti and coworkers performed a retrospective randomized evaluation of a modified Racz adhesiolysis protocol in 232 patients with low back pain.[24] The study involved lesion-specific catheter placement, but the usual 3-day procedure was reduced to a 2-day (group I) or 1-day (group II) procedure. Group I had 103 patients and group II had 129 patients. Other changes included changing the local anesthetic from bupivacaine to lidocaine, substituting methylprednisolone acetate or betamethasone acetate and phosphate for triamcinolone diacetate, and reduction of the volume of injectate. Of the patients in groups I and II, 62% and 58 % had >50% pain relief at 1 month, respectively—with these percentages decreasing to 22% and 11% at 3 months; 8% and 7% at 6 months; and 2% and 3% at 1 year. Of significant interest is that the percentage of patients receiving >50% pain relief after four procedures increased to 79% and 90% at 1 month; 50% and 36% at 3 months; 29% and 19% at 6 months; and 7% and 8% at 1 year for groups I and II, respectively. Short-term relief of pain was demonstrated, but long-term relief was not.

In a randomized, prospective study, Manchikanti and colleagues evaluated a 1-day epidural adhesiolysis procedure against a control group of patients who received conservative therapy.[25] Results showed that cumulative relief, defined as relief greater than 50% with one to three injections, in the treatment group was 97% at 3 months; 93% at 6 months; and 47% at 1 year. The study also showed that overall health status improved significantly in the adhesiolysis group.

Recently, Manchikanti and colleagues published their results of a randomized, double-blind, controlled study on the effectiveness of 1-day lumbar adhesiolysis and hypertonic saline neurolysis in treatment of chronic low back pain.[26] Seventy-five patients whose pain was unresponsive to conservative modalities were randomized into one of three treatment groups. Group I (control group) underwent catheterization without adhesiolysis, followed by injection of local anesthetic, normal saline, and steroid. Group II consisted of catheterization and adhesiolysis, followed by injection of local anesthetic, normal saline, and steroid. Group III consisted of adhesiolysis, followed by injection of local anesthetic, hypertonic saline, and steroid. Patients were allowed to have additional injections based on the response, either after unblinding or without unblinding after 3 months. Patients without unblinding were offered either the assigned treatment or another treatment based on their response. If the patients in groups I or II received adhesiolysis and injection of hypertonic saline, they were considered withdrawn, and no subsequent data was collected. Outcomes were assessed at 3, 6, and 12 months using visual analog scale pain scores, Oswestry Disability Index, opioid intake, range-of-motion measurement, and P-3. Significant pain relief was defined as average relief of 50% or greater. Seventy-two percent of patients in group III; 60% of patients in group II; and 0% in group I showed significant pain relief at 12-months. The average number of treatments for 1 year were 2.76 in group II and 2.16 in group III. Duration of significant relief with the first procedure was 2.8 ± 1.49 months and 3.8 ± 3.37 months in groups II and III, respectively. Significant pain relief (≥50%) was also associated with improvement in Oswestry Disability Index, range of motion, and psychological status.

CONCLUSION

Epidural adhesiolysis has evolved over the years as an important treatment option for patients with intractable cervical, thoracic, and low back and leg pain. Studies show that patients are able to enjoy significant pain relief and restoration of function over several months. Manchikanti's studies show that the amount and duration of relief can be achieved by repeat procedures. Endoscopy offers direct visualization of the affected nerve roots in addition to mechanical adhesiolysis, and may become more mainstream as the technique is refined. More prospective, randomized, controlled studies need to be performed to further solidify the role of epidural adhesiolysis in the treatment algorithm of patients with intractable pain that is refractory to previous treatments.

References

1. Lawrence R, Helmick C, Arnett F, et al: Estimates of the prevalence of arthritis and selected musculoskeletal disorders in the United States. Arthritis Rheum 41(5):778, 1998.
2. Straus B: Chronic pain of spinal origin: The costs of intervention. Spine 27(22):2614, 2002.
3. National Center for Health Statistics: National Hospital Discharge Survey. Report No. PB92-500818. Washington DC: U.S. Department of Health and Human Services, Center for Disease Control, 1990.
4. Viesca C, Racz G, Day M: Special techniques in pain management: Lysis of adhesions. Anesthesiology Clin North Am 21:745, 2003.
5. Hatten H, Jr. Lumbar epidurography with metrizamide. Radiology 137:129, 1980.
6. Stewart H, Quinnell R, Dann N: Epidurography in the management of sciatica. Br J Rheumatol 26(6):424, 1987.
7. Devulder J, Bogaert L, Castille F et al: Relevance of epidurography and epidural adhesiolysis in chronic failed back surgery patients. Clin J Pain 11:147, 1995.
8. Manchikanti L, Bakhit C, Pampati V: Role of epidurography in caudal neuroplasty. Pain Digest 8:277, 1998.
9. Day M, Racz G: Technique of caudal neuroplasty. Pain Digest 9(4):255, 1999.
10. Horlocker T, Wedel D, Benzon, et al: Regional anesthesia in the anticoagulated patient: Defining the risks (the second ASRA Consensus Conference on Neuraxial Anesthesia and Anticoagulation). Reg Anesth Pain Med 28:172, 2003.
11. Kaye A, Sabar R, Vig S, et al: Nutraceuticals—current concepts and the role of the anesthesiologist. Part 1. Echinacea, garlic, ginger, gingko, and St. John's wort. Am J Anesthesiol 27(7):405, 2000.
12. Kaye A, Sabar R, Vig S, et al: Nutraceuticals—current concepts and the role of the anesthesiologist. Part 2. Panax ginseng, kava kava, feverfew, and ma huang. Am J Anesthesiol 27(8):467, 2000.
13. Omnipaque product insert. Princeton, NJ, Nycomed, Inc.
14. Isovue product insert. Princeton, NJ, Bracco Diagnostics, Inc.
15. Hypaque product insert. Princeton, NJ, Amersham Health, Inc.
16. Conray product insert. Phillipsburg, NJ, Mallinckrodt, Inc.
17. Manchikanti L: Role of neuraxial steroids in interventional pain management. Pain Physician 5(2):182, 2002.
18. Racz G, Holubec J: Lysis of adhesions in the epidural space. In Raj P (ed): Techniques of Neurolysis. Boston, Kluwer, 1989, p 57.
19. Arthur J, Racz G, Heinrich, et al: Epidural space: Identification of filling defects and lysis of adhesions in the treatment of chronic painful conditions. Abstracts of the 7th World Congress on Pain, Paris, IASP, 1993.
20. Stolker R, Vervest A, Gerbrand J: The management of chronic spinal pain by blockades: A review. Pain 58:1, 1994.
21. Devulder J, Bogaert L, Castille F, et al: Relevance of epidurography and epidural adhesiolysis in chronic failed back surgery patients. Clin J Pain 11:147, 1995.
22. Racz G, Heavner J: In response to article by Drs. Devulder, et al. Clin J Pain 11:151, 1995.
23. Heavner J, Racz G, Raj P: Percutaneous epidural neuroplasty: Prospective evaluation of 0.9% saline versus 10% saline with or without hyaluronidase. Reg Anesth Pain Med 24:202, 1999.
24. Manchikanti L, Pakanati R, Bakhit C, Pampati V: Role of adhesiolysis and hypertonic saline neurolysis in management of low back pain: Evaluation of modification of the Racz protocol. Pain Digest 9:91, 1999.
25. Manchikanti L, Pampati V, Fellow B, et al. Role of one day epidural adhesiolysis in management of chronic low back pain: A randomized clinical trial. Pain Physician 4:153, 2001.
26. Manchikanti L, Rivera J, Pampati V, et al: One day lumbar adhesiolysis and hypertonic saline neurolysis in treatment of chronic low back pain: A randomized, double-blind trial. Pain Physician 7:177, 2004.

chapter 161

Hypogastric Plexus Block and Impar Ganglion Block

Steven D. Waldman

HYPOGASTRIC PLEXUS BLOCK

Hypogastric plexus block continues to gain favor as a technique in the evaluation and treatment of sympathetically mediated pain emanating from the pelvic viscera. Recently repopularized by Patt and Plancarte, this useful regional anesthesia block provides the clinician with new options when faced with a patient presenting with pelvic pain.[1] Recent advances in the use of fluoroscopic and computerized tomographic guidance have contributed greatly to the understanding of the functional anatomy of this anatomic region and have led to the development of several variations of the technique including both a single- and a two-needle approach.

Clinically Relevant Anatomy

In the context of neural blockade, the hypogastric plexus can simply be thought of as a continuation of the lumbar sympathetic chain that can be blocked in a manner analogous to lumbar sympathetic nerve block. The preganglionic fibers of the hypogastric plexus find their origin primarily in the lower thoracic and upper lumbar region of the spinal cord. These preganglionic fibers interface with the lumbar sympathetic chain via the white communicantes. Postganglionic fibers exit the lumbar sympathetic chain and, together with fibers from the parasympathetic sacral ganglion, make up the superior hypogastric plexus. The superior hypogastric plexus lies in front of L4 as a coalescence of fibers. As these fibers descend, at a level of L5, they begin to divide into the hypogastric nerves following in proximity the iliac vessels (Fig. 161–1). As the hypogastric nerves continue their lateral and inferior course, they are accessible for neural blockade as they pass in front of the L5-S1 interspace. The hypogastric nerves pass downward from this point, following the concave curve of the sacrum and passing on each side of the rectum to form the inferior hypogastric plexus. These nerves continue their downward course along each side of the bladder to provide innervation to the pelvic viscera and vasculature.

Single-Needle Approach to Hypogastric Plexus Block

Hypogastric plexus block with the single-needle technique is useful in the evaluation and management of sympathetically mediated pain of the pelvic viscera.[2] Included in this category are pain secondary to malignancy, endometriosis, reflex sympathetic dystrophy, causalgia, proctalgia fugax, or radiation enteritis.[3] Hypogastric plexus block is also useful in the palliation of tenesmus secondary to radiation therapy to the rectum. Hypogastric plexus block with local anesthetic can be used as a diagnostic tool when performing differential neural blockade on an anatomic basis in the evaluation of pelvic and rectal pain. If destruction of the hypogastric plexus is being considered, this technique is useful as a prognostic indicator of the degree of pain relief that the patient may experience. Hypogastric plexus block with local anesthetic is also useful in the treatment of acute herpes zoster and postherpetic neuralgia involving the sacral dermatomes. Destruction of the hypogastric plexus is indicated for the palliation of pain syndromes that have temporarily responded to blockade of the hypogastric plexus with local anesthetic and have not been controlled with more conservative measures.[4,5]

Blind Technique

The patient is placed in the prone position with a pillow placed under the lower abdomen to gently flex the lumbar spine and maximize the space between the transverse process of L5 and the sacral alae. The L4-L5 interspace is located by identifying the iliac crests and finding the interspace at that level. The skin at this level is prepared with antiseptic solution. A point 6 cm from the midline at this level is identified, and the skin and subcutaneous tissues are anesthetized with 1.0% lidocaine. A 20-gauge, 13-cm needle is then inserted through the previously anesthetized area and directed approximately 30 degrees caudad and 30 degrees mesiad toward the anterolateral portion of the L5-S1 interspace. If the transverse process of L5 is encountered, the needle is withdrawn and redirected slightly more caudad. If the vertebral body of L5 is encountered, the needle is withdrawn and redirected slightly more lateral until, in a manner analogous to lumbar sympathetic block, the needle is walked off the anterolateral aspect of the vertebral body.

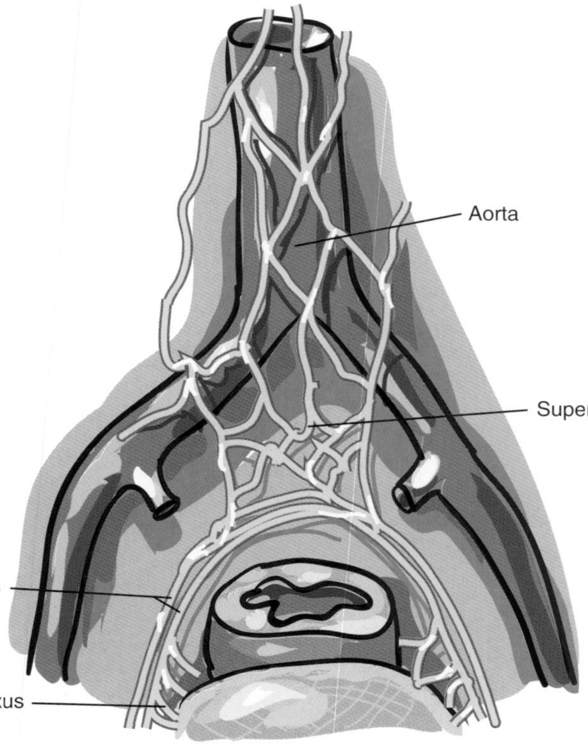

FIGURE 161–1 ■ Clinically relevant anatomy of the hypogastric plexus.

A 5-mL glass syringe filled with preservative-free saline is then attached to the needle. The needle is then slowly advanced into the prevertebral space while maintaining constant pressure on the plunger of the syringe in a manner analogous to the loss-of-resistance technique used for identification of the epidural space. A "pop" and loss of resistance will be felt as the needle pierces the anterior fascia of the psoas muscle and enters the prevertebral space (Fig. 161–2). After careful aspiration for blood, cerebrospinal fluid, and urine, 10 mL of 1.0% preservative-free lidocaine is slowly injected in incremental doses while observing the patient closely for signs of local anesthetic toxicity. If there is believed to be an inflammatory component to the pain, the local anesthetic is combined with 80 mg of methylprednisolone and is injected in incremental doses. Subsequent daily nerve blocks are carried out in a similar manner, substituting 40 mg of methylprednisolone for the initial 80-mg dose. The needle is then removed, and an ice pack is placed on the injection site to decrease post-block bleeding and pain.

CT-Guided Technique

The patient is placed in the prone position on the computed tomography (CT) gantry with a pillow placed under the lower abdomen to gently flex the lumbar spine and maximize the space between the transverse process of L5 and the sacral alae. A CT scout film of the lumbar spine is taken, and the L4-L5 interspace is identified. The skin overlying the L4-L5 interspace is prepared with antiseptic solution, and sterile drapes are placed. At a point approximately 6 cm from midline, the skin and subcutaneous tissues are anesthetized with 1% lidocaine using a 25-gauge, 3.8-cm needle. A 20-gauge, 13-cm needle is then inserted through the previously anesthetized area and directed approximately 30 degrees caudad and 30 degrees mesiad toward the anterolateral portion of the L5-S1 interspace.[6] If the transverse process of L5 is encountered, the needle is withdrawn and redirected slightly more caudad. If the vertebral body of L5 is encountered, the needle is withdrawn and redirected slightly more lateral and "walked off" the anterolateral aspect of the vertebral body in a manner analogous to lumbar sympathetic block. A 5-mL glass syringe filled with preservative-free saline is then attached to the needle. The needle is then slowly advanced into the prevertebral space while maintaining constant pressure on the plunger of the syringe. A "pop" and loss of resistance will be felt as the needle pierces the anterior fascia of the psoas muscle. After careful aspiration, 2 to 3 mL of water-soluble contrast medium is injected through the needle and a CT scan is taken to confirm current retroperitoneal needle placement (Fig. 161–3). Because of contralateral spread of the contrast medium in the prevertebral space, it is often unnecessary to place a second needle as is advocated by some pain specialists. A total volume of 10 mL of 1.0% preservative-free lidocaine is then injected in divided doses after careful aspiration for blood, cerebrospinal fluid, and urine. If adequate pain relief is obtained, incremental doses of absolute alcohol or 6.5% aqueous phenol may be injected in a similar manner after it is ascertained that the patient is experiencing no untoward bowel or bladder effects from blockade of the hypogastric plexus.

Classic Two-Needle Technique

Hypogastric plexus block using the classic two-needle technique is reserved for those patients in whom presacral tumor mass or adenopathy prevents contralateral spread of solutions

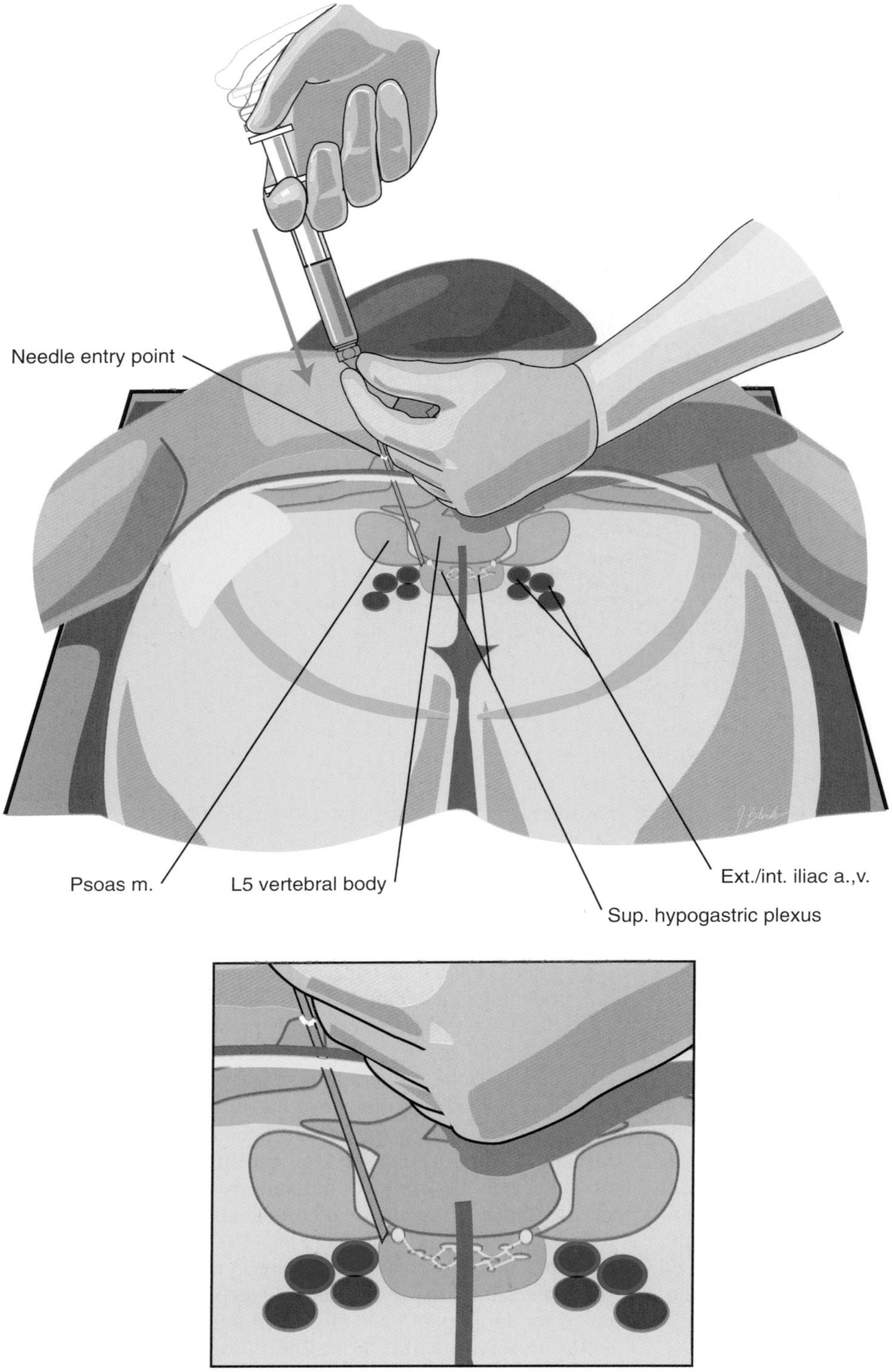

FIGURE 161–2 ■ Blind single-needle technique for hypogastric plexus block. (From Waldman SD: Atlas of Interventional Pain Management, 2nd ed. Philadelphia, Saunders, 2003, p 413, Fig. 89–1.)

injected through a single needle. This technique is useful in the evaluation and management of sympathetically mediated pain of the pelvic viscera.[6] Included in this category are pain secondary to malignancy, endometriosis, reflex sympathetic dystrophy, causalgia, proctalgia fugax, and radiation enteritis. Hypogastric plexus block is also useful in the palliation of tenesmus secondary to radiation therapy to the rectum. Hypogastric plexus block with local anesthetic can be used as a diagnostic tool when performing differential neural blockade on an anatomic basis in the evaluation of pelvic and rectal pain. If destruction of the hypogastric plexus is being considered, this technique is useful as a prognostic indicator of the degree of pain relief that the patient may experience. Hypogastric plexus block with local anesthetic is also useful in the treatment of acute herpes zoster and postherpetic neuralgia involving the sacral dermatomes. Destruction of the

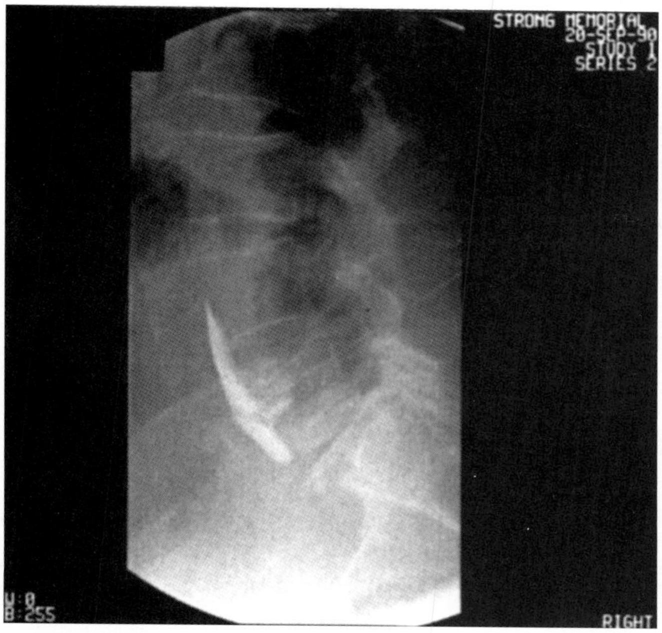

FIGURE 161–3 ■ Lateral radiograph demonstrates verification of correct needle placement for unilateral superior hypogastric plexus block. Note smooth margins of opacity formed by contrast medium anterior to the psoas fascia, which suggests retroperitoneal placement. (From Plancarte R, Amescua C, Patt RB: Sympathetic neurolytic blockade. In Patt RB (ed): Cancer Pain. Philadelphia, JB Lippincott, 1993, pp 377-425.)

hypogastric plexus is indicated for the palliation of pain syndromes that have temporarily responded to blockade of the hypogastric plexus with local anesthetic and have not been controlled with more conservative measures.[7]

Blind Technique

The patient is placed in the prone position with a pillow placed under the lower abdomen to gently flex the lumbar spine and maximize the space between the transverse process of L5 and the sacral alae. The L4-L5 interspace is located by identifying the iliac crests and finding the interspace at that level. The skin at this level is prepared with antiseptic solution. A point 6 cm from the midline at this level is identified, and the skin and subcutaneous tissues are anesthetized with 1.0% lidocaine. A 20-gauge, 13-cm needle is then inserted through the previously anesthetized area and directed approximately 30 degrees caudad and 30 degrees mesiad toward the anterolateral portion of the L5-S1 interspace (Fig. 161–4). If the transverse process of L5 is encountered, the needle is withdrawn and redirected slightly more caudad. If the vertebral body of L5 is encountered, the needle is withdrawn and redirected slightly more lateral until, in a manner analogous to lumbar sympathetic block, the needle is walked off the anterolateral aspect of the vertebral body.

A 5-mL glass syringe filled with preservative-free saline is then attached to the needle. The needle is then slowly advanced into the prevertebral space while maintaining constant pressure on the plunger of the syringe in a manner analogous to the loss-of-resistance technique used for identification of the epidural space. A "pop" and loss of resistance will be felt as the needle pierces the anterior fascia of the psoas muscle and enters the prevertebral space. A contralateral needle is then inserted in a similar manner using the trajectory and depth of the first needle as a guide (see Fig. 161–1). After careful aspiration for blood, cerebrospinal fluid, and urine, 5 mL of 1.0% preservative-free lidocaine is slowly injected in incremental doses while observing the patient closely for signs of local anesthetic toxicity. If there is believed to be an inflammatory component to the pain, the local anesthetic is combined with 80 mg of methylprednisolone and is injected in incremental doses. Subsequent daily nerve blocks are carried out in a similar manner, substituting 40 mg of methylprednisolone for the initial 80-mg dose. Each needle is then removed, and an ice pack is placed on the injection site to decrease post-block bleeding and pain.

CT-Guided Technique

The patient is placed in the prone position on the computed tomography (CT) gantry with a pillow placed under the lower abdomen to gently flex the lumbar spine and maximize the space between the transverse process of L5 and the sacral alae. A CT scout film of the lumbar spine is taken, and the L4-L5 interspace is identified. The skin overlying the L4-L5 interspace is prepared with antiseptic solution, and sterile drapes are placed. At a point approximately 6 cm from midline, the skin and subcutaneous tissues are anesthetized with 1% lidocaine using a 25-gauge, 3.8-cm needle. A 20-gauge, 13-cm needle is then inserted through the previously anesthetized area and directed approximately 30 degrees caudad and 30 degrees mesiad toward the anterolateral portion of the L5-S1 interspace. If the transverse process of L5 is encountered, the needle is withdrawn and redirected slightly more caudad. If the vertebral body of L5 is encountered, the needle is withdrawn and redirected slightly more lateral and walked off the anterolateral aspect of the vertebral body in a manner analogous to lumbar sympathetic block. A 5-mL glass syringe filled with preservative-free saline is then attached to the needle. The needle is then slowly advanced into the prevertebral space while maintaining constant pressure on the plunger of the syringe. A "pop" and loss of resistance will be felt as the needle pierces the anterior fascia of the psoas muscle. After careful aspiration, 2 to 3 mL of water-soluble contrast medium is injected through the needle and a CT scan is taken to confirm current retroperitoneal needle placement. If no contralateral spread of the contrast medium in the prevertebral space is observed, a contralateral needle is inserted in a similar manner using the trajectory and depth of the first needle as a guide. A total volume of 5 mL of 1.0% preservative-free lidocaine is then injected in divided doses after careful aspiration for blood, cerebrospinal fluid, and urine. If adequate pain relief is obtained, incremental doses of absolute alcohol or 6.5% aqueous phenol may be injected in a similar manner after it is ascertained that the patient is experiencing no untoward bowel or bladder effects from blockade of the hypogastric plexus. Each needle is then removed, and an ice pack is placed on the injection site to decrease post-block bleeding and pain.

Side Effects and Complications

The proximity of the hypogastric nerves to the iliac vessels means that the potential for bleeding or inadvertent intravascular injection remains a distinct possibility.[8] The relationship of the cauda equina and exiting nerve roots makes it impera-

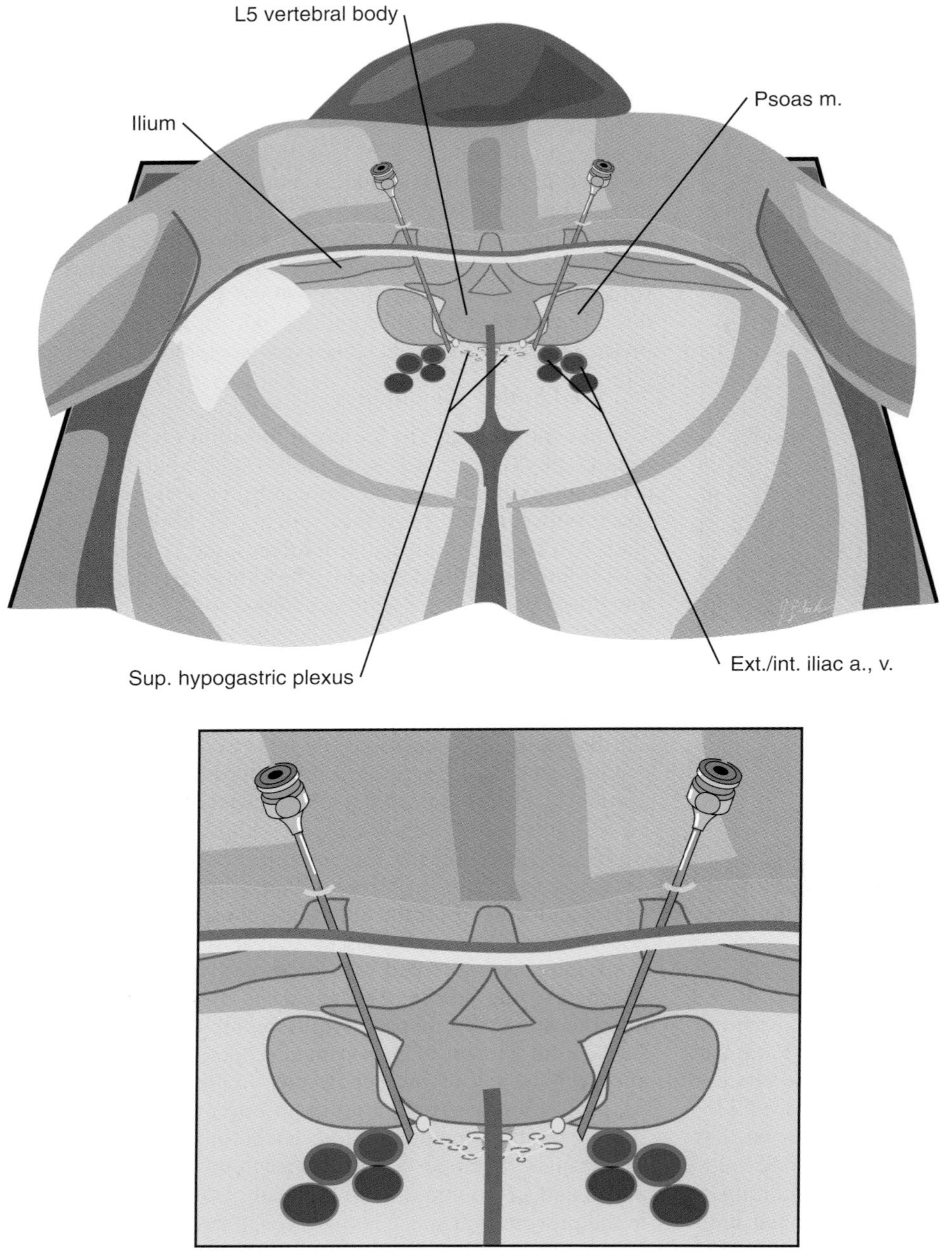

FIGURE 161–4 ■ Blind two-needle technique for hypogastric plexus block. (From Waldman SD: Atlas of Interventional Pain Management, 2nd ed. Philadelphia, Saunders, 2003, p 417, Fig. 90-1.)

tive that this procedure be carried out only by those well versed in the regional anatomy and experienced in performing lumbar sympathetic nerve block. Given the proximity of the pelvic cavity, damage to the pelvic viscera including the ureters during hypogastric plexus block is a distinct possibility. The incidence of this complication will be decreased if care is taken to place the needle just beyond the anterolateral margin of the L5-S1 interspace. Needle placement too medial may result in epidural, subdural, or subarachnoid injections or trauma to the intervertebral disk, spinal cord, and exiting nerve roots. Although uncommon, infection remains an ever-present possibility, especially in the immunocompromised cancer patient. Early detection of infection, including diskitis, is crucial to avoid potentially life-threatening sequelae.

GANGLION OF WALTHER (IMPAR) BLOCK

Ganglion of Walther (also known as the *impar ganglion*) block is useful in the evaluation and management of sympathetically mediated pain of the perineum, rectum, and genitalia.[9] This technique has been used primarily in the treatment of pain secondary to malignancy, although theoretical applications for benign pain syndromes including pain secondary to endometriosis, reflex sympathetic dystrophy, causalgia, proctalgia fugax, and radiation enteritis can be considered if the pain has failed to respond to more conservative therapies.[10] Impar ganglion block with local anesthetic can be used as a diagnostic tool when performing differential neural blockade on an anatomic basis in the evaluation of pelvic and rectal pain. If destruction of the impar ganglion is being considered, this technique is useful as a prognostic indicator of the degree of pain relief that the patient may experience. Destruction of the impar ganglion is indicated for the palliation of pain syndromes that have temporarily responded to blockade of the ganglion with local anesthetic and have not been controlled with more conservative measures.

Clinically Relevant Anatomy

In the context of neural blockade, the impar ganglion can simply be thought of as the terminal coalescence of the sympathetic chain. The impar ganglion lies in front of the sacrococcygeal junction and is amenable to blockade at this level. The ganglion receives fibers from the lumbar and sacral portions of the sympathetic and parasympathetic nervous system and provides sympathetic innervation to portions of the pelvic viscera and genitalia.

Blind Technique

The patient is placed in the jackknife position to facilitate access to the inferior margin of the gluteal cleft. The midline is identified, and the skin just below the tip of the coccyx that overlies the anococcygeal ligament is prepared with antiseptic solution. The skin and subcutaneous tissues at this point are anesthetized with 1.0% lidocaine. A $3\frac{1}{2}$-inch spinal needle is then bent at a point 1 inch from its hub to a 30-degree angle to allow placement of the needle tip in proximity to the anterior aspect of the sacrococcygeal junction. The needle may be bent again at a point 2 inches from the hub to accommodate those patients with an exaggerated coccygeal curve to allow placement of the needle tip to rest against the sacrococcygeal junction.

The bent needle is then placed through the previously anesthetized area and is advanced until the needle tip impinges on the anterior surface of the sacrococcygeal junction (Fig. 161–5). After careful aspiration for blood, cerebrospinal fluid, and urine, 3 mL of 1.0% preservative-free lidocaine is slowly injected in incremental doses. If there is believed to be an inflammatory component to the pain, the local anesthetic is combined with 80 mg of methylprednisolone and is injected in incremental doses. Subsequent daily nerve blocks are carried out in a similar manner, substituting 40 mg of methylprednisolone for the initial 80-mg dose. The needle is then removed, and an ice pack is placed on the injection site to decrease post-block bleeding and pain.

CT-Guided Technique

The patient is placed in the prone position on the computed tomography (CT) gantry with a pillow placed under the pelvis to facilitate access to the inferior gluteal cleft. A CT scout film is taken, and the sacrococcygeal junction and the tip of the coccyx are identified. The midline is also identified, and the skin just below the tip of the coccyx that overlies the anococcygeal ligament is prepared with antiseptic solution. The skin and subcutaneous tissues at this point are anesthetized with 1.0% lidocaine. A $3\frac{1}{2}$-inch spinal needle is then bent at a point 1 inch from its hub to a 30-degree angle to allow placement of the needle tip in proximity to the anterior aspect of the sacrococcygeal junction (Fig. 161–6A). The needle may be bent again at a point 2 inches from the hub to accommodate patients with an exaggerated coccygeal curve to allow the needle tip to rest against the anterior sacrococcygeal junction.

The needle is then placed through the previously anesthetized area and is advanced until the needle tip impinges on the anterior surface of the sacrococcygeal junction. After careful aspiration for blood, cerebrospinal fluid, and urine, 2 to 3 mL of water-soluble contrast medium is injected through the needle and a CT scan is taken to confirm the spread of contrast medium just anterior to the sacrococcygeal junction (see Fig. 161–6B and C). After correct needle placement is confirmed, a total volume of 3 mL of 1.0% preservative-free lidocaine is injected in divided doses after careful aspiration

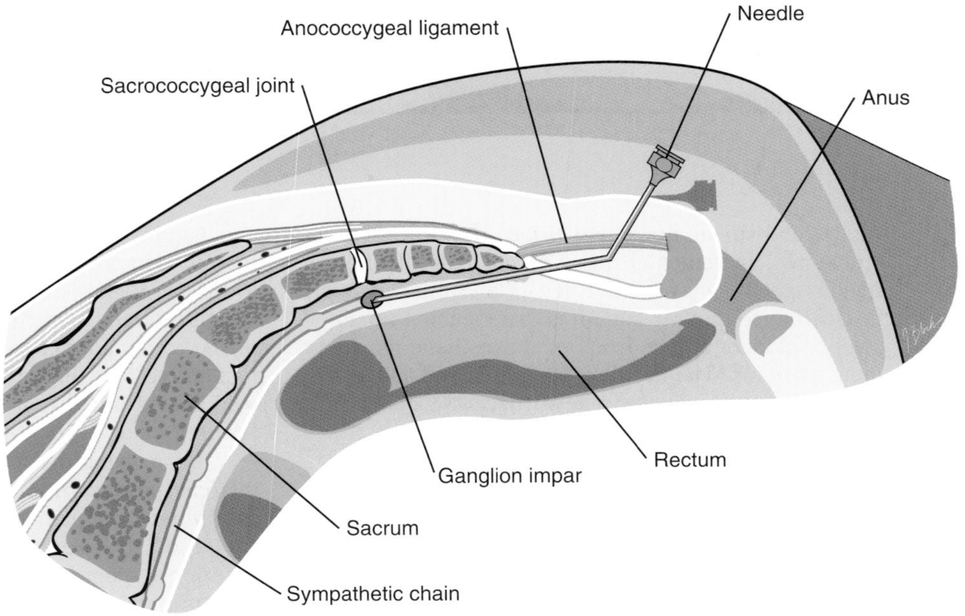

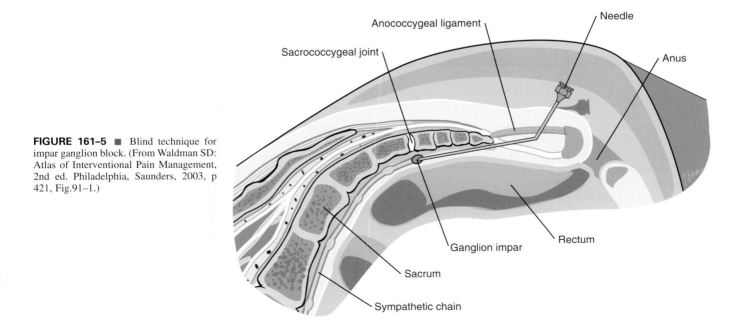

FIGURE 161–5 ■ Blind technique for impar ganglion block. (From Waldman SD: Atlas of Interventional Pain Management, 2nd ed. Philadelphia, Saunders, 2003, p 421, Fig.91–1.)

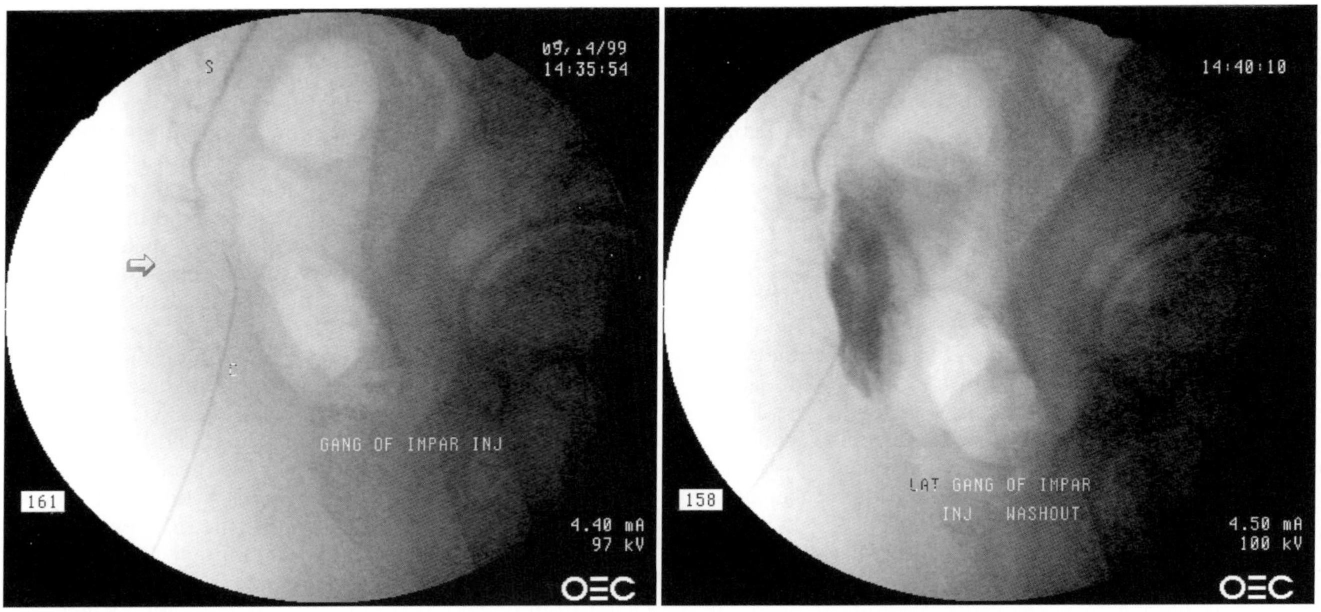

A

B

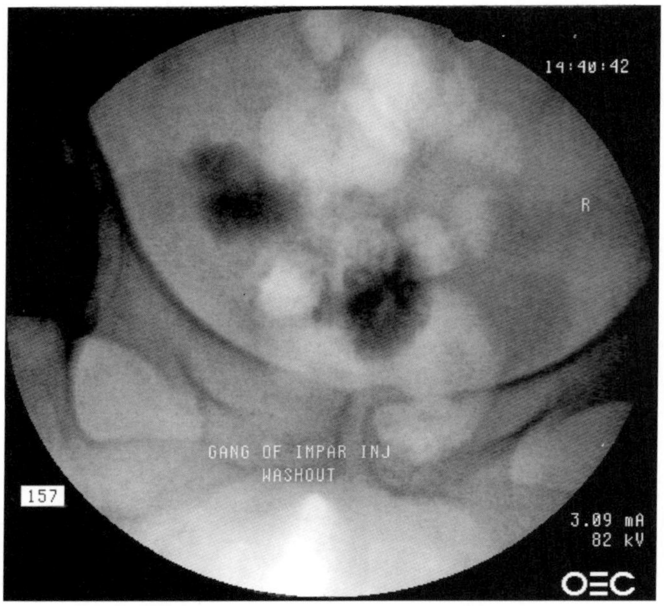

C

FIGURE 161–6 ■ CT-guided technique for impar ganglion block. **A,** Tip of the spinal needle is positioned in proximity to the anterior aspect of the sacrococcygeal junction. **B,** The needle is advanced until the tip impinges on the anterior surface of the sacrococcygeal junction. **C,** CT scan confirming the spread of contrast medium just anterior to the sacrococcygeal junction. (From Waldman SD: Atlas of Interventional Pain Management, 2nd ed. Philadelphia, Saunders, 2003, pp 421-422, Figs. 91–2, 91–3, 91–4.)

for blood, cerebrospinal fluid, and urine. If adequate pain relief is obtained, incremental doses of absolute alcohol or 6.5% aqueous phenol may be injected in a similar manner, after it is ascertained that the patient is experiencing no untoward bowel or bladder effects from local anesthetic blockade of the impar ganglion. The needle is then removed and an ice pack is placed on the injection site to decrease post-block bleeding and pain.

Side Effects and Complications

The proximity of the impar ganglion to the rectum makes perforation and tracking of contaminants back through the needle track during needle removal a distinct possibility. Infection and fistula formation, especially in those patients who are immunocompromised or who have received radiation therapy to the perineum, can represent a devastating and potentially life-threatening complication to this block. The relationship of the cauda equina and exiting sacral nerve roots makes it imperative that this procedure be carried out only by those well versed in the regional anatomy and experienced in performing interventional pain management techniques.

Impar ganglion block is a straightforward technique that can produce dramatic relief for patients suffering from the aforementioned pain complaints. Given the localized nature of this neural structure when compared with the superior hypogastric plexus, neurolytic block with small quantities of absolute alcohol or phenol in glycerin or by cryoneurolysis or radiofrequency lesioning may be a reasonable choice over superior hypogastric plexus block—at least insofar as bowel and bladder dysfunction is concerned. Destruction of the impar ganglion has been shown to provide long-term relief for patients suffering from sympathetically maintained pain that has been relieved with local anesthetic. Computed tomographic guidance allows visualization of the regional anatomy and the relationship of the rectum to the needle. This is a significant advance over blind or fluoroscopically guided techniques.

References

1. Plancarte R, Amescua C, Patt R, et al: Superior hypogastric plexus block for pelvic cancer pain. Anesthesiology 73:236, 1990.
2. Waldman SD: Hypogastric plexus block—single needle technique. In Waldman SD: Atlas of Interventional Pain Management, 2nd ed. Philadelphia, Saunders, 2004, p 441.
3. Dargent M: Role of sympathetic nerve in cancerous pain. Br Med J 1:440, 1948.
4. Lee RB, Stone K, Magelssen D, et al: Presacral neurotomy for chronic pelvic pain. Obstet Gynecol 68:517, 1986.
5. De Leon-Casasola OA, Kent E, Lema MJ: Neurolytic superior hypogastric plexus block for chronic pelvic pain associated with cancer. Pain 54:145, 1993.
6. Waldman SD, Wilson WL, Kreps RD: Superior hypogastric plexus block using a single needle and computed tomography guidance: Description of a modified technique. Reg Anesth 16:286, 1991.
7. Waldman, SD: Hypogastric plexus block: Classic two-needle technique. In Waldman SD: Atlas of Interventional Pain Management, 2nd ed. Philadelphia, Saunders, 2004, p 415.
8. Brass A: Anatomy and physiology: Autonomic nerves and ganglia in pelvis. In Netter FH (ed): The Ciba Collection of Medical Illustrations, vol 1. Nervous System. Summit, NJ, Ciba Pharmaceutical, 1983, p 85.
9. Plancarte R, Amescua C, Patt RB, et al: Presacral blockade of the ganglion of Walther (ganglion impar). Anesthesiology 73:A751, 1990.
10. Waldman SD: Ganglion of Walther (impar) block. In Waldman SD: Atlas of Interventional Pain Management, 2nd ed. Philadelphia, Saunders, 2004, p 419.

chapter 162

Injection of the Sacroiliac Joint

Steven D. Waldman

The sacroiliac joint is a diarthrodial joint that is susceptible to the development of arthritis from a variety of conditions that have in common the ability to damage the joint cartilage.[1] The sacroiliac joint is also susceptible to the development of strain from trauma or misuse. Osteoarthritis of the joint is the most common form of arthritis that results in sacroiliac joint pain. However, rheumatoid arthritis and posttraumatic arthritis are also common causes of sacroiliac pain. Less frequent causes of arthritis-induced sacroiliac pain include collagen vascular diseases such as ankylosing spondylitis, infection, and Lyme disease. Acute infectious arthritis is usually accompanied by significant systemic symptoms, including fever and malaise, and should be easily recognized by an astute clinician and treated appropriately with culture and antibiotics rather than injection therapy. The collagen vascular diseases are generally manifested as a polyarthropathy rather than a monoarthropathy limited to the sacroiliac joint, although sacroiliac pain secondary to the collagen vascular disease ankylosing spondylitis responds exceedingly well to the intra-articular injection technique described later.[2] Occasionally, the clinician will encounter patients with iatrogenically induced sacroiliac joint dysfunction caused by overaggressive bone graft harvesting for spinal fusion.

The majority of patients with sacroiliac pain secondary to strain or arthritis will complain of pain localized around the sacroiliac joint and upper part of the leg.[3] The pain associated with sacroiliac joint strain or arthritis radiates into the posterior of the buttocks and back of the legs (Fig. 162–1). The pain does not radiate below the knees.[4] Activity makes the pain worse, with rest and heat providing some relief. The pain is constant and characterized as aching. It may interfere with sleep. On physical examination there will be tenderness to palpation of the affected sacroiliac joint. The patient will often favor the affected leg and exhibit a list to the unaffected side.[5] Spasm of the lumbar paraspinal musculature is often present, as is limitation of range of motion of the lumbar spine in the erect position that improves in the sitting position because of relaxation of the hamstring muscles.[6] Patients with pain emanating from the sacroiliac joint will exhibit a positive pelvic rock test. The pelvic rock test is performed by placing the hands on the iliac crests and the thumbs on the anterior superior iliac spines and then forcibly compressing the pelvis toward the midline (Fig. 162–2). A positive test is indicated by the production of pain around the sacroiliac joint.

Plain radiographs are indicated in all patients with sacroiliac pain. Based on the patient's clinical findings, additional testing, including a complete blood count, sedimentation rate, and HLA-B27 antigen and antinuclear antibody testing may be indicated (Fig. 162–3).

CLINICALLY RELEVANT ANATOMY

The sacroiliac joint is formed by the articular surfaces of the sacrum and iliac bones (Fig. 162–4). These articular surfaces have corresponding elevations and depressions that give the joints their irregular appearance on radiographs. The strength of the sacroiliac joint comes primarily from the posterior and interosseous ligaments rather than the bony articulations. The sacroiliac joints bear the weight of the trunk and are thus subject to the development of strain and arthritis.[7] As the joint ages, the intraarticular space narrows, thus making intraarticular injection more challenging. The ligaments and the sacroiliac joint itself receive their innervation from the L3 to S3 nerve roots, with L4 and L5 providing the greatest contribution to innervation of the joint. This diverse innervation may help explain the ill-defined nature of sacroiliac pain. The sacroiliac joint has very limited range of motion, and that motion is induced by changes in the force placed on the joint by shifts in posture and joint loading.

TECHNIQUE

The goals of the injection technique are explained to the patient. The patient is placed in the supine position, and proper preparation with antiseptic cleansing of the skin overlying the affected sacroiliac joint space is carried out. A sterile syringe containing 4.0 mL of 0.25% preservative-free bupivacaine and 40 mg of methylprednisolone is attached to a 3½-inch, 25-gauge needle under strict aseptic technique. Also with strict aseptic technique, the posterior superior spine of the ilium is identified. At this point the needle is carefully advanced through the skin and subcutaneous tissue at a 45-degree angle toward the affected sacroiliac joint (Fig. 162–5). If bone is encountered, the needle is withdrawn into the subcutaneous tissue and redirected superiorly and slightly more laterally.[8] After entering the joint space, the contents of the syringe is gently injected. There should be little resistance to injection. If resistance is encountered, the needle is

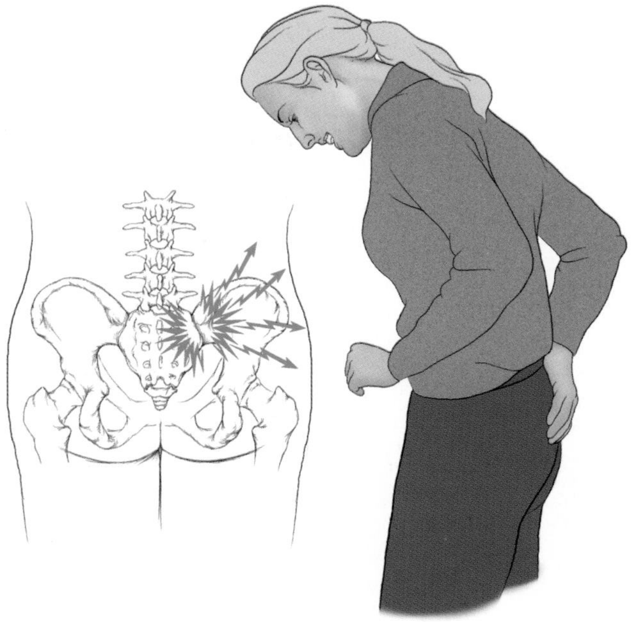

FIGURE 162–1 ■ Sacroiliac joint pain radiates into the buttock and upper part of the leg. (From Waldman SD: Atlas of Common Pain Syndromes. Philadelphia, WB Saunders, 2002, p 213.)

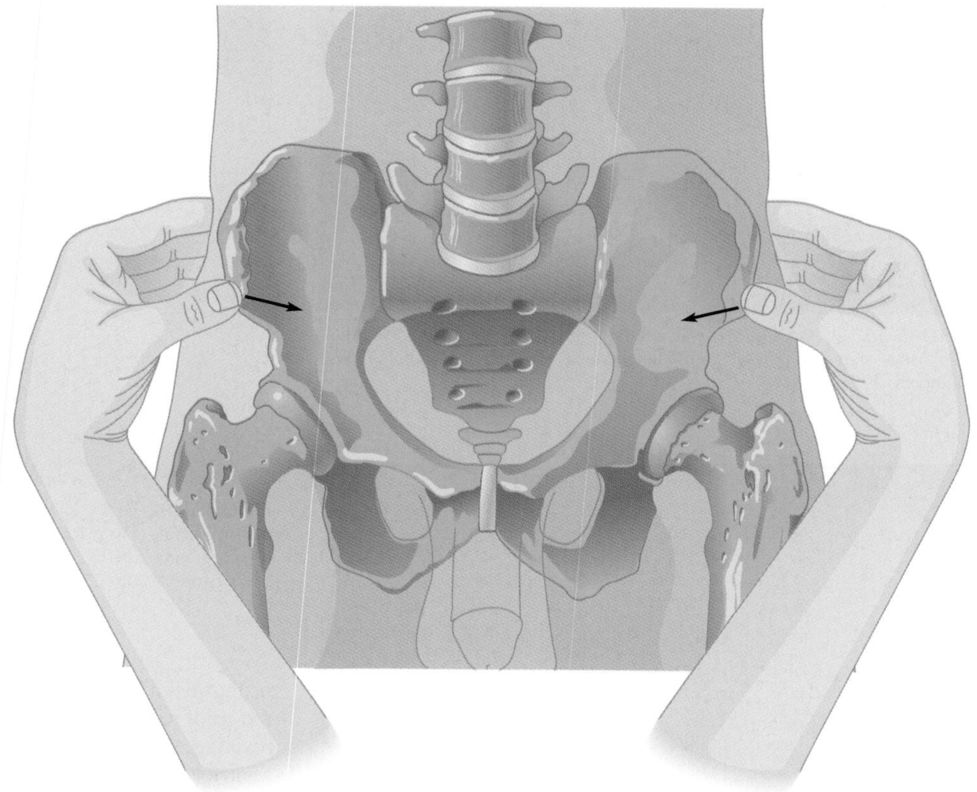

FIGURE 162–2 ■ Pelvic rock test. (From Waldman SD (ed): Atlas of Interventional Pain Management, 2nd ed. Philadelphia, WB Saunders, 2003, p 430.)

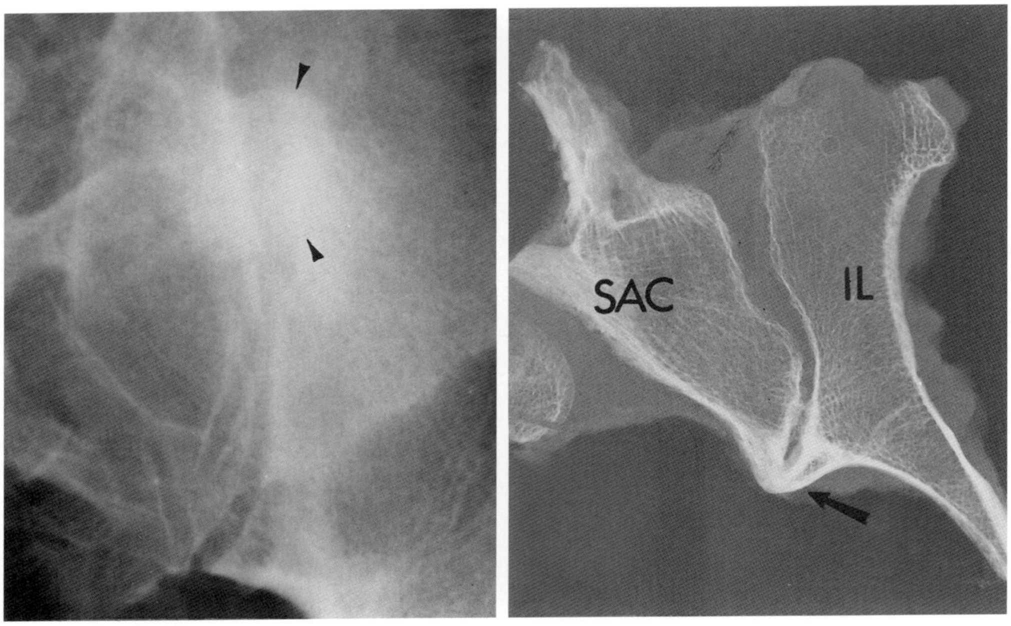

FIGURE 162–3 ■ Ankylosing spondylitis as indicated by the black arrows. (From Resnick D: Diagnosis of Bone and Joint Disorders, 4th ed. Philadelphia, WB Saunders, 2002, p 1325.)

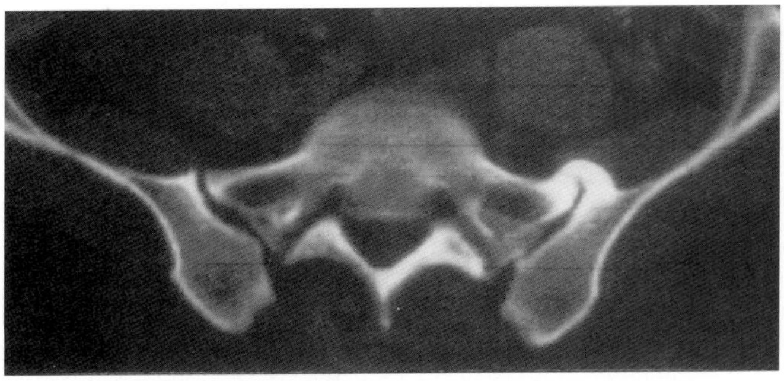

FIGURE 162–4 ■ Radiographic anatomy of the SI joint. (From Waldman SD: Atlas of Interventional Pain Management, 2nd ed. Philadelphia, WB Saunders, 2003, p 430.)

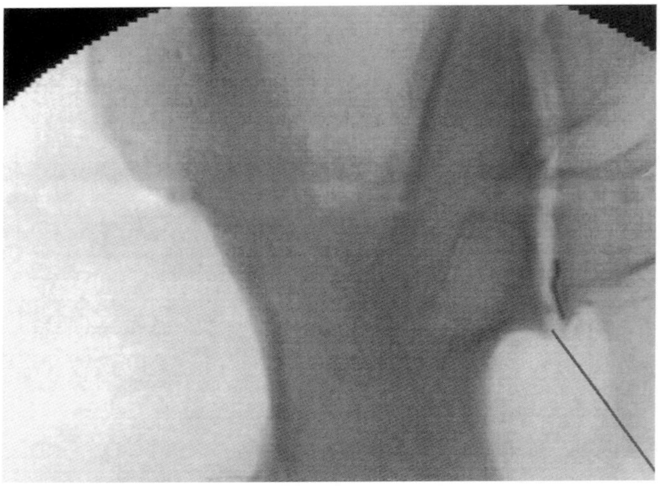

FIGURE 162–5 ■ Sacroiliac joint enhanced fluoroscopically by oblique positioning of the C-arm. (From Raj PP, Lou L, Erden S, et al: Radiographic Imaging for Regional Anesthesia and Pain Management. Philadelphia, Churchill Livingstone, 2003, p 243.)

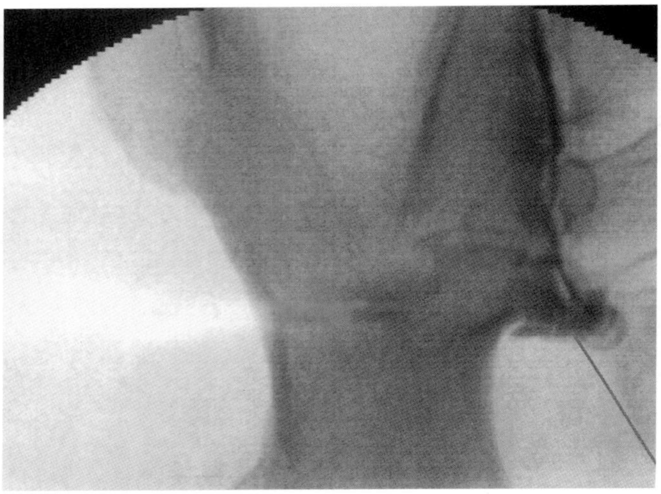

FIGURE 162–6 ■ Sacroiliac joint fluoroscopically enhanced with contrast material. (From Raj PP, Lou L, Erden S, et al: Radiographic Imaging for Regional Anesthesia and Pain Management. Philadelphia, Churchill Livingstone, 2003, p 244.)

probably in a ligament and should be advanced slightly into the joint space until the injection proceeds without significant resistance. Fluoroscopic guidance and the use of iodinated contrast may aid in the performance of this technique in selected patients (Fig. 162–6). The needle is then removed, and a sterile pressure dressing and ice pack are placed at the injection site.

The major complication of intraarticular injection of the sacroiliac joint is infection. This complication should be exceedingly rare if strict aseptic technique is followed. Approximately 25% of patients will complain of a transient increase in pain after intraarticular injection of the sacroiliac joint and should be warned of such. Care must be taken to avoid injection too laterally or the needle may traumatize the sciatic nerve.

References

1. Resnick D: Degenerative disease of extraspinal locations. In Resnick D (ed): Diagnosis of Bone and Joint Disorders, 4th ed. Philadelphia, WB Saunders, 2002, p 1323.
2. Maugars Y, Mathis C, Berthelot JM, et al: Assessment of the efficacy of sacroiliac corticosteroid injections in the spondyloarthropathies: A double-blind study. Br J Rheumatol 35:767, 1996.
3. Waldman SD: Sacroiliac joint pain. In Waldman SD (ed): Atlas of Common Pain Syndromes. Philadelphia, WB Saunders, 2002, p 212.
4. Fortin JD, Dwyer AP, West S, Pier J: Sacroiliac joint: Pain referral maps upon applying a new injection/arthrography technique. Part I: Asymptomatic volunteers. Spine 19:1475, 1994.
5. Snijders CJ, Vieeming A, Stoeckart R, et al: Transfer of lumbosacral load to iliac bones and legs. Part I: Biomechanics of self-bracing of the sacroiliac joints and its significance for treatment and exercise. Part II: Loading of the sacroiliac joints when lifting in a stooped posture. Clin Biomech 8:285, 1993.
6. Lavignolle B, Vital JM, Senegas J, et al: An approach to the functional anatomy of the sacroiliac joints in vivo. Anat Clin 5:169, 1983.
7. Thorstensson A, Nilsson J, Carlson H, Zomlefer MR: Trunk movements in human locomotion. Acta Physiol Scand 121:9, 1984.
8. Waldman SD: Sacroiliac joint injection. In Waldman SD (ed): Atlas of Interventional Pain Management. Philadelphia, WB Saunders, 2004, p 4291.

chapter 163

Neural Blockade of the Peripheral Nerves of the Lower Extremity

Debra A. DeAngelo and Vitaly Gordin

HISTORICAL CONSIDERATIONS

Neural blockade of the lower extremity is not a new technique. Braun mentions that blockade of the lateral cutaneous femoral nerve was described by Nystrom in 1909.[1] Laewen expanded on this technique by describing the additional blockade of the anterior crural nerve, and Keppler improved both techniques by advocating the elicitation of paresthesias.[2] Earlier than all of this activity—around 1887—Crile performed amputations by exposing the sciatic nerve in the gluteal fold and the femoral nerve in the inguinal fold and injecting cocaine intraneurally. Subsequently, no fewer than six others advocated percutaneous approaches to the sciatic nerve alone.[3]

Many of the old techniques are still used today, some with modifications such as the use of a peripheral nerve stimulator. Adequate peripheral nerve blockade still hinges on one's knowledge of the anatomy as emphasized by Labat: "Anatomy is the foundation upon which the entire concept of regional anesthesia is built"; that "landmarks are anatomic guideposts of the body which are used to locate the nerves"; that "superficial landmarks are distinguishing features of the surface of the body which can be easily recognized and identified by sight or palpation. Bones and their prominences, blood vessels and tendons serve as deep landmarks. Deep landmarks can be defined only by the point of the needle. They are the only reliable guide for advancing the needle in attempting to reach the vicinity of the nerve"; and that "the anesthetist should attempt to visualize the anatomic structures traversed by the needle and utilize the tactile senses to determine the impulses transmitted by the point of the needle as it approaches a deep landmark (e.g., bone)."[4]

Although peripheral neural blockade of the lower extremity has been described for greater than a century, its use is still limited in most practices when compared with blockade of the upper extremity. This limited use is most likely due to the ability to provide rapid, complete, and safe anesthesia of the lower extremity with neuraxial blockade. In addition, neural blockade of the upper extremity is accomplished with a single injection, which is not the case with the lower extremity. Despite these facts, neural blockade of the peripheral nerves of the lower extremity does have advantages and should be considered when deciding on an anesthetic technique.

INDICATIONS

Indications for neural blockade of the peripheral nerves of the lower extremity include management of acute pain, as well as diagnostic management of chronic pain syndromes. Regional anesthesia allows the surgical site to be anesthetized without the hemodynamic instability associated with neuraxial anesthesia and also gives the provider the ability to avoid general anesthesia if so desired. In addition, varying approaches to neural blockade add flexibility to accommodate the surgery in case of swelling or infection, for example, performing sciatic or popliteal blocks with or without a femoral nerve block if the surgical site is a swollen or infected foot. When deciding on regional anesthesia, one must be cognizant of the site, degree, and duration of the procedure and the requirements for pain control in the postoperative period in order to deliver safe and efficient anesthesia.

SCIATIC NERVE BLOCK

Indications

Blockade of the sciatic nerve is indicated when the distal part of the lower extremity and foot, with the exception of the medial aspect of the leg, needs to be anesthetized. Because of the sensory and cutaneous distribution of the sciatic nerve, few surgical procedures could be accomplished with a sciatic nerve block as the sole anesthetic. If combined with a saphenous nerve block, any surgery below the level of the knee may be performed.

Blockade of the sciatic nerve is also used to manage postoperative pain after surgery on the lower extremity performed under general anesthesia.

Clinically Relevant Anatomy

The sciatic nerve is formed from the anterior divisions of the L4, L5, and S1-3 nerves. These nerves fuse and exit the pelvis through the greater sciatic notch and then pass between the greater trochanter and ischial tuberosity.[5] The nerve becomes superficial at the lower border of the gluteus maximus muscle. From there, it courses down the posterior aspect of the thigh to the popliteal fossa, where it divides into the tibial and common peroneal nerves.[3] The sciatic nerve is both a sensory and a motor nerve and will include some sympathetic fibers originating in the lumbosacral plexus.[5] It is the largest of the four major nerves supplying the leg.

Technique

The sciatic nerve can be blocked by several techniques. The least complicated, most common, and most widely recognized is the peripheral approach, also known as the classic Labat technique. The patient is placed in a lateral position with the operative extremity uppermost. The extremity should be flexed at the knee and rest on the dependent extremity. The greater trochanter and the posterior superior iliac spine (PSIS) are identified, and the midpoint between the greater trochanter and PSIS is marked. A perpendicular line is drawn from the midpoint 4 cm caudad, and this point is marked as the entry site.[5] The skin is cleansed with iodine solution and prepared in sterile fashion.

The skin should be anesthetized over the entry site midway between the two landmarks with 1 to 2 mL of 0.5% lidocaine injected through a 1½-inch, 25-gauge needle. A 100-mm insulated stimulating needle is connected to a nerve stimulator (initial current, 1.5 mA, 2 Hz) and inserted perpendicular to all planes. As the needle is inserted, the gluteal muscles will contract. Once these contractions disappear and the needle is advanced further, stimulation of the sciatic nerve is achieved. The stimulation can be hamstrings twitches or the tibial or common peroneal nerves. Typically, twitch of the hamstrings muscles is observed first. With minimal further needle advancement, twitches of the foot are readily observed. When this maneuver fails to localize the sciatic nerve, the needle is withdrawn to the skin and redirected 15 degrees toward the greater trochanter. If this is also unsuccessful, the needle is again withdrawn to the skin and redirected in the opposite direction, 15 degrees toward the PSIS. The sciatic nerve is typically located at a depth of 5 to 8 cm in an average-sized adult patient. Once stimulation of the foot is achieved at 0.20 to 0.40 mA or less, 20 mL of local anesthetic is injected.[5] The local anesthetic used is determined by the length of blockade required: 1.5% mepivacaine or 1% to 2% lidocaine for intermediate-acting effect (onset time, 5 to 15 minutes and lasting approximately 1 hour) or 0.5% to 0.75% ropivacaine or 0.5% bupivacaine for long-acting effect (onset time, 20 to 30 minutes and lasting 2 to 3 hours). A combination of 0.5% bupivacaine and 1.5% mepivacaine in a 2 : 1 mixture can be used for quicker onset but longer duration of action. It is *not* recommended that epinephrine be added to this injection because of the lack of a prominent blood supply to the sciatic nerve, which would increase the risk for ischemia if vasoconstricted.

An alternative approach is to identify the greater trochanter and ischial tuberosity, insert the needle as described earlier, and advance the needle until a twitch is obtained. This technique eliminates the requirements of drawing lines on the patient but may be difficult in obese patients, in whom the landmarks are not readily identified.

Side Effects and Complications

The most common complication of sciatic nerve blockade is failure of the block. One must observe stimulation of the sciatic nerve and watch for foot twitches. Observing foot stimulation at 0.40 mA or less will greatly increase the success rate of the block. Stimulation at 0.20 mA or less indicates needle placement in too close proximity to the nerve and may result in paresthesias or intraneural injection. Other complications include hematoma formation in the gluteal region and local anesthesia toxicity as a result of rapid absorption. The speed of injection should not exceed 20 mL/min because of this risk for rapid absorption. As with any injection, there is a risk for infection, and thus sterile technique should always be used.

FEMORAL NERVE BLOCK

Indications

Blockade of the femoral nerve is indicated for both anesthesia and analgesia. Examples include situations in which the anterior aspect of the thigh needs to be anesthetized, such as for muscle biopsy or skin grafting, knee surgery such as arthroscopy or patella tendon repair, or repair of lacerations. It also may be used to provide relief of femoral shaft and neck fractures, as well as for postoperative pain relief after operations on the thigh, patella, and knee.[7] In addition, it is used as an adjunct to sciatic or popliteal nerve blocks to provide anesthesia to the entire lower extremity or the lower part of the leg.

Blockade of the femoral nerve has been shown to be an effective adjunct to general anesthesia for knee joint surgery. Postoperative opiate administration was reduced by 80% in the recovery room and by 40% in the first 24 hours postoperatively in patients receiving nerve blocks.[8]

Clinically Relevant Anatomy

The femoral nerve is the largest branch of the lumbar plexus. It emerges through the fibers of the psoas muscle and descends between the psoas and iliacus muscles. It passes under the inguinal ligament lateral to the femoral artery. It then divides into a superficial bundle, which is primarily sensory and innervates the skin of the anterior aspect of the thigh with a motor branch to the sartorius muscle, and a deep bundle, which is primarily motor and innervates the quadriceps muscle with some sensory fibers to the knee joint and medial aspect of the lower extremity. The femoral nerve terminates as the purely sensory saphenous nerve.[7] Therefore, the femoral nerve supplies sensation to the skin over the medial, anterior medial, and posterior medial aspects of the leg, from just above the knee to the great toe.

Technique

The patient is positioned in the supine position with the lower extremities fully extended. The femoral artery is identified and a point immediately lateral, along the femoral crease, is marked as the entry site.[6] The skin is prepared with iodine solution and draped in sterile fashion.

The skin overlying the entry site is anesthetized with 1 to 2 mL of 0.5% lidocaine injected through a 25-gauge, 1½-inch needle. A 22-gauge, 50-mm insulated short-beveled needle is attached to a stimulator (initial current, 1.0 mA, 2 Hz). The needle is inserted immediately lateral to the pulse while palpating the femoral artery pulse and advanced at a 60-degree angle posteriorly and cephalad. Contraction of the quadriceps muscle is the goal of this stimulation. The needle is redirected laterally in progressive fashion until the nerve is identified. Quadriceps contraction is not to be confused—and very commonly results in failure of this block—with contraction of the sartorius muscle. If sartorius contraction is obtained, the needle is redirected 15 degrees laterally and 1 to 2 mm deeper until the femoral nerve is identified. The ultimate goal is to achieve quadriceps muscle stimulation (patella twitches) at 0.4 mA or less. After negative aspiration for blood, 15 to 30 mL of local anesthetic is injected.[6] Local anesthetics used are again 1.5% mepivacaine or 1% to 2% lidocaine for intermediate-acting effect (onset time, 5 to 15 minutes) or 0.5% to 0.75% ropivacaine or 0.5% bupivacaine for long-acting effect (onset time, 20 to 30 minutes). Again, a combination of 0.5% bupivacaine and 1.5% mepivacaine in a 2:1 mixture can be used for quicker onset but longer duration of action. Epinephrine can be added at 1:300,000 to prolong this nerve block.

Side Effects and Complications

Complications of a femoral nerve block may include intravascular injection, either intraarterial or intravenous in the femoral artery or vein because of their close proximity to the femoral nerve. Care should be taken to aspirate for heme before injection of local anesthetic. Hematoma formation is also a risk associated with this injection because of the anatomic situation of the vasculature as compared with the nerve. The anesthesiologist should be alert for the presence of vascular grafts of the femoral artery, which would be a relative contraindication to elective femoral nerve block. Nerve injury is a possibility with intraneural injection. Needle positioning should be adjusted if stimulation is achieved at 0.20 mA or less.

Blockade of the obturator and lateral femoral cutaneous nerves may occur (3-in-1 block) with femoral nerve blockade. As with any injection, there is a risk for infection, and thus sterile technique should always be used.

LATERAL FEMORAL CUTANEOUS NERVE BLOCK

Indications

Blockade of the lateral femoral cutaneous nerve is indicated in conjunction with blockade of other nerves or by itself for skin grafting sites or for the treatment of meralgia paresthetica. It can also be useful for providing pain relief associated with the use of tourniquets.

Meralgia paresthetica is a pain syndrome believed to be caused by compression or injury to the lateral femoral cutaneous nerve. It causes pain emanating from the skin of the lateral aspect of the thigh. Meralgia paresthetica can be diagnosed and treated with a nerve block and neural destruction, if needed, of the lateral femoral cutaneous nerve.

Clinically Relevant Anatomy

The lateral femoral cutaneous nerve is derived from the L2-3 nerve roots and is purely a sensory nerve. It runs through the pelvis along the lateral border of the psoas muscle, deep to the iliac fascia and anterior to the iliacus muscle. It emerges through the fascia inferior and medial to the anterior superior iliac spine (ASIS) and divides into anterior and posterior branches. The anterior branch innervates the lateral aspect of the front of the thigh down to the knee. The posterior branch innervates the skin overlying the lateral portion of the buttock distal to the greater trochanter to approximately the middle of the thigh.

Technique

The patient is placed in the supine position. The ASIS is identified and a point 2 cm medial and 2 cm inferior is selected as the entry site. The skin is cleansed with alcohol.

The skin is anesthetized with 1 to 2 mL of 0.5% lidocaine injected through a 25-gauge, 1½-inch needle. A 3- to 4-cm needle is inserted perpendicular to the skin through the fascia lata. The fascia lata is identified when the operator feels a "pop" or a "release" as the needle passes through it. After careful aspiration, 10 to 15 mL of local anesthetic is injected above and below the fascia in a medial-to-lateral fan-like distribution to ensure covering the nerve branches. If performing this block for surgical anesthesia, 0.5% bupivacaine or 0.5% ropivacaine is used. For treatment of meralgia paresthetica, a mixture of 5 mL of 0.5% bupivacaine, 4 mL of Sarapin, and 40 mg of methylprednisolone (Depo-Medrol) can be used.

Side Effects and Complications

Complications are quite rare with blockade of the lateral femoral cutaneous nerve. Theoretically, direct nerve injury may result from intraneural injection but is unlikely. Local hematoma may occur but is very unlikely because of the lack of large blood vessels in the area. As with any injection, there is a risk for infection and therefore sterile technique should always be used.

OBTURATOR NERVE BLOCK

Indications

Obturator nerve blockade is indicated in conjunction with blockade of other nerves such as the lateral femoral cutaneous, the femoral, and the sciatic for surgical procedures on the lower extremity. It can be used alone to alleviate adductor spasms of the hip and reduce pain in the hip joint. It can be perfromed as a diagnostic tool for pain syndromes in the hip joint, inguinal area, or lumbar spine.

Clinically Relevant Anatomy

The obturator nerve is derived from L2-4 and travels along the medial border of the psoas muscle; it is both a motor and a sensory nerve. It travels through the obturator foramen with the obturator artery and vein into the thigh. The obturator nerve divides into anterior and posterior branches. The anterior branch provides motor innervation to the superficial adductors and sensory innervation to the hip joint and medial aspect of the distal part of the thigh. The posterior branch provides motor innervation to the deep adductors and sensory innervation to the posterior knee joint.

Technique

The patient is placed in the supine position with the affected extremity slightly abducted and the knee slightly flexed. The pubic tubercle on the side to be anesthetized is identified. Two centimeters lateral and 2 cm caudad to the pubic tubercle is the entry site. The skin is prepared with iodine solution and draped in sterile fashion.

The skin overlying the entry site is anesthetized with 1 to 2 mL of 0.5% lidocaine injected through a 25-gauge, 1½-inch needle. A 22-gauge, 100-mm insulated stimulating needle is connected to a nerve stimulator (initial current, 2 to 3 mA, 2 Hz) and inserted perpendicular to the skin until the inferior border of the superior ramus of the pubic bone is contacted at a depth of approximately 1.5 to 4 cm.

The needle is then slightly withdrawn and redirected posteriorly and laterally to walk off the inferior margin of the superior pubic ramus. At 2 to 3 cm, the needle is in close proximity to the obturator canal. The adductor muscles twitches should be seen and felt at a current intensity of 0.5 mA or less, at which point 10 mL of local anesthetic is injected. Local anesthetics used are again 1.5% mepivacaine or 1% to 2% lidocaine for intermediate-acting effect (onset time, 5 to 15 minutes) or 0.5% to 0.75% ropivacaine or 0.5% bupivacaine for long-acting effect (onset time, 20 to 30 minutes). Again, a combination of 0.5% bupivacaine and 1.5% mepivacaine in a 2 : 1 mixture can be used for quicker onset but longer duration of action.

Alternative approaches can also be used for an obturator nerve block:

- Interadductor approach—The patient is placed in the supine position, and a mark is made on the skin 1 to 2 cm medial to the femoral artery and immediately below the inguinal ligament to denote the direction of the needle toward the obturator canal. The adductor longus tendon is identified near its pubic insertion. A 22-gauge, 100-mm insulated stimulating needle is introduced behind the adductor longus tendon and directed laterally, with slight posterosuperior inclination, toward the skin mark. The needle is advanced toward the obturator canal until stimulation of the adductor muscles is still visible at a current of 0.5 mA or less.
- Three-in-one block—This block is similar to a femoral nerve block except that digital pressure is applied distal to the site of injection and large volumes of local anesthetic (30 mL or more) are used. This results in substantial cephalad spread of local anesthetic under the fascia iliaca and blocks the remaining branches of the lumbar plexus: the femoral, obturator, and lateral femoral cutaneous nerves of the thigh.

Side Effects and Complications

Because intravascular injection into the obturator artery or vein may occur, careful aspiration before injection should be performed. Damage to the pelvic organs, such as the bladder, rectum, vagina, or spermatic cord, can occur. The depth of needle placement should be noted, and the needle should not be advanced more than 3 cm into the pelvis to decrease the incidence of this complication. As with any injection, there is a risk for infection and thus sterile technique should always be used.

NERVE BLOCKS AROUND THE KNEE

Three major nerve trunks can be blocked at the level of the knee: the posterior tibial, the common peroneal, and the saphenous. When the posterior tibial and the common peroneal nerves are blocked at the popliteal fossa, it is referred to as a popliteal block.

Indications

Blockade of the posterior tibial, common peroneal, and saphenous nerves can be performed at the popliteal fossa to provide surgical analgesia from the knee down. Lack of access to these nerves more proximally and reduced doses of local anesthetic make them valuable to justify one's familiarity with these techniques. A wide variety of procedures can be performed with this technique, including removal of soft and bony tumors, ankle procedures, and operations on the foot requiring a tourniquet.

Clinically Relevant Anatomy

The sciatic nerve bifurcates in the distal part of the thigh into the tibial nerve and the common peroneal nerve. The tibial nerve often arises at the upper end of the popliteal fossa, although the sciatic nerve can bifurcate more superiorly. The tibial nerve is the larger of the two terminal branches of the sciatic nerve and has both a muscular branch to the back of the leg and cutaneous branches in the popliteal fossa and down the back of the leg to the ankle. The common peroneal nerve is about half the size of the tibial nerve and provides articular innervation to the knee joint; cutaneous innervation to the lateral side of the leg, heel, and ankle; and motor innervation to the muscles of the anterior lateral compartment of the lower part of the leg.[9]

The posterior tibial nerve provides motor innervation to the back of the lower part of the leg and cutaneous innervation from the popliteal fossa to the ankle, as well as the sole of the foot. The posterior tibial nerve then divides into the plantar digital nerves.[9]

Technique

Three different approaches for performing a popliteal block have been described. The posterior approach requires the patient to be placed in the prone position. The lateral approach requires contact with periosteum but allows the patient to remain in the supine position. The lithotomy approach again allows the patient to remain in the supine position and uses the same landmarks as for the posterior approach. It should be remembered than none of the popliteal blocks anesthetize the saphenous nerve; therefore, this nerve must be blocked separately.

Posterior Approach

The patient is placed in the prone position with the feet extending beyond the edge of the table to allow interpretation of the twitches. The landmarks identified are the popliteal fossa crease, the tendon of the biceps femoris laterally, and the tendons of the semitendinosus and semimembranosus medially. These landmarks can easily be identified in all patients, even obese ones, by asking the patient to flex the leg at the knee joint. The entry site is the midpoint between the two tendons, 7 cm above the popliteal fossa crease.[6] The skin is prepared with iodine solution and draped in sterile fashion.

The skin overlying the entry site is anesthetized with 1 to 2 mL of 0.5% lidocaine injected through a 25-gauge, 1½-inch needle. A 22-gauge, 50-mm insulated short-beveled needle is attached to a stimulator (initial current, 1.5 mA, 2 Hz). The stimulating needle is inserted perpendicular to the skin while observing for plantar flexion *or* dorsiflexion of the foot with currents of 0.4 mA or less. If stimulation cannot be achieved with currents of 0.4 mA, the tibial twitch (plantar flexion) is more reliable in achieving blockade of both branches of the sciatic nerve. If no stimulation is elicited, the needle should be withdrawn and redirected laterally because more medial insertion is less likely to result in nerve localization and carries a risk of puncturing the popliteal artery and vein. If no stimulation is observed after redirection of the needle, the injection should be repeated through a new insertion site 5 mm laterally until the desired response is obtained. If stimulation of the biceps femoris muscle occurs, the needle is in too lateral a position and the needle should be redirected slightly medially. Once the tibial nerve (plantar flexion) or the common peroneal nerve (dorsiflexion) is stimulated, 40 to 50 mL of local anesthetic is injected.[6] Local anesthetics used are 1.5% mepivacaine for intermediate-acting effect (onset time, 5 to 15 minutes) or 0.5% to 0.75% ropivacaine for long-acting effect (onset time, 20 to 30 minutes). Again, a combination of 0.5% bupivacaine and 1.5% mepivacaine in a 2:1 mixture can be used for quicker onset but longer duration of action. Epinephrine can be added at 1:300,000 to prolong this nerve block.

Lateral Approach

The patient is placed in the supine position. The leg is extended and the foot is positioned at a 90-degree angle relative to the table. Landmarks include the lateral femoral epicondyle and the biceps femoris and vastus lateralis muscles. The entry site is 7 cm cephalad to the most prominent point of the lateral femoral epicondyle and in the groove between the two muscles. The skin is prepared with iodine solution and draped in sterile fashion.[6]

The skin overlying the entry site is anesthetized with 1 to 2 mL of 0.5% lidocaine injected through a 25-gauge, 1½-inch needle. A 100-mm insulated stimulating needle is connected to a nerve stimulator (initial current, 1.5 mA, 2 Hz) and inserted in a horizontal plane until the shaft of the femoral bone is contacted. Once the femoral bone is contacted, the needle is withdrawn to the skin and redirected posteriorly at a 30-degree angle to the horizontal plane. Again, the operator is watching for stimulation of either the tibial or the common peroneal nerve at a current of 0.4 mA or less. If no stimulation is achieved, the needle should be redirected first 5 to 10 degrees anterior and then 5 to 10 degrees posterior through the same skin puncture. If this does not lead to nerve localization, the same technique is repeated through new skin punctures in 5-mm increments posterior to the initial insertion plane. Once the tibial nerve (plantar flexion) or the common peroneal nerve (dorsiflexion) is stimulated, 40 to 50 mL of local anesthetic is injected.[6] Local anesthetics used are 1.5% mepivacaine for intermediate-acting effect (onset time, 5 to 15 minutes) or 0.5% to 0.75% ropivacaine for long-acting effect (onset time, 20 to 30 minutes). Again, a combination of 0.5% bupivacaine and 1.5% mepivacaine in a 2:1 mixture can be used for quicker onset but longer duration of action. Epinephrine can be added at 1:300,000 to prolong this nerve block.

Lithotomy Approach

The patient is placed in the supine position. The leg is flexed at both the hip and knee joints and supported by an assistant. Landmarks are the same as for the posterior approach: the popliteal fossa crease, the tendon of the biceps femoris (laterally), and the tendons of the semitendinosus and semimembranosus medially. The entry site is the midpoint of the two tendons, 7 cm above the popliteal fossa crease. The skin is prepared with iodine solution and draped in sterile fashion.

The skin overlying the entry site is anesthetized with 1 to 2 mL of 0.5% lidocaine injected through a 25-gauge, 1½-inch needle. A 22-gauge, 50-mm insulated short-beveled needle is attached to a stimulator (initial current, 1.5 mA, 2 Hz). The stimulating needle is inserted at a 45-degree angle cephalad while observing for plantar flexion *or* dorsiflexion of the foot with currents of 0.4 mA or less. If no stimulation is observed, the needle is withdrawn and redirected 5 to 10 degrees laterally until the desired response is obtained. If no stimulation is achieved, the needle is removed and reinserted through another entry site 5 mm lateral to the initial site. Once the tibial nerve (plantar flexion) or the common peroneal nerve (dorsiflexion) is stimulated, 40 to 50 mL of local anesthetic is injected. Local anesthetics used are 1.5% mepivacaine for intermediate-acting effect (onset time, 5 to 15 minutes) or 0.5% to 0.75% ropivacaine for long-acting effect (onset time, 20 to 30 minutes). Again, a combination of 0.5% bupivacaine and 1.5% mepivacaine in a 2 : 1 mixture can be used for quicker onset but longer duration of action. Epinephrine can be added at 1 : 300,000 to prolong this nerve block.

The saphenous nerve may be blocked by injecting 5 mL of local anesthetic (any of the aforementioned mixtures) in a subcutaneous ring from the medial aspect of the tibia to the border of the patellar tendon.

Side Effects and Complications

Complications with these nerve blockades are extremely rare. Careful aspiration should be performed to prevent intravascular injection. Nerve injury is a possibility with intraneural injection. Needle positioning should be adjusted if stimulation is obtained at 0.20 mA or less. As with any injection, there is a risk for infection and therefore sterile technique should always be used.

NERVE BLOCKS AT THE ANKLE

Five branches of the principal nerve trunks supply the ankle and foot: the posterior tibial, sural, superficial peroneal (musculocutaneous), deep peroneal (anterior tibial), and saphenous. These nerves are relatively easy to block at the ankle.

Indications

The posterior tibial, sural, superficial peroneal, deep peroneal, and saphenous nerves can be blocked at the ankle to provide surgical analgesia of the foot for procedures such as treatment of Morton neuroma, operations on the great toe, amputation of the midfoot and toes, and incision and drainage. An adjunct nerve block may be required if a tourniquet is being used.

Clinically Relevant Anatomy

The tibial nerve is the larger of the two branches of the sciatic nerve and reaches the distal part of the leg from the medial side of the Achilles tendon, where it lies behind the posterior tibial artery. It divides into medial and lateral branches, with the medial branch supplying the medial two thirds of the sole and the plantar portion of the medial 3½ toes up to the nail. The lateral branch supplies the lateral third of the sole and the plantar portion of the lateral 1½ toes.[3]

The sural nerve is a cutaneous nerve that arises through the union of a branch from the tibial nerve and one from the common peroneal nerve. It becomes subcutaneous distal to the middle of the leg and proceeds along with the short saphenous vein behind and below the lateral malleolus to supply the lower posterolateral surface of the leg, the lateral side of the foot, and the lateral part of the fifth toe.[3]

The common peroneal divides into the superficial and deep peroneal nerves. The superficial peroneal nerve perforates the deep fascia on the anterior aspect of the distal two thirds of the leg and runs subcutaneously to supply the dorsum of the foot and toes, except for the contiguous surfaces of the great and second toes.[3]

The deep peroneal nerve descends down the anterior aspect of the interosseous membrane of the leg and continues midway between the malleoli onto the dorsum of the foot. Here it divides into medial and lateral branches of the plantar nerves, with the medial branch dividing into two dorsal digital branches that innervate the adjacent sides of the first and second digits. At the level of the foot, the anterior tibial artery lies medial to the nerve, as does the tendon of the extensor hallucis longus muscle.[3]

The saphenous nerve, which is the sensory terminal branch of the femoral nerve, becomes subcutaneous at the lateral side of the knee joint. It then follows the great saphenous vein to the medial malleolus and supplies the cutaneous area over the medial side of the lower part of the leg, anterior to the medial malleolus and the medial part of the foot and as far forward as the midportion.[3]

Technique

The patient is placed in the supine position with the foot on a footrest. The posterior tibial nerve is located just behind and distal to the medial malleolus. The pulse of the posterior tibial artery can be felt at this location; the nerve is just posterior to the artery.[6]

The deep peroneal nerve is located immediately lateral to the tendon of the extensor hallucis longus muscle. The pulse of the anterior tibial artery (dorsalis pedis) can be felt at this location; the nerve is immediately lateral to the artery.[6]

The superficial peroneal, sural, and saphenous nerves are located in subcutaneous tissue along a circular line stretching from the lateral aspect of the Achilles tendon across the lateral malleolus, anterior aspect of the foot, and medial malleolus to the medial aspect of the Achilles tendon.[6]

The skin of the entire foot is prepared with iodine solution and draped in sterile fashion. This procedure should begin with the two deep nerves because subcutaneous injections for the superficial blocks inevitably deform the anatomy.

Deep Peroneal Block

After palpation of the groove just lateral to the extensor hallucis longus with a finger, a 25-gauge, 1½-inch needle with 5 mL of lidocaine is inserted under the skin and advanced until stopped by bone. The needle is then withdrawn 1 to 2 mm and the previously listed anesthetic is injected after a negative aspiration.[6]

Posterior Tibial Block

A 25-gauge, 1½-inch needle with 5 mL of lidocaine is inserted in the groove behind the medial malleolus and advanced until contact is made with bone. The needle is withdrawn 1 to 2 mm and the aforementioned medication is injected after a negative aspiration.[6]

Saphenous Block

A 25-gauge, 1½-inch needle with 5 mL of lidocaine is inserted at the level of the medial malleolus, and a "ring" of local anesthetic is raised from the point of needle entry to the Achilles tendon and anteriorly to the tibial ridge.[6]

Superficial Peroneal Block

A 25-gauge, 1½-inch needle with 5 mL of lidocaine is inserted at the tibial ridge and extended laterally toward the lateral malleolus. It is important to raise a subcutaneous "wheal" during injection, which indicates a proper, superficial plane.[6]

Sural Block

A 25-gauge, 1½-inch needle with 5 mL of lidocaine is inserted at the level of the lateral malleolus, and the local anesthetic is infiltrated toward the Achilles tendon. The previously mentioned medication is injected is a circular fashion to raise a skin wheal.[6]

Side Effects and Complications

Complications from ankle blocks are rare, but residual paresthesias can occur as a result of inadvertent intraneuronal injection. Epinephrine-containing solutions should be avoided because of the risk for ischemia. As with any injection, there is a risk for infection and thus sterile technique should always be used.

DIGITAL NERVE BLOCK OF THE FOOT

Indications

A digital nerve block of the foot is indicated for limited procedures involving one or two digits or for postoperative pain relief.

Clinically Relevant Anatomy

Each nerve passes through the intermetatarsal space alongside each toe. The sole of the foot is innervated primarily by the posterior tibial nerve. After passing behind the medial malleolus, the posterior tibial nerve divides into the plantar digital nerves. The plantar digital nerves are larger than the dorsal digital nerves and terminally send twigs onto the dorsum of the phalanx. The digital branch of the lateral plantar nerve supplies the lateral $1\frac{1}{2}$ toes. The digital branch of the medial plantar nerve supplies the medial $3\frac{1}{2}$ toes. The dorsum of the foot is innervated by the superficial and deep peroneal nerves. The deep peroneal nerve divides at the extensor retinaculum into medial and lateral branches. The medial branch divides into two dorsal digital branches that innervate adjacent sides of the first and second digits. The superficial peroneal nerve innervates the dorsum of the rest of the toes.[9]

Technique

The patient is placed in the supine position, and the skin is prepared with iodine solution and draped in sterile fashion. Skin wheals are raised over the distal intermetatarsal space. A total of 2 to 3 mL of a non–epinephrine-containing local anesthetic solution such as 0.5% lidocaine or 0.25% bupivacaine is injected in a fan-like fashion subcutaneously, as well as deep to the metatarsals, to ensure blockade of both the dorsal and plantar digital nerves. Blockade can also be performed at the level of the digits by injecting skin wheals into the web space of the dorsal surface on either side of the digit to be blocked.[9]

Side Effects and Complications

Complications are extremely rare. Large volumes of local anesthetic– and epinephrine-containing solution should not be used to avoid the risk of vascular compromise to the digits. As with any injection, there is a risk for infection and therefore sterile technique should always be used.

CONCLUSION

Neural blockade of the lower extremity can be a very useful tool in an anesthesiologist's armamentarium. It is easily accomplished, with minimal side effects, and can provide complete anesthesia of the lower extremity. To obtain good anesthesia when performing these procedures, several important facts must be kept in mind. First, when using a peripheral nerve stimulator, obtaining a nonspecific twitch at high milliamperage may result in a failed block. Second, one must remember not only the dermatomes but also the myotomes and osteotomes for the surgical procedures to be performed. Finally, appropriate local anesthetic to last the duration of the procedure should be used and enough time allowed for the block to fully function before surgical intervention.

As stated earlier, peripheral blockade of the lower extremity is not a new technique. For more than a century physicians have been anesthetizing the nerves of the lower extremity. The difference has occurred in the technology and pharmacology through the years, both of which have only been improving the results of our forefathers.

References

1. Braun H: Anesthesia—Its Scientific Basis and Practical Use, 2nd ed. Philadelphia, Lea & Febiger, 1924, p 3.
2. Lawen A: Ueber segmentare Schmerzaufhebung durch papavertebrale Novokaininjektionen zur Differentialdiagnose intra-abdominaler Erkrankungen. Med Wochenschr 69:1423, 1922.
3. Bridenbaugh P, Wedel D, Cousins MJ: Neural Blockade in Clinical Anesthesia and Management of Pain, 3rd ed. Philadelphia, Lippincott-Raven, 1998, p 373.
4. Labat G: Regional Anesthesia: Its Technic and Clinical Application. Philadelphia, WB Saunders, 1924, p 45.
5. Broadman L: The sciatic nerve. In Hahn MB, McQuillan PM, Sheplock GJ (eds): Regional Anesthesia, An Atlas of Anatomy and Techniques. St Louis, CV Mosby, 1996, p 127.
6. Hadzic A, Vloka J: Peripheral Nerve Blocks, Principles and Practice. New York, McGraw-Hill, 2004, p 234.
7. McQuillan P: The femoral nerve. In Hahn MB, McQuillan PM, Sheplock G (eds): Regional Anesthesia, An Atlas of Anatomy and Techniques. St Louis, CV Mosby, 1996, p 139.
8. Edwards ND, Wright EM: Continuous low-dose 3-in-1 nerve blockade for postoperative pain relief after total knee replacement. Anesth Analg 75:265, 1992.
9. Keifer J, McQuillan P, Hahn M, Sheplock G: Peripheral nerves at the ankle. In Hahn MB, McQuillan PM, Sheplock GJ (eds): Regional Anesthesia, An Atlas of Anatomy and Techniques. St Louis, CV Mosby, 1996, p 151.

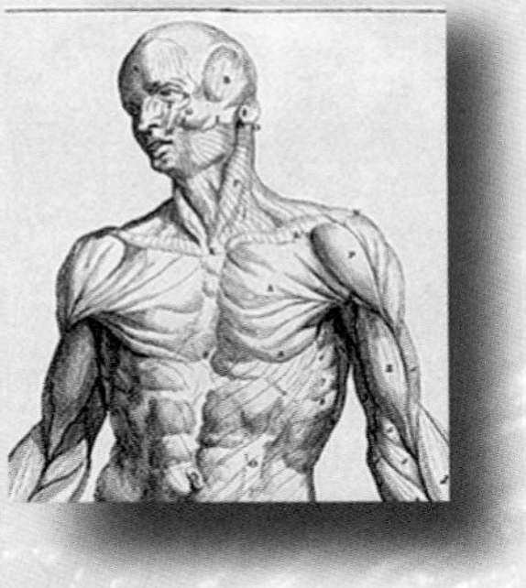

Part E

Neuroaugmentation and Implantable Drug Delivery Systems

chapter 164

Peripheral Nerve Stimulation

Matthew P. Rupert, Miles Day, and Gabor Racz

HISTORICAL CONSIDERATIONS

The application of electricity to treat pain dates back to ancient times, although its modern use began in the 1960s. Egyptians and Greeks were known to place electrogenic torpedo fish over painful areas in hopes of eliciting a cure. Along with the introduction of the gate-control theory of pain in 1965, peripheral nerve stimulation was implemented by placing cuffed electrodes around the affected nerve.[1,2] Cuffed electrodes soon gave way to flat, paddle electrodes.[3] Paddle-type electrodes are less constrictive and have the advantage of less scarring and nerve injury.[4] Nerve stimulation technology has advanced to include a variety of multicontact flat electrodes powered by internal and radiofrequency systems. Peripheral nerve stimulation has found its niche in treating patients with identifiable nerve injuries who have failed conservative and less invasive interventional therapies.

The mechanism of action of peripheral nerve stimulation is not entirely understood, but peripheral and central theories have been proposed. Campbell and Taub[5] showed a sensory loss in human subjects in the distribution of a peripherally stimulated nerve that was associated with a loss in the A-δ component of the afferent action potential. Wall and Gutnick[6] showed a reduction in the rate of spontaneous neuroma firing that outlasted a peripherally applied electrical stimulus. Based on a central gate-control theory, Chung and associates[7] showed inhibition of spinothalamic tract transmission in primates after applying a peripheral electrical stimulation. This central response also was shown to outlast the initiating peripheral stimulus. A better understanding of multicontact electrodes allows some adjustment of the applied electrical field.[8]

INDICATIONS

Peripheral nerve stimulation is indicated for neuropathic pain in a single nerve distribution that failed less invasive treatments. This technology most commonly has been used to treat painful conditions of the median, radial, ulnar, sciatic, posterior tibial, and common peroneal nerves. It also has been used to treat neuralgias of the intercostal, ilioinguinal, occipital, superior cluneal, supraorbital, and supratrochlear.[9,10] Other indications include complex regional pain syndromes, plexus avulsions, and electrical injuries.[11] Cancer pain, idiopathic pain, and nerve root injury pain have generally been found unresponsive to peripheral nerve stimulation.[12]

As with any implantable technology, patient selection is multifactorial. It is important to rule out correctable pathology, such as nerve entrapment. Complete patient evaluation should include psychological assessment, and there should be no evidence of drug abuse. A trial with transcutaneous electrical nerve stimulation is suggested, although not required.[13] A positive diagnostic block of the suspected nerve with local anesthetic is likewise suggested. Temporary relief with such a block does not guarantee peripheral nerve stimulation will work, but a negative diagnostic block suggests that peripheral nerve stimulation is unlikely to help.[2] Adherence to these criteria may improve success rates.

CLINICALLY RELEVANT ANATOMY

The key to peripheral nerve stimulation implantation is correct identification of the offending peripheral nerve through history, physical examination, and diagnostic blockade. There is no specific limitation as to what nerves can be targeted for stimulation. When identified, exposure and electrode placement can be performed by a qualified surgeon. Physical constraints include size of electrode, anatomic restrictions, and proximity of other nerves. Hardware placement should not impinge on surrounding structures through ranges of motion. It also is undesirable to stimulate nontargeted nerves. Some superficial nerves can be approached by percutaneous placement of cylindrical leads. Examples include occipital, supraorbital, supratrochlear, and superior cluneal nerves.

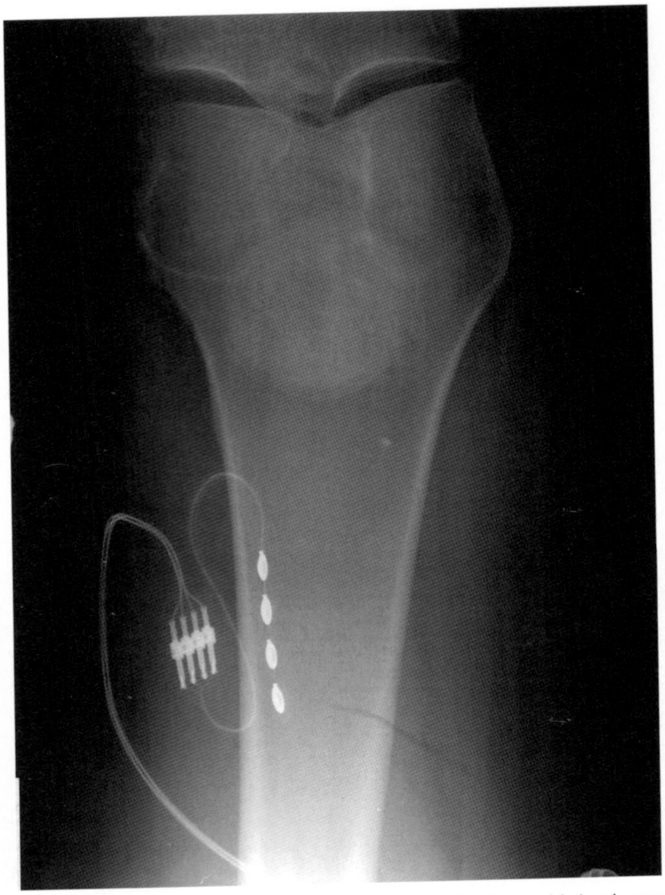

FIGURE 164–1 ■ Left sciatic peripheral nerve stimulator with 1 × 4 array OnPoint lead.

TECHNIQUE

Peripheral nerve stimulator placement is a two-stage procedure: a trial and a permanent implantation. The trial can be performed via a surgical incision or percutaneously. Both can be implanted with an extension lead for immediate conversion to a permanent lead if the trial is positive. An externalized percutaneous trial lead also can be performed so that a negative trial can be removed without a second surgery. The surgical trial and permanent pulse generator placement are described first (Figs. 164–1 and 164–2).

The site for electrode placement is usually proximal to the site of injury. An intimate understanding of the surgical anatomy is imperative. The surgical incision and dissection are taken down to the neurovascular bundle. A 2-inch section of the nerve is freed from surrounding tissues, taking care not to disrupt any blood supply. The selected electrode is secured with sutures immediately below the nerve with the active leads facing the nerve. Next, a piece of fascia is sutured directly to the electrode covering the active leads (Fig. 164–3). This step is recommended to minimize irritation and scarring of the nerve to the electrode. The nerve is allowed to rest in its normal position, and overlying tissue is loosely secured to maintain proximity of the nerve to the electrode. The lead is connected to an extension set and secured below the skin. The limb is taken through a full range of motion to rule out impingement or increased tension before the primary incision is closed. The extension lead is externalized for trial with a temporary stimulator (standard Medtronic screener 7431), usually for 2 to 3 days.

If the trial is positive, the patient returns to the operating room for implantation of the permanent pulse generator. Upper extremity and occipital nerve generators can be placed on the upper chest wall. Lower extremity generators can be placed over the medial thigh or the lateral buttocks. The generator is secured to the underlying fascia with suture. A new extension set is connected from the lead to the generator through a new subcutaneous tunnel. The old extension is then removed, either by preparing and cutting it at the skin and pulling inward or by cutting at the connection and pulling outward. If the trial is ineffective or uncomfortable, the patient requires a second surgery for hardware removal.

Percutaneous cylindrical leads can be placed for terminal branches of peripheral nerves. The lead can be placed with an extension as above or by itself as a trial. The advantage of a single lead wire is the ease of removal if the trial is negative. If positive, this requires a second surgery at a later date for the permanent lead. The inability to visualize the proximity of the electrode and the nerve is the main disadvantage. Placement is confirmed with on-table stimulation and patient confirmation.

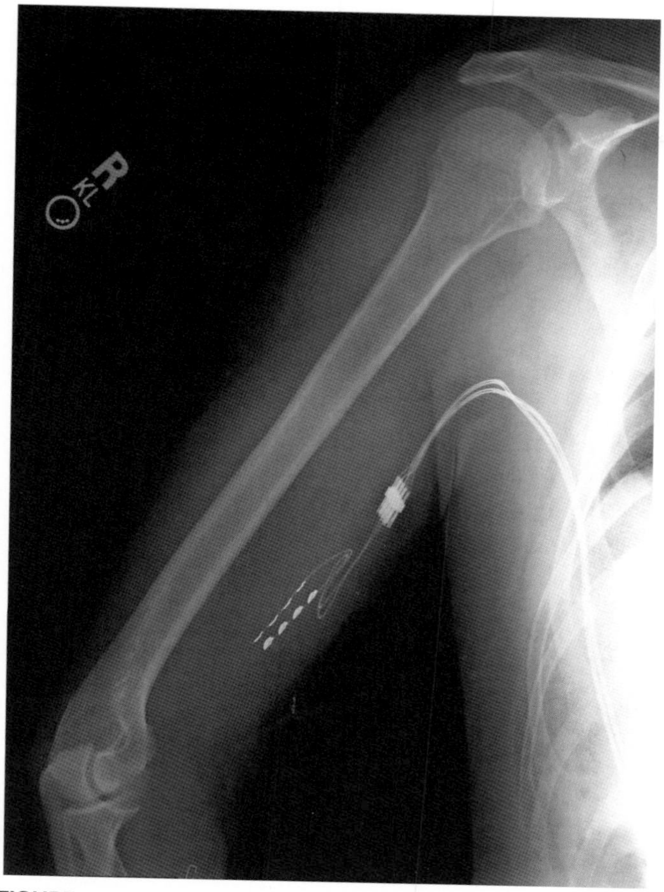

FIGURE 164–2 ■ Right ulnar peripheral nerve stimulator with 2 × 4 array lead.

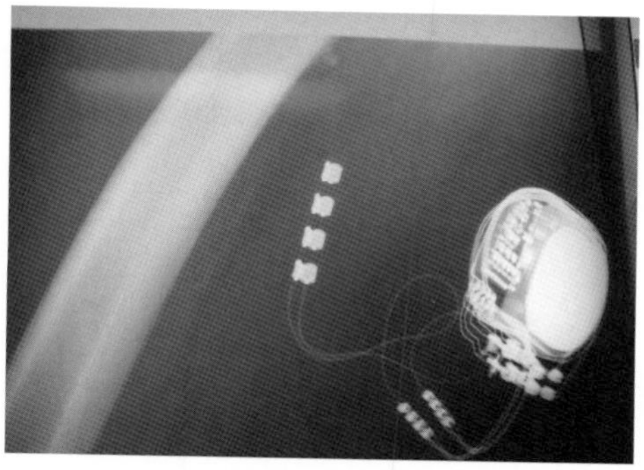

FIGURE 164–3 ■ Peripheral nerve stimulating electrode applied to the sciatic nerve above the bifurcation. Two on-point Medtronic electrodes are sutured together in a saddle shape with nonabsorbable sutures. The active electrodes are covered with a thin layer of harvested fascia and the Dacron skirt of the electrode loosely stitched around the nerve with an absorbable suture. The appropriate location of the electrodes is verified by motor or tetanic stimulation in order to cover the targeted tibialis and/or peroneal nerves.

SIDE EFFECTS AND COMPLICATIONS

Potential complications associated with peripheral nerve stimulators are similar to complications associated with other implantable technology. Infection and bioincompatibility are possible. Nerve injury, scarring, and associated ischemia have occurred, but the use of longitudinal rather than cuffed electrodes and an overlying fascial flap are believed to minimize these risks. It is possible the patient may have no response, an uncomfortable response, or aberrant sensory or motor stimulation. The use of multicontact electrodes allows some titration of effect. Mechanical problems, such as lead fractures, electrode shorts, lead migration, and battery depletion, are possible. Implanted batteries can interfere with pacemakers and can channel electrical and magnetic fields. The units should be turned off when electrocautery or electrocardiogram is to be performed. An implanted generator is a contraindication for MRI.

CONCLUSION

Peripheral nerve stimulators have shown efficacy in many clinical settings of chronic neuropathic pain in a single nerve distribution. Implantable technology is invasive and expensive; adequate conservative and less invasive methods should be tried first. Peripheral and central mechanisms of action have been postulated. Patient selection is multifactorial and should include a psychological assessment and absence of correctable pathology. Patients should have positive screening procedures such as diagnostic nerve blockade and a period of trial stimulation before placement of permanent equipment. The use of transcutaneous nerve stimulation can be helpful but is not diagnostic or prognostic for the use of peripheral nerve stimulation. Electrode implantation is dictated by the specific nerve anatomy, which may require surgical exposure or may be amenable to percutaneous placement. Advances in clinical strategies, electrode design, and neuroscience research are likely to pave the road for future changes. Treatment of mononeuropathy is more effective with peripheral nerve stimulation than with spinal cord stimulation.[14] In the modern treatment of chronic regional pain syndrome, the earlier use of neuromoducation techniques is recommended.[15,16]

References

1. Wall PD, Sweet WH: Temporary abolition of pain in man. Science 155:108, 1967.
2. Sweet WH: Control of pain by direct electrical stimulation of peripheral nerves. Clin Neurosurg 23:103, 1976.
3. Racz GB, Browne T, Lewis R: Peripheral nerve stimulator for treatment of nerve injury (causalgia) caused by electrical burns. Report of two cases. Texas Med 84:45, 1988.
4. Nielson D, Watts C, Clark W: Peripheral nerve injury from implantation of chronic stimulating electrodes for pain control. Surg Neurol 5:51, 1976.
5. Campbell JN, Taub A: Local analgesia from percutaneous electrical stimulation: A peripheral mechanism. Arch Neurol 28:347, 1973.
6. Wall PD, Gutnick M: Properties of afferent nerve impulses originating from a neuroma. Nature 248:740, 1974.
7. Chung JM, Lee K, Hori Y, et al: Factors influencing peripheral nerve stimulation produced inhibition of primate spinothalamic tract cells. Pain 19:277, 1984.
8. Alo KM, Holsheimer J: New trends in neuromodulation for the management of neuropathic pain. Neurosurgery 50:690, 2004.

9. Weiner RL, Reed KL: Peripheral neuromodulation for control of intractable occipital neuralgia. Neuromodulation 2:217, 1999.
10. Eisenburg E, Waisbrod H, Gerbershagen HU: Long term peripheral nerve stimulation for painful nerve injuries. Clin J Pain 20:143, 2004.
11. Racz GB, Lewis R, Heavner JE, Scott J: Peripheral nerve stimulator implant for treatment of causalgia. In Stanton-Hicks M (ed): Pain and the Sympathetic Nervous System. Boston, Kluwer Academic Publishers, 1990, p 225.
12. Nashold BS, Goldner JL, Mullen JB, Bright DS: Long-term pain control by direct peripheral nerve stimulation. J Bone Joint Surg Am 64:1, 1982.
13. Picaza JA, Hunter SE, Canon BW: Pain suppression by peripheral nerve stimulation. Appl Neurophysiol 52:482, 1977/78.
14. Calvillo O, Racz GB, Diede J, Smith K: Neuroaugmentation in the treatment of complex regional pain syndrome of the upper extremity. Acta Orthopa Belg 64:57, 1998.
15. Stanton-Hicks MD, Racz GB, et al: Interdisciplinary clinical pathway for CRPS: Report of an expert panel. World Institute of Pain, Pain Practice 2:1, 2002.
16. Shetter AG, Racz GB, Lewis R, Heavner JE: Peripheral nerve stimulation. In North R (ed): Neurosurgical Management of Pain. New York, Springer-Verlag, 1997

chapter 165

Spinal Cord Stimulation

Allen W. Burton

Spinal cord stimulation (SCS) describes the use of pulsed electrical energy near the spinal cord to control pain.[1,2] This technique was first applied in the intrathecal space and finally in the epidural space as described by Shealy in 1967.[2] In the present day, most commonly SCS involves the implantation of leads in the epidural space to transmit this pulsed energy across the spinal cord or near the desired nerve roots. This technique has notable analgesic properties for neuropathic pain states, anginal pain, and peripheral ischemic pain. The same technology can be applied in deep brain stimulation, cortical brain stimulation, and peripheral nerve stimulation (PNS).[3-6]

MECHANISM OF ACTION

Neurostimulation began shortly after Melzack and Wall proposed the gate control theory in 1965.[6] This theory proposed that painful peripheral stimuli carried by C-fibers and lightly myelinated A-delta fibers terminated at the substantia gelatinosa of the dorsal horn (the gate). Large myelinated A-beta fibers responsible for touch and vibratory sensation also terminated at "the gate" in the dorsal horn. It was hypothesized that their input could be manipulated to "close the gate" to the transmission of painful stimuli. As an application of the gate control theory, Shealy implanted the first spinal cord stimulator device for the treatment of chronic pain.[2] This technique was noted to control pain, and has undergone numerous technical and clinical refinements in the ensuing years. Although the gate theory was initially proposed as the mechanism of action, the underlying neurophysiologic mechanisms are not clearly understood.

The neurophysiologic mechanisms of action of spinal cord stimulation are not completely understood; however, recent research has given us insight into effects occurring at the local and supraspinal levels, and through dorsal horn interneuron and neurochemical mechanisms.[7,8] Linderoth and others have noted that the mechanism of analgesia when SCS is applied in neuropathic pain states may be very different from that involved in analgesia due to limb ischemia or angina. Experimental evidence points to SCS having a beneficial effect at the dorsal horn level by favorably altering the local neurochemistry in that zone, thereby suppressing the hyperexcitability of the wide dynamic range interneurons. Specifically, there is some evidence for increased levels of GABA release and serotonin, and perhaps suppression of levels of some excitatory amino acids including glutamate and aspartate. In the case of ischemic pain, analgesia seems to be obtained through restoration of a favorable oxygen supply and demand balance—perhaps through a favorable alteration of sympathetic tone.

TECHNICAL CONSIDERATIONS

SCS is a technically challenging interventional/surgical pain management technique. It involves the careful placement of an electrode array (leads) in the epidural space, a trial period, anchoring the lead(s), positioning and implantation of the pulse generator or radiofrequency (RF) receiver, and the tunneling and connection of the connecting wires. This author advocates a collaborative effort between neurosurgeon and anesthesiologist for optimal success with neurostimulation.

Electrodes are of two types, catheter or percutaneous versus paddle or surgical (Fig. 165–1). These electrodes are connected to an implanted pulse generator (IPG) or a RF unit (Fig. 165–2). Currently, three companies, Medtronic Inc., American Neuromodulation Systems Inc., and Advanced Bionics, Inc., manufacture neurostimulation equipment (Table 165–1). Interested readers are directed to these companies for further specific information on the equipment.

A stimulator trial may be accomplished in two ways: "straight percutaneous" or "implanted lead." In both trial methods, under fluoroscopy and sterile conditions, a lead is introduced into the epidural space with the standard epidural needle placement. The lead is steered under fluoroscopic imaging into the posterior paramedian epidural space up to the desired anatomic location. Trial stimulation is undertaken to attempt to "cover" the painful area with an electrically induced paresthesia. After the painful area is "captured" with either one or two leads, the two techniques diverge.

In the straight percutaneous trial, the needle is withdrawn, an anchoring suture is placed into the skin, and a sterile dressing is applied. When the patient returns after a trial of several days, the dressing is removed, the suture is clipped, and the lead is removed and discarded *regardless* of the success of the trial. When the patient returns for implant, a new lead is placed in the location of the trial lead and connected to an implanted IPG.

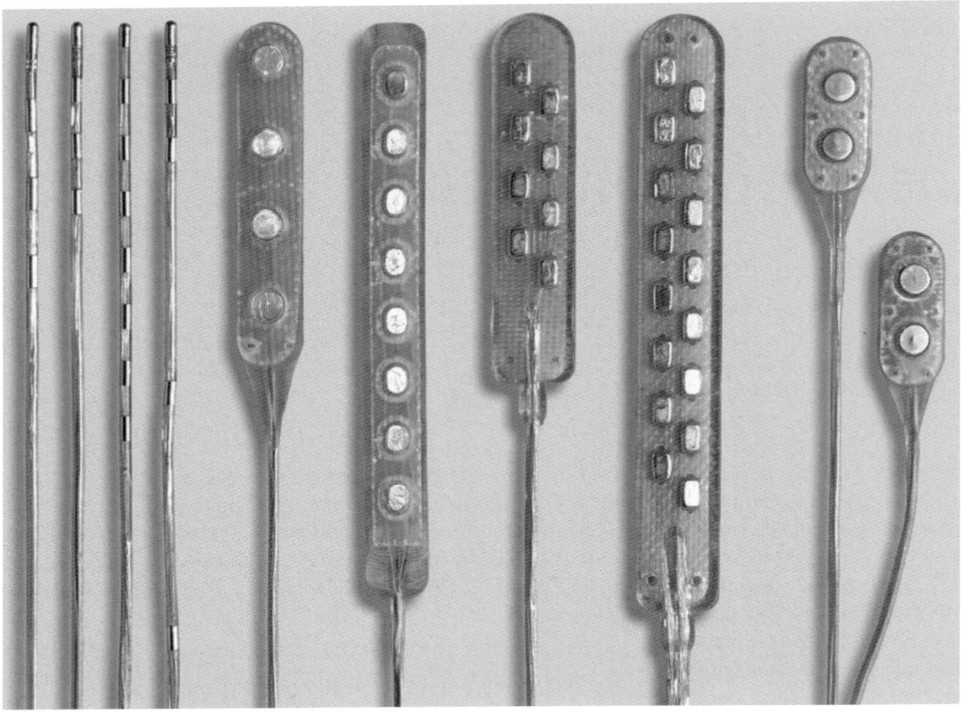

FIGURE 165–1 ■ Neurostimulator leads *(left to right)*: percutaneous type to paddle type (Courtesy of ANS, Inc.).

Table 165–1

Manufacturers of Neurostimulation Equipment

Medtronic Inc, 710 Medtronic Parkway, Minneapolis, MN, 55432, USA. 763-514-5604. www.medtronic.com

American Neuromodulation Systems, Inc, 6501 Windcrest Dr, Ste 100, Plano, TX, 75024, USA. 800-727-7846. www.ans-medical.com

Advanced Bionics, Inc. 12740 San Fernando Road, Sylmar, California 91342, USA. 800-678-2575. www.advancedbionics.com

In the "implanted lead" trial, after successful positioning of the trial lead(s), local anesthetic is infiltrated around the needle(s) and an incision is made, cutting down to the supraspinous fascia to anchor the leads securely using nonabsorbable suture. Then, a temporary extension piece is tunneled away from the back incision and out through the skin. This exiting piece is secured to the skin using a suture, antibiotic ointment, and a sterile dressing. If the trial is successful at the time of implant, the back incision is opened up, the percutaneous lead is cut, pulled out through the skin site, and discarded. The permanent lead(s) that were used for the trial are hooked to new extension(s) and are tunneled to an IPG.

The "implanted lead" method has the advantages of saving the cost of new electrodes at implant and ensuring that the implanted lead position matches the trial lead position. Differences of the "percutaneous lead" approach include (1) avoiding the costs of two trips to the operating room (even for an unsuccessful trial to remove the anchored trial lead); (2) avoiding an incision and postoperative pain during the trial, which may confuse trial interpretation by the patient; and (3) the percutaneous temporary extension is a risk for infection. The percutaneous extension must be anchored and meticulously dressed or the risk of infection may be higher than with the straight percutaneous technique.[9] Most clinicians consider 50% or more pain relief to be indicative of a successful trial, although the ultimate decision also should include other factors such as activity level and medication intake. To paraphrase, some combination of pain relief, increased activity level, and decreased medication intake is indicative of a favorable trial.

A trial with paddle-type electrodes requires the "implanted lead" approach—with the significant addition of a laminotomy to slip the flat plate electrode into the epidural space. Some physicians try the patient with the "straight percutaneous" approach and, if successful, will send the patient to a neurosurgeon for a paddle-type implant. The author's preference is to do a "straight percutaneous" trial, with an implant using non-paddle-type electrodes.

The IPG/RF unit is generally implanted in the lower abdominal area or in the posterior superior gluteal area. It should be in a location the patient can access with their dominant hand for adjustment of their settings with the patient-held remote control unit. The decision to use a fully implantable IPG or an RF unit depends on several considerations. If the patient's pain pattern requires the use of many anode/cathode settings with high power settings during the

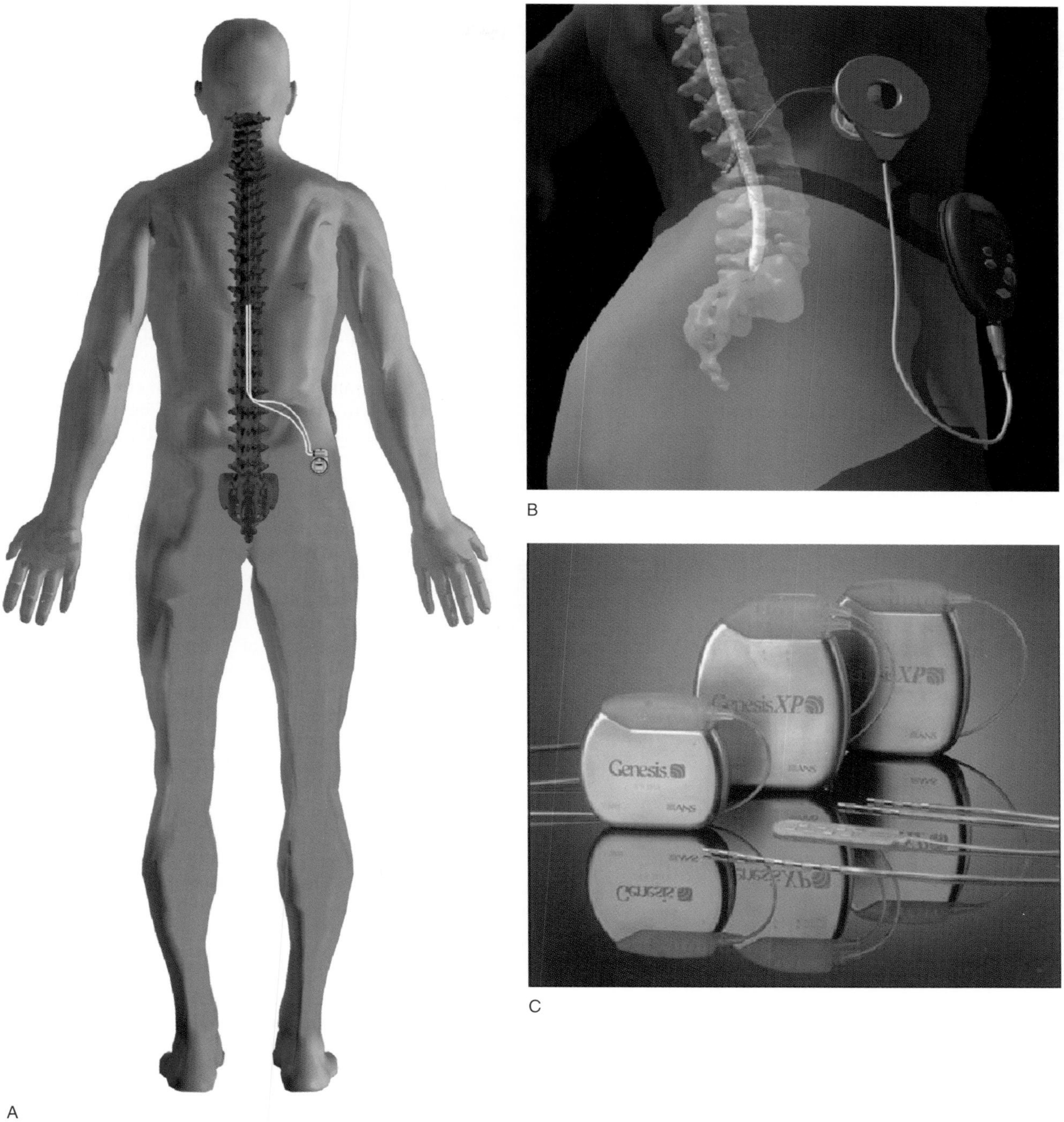

FIGURE 165–2 ■ **A,** Schematic view of an IPG system implanted. **B,** Schematic view of an implanted RF SCS system. **C,** IPG neurostimulation units with leads. IPG, implanted pulse generator; RF SCS, radiofrequency spinal cord stimulation. (**A,** courtesy of Medtronic, Inc.; **B** and **C,** courtesy of ANS, Inc.)

trial, an RF unit should be condiered. The IPG battery life will largely depend on the power settings used, but the newer IPG units (Synergy or Genesis XP) will generally last several years at average power settings.

PATIENT SELECTION

Appropriate patients for neurostimulation implant must meet the following criteria: the patient has a diagnosis amenable to this therapy (i.e., neuropathic pain syndromes); the patient has failed conservative therapy; significant psychological issues have been ruled out; and a trial has demonstrated pain relief.[10] However, pure neuropathic pain syndromes are relatively less common than the mixed nociceptive/neuropathic disorders—including failed back surgery syndrome (FBSS). Also, many patients with chronic pain will have some depressive symptomatology; however, psychological screening can be extremely helpful to avoid implanting patients who have major psychological disorders. An interesting study by Olson and colleagues revealed a high correlation between many items on a complex psychological testing battery and favorable response to trial stimulation.[11] This is to say that overall mood state is an important predictor of outcomes.

A careful trial period is advocated to avoid a failed implant. Trials of different lengths have been advocated. The main risk of a longer trial is infection, whereas the risk of too short a trial is misreading success. The author uses a 5- to 7-day trial with the use of oral antibiotics. We encourage the patient to be as active as possible in their usual environment, with the exception of limiting bending/twisting movements. In spite of advances in the understanding of diagnoses that respond to neurostimulation, increased understanding of and improved psychological screening, and improved multi-lead systems, clinical failures of implanted neurostimulator devices remain too common and pain practitioners must critically evaluate their own outcomes and adhere to strict selection criteria discussed earlier.

COMPLICATIONS

Complications with spinal cord stimulation range from simple, easily correctable problems, such as lack of appropriate paresthesia coverage, to devastating complications, such as paralysis, nerve injury, and death. Prior to the implantation of the trial lead, an educational session should occur with the patient and significant family members. This meeting should include a discussion of possible risks and complications. In the postoperative period, the caregiver should be involved in identifying problems and alerting the healthcare team.

North and colleagues reported their experience in 320 consecutive patients treated with SCS between 1972 and 1990.[12] A 5% rate of subcutaneous infection was seen and is consistent with the literature. The predominant complication consisted of lead migration or breakage. This remains the "Achilles' heel" of neurostimulation. In an earlier series, bipolar leads required electrode revision in 23% of patients. The revision rate for patients with multichannel devices was 16%. Failure of the electrode lead was observed in 13% of patients and steadily declined over the course of the study.When analyzed by implant type (single-channel percutaneous, single-channel laminectomy, and multichannel), the lead migration rate for multichannel devices was approximately 7%. Analysis of hardware reliability for 298 permanent implants showed that technical failures (particularly electrode migration and malposition) and clinical failures had become significantly less common as implants evolved into programmable, "multichannel" devices.

More recent studies by Barolat and May reported lead revision rates due to lead migration of 4.5% and 13.6% and breakage of 0% and 13.6%, respectively.[13,14] Infections occurred in 7% and 2.5% of cases, respectively. No serious complications were seen in either study. These studies are representative of the complication rates of neurostimulation therapy.

Infections range from simple infections at the surface of the wound to epidural abscess. The patient should be instructed on wound care and recognition of signs and symptoms indicative of infection. Many superficial infections can be treated with oral antibiotics or simple surgical exploration and irrigation. At the author's center, the standard includes prophylactic intraoperative antibiotics and oral coverage postoperatively for 10 days.

If infection reaches the tissues involving the devices, in most cases the implant should be removed. In such cases, one should have a high index of suspicion for an epidural abscess. Abscess of the epidural space can lead to paralysis and death if not identified quickly and treated aggressively. In the case of temporary epidural catheters (somewhat analogous to a percutaneous stimulator trial), Sarubbi discovered only 20 well-described cases.[14] The mean age of these 22 patients was 49.9 years, the median duration of epidural catheter use was 3 days, and the median time to onset of clinical symptoms after catheter placement was 5 days. The majority of patients (63.6%) had major neurologic deficits; 22.7% also had concomitant meningitis. *Staphylococcus aureus* was the predominant pathogen. Despite antibiotic therapy and drainage procedures, 38% of the patients continued to have neurologic deficits. These unusual but serious complications of temporary epidural catheter use require efficient and accurate diagnostic evaluation, and treatment, as the consequences of delayed therapy can be substantial. Schuchard reported an infection with *Pasteurella* during an "implanted lead" trial, which required explanting the system.[15] The author (AB) has experienced one similar case with *S. aureus* requiring explant of the entire system (unpublished).

PROGRAMMING

There are four basic parameters in neurostimulation that may be adjusted to create stimulation paresthesias in the painful areas, thereby mitigating the patient's pain. They are: amplitude, pulse width, rate, and electrode selection.[16]

Amplitude is the intensity or strength of the stimulation measured in volts (V). The voltage may be set from 0 to 10 V, with lower settings typically used over peripheral nerves and with paddle type electrodes. Pulse width is a measure in microseconds (μsec) of the duration of a pulse. Pulse width is usually set between 100 and 400 μsec. A larger pulse width will typically give the patient a broader coverage. Rate is measured in hertz (Hz) or cycles per second, between 20 and 120 Hz. At lower rates, the patient feels more of a thumping, whereas at higher Hz, the feeling is more of a buzzing. Electrode selection is a complex topic that has been the subject of some research by Barolet and colleagues who provided mapping data of coverage patterns based on lead location in 106 patients.[17] The primary target is the negative cathode, from which electrons flow to the positive anode(s). Most patients' stimulators are programmed with electrode selection changed until the patient obtains anatomic coverage; then the pulse width and rate are adjusted for maximal comfort. The patient is left with full control of turning the stimulation off and on, and the voltage up and down to comfort.

We use an analogy of a stereo to discuss programming with patients. Amplitude is the "volume control," the pulse width is "how many speakers are on mono- versus surround sound," and the rate is the "bass or treble control." The lowest acceptable settings on all parameters are generally used to conserve battery life. Other programming modes that save battery life include a cycling mode during which the stimulator cycles full on/off at patient-determined intervals (minutes, seconds, or hours). The patient's programming may change over time and reprogramming needs are common. Both neurostimulator manufacturing companies are very helpful to clinicians with patient reprogramming assistance. Many busy pain practices designate a nurse who specializes in stimulators to handle patient reprogramming needs.

OUTCOMES

The most common use for SCS in the United States is FBSS, whereas in Europe, peripheral ischemia is the predominant indication. It makes sense to subdivide clinical outcomes based on diagnosis. In a review of the available SCS literature, most evidence falls within the level IV (limited) or level V (indeterminate) category owing to the invasiveness of the modality and the inability to provide blinded treatment. Recognition must also be given to the time frame within which a study was performed owing to rapidly evolving SCS technology. Basic science knowledge, implantation techniques, lead placement locations, contact array designs, and programming capabilities have changed dramatically from the time of the first implants. These improvements have led to decreased morbidity and much greater probability of obtaining adequate paresthesia coverage with subsequent improved outcomes.[13] Thus, even a level II review study, such as the one by Turner with FBSS patients from 1966 to 1994, reported fewer positive outcomes than Barolat's level IV FBSS study in 2001.[18,19] The author believes this represents the effect of improving technology.

Failed Back Surgery Syndrome

There has been one recent prospective, randomized study of FBSS. North and colleagues[20] selected 50 patients as candidates for repeat laminectomy. All the patients had undergone previous surgery and were excluded from randomization if they presented with severe spinal canal stenosis, extremely large disk fragments, a major neurologic deficit such as foot drop, or radiographic evidence of gross instability. In addition, patients were excluded for untreated dependency on narcotic analgesics or benzodiazepines, major psychiatric comorbidity, the presence of any significant or disabling chronic pain problem, or a chief complaint of low back pain exceeding lower extremity pain. Crossover between groups was permitted after the 6-month follow-up. Of the 26 patients who had undergone reoperation, 54% (14 patients) crossed over to SCS. Of the 24 who had undergone SCS, 21% (5 patients) opted for crossover to reoperation. For 90% of the patients, long-term (3-year) follow-up evaluation has shown that SCS continues to be more effective than reoperation, with significantly better outcomes by standard measures and significantly lower rates of crossover to the alternate procedure. Additionally, patients randomized to reoperation used significantly more opioids than those randomized to SCS. Other measures assessing activities of daily living and work status did not differ significantly.

Two recent, prospective case series have been done. The first, by Barolat examined the outcomes of patients with intractable low-back pain treated with epidural SCS using paddle electrodes and an RF stimulator.[21] In four centers, 44 patients were implanted and followed with the visual analog scale (VAS), the Oswestry Disability Questionnaire, the Sickness Impact Profile (SIP), and a patient satisfaction rating scale. All patients had back and leg pain, and all had at least one previous back surgery, with most (83%) having two or more back surgeries, and 51% having had a spinal fusion. Data were collected at baseline, at 6 months, at 12 months, and at 2 years.

All patients showed a reported mean decrease in their 10-point VAS scores compared to baseline. The majority of patients reported fair to excellent pain relief in both the low back and legs. At 6 months, 91.6% of the patients reported fair to excellent relief in the legs and 82.7% of the patients reported fair to excellent relief in the low back. At 1 year, 88.2% of the patients reported fair to excellent relief in the legs and 68.8% of the patients reported fair to excellent relief in the low back. Significant improvement in function and quality of life was found at both the 6-month and 1-year follow-up using the Oswestry and SIP, respectively. The majority of patients reported that the procedure was worthwhile (92% at 6 months; 88% at 1 year). The authors concluded that SCS proved beneficial at 1 year for the treatment of patients with chronic low back and leg pain.

The second multicenter prospective case series was published by Burchiel in 1996.[22] The study included 182 patients with a permanent system after a percutaneous trial. Patient evaluation of pain and functional levels was performed before and 3, 6, and 12 months after implantation. Complications, medication usage, and work status also were monitored. A 1-year follow-up, evaluation was available for 70 patients. All pain and quality-of-life measures showed statistically significant improvement, whereas medication usage and work status did not significantly improve during the treatment year. Complications requiring surgical interventions were experienced by 17% (12 of 70) of the patients.

There have been two systematic review articles on neurostimulation. Turner completed a meta-analysis from the articles related to the treatment of FBSS by SCS from 1966 to 1994.[23] They reviewed 39 studies that met the inclusion criteria. The mean follow-up period was 16 months with range of 1 to 45 months. Pain relief exceeding 50% was experienced by 59% of patients with a range of 15% to 100%. Complications occurred in 42% of patients, with 30% of patients experiencing one or more stimulator-related complications. However, all the studies were case control investigations. Based on this review, the authors concluded that there was insufficient evidence from the literature for drawing conclusions about the effectiveness of SCS relative to no treatment or other treatments, or about the effects of SCS on patient work status, functional disability, and medication use.

The second study by North and Wetzel consisted of a review of case-control studies and two prospective control studies.[24] They concluded that if a patient reports a reduction in pain of at least 50% during a trial, as determined by standard rating methods, and demonstrates improved or stable analgesic requirements and activity levels, significant benefit may be realized from a permanent implant. The authors conclude the bulk of the literature appears to support a role for SCS (in neuropathic pain syndromes), but caution that the quality of the existing literature is marginal—largely case series.

Complex Regional Pain Syndrome

Research of high quality regarding SCS and complex regional pain syndrome (CRPS) is limited, but existing data are overwhelmingly positive in terms of pain reduction, quality of life, analgesic usage, and function. Kemler and colleagues published a prospective, randomized, comparative trial of SCS versus conservative therapy for CRPS.[25] Patients with a 6-month history of CRPS of the upper extremities were randomized to undergo trial SCS (and implant if successful) plus physiotherapy versus physiotherapy alone. In this study, 36 patients were assigned to receive a standardized physical therapy program together with SCS, whereas 18 patients were assigned to receive therapy alone. In 24 of the 36 patients, randomized to SCS, along with physical therapy, the trial was successful, and permanent implantation was performed. At a 6-month follow-up assessment, the patients in the SCS group had a significantly greater reduction in pain, and a significantly higher percentage was graded as much improved for the global perceived effect. However, there were no clinically significant improvements in functional status. The authors concluded that in the short-term, SCS reduces pain and improves the quality of life for patients with CRPS involving the upper extremities.

Several important case series have been published on the use of neurostimulation in the treatment of CRPS. Calvillo reported a series of 36 patients with advanced stages of CRPS (at least 2 years' duration) who had undergone successful SCS trial (>50% reduction of pain).[26] They were treated with either SCS or PNS—and in some cases with both modalities. The reported pain measured on visual analog scales 36 months after implantation was an average of 53% better; this change was statistically significant. Analgesic consumption decreased in the majority of patients and 41% of patients had returned to work on a modified duty. The authors concluded that in late stages of CRPS, neurostimulation (with SCS or PNS) is a reasonable option when alternative therapies have failed.

Another case series reported by Oakley is remarkable in that it used a sophisticated battery of outcomes tools to evaluate treatment response in CRPS using SCS.[27] The study followed 19 patients and analyzed the results from the McGill Pain Rating Index, the Sickness Impact Profile, Oswestry Disability Profile, Beck Depression Inventory, and Visual Analog Scale. Nineteen patients were reported as a subgroup enrolled at two centers participating in a multicenter study of efficacy/outcomes of SCS. Specific pre-implant and post-implant tests to measure outcome were administered. Statistically significant improvement in the Sickness Impact Profile physical and psychosocial subscales was documented. The McGill Pain Rating Index words chosen and sensory subscale also improved significantly as did Visual Analog Scale scores. The Beck Depression Inventory trended toward significant improvement. All patients received at least partial relief and benefit from their device, with 30% receiving full relief. Eighty percent of the patients obtained at least 50% pain relief through the use of their stimulators. The average percent of pain relief was 61%. The authors concluded that patients with CRPS benefitted significantly from the use of SCS based on average follow-up of 7.9 months.

A literature review by Stanton-Hicks of SCS for CRPS consisted of seven case series. These studies ranged in size from 6 to 24 patients. Results were noted as "good to excellent" in greater than 72% of patients over a time period of 8 to 40 months. The review concluded that SCS proved to be a powerful tool in the management of patients with CRPS.[28]

A retrospective, 3-year, multicenter study of 101 patients by Bennett evaluated the effectiveness of SCS applied to CRPS I and compared the effectiveness of octapolar versus quadripolar systems, as well as high-frequency and multiprogram parameters.[29] VAS was significantly decreased in the group using the dual-octapolar system with reductions in overall VAS approaching 70%. Of the dual-octapolar group, 74.8% used multiple arrays to maximize paresthesia coverage. VAS reduction in the group using quadripolar systems approached 50%. Of the quadripolar systems and dual-octapolar systems, 86.3% and 97.2% continued to be used, respectively. Overall satisfaction with stimulation was 91% in the dual-octapolar group and 70% in the quadripolar group ($P < .05$). The authors concluded that SCS is effective in the management of chronic pain associated with CRPS I and that use of dual-octapolar systems with multiple-array programming capabilities appeared to increase the paresthesia coverage and thus, further reduce pain. High-frequency stimulation (>250 Hz) was found to be essential in obtaining adequate analgesia in 15% of the patients using dual-octapolar systems (this frequency level was not available to those with quadripolar systems).

Peripheral Ischemia and Angina

Cook reported in 1976, that SCS effectively relieved pain associated with peripheral ischemia.[30] This result has been repeated and noted to have particular efficacy in conditions associated with vasospasm—such as Raynaud disease.[31] Many studies have shown impressive efficacy of SCS in treating intractable angina.[32] Reported success rates are consistently greater than 80% and these indications, already widely used outside of the United States are certain to expand within the United States.

COST EFFECTIVENESS

Cost effectiveness of SCS (in the treatment of chronic back pain) was evaluated by Kumar and colleagues in 2002.[33] They prospectively followed 104 patients with FBSS. Of the 104 patients, 60 were implanted with an SCS using a standard selection criterion. Both groups were monitored over a period of 5 years. The stimulation group's annual cost was $29,000 versus $38,000 in the control group. The authors found 15% of subjects returned to work in the stimulation group versus 0% in the control group. The higher costs in the nonstimulator group were in the categories of medications, emergency center visits, radiographs, and ongoing physician visits.

Bell performed an analysis of the medical costs of SCS therapy in the treatment of patients with FBSS.[34] The medical costs of SCS therapy were compared with an alternative regimen of surgeries and other interventions. Externally powered (external) and fully internalized (internal) SCS systems were considered separately. No value was placed on pain relief or improvements in the quality of life that successful SCS therapy can generate. The authors concluded that by reducing the demand for medical care by FBSS patients, SCS therapy can lower medical costs and found that, on average, SCS therapy pays for itself within 5.5 years. For those patients for whom SCS therapy is clinically efficacious, the therapy pays for itself within 2.1 years.

Kemler performed a similar study by looking at "chronic reflex sympathetic dystrophy (RSD)" using outcomes and costs of care before and after the start of treatment.[35] This essentially is an economic analysis of the Kemler RSD outcomes paper. Fifty-four patients with chronic RSD were randomized to receive either SCS with physical therapy (SCS + PT; $n = 36$) or physical therapy alone (PT; $n = 18$). Twenty-four SCS + PT patients responded positively to trial stimulation and underwent SCS implantation. During 12 months of follow-up, costs (routine RSD costs, SCS costs, out-of-pocket costs), and effects (pain relief by visual analog scale, health-related quality of life [HRQL] improvement by a validated quality of life instrument) were assessed in both groups. Analyses were carried out up to 1 year and up to the expected time of death. SCS was both more effective and less costly than the standard treatment protocol. As a result of high initial costs of SCS in the first year, the treatment per patient is $4,000 more than control therapy. However, in the lifetime analysis, SCS per patient is $60,000 cheaper than control therapy. In addition, at 12 months, SCS resulted in pain relief (SCS + PT [−2.7] versus PT [0.4] [$P < .001$]) and improved HRQL (SCS + PT [0.22] versus PT [0.03] [$P = .004$]). The authors found SCS to be more effective and less expensive when compared with the standard treatment protocol for chronic RSD.

Table 165–2

Principles of Spinal Cord Stimulation

1. SCS mechanism of action is not completely understood but influences multiple components and levels within the CNS with both interneuron and neurochemical mechanisms.
2. SCS therapy is effective for many neuropathic pain conditions. Stimulation-evoked paresthesia must be experienced in the entire painful area. No consistent evidence exists for the efficacy of neurostimulation in primary nociceptive pain conditions.
3. Stimulation should be applied with low intensity, just suprathreshold for the activation of the low-threshold, large-diameter fibers, and should be of nonpainful intensity. To be effective SCS must be applied continuously (or in cycles) for at least 20minutes prior to the onset of analgesia. This analgesia develops slowly and typically lasts several hours after cessation of the stimulation.
4. SCS has demonstrated clinical and cost effectiveness in FBSS and CRPS. Clinical effectiveness has also been shown in peripheral ischemia and angina.
5. Multicontact, multiprogram systems improve outcomes and reduce the incidence of surgical revisions. Insulated paddle-type electrodes *probably* decrease the incidence of lead breakage, prolong battery life and show early superiority in quality of paresthesia coverage and analgesia in FBSS as compared to permanent percutaneous electrodes.
6. Serious complications are exceedingly rare but can be devastating. Meticulous care must be taken during implantation to minimize procedural complications. The most frequent complications are wound infections (approximately 5%) and lead breakage or migration (approximately 13% each for permanent percutaneous leads and 3%-6% each for paddle leads).

CRPS, complex regional pain syndrome; FBSS, failed back surgery syndrome; SCS, spinal cord stimulation.
Adapted from Linderoth B, Meyerson BA: Spinal cord stimulation: Mechanisms of action. In Burchiel K (ed): Surgical Management of Pain. New York, Thieme, 2002, p 505.

PERIPHERAL, CORTICAL, AND DEEP BRAIN STIMULATION

Besides stimulation of the spinal cord, neurostimulation can successfully be used at other locations in the peripheral and central nervous systems to provide analgesia. Peripheral nerve stimulation was introduced by Wall, Sweet, and others in the mid-1960s.[36] This technique has shown efficacy for peripheral nerve injury pain syndromes as well as CRPS, with the use of a carefully implanted paddle lead using a fascial graft to help anchor the lead without traumatizing the nerve.[37]

Motor cortex and deep brain stimulation are techniques that have been explored to treat highly refractory neuropathic pain syndromes including central pain, deafferentation syndromes, trigeminal neuralgia, and others.[38] Deep brain stimulation has become a widely used technique for movement disorders, and much less so for painful indications, although there have been many case reports of utility in treating highly refractory central pain syndromes.[39]

CONCLUSION

SCS is an invasive, interventional surgical procedure. Linderoth and Meyerson wrote some principles of neurostimulation that are cornerstones of SCS theory and practice (Table 165–2).[40] The difficulty of randomized clinical trials in such situations is well recognized. Based on the present evidence with two randomized, one prospective trial, and multiple retrospective trials, the evidence for SCS in properly selected populations with neuropathic pain states is moderate. Clearly, this technique should be reserved for patients who have failed more conservative therapies. With appropriate patient selection and careful attention to technical issues, the clinical results are overwhelmingly positive.

References

1. Kumar K, Nath R, Wyant GM: Treatment of chronic pain by epidural spinal cord stimulation: A 10-year experience. J Neurosurg 5:402, 1991.
2. Shealy CN, Mortimer JT, Resnick J: Electrical inhibition of pain by stimulation of the dorsal columns: Preliminary reports. J Int Anesth Res Soc 46:489, 1967.
3. Kumar K, Toth C, Nath RK: Deep brain stimulation for intractable pain: A 15 year experience. Neurosurgery 40(4):736, 1997.
4. Nguyen JP, Lefaucher JP, Le Guerinel C, et al: Motor cortex stimulation in the treatment of central and neuropathic pain. Arch Med Res 31(3):263, 2000.
5. Campbell JN, Long DM: Stimulation of the peripheral nervous system for pain control. J Neurosurg.45:692, 1976.
6. Melzack R, Wall PD: Pain mechanisms: A new theory. Science 150:971, 1965.
7. Oakley J, Prager J: Spinal cord stimulation: Mechanism of action. Spine (27):22:2574, 2002.
8. Linderoth B, Foreman R: Physiology of spinal cord stimulation: Review and update. Neuromodulation 2(3):150, 1999.
9. May MS, Banks C, Thomson SJ: A retrospective, long-term, third-party follow-up of patients considered for spinal cord stimulation. Neuromodulation 5(3):137, 2002.
10. Burchiel KJ, Anderson VC, Wilson BJ, et al: Prognostic factors of spinal cord stimulation for chronic back and leg pain. Neurosurgery 36:1101, 1995.
11. Olson KA, Bedder MD, Anderson VC, et al: Psychological variables associated with outcome of spinal cord stimulation trials. Neuromodulation1:6, 1998.
12. North RB, Kidd DH, Zahurak M, et al: Spinal cord stimulation for chronic, intractable pain: Two decades' experience. Neurosurgery 32:384, 1993.
13. Barolat G, Oakley J, Law J, North R: Epidural spinal cord stimulation with a multiple electrode paddle lead is effective in treating low back pain. Neuromodulation 4(2):59, 2001.
14. Sarubbi F, Vasquez J: Spinal epidural abscess associated with the use of temporary epidural catheters: Report of two cases and review. Clin Infect Dis 25(5):1155, 1997.
15. Schuchard M, Clauson W: An interesting and heretofore unreported infection of a spinal cord stimulator: Smitten by a kitten revisited. Neuromodulation 4(2):67, 2001.
16. Alfano S, Darwin J, Picullel B: Programming principles in spinal cord stimulation: Patient management guidelines for clinicians, Medtronic, Minneapolis, Minn, 2001, p 27.
17. Barolat G, Massaro F, He J, et al: Mapping of sensory responses to epidural stimulation of the intraspinal neural structures in man. J Neurosurg 78(2):233, 1993.
18. Turner JA, Loeser JD, Bell KG: Spinal cord stimulation for chronic low back pain: A systematic literature synthesis. Neurosurgery 37(6):1088, 1995; discussion 1095.
19. Barolat G, Oakley J, Law J, North RB: Epidural spinal cord stimulation with a multiple electrode paddle lead is effective in treating low back pain. Neuromodulation (4):2:59, 2001.
20. North RB, Kidd DH, Farrokhi F, Piantadosi SA: Spinal cord stimulation versus repeated lumbosacral spine surgery for chronic pain: A randomized, controlled trial. Neurosurgery. 56(1):98, 2005; discussion 106.
21. Barolat G, Oakley J, Law J, North R: Epidural spinal cord stimulation with a multiple electrode paddle lead is effective in treating low back pain. Neuromodulation (4):2:59, 2001.
22. Burchiel KJ, Anderson VC, Brown FD, et al: Prospective, multicenter study of spinal cord stimulation for the relief of chronic back and extremity pain. Spine 21(23):2786, 1996.
23. Turner JA, Loeser JD, Bell KG: Spinal cord stimulation for chronic low back pain: A systematic literature synthesis. Neurosurgery Dec;37(6): 1088, 1995.
24. North R, Wetzel T: Spinal cord stimulation for chronic pain of spinal origin. Spine 27(22):2584, 2002.
25. Kemler MA, Barendse GA, van Kleef M, et al: Spinal cord stimulation in patients with chronic reflex sympathetic dystrophy. N Engl J Med 343(9):618, 2000.
26. Calvillo O, Racz G, Didie J, Smith K: Neuroaugmentation in the treatment of complex regional pain syndrome of the upper extremity. Acta Orthop Belg 64(1):57, 1998.
27. Oakley J, Weiner R: Spinal cord stimulation for complex regional pain syndrome: A prospective study of 19 patients at two centers. Neuromodulation (2);1:47, 1999.
28. Stanton-Hicks M: Spinal cord stimulation for the management of complex regional pain syndromes. Neuromodulation (2);3:193, 1999.
29. Bennett D, Alo K, Oakley J, Feler C: Spinal cord stimulation for complex regional pain syndrome i (rsd): A retrospective multicenter experience from 1995-1998 of 101 patients. Neuromodulation (2);3:202, 1999.
30. Cook AW, Oygar A, Baggenstos P, et al: Vascular disease of extremities: Electrical stimulation of spinal cord and posterior roots. NY State J Med 76:366, 1976.
31. Broseta J, Barbera J, De Vera JA: Spinal cord stimulation in peripheral arterial disease. J Neurosurg 64:71, 1986.
32. Eliasson T, Augustinsson LE, Mannheimer C: Spinal cord stimulation in severe angina pectoris—presentation of current studies, indications, and clinical experience. Pain 65:169, 1996.
33. Kumar K, Malik S, Demeria D: Treatment of chronic pain with spinal cord stimulation versus alternative therapies: Cost-effectiveness analysis. Neurosurgery 51(1):106, 2002.
34. Bell G, North R: Cost-effectiveness analysis of spinal cord stimulation in treatment of failed back surgery syndrome. J Pain Symptom Manage 13(5):285, 1997.
35. Kemler M, Furnee C: Economic evaluation of spinal cord stimulation for chronic reflex sympathetic dystrophy. Neurology 59(8):1203, 2002.
36. Wall PD, Sweet WH: Temporary abolition of pain in man. Science 155:108, 1967.

37. Hassenbusch SJ, Stanton-Hicks M, Shoppa D: Long-term results of peripheral nerve stimulation for reflex sympathetic dystrophy. J Neurosurg 84:415, 1996.
38. Tsubokawa T, Katayama Y, Yamamoto T, et al: Chronic motor cortex stimulation in patients with thalamic pain. J Neurosurg 78:393, 1993.
39. Limousin P, Krack P, Pollack P, et al. Electrical stimulation of the subthalamic nucleus in advanced Parkinson's disease. N Engl J Med 339:1105, 1998.
40. Linderoth B, Meyerson BA: Spinal cord stimulation: Mechanisms of action. In Burchiel K (ed): Surgical Management of Pain. New York, Thieme, 2002, p 505.

chapter 166

Implantable Drug Delivery Systems: Practical Considerations

Steven D. Waldman

Spinal opioids have dramatically changed the way acute, obstetric, non-malignant chronic pain and pain of malignant origin are managed. The development of various implantable drug delivery systems (IDDSs) has complemented and facilitated the growth of this treatment modality. By interfacing appropriate patient selection with the unique advantages and disadvantages of each type of IDDS, improved results in terms of both pain relief and patient satisfaction can be achieved.

HISTORY

In the late 1970s, a group of cancer patients at the Mayo Clinic underwent spinal administration of morphine in the hope of finding an alternative to neurodestructive procedures for relief of intractable pain of malignant origin. This brilliant clinical application by Wang and Nauss[1] of the basic research of Yaksh[2] heralded a new era in the specialty of pain management. This development not only dramatically changed the management of cancer pain but also triggered an entirely new way of looking at the route of drug administration. The years since this landmark event have yielded vast clinical experience with this powerful new modality, which in turn has resulted in the publication of an extensive literature describing the use of spinal opioids in a variety of clinical situations.[3] As clinicians gained more experience in the use of spinal opioids for the management of cancer pain, they began to apply this modality to non-malignant acute pain and experiment with the spinal administration of drugs other than opioids. This experimentation has not been without its critics, but by and large, the use of spinal opioids for acute pain has been a great advance. Clinicians have successfully adapted this technique to relieve postoperative and other acute pain syndromes, obstetric pain, non-malignant chronic pain, and cancer pain in thousands of patients. In tandem, the development of various IDDSs has occurred and facilitated this expanded role of spinal drugs in the palliation of pain and, more recently, spasticity.[4]

THE ROLE OF PATIENT SELECTION WHEN CONSIDERING IMPLANTABLE DRUG DELIVERY SYSTEMS

Does a Spinally Administered Drug Relieve the Symptoms Being Treated?

The first factor to consider when determining whether a patient is an appropriate candidate for implantation of an IDDS is whether spinal opioids adequately relieve the patient's pain and whether spinal administration of baclofen adequately relieves the patient's spasticity. Not all pain is relieved by spinal opioids, and not all spasticity is relieved by spinally administered baclofen.[5,6] For this reason, an IDDS should never be implanted without first verifying the ability of the intended drug to relieve the patient's pain or spasticity on at least two occasions. Failure to do so could subject the patient to implantation of a delivery system that fails to achieve the desired result—namely, pain relief.

The Preimplantation Trial

Table 166–1 outlines a suggested protocol for the preimplantation trial for spinal opioids. The expected result of the preimplantation trial of spinal opioids is adequate pain relief as perceived by the patient. This relief should be of appropriate duration for the narcotic analgesic injected.[7] Other variables that should be quantified include the level of activity, the use of narcotics by other routes, and the amount and quality of sleep. This same approach should be used to verify that spinally administered baclofen adequately relieves the patient's spasticity.

Side Effects

Side effects secondary to spinal opioids, including pruritus, urinary retention, and respiratory depression, must be noted. Side effects secondary to spinally administered baclofen, including weakness and sedation, must also be noted. These side effects must be acceptable to the patient before implantation can be considered. Any inconsistency in the expected versus the observed results should alert the clinician to strongly consider delaying implantation of the delivery

Table 166–1

Protocol for Preimplantation Trials of Spinal Opioids

1. Explain the procedure, expected goals, and potential side effects to the patient and family.
2. Select an appropriate narcotic for intraspinal administration.
3. Determine the appropriate dosage and volume of diluent expected to relieve the pain.
4. Administer the intraspinal narcotic and diluent via the intended route of delivery, i.e., epidural or subarachnoid.
5. Quantify on a flow sheet the duration of pain relief, level of activity, amount of sleep, and need for additional narcotic analgesics.
6. Quantify the side effects of intraspinal narcotics.
7. Repeat the trial to quantify the results.
8. Observe 24 hours after intraspinal narcotics and requantify the variables listed in item 5 before proceeding with an implantable drug delivery system.

system. Careful evaluation of the patient's ability to assess pain relief, as well as reevaluation of other behavioral or psychosocial factors at play, should be undertaken before implantation of an IDDS.

The Patient's Ability to Assess the Results of the Preimplantation Trial

The ability of the patient to accurately assess the adequacy of pain relief or relief of spasticity is essential to avoid the implantation of an IDDS that will be deemed useless. Impairment of this ability may be either physiologic or behavioral in origin.

Physiologic abnormalities that may impair the patient's ability to assess the adequacy of pain relief or relief of spasticity are listed in Table 166–2. Most occur in patients with significant multi-system disease, but occasionally, seemingly otherwise healthy patients may suffer significant impairment of mentation that is not obvious to the clinician. Many of these abnormalities are reversible, and every attempt should be made to correct them before a trial of spinal opioids is undertaken. It should be remembered that the central nervous system symptoms caused by these abnormalities may be incorrectly interpreted as uncontrolled pain by the patient and clinician alike.

Behavioral factors that may affect the patient's ability to assess the adequacy of pain relief or relief of spasticity (Table 166–3) are often difficult to identify. They may coexist with physiologic factors, but care must be taken to not attribute inadequate pain relief solely to behavioral factors until all other reasons have been explored. A patient who received adequate pain relief during the preimplantation trial may be a candidate for implantation of an IDDS. Adequacy of patient motivation, the patient's support system, concurrent therapy, systemic infection, life expectancy, and the cost of spinal opioids must also, however, be evaluated before referring a patient for implantation.

Table 166–2

Common Physiologic Abnormalities That May Interfere with the Patient's Ability to Assess Pain Relief

Metabolic encephalopathy
Hypercalcemia
Hyponatremia
Hypoxemia
Hypercapnia
Azotemia
Hepatic encephalopathy
Paraneoplastic syndrome
Drug-induced organic brain syndrome
Narcotics
Minor tranquilizers
Barbiturates
Phenothiazine reactions
Cimetidine
Structural brain disease
Metastatic tumor
Increased intracranial pressure
Preexisting structural abnormality
Cerebral infarction
Cerebral hemorrhage
Abscess
Preexisting neurodegenerative disorders
Alzheimer disease

Table 166–3

Common Behavioral Abnormalities That May Interfere with the Patient's Ability to Assess Symptom Relief

Preexisting psychiatric illness
Preexisting chemical dependence
Use of pain as a controlling device
Use of pain to obtain more medication to alter the sensorium
Use of pain as an attention-seeking device
Patient's refusal to accept the person designated as caregiver
Patient's use of pain to punish certain caregivers within the support system

The Patient's Support System

An IDDS requires a baseline level of commitment not only from the patient but also from the support system. The person or persons designated as the patient's support system must be acceptable to the patient in the role of care provider. If such is not the case, problems may arise. This person must be available night and day to care for and, if a Type I to III delivery system is used, be available to inject medication into the delivery system should the patient be unable to do so. It should be remembered that patients who inject narcotics into their own delivery system initially may be unable to do so later in the course of the disease. If the support system is unable or unwilling to care for the delivery system, a continuous infusion pump may be a better option; however, someone must be available to bring the patient to the pain center to have the pump refilled. It is important to also consider the possibility that there may be family members who will divert the patient's drugs for illicit purposes.

Unique Problems When Managing Patients with Cancer Pain

Before proceeding with implantation of an IDDS, a review of concurrent primary therapy and its potential to relieve the pain is indicated. In this author's opinion, long-term administration of spinal opioids should be reserved for patients with pain of malignant origin. Our experience with the use of spinal opioids for non-malignant chronic pain has been disappointing. However, other clinicians have reported more satisfactory results with this group of patients. Currently, I reserve implantation of an IDDS for the following groups of patients: (1) cancer patients in whom primary modes of tumor eradication (surgery, chemotherapy, and radiation therapy) did not relieve the pain; (2) patients with spasticity uncontrolled by aggressive oral drug therapy; and (3) rare patients with non-malignant chronic pain whose disease process is so devastating that it is analogous to cancer pain, such as those with end-stage connective tissue disease or advanced demyelinating disease. It is my opinion that one of two things need to happen before the use of spinal opioids for non-malignant chronic pain can be routinely recommended: (1) a better way to identify patients who will experience long-term satisfactory results with this modality or (2) release of new drugs suitable for spinal administration that do not cause tolerance or the myriad behavioral issues associated with the long-term use of opioids administered spinally or systemically for non-malignant chronic pain.

In determining whether a specific patient is suitable for the implantation of an IDDS, it should be recognized that patients suffering from pain of malignant origin present some specific challenges. A cancer patient may have quantitative and qualitative problems with clotting that may be further compromised by chemotherapy and radiation therapy.[8] In my experience, this rarely presents any practical problems as long as the patient's clotting parameters are brought into acceptable range before implantation takes place. However, in a cancer patient receiving systemic anticoagulants, the risk for epidural hematoma is an ever-present possibility. In these patients, the risk-to-benefit ratio of the anticoagulants must be weighed carefully.

In an immunocompromised cancer patient, ongoing infection is not uncommon. Epidural abscess formation, as well as spondylitis and diskitis, have been reported in some cases when percutaneous catheters were advanced into the epidural space without subcutaneous tunneling and left in place for as little as 6 days.[9,10] It appears that for long-term use, an IDDS that is totally implanted or subcutaneously tunneled is superior to a percutaneous indwelling epidural catheter. Common sense dictates against placing an indwelling foreign body in a septic patient.

A realistic appraisal of life expectancy is necessary to determine the appropriateness of an invasive and relatively expensive procedure for pain relief. For cancer patients with limited life expectancy, it may be more reasonable to simply percutaneously place an epidural or subarachnoid catheter with subcutaneous tunneling rather than a more expensive type III to V system.

Cost of the Implantable Drug Delivery System, Drugs, and Supplies

When evaluating the cost of an IDDS, it is necessary to consider the cost of both the system and the drugs to be administered through it. The hardware for an IDDS can amount to more than $10,000 for a totally implantable infusion pump, exclusive of professional fees and hospital charges. The cost of the narcotics or adjuvant drugs, or both, is not insubstantial, nor is the cost of antiseptic solutions, sterile preparation swabs, gauze, and so forth needed for patients who are self-administering opioids via a type I to III system. Some patients simply cannot afford the daily expense. Cost must be considered before implanting a delivery system that will ultimately not be used.

CLASSIFICATION OF IMPLANTABLE DRUG DELIVERY SYSTEMS

Table 166–4 describes the five basic types of IDDS. The type I system, a simple percutaneous catheter analogous to those used for obstetric pain control, is one with which clinicians are most familiar. The type II system is simply a catheter suitable for percutaneous placement and tunneling. The type III system consists of a totally implantable injection port that is attached to a type II tunneled catheter. The type IV system is a totally implantable continuous infusion pump that is connected to a type II tunneled catheter. The type V system is a totally implantable programmable infusion pump attached to a type II tunneled catheter. The programmable feature of a type V IDDS allows a broad spectrum of delivery rates and modes, including occasional bolus injections.

Each of these drug delivery systems has its own unique profile of advantages and disadvantages. The clinician must be familiar with the particular merits of each system if optimal selection is to be made. In this time of increasing pressure to control the cost of health care, economic factors must also play a role in the selection of an IDDS. The cost of both the intended delivery system and the drugs to be administered through the delivery system must be considered before

Table 166–4

Spinal Drug Delivery Systems

Type I: Percutaneous epidural or subarachnoid catheter
Type II: Percutaneous epidural or subarachnoid catheter with subcutaneous tunneling
Type III: Totally implanted epidural or subarachnoid catheter with a subcutaneous injection port
Type IV: Totally implanted epidural or subarachnoid catheter with an implanted infusion pump
Type V: Totally implanted epidural or subarachnoid catheter with an implanted programmable infusion pump

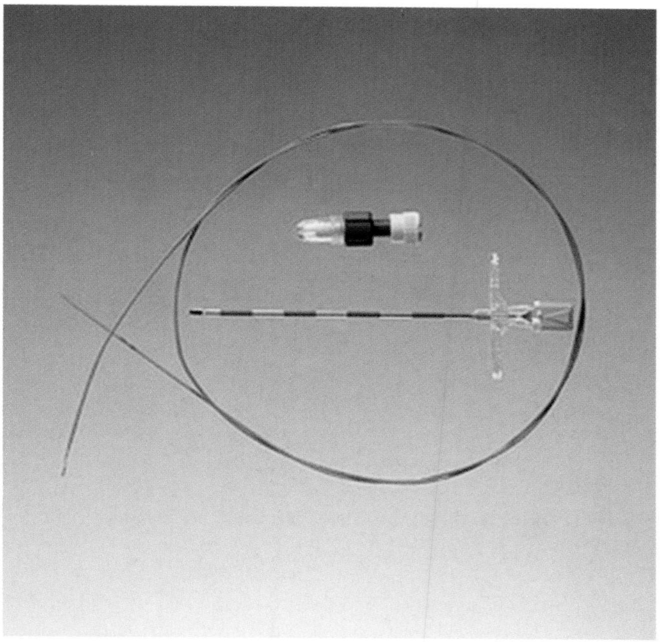

FIGURE 166–1 ■ Type I percutaneous catheter.

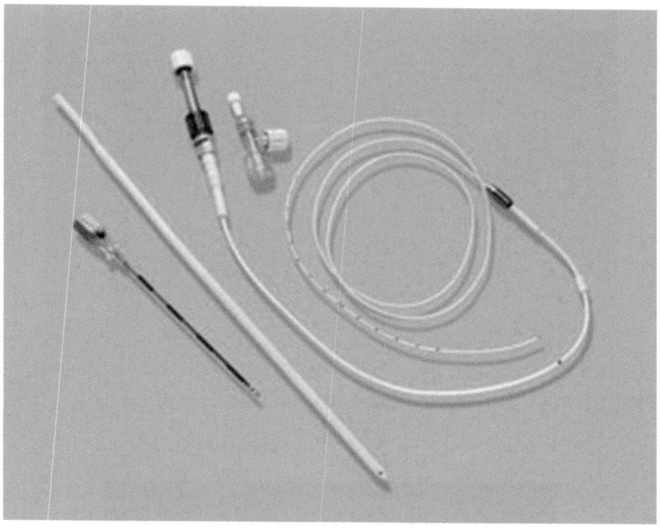

FIGURE 166–2 ■ Type II subcutaneous tunneled catheter.

implantation of an IDDS. A perfectly functioning IDDS is of no value to a patient who is unable to pay for the drugs, special needles, and supplies needed to use the delivery system. Similarly, implanted systems may superimpose financial hardship on a difficult terminal course. With prior planning, the financial issues can be individualized and resolved.

Type I: Percutaneous Catheter

The type I percutaneous catheter has gained wide acceptance for the short-term administration of spinal opioids or local anesthetics, or both, for the palliation of acute pain, including obstetric and postoperative pain (Fig. 166–1). The type I system also has three applications in cancer pain management. The first is in the acute setting, in which the delivery of opioids into the epidural or subarachnoid space can provide temporary palliation of pain postoperatively or until other concurrent treatments, such as radiotherapy, become effective. The second is in imminently dying patients too ill for more invasive procedures. The third is the use of a percutaneous catheter to administer test doses of spinal opioids before placement of a more permanent IDDS. In many centers, the use of a percutaneous catheter for the delivery of epidural and especially subarachnoid opioids is limited because of the ease with which catheters can be tunneled. The improved catheter fixation and reduced risk for infection associated with subcutaneous tunneling, combined with the relative ease of tunneling, have led many pain specialists to tunnel the spinal catheter to the flank, abdomen, or chest wall. In view of the potentially devastating and life-threatening consequences of catheter-induced spinal infection, as well as the highly favorable risk-to-benefit ratio of the type II tunneled catheter, use of the type I system should in my opinion be limited solely to the acute setting.

Type II: Subcutaneous Tunneled Catheter

Subcutaneously tunneled catheters are usually selected for patients who will have a finite need for spinally administered opioids (Fig. 166–2). Patients with pain secondary to major trauma, such as pelvic and long bone fractures and flail chest, are appropriate candidates for a type II system, as are cancer patients with life expectancies of weeks to months who have experienced excellent palliation of symptoms with trial doses of spinal drugs.[11,12] The type II system carries significantly less risk for infection than percutaneous catheters do.[12] The simplified catheter care and the ease of injection by both medical and non-medical personnel are also significant advantages of the type II system. The type II system can also be attached to an external continuous infusion pump.

Type III: Totally Implantable Reservoir/Port

The totally implantable reservoir is often chosen for cancer patients with life expectancies of months to years who have had excellent relief of symptoms with trial doses of spinal drugs (Fig. 166–3). Significantly less expensive that the type IV or V system, the type III system is a reasonable choice for patients who do not have a third party to cover the cost of a most sophisticated system.[13] The type III system is associated with potentially less risk of infection than is the case with type I and II systems, as well as a decreased risk of catheter failure.

Injection of the type III system is more difficult than with type I and II systems, and this disadvantage can have significant import when training lay people to inject and care for this system. Furthermore, removal or replacement requires a surgical incision.

Type IV: Totally Implantable Infusion Pump

The totally implantable infusion pump is also used in patients with life expectancies of months to years who obtained relief

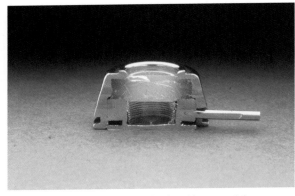

FIGURE 166–3 ■ Type III totally implantable reservoir/port.

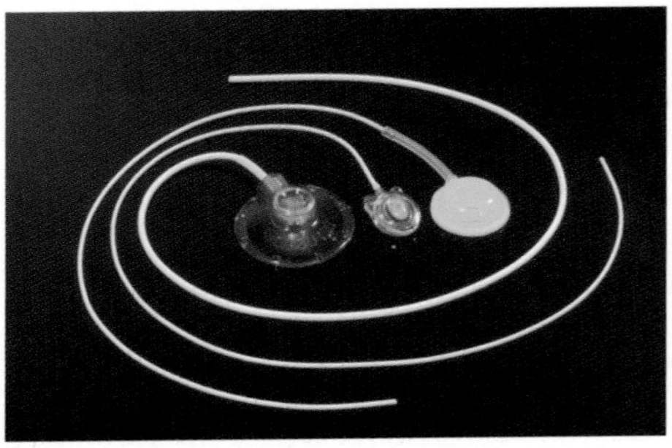

FIGURE 166–4 ■ Type IV totally implantable infusion pump.

of symptoms after trial doses of spinal drugs (Fig. 166–4). Type IV delivery systems may also be indicated in a cancer patient with a shorter life expectancy who experiences intermittent confusion secondary to metabolic abnormalities or systemically administered drugs. Clinical experience suggests that such patients may obtain analgesia with fewer side effects with low-dose continuous spinal opioid infusion than with repeated bolus injections into a spinal catheter. Alternatively, a type III implanted port with an external infusion pump may suffice in this situation, although such a system may be more inconvenient and require more support.

Because type IV systems require infrequent refills and run continuously, they are ideal for patients with limited medical or non-medical family support services. The type IV system is usually selected with an auxiliary bolus injection port to take advantage of potential drug options, such as injection of local anesthetics and the ability to inject contrast to troubleshoot the system.

Advantages of the type IV system include minimal risk for infection after the perioperative period and the need to inject the pump very infrequently relative to other IDDSs (the pump reservoir needs to be refilled approximately every 7 to 20 days). The overall high cost of the type IV system is a disadvantage and may occasionally result in the selection of a less effective or more inconvenient analgesic technique.

Type V: Totally Implantable Programmable Infusion Pump

The type V totally implantable programmable infusion pump is implanted with the same ease as the type IV system[14] (Fig. 166–5). These systems allow a broad spectrum of delivery rates and modes, including occasional bolus injections. Their principal application to date has been intrathecal infusion, especially for the treatment of spasticity in multiple sclerosis and spinal cord–injured patients, but the type V IDDS is also gaining increasing acceptance as the preferred type of IDDS for the long-term administration of spinal opioids.

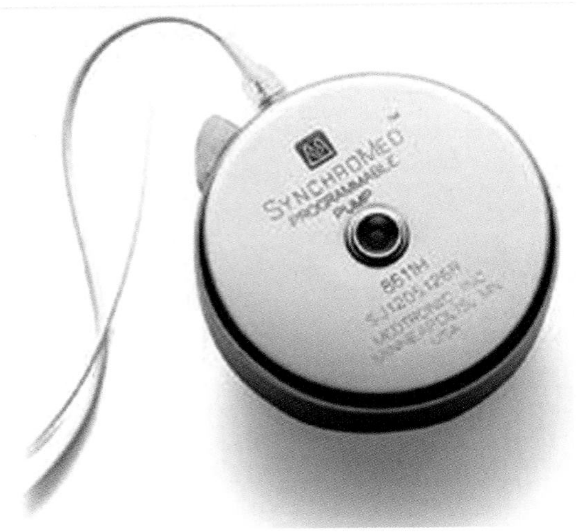

FIGURE 166–5 ■ Type V totally implantable programmable infusion pump.

CONCLUSION

The administration of spinal drugs via an IDDS is a useful addition to the armamentarium of clinicians treating patients with pain or spasticity that does not respond to conventional means. Proper selection of the patient and an appropriate delivery system are crucial if optimal results are to be achieved. It should be recognized that the chronic administration of opioids and other drugs into the epidural or subarachnoid space is evolving. Advances in the pharmacology of spinal drugs and the development of new delivery system technology will in time no doubt expand the options available for the relief of uncontrolled pain and spasticity.[6]

References

1. Wang JK, Nauss LE, Thomas JE: Pain relief by intrathecally applied morphine in man. Anesthesiology 50:149, 1979.
2. Yaksh TL: Opiate receptors for behavioral analgesia resemble those related to the depression of spinal nociceptive neurons. Science 199:1231, 1978.
3. Smith TJ, Staats PS, Deer T, et al: Randomized clinical trial of an implantable drug delivery system compared with comprehensive medical management for refractory cancer pain: Impact on pain, drug-related toxicity, and survival. J Clin Oncol 20:4040, 2002.
4. Korenkov AI, Niendorf WR, Darwish N, et al: Continuous intrathecal infusion of baclofen in patients with spasticity caused by spinal cord injuries. Neurosurg Rev 25:228, 2002.
5. Holmfred A: Failed intrathecal analgesia following severe, terminal cancer pain. Acta Anaesthesiol Scand 48:796, 2004.
6. Vaidyanthan S, Soni BM, Oo T, et al: Bladder stones—red herring for resurgence of spasticity in a spinal cord injury patient with implantation of Medtronic Synchromed pump for intrathecal delivery of baclofen—a case report. BMC Urol 3:3, 2003.

7. Waldman SD, Feldstein GS, Allen ML: Selection of patients for implantable spinal narcotic delivery systems. Anesth Analg 65:883, 1986.
8. Waldman SD, Feldstein GS, Waldman HJ, et al: Caudal administration of morphine sulfate in anti-coagulated and thrombocytopenic patients. Anesth Analg 66:267, 1987.
9. Mercandante S: Problems of long-term spinal opioid treatment in advanced cancer patients. Pain 79:1, 1999.
10. Datta S, Hurford W: Transverse myelitis associated with *Acinetobacter baumanii* intrathecal pump catheter–related infection. Where was the source of the infection? Reg Anesth Pain Med 29:503, 2004.
11. Waldman SD: Implantation of subcutaneously tunneled one piece epidural catheters. In Atlas of Interventional Pain Management, 2nd ed. Philadelphia, WB Saunders, 2004, p 534.
12. Waldman SD: Implantation of subcutaneously tunneled two piece epidural catheters. In Atlas of Interventional Pain Management, 2nd ed. Philadelphia, WB Saunders, 2004, p 538.
13. Waldman SD: Implantation of totally implantable reservoirs and injection ports. In Atlas of Interventional Pain Management, 2nd ed. Philadelphia, WB Saunders, 2004, p 607.
14. Waldman SD: Implantation of totally implantable infusion pumps. In Atlas of Interventional Pain Management, 2nd ed. Philadelphia, WB Saunders, 2004, p 612.

chapter 167

Complications of Implantable Technology for Pain Control

Richard B. Patt and Samuel J. Hassenbusch III

The use of implantable technology for controlling pain is new enough that data are still insufficient to make authoritative statements about the incidence and nature of complications and the definitive means of their prevention and management. The content of this review is derived in large part from clinical experience and a comprehensive review chapter.[1] Although we anticipate that standardized protocols will emerge over time, the recommendations provided here, unless stated otherwise, should be considered, at most, guidelines intended to assist the clinician in decision making.

DEFINITION OF TERMS

At the outset, it is useful to make a distinction among side effects, corollary effects, and complications.[2] Side effects and corollary effects are similar phenomena and differ from complications in that they are anticipated, at least in a large proportion of cases. According to Webster's Dictionary,[3] a *corollary effect* is one that "follows as a normal result," and a *side effect* is a "secondary and usually adverse effect." In contrast, although the risk for a *complication* may be known, it is unanticipated and a "difficult factor or issue, often appearing unexpectedly."[3] The term *complication* further implies an adverse outcome, which may or may not apply to a corollary effect or side effect.

It is important that the distinction between anticipated and unanticipated events (corollary and side effects versus complications) be appreciated so that the outcome can be characterized accurately. Furthermore, this distinction is important to invoke in discussions with patients, their families, and referring physicians to ensure that they understand the potential risks and benefits associated with a treatment and its alternatives.

The term *complication* implies an unanticipated adverse outcome. Although complications are by definition iatrogenic (caused by treatment), the occurrence of a complication or an adverse outcome does not, in and of itself, imply negligence. An injury stemming from *negligence* is one caused by a breach of duty, by a preventable error associated with a poor outcome.[4] A variety of factors predispose to such outcomes, independent of physician competence. Such factors include passage of sharp needles through tissue, the potential for movement of the needle or the patient, dependence on some degree of inference to determine actual needle placement (even with the benefit of radiologic guidance), normal anatomic variations, distortion of normal tissues by a tumor mass, failure of mechanical devices, and normal incidences of perioperative infection and other complications. Because of such factors, even independent of any contribution from physician error, if a sufficient number of procedures are undertaken, some complications are inevitable.

Regrettably, in addition to the factors just listed, physician error contributes to many adverse outcomes, although the actual incidence is not known. Given the potentially serious nature of complications, every conceivable effort obviously should be made to eliminate preventable errors. In addition, it is essential that once a complication has occurred, it be recognized promptly so that treatment or rehabilitation can be instituted. To achieve the most successful outcome, a fundamental knowledge of the pertinent anatomy, physiology, and pharmacologic effects related to the procedure is essential. A thorough understanding of the possible complications of a given procedure and strategies aimed at their prevention is also essential. Access to monitoring and resuscitation equipment and knowledge of their use are required. A comprehensive quality assurance program that includes a process for credentialing physicians and nurses, establishing protocols, monitoring outcome, and providing in-service training workshops is an essential component of any implantation program.

Unfortunately, standards of training for pain specialists have not been established. Some level of experience with the given procedure or a related one is assumed. Physicians with limited or accruing experience do well to consult with a more expert authority. Even with ample experience, a review of reference materials is prudent before undertaking a procedure.

COMPLICATIONS ASSOCIATED WITH IMPLANTABLE DEVICES

Technical Problems Common to Implantable Infusion and Stimulation Technology

Bleeding

Bleeding may occur intraoperatively or postoperatively, may be superficial or deep, and may be due to mechanical or systemic factors.

Intraoperative Bleeding

Systemic Sources of Bleeding

Systemic factors may produce diffuse bleeding in the surgical field that is difficult to control until the factors that predisposed to the bleeding are identified and corrected. It is essential that patients scheduled for surgery (particularly that involving the CNS) undergo screening for risk factors for bleeding of systemic origin. There is considerable debate about what screening methods strike a reasonable balance between clinical prudence and cost-effectiveness. There is no doubt that a careful interview is a sensitive screening tool and should be conducted in every case. The history taking should include elicitation of easy bruising, difficulty stopping bleeding once it has started, epistaxis, rectal bleeding, use of anticoagulants, including aspirin and nonsteroidal antiinflammatory drugs, and a family history of bleeding disorders. Some authorities argue that such a history is sufficient to rule out systemic factors that might predispose to surgical bleeding, especially in young patients. Given that implantation of pain control devices involves the potential for occult CNS hemorrhage, however, it may be prudent to require laboratory tests (prothrombin time, partial thromboplastin time, platelet count, and bleeding time) for all surgical candidates.

In summary, the strategy for management of bleeding induced by systemic factors is prevention. Management of intraoperative bleeding suspected to be related to systemic factors is reviewed elsewhere. Krames recommends discontinuing anticoagulant therapy 3 to 7 days before surgery and insisting on an increase in the prothrombin time to 75% of normal before surgery is undertaken.[5]

Intraoperative Bleeding Secondary to Mechanical Causes

Superficial Bleeding

Intraoperative bleeding is most often due to simple mechanical factors (i.e., ineffective local hemostasis). Requisites for the management of superficial bleeding related to mechanical causes are vigilance, patience, and experience. Excessive bleeding is uncommon because implantation of pain control devices does not require extensive surgery, nor are the contiguous anatomic areas densely vascular.

Regardless of the type of anesthesia that is chosen, infiltration with a local anesthetic containing 1:200,000 epinephrine is strongly recommended to reduce the risk for surgical bleeding. An important technical means of reducing the likelihood of bleeding is the use of electrocautery instead of sharp surgical instruments. A sharp scalpel should be used to incise the skin; after that, electrocautery may be used extensively. When further dissection is needed, blunt dissection is preferred. When sharp dissection is required, scissors are preferable to the scalpel, and care must be taken to spread the blades beneath each tissue plane before cutting and to keep the tips of the scissors constantly in view.

When bleeding does occur, the field should be kept as dry as possible with suction and dry gauze wielded by an assistant while the source is calmly identified. The most effective method of identifying the source of bleeding and reducing or eliminating it is firm pressure applied with dry gauze pads. The pads should be pressed directly onto the surface of the wound and never rubbed because rubbing increases bleeding. An initial trial of simple pressure applied for 30 to 60 seconds may be all that is required to stop the bleeding by promoting local vasoconstriction and clot formation. If bleeding persists, the area should be irrigated, and when a source of bleeding is identified, the coagulation mode of the electrocautery should be applied, but sparingly. The current should not be so high that an arc is created between the cautery tip and tissue. Extensive cauterization distorts anatomic detail, creates friable tissue, and by generating a large area of devitalized tissue, may produce a nidus for infection. Rarely, a larger vessel is incised or transected, in which case it may be ligated with an absorbable suture or metal clip.

Deep Bleeding

Bleeding into the subarachnoid or epidural space is a more worrisome problem because such bleeding is often occult and may be associated with neurologic morbidity. Fortunately, the incidence of clinically significant neuraxial hemorrhage after implantation is extremely low. The key strategy is again prevention: (1) identifying and correcting systemic factors that might predispose to bleeding, (2) using good surgical technique, and (3) promptly recognizing the problem and applying aggressive intervention.

Access to the epidural or subarachnoid space should be gained with as few passages of the large Tuohy needle as possible. This is facilitated by the judicious use of fluoroscopy. Periosteum is an important potential source of hemorrhage, so contact with bone should be appreciated immediately to minimize trauma. If access is difficult, a 22-gauge pilot needle may be used to identify an appropriate trajectory. Tumor is another important source of potential hemorrhage, so particular caution should be exercised in patients with bony metastases. In our experience, it is not uncommon to encounter frank bleeding from the epidural or subarachnoid space when entry has been difficult, especially if multiple passages of a guidewire have been necessary to clear a tract for the catheter or lead. Although this has not been associated with postoperative problems in our experience, it calls for careful postoperative observation. Bleeding is usually sparse and ultimately ceases after irrigation with saline through the Tuohy needle. Patients should be observed particularly carefully for new back pain and neurologic abnormalities (altered sensation, motor or sphincter weakness) in the postoperative period. If bleeding persists, it is prudent to obtain an intraoperative consultation with a neurosurgeon for consideration of laminotomy to identify and eliminate the source of hemorrhage.

Postoperative Bleeding

Deep Bleeding: Subarachnoid or Epidural Hemorrhage

In the rare instance when a clinically significant subarachnoid or epidural hemorrhage occurs, it is usually manifested by the onset of back pain and rapidly progressive neurologic abnormalities in the postoperative period. To identify such changes, it is essential that the results of a careful neurologic examination be documented preoperatively. Patients should routinely undergo a neurologic examination during the recovery phase. Subjective complaints of new back pain, weakness, and sensory changes should be elicited and taken seriously. New neurologic abnormalities (subjective or objective) suggest a space-occupying collection of blood and warrant further investigation. Fever and nuchal rigidity may result from blood in the subarachnoid space. The results of closely spaced, serial neurologic examinations determine whether these findings are transient. If they persist or progress, urgent consultation with a neurologist or neurosurgeon should be sought, and patients should undergo urgent radiologic screening—with MRI, CT, or myelography, depending on the clinical scenario. MRI is contraindicated in patients with a spinal stimulator and requires that special precautions be exercised if a drug-infusion device has been implanted. Testing of the implanted device may provide indirect evidence of a fluid collection. Clotted blood may interfere with function by impeding flow through an infusion device (tested by accessing the side port) or by a reduction in electrical contact manifested as loss of stimulation or increased impedance.

Epidural or subarachnoid hemorrhage is a surgical emergency. Symptoms (back pain, altered sensation, bowel or bladder incontinence) characteristically progress over a period of hours, and permanent neurologic injury is likely if decompressive surgery is delayed.

Superficial Bleeding: Wound Hematoma or Seroma

Superficial bleeding is manifested as a *hematoma*, a collection of coagulated blood, or a *seroma*, a collection of serum. The incidence of these problems can be reduced by meticulous attention to maintaining intraoperative hemostasis. The first sign of such problems is usually a sensation of local pressure or pain during the recovery period, with or without the leakage of sanguineous or serosanguineous material from the wound edges. It ordinarily resolves with the application of local pressure and ice, but occasionally, re-exploration or reversal of systemic clotting abnormalities is required.

Often, hematoma or seroma is not identified until after the immediate postoperative period, in which case it is manifested as a diffuse bruise or a fluctuant collection, respectively. Both conditions are usually self-limited and resolve with time, during which analgesics may be provided and hot packs applied for comfort. Some authorities believe that a pocket seroma may occur in as many as 80% of patients, whereas others report seroma in less than 10% of cases. Generally, seromas are a self-limited problem that resolve over time and should be managed with simple observation and reassurance. Treatment of excessive or chronic collections is controversial. Because a chronic seroma or hematoma is an ideal medium for infection, conventional surgical texts recommend fine-needle aspiration and even insertion of a polyethylene catheter when collections repeatedly re-form. Others caution that aspiration may result in bacterial contamination.[6] Large postoperative seromas and liquefied hematomas should probably be aspirated, but under strict sterile conditions. Early and frequent pump refills should be minimized when such a collection is present to reduce the risk for contamination. In addition, such collections may increase the difficulty of accurately locating the access port of an infusion device,[7,8] an obstacle that predisposes to accidental subcutaneous or intrathecal deposition of drug during attempts at pump refilling.

Infection

Fortunately, the incidence of infection after implant surgery for pain and spasticity is low. Most authorities advocate the use of prophylactic antibiotics. The most common recommendation is vancomycin, 500 mg 2 hours before surgery, and copious irrigation of all wounds with fluid containing antibiotics. The same fluid may be used to bathe hardware before insertion. Other authorities recommend intravenous cephalothin, 2 g preoperatively and then every 6 hours for 24 hours. The incidence of infection is probably highest in the immediate postoperative period, which is when vigilance should be greatest. Problems range from local infections of the pocket or subcutaneous tract to meningitis and epidural abscess.

Local Infection

Local subcutaneous infection is usually heralded by fever, leukocytosis, and inflammatory skin changes (erythema, tenderness, fluctuance, drainage) overlying the infected region. Leukocytosis is often observed on Gram stain of fluid aspirated from the subcutaneous pocket in patients with simple seroma (see earlier), so a pathogen should be sought if infection is suspected.

When infection is suspected, concerns relate both to resolving the local process and to guarding against extension of the infectious process to the CNS. What is the best treatment is controversial. Some authorities advocate vigorous conservative management for 1 to 2 weeks with intravenous antibiotics and local wound care while observing for signs of CNS involvement. Local ("intrapocket") deposition of antibiotics has also been advocated. Others believe that removal of all hardware is always indicated. An infectious disease consultation may be warranted, although the implant surgeon should be aware that such a consultation is usually accompanied by a recommendation that the hardware be removed.

Central Nervous System Infection

Meningitis

Meningitis is inflammation of the meninges of the brain or spinal cord. After surgical implantation, meningitis is more likely to be a relatively focal process involving the spinal cord, although with encephalitis, more diffuse involvement is a possibility.

Meningitis is usually heralded by fever, chills, leukocytosis, malaise, headache, vomiting, and back or neck pain and stiffness, and it tends to be accompanied by signs of meningeal irritation. The Kernig sign is pain associated with simultaneous flexion of the hip and extension of the knee in a supine patient. The Brudzinski sign is involuntary flexion of the knee when a supine patient's neck is abruptly flexed. Although it is difficult to quantify, a key diagnostic finding is that affected patients tend to look extremely ill or "septic." Progression of signs and symptoms is typically rapid. Patients may become confused, stuporous, and dehydrated, and unstable hemodynamics may develop. Classically, cerebral involvement is manifested by cranial nerve abnormalities (including loss of auditory acuity), seizures, focal cerebral signs (hemiparesis, visual field defects), and signs of elevated intracranial pressure, although these findings are unusual in patients with infection involving implanted intraspinal devices.

Early recognition is essential, and consultation with a neurologist or infectious disease specialist is recommended. Laboratory examinations of blood and CSF help confirm a diagnosis, although culture results are affected if empirical antibiotic treatment has already been instituted. Recovery is usually complete when diagnosis and treatment with intravenous antibiotics are rendered promptly. Removal of all implanted hardware is necessary. The only possible exception to this dictum involves a patient with imminently terminal cancer whose pain is well controlled. In this case, considerations of comfort may prevail, and treatment with intrathecal antibiotics may be considered.

Epidural Abscess

Signs and symptoms of epidural abscess are similar to those described for epidural hematoma, but if the abscess is allowed to progress, findings consistent with meningitis may become more prominent. The initial signs are usually localized back pain and deep tenderness. Symptoms may be radicular in nature and, depending on the size and location of the lesion, may be associated with neurologic abnormalities (focal weakness, sensory abnormalities, incontinence). Progression of symptoms, especially weakness in a paraplegic or root distribution, generally occurs over a course of hours or days, with a slower progression of symptoms than that seen with postoperative hemorrhage. Fever and meningeal signs may be present but are less prominent than in patients with frank meningitis. Laboratory studies should include blood work and examination of CSF, but ultimately, myelography is required for diagnosis and localization. Treatment is prompt surgical decompression and removal of all implanted hardware. Ideally, intravenous antibiotics should be started after specimens for cultures and Gram stain have been obtained. *Staphylococcus aureus* is often the infecting bacterium; therefore, the initial antibiotic should be effective against it.

Postoperative Fever

Postoperative fever should always generate concern and a high index of suspicion of underlying local or systemic infection, especially in view of the serious consequences of the conditions already described, although they are relatively uncommon. It should be recognized that in the initial days after implantation (particularly of an intrathecal catheter), fever develops in a large proportion of patients in the absence of signs of local, systemic, or meningeal infection. In this scenario, low-grade fever (38° C to 38.5° C) is usually associated with a normal WBC count and a CSF that is remarkable only for pleocytosis and elevated protein content. Treatment is conservative, and administration of antibiotics is unwarranted. Indiscriminate early use of antibiotics makes the selection of effective therapy much more problematic later if cultures eventually yield positive results.

Cerebrospinal Fluid Leak, Post–Dural Puncture Headache, and Hygroma

CSF leak is definitely a risk after puncture of the dura with a large (15-gauge) Tuohy needle. It can occur during placement of a spinal cord stimulator if the dura is accidentally punctured during efforts to identify the epidural space or if the guidewire or lead pierces the dura. CSF leak may occur after subarachnoid catheter placement under two circumstances. First, leakage can occur by the same mechanism cited earlier if successful dural puncture is followed by an inability to advance the catheter and a second puncture becomes necessary. Second, CSF leakage can occur around the implanted catheter because the tract created by the needle slightly exceeds the caliber of the catheter. Many surgeons routinely create a purse-string suture in the ligament surrounding the catheter's entrance into the dura, usually with absorbable material. In addition to possibly reducing the risk for CSF leak, this measure may also discourage catheter extrusion. If a purse-string suture is chosen, care must be taken to ensure that (1) the needle does not damage the catheter and (2) the suture is not pulled so tight that it occludes the lumen of the catheter. The risk for catheter occlusion may be reduced by creating the purse-string suture when the catheter is still within the needle and by periodically verifying free flow of CSF.

CSF leak is usually heralded by a classic postural post–dural puncture headache, although other causes of headache should still be considered. Many headaches resolve with conservative management. Even though what constitutes proper conservative management of post–dural puncture headache is still debated, several days' bed rest, fluids, and an abdominal binder are recommended. Persistent postural headache may be treated with an epidural blood patch consisting of 5 to 15 mL of autologous blood. The blood patch should be performed under the strictest of aseptic conditions and with fluoroscopy to avoid damaging the catheter or lead. Rarely, when headaches persist, surgical exploration and placement of a fat graft may be necessary.

Hygroma typically refers to a benign, distended, lymph-filled cavity, usually in a child, but the word is also used for a postoperative collection of CSF. Hygroma can develop after a large CSF leak and is eventually manifested as a subcutaneous bulge near the dorsal incision. The mechanism may even be disruption of the pia arachnoid membrane and formation of a subdural collection through a ball-valve effect. Theoretically, such a collection may produce focal neurologic deficits in the same way that an epidural abscess does, but in general, such signs have little clinical significance. The diagnosis is based on clinical findings and radiologic studies. Most authorities recommend that such collections not be aspirated because of the risk for infection; rather, they advise waiting for it to resolve or reoperating. Large collections occasionally require aspiration, although care must be taken to avoid damaging the underlying apparatus. An infected hygroma should be treated in the same way as meningitis. A frank percutaneous CSF leak requires revision of the wound with primary closure.

Malposition of the Subcutaneous Pocket

Care should be taken to ensure that the subcutaneous position of the infusion device or pulse generator does not impinge on the ribs superiorly or the iliac crest inferiorly. Such bony impingement is a cause of chronic postoperative pain and usually requires reoperation. It can generally be avoided by marking the patient's skin before surgery and observing where the marks fall when the patient is supine, standing, and sitting. A pocket positioned too far cephalad or caudad or too close to the skin surface can also impair wound healing and predispose to erosion through the skin. Patients who are cachectic, diabetic, or taking steroids are at increased risk for these complications. A pocket placed too deep (>2.5 cm) can also create problems during refills.

When implanting a spinal cord stimulator, it should be ascertained that the pulse generator is placed with the Medtronic trademark facing outward to avoid problems with programming. Care should be taken to tighten the set screws snugly to avoid disconnection but not so tight that the threads become stripped. With an infusion device, care must be taken to properly anchor the Dacron sleeve to avoid rotation of the pump, which could put enough traction on the catheter to cause it to withdraw from the intrathecal space.

Technical Problems Specific to Implantable Infusion Devices

Contamination of the Pump Reservoir

The pump reservoir can be contaminated by seeding with skin flora during refills. Although the Medtronic's 0.22-μm filter would be expected to prevent extension of an infection from the reservoir to the CNS, prudence dictates that documentation of an infected aspirate be followed by removal of the system.

Catheter Care

Silastic catheters are extremely fragile and ideally should be handled only with the fingers. If such a catheter must be manipulated with forceps, rubber shods should be used. The catheter may become difficult to manipulate because of the lubricity of body fluids, in which case the field should be irrigated. Dry gauze also provides excellent traction and causes no trauma. The catheter should never be forced into the epidural or subarachnoid space because the guidewire would develop a "memory" that would make further passage difficult. The catheter should be stabilized with an anchoring sleeve and should not be sutured directly. Nicking or cutting of the catheter should be avoided. Excess length of catheter should be coiled behind the infusion device, well away from the access port.

Pump Care

The pump reservoir should be emptied before instillation of drug (10 mL) and should be programmed to deliver at least 0.096 mL/day. The necessity of initially filling the reservoir only partially cannot be overemphasized because excess pressurization can be associated with erratic infusion rates (the total reservoir capacity is 18 mL). The incision for the subcutaneous pocket should be positioned eccentrically so that it is not directly over the access port.

Failure of Analgesia in Patients with Infusion Devices

Immediate Postoperative Failure

Failure as a result of mechanical causes most often occurs in the immediate postoperative period. Uncontrolled postoperative (nonsurgical) pain in a patient who was previously comfortable during a trial of intraspinal opioids suggests some error during implantation. Such difficulties may relate to failure to cannulate the epidural or subarachnoid space; a disconnected, kinked, or leaking catheter; or programming or pharmacy error. Problems can usually be avoided by careful confirmation of the location of the catheter tip, gentle handling of the catheter, careful suturing, and verification of the accuracy of the program and the prescription. Before the spinal catheter is connected to the infusion device, if it is intrathecal, free flow of CSF should be confirmed, and if it is epidural, the catheter should be checked for obstruction or occlusion. The same procedures should be performed through the infusion device's side port once the catheter has been connected.

Late Failure

Failure of analgesia after apparently successful implantation is not uncommon, but it is usually due to the development of anesthetic tolerance or new foci of pain and rarely to mechanical malfunction. Because physiologic rather than mechanical causes are most often responsible, it is reasonable to respond initially by increasing the rate of the infusion to determine whether pain control can be regained. Although this is often ultimately a correct and effective approach, intervention should be individualized and predicated on the findings of a careful history and examination.

Differential Diagnosis

The differential diagnosis of late failure of analgesia includes the development of tolerance, new foci of pain, an incorrect prescription, failure to properly load the pump, pump malfunction,[9] disconnection, and obstruction or migration of the catheter system.[10] A careful history and physical examination should be performed and, when indicated, supplemented by communication with the family, primary care physician, oncologist, and home nursing and pharmacy services. Assessment is undertaken to rule out a new pain-generating lesion or extension of underlying disease. Pain is multifactorial; because the pain threshold is influenced by a variety of factors, new psychosocial causes should be sought as well.

Progression of Disease

Local extension, distant metastases, or an unrelated pain problem should be confirmed or excluded by the history and physical examination, appropriate laboratory and radiologic investigations, and when indicated, consultation.

Tolerance

Tolerance is manifested as the need for progressively higher doses of a drug over time to achieve a given degree of effect. If problems related to the integrity of the delivery system and demonstrable new underlying disease (physical and psychological) have been excluded, the most likely explanation for increased pain is tolerance. In the past, loss of analgesia had been assumed to be rather uniformly related to the development of tolerance. More recently, it has been accepted that loss of analgesia is more often related to undetected progression of cancer and more extensive tissue damage.[11] Nerve injury of new onset often produces neuropathic pain, which may be less opioid responsive. Tolerance remains an important cause of failed analgesia. Tolerance does not usually develop equally to all effects of a drug at the same rate, and fortunately, tolerance to a drug's undesirable effects can also develop.[12] Management of tolerance is discussed later.

Mechanical Failure

Examination of the infusion system is approached logically and simply by working sequentially from the periphery of the system toward the center:

1. Examination of the drug prescription and confirmation of its accuracy.
2. Examination of the infusion device and verification that the program and prescription are correct. Verification of proper battery function and that the volume in the reservoir corresponds to the expected and actual volume of drug delivered (≤15%).
3. Examination of external portions of the system for kinking and to confirm that the drug is actually exiting the pump tubing.
4. Examination of the tunneled portion of the catheter to detect kinks or rents in the tubing or evidence of infection or subcutaneous drug deposition.
5. In the absence of demonstrable defects in the integrity of the delivery system, injection of radiopaque contrast medium and radiography. The results of these studies provide more definitive data on the system's integrity and help identify catheter migration or diminished drug delivery because of tumor or deposition of fibrous tissue around the catheter outlet. MRI is a potentially useful adjunct to assessment, although the device may create artifacts. MRI is not contraindicated, but it requires that the device first be emptied and turned off. Myelography may be performed after injection of contrast medium through the device's access port, and subsequently, CT can be performed.

Radiography, Myelography, and Epidurography or Test Doses

The radiopacity of the system's catheter facilitates radiologic visualization, although filling the catheter lumen with contrast medium is often useful to enhance image quality. The Model 8615 device (Medtronic, Minneapolis) has a second port that is eccentrically located and bypasses the pump for myelography or epidurography. If a model without a bypass port (Medtronic 8611-H) has been implanted, the reservoir may be filled with contrast medium and the rate of infusion can be increased, after which films can be obtained. A water-soluble, non-ionic contrast medium should be used in all cases,[13] and the patient should first be screened for a history of allergy. If further information is needed, post-contrast CT may be performed. Although their use is not encouraged because of considerations of safety, the same means can be used for the administration of test doses of local anesthetics.

Treatment Strategies for Opioid Tolerance

Tolerance is implied by failure of analgesia in the absence of new disease or equipment failure. Obviously, the approach to tolerance depends on the baseline treatment protocol. In general, a reasonable approach when tolerance is suspected involves sequentially increasing the dose by 10% to 30% per day. If this strategy would require administering excessive volumes of drug, the solution may need to be reformulated. What constitutes an excessive flow rate is still not known, although Leak and colleagues[14] propose 10 to 15 mL/hr for epidural infusion and a daily rate that does not exceed 10% of a given patient's calculated CSF volume for intrathecal devices. Morphine can readily be concentrated to 50 mg/mL and hydromorphone to about 200 mg/mL.[15] Long-term infusions of high concentrations of morphine have not been associated with neurotoxicity or CNS lesions, although collection of more animal and human data is warranted before definitive conclusions can be drawn about neurotoxicity.[16] Maximum daily doses cited in the literature range from 60 to 480 mg for epidural morphine[17] and up to 150 mg for intrathecal morphine.[18]

Titration-Resistant Tolerance

Tolerance may make it impossible to regain analgesia by simple dose titration, although it is not clear to what extent titration-resistant tolerance represents tolerance per se or the emergence of a relatively opioid-resistant neuropathic focus of pain.

Preventing Tolerance

The emergence of true, pharmacodynamically based tolerance can be managed in several ways, none entirely satisfactory. One approach is prophylaxis. It has been suggested that tolerance appears to be less troublesome when intraspinal opioids are administered by continuous infusion rather than by intermittent boluses,[19-22] although this theory has not been proved conclusively. It has also been suggested that the use of a more potent opioid, such as sufentanil, may result in slower receptor down-regulation.[23-25]

Use of Non-opioid Substances

Once tolerance develops, theoretically, other spinal antinociception-modulating systems can be used, either temporarily, to "rest" and "recruit" receptors (a drug holiday), or over the long term as an alternative or supplement to opioid therapy. A variety of disparate substances have been administered intraspinally in an effort to produce safe, reliable analgesia. Even encouraging reports warrant cautious interpretation because animal and human studies of toxicology and efficacy are inadequate in many cases. No substances other than morphine and baclofen are currently approved for administration via an implanted Medtronic infusion device.

Clonidine

The α_2-adrenergic agonist clonidine is perhaps the best studied of these agents. Successful management of both cancer pain and postoperative pain has been reported with epidural and intrathecal clonidine.[26-28] Through its action on postsynaptic receptors in the dorsal horn, clonidine appears to produce spinally mediated antinociception by activation of descending noradrenergic inhibitory systems.[29] Analgesia is reversible with α-antagonist agents but is not affected by naloxone. Hypotension is the main potential adverse effect. When clonidine is used in combination with opioids, opioid-mediated respiratory depression may be potentiated, especially in opioid-naive patients. Clonidine does not appear to cause local toxicity.[30] Reporting on 52 patients with chronic cancer pain, Glynn and associates[28] observed consistently adequate analgesia in 20 patients with a low incidence of side effects, and Eisenach and colleagues[26] treated patients successfully with intrathecal clonidine and morphine for as long as 5 months. It has been suggested that intraspinal clonidine may have a particularly important role in the management of opioid-resistant neuropathic pain syndromes. Preliminary evaluation of the α-adrenergic agonists tizanidine and dexmedetomidine is ongoing.

Droperidol

Droperidol appears to be a safe and effective adjunct to intraspinal opioid therapy. Animal experiments have demonstrated that intrathecal morphine analgesia is prolonged and potentiated by the addition of droperidol and that tolerance is delayed.[31] The pooled results of clinical series suggest that the addition of 2.5 mg of droperidol to epidural or intrathecal morphine may potentiate analgesia, reduce a range of side effects (nausea, vomiting, pruritus, urinary retention, hypotension), and delay tolerance, although sedative effects may occur.[32,33]

Somatostatin and Calcitonin

Chrubasik and coworkers[34,35] have reported that somatostatin, an endogenous neuropeptide, when injected intrathecally, epidurally, or intraventricularly, produces analgesia equal to that of intrathecal morphine in patients with postoperative or cancer pain. On the basis of these findings, somatostatin is another potential means of limiting or managing opioid tolerance, although expense and suggestions of local neurotoxicity are barriers to more widespread trials.[36,37] Octreotide, a synthetic somatostatin analog, may ultimately prove to be a safer and more useful compound.[38,39] Intrathecal salmon calcitonin, though probably ineffective alone as an analgesic agent, has an opioid-sparing effect when used in conjunction with morphine.[36,40] The currently available data from animal research are insufficient to recommend routine clinical use of intrathecal or epidural calcitonin.[41]

Antinociceptive Agents

Stein and Brechner[42] administered epidural norepinephrine, 50 to 250 μg, combined with morphine in a tolerant patient and consequently were able to reduce the dose of opioid by 50% without altering analgesia. Russell and Chang demonstrated in rats that alternating administration of a relatively receptor-specific agent modifies tolerance favorably.[43] (Morphine affects predominantly mu receptors; D-Ala2-D-Leu5-enkephalin [DADL] predominantly affects delta receptors.) Anecdotal reports of analgesia in morphine-tolerant patients given intrathecal DADL, a synthetic enkephalin analog, have also appeared in the literature.[44,45] Other substances with potential antinociceptive activity at the level of the neuraxis are ketamine,[46] midazolam,[47] baclofen,[48] an injectable form of aspirin (lysine acetylsalicylate), and various α-adrenergic adenosine analogs.[36]

Use of a Different Opioid

Cross-tolerance is the phenomenon whereby tolerance to one drug induces tolerance to another. The issue of cross-tolerance among the various subsets of opioid receptors and different receptor systems is an important one. There is some evidence for incomplete cross-tolerance,[39,49,50] and that is a rationale for substituting one opioid for another, although additional research is required to gain a better understanding of the nature of incomplete cross-tolerance among otherwise similar drugs.

Substitution of Local Anesthetics

An alternative strategy for reversing tolerance or delaying its development involves the administration of epidural or even intrathecal local anesthetic. Local anesthetic may be substituted for opioids to provide an opioid-free interval (a drug holiday), during which receptor activity may revert toward normal, once again rendering the patient opioid sensitive.[51] This strategy should be used only in a closely supervised setting to monitor for adverse sequelae of opioid withdrawal (abstinence syndrome) or local anesthetics (hypotension).

Combining Opioid with Other Agents

Alternatively, dilute concentrations of local anesthetic (0.012% to 0.25% bupivacaine) can be added to an epidural opioid infusion. Such combinations are often used successfully to manage acute pain and have well-established safety profiles in the acute care setting. Du Pen[52] has demonstrated the safety of administering a combination of epidural morphine and dilute bupivacaine to patients in their homes. In a series of 105 patients treated with epidural morphine, 7.6% (8 patients) required further analgesia with bupivacaine for new bone or nerve pain. In addition to epidural morphine, these patients received epidural bupivacaine, 0.125% to 0.5%, with epinephrine, administered at 6 mL/hr. Clinically significant hypotension did not develop, and many patients remained ambulatory. Patients receiving this treatment should be well hydrated and restricted to bed rest during the initial stages of therapy. Such combination therapy may minimize the adverse side effects of each type of agent[53] and may be particularly efficacious for sharp, incident pain caused, for example, by a pathologic fracture or a neurogenic process. Animal evidence of synergistic effects after the administration of combinations of opioids with distinctive receptor affinities[54] or an opioid and an α-agonist[55] suggests that combining such agents is another means of reducing or offsetting opioid tolerance.

Summary

Careful assessment helps determine the relative contributions of each of the factors that might be responsible for loss of analgesia after previously reliable intraspinal opioid therapy. The system's integrity and the patient's physiologic and psychological status should be evaluated. Subsequent management must be expressly individualized.

Psychological and emotional adjustments to progressive cancer, disability, and impending death sometimes color subjective reports of pain and must be addressed. Increased complaints of pain may signal the need for counseling or treatment with psychotropic agents, including antidepressants and sleep-restoring medications. Any new lesions (bowel obstruction, pathologic fracture, spinal cord compression) should be identified and, when appropriate, managed with alternative palliative interventions (e.g., radiation therapy, surgery, steroids). Neuropathic pain is often resistant to intraspinal opioid therapy but may be effectively managed with oral adjuvants (antidepressants, anticonvulsants, sodium channel blockers) or local anesthetic blockade. Intermittent regional blocks or the addition of a local anesthetic to the intraspinal opioid infusion may be particularly efficacious when symptoms are sympathetically maintained. Incident pain can often be effectively managed by supplementing the continuous intraspinal opioid infusion with oral opioids. Depending on the system in use, patient-controlled analgesia (PCA) or the addition of a preprogrammed bolus schedule may be useful. As clinical experience with new agents and methods of administration accrues, better-defined roles for these interventions are anticipated.

Problems with Refills of Infusion Devices

Accidental overdose of morphine in the course of refilling an intrathecal infusion device is an uncommon event but has been known to occur (Medtronic, personal communication, 1991). The potential for accidental overdose as a result of equipment malfunction or human error has been cited as a possible disadvantage of implantable systems.[56] Accidental massive overdoses of opioids in other settings have been reported, including malfunction of a PCA device (administration of 495 mg meperidine within 20 minutes, which resulted in respiratory arrest),[57] as well as overdoses of epidural[58] and intrathecal morphine.[59] Independent of the route of administration, excessive doses of opioids may result in a variety of adverse outcomes, including respiratory depression, hypothermia, myoclonic seizures, pulmonary edema, coma, and death.[36,60]

Accidental Subcutaneous Administration

In a case reported in 1992, a patient accidentally received a subcutaneous bolus injection of 480 mg morphine that was supposed to be instilled into the reservoir of an infusion pump and administered continuously over a period of 6 to 8 weeks.[7] Mild respiratory depression and confusion developed approximately 2 hours afterward, but no significant cardiovascular effects or lasting neurologic deficits resulted. The patient was treated with 0.16 mg of naloxone intravenously, predominantly for diagnostic purposes. After 20 hours of observation, the patient was discharged without sequelae. This relatively innocuous outcome was probably related to a constellation of factors, including opioid tolerance, early recognition, and prompt management. Given the patient's stable course, the emergency medicine house staff involved in the case were reluctant to believe that such an overdose actually occurred, but tolerance to high doses of opioids after long-term exposure to these drugs is well known in the cancer pain literature.[61] Reversal of respiratory depression with an opioid antagonist is warranted in such cases, but it should be accomplished with small, incremental doses to avoid severe hypertension, dysrhythmia, and pulmonary edema, which presumably result from the rapid increases in sympathetic tone that may accompany the sudden return of pain when opioid effects are antagonized too rapidly.[62]

The Medtronic SynchroMed infusion pump is a titanium device about the size of a hockey puck that is usually implanted in the subcutaneous tissue of the flank. In the center of the pump's ventral surface is a small silicone injection port that must be palpated through intact skin. Identification of the septum may be difficult shortly after surgery because of swelling and inflammation. Passage of a 22-gauge, eccentrically tipped needle is marked by a characteristic giving way and ready return of clear fluid. Postoperative edema, obesity, or a deep implant may interfere with easy palpation of the port. It is possible that in the case just cited, the curved tip of the Huber needle slid over the pump's metal surface, thereby mimicking the anticipated "give." Serous extravasation or seroma (usually clear) has been noted as one of the most common complications after surgery on subcutaneous tissue[63]; thus, in the postoperative patient described in this case, aspiration of a seroma mimicked return of drug.

Accidental Intrathecal Bolus Administration during Intended Refill

Two models of the Medtronic SynchroMed infusion pump are currently available. The older Model 8611H pump has a single refill port located centrally and no accessory port, whereas the newer Model 8615 has a central port for refill and an eccentric accessory port. The accessory port bypasses the reservoir and pump mechanism and is intended to facilitate myelography and to allow for planned intraspinal boluses or test doses of drug. At least four cases of accidental administration of large doses of morphine into accessory ports have been reported; two were fatal.[8] Accidental administration of baclofen into accessory ports has also been reported. These incidents prompted issuance of an FDA-required "Urgent Medical Device Safety Alert" (June 15, 1992) by Medtronic that should be required reading for all healthcare professionals involved in maintenance of implantable intraspinal infusion systems.

Avoiding and Managing Problems during Refill of a Medtronic Reservoir

The potentially devastating events just described seem to not be the result of faulty design or system malfunction; rather, they are directly attributable to human error. Thus, they should be reliably preventable by careful observation of the precautions and guidelines related to replenishing the pump as they are set forth in the SynchroMed pump and refill kit technical manuals and reviewed here. The most important and essential precautionary measure is to use the Medtronic Model 8551 refill kit *each time* a pump's reservoir is replenished. The pump model is first identified so that the proper template[7] will be used to pinpoint the refill port, which is located centrally. A Huber needle is then inserted, with sterile technique, through the template's center hole and advanced through the skin, subcutaneous tissue, and pump septum until the rigid needle stop arrests the needle's progress. The reservoir's residual volume should be emptied by applying continuous, gentle negative pressure to the plunger of the syringe. Proper needle placement is evidenced by air bubbles, which are not normally seen if the accessory port has accidentally been entered. Tubing and a three-way stopcock are provided in the kit to avoid entraining air into the reservoir. Resuscitation equipment, including naloxone (for morphine infusions) and physostigmine (for baclofen infusions), should be immediately available. Algorithms for both contingencies are included in the FDA-mandated safety alert already cited. Guidelines call for support of the airway, breathing, and circulation; serial intravenous administration of naloxone or physostigmine (when indicated); and (when not contraindicated) withdrawal of CSF.

Risk factors for problems during refilling include obesity, a "deep" implant, and particularly early after implantation, local edema. If needed, fluoroscopy may be used to locate the proper port. Air bubbles are not normally obtained when the accessory port has been entered accidentally (CSF is returned). If a question remains about which port has been entered, CSF can be identified by chemically testing the aspirate for glucose. Given the serious nature of an error, routine dipstick examination would not be imprudent. Our report recommends that during refilling of the reservoir, its entire volume be intermittently aspirated to verify that the residual volume is equal to what has been instilled during the intended refill.

An alternative safety measure that we recently adopted is to empty the pump and then inject preservative-free saline and aspirate it before loading the reservoir with fresh morphine. We believe that the theoretical disadvantage of diluting the ultimate dose of morphine slightly (by mixing saline within the pump's dead space volume) is offset by the reduced risk of injecting even a few milliliters of concentrated morphine (25 to 50 mg/mL) intrathecally.

A final precaution concerns pump selection. Although an accessory port is often desirable, the option of the Medtronic Model 8611H (without an accessory port) should be seriously considered for patients who are likely to be residing outside the geographic area of the implanting physician.

Summary

Although several regrettable incidents of patient injury have occurred in association with the use of an intraspinal infusion pump, it appears to be a reliable and safe device. More such incidents can be prevented by the institution of several simple precautions and the implementation of pump training programs for all involved healthcare professionals.

Physiologic and Pharmacologic Side Effects

Unlike their opioid-naive counterparts, cancer patients with long-term exposure to systemic opioids rarely have dose-limiting side effects.[64,65] This distinction provides a tremendous measure of safety. Because a cardinal rule for instituting intraspinal therapy is documented failure of conservative pharmacotherapy, it would be unusual to institute long-term intraspinal therapy in an opioid-naive patient.

Potential side effects of intraspinal opioids that occur with clinically significant frequency include respiratory depression, gastrointestinal hypomotility, inhibition of micturition, nausea, vomiting, pruritus, and CNS toxicity (usually manifested as sedation).[66] DeCastro and colleagues[64] list a multitude of other side effects that occur much more rarely or have been reported only anecdotally but of which the clinician should be aware. These side effects include dysphoria, hypothermia, oliguria, failure of ejaculation, headache, erythema, agitation, miosis, muscle weakness, hallucinations, catatonia, abdominal spasm, diarrhea, shivering, hypotension, abstinence syndrome, and (in a patient with intracranial hypertension) seizure.[67] Treatment of side effects is generally symptomatic, but persistent or severe ones can usually be countered with intravenous or intramuscular naloxone, often with preservation of analgesia.[68,69]

Respiratory Depression

Of all potential complications, the risk for respiratory depression generates the most clinical concern. Respiratory depression may be an early (<2 hours after initial administration) or late (4 to 24 hours after administration) phenomenon.[25,70-72] Activity at both the mu and delta receptors has been demonstrated to be associated with both types of respiratory depression.[73,74] Kappa receptor activation may not be associated with significant respiratory depression,[75] but a pure kappa agonist with reliable analgesic properties is not yet available.[25,71]

Management of Respiratory Depression

Factors that predispose to respiratory depression include accidental overdose, absence of severe pain, advanced age or debility, coexisting pulmonary disease, sleep apnea, intercurrent opioid analgesic dosing by alternative routes, and opioid naiveté.[36] Respiratory depression is significantly more likely to occur in opioid-naive patients, and there are few or no reports of late respiratory depression in patients previously maintained on systemic opioids for even short periods. Reversal of respiratory depression can be accomplished with the administration of a mu antagonist (naloxone) or the kappa agonist–mu antagonist nalbuphine.[64,76-80] Oral administration of naltrexone (prophylactically) to surgical patients reduces pruritus, nausea, and somnolence but may be associated with a decrement in analgesia.[81] That these agents must be administered cautiously and in small increments is supported by reports of cardiogenic shock, irreversible ventricular fibrillation, and pulmonary edema associated with the sudden reversal of systemic and intraspinal opioids.[53,73,82,83] A report of successful reversal of respiratory depression by the replacement of aspirated CSF with normal saline suggests another intriguing therapeutic approach.[84]

Gastrointestinal Side Effects

Constipation

Maintenance of gastrointestinal motility and avoidance of constipation are of particular concern in cancer patients. Systemic opioids delay gastric emptying and decrease lower gastrointestinal tract motility, presumably by their action on opioid receptors in the gut. Experimental work suggests that intrathecal morphine does not decrease peristalsis,[85,86] but systematic studies in humans have not been reported.[53] Clinically, gastrointestinal motility seems to be better preserved with intraspinal than with systemic opioids but may still be adversely affected as intraspinal doses increase. Studies in postoperative patients do, however, confirm that postoperative ileus persists longer when pain is treated with epidural morphine than with bupivacaine.[22]

Management of Constipation

Constipation in a cancer patient is commonly multifactorial. Reversible causes should be identified and treated; in addition, a prophylactic symptomatic approach using a sliding-scale regimen of cathartics should be adopted. The pharmacology of these agents and rationale for their use are reviewed elsewhere.[87] The tendency toward less constipation with intraspinal opioids may provide a rationale for a transition from systemic to intraspinal therapy when intractable constipation complicates management with systemic opioids.[88]

Nausea and Vomiting

Epidural morphine has been observed to reduce gastric emptying and small intestinal transit in volunteers.[89] The incidence of nausea and vomiting associated with the administration of intraspinal opioids may range as high as 25% to 30% in opioid-naive subjects but is very low in patients with previous long-term exposure to opioids. Like nausea and vomiting induced by oral opioids, these effects generally resolve rapidly with continued administration.[90,91] Nausea and vomiting are believed to be related to activity at the chemoreceptor trigger zone and vomiting center; that the vestibular system is often involved as well is suggested by a higher incidence of nausea and vomiting in ambulatory patients than in bedbound ones.[92]

Management of Nausea and Vomiting

Nausea and vomiting may be reversed with the administration of nalbuphine or naloxone (see earlier), but this therapy is usually unnecessary because symptoms generally subside with time. If symptoms persist, patients should first be treated symptomatically with standard antiemetics, such as a phenothiazine, a butyrophenone, hydroxyzine, metoclopramide, or dexamethasone. Alternatively, patients may benefit from a trial of a more lipophilic opioid.[36] In a double-blind, placebo-controlled study that targeted patients receiving epidural morphine (postoperatively), transdermal scopolamine was shown to be more effective than either placebo or a combination of metoclopramide and droperidol.[93]

Urinary Side Effects

Intraspinally administered morphine may be associated with naloxone-reversible urinary retention, principally because of decreased detrusor muscle tone and detrusor-urethral sphincter dyssynergia.[61,94,95] Such effects on the urinary tract appear to be mediated by mu and delta, but not kappa receptors.[96] Urinary retention has not been reported after the intraventricular administration of morphine, which suggests that a spinally mediated mechanism is responsible. Despite an incidence of 20% to 40% and higher in male patients after an initial dose of intraspinal opioids,[97] retention is rarely observed in opioid-tolerant cancer patients or in women.

Management

Tolerance often develops after 24 to 48 hours of continued treatment, during which time treatment with small doses of an opioid antagonist[93] or intermittent bladder catheterization may be undertaken. Alternative approaches include conversion to treatment with a more lipid-soluble opioid (especially methadone, which has been observed to actually increase detrusor tone, or buprenorphine, which seems to have little or no effect) and a trial of phenoxybenzamine.[98-101]

Pruritus

Pruritus can be very disturbing to patients. Fortunately, though extremely common in opioid-naive subjects, especially after intrathecal administration, pruritus is extremely uncommon in cancer patients. Diphenhydramine, antihistamines, opioid antagonists,[76] and droperidol have all been recommended, but all interventions yield mixed results at best.[36,61] The optimal solution may be to embark on a therapeutic trial of alternative opioids in an attempt to find a compatible agent based on incomplete cross-tolerance.

Opioid Withdrawal (Abstinence Syndrome)

The abrupt conversion from systemic to intraspinal administration of opioids may result in opioid withdrawal with its classic signs and symptoms,[102] such as lacrimation, rhinorrhea, mydriasis, diaphoresis, pilomotor erection, restlessness, irritability, tremor, nausea, vomiting, diarrhea, and abdominal cramping.[12] Episodes of heightened pain, pulmonary edema, and cardiovascular collapse have also been reported.[82,103] The development of this syndrome is attributed to reductions in the total dose of drug and subsequent delivery of reduced quantities of opioid to rostral CNS sites. The administration of an opioid antagonist or agonist-antagonist drug to an opioid-dependent patient, systematically or at the neuraxial level, can also induce profound withdrawal and even shock.[61,104] Prevention of this syndrome is facilitated by tapering systemic opioids and cautious introduction of drugs with antagonist properties, should they be indicated. Guidelines for these procedures have been published.[105]

Anaphylaxis

Despite a high incidence of patients with so-called morphine allergy, true allergic reactions to morphine and its congeners are rare.[106,107] Such a history is usually more consistent with an unpleasant side effect.

Miscellaneous Problems

Misinjections

There is no question that a fully internalized system that needs to be replenished only from time to time reduces the likelihood of accidental injection of other drugs. Various substances have been accidentally injected through (mostly externalized) epidural and intrathecal catheters, including thiopental, methohexital, diazepam, pancuronium, gallamine, potassium chloride, magnesium sulfate, ephedrine, ranitidine, cefazolin, paraldehyde, total parenteral nutrition solutions, hypertonic contrast medium, hypertonic saline, and collodion.[108] Most cases involved infusion of dilute solutions that resulted in self-limited back pain and spasm, although severe permanent neurologic injury has occurred in several cases.[104] Prevention of such incidents by applying special care in affixing distinctive labels to intraspinal catheters, lines, and infusion devices, occluding accessory ports, and reducing the proximity of ports by thoughtful routing cannot be overemphasized. Various interventions have been undertaken once an injection error has occurred, including injection of epidural steroids, dilution with epidural saline, and aspiration and dilution of the injectate via an intrathecal catheter.

Travel, Security Systems, and High Altitudes

Patients should be provided with identification cards to alert security personnel to the probability that their implanted drug delivery systems will activate metal detectors. These systems may also trigger some of the newer antitheft detectors. Neither high altitude within a pressurized cabin nor relocation to areas up to 10,000 ft above sea level should affect flow rates.

Magnetic Resonance Imaging and Other Therapeutic Devices

Despite early controversy about the safety of MRI in patients with implanted drug delivery systems, most authorities now agree that because the only portions of the SynchroMed pump that are ferrous are the rotors, MRI can be performed safely. Current recommendations call for turning the device off before the examination. Although it is probably unnecessary, it may also be prudent to empty the reservoir as well. Once the examination has been completed, the reservoir should be refilled and the pump carefully reprogrammed. There is still the potential for a poor image as a result of artifact. MRI should not be used in patients with a spinal cord stimulator because of the potential for lead movement and consequent trauma.

Certain physical therapy devices (diathermy and ultrasound) should not be permitted near the site of the device. The lithotripter should be directed away from the device.

Alarms

The infusion device has alarms that signal low battery reserve and low capacity (recommended setting, 2 mL). The infusion rate may decrease spontaneously when the 2-mL limit is reached (by ≤15%), and therefore, devices should be refilled before that point.

Hyperbaric Therapy, Hot Tubs, and Scuba Diving

Hyperbaric therapy may lead to under-infusion and should not be carried out while an infusion pump is operational. Hot tubs (temperature ≤110° F or 43° C) do not the affect the infusion rate, but scuba diving to depths greater than 20 ft may be associated with under-infusion.

Disposition after the Patient's Death

Because of the risk for explosion, implanted drug infusion devices should be removed by funeral personnel before cremation. Explanted pumps should *not* be resterilized and reused.

Technical Problems Specific to Spinal Cord Stimulation

Surgical Complications

Many of the potential complications related to the surgical implantation of a spinal cord stimulator are similar to those encountered with pump implantation and include intraoperative bleeding, epidural hematoma, wound hematoma, seroma, wound infection, meningitis, epidural abscess, CSF leak, post–dural puncture headache, and malposition of the subcutaneous pocket, all of which have been described in the preceding section.

Failed Analgesia

Failed analgesia may be due to myriad causes. Problems may be patient related, disease related, mechanical, or a combination of these factors. Patient selection, education, and preparation are key issues that must be addressed to avoid difficulties. Considerations related to the patient's psychological status and the nature of the disease that is causing the pain are discussed in depth elsewhere in this volume. The emphasis here is on mechanical problems and how to avoid them.

Preoperative Check of Equipment to Be Implanted

Before implantation, the surgeon or pain management specialist should take the following measures:

- Confirm that a screening device with a fresh battery is available and functional.
- Ensure that the proper equipment is available and that the lead and extension match. It is wise to have additional stock of each item in case of contamination, damage, or defects. (If the equipment budget is tight, additional units should be ordered just before surgery; any that are not used can replace those used for surgery.)
- Ascertain that the patient has been properly oriented to the procedure to maximize compliance.
- Obtain informed patient consent.
- Discuss the procedure with the anesthesiologist to ensure that the patient will be both comfortable and cooperative.

Difficult Lead Placement

Though not a complication per se, difficulty placing leads is a potentially troublesome and critical problem that may ultimately be a source of complications. Positioning of the patient is often overlooked but is key to facilitating lead placement. Before the patient is prepared for surgery, the surgeon should verify that fluoroscopic access is not impaired by radiolucent components of the operating room table and that mechanical passage of the C-arm is unimpeded. Fluoroscopy is an essential adjunct to placement and should be used freely throughout the procedure rather than being reserved until the conclusion. Non-ionic contrast medium should be available to confirm localization of the epidural space and to distinguish between subarachnoid and epidural lead placement. Whether a prone or lateral position is selected, patients should be positioned precisely so that true anteroposterior and lateral films can be obtained. Most clinicians prefer the prone position, in which case the table should be flexed and padded to minimize lumbar lordosis. The back should be flexed, and consideration should be given to securing the patient in position with adhesive tape and a safety belt.

During needle placement, care should be taken to think three-dimensionally, particularly if a slightly paramedian approach is selected, which is preferred by most physicians. A steep angle in the cephalocaudad plane should be adopted to facilitate the lead's passage. Ten milliliters of preservative-free saline may be injected before passage of the lead to expand the epidural space. If advancing the lead is difficult, epidural positioning should be verified. Passage may be facilitated by rotating the bevel of the needle carefully up to 45 degrees to either side (with the lead retracted), and the lead may be gently rotated between the thumb and forefinger while it is advanced in an effort to "steer" its tip. Finally, if problems persist, a guidewire may be gently advanced under fluoroscopic guidance to create a tract, or alternatively, another needle trajectory or interspace may be selected. Occasionally, the entry point is so far from the pain-generating site that the electrode portion of the lead does not extend to the intended target and the boot cannot be placed. In implantation planning, the guidelines shown in Table 167–1 may be useful. The lead and, indeed, all component parts should be handled carefully. Kinking, bending, and tension on the lead should be avoided. The lead should not be forced into the epidural space against resistance, and sutures should not be tied directly to

Table 167–1

Spinal Levels for Catheter Entry and Lead Tip Location according to Pain Distribution

Pain Distribution	*Entry Level*	*Lead Tip Level*
Foot only	L2-3	T11-12
Lower extremity with hip and back involvement	T12-L1	T9-10
Upper chest wall (intercostals)	T4-6	T1-2
Upper extremity	T1-3	C3-T5

it. Extreme caution should be exercised when sharp instruments are used around the lead. The lead should be handled only with the fingers; when it is necessary to manipulate it with instruments, rubber shods should be used.

If the lead needs to be repositioned once it has been inserted, care should be taken to withdraw it gently and carefully through the needle to avoid damaging the lead. If resistance is met, the lead and needle should be removed simultaneously and the epidural space approached anew. Once the lead is optimally positioned, it must be stabilized while the needle is removed. Intermittent or continuous fluoroscopy is useful to confirm that the tip of the lead does not move during this process.

Accidental Dural Puncture

Dural puncture is usually heralded by frank flow of CSF. If this problem occurs, a neighboring interspace should be selected, and treatment of post–dural puncture headache should be anticipated.

Subarachnoid Lead Placement

Occasionally, dural puncture occurs in the absence of obvious CSF leakage because of either the catheter or guidewire breaching the dura or altered CSF mechanics secondary to scarring from earlier surgery. Dural puncture is usually manifested as unexpectedly low stimulation thresholds (often ≤1 V) and can be confirmed if anterior displacement of the lead is noted on fluoroscopy and if injection of contrast material through the needle produces a radiographic image more characteristic of a myelogram than an epidurogram. Even if adequate stimulation is obtained, the risk for migration and scarring requires that the lead be removed and reinserted at another interspace.

Neurologic Injury

Significant neurologic injury is unusual. Occasionally, patients experience radicular pain coincident with advancement of the lead, in which case it should be withdrawn. If new pain or new neurologic signs emerge in the immediate postoperative period, the patient should be investigated for epidural hematoma. If signs and symptoms occur later in the postoperative period, infection must be ruled out. It is not uncommon for new, well-localized paresthesias to develop with minor nerve root injury, but they usually resolve over a period of days or weeks. Lead removal is not generally necessary, although CT may be indicated.

Lead Migration and Positional Stimulation

When a patient describes a change in the stimulation pattern that consists of either the perception of adequate stimulation in a body part other than the painful area or a stimulation pattern that changes with posture, lead migration is probably responsible. Unfortunately, this complication occurs with some frequency. It is inherent in the procedure because adequacy of pain relief depends in large part on localization of the lead within a living, moving human being. A process of "scarring down" is generally thought to occur during the first weeks after surgery; restricting movements (bending, reaching) during this period may promote immobilization of the lead. Some clinicians require a short period of bed rest or even a soft cervical collar as a reminder to patients to limit their activity.

Stimulation can often be recaptured by meticulous reprogramming. Problems may, to an extent, be forestalled by initially locating the lead directly over the involved dermatomes to give some margin for readjustment on either side. A change in stimulation pattern warrants anteroposterior and lateral radiographs, which should be compared with postoperative films to document lead movement. If proper stimulation cannot be recaptured, elective surgical revision is indicated, with consideration of substituting a plate-type (Resume) electrode for the original lead.

Truncal Stimulation

Occasionally, patients experience truncal stimulation either in addition to or in place of the topically desired therapeutic stimulation. This complication is manifested by paresthesias and muscle twitching, usually along the myotomes of the flank. It may be related to current leak or to stimulation of a nerve root as a result of a lateral shift in lead position. It can often be averted by reprogramming but sometimes requires surgical revision.

Insulation Failure, Fracture, or Disconnection

Failure of insulation or fracture or disconnection of wires may be manifested as total loss of stimulation or a combination of loss of the usual stimulation pattern or intermittent stimulation coupled with focal pain that ultimately corresponds to the site of the short circuit. Some authorities advocate applying either bone wax or cyanoacrylate to connections prophylactically. In cases of suspected electrical leak or discontinuity, an electronic survey should be performed to exclude pulse generator failure and to detect abnormally high impedance. A battery-operated portable radio may be used as an adjunct; an AM radio, tuned between stations to produce static, is applied to the skin overlying the system. The radio is then passed gently over the skin along the path of the system from the pocket to the back, over the lead tips. Increased static usually correlates with a site of current leakage. Radiographs should be reviewed to detect disconnection or a break in wiring, although such films generally look normal. Elective revision is indicated. At surgery, the system can be tested sequentially, usually starting at the pocket and moving proximally.

Painful Connector or Transmitter Site

Pain at the site of a connector or transmitter may be due to mechanical causes, as when a generator impinges on the ribs or iliac crest, or to electrical leakage, in which case patients typically complain of a local sensation of burning.

Pacemakers, MRI, and Security Systems

Insertion of a spinal cord stimulator may be contraindicated in patients with pacemakers. Demand pacemakers may mistake the pulse generator's impulses for those originating in the heart. Theoretically, patients with fixed-rate devices do not have problems, but consultation with the stimulator manufacturer is recommended before considering implantation in a patient with any type of pacemaker. Although infusion devices need only be emptied and turned off, MRI is still contraindicated for patients with stimulators because of the potential for damage to the device and electrical and mechanical injury to the patient. A stimulating system may also activate airport boarding gate alarms and certain other alarms intended to detect theft.

Published Data on Complications

Spinal Cord Stimulation

Regrettably, there is a paucity of good, controlled studies that provide detailed descriptions of patient selection, outcome, and morbidity. This status is characteristic of interventions for pain in general and should not be regarded as an indictment of spinal cord stimulation (SCS). The quality of later literature is markedly superior to that associated with earlier eras. It is essential that this literature be scrutinized extremely carefully. The reader must bear in mind that data from earlier studies are influenced by less sophisticated patient selection methods and equipment that was far cruder and more prone to failure than contemporary systems are. In addition there is considerable delay between submission of a study and its publication; thus, a large study population usually means that the data were collected over a period of several years before the paper was submitted. There is also widespread agreement that the results of treatment are very specific to the practitioner, the technique, and the disorder being treated, so the reader should be aware that outcome reflects the skill and experience of the implant surgeon and the technique and study population.

The following brief review of the literature is, admittedly, incomplete, but it gives a sense of the variety and incidence of complications that have been reported for SCS. In a 1982 European study, Siegfried and Lazorthes[109] reported on 191 patients with chronic low back pain who underwent trials of SCS, 89 of whom had an implant. It is noteworthy that the study population was characterized by patients with histories of long-standing pain, multiple laminectomies, and oil-based myelography. Most systems were placed via laminectomy, and it is again noteworthy that a proportion of them underwent deliberate subarachnoid, subdural, or endodural placement of leads. At 1 year, among the 89 patients, 21 failures (24%) were attributed to nonmechanical failure—"psychiatric causes" in 9 cases, "narcotic dependency" in 5, and idiopathic in 7. Another 21 failures (24%) were due to mechanical causes—electrode migration in 9 cases, defects in the stimulating system in 3, necrosis and infection in 7, and receiver rejection in 2.

In 1983, de la Porte and Siegfried[110] reported on 94 patients who underwent trials of SCS for "lumbosacral spinal fibrosis (spinal arachnoiditis)," 38 of whom (40%) underwent implantation. In these 38 patients, 50 more procedures were performed because of problems with wound healing (10 cases), removal or reimplantation (5 cases), and other complications (23 cases). Only 12 of the implanted devices were Medtronic systems, and these were implanted by laminectomy. A total of 26 complications occurred in this subgroup (skin erosion, 7; incisional pain, 3; receptor site pain, 2; lead migration, 6; electrode malfunction, 2; and system malfunction, cable or connection disruption, and antenna malfunction, 1 each). In this admittedly antiquated study, no complications were encountered in 50% of patients and no re-intervention was required for 60% of patients. An interesting conclusion was that the occurrence of postoperative problems increased the chance of further problems enormously. Again, the study's vintage must be taken into account, as must its population (patients with pain from failed back surgery).

In a brief report that lacks detailed descriptions, Romy and Sussman[111] described 19 patients who underwent implantation of Cordis SCS systems. Of these, two systems were removed (11%) and 11 (58%) required at least one revision for reasons that were not reported. Murphy and Giles,[112] reporting on implantation of Medtronic systems in a group of 10 patients treated for angina, fared considerably better. A faulty signal receiver was replaced in one patient, and another required revision because of posturally related changes in stimulation.

Meglio and Cioni[113] reported on 26 patients who received permanent percutaneous implants (Medtronic, Sigma lead) between 1978 and 1981. Thirteen of their patients (50%) had vascular disease, only 6 had arachnoiditis, and the rest had other problems (e.g., herpes zoster, cancer). Eight patients (31%) experienced complications, seven of whom required corrective procedures. Reported complications were subcutaneous hematoma (three), inadequate paresthesia (two), receiver malfunction (one), subcutaneous lead rejection (one), and aseptic meningitis (one). Side effects that did not require reoperation included headache, asthenia, dizziness, and radicular muscle twitch.

Meglio and colleagues[114] reported on 167 patients who underwent implantation with Medtronic systems. Low back pain was the indication for treatment in only a small proportion of patients, and in all but five, a percutaneous approach was used. These authors reported complications in 26 patients and side effects in 11, although it is not clear whether the problems occurred in the implanted group only (167) or in the group who underwent trials (109). Complications included four cases of aseptic meningitis (two of which resolved within days without system removal), bacterial infection at the electrode site (two) and pocket (one), lead rejection (two), CSF leak (three), subcutaneous hematoma (three), pain at the electrode site (two), accidental removal of the system by the patient (one), and "suspected system failure" (four). In one of the patients with bacterial infection at the lead site, paraplegia developed within a few days despite removal of the system and treatment with antibiotics. Re-exploration revealed an extradural-intradural bacterial abscess, and the result was "good but incomplete" recovery.

Krainick and associates[115] reported on 84 patients who received implants between 1972 and 1974, 64 of whom were amputees with lower extremity pain. Four patients experienced partial transverse spinal lesions, three of which resolved after system removal. Disagreeable thoracic radicular paresthesias were "common," especially with unipolar systems, but they usually improved after alteration of the stimulation parameters. Interestingly, CSF leakage occurred in three patients who were among the first few to undergo subdural placement, and this complication did not recur once the protocol was altered to one of exclusive epidural placement, thus suggesting the superiority of the latter approach. Removal of the system as a result of technical failure was necessary in three cases, but the exact causes were not specified (because of lead damage during removal). One patient with cervical placement experienced symptoms consistent with spinal cord compression 2 years after surgery and, during system removal, was found to have a severe tissue reaction.

In 1986, Kumar and colleagues[116] reported on the implantation of 65 Medtronic systems, most in patients with back pain. Complications were reported in 23 cases (35%): wound infection (3, only 1 requiring removal), CSF leak (1, resolved with bed rest), electrode displacement (12), electrode fracture (2), lead fibrosis (3), and a sensation of burning over the receiver site (2). In a 1991 follow-up study reporting on 94 patients (60% with back problems) who had implants (mostly Medtronic systems), the same group reported 43 complications (46%)[117]: electrode displacement (25), infection (8, with 7 requiring system removal), lead fracture (4, usually at the entrance to the epidural space), battery depletion (2), electrical leak (2, usually at the junction of extension and receiver), and CSF leak (2, resolved with bed rest). Patients with scoliosis or "similar spinal deformities" were found to have a threefold greater increase in the rate of electrode displacement.

A group of Spanish investigators reported, in abstract form, on a single case of transient tetraplegia after implantation in a patient with mediastinal sarcoma and herpes zoster.[118] The system was removed, and the authors concluded that under certain circumstances (osteolytic metastases), the lead and associated edema could act like a space-occupying lesion. Preliminary results of a Medtronic-sponsored multicenter trial of their original Itrel system were published in 1984.[119] They reported on 116 implants in patients with low back pain, leg pain, or both. Twenty-three systems (20%) were explanted for various reasons. Problems at implantation included a malfunctioning portable programmer (one), stripped set screw (one), ineffective stimulation (one), "medicine reaction" (one), device accidentally removed by the patient (one), and electrode failure (one). Subsequent problems were infection at the site of the pulse generator (six, four requiring surgery), burning near the generator site (three), radicular stimulation (three), positional stimulation (two), dislodged leads (six), difficulty programming (three, requiring replacement), and flank pain (one). In one of the cases of infection, the generator was sterilized and reimplanted without apparent problems, although this procedure is not recommended by Medtronic.

In 1991, North and colleagues[120] reported on implantation (64% percutaneous, mostly Medtronic) in 50 patients with failed back surgery (average of 3.1 operations) with 2- and 5-year follow-up. All together, 48% of patients required some secondary procedure (mostly repositioning). Superficial *Staphylococcus* infection that required system removal developed in six patients (12%). Other problems were spontaneous migration (1, or 2%), revision to enhance the stimulation pattern (14, or 28%), lead fracture (7, or 14%), and receiver failure (4, or 8%). Of note is that secondary procedures were required in only 34% of the subset of patients treated with four-channel systems. In a follow-up report, North and colleagues[121] documented similar findings that emphasized the superiority of multichannel systems. Of patients treated with multichannel systems, only 16% required revision because of inadequate topographic stimulation as compared with 23% of patients who had bipolar systems.

In a 1989 study, Racz and associates[122] reported on 26 patients (predominantly with back pain and having undergone an average of 21 previous procedures) after implantation of a Medtronic spinal cord stimulator. Twenty-seven complications occurred: lead migration (18), lead fracture (6), infected hematoma (1), and wound infection (2). The authors observed that electrode migration was far more likely to occur early, "probably before fibrous tissue was able to form," and that it was usually from a dorsal to a more anterolateral position. Migration was generally manifested by the appearance of a radicular, intercostal pattern of stimulation and little change in electrode position on radiographs.

Infusion Systems

Because of the relatively new technology with narrow indications, the data available on problems related to the implantation of long-term drug infusion systems are even more meager than those for SCS. In a series of 18 patients undergoing implantation for baclofen infusion,[123] there were three instances of extrusion of the intrathecal portion of the Silastic catheter. One instance of device malfunction resulted in an overdose in a system that had been operable for 1 year. Interestingly, there were seven infectious complications (four cases of local sepsis and three of transient meningitis) in patients treated with an implanted port that required regular percutaneous access and none in patients who received a SynchroMed implant. Similarly, in Penn and Kroin's series of seven spastic patients treated with the SynchroMed system, no infectious complications occurred.[124] Two devices were explanted for apparent malfunction (overdose and beeping) but were subsequently found to be functional ex vivo. Two catheters were replaced, one for a kink that occurred at its junction with the pump and a second for a nick produced during surgery. One incident of erosion of the pocket incision occurred, and there were several instances of self-limited (7 to 10 days) seroma.

SUMMARY

If one uses a broad definition of *complication*, spinal cord–stimulating systems are subject to a relatively high rate of complications that despite often requiring another intervention, tend by far to be benign. Implanted infusion devices are associated with a relatively low incidence of such problems.

References

1. Waldman S, Leak D, Kennedy D, Patt RB: Intraspinal opioid analgesia in the management of oncologic pain. In Patt RB (ed): Cancer Pain. Philadelphia, JB Lippincott, 1993, p 285.
2. Bridenbaugh PO: Complications of local anesthetic neural blockade. In Cousins MJ, Bridenbaugh PO (eds): Neural Blockade, 2nd ed. Philadelphia, JB Lippincott, 1988, p 695.
3. Webster's Dictionary.
4. Quimby CW: Medicolegal hazards of destructive nerve blocks. In Abram SE (ed): Cancer Pain. Boston, Kluwer Academic, 1989, p 137.
5. Krames E: Faculty Handbook. Minneapolis, Medtronic, 1992.
6. Hahn M: Faculty Handbook. Minneapolis, Medtronic, 1992.
7. Wu C, Patt RB: Accidental overdose of systemic morphine during intended refill of intrathecal infusion device. Anesth Analg 75:130, 1992.
8. Patt RB, Wu C, Bressi J, Catania J: Accidental intraspinal overdose revisited. Anesth Analg 76:202, 1993.
9. Penn RD, Paice JA, Gottschalk W, et al: Cancer pain relief using chronic morphine infusions: Early experience with a programmable implanted drug pump. J Neurosurg 61:302, 1984.
10. Hirsch LF, Thanki A, Nowak T: Sudden loss of pain control with morphine pump due to catheter migration. Neurosurgery 17:965, 1985.
11. Portenoy R: Practical aspects of pain control in the patient with cancer. CA Cancer J Clin 38:327, 1988.
12. Jaffe JH, Martin WR: The opioid analgesics and antagonists. In Gillman AG, Rall TW, Nies AS, et al (eds): The Pharmacologic Basis of Therapeutics, 8th ed. New York, Pergamon, 1980.
13. Catania JA, Patt RB: Radiologic guidance, contrast medium and untoward reactions. In Patt RB (ed): Cancer Pain. Philadelphia, JB Lippincott, 1994, p 616.
14. Leak WD, Kennedy LD, Graef W: Clinical experience with implantable, programmable pumps: The Medtronic SynchroMed pump. Clin J Pain 7:44, 1991.
15. Swenson C, Patt RB: Manufacturing processes. In Patt RB (ed): Cancer Pain. Philadelphia, JB Lippincott, 1994, p 612.
16. Yaksh TL, Onofrio BM: Retrospective consideration of the doses of morphine given intrathecally by chronic infusion in 163 patients by 19 physicians. Pain 31:211, 1987.
17. Amer S, Rawal N, Gustafsson LL: Clinical experience of long-term treatment with epidural and intrathecal opioids, a nationwide survey. Acta Anaesthesiol Scand 32:253, 1988.
18. Ventafridda V, Spoldi E, Caraceni A, et al: Intraspinal morphine for cancer pain. Acta Anaesthesiol Scand 85:47, 1987.
19. Coombs DW, Saunders RL, Harbaugh R, et al: Relief of continuous chronic pain by intraspinal narcotics infusion via an implanted reservoir. JAMA 250:2336, 1983.
20. Shetter AG, Hadley MH, Wilkinson E: Administration of intraspinal morphine sulfate for the treatment of intractable cancer pain. Neurosurgery 18:740, 1986.
21. Pasqualucci V: Advances in the management of cardiac pain. In Benedetti C, Chapman RC, Moricca G (eds): Advances in Pain Research and Therapy, vol 7. New York, Raven Press, 1984.
22. Sundberg TT, Wattwil M, Garvill JE, et al: Effects of epidural bupivacaine and epidural morphine on bowel function and pain after hysterectomy. Acta Anaesthesiol Scand 33:181, 1989.
23. Stevens CW, Yaksh TL: Potency of spinal antinociceptive agents is inversely related to magnitude of tolerance after continuous infusion. J Pharmacol Exp Ther 250:1, 1989.
24. Sosnowski M, Stevens CW, Yaksh TL: Comparison of magnitude of tolerance development observed after continuous spinal intrathecal infusions in rats. Reg Anesth 14:76, 1989.
25. Baskoff JD, Watson RL, Muldoon SM: Respiratory arrest after intrathecal morphine. Anesthesiology 7:12, 1980.
26. Eisenach JC, Rauck RL, Buzzanell C, et al: Epidural clonidine analgesia for intractable cancer pain: Phase I. Anesthesiology 71:1677, 1989.
27. Coombs DW, Saunders RL, LaChance D, et al: Intrathecal morphine tolerance: Use of intrathecal clonidine, DADL and intravenous morphine. Anesthesiology 62:358, 1985.
28. Glynn CJ, Jamous A, Dawson D, et al: The role of epidural clonidine in the treatment of patients with intractable pain. Pain Suppl 4:45, 1987.
29. Yaksh TL, Reddy SV: Studies in the primate on the analgesic effects associated with intrathecal actions of opiates, alpha-adrenergic agonists and baclofen. Anesthesiology 54:451, 1981.
30. Coombs DW, Allen C, Meier FA, et al: Chronic intraspinal clonidine in sheep. Reg Anesth 9:47, 1994.
31. Kim KC, Stoelting RK: Effect of droperidol on the duration of analgesia and development of tolerance to intrathecal morphine. Anesthesiology 35(Suppl):S219, 1980.
32. Naji P, Farschtschian M, Wilder-Smith O, et al: Epidural droperidol and morphine for postoperative pain. Anesth Analg 70:583, 1990.
33. Bach V, Carl P, Ravlo ME, et al: Potentiation of epidural opioids with epidural droperidol. Anaesthesia 41:1116, 1986.
34. Chrubasik J, Meynadier J, Blond S, et al: Somatostatin, a potent analgesic. Lancet 2:1208, 1984.
35. Meynadier J, Chrubasik J, Dubar M, Wünsch E: Intrathecal somatostatin in terminally ill patients: A report of two cases. Pain 23:9, 1985.
36. Bruera E: Narcotic-induced pulmonary edema. J Pain Symptom Manage 5:55, 1990.
37. Gaumann DM, Yaksh TL, Post C, et al: Intrathecal somatostatin in cat and mouse studies on pain, motor behavior and histopathology. Anesth Analg 68:623, 1989.
38. Penn RD, Paice JA, Kroin JS: Octreotide: A potent new non-opiate analgesic for intrathecal infusion. Pain 49:13, 1992.
39. Candrina R, Galli G: Intraventricular octreotide for cancer pain. J Neurosurg 76:336, 1992.
40. Fiore CE, Castolina F, Malatino LS, et al: Antalgic activity of calcitonin: Effectiveness of the epidural and subarachnoid routes in man. Int J Clin Pharmacol Res 3:257, 1983.
41. Eisenach JC: Demonstrating safety of subarachnoid calcitonin: Patients or animals. Anesth Analg 67:298, 1988.
42. Stein C, Brechner T: Epidural morphine tolerance: Use of norepinephrine. Clin J Pain 2:267, 1987.
43. Russell RD, Chang KJ: Alternated delta and mu receptor activation: A strategy for limiting opioid tolerance. Pain 36:381, 1989.
44. Krames ES, Wilkie DJ, Gershow J: Intrathecal D-ala2-D-leu5enkephalin (DADL) restores analgesia in a patient analgetically tolerant to intrathecal morphine sulfate. Pain 24:205, 1986.
45. Onofrio BM, Yaksh TL: Intrathecal delta-receptor ligand produces analgesia in man. Lancet 2:1386, 1983.
46. Naguib M, Adu-Gyamfi Y, Absood GH, et al: Epidural ketamine for postoperative analgesia. Anesth Analg 67:798, 1988.
47. Cripps TP, Goodchild CS: Intrathecal midazolam and the stress response to upper abdominal surgery. Br J Anaesth 58:1324, 1986.
48. Wilson PR, Yaksh TL: Baclofen is anti-nociceptive in the spinal intrathecal space of animals. Eur J Pharmacol 51:323, 1978.
49. Yaksh TL: Spinal opiates: A review of their effect on spinal function with an emphasis on pain processing. Acta Anaesthesiol Scand Suppl 85:25, 1987.
50. Coombs DW: Effect of spinal adrenergic analgesia on opioid resistant pain. Acta Anaesthesiol Scand 91:37, 1989.
51. Coombs DW: Intraspinal narcotics for intractable cancer pain. In Abrams S (ed): Cancer Pain. Boston, Kluwer Academic, 1989, p 82.
52. Du Pen SL: After epidural narcotics: What next? Anesth Analg 66(Suppl):S46, 1987.
53. Taff RH: Pulmonary edema following a naloxone administration in a patient without heart disease. Anesthesiology 59:576, 1983.
54. Omote K, Nakagawa I, Kitahata LM, et al: The antinociceptive role of mu and delta opiate receptors and their interactions in the spinal dorsal horn of cats. Anesth Analg 68(Suppl):S215, 1989.
55. Omote K, Nakagawa I, Kitahata LM, et al: Spinal delta but not mu opiate receptors appear to interact with noradrenergic systems in the cat's spinal dorsal horn. Anesth Analg 68(Suppl):S216, 1989.
56. Waldman SD, Coombs DW: Selection of implantable narcotic delivery systems. Anesth Analg 68:377, 1989.
57. Kreitzer JM, Kirschenbaum LP, Eisenkraft JB: Safety of PCA devices. Anesthesiology 70:881, 1989.
58. Dahl JB, Jacobsen JB: Accidental epidural narcotic overdose. Anesth Analg 70:321, 1990.
59. Kaiser KG, Bainton CR: Treatment of intrathecal morphine overdose by aspiration of cerebrospinal fluid. Anesth Analg 66:475, 1987.
60. Parkinson SK, Bailey SL, Little WL, Mueller JB: Myoclonic seizure activity with chronic high-dose spinal opioid administration. Anesthesiology 72:743, 1990.
61. Ventafridda V, Spoldi E, Caraceni A, et al: Intraspinal morphine for cancer pain. Acta Anaesthesiol Scand Suppl 85:47, 1987.

62. Flacke JW, Flacke WE, Williams GD: Acute pulmonary edema following naloxone reversal of high-dose morphine anesthesia. Anesthesiology 47:376, 1977.
63. Gurdin MM, Carlin GA: Aesthetic surgery of the breast. In Masters FW, Lewis JR (eds): Symposium on Aesthetic Surgery of the Face, Eyelid, and Breast, vol 4. St Louis, CV Mosby, 1972, p 160.
64. De Castro J, Meynadier J, Zenz M: Regional Opioid Analgesia. Dordrecht, Germany, Kluwer Academic, 1991.
65. Cousins MJ, Mather LE: Intrathecal and epidural administration of opioids. Anesthesiology 61:276, 1984.
66. Ventafridda V, Spoldi E, Caraceni A, et al: Intraspinal morphine for cancer pain. Acta Anaesthesiol Scand Suppl 85:47, 1987.
67. Arai T, Dote K, Senda T, et al: Convulsion after epidural injection in a patient with increased intracranial pressure. Pain Clin 3:195, 1987.
68. Korbon GA, James DJ, Verlander JM, et al: Intramuscular naloxone reverses the side effects of epidural morphine while preserving analgesia. Reg Anesth 10:16, 1985.
69. Rawal N, Schott U, Dahlstrom B: Influence of naloxone infusion on analgesia and respiratory depression following epidural morphine. Anesthesiology 167:194, 1986.
70. Davies GK, Tolhurst-Cleaver CL, James TL: CNS depression from intrathecal morphine. Anesthesiology 52:280, 1980.
71. Glynn CJ, Mather LE, Cousins, MJ, et al: Spinal narcotics and respiratory depression. Lancet 1:356, 1979.
72. Christensen V: Respiratory depression after extradural morphine. Br J Anaesth 52:841, 1980.
73. Sosnowski M, Yaksh TL: Spinal administration of receptor-selective drugs as analgesics: New horizons. J Pain Symptom Manage 5:204, 1990.
74. Pazos A, Florez J: Interaction of naloxone with agonists on the respiration of rats. Eur J Pharmacol 87:309, 1983.
75. Abboud TK, Moore M, Zhu J, et al: Epidural butorphanol or morphine for the relief of post cesarean section pain: Ventilatory responses to carbon dioxide. Anesth Analg 66:887, 1987.
76. Latasch L, Probst S, Dudziak R: Reversal by nalbuphine of respiratory depression caused by fentanyl. Anesth Analg 63:814, 1984.
77. Baise A, McMichan JC, Nugent M, et al: Nalbuphine produces side effects while reversing narcotic induced respiratory depression. Anesth Analg 65(Suppl):S19, 1986.
78. Hammond JE: Reversal of opioid associated late onset respiratory depression by nalbuphine hydrochloride. Lancet 2:1208, 1984.
79. Schmauss C, Doherty C, Yaksh TL: The analgesic effects of an intrathecally administered partial opiate agonist, nalbuphine hydrochloride. Eur J Pharmacol 86:1, 1983.
80. Wakefield RD, Mesaros M: Reversal of pruritus secondary to epidural morphine with a narcotic agonist/antagonist nalbuphine (Nubain). Anesthesiology 63(Suppl):A255, 1985.
81. Abboud TK, Lee K, Zhu J, et al: Prophylactic oral naltrexone with intrathecal morphine for cesarean section: Effects on adverse reactions and analgesia. Anesth Analg 71:367, 1990.
82. Prough BS, Roy R, Bumgamer J, et al: Acute pulmonary edema in healthy teenagers following conservative doses of intravenous naloxone. Anesthesiology 60:485, 1984.
83. DesMarteau JK, Cassot AL: Acute pulmonary edema resulting from nalbuphine reversal of fentanyl-induced respiratory depression. Anesthesiology 65:237, 1986.
84. Kaiser KG, Bainton CR: Treatment of intrathecal morphine overdose by aspiration of cerebrospinal fluid. Anesth Analg 66:475, 1987.
85. Cousins MJ, Cherry DA, Gourlay GK: Acute and chronic pain: Use of spinal opioids. In Cousins MJ, Bridenbaugh PO (eds): Neural Blockade, 2nd ed. Philadelphia, JB Lippincott, 1988, p 955.
86. Yaksh TL, Noueihed R: The physiology and pharmacology of spinal opioids. Annu Rev Pharmacol Toxicol 25:433, 1985.
87. Twycross RG, Harcourt JMV: The use of laxatives at a palliative care center. Palliat Med 5:27, 1991.
88. Patt R, Jain S: Long term management of a patient with perineal pain secondary to rectal cancer. J Pain Symptom Manage 5:127, 1990.
89. Thom T, Tanhhoj H, Jarnerot G: Epidural morphine delays gastric emptying time and small intestinal transit in volunteers. Acta Anaesthesiol Scand 33:174, 1989.
90. Benedetti C: Intraspinal analgesia: An historical overview. Acta Anaesthesiol Scand 85:17, 1987.
91. Watson RL, Rayburn RL, Muldoon SM, et al: The mechanism of action and utility of epidurally administered morphine. In Wain HJ (ed): Treatment of Pain. New York, Aaronson, 1982.
92. Calvey TN: Side effect problems of the mu and kappa agonists in clinical use. Update Opioids 1:803, 1987.
93. Loper KA, Ready LB, Dorman BH: Prophylactic transdermal scopolamine patches reduce nausea in postoperative patients receiving epidural morphine. Anesth Analg 68:144, 1989.
94. Rawal N, Mollefors K, Axelsson K, et al: An experimental study of urodynamic effects of epidural morphine and of naloxone reversal. Anesth Analg 62:1671, 1983.
95. Dray A: Epidural opiates and urinary retention: New models provide new insights. Anesthesiology 68:323, 1988.
96. Durant PAC, Yaksh TI: Drug effects on urinary bladder tone during spinal morphine-induced inhibition of the micturition reflex in unanesthetized rats. Anesthesiology 68:325, 1988.
97. Rawal N, Mollefors K, Axelsson K, et al: Naloxone reversal of urinary retention after epidural morphine. Lancet 2:1411, 1981.
98. Evron S, Samueloff A, Simon A, et al: Urinary function during epidural analgesia with methadone and morphine in post–cesarean section patients. Pain 23:135, 1985.
99. Drenger B, Magora F, Evron S, et al: The action of intrathecal morphine and methadone on lower urinary tract in dog. J Urol 135:852, 1986.
100. Drenger B, Pikarsky AJ, Magora F: Urodynamic studies after intrathecal fentanyl and buprenorphine in the dog. Anesthesiology 67(Suppl):A240, 1987.
101. Evron S, Magora E, Sadovsky E: Prevention of urinary retention with phenoxybenzamine during epidural morphine. BMJ 288:190, 1984.
102. Messahel FM, Tomlin PJ: Narcotic withdrawal syndrome after intrathecal administration of morphine. BMJ 283:471, 1981.
103. Delander GE, Takemori AE: Spinal antagonism of tolerance and dependence induced by systemically administered morphine. Eur J Pharmacol 94:35, 1983.
104. Christensen FR, Anderson LW: An adverse reaction to extradural buprenorphine. Br J Anaesth 54:476, 1982.
105. American Pain Society: Principles of Analgesia Use in the Treatment of Acute and Chronic Cancer Pain: A Concise Guide to Medical Practice, 2nd ed. Skokie, IL, American Pain Society, 1989.
106. Fisher MM: The diagnosis of acute anaphylactoid reactions to drugs. Anaesth Intensive Care 9:234, 1981.
107. Zucker-Pinchoff B, Ramanathan S: Anaphylactic reaction to epidural fentanyl. Anesthesiology 71:599, 1989.
108. Kopacz DJ, Slover RB: Accidental epidural cephazolin injection: Safeguards for patient controlled analgesia. Anesthesiology 72:944, 1990.
109. Siegfried J, Lazorthes Y: Long-term follow-up of dorsal cord stimulation for chronic pain syndrome after multiple lumbar operations. Appl Neurophysiol 45:201, 1982.
110. de la Porte C, Siegfried J: Lumbosacral spinal fibrosis (spinal arachnoiditis): Its diagnosis and treatment by spinal cord stimulation. Spine 8:593, 1983.
111. Romy M, Sussman M: Intraspinal neural stimulation for relief of intractable pain: Introduction and technique of insertion. J Neurol Orthop Med Surg 5:33, 1984.
112. Murphy DF, Giles KE: Dorsal column stimulation for pain relief from intractable angina pectoris. Pain 28:365, 1987.
113. Meglio M, Cioni B: Personal experience with spinal cord stimulation in chronic pain management. Appl Neurophysiol 45:195, 1982.
114. Meglio M, Cioni B, Rossi GF: Spinal cord stimulation in the management of chronic pain. J Neurosurg 70:519, 1989.
115. Krainick JU, Thoden U, Traugott R: Pain reduction in amputees by long-term spinal cord stimulation. J Neurosurg 52:346, 1980.
116. Kumar K, Wyant GM, Ekong CEU: Epidural spinal cord stimulation for relief of chronic pain. Pain Clin 1:91, 1986.
117. Kumar K, Nauth R, Wyant GM: Treatment of chronic pain by epidural spinal cord stimulation: A 10 year experience. J Neurosurg 75:402, 1991.
118. Miranda-Casas JA, Garcia-Ferrando V, Seller-Losada JM: Transitory tetraplegia after electrocatheter implantation in the cervical epidural space. Paper presented at a meeting of the World Congress of Pain, November 1990, Adelaide, Australia.
119. Dooley DM, Heimburger RF, Hunter SE, et al: Medronic Itrel Spinal Cord Stimulation System: Preliminary Clinical Results. Minneapolis, Medtronics, 1984, p 1.
120. North RB, Ewend MG, Lawton, MT, et al: Failed back surgery syndrome: 5 year follow-up after spinal cord stimulator implantation. Neurosurgery 28:692, 1991.

121. North RB, Ewend MG, Lawton MT, Piantadosi S: Spinal cord stimulation for chronic, intractable pain: Superiority of multichannel devices. Pain 44:119, 1991.
122. Racz GB, McCarron RF, Talboys P: Percutaneous dorsal column stimulator for chronic pain control. Spine 14:1, 1989.
123. Lazorthes Y, Sallerin-Caute B, Verdie JC, et al: Chronic intrathecal baclofen administration for control of severe spasticity. J Neurosurg 72:393, 1990.
124. Penn RD, Kroin JS: Long-term intrathecal baclofen infusion for treatment of spasticity. J Neurosurg 66:181, 1987.

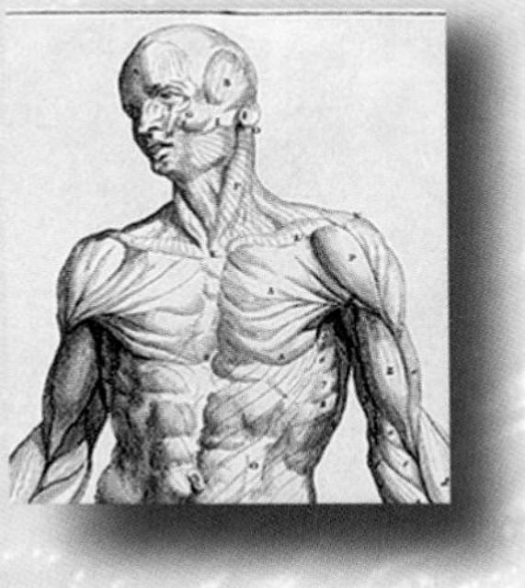

Part F

Advanced Pain Management Techniques

chapter 168

Neuroadenolysis of the Pituitary

Steven D. Waldman

HISTORY

Surgery has been used to palliate pain secondary to hormone-dependent tumors since the late 1800s. Early surgical efforts were directed primarily at surgical castration.[1] The addition of adrenalectomy followed, as the importance of this gland in the secretion of sex hormones became better understood.[2] Advances in the field of endocrinology in the 1950s led to an increasing focus on the pituitary gland. To this end, transcranial hypophysectomy was performed in an effort to induce regression of hormone-dependent tumors and to palliate symptoms. Investigators became aware that pain relief was a more consistent finding than actual tumor regression.[3]

Unfortunately, transcranial hypophysectomy was a major procedure with significant surgical risk that precluded its use in many of the patients who could most benefit, namely, patients suffering from advanced malignancy. Consequently, less-invasive means of pituitary destruction were undertaken. These attempts included radiation therapy, implantation of radon seeds, and, ultimately, chemical neurolysis of the pituitary.[4]

Neuroadenolysis of the pituitary (NALP) was first described by Moricca in 1958 as a technique to relieve pain of malignant origin by placing multiple needles into the pituitary gland and then injecting small amounts of absolute alcohol.[5] Moricca's early reports led other investigators to adopt and modify this procedure. To date, more than 14,000 patients suffering from intractable pain have been treated with NALP.[6]

INDICATIONS AND CONTRAINDICATIONS

Indications for NALP are summarized in Table 168–1.

NALP is an appropriate treatment for patients who suffer from bilateral facial or upper body cancer pain, bilateral diffuse cancer pain, intractable visceral pain, or pain secondary to compression of neural structures after all antiblastic methods and other analgesic measures have been exhausted. When medical hormonal control of pain no longer works, patients may also benefit from the procedure.[4] Most investigators observe better results in patients whose pain is secondary to hormone-dependent tumors, although the procedure is also effective for palliation of pain from hormone-unresponsive malignancies.[7] Contraindications to neuroadenolysis

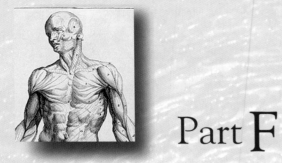

Table 168–1

Indications for Neuroadenolysis of the Pituitary

- Failure of all antiblastic treatments
- Failure of all other appropriate pain-relieving measures
- Bilateral facial or upper body cancer pain
- Bilateral diffuse cancer pain
- Intractable visceral pain
- Pain secondary to compression of neural structures
- Loss of hormonal control of pain

Table 168–2

Contraindications to Neuroadenolysis of the Pituitary

- Local infection
- Sepsis
- Coagulopathy
- Increased intracranial pressure
- Empty sella syndrome

of the pituitary are summarized in Table 168–2. Local infection, sepsis, coagulopathy, significantly increased intracranial pressure, and empty sella syndrome are absolute contraindications to NALP.[4,7] Relative contraindications to NALP include poor anesthesia risk, disulfiram therapy, and significant behavioral abnormalities. Obviously, owing to the desperate circumstances of most patients considered for NALP, the risk-benefit ratio is shifted toward performing the procedure on both ethical and humanitarian grounds.

CLINICALLY RELEVANT ANATOMY AND TECHNIQUE

In an effort to improve on Moricca's original technique, Corssen and associates[8] and other investigators have modified it by decreasing the number of needles used. Levin and colleagues[9] further modified the technique by utilizing a stereotactic head frame. Attempting to reduce the incidence of postoperative cerebrospinal fluid (CSF) leakage, these investigators suggested initially placing an 18-gauge, 6-inch spinal needle through the floor of the sphenoidal sinus. The needle was then removed, and a smaller, 20-gauge, 6-inch spinal needle was placed through the hole left by the 18-gauge needle. The 20-gauge needle was then advanced into the sella turcica. On occasion, these investigators found it necessary to drill through the floor of the sella turcica with a Kirschner wire because the needle would not pass through dense bone. They also noted the occasional occurrence of CSF leakage until they instituted the injection of ethyl alpha cyanomethacrylate resin through the spinal needles.

Waldman and Feldstein[10] further modified NALP by using a needle-through-needle technique, thus eliminating the need for the stereotactic frame or drilling. These modifications made the procedure more suitable for use in the community hospital.

Phenol, cryoneurolysis, radiofrequency lesioning, and electrical stimulation in place of alcohol all have been advocated for NALP.[11-13] More experience is needed with each of these modalities to determine whether some of the theoretical advantages and disadvantages of each modification translate into clinically relevant benefits.

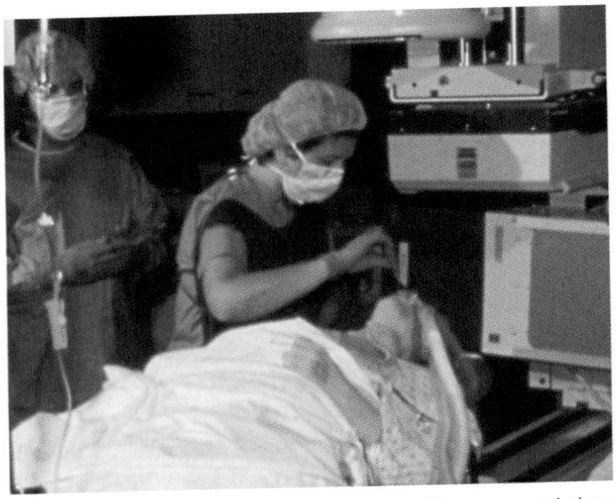

FIGURE 168–1 ■ The nose is packed to provide vasoconstriction and mucosal shrinkage.

Preoperative Preparation

Screening laboratory tests, consisting of a complete blood cell count, chemistry profile, electrolyte determination, urinalysis, coagulation profile, chest radiography, and electrocardiography, are performed as for any other patient undergoing general anesthesia. Anteroposterior and lateral skull films are also obtained to evaluate the size and relative position of the sella turcica and to rule out sphenoidal sinus infection, which may be clinically silent.[4,10]

Preoperative treatment of all patients with an intravenous dose of a cephalosporin and aminoglycoside antibiotic 1 hour before induction of anesthesia is indicated to reduce the risk of infection in these immunocompromised patients.[10] Most investigators perform NALP with the patient under general endotracheal anesthesia, although, because the procedure is relatively painless, it can be performed with local anesthesia.[14] Opioids are avoided before and during the operation to avoid pupillary miosis, which might obscure the pupillary dilatation observed when alcohol spills out of the sella onto the oculomotor nerve (see later).[7,10]

Technique

With the intubated patient in the supine position on a biplanar fluoroscopy table, the nose is packed with pledgets soaked in 7.5% cocaine solution to provide vasoconstriction and shrinkage of the nasal mucosa (Fig. 168–1). After 10 minutes, the packs are removed and the anterior nasal mucosa and face are prepared with povidone iodine solution. Sterile drapes are placed over the nose and face. The anterior medial mucosa and deep tissues are infiltrated with a solution of 1.0% lidocaine and 1:200,000 epinephrine. During infiltration and subsequent needle placement, care must be taken to avoid Kesselback's plexus lest vigorous bleeding ensue. It is imperative that the head be kept precisely in the midline to allow accurate needle placement.

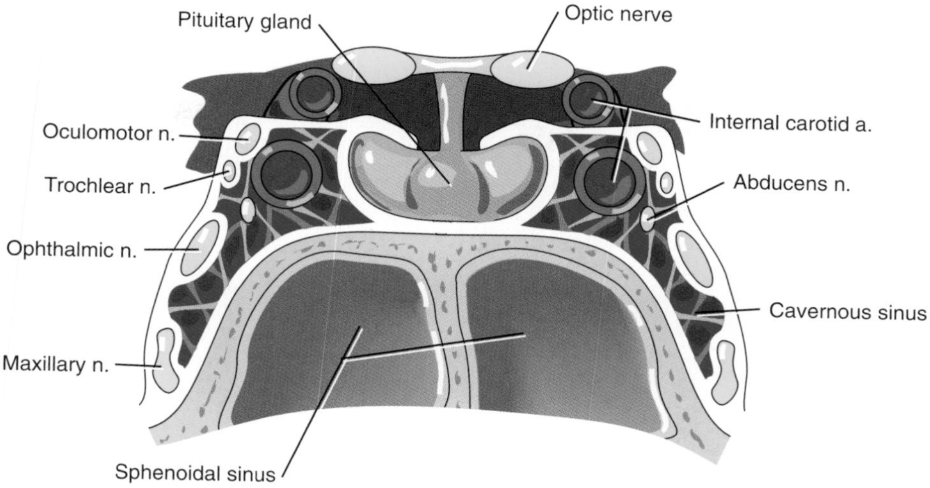

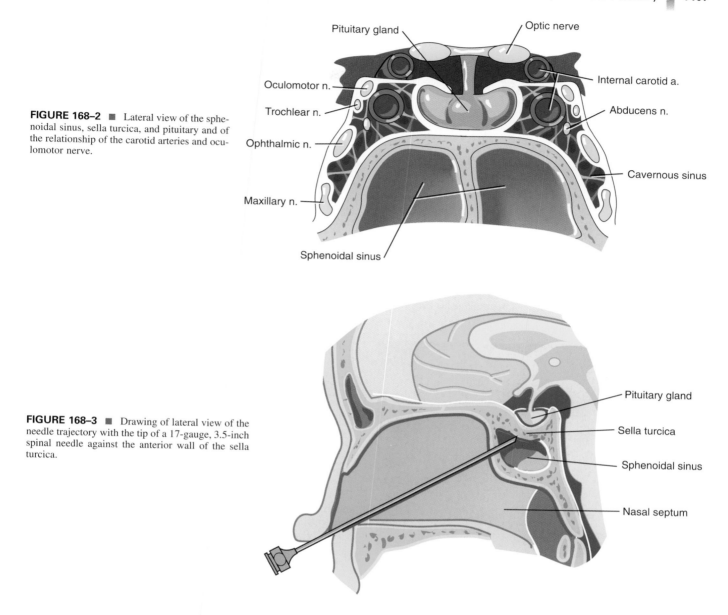

FIGURE 168–2 ■ Lateral view of the sphenoidal sinus, sella turcica, and pituitary and of the relationship of the carotid arteries and oculomotor nerve.

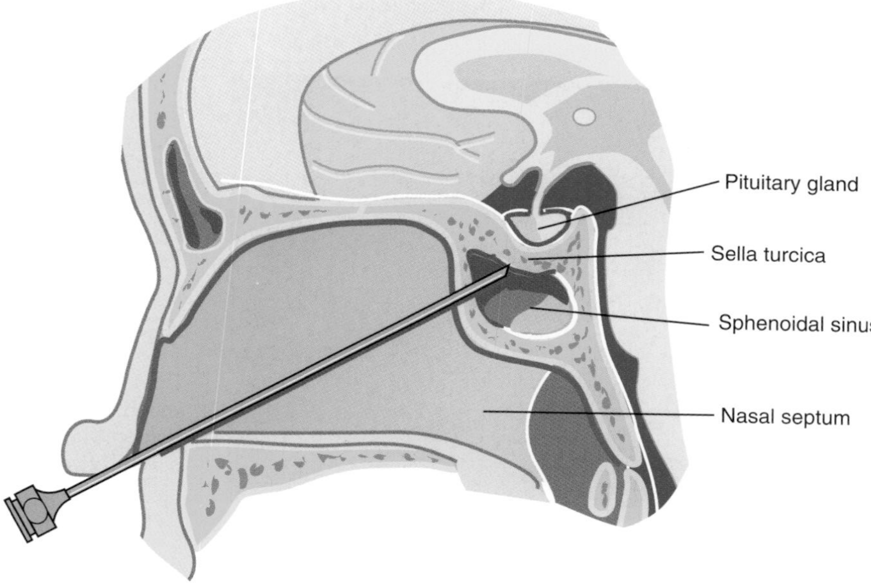

FIGURE 168–3 ■ Drawing of lateral view of the needle trajectory with the tip of a 17-gauge, 3.5-inch spinal needle against the anterior wall of the sella turcica.

A 17-gauge, 3.5-inch spinal needle with the stylet in place is advanced under biplanar fluoroscopic guidance, with care being taken to ensure that the needle remains exactly in the midline to avoid trauma to the adjacent structures, including the carotid arteries (Fig. 168–2). The needle is advanced until its tip rests against the anterior wall of the sella turcica (Fig. 168–3). At this point, plain radiographs are taken to confirm the needle position (Fig. 168–4). After satisfactory positioning is verified, the stylet is removed from the 17-gauge needle. A 20-gauge, 13-cm styleted Hinck needle (Cook Incorporated, Bloomington, IN) is placed through the 17-gauge needle and is carefully advanced through the anterior wall of the sella turcica (Fig. 168–5). This process feels like passing a needle through an eggshell. The Hinck needle is then further advanced under biplanar fluoroscopic guidance through the substance of the pituitary gland, until the tip rests against the posterior wall of the sella turcica (Fig. 168–6). Needle position is again confirmed with plain radiographs (Fig. 168–7).

The patient's eyes are then exposed, and alcohol in aliquots of 0.2 mL is injected as the Hinck needle is gradually withdrawn back through the pituitary gland (Fig. 168–8). Depending on the size of the sella, a total of 4 to 6 mL of alcohol is injected. During the injection process, the pupils are constantly monitored for dilatation. Pupillary dilatation indicates that the alcohol has spilled outside the sella turcica and has come in contact with an oculomotor nerve. If pupillary dilatation is observed, injection of alcohol is discontinued and the needle is withdrawn to a more anterior position. The injection process then resumes. In most instances, if the alcohol injection is discontinued at the first sign of pupillary dilatation, any resultant visual disturbance is transitory.[15] It has been suggested that monitoring with visual evoked responses during alcohol injection may be a more sensitive test for visual complications than pupillary dilatation is.[4]

After the injection of alcohol is completed, 0.5 mL of cyanomethacrylate resin is injected via the Hinck needle to seal the hole in the sella turcica and to prevent CSF leakage.

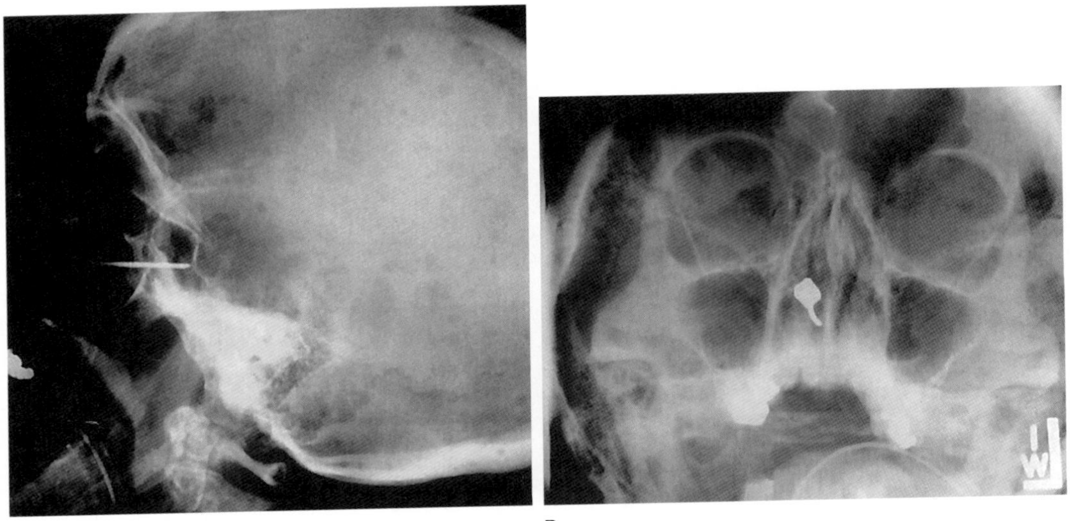

A B

FIGURE 168–4 ■ Plain radiographs confirming placement of the 17-gauge, 3.5-inch needle in a midline position with the tip resting against the anterior wall of the sella turcica. **A**, Lateral view. **B**, Anteroposterior view. (From Waldman SD [ed]: Interventional Pain Management, 2nd ed. Philadelphia, WB Saunders, 2001, p 679.)

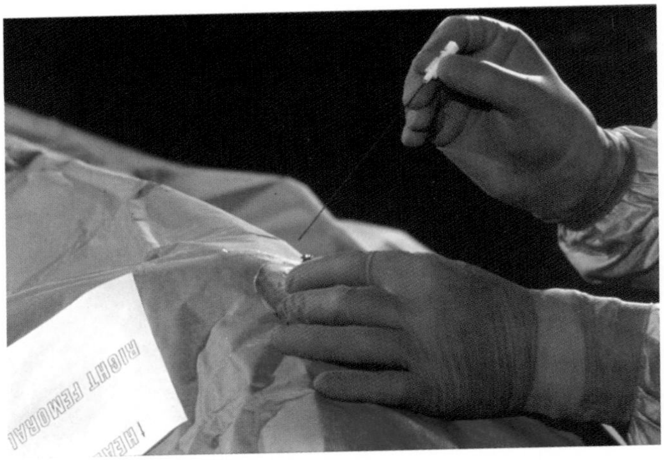

FIGURE 168–5 ■ A 20-gauge, 13-cm Hinck needle is introduced through the 17-gauge needle.

Both needles are removed. The nasal mucosa is observed for bleeding or CSF leakage. Nasal packing is not generally required with this modified procedure. The patient is then extubated and taken to the recovery room. Approximately 30 minutes is required to perform NALP.

POSTOPERATIVE CARE

All patients are continued on antibiotics for 24 hours. Endocrine replacement, consisting of 15 mg of prednisone and 0.15 mg of levothyroxine sodium (Synthroid) every morning, is required for every patient.[10]

Accurate monitoring of intake and output is mandatory because transient diabetes insipidus occurs in approximately 40% of patients undergoing NALP.[16] In most instances, the diabetes insipidus is self-limited but vasopressin administration should be considered for patients who are unable to drink as much as they excrete or whose urinary output exceeds 2.5 L/day.[4] Failure to identify and treat diabetes insipidus is the leading cause of morbidity and mortality in patients who undergo NALP.

All patients are continued on preoperative levels of oral narcotics for 24 hours, and then doses are tapered. Patients generally resume their normal diet and activities the day of the procedure.

MECHANISMS OF PAIN RELIEF

Levin and Ramirez[15] and Bonica[7] have reviewed the proposed mechanisms of pain relief after NALP. Early investigators centered their theories on the concept of pain relief secondary to elimination of the pituitary hormones responsible for enhancement of nocioceptive transmission. Later, Yanagida and colleagues[11] suggested that pain appears to be independent of the extent of pituitary damage and may be caused by reactionary hyperactivity of the hypophyseal system exerting inhibitory influences on the pain pathways of the brain. In spite of extensive research, the exact mechanism of pain relief after NALP remains unclear, as does whether the procedure produces pain relief by neurodestruction or neuroaugmentation.[13]

RESULTS

Incidence of Pain Relief

In 1990, Bonica[7] reviewed the world literature on NALP and summarized the data and conclusions. The world literature suggests a success rate (pain relief rated complete to good) of approximately 63%. An additional 23% of patients described their pain relief as fair. Fourteen percent of patients reported poor to no relief of pain after NALP. A closer look at this patient population reveals that patients with hormone-dependent tumors experienced better pain relief than did those with non–hormone-dependent tumors.[7] Furthermore, it appears that investigators who injected larger volumes of

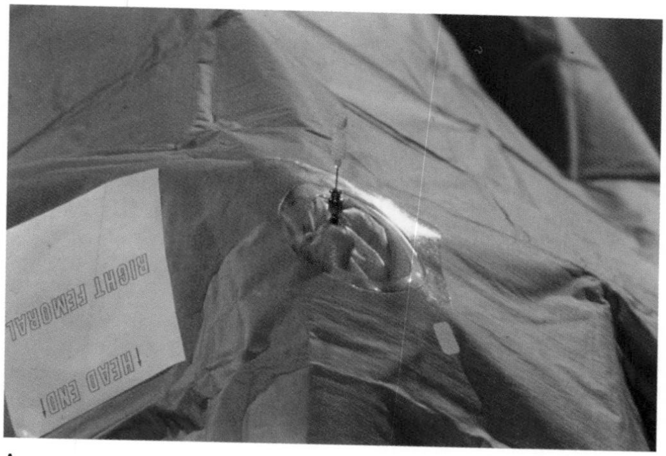

A

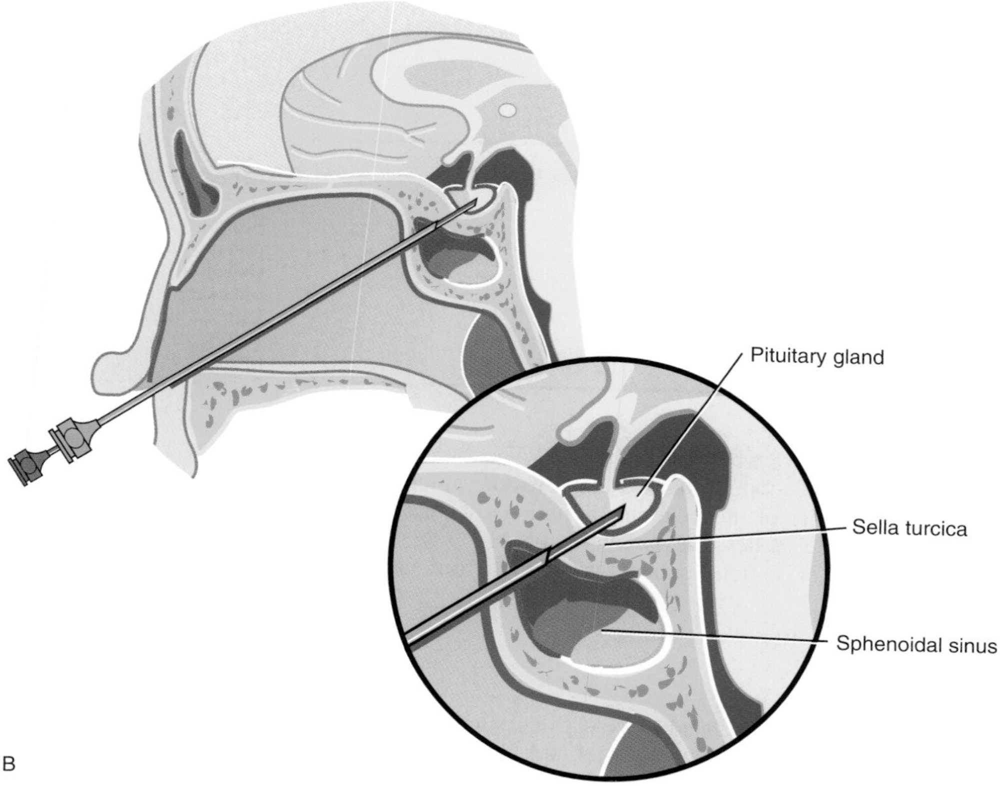

B

FIGURE 168–6 ■ **A,** The Hinck needle has been placed through the 17-gauge needle, and the Hinck needle's tip is resting against the posterior wall of the sella turcica. **B,** Drawing of a lateral view of the needle trajectory with the tip of the 17-gauge spinal needle against the anterior wall of the sella turcica and the Hinck needle through it into the substance of the pituitary.

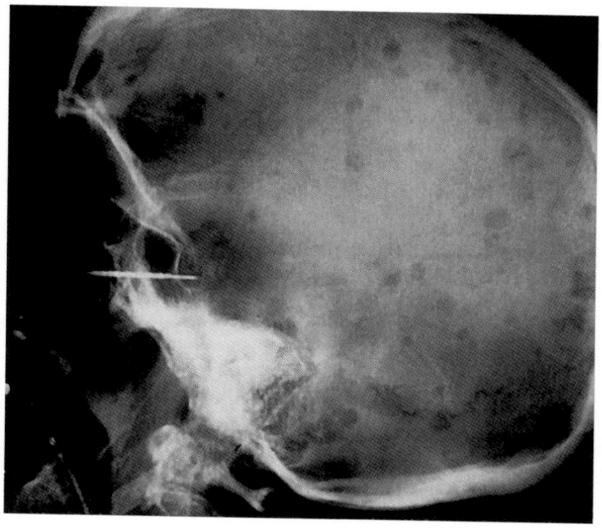

FIGURE 168–7 ■ Plain radiograph confirms that the tip of the Hinck needle is resting against the posterior wall of the sella turcica. (From Waldman SD [ed]: Interventional Pain Management, 2nd ed. Philadelphia, WB Saunders, 2001, p 680.)

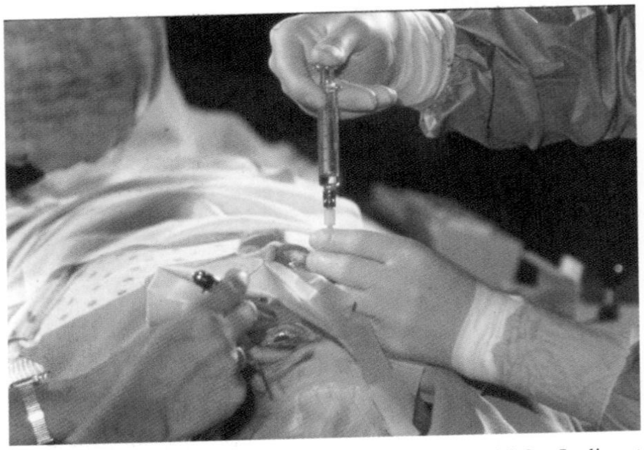

FIGURE 168–8 ■ The patient's eyes are exposed, and 0.2-mL aliquots of alcohol are injected as the Hinck needle is gradually withdrawn.

Table 168–3

Complications of Neuroadenolysis of the Pituitary

- Bilateral frontal headache
- Diabetes insipidus
- Abnormal temperature regulation
- Increased pulmonary secretion
- Ocular disturbances

alcohol (4 to 6 mL) or who repeated NALP when the first procedure was not successful obtained better results in terms of pain relief. In spite of the inherent limitations of analyzing data from multiple studies, it is obvious that NALP is an effective treatment for certain patients suffering from cancer pain.[7,10,17,18]

Complications

Complications directly related to NALP are summarized in Table 168–3. Virtually all patients who undergo NALP complain of a bilateral frontal headache that resolves spontaneously within 24 to 48 hours.[10] Diabetes insipidus develops in approximately 40% of patients who undergo the procedure. Approximately 35% of patients experience transient temperature increases up to 1.5°C after NALP.[10,16] These temperature aberrations are attributed to disturbance of the temperature-regulating mechanism of the hypothalamus.[10] About 20% of patients experience an increase in pulmonary secretions and mild orthopnea that clinically resembles congestive heart failure.[10] This problem is self-limited if careful attention is paid to the patient's fluid status. It has been postulated that this phenomenon is centrally mediated. Although the potential exists for serious ocular disturbances, a review of the literature suggests that transient visual disturbances, including diplopia, blurred vision, and loss of visual field, occur in fewer than 10% of patients who undergo neuroadenolysis of the pituitary gland.[4,7,16] Permanent visual disturbances occur much less often, with an average incidence of approximately 5%.[4,7,10,16] CSF leakage, infection, and pituitary hemorrhage develop in fewer than 1% of patients reported but are some of the most devastating complications. If they are not recognized immediately and treated, death can result.[4,7,10]

CONCLUSION

Neuroadenolysis of the pituitary gland is a safe, effective method for palliating diffuse cancer pain that does not respond to conservative treatment modalities. Its technical simplicity and relative safety make NALP an ideal procedure for cancer patients who have undergone a vast array of treatments. Although spinal administration of opioids has replaced NALP as the procedure of choice for many cancer pain syndromes, it is the belief of many cancer pain specialists that NALP is still underutilized today. With the needle-through-needle modification described, a more favorable risk-benefit ratio is expected. As Bonica[7] has stated, "NALP is one of the most, if not the most, effective ablative procedures for the relief of severe diffuse cancer pain."

References

1. Beatson GT: On the treatment of inoperable cases of cancer of the mamma. Lancet 2:104, 1896.
2. Huggins C, Hodges CV: Inhibition of mammary and prostate cancers by adrenalectomy. Cancer 12:131, 1952.
3. Luft R, Olivercrona H: Experiences with hypophysectomy. J Neurosurg 10:301, 1953.
4. Lipton S: Pituitary adenolysis. In Raj PP (ed): Practical Management of Pain, 2nd ed. St. Louis, CV Mosby, 1992, p 908.
5. Ventifredda V, DeConno F: Moricca's operation at the National Cancer Institute of Milan. In Ischia S, Lipton S, Maffezzoli GF (eds): Pain Treatment. New York, Raven, 1993, pp 85-90.
6. Gianasi G: Neuroadenolysis of the pituitary of Moricca: An overview of development, mechanisms, technique, and results. Adv Pain Res Ther 7:647, 1984.
7. Bonica JJ: Neurolytic block and hypophysectomy. In Bonica JJ: The Management of Pain. Philadelphia, Lea & Febiger, 1990, vol 2, pp 2028-2034.
8. Corssen G, Holcomb MA, Moustapha I, et al: Alcohol-induced adenolysis of the pituitary gland: A new approach to control of intractable cancer pain. Anesth Analg 56:414, 1977.
9. Levin AB, Katz J, Benson RC, Jones AG: Treatment of pain of diffuse metastatic cancer by stereotactic chemical hypophysectomy: Long-term results and observations on mechanisms of action. Neurosurgery 6:258, 1980.
10. Waldman SD, Feldstein GS: Neuroadenolysis of the pituitary: Description of a modified technique. J Pain Symptom Manage 2:45, 1987.
11. Yanagida H, Corssen G, Trouwborst A, Erdman W: Relief of cancer pain in man: Alcohol-induced neuroadenolysis vs. electrical stimulation of the pituitary gland. Pain 19:133, 1984.
12. Duthie AM: Pituitary cryoablation. Anaesthesia 38:495, 1983.
13. Patt RB: Neurosurgical and neuroaugmentative intervention. In Patt RB (ed): Cancer Pain. Philadelphia, JB Lippincott, 1993, p 489.
14. Lipton S: The injection of alcohol into the pituitary fossa (Moricca's operation). In Lipton S: Relief of Pain in Clinical Practice. Oxford, Blackwell Scientific, 1979, pp 179-220.
15. Levin AB, Ramirez LL: Treatment of cancer pain with hypophysectomy: Surgical and chemical. Adv Pain Res Ther 7:631, 1984.
16. Gianasi GC: Pituitary neuroadenolysis: An analysis of the clinical results in a group of high-risk patients. In Ischia S, Lipton S, Maffezzoli GF (eds): Pain Treatment. New York, Raven, 1993, pp 91-95.
17. Takeda F: Results of cancer pain relief and tumour regression by pituitary neuroadenolysis and surgical hypophysectomy. In Ischia S, Lipton S, Maffezzoli GF (eds): Pain Treatment. New York, Raven, 1993, pp 103-113.
18. Waldman SD: Neuroadenolysis of the pituitary. In Waldman SD: Atlas of Interventional Pain Management Techniques. Philadelphia, WB Saunders, 1998, pp 513-515.

chapter 169

Radiofrequency Techniques

Matthew T. Kline

The application of radiofrequency (RF) lesions generated in the nervous system for a variety of therapeutic purposes has had excellent success. Compared with other selective lesioning techniques, modern RF methods afford several clinical and practical advantages.

METHODS OF CREATING NERVOUS SYSTEM LESIONS

Historically, numerous techniques have been used to destroy nerve tissue selectively in the brain and elsewhere in the body; the most important of these techniques include cryogenic surgery, focused ultrasound, chemical destruction, ionizing radiation, mechanical methods, lasers, RF heating method, and direct current (DC) heating method. A brief critique of these methods is given here, with a view of their relative merits compared with the RF heating method. The RF and DC heating methods involve the passage of current from an electrode placed in the target zone through the surrounding tissue, heating and destroying the tissue in the vicinity of the electrode.

Cryogenic Surgery

Cryogenic surgery typically has involved inserting a probe into the brain or other body tissue and cooling the tip of the probe to extremely low temperatures to freeze a region of tissue around the tip. Technically, this has been accomplished with ingenious cryogenic devices, usually cannulas with internal channels to circulate extremely cold liquids such as liquid nitrogen or rapid expansion of gas, creating extremely low temperatures at the probe tip, but not along its shaft. The cryogenic surgery technique has been applied extensively for intracranial stereotaxy in past decades, but its use has declined in recent years. Cryofreezing techniques using similar modern instrumentation have become popular for freezing tumors elsewhere in the body, as in the liver and prostate.[1,2] Several difficulties in using the cryogenic technique in the brain and elsewhere in the body have become apparent. Cryogenic probes usually have diameters of 3 mm or larger, a size that tends to be unacceptable for many procedures in the brain and the peripheral nervous system. There is also the potential for the frozen tissue to stick to the tip of the probe as it is being withdrawn from the brain or other tissue if defreezing is not done carefully and completely. Cryogenic probes, which have had a prominent place in neurosurgery, are not adapted easily to percutaneous procedures owing to their intrinsic construction.

Focused Ultrasound

Focused ultrasound has the advantage of making a trackless lesion and has the potential to be totally noninvasive. Ultrasound was used in the 1950s for neurosurgical functional lesions made in the brain. Significant mechanical disadvantages of the ultrasound technique include (1) the scatter of ultrasound from surrounding bony structures, making it difficult to control fully; (2) the necessity, for achieving trackless lesions in the brain, of making a large craniotomy to couple the ultrasonic transducer properly to the brain tissue; and (3) the inability to quantify the temperature distribution at the ultrasound focal site, leaving the technique without adequate monitoring.

Induction Heating

Disadvantages of induction heating, using implanted pellets of metal or highly intense electromagnetic fields, are the lack of knowledge about the thermal distribution near the lesion site and the inability to control lesion size reproducibly and quantitatively. Induction heating, similar to ultrasound, seems to have more applicability in hyperthermia therapy, in which more diffuse, nonlethal thermal elevations of tissue temperature are the desired objective.

Chemical Destruction

Chemical destruction, as by injection of alcohol, phenol, or glycerol, often has been used primarily for peripheral nerve denervation. Controversy exists regarding the merits of chemical injection techniques versus the RF heating method. The obvious advantage of chemical injection is its simplicity, an attribute illustrated by the widespread use of nerve blocks and of glycerol injections in the treatment of trigeminal neuralgia. The most obvious and commonly reported disadvantage is that the spread of the injected material in the target tissue region is impossible to control, leading to lesions that are irregular and variable in size and shape and inconsistent in therapeutic effects.

Ionizing Radiation

The use of ionizing radiation, whether internally implanted or with external beam arrays, has played a major role in the treatment of tumors. This modality also has been used for destruction of smaller functional targets. External beam radiation has the advantage of being noninvasive.

Brachytherapy

Brachytherapy—the implantation of radioactive seeds, such as iodine 125 (^{125}I) or iridium 1692 (^{1692}Ir)—is widely practiced in neurosurgery.[3-11] Focal external beam irradiation employing radioactive sources such as cobalt 60 (^{60}Co) and linear accelerators in techniques called *stereotactic radiosurgery* and *stereotactic radiotherapy* has become popular. Radiosurgery using linear accelerators is able to ablate targets a few millimeters in diameter with submillimeter precision. Sophisticated computer graphic workstations and three-dimensional treatment planning systems enable highly controlled planning so that the external photon beams avoid critical structures.[12-14] It is possible to make very small therapeutic lesions noninvasively by stereotactic radiosurgery methods. Time fractionation may augment effectiveness and safety further. The difficulties with these methods compared with the RF technique are that they do not afford interactive target identification by means of stimulation and other methods, and that the extent of circumscription of the radiation and the uncertainty about radiation to normal surrounding tissues may be problematic.

Mechanical Methods

Mechanical methods for making lesions in the nervous system, including the use of the lucotome and other tools, have been effective in some settings. Extremely small lesions can be made in this way. The dangers of these techniques are primarily hemorrhage and the lack of quantitative controls. Focused electromagnetic radiation with large, external arrays of microwaves has not been used widely to date. This technology has potential, but has the same disadvantage as induction heating and focused ultrasound—the inability to monitor the temperature distribution as the lesions are being made without the direct implantation of temperature sensors.

Lasers

Lasers have been used to make lesions in the brain, spinal cord, and elsewhere in the body. Although much work has been done comparing laser and RF heating methods, it is difficult to quantify the extent and rapidity of tissue destruction using the laser because it is not amenable to adequate temperature monitoring and produces varying effects, depending on tissue parameters such as blood flow and thermoconductivity. Laser light of different wavelengths and differing photon delivery systems also may affect significantly the size and controllability of a laser-generated lesion. The use of lasers for making therapeutic lesions in the dorsal root entry zone lesion procedure has come under some criticism compared with the RF technique because of the lack of quantification and consistency and the production of defects.[15]

BRAIN LESIONING WITH ELECTRIC CURRENT

Direct Current Electrolytic Lesion

Many 19th century workers experimented with making lesions in neural tissue using DC. Because the brain is composed largely of electrolytes, it was natural to place electrodes in it and to see what happens when current is passed between them. In this way, Beaunis (1868), Fournie (1873), and others made the first electrolytic brain lesions in animals using bipolar DC electrodes. Golsinger (1895) did the same with monopolar brain electrodes. Horsley and Clarke (1905), who carefully studied the quality of lesions as a function of electrode polarity and material, concluded that the anodal (positive electrode) lesion was superior because it generated less gas. They put forward empirical rules for "incrementing" anodal lesion size on the basis of current and time parameters. The first stereotactic DC brain lesions were described in 1947.

DC lesions can vary in size to a factor of 4:1 for a fixed electrode geometry, lesion current, and lesion time.[16] The reason for the erratic nature of DC lesions is that they depend strongly on electrolysis, with its inherent polarization and gas formation, and on the specific anatomy of tissue planes and vascular interruptions. These factors make DC electrolytic lesions ragged at the circumference and variable in size and unacceptable for accurate lesion making.

Radiofrequency Electrolytic Lesion

The first practical and commercially available RF lesion generators were built in the early 1950s using continuous-wave RF in the 1-MHz range. The brain lesions made with these machines using the controls of current and power level had smooth borders, an immediate improvement over DC lesions.[17,18]

Advantages of Radiofrequency Heating Method

RF lesion technology has advantages over other techniques for making discrete therapeutic or functional lesions in the brain and elsewhere in the body. With the advent of temperature control, *quantifiable lesions* could be made consistently from one patient to another, with the added safety factor of *avoiding unwanted and uncontrolled side effects,* such as sticking, charring, and formation of explosive gas. The concept of *differential selection of pain fibers* (versus other neural fibers) has been suggested, and there is some indication from clinical experience that it is achievable using the RF method. Because of the nature of the RF electrode, it is directly amenable to *stimulation, impedance monitoring,* and *recording,* all of which greatly enhance the surgeon's ability to know that the electrode is at the appropriate target for making the lesion. Because the RF lesion electrode is an electric connection, it automatically provides these secondary target benefits. RF electrodes adapt to stereotactic technique and to other fixation devices because of their *convenient, cylindrical, narrow* geometry. They can be made in a variety of elaborate shapes with extremely small tips (0.25 mm) or with side-issue tips for searching space near the target volume

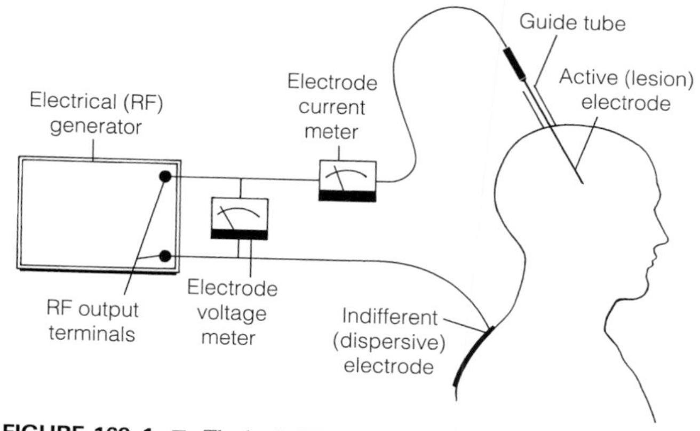

FIGURE 169–1 ■ The basic RF lesioning circuit.

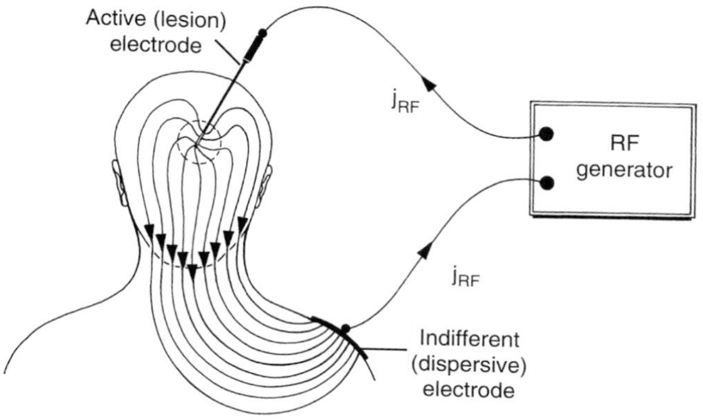

FIGURE 169–2 ■ The spread of the RF current density (j_{RF}) in the tissue between the active and dispersive electrodes.

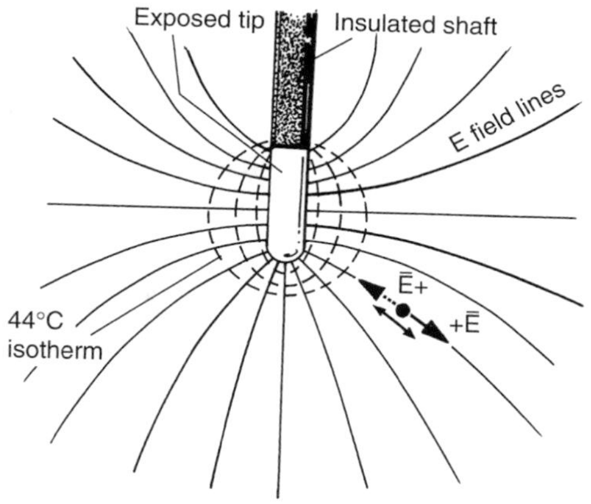

FIGURE 169–3 ■ A typical electric field line pattern *(solid lines)* around the exposed tip of an RF lesion electrode in a uniform medium, with typical isotherms *(dashed lines)*. The 44°C isotherm is at the outer limits of the permanent lesion zone.

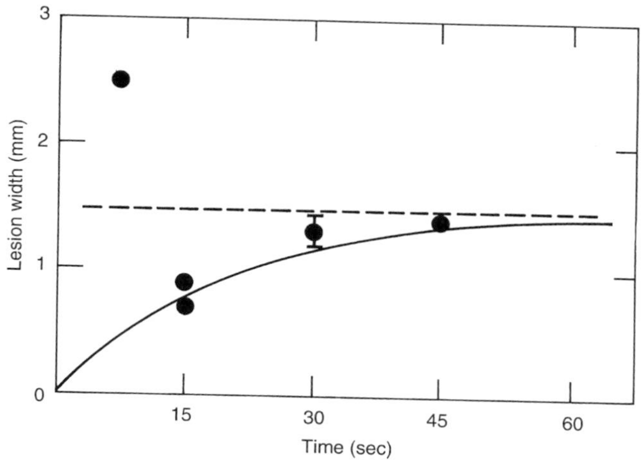

FIGURE 169–4 ■ A plot of dorsal root entry zone lesion width over time. In this experiment, the temperature was 75°C.

for the appropriate target point. The electrodes can be made very robust and in a nearly endless variation of shapes and configurations. This is another of the decisive advantages of the RF lesioning technique. Perhaps, overall, the most telling attributes of the RF lesion method are that it has been safe, effective, and simple to use.

PHYSICAL PRINCIPLES OF LESION GENERATION

Basic Concepts of Heat Lesioning and Monitoring

The basic RF lesioning circuit is shown schematically in Figure 169–1. The RF generator is the source of RF voltage across its output terminals. When it is connected to electrodes placed on the body, current flows between them through the tissue. The body becomes an element of the complete electric circuit. The *active* electrode is positioned where the heat lesion is to be made, and the *dispersive* or *indifferent* electrode is a larger area electrode that usually is not intended to produce tissue heating. The path of the electric current lines in the body between the active and dispersive electrodes is illustrated in Figure 169–2.

Field patterns near a straight-tipped active electrode are shown in Figure 169–3. The mechanism for tissue heating in the 1-MHz range is primarily ionic, rather than dielectric, and is qualitatively simple to understand. The RF voltage on the tip sets up electric field lines in space around the exposed electrode tip according to the basic laws of electrostatics. The heat is generated in the tissue, not in the electrode tip. Because the tip is lying in the heated tissue, the tip absorbs heat from the tissue. If the electrode is designed properly, it does not absorb much heat at equilibrium, and the tip temperature is approximately equal to that of the hottest tissue adjacent to it. Because temperature is the fundamental lesion parameter, it must be measured; and monitoring tip temperature makes it possible to control the lesion's size. For consistent prediction of lesion size, the correct electrode tip size and lesion temperature at the tip must be selected.

Consistency of lesion size also depends on eliminating the time dependence on the lesion's size. This is done easily by letting the lesion come to thermal equilibrium. Lesion size in relation to time for a given tip temperature or RF current is illustrated in Figure 169–4, based on experimental data.[19]

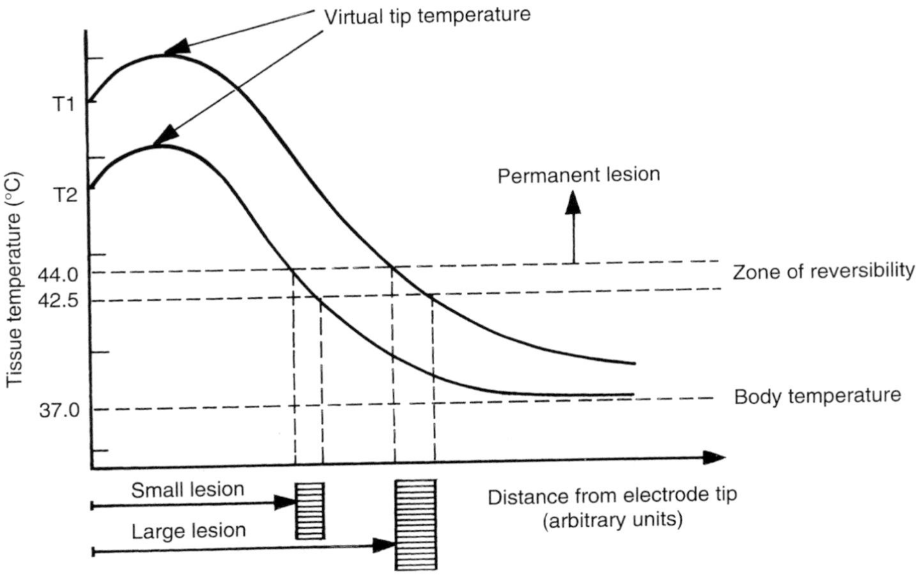

FIGURE 169–5 ■ The distribution of tissue temperature as a function of distance from the active electrode tip. The actual function depends on the shape of the tip and the point on the tip from which the distance is measured.

The nominal radius of the lesion approaches a maximum value as equilibrium between the RF heat into and the heat conduction away from the tissue around the tip is established. Equilibrium size is reached in about 60 seconds and very nearly so in 30 seconds. During the first 30 seconds, the lesion size is increasing. One can make a "time-dependent" lesion, whose size increases nearly linearly over time for about the first 15 seconds. In this way, the lesion volume can be increased gradually. The current needed to achieve a given tip temperature depends, however, on variables such as resistance, heat conduction, and tip geometry. The time versus lesion size curve shown in Figure 169–4 depends on other variables, such as vascularity and proximity to CSF, bone, and other heat sinks. It is preferable to eliminate uncertainties of the time-current prescription by choosing an appropriate tip size and temperature and allowing the lesion size to reach its equilibrium value by means of a 30- to 60-second exposure.

There is a narrow zone of reversibility for lesions in the brain. Brain tissue can withstand temperatures of about 42.5°C without injury for minutes. Temporary cessation of certain neural functions may occur between 42.5°C and 44°C, whereas temperatures greater than 45°C result in some form of permanent damage.[20] There should be a thin zone of reversibility on the perimeter of the zone of permanent destruction (Fig. 169–5). Practical use of this zone has not yet been exploited in clinical lesion making, but anyone performing RF stereotaxy must be aware of how critical these temperatures are in the brain.

In the peripheral nervous system, a promising aspect of RF lesion making is the possibility of accurate and highly selective destruction of pain-carrying nerve fibers. An apparent example is in the trigeminal ganglion, where, at temperatures near 60°C to 70°C, the highly myelinated A beta fibers seem to survive better than the unmyelinated A delta and C fibers. This observation derives from clinical experience: Trigeminal neuralgia can be specifically eliminated, but tactile and motor innervation is preserved. The importance of temperature as the fundamental lesion parameter is underscored.

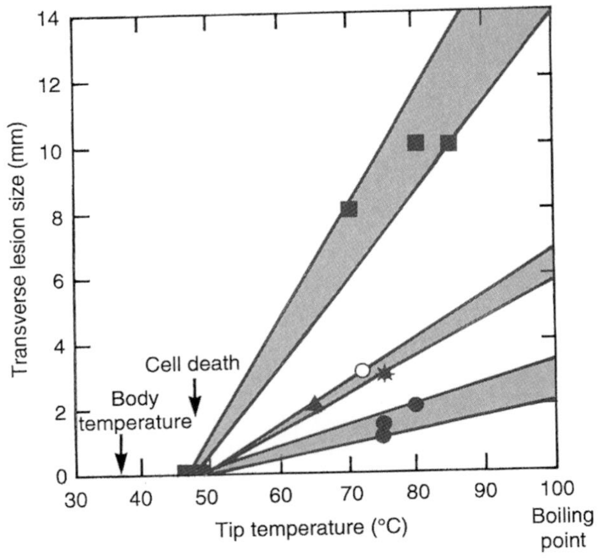

FIGURE 169–6 ■ Plot of lesion width versus electrode tip diameter and temperature. Area bounding squares represents tip diameter of 1.6 mm; area bounding solid circles represents tip diameter of 0.25 mm; area bounding triangle represents tip diameter of 1.1 to 1.2 mm. (*Open circle* and *asterisk* are the same values as *triangle*.)

"Golden Rules" for Lesion Generation (for Homogeneous Conductive Medium)

Temperature is the fundamental lesion parameter (Fig. 169–6). Measurement of temperature not only ensures quantification and consistency of lesion size, but also is essential for safety, to avoid the boiling point and to ensure that the lesion is being made at the electrode tip and not elsewhere.

Other aspects of temperature monitoring, such as dynamic response and automatic overheating control, are addressed later in this chapter.

The RF current heats the tissue, and the tissue heats the electrode tip. This fundamental concept enables accurate monitoring of tissue temperature. A common misconception is that the electrode tip itself becomes hot because power dissipates through it. The converse is true: The tissue becomes hot because of power dissipation in the tissue itself; the heat flows *back* to the electrode tip and heats it. An accurate representation of tissue temperature can be gained by monitoring the temperature at the electrode tip. There are engineering subtleties to proper temperature monitoring of an RF lesion electrode tip, however. If the electrode tip has a high thermal mass, or if the temperature sensor is not located in intimate thermal conduction connection to the surface of the electrode, time delays and inaccuracies can result, which can lead to serious adverse effects in the lesioning process. Properly designing an RF electrode so that it adequately measures the temperature of the tissue is essential.

Consistent lesion size is determined by proper choice of electrode tip size and temperature. This is an important concept. Selection of the proper tip size, shape, and configuration and the achievement of a desired electrode tip temperature are key factors in achieving consistent RF lesioning for any given procedure in a given anatomic area. Prescriptions of lesion making based on power, time, current, voltage, or other parameters have variable results, are unpredictable, and often produce uncontrolled effects and unsatisfactory clinical results. Although temperature is the most important *observable* parameter in the clinical process, it is wise clinical practice to monitor and record other parameters, such as power, current, voltage, and impedance. If these other parameters are in acceptable ranges of normal, the lesioning process is going satisfactorily; if they are not in acceptable ranges, something is grossly wrong with the setup, such as a short circuit, open circuit, or misplaced electrode tip.

Equilibrium lesions should be made by sustaining the proper tip temperature for 30 to 60 seconds. This rule embodies the process of the equilibrium or asymptotic lesion and circumvents variability secondary to the lesion-time build-up curve, which can be a function of other parameters in the environment. The time constant for any given tip geometry or physical location can differ, but in most settings, in homogeneous tissue, 30 to 60 seconds is adequate to approximate the maximum of the exponential asymptotic curve.

Unpredictable Factors in the Lesioning Process

Although the general rules just described have given excellent results, some are difficult to predict or quantify and can cause deviations in the RF lesion process. Most important among them is the nonhomogeneous tissue in the medium itself (Fig. 169–7). Proximity of the electrode to a CSF cistern or ventricle can present a low-impedance shunt pathway for RF current and draw the lesion heat to *it,* rather than to neighboring tissue. Such an effect is commonly seen during lesion making in the trigeminal ganglion. Even more dramatic might be the effect of a large nearby blood vessel, which can sink heat away from the surrounding tissue and produce asymmetry in lesion shape.

Proximity to bone is another significant environmental variable. Bone has a lower conductivity for heat and current and creates discontinuity, especially in procedures such as facet denervation and ganglion RF procedures, in which the nerves to be heated lie next to large bones. In this situation, there is a complex of slower heating of the bone itself and a tendency for thermal insulation against the bone mass. The RF heating most likely is shunted to the tissue and away from bone. As the bone warms up, however, it becomes a reservoir of heat and affects the time constants (see Fig. 169–4).

Empirical Lesion Sizes and Recommended Electrode Geometries and Lesion Parameters in the Brain and Spinal Cord

Overall, the experience with RF lesioning using acceptable lesion parameters has yielded excellent and consistent results (see Fig. 169–6). It is unknown how lesion size changes between the first few weeks after lesioning and death. It seems that with thalamotomies, electrode tips of about 1.1 mm in diameter and 3 to 5 mm in length at temperatures of 65°C to 75°C produce lesions about 3 mm in circumference or diameter and 4 to 7 mm in length. Lesion shapes are typically prolate ellipsoids of revolution for simple cylindrical electrodes. Lesions made in the cingulum with electrodes of 1.6-mm tip diameter and 10-mm tip length at 80°C to 90°C are typically 10 mm in diameter and 12 mm long.

Information also has been accumulated on small lesions in the spinal cord using very fine–gauge electrodes.[21] Empirical information on dorsal root entry zone–type electrodes,

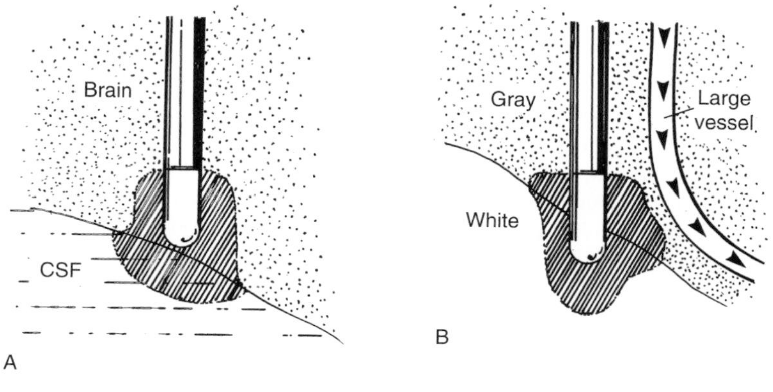

FIGURE 169–7 ■ Conditions affecting the size and shape of an RF lesion. **A,** Low-resistance shunting of RF current. **B,** Nonuniform impedances, large blood vessels. (See text for discussion.)

which are 0.25 mm in diameter with 2-mm tips, was gathered from experiments in the spinal cords of cats. Lesioning at 75°C for 15 seconds gave rise to lesion sizes of 0.7 to 0.9 mm in diameter and 1.8 to 2.2 mm in length. Increasing the lesioning time to 45 seconds increased the lesion's size to 1.4 mm in diameter and 2.3 mm in length. Lesioning at 80°C for 15 seconds produced lesions of 2 mm in diameter and approximately 2 mm long. These data are consistent with indirect information on similar-sized electrodes used in percutaneous cordotomy. Lesions of 2 to 3 mm in diameter by 2 to 3 mm in length were seen to occur when an electrode of 0.5 mm in diameter and 2 to 2.5 mm in length was placed in the lateral spinal thalamic tract.[19,22-24] This electrode size seems to be satisfactory when properly placed for percutaneous cordotomy procedures with the objective of pain relief in cancer patients. These measurements were made at a time when current and time lesion parameter prescriptions were used, but not temperature monitoring. It also is known, however, that using the Type LCE Levin Cordotomy Electrode with tip dimensions of 0.25 mm diameter and 2 mm length produces adequate percutaneous cordotomy lesions at 80°C to 85°C for 30 seconds.[25]

A summary of empirical lesion size data gathered in this way is shown in Figure 169–6. These graphs may serve as "canonical curves" for estimating the lesion size of a given tip size and tip temperature. In Figure 169–6, the transverse lesion diameter (the width or girth of the lesion) is plotted as a function of the tip temperature of the electrode (measured in °C). Each of the graphs is drawn for different tip diameters, based on the data cited. The long axis of the lesion can be assumed to be approximately 1 to 3 mm longer than the tip of the electrode for an axially symmetric and approximately cylindrical electrode geometry. These curves are based on lesion data in the brain and spinal cord and may not apply in extremely inhomogeneous tissues or in close proximity to large bony masses.

Practical Aspects of Radiofrequency Lesion Making

The modern RF lesion generator system includes not only the means to make the lesion and display the temperature of the electrode tip, but also auxiliary electronic aids to improve target determination, safety, and ease of operation. A modern RF lesion generator system is a sophisticated microprocessor-based apparatus with multiple functions to enhance the lesion generation process. It has a built-in advanced impedance monitor, a wide parameter stimulator, a lesion generator, and digital readout of all relevant parameters—impedance, stimulation parameters, power, voltage, current, time, and device function status. Its advanced temperature-monitoring system not only has thermistor and thermocouple readouts, but also analog and digital displays of temperature (both important, for reasons discussed later) and an automatic overheating control system, which enables automatic locking onto a lesion temperature when the desired electrode tip temperature has been achieved. Because the system is based on a microprocessor, many functions can be monitored simultaneously, and an alpha-numeric status display on the front panel gives the operator an instant report of the status of the generator and problems, should they arise, such as short circuit or open circuit.

Recording Parameters

It is good practice to record voltage, current power, temperature, time, and electrode type for each lesion. Such data are useful in analyzing any problem that might arise and in evaluating the operator's awareness of what these values should be under normal conditions. Erratic behavior of temperature, voltage, or current readings (a too rapid or too slow response for a given RF power increase) should be regarded as a warning of possible trouble.

Temperature Readings

The operator always should ensure, before lesioning, that the temperature meter reads body temperature at about 37°C. This is the simplest check to ensure that the electrode, thermistor, and temperature monitoring circuitry are functioning properly. The RF power should be increased slowly, and the operator should ensure that the temperature increase is normal; if it is not, the operator should not continue to increase the power and should check the system carefully. With any reading greater than 80°C, close attention must be paid because in that range a rapid "runaway" to boiling (100°C) is possible.

Electrode tip temperature may be controlled by a direct temperature control mechanism. The operator manually increases the RF voltage on the electrode. Output always should be increased gradually and carefully while the operator observes the increase in tip temperature reading as the tissue begins to heat up. As the desired tip temperature is approached, the RF control knob should be attended to, and the temperature meter should be watched to prevent drift of tip temperature from the desired lesion temperature.

Cables

Most equipment problems in RF lesioning arise from faulty cables. The cable is vulnerable to damage during handling and sterilizing. It is advisable to have sterilized spare cables on hand during the operation. The operator should remember that switching to the impedance monitor can allow an instant check of cable and electrode continuity during the procedure.

Electrode Insulation

Insulation on the electrode should be checked for cracks or breaks before each procedure. Broken insulation can cause current to flow somewhere other than to the target region and to cause unwanted tissue damage.

Dispersive Electrodes

Skin burns at the dispersive electrode arise because it has too small an area relative to that of the active electrode tip. To be maximally safe, a large-area dispersive electrode is recommended, rather than spinal needles placed in muscle or fatty tissue. A stainless steel, large-area dispersive electrode with area of at least 150 cm^2 and an ample coating of conductor gel for good electrical conductivity are recommended. Such an electrode can be taped onto the arm, hip, or another area near muscle for an adequate, low-impedance dispersive connection.

CLINICAL APPLICATIONS OF LESIONING

Only modern, thermally coupled electrode systems should be used, and it is recommended that disposable cannulas be used whenever possible. The electrode systems and the associated wires should be gas sterilized before each operative procedure. Heat sterilization is not recommended because it decreases the life expectancy of the reusable electrode systems. The safest way to maintain the long-term integrity of the electrode systems is to allow for adequate sterilization using a cool-gas sterilization cycle. Multiple wires and electrode systems need to be kept on hand if RF procedures are to be performed on a regular basis.

Regardless of the RF unit chosen, the lesion generator must be able to stimulate at multiple frequencies; monitor impedance, voltage, amperage, and temperature; allow for gradual increases in lesion temperature; and use modern, thermally coupled electrodes. For component maintenance, it is recommended that at least two electrode systems with lengths of 50 mm, 100 mm, and 150 mm be kept in sterile packages. It also is recommended that cannula systems in the 50-mm, 100-mm, and 150-mm lengths with 5-mm and 2-mm active tip exposures be kept in stock. These are the electrode and cannula systems most often used for most spinal rhizotomy procedures. The 150-mm cannula with 10-mm and 15-mm active tip exposures is useful for lumbar disk, sacroiliac joint, and lumbar sympathectomy procedures. Other specialized electrodes worthy of general consideration are blunt, curved-tip electrodes in 100-mm and 150-mm lengths with 10-mm active tips.

Lumbar Spine Disorders

Lumbar spinal disease is a common problem and often difficult to treat. To understand properly the use of RF lesions in the treatment of chronic pain of the low back, one must be familiar with the anatomy and pathophysiology of the lumbar spine.

The lumbar spine has many potential pain generators. Some areas that have been identified by neuroanatomic dissections are the anulus of the disk, the posterior longitudinal ligament, portions of the dural lining, the facet joints and capsules, the spinal nerve roots and their associated dorsal root ganglia, the sacroiliac joint and its capsule and ligaments, and the associated musculature.[26-32] Specific RF techniques have been devised for the treatment of pain emanating from the facet joints, nerve roots, anulus fibrosus, and sacroiliac joint.[33-38] No specific RF techniques have been devised for the treatment of pain emanating from the dural lining, the posterior longitudinal ligament, or myofascial trigger points. The lumbar facet joints receive innervation from multiple levels of the lumbar spine. To denervate a lumbar facet joint properly, two levels must be lesioned (Fig. 169–8).[26,35,38]

Lumbar Facet Joint Pain

The role of the facet joint in the production of chronic pain has been known since 1911,[39-41] although Ghormely[42] was the first clinician to use the term *facet syndrome.* Many authors have reported on facet joint pain[43] and its treatment with selective RF lesions.[34,35,37,44-73] Approximately 50% to 67% of properly selected patients with chronic, mechanical low back pain realize moderate to significant reduction in pain or improvement in range of motion after RF facet rhizotomy.[34,36,38,44-73] In one controlled, meticulously performed clinical study, 87% of patients reported greater than 60% pain relief (60% reported >90% relief) 1 year after RF lumbar facet denervation.[74]

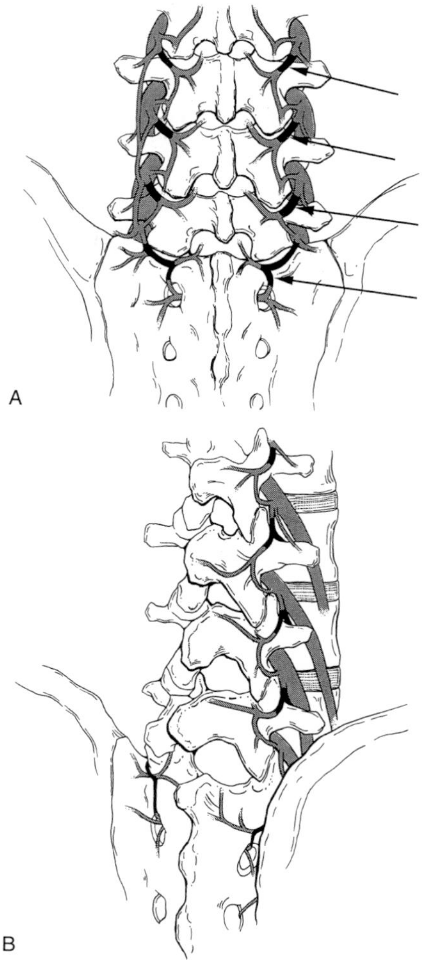

FIGURE 169–8 ■ Drawings of the nerve supply to the lumbar facet joints *(arrows).* **A,** Anteroposterior. **B,** Oblique views.

Lumbar facet joint pain can be manifested as an acute or chronic problem. It can be secondary to long-term degenerative changes or to acute trauma, as in a motor vehicle accident.[75,76] Imaging studies frequently show a normal-looking facet joint, and the x-ray status of the joint bears no relationship to the joint's pain status.[77]

Patients with facet joint pain commonly present with deep, aching pain in the paravertebral regions of the low back. They often have a somatic referral pattern of pain into the buttocks, posterior or anterior thigh, or knee region and aching in the area of the hip.[48,77] On physical examination, there is usually palpable tenderness over the facet joints. This is often associated with back pain when the lumbosacral junction is extended or flexed to the side. In patients who have facet joint pain alone, the neurologic examination is normal. Straight leg raising may not be painful, and the deflexion maneuver is uniphasic. The diagnosis of facet joint pain cannot be made on the basis of history and manual examination alone. Relief from intra-articular or medial branch local anesthetic block is an important indicator of the diagnosis of facet joint pain, but results can be false positive, and blockade is not a substitute for careful history taking and a detailed and focused manual examination.[78]

Lumbar Facet Joint Rhizotomy

A patient with facet joint pain (emanating from the L5-S1 and L4-5 joints) first is placed prone on the fluoroscopy table. A small amount of intravenous sedation is given. The patient needs to remain awake enough to cooperate throughout the procedure because it is crucial that he or she respond properly to electrical stimulation. The stimulation process allows for accurate electrode placement with a high level of safety.

After the patient's back is antiseptically prepared, the C-arm fluoroscopic device is used to identify the junction of the sacral ala with the superior articulating process of S1. The groove formed by this junction is the site of the L5 dorsal ramus. The second and third targets are the superior and medial aspects of the transverse processes at L5 and L4 (junction of transverse process with superior articulating process).

The skin and subcutaneous tissues are anesthetized with 0.5% lidocaine before placement of the RF cannulas. The first cannula is placed so that it just touches the target point for the L5 dorsal ramus (in the groove between the sacral ala and the superior articulating process of S1). The remaining cannulas are placed so that they just touch the superomedial aspects of the transverse processes at L5 and L4. At the level of the sacral ala and the transverse processes, the cannula is slipped over the leading edge of the periosteum and advanced approximately 2 mm; this allows more precise alignment of the RF cannula with the long axis of the facet joint nerve.

Correct use of the fluoroscopy unit enables the clinician to image the periosteal target points adequately. At the level of the sacral ala, a direct posterior view with 5 to 10 degrees of angulation usually shows the anatomy accurately. At the level of the transverse processes of L5 and L4, an oblique view (5 to 15 degrees) is usually necessary to show the most mediad aspect of the transverse process. Sometimes craniad or caudad movement of the fluoroscopy tube is necessary to sharpen the image of the edge of the transverse process, especially to avoid superimposed osteophytes that can block the correct view (Fig. 169–9).

The RF cannulas should lie parallel to the nerve to be lesioned whenever possible. Because the length of the lesion corresponds to the length of the bare metal tip exposed, a larger portion of the nerve is lesioned when the cannula is placed parallel to the nerve.

After the cannulas have been placed, it is wise to check the electrical impedance, which is usually between 300 Ω and 700 Ω when the cannulas are positioned correctly. Checking the impedance is a good method for measuring the overall integrity of the RF system. After the impedance has been checked, a lateral view further confirms correct placement of the cannulas, with the tips posterior to the respective foramina. The next step involves electrical stimulation at 50 Hz. Stimulation in the paravertebral and hip areas should be noted when the medial branches are stimulated at this frequency. Strong stimulation should be noted at less than 1 V at 50 Hz when the cannula is in correct alignment with the facet joint nerve. Next, stimulation is performed at 2 Hz, and lower extremity motor fasciculations should be absent at 2.5 V. Multifidus muscle stimulation usually is noted at the 2-Hz point. After confirmation of correct placement with fluoroscopy and stimulation, 1 mL of 2% lidocaine is injected through each of the cannulas. After allowing 30 seconds to pass, lesions are created at a temperature of 80°C applied for 60 seconds. After the lesions are completed, the cannulas are removed and sterile bandages are placed at the puncture sites.

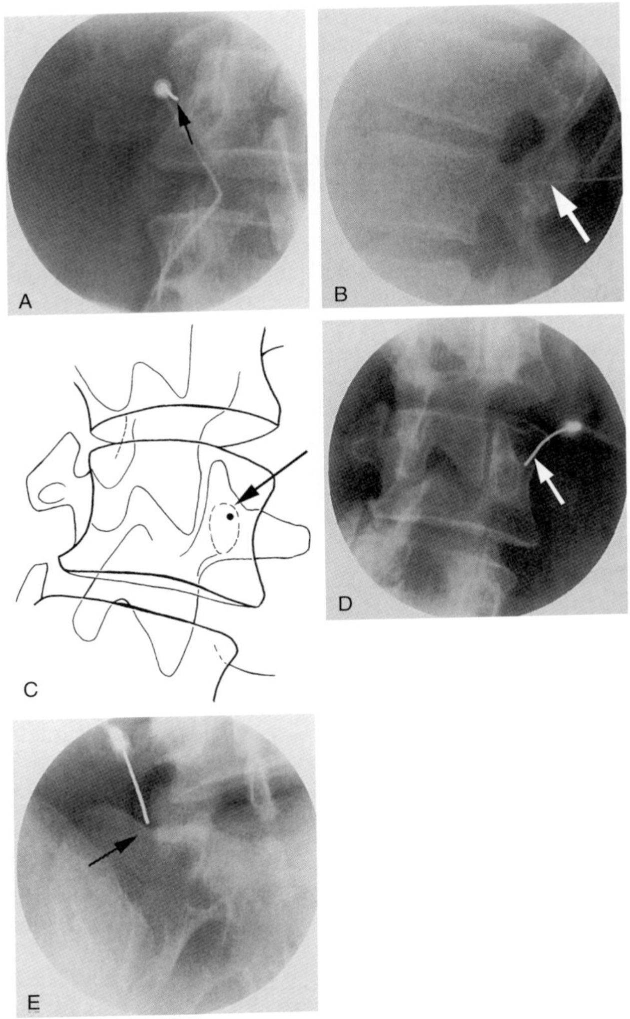

FIGURE 169–9 ■ Lumbar facet joint rhizotomy. **A,** Posteroanterior view of lumbar medial branch lesion. **B,** Lateral view of lumbar medial branch lesion. **C,** Lumbar medial branch target point, oblique view. **D,** Lumbar medial branch target point, oblique view. **E,** Lesion point for L5 dorsal ramus. (From Waldman SD: Interventional Pain Management, 2nd ed. Philadelphia, WB Saunders, 2001, p 251.)

The risks of the lumbar facet rhizotomy include numbness and weakness in the lower extremities, although long-term sensory or motor deficits are rare. Accurate stimulation during the operative procedure prevents nerve root injury. Occasionally, patients develop mild dysesthesia or short-term motor and sensory changes; this is unusual, however, and most patients have no complications involving neurologic changes.

Some patients notice motor extremity weakness immediately after the procedure, which is usually due to extravasation of local anesthetic onto the main nerve root during the procedure. This phenomenon usually resolves within 1 to 2 hours postoperatively. Most patients are fit to go home 2 hours after the procedure. Patients can expect to have 1 to 2 weeks of perioperative discomfort—pain in the paravertebral regions and the upper buttock. Hip pain can be bothersome after this procedure. It usually begins on postoperative day 3 and can last 10 days. If the pain is severe enough, appropriate analgesics and a short course of oral steroids can be helpful. The cause of the hip pain is unclear, but might be related to spasm of the quadratus lumborum.

It is important to bear in mind that mechanical low back pain frequently is associated with multiple pain generators. More than one facet joint can be involved, or the problem may involve disks and facets. A careful physical examination is crucial to explore for signs of combined involvement of any of the previously mentioned pain generators.

Functional Stereotactic Identification of Symptomatic Levels and Subsequent Radiofrequency Lesioning

As advances are made in the techniques of lesion-specific therapies for chronic pain, the opportunity to ascertain definitively, in real time, the relative contribution of any purported and identifiable pain generator becomes extremely attractive. A functional stereotactic approach, in which electrode proximity to the target nerve tissue may be assessed objectively with patient-blinded sensory or motor stimulation, has broad application in percutaneous RF techniques. Maximizing the proximity of the electrode to the target nerve tissue increases the likelihood that a therapeutic lesion would encompass the structures that are causing symptoms.

Sensory and motor stereotaxy guides several RF procedures currently performed (most notably dorsal root ganglion partial rhizotomy, gasserian rhizotomy, and sphenopalatine ganglionolysis), but may be applied to virtually any RF procedure currently performed. The adoption of a functional stereotactic approach minimizes the risk that "innocent" structures would be lesioned and may give the physician a more objective assessment of the relative contributions of any particular pain generator to the patient's overall pain picture. Sensory stereotaxy also may be used to confirm clinical suspicions that a given structure may or may not be involved in the primary pain complaint.

We recommend that the functional RF lesioning procedure be guided by precise fluoroscopic imaging in conjunction with a sound functional stereotactic approach. Functional stereotaxy has become invaluable in determining the symptomatic levels of involvement in facet-related pain and ganglion rhizotomy and reliably reproduces sympathetic ganglion-mediated and splanchnic pain. If concordant symptoms are not reproduced with low-voltage sensory stimulation, either the electrode is positioned improperly or the target structure is not involved in the patient's symptom complex. In either of these cases, no lesioning should be performed. With few exceptions, patients undergoing functional stereotactic RF procedures should be *awake. Minimal supplemental reversible analgesic medication* (e.g., alfentanil, fentanyl) may be administered judiciously, but only when absolutely required. Any alteration in the patient's ability to differentiate responses to stereotactic stimulation can compromise the efficacy and safety of the procedure.

Example 1

If facet joint pain is suspected on the basis of a careful history and physical examination, confirmation of the clinical diagnosis is mandatory before RF denervation is considered. Despite the most carefully performed physical examination, the presence of other active lumbar pain generators may confound definitive diagnosis that relies on clinical examination findings alone. Selective medial branch or intra-articular facet joint injections are invaluable in determining the *presumptive* levels of facet involvement and in identifying the relative contribution of facet-related pain to the patient's overall pain picture. The use of corticosteroid medications (e.g., triamcinolone, concentration 4 to 8 mg/mL) in conjunction with small (diagnostic) doses of local anesthesia (0.5 to 0.7 mL total volume) may prolong the benefit experienced by the patient (and, in a reasonable percentage of patients, be sufficiently therapeutic as to provide long-term relief), and a reproducible response with high-grade improvement of pain must be documented before consideration of RF denervation.

Despite the most carefully performed physical examination and meticulous injection technique, however, the precise distribution of medial branch–mediated pain is impossible to determine by diagnostic injection alone. If the patient's pain is dramatically or completely reduced after diagnostic or confirmatory local anesthetic or steroid injection, the physician can only surmise that an adequate number of levels has been injected, without knowing if asymptomatic levels also have been injected.

Using sensory stereotaxy during the RF facet denervation procedure ensures that only—and all—symptomatic levels are denervated and avoids unnecessary lesioning of asymptomatic levels. Because the medial branch of the posterior primary rami provides primary facet capsular sensory innervation (along with segmental ipsilateral multifidus motor innervation), sensory stereotaxy may be used to verify proximity of the RF electrode to the symptom-producing nerves, maximizing the likelihood that the target nerve would lie within the 45°C isotherm, or "kill zone," of the lesion.

When the electrodes have been placed in the approximate location of the medial branch nerves under fluoroscopic guidance, precise final electrode positioning may be guided by the patient's subjective and objective responses to low-voltage sensory stimulation. Low-voltage sensory stimulation between 0.2 and 0.5 V (1 msec pulse duration, frequency 50 Hz) should reproduce concordant pain, in conjunction with simultaneous segmental ipsilateral multifidus contraction. Stimulation of nonsymptomatic levels would produce segmental multifidus contraction *without* reproducing concordant pain, generally described by patients as a sensation of light paresthesia, or "tightness," in the back and areas of sensory referral.

Before RF denervation is undertaken, attempts should be made to reproduce selectively concordant pain at the lowest stimulation voltage possible (0.15 to 0.3 V). This correlates with proximity of the electrode to the target nerve, which maximizes the likelihood of successful denervation. No radiating paresthesias should be experienced in the distribution of the anatomically related spinal nerve root. Stimulation should be performed with the patient blinded, to eliminate observational bias.

Example 2

Sensory stereotaxy may play a vital role in the diagnosis of complex pain problems. In the case of a 29-year-old woman with a history of iatrogenic chronic celiac plexopathy secondary to pancreatic duct outlet obstruction after an exploratory laparotomy, an alcohol celiac plexus block was performed at another institution. After the lytic block, the patient had intractable diarrhea and had been managed by another practitioner with steroid and local anesthetic celiac plexus blocks. After 9 months, the local anesthetic/steroid injections were no longer effective, and the patient was referred to one of the authors (W.Y.) for further evaluation and management. A stereotactic RF splanchnic denervation procedure was performed, which reduced the patient's symptoms approximately 50%. The patient still required a significant opioid analgesic supplement. Stereotactic thoracic sympathetic stimulation subsequently was performed. Findings were significant thoracic sympathetic involvement and reproduction of concordant pain with bilateral sympathetic ganglionic stimulation to T8. Stereotaxy-guided RF lesions were created over the symptomatic sympathetic ganglia, and the patient remained completely pain-free for 9 weeks (i.e., she needed no prescription or over-the-counter analgesics). The patient's pain began to return 10 weeks after the RF procedure. The patient was referred for bilateral surgical thoracoscopic sympathectomy at T8-12. The patient experienced complete pain relief after surgical sympathectomy and remained completely pain-free and without medication for more than 2 years.

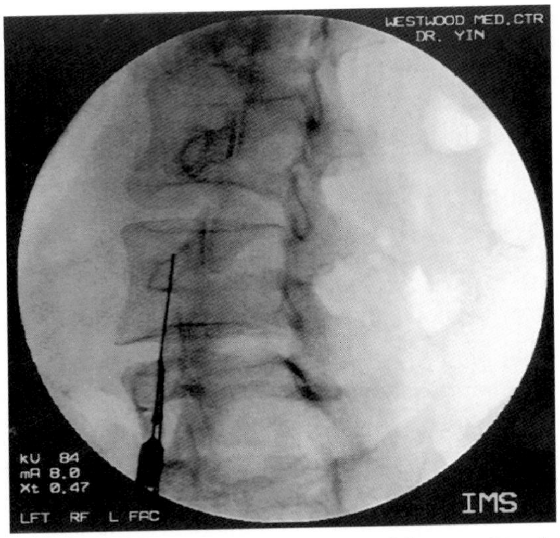

FIGURE 169–10 ■ Oblique images of caudal posterolateral lumbar medial branch RF denervation. Note electrodes overlapping Burton's point at L3 and L4. (From Waldman SD: Interventional Pain Management, 2nd ed. Philadelphia, WB Saunders, 2001, p 253.)

Caudal Approach to Lumbar Medial Branch Denervation

To maximize the success of any RF procedure, every effort must be made to place the active tip of the electrode as close to the target nerve as possible. The effective size of the nerve lesion also is increased if the cannula is placed as nearly parallel to the nerve as possible. Commercially available blunt-tipped RF cannulas (Radionics, Inc, Burlington, Mass) combined with a slight curve (10 to 15 degrees) involving the active distal tip have augmented the safety and technical efficacy of many RF procedures. For many lumbar facet denervation procedures, especially in larger patients or patients who have undergone previous surgical interventions, 20-gauge, 100-mm long blunt, curved-tip RF cannulas with a 10-mm active tip may be used to great effect. These 20-gauge cannulas produce quantitatively larger thermal lesions than 22-gauge electrodes, the diameter of the lesion being roughly related to the square of the radius of the electrode and linearly related to the length of the active tip.

The caudal approach using a blunt-tipped electrode differs from the posterolateral approach in several ways. The patient is positioned in the prone position, and anteroposterior fluoroscopic images are obtained to identify lumbar levels. The caudal posterior oblique approach may be used for the lumbar medial branches of T12-L5 because it most closely parallels the course of the medial branch nerve as it wraps around the superomedial aspect of the transverse process beneath the mammilloaccessory ligament before it divides into separate articular branches. Any given lumbar medial branch crosses over the superomedial aspect of the transverse process of the next level *below* (i.e., the L2 medial branch would be found crossing over the superomedial aspect of the L3 transverse process). Posterior oblique fluoroscopic projections are obtained (30 to 40 degrees) to identify the junction of the superomedial aspect of the transverse process with the superior articulating process (Burton's point), and the skin is marked over this radiographic landmark. The electrode entry sites for the caudal posterior oblique approach start at the skin markings *one level below* each respective level. The entry sites are anesthetized with a small volume of local anesthetic, and short (1¼-inch), 16-gauge intravenous cannulas are placed through the skin and subcutaneous fascia to facilitate passage of the blunt-tipped electrodes.

The electrodes are advanced in a posterolateral and cephalad approach toward Burton's point one level above the skin entry site under posterior oblique fluoroscopic guidance (Fig. 169–10). When bone contact is made with the transverse process, the cannula tip is rotated to overlie the superomedial aspect of the transverse process under anteroposterior fluoroscopic imaging (Fig. 169–11). Lateral images are taken to verify that the cannula tips do not approach the intervertebral neural foraminal apertures (Fig. 169–12).

The caudal approach to the L5 posterior primary ramus differs from the approach to T12-L4, in that it is a posterior parasagittal approach (the iliac wing obstructs a posterolateral approach). Under anteroposterior fluoroscopic imaging, the superomedial aspect of the sacral ala (which corresponds developmentally to the transverse process of S1) is identified, and a skin entry site is marked and anesthetized approximately 2 to 3 cm caudad. The blunt-tipped electrode is advanced toward the superomedial aspect of the sacral ala, the tip of the electrode overlapping this structure as it is at other levels (Fig. 169–13).

Sensory stereotactic localization of the medial branch nerves is performed (as described earlier). No segmental multifidus contraction is generally observed on stimulation of the L5 posterior primary ramus. Before RF denervation, 1 mL of 2% lidocaine is injected, and thermal lesioning is performed (at 80°C to 85°C for 60 seconds).

Thoracic Facet Joint Pain

Thoracic facet joint pain also can be treated with RF neurotomy. The course of the medial branch differs from that in the lumbar region, but the technique can be similar. Detailed

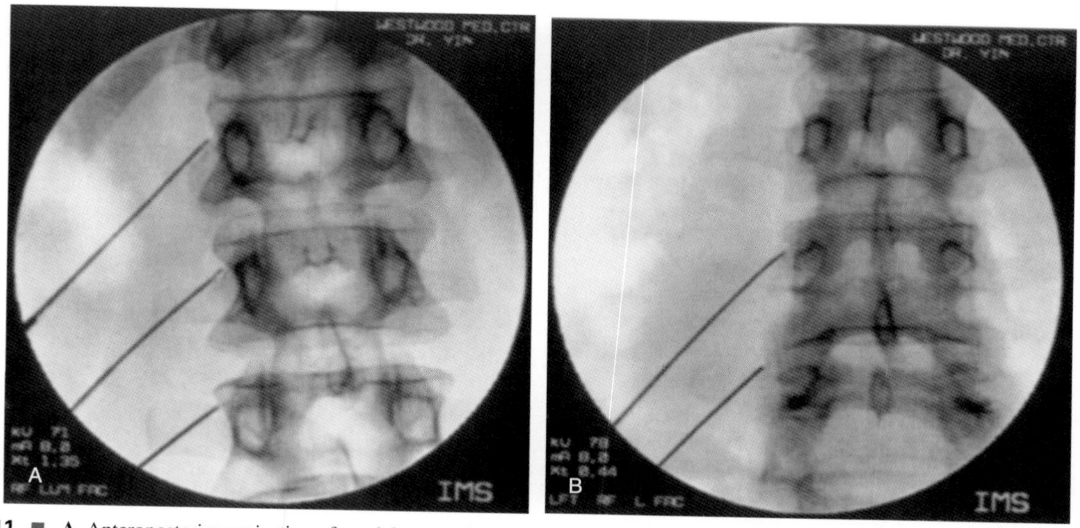

FIGURE 169–11 ■ **A,** Anteroposterior projection of caudal posterolateral lumbar medial branch RF denervation using curved blunt electrode, left T12, L1, and L2 medial branch nerves. **B,** Anteroposterior projection of caudal posterolateral lumbar medial branch RF denervation, left L3 and L4 medial branch nerves. (From Waldman SD: Interventional Pain Management, 2nd ed. Philadelphia, WB Saunders, 2001, p 253.)

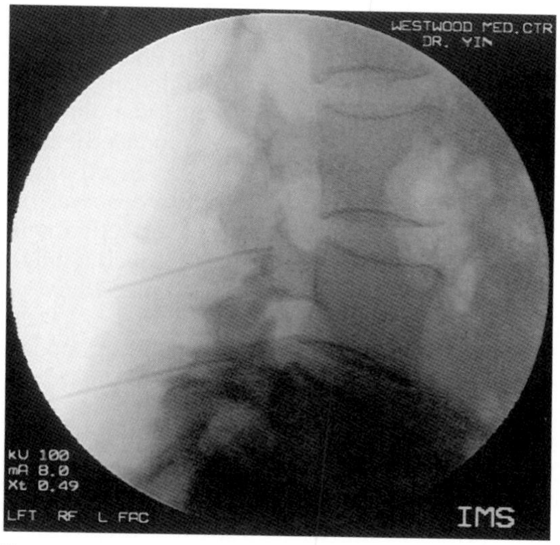

FIGURE 169–12 ■ Lateral radiograph of caudal posterolateral lumbar facet RF denervation using curved blunt electrodes, L4 medial branch and L5 posterior primary ramus. Note electrode tip position relative to intervertebral neural foramina. (From Waldman SD: Interventional Pain Management, 2nd ed. Philadelphia, WB Saunders, 2001, p 254.)

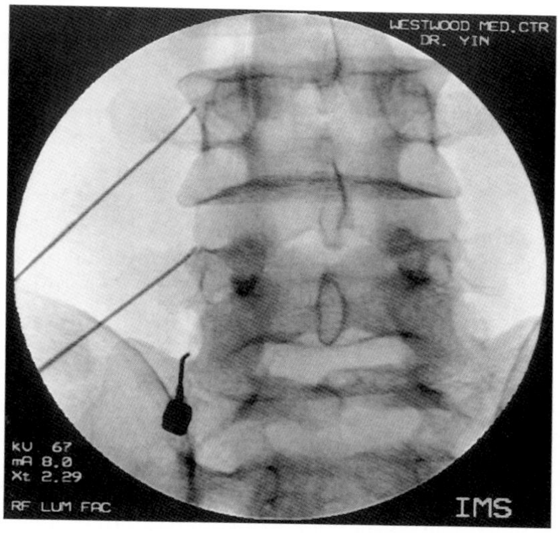

FIGURE 169–13 ■ Anteroposterior radiograph of caudal posterolateral lumbar medial branch RF denervation of left L3, L4, and left L5 posterior primary ramus. (From Waldman SD: Interventional Pain Management, 2nd ed. Philadelphia, WB Saunders, 2001, p 254.)

dissections of the medial branches of the dorsal rami were performed by Chua.[79,85] The typical courses of the medial branches in the upper (T1-4) and lower thoracic levels (T9-10) exited the intertransverse space in a mediolateral direction, crossing the superolateral corners of the transverse process at their inflection point. From the inflection point, the nerve moved mediad and downward across the posterior surface of the transverse process. Exceptions were noted at the midthoracic levels (T5-8), where the nerve follows a parallel course, but at times is displaced superiorly and may not contact the inflection point of the transverse process. At the T11-12 levels, the nerve follows a course analogous to that of the lumbar region. Stimulation can be achieved at the inflection point and at the more traditional "medial position" described for the lumbar medial branches. Good results have been noted after RF lesioning in either position, which indicates that the fibers of the medial branch may find their way back to the superomedial position, as it crosses medially from the inflection point.[79,80,85] The fluoroscopy tube may need to be angled craniad or caudad to show separation of the transverse process from its associated rib. If the medial approach is chosen, the facet rhizotomy in the thoracic region is similar to that of the lumbar region. Otherwise, the nerve can be lesioned at the inflection point. Among other potential complications in the thoracic region is a small risk of pneumothorax (Fig. 169–14).

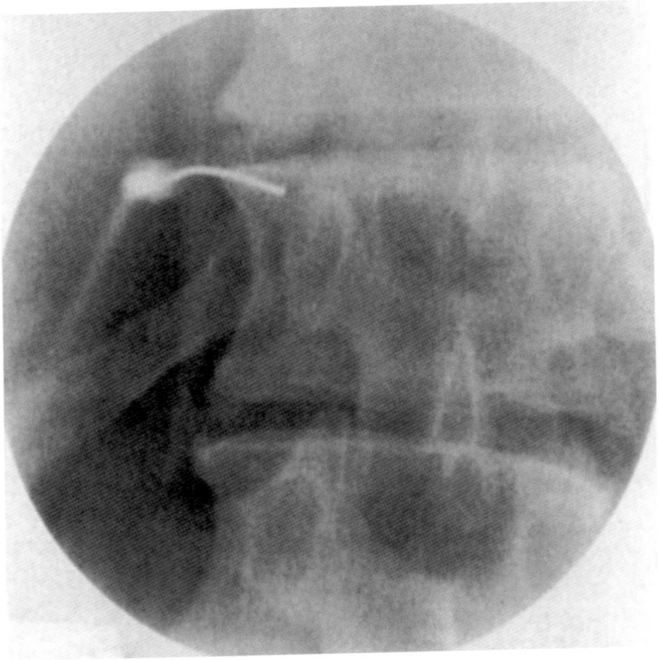

FIGURE 169–14 ■ Posterior view of a thoracic facet RF rhizotomy procedure shows the correct cannula position for a lesion of the T11 facet joint nerve. (From Waldman SD: Interventional Pain Management, 2nd ed. Philadelphia, WB Saunders, 2001, p 254.)

Sacroiliac Joint Pain

Biomechanical analysis reveals the principal function of the sacroiliac joint complex to be stress reduction, as opposed to active movement.[81] The deep and superficial sacroiliac joint ligaments serve a vital function in maintaining the integrity of the joint complex, binding the sacrum to the ilia. Unusual stress on the ligaments because of abnormalities in axial loading may result in the development of chronic sacroiliac joint complex pain.

The sacroiliac joint can produce symptoms similar to facet joint abnormalities. Pain emanating from the sacroiliac joint usually causes buttock pain and referred mechanical symptoms. Areas of referral include the hip, groin, anterior thigh, and calf. Examination usually detects distinct tenderness over the middle and lower sacroiliac joint. Compression tests are frequently painful, and distraction tests often reveal poor joint mobility. Patients with sacroiliac joint pain frequently report that their pain is at its worst when they first arise in the morning and abates over the next several hours. Typically, sacroiliac joint pain is exacerbated with prolonged sitting or standing, is relieved with lumbosacral flexion, and is accompanied by findings of reproducible tenderness directly over the posterior ligamentous structures. Details of the examination of a painful sacroiliac joint have been reviewed in the literature.[82] The clinical suspicion of sacroiliac joint intra-articular or ligament pain may be confirmed by differential, fluoroscopically guided interosseous ligament or intra-articular injection of local anesthetic, with or without steroid. The reported prevalence of sacroiliac joint pain (15%)[83] may underestimate the true prevalence in the population with chronic back pain.[84] Overlapping patterns of referred mechanical or somatic pain of diskogenic origin (especially in the L4-5 and L5-S1 intervertebral disks) further confound the clinical diagnosis.

The sensory innervation of the sacroiliac joint complex remains to be described definitively. The need to distinguish posterior from anterior sacroiliac pain and intra-articular pain from ligamentous pain further complicates the issue. Approximately 50% to 60% of patients with intractable posterior ligamentous or intra-articular pain experience prolonged high-grade relief from sensory stereotactic sacral posterior primary ramus rhizotomy.

Rhizotomy of the Sacroiliac Joint

The patient is placed in the prone position on the fluoroscopy table. The fluoroscopy unit is angled in so that the lines of the posterior aspects of the joint are seen. The tube is angled caudad and obliquely from the side opposite the joint to be lesioned; that is, an oblique view at 15 to 20 degrees from the opposite side of the body is used to visualize the posterior joint lines correctly.

One technique used to denervate the sacroiliac joint involves the formation of bipolar lesions using two electrode systems, the first being the active electrode and the second being a ground system. Bipolar electrode wires can be obtained from the manufacturer of the RF generator so that the second cannula can attach directly to the ground plug. Lesioning can be performed between points A and B to produce a linear lesion. As long as the distance between the two cannulas does not exceed five times the diameter of an individual cannula, a linear lesion is produced between the two electrodes. Multiple linear lesions can be produced along the entire length of the sacroiliac joint to denervate the posterior aspect of the joint and its capsule effectively. Because the bipolar method produces multiple, overlapping, linear lesions, stimulation before lesioning is unnecessary with this technique (Fig. 169–15).

The clinician is able to anesthetize the skin, subcutaneous tissues, and joint before performing the procedure. This rhizotomy technique is almost painless. Usually, 15 to 20 connecting linear lesions are produced along the posterior sacroiliac joint. Each bipolar lesion is created at a temperature of 80°C for 60 seconds (using two cannulas, each 150 mm long with 10-mm active tips). It is important to ensure that the lesions overlap slightly so that a complete linear lesion is produced along the entire posterior joint line. As one moves farther craniad, the cannula's entry must be farther mediad to be positioned beneath the posterior iliac crest.

The S2 level contributes much to the innervation of the sacroiliac joint. An S2 ganglionotomy can be an important adjunct to the sacroiliac joint rhizotomy (if the S2 analgesic test block gives good relief). Some patients have residual buttock, referred posterior thigh, or hip pain after sacroiliac joint rhizotomy, and if the S2 test block temporarily relieves the residual pain, an S2 ganglionotomy often ameliorates the residual symptoms. Patients usually experience 2 weeks of buttock discomfort after sacroiliac joint rhizotomy. Patchy decreased skin sensation in the buttock is seen sometimes, and it usually resolves in 2 to 6 weeks.

Sacroiliac Joint Stereotactic Posterior Primary Ramus Rhizotomy

The stereotactic sacroiliac denervation procedure differs from the bipolar technique in that individual posterior primary rami

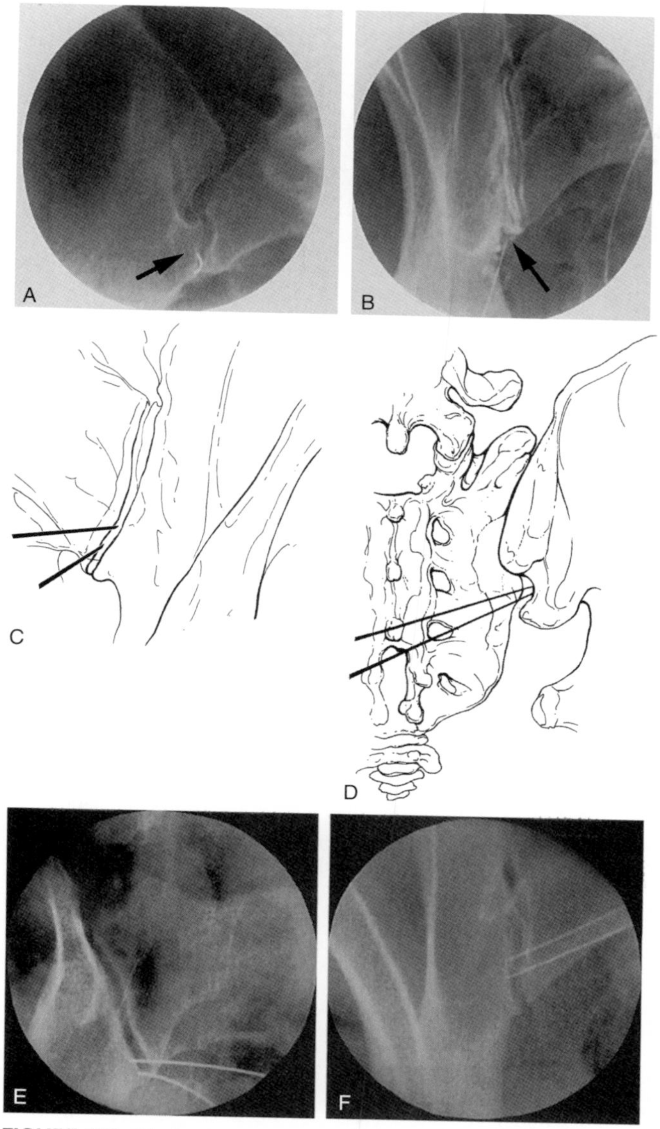

FIGURE 169–15 ■ **A,** Radiograph shows the needle position *(arrow)* for entry into the posteroinferior aspect of the sacroiliac joint. **B,** Arthrogram of the sacroiliac joint; note the needle entry into the inferior aspect of the joint *(arrow)*. **C** and **D,** Drawing of two RF cannulas in parallel alignment for a bipolar lesion at the posteroinferior aspect of the sacroiliac joint. **E** and **F,** Radiographs show the RF cannula positions for bipolar lesions at the inferoposterior aspect of the sacroiliac joint. (**A**, **B**, **E**, and **F** from Waldman SD: Interventional Pain Management, 2nd ed. Philadelphia, WB Saunders, 2001, p 255.)

are localized near their decussation at the level of the dorsal sacral foraminal apertures. Reproduction of concordant pain guides the rhizotomy procedure. The preferred technique uses a 20-gauge, 100-mm blunt-tipped, 10-mm active tip, curved-tip RF electrode.

As with the bipolar technique, the patient is placed prone on the fluoroscopy table. The fluoroscopy unit is angled so that the sacrum is seen en face (i.e., the L5-S1 disk space is seen "crisply"), the objectives being maximal visualization of the lateral border of the dorsal foraminal apertures of S1 and S2 and clear delineation of the superomedial aspect of the sacral ala. A skin entry site is marked and anesthetized over

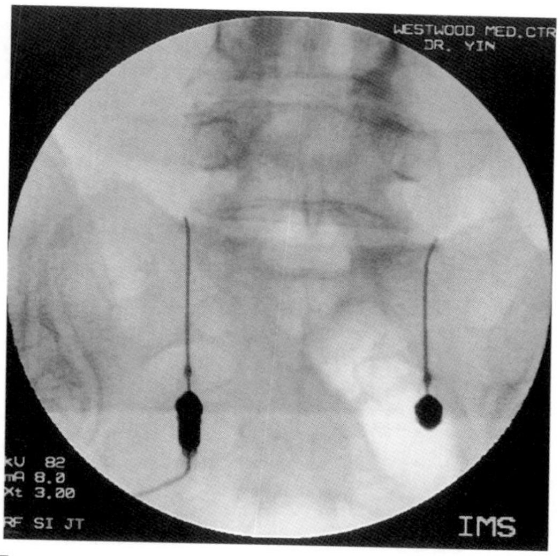

FIGURE 169–16 ■ Anteroposterior image illustrates electrode placement for bilateral L5 posterior primary ramus stereotactic lesion for sacroiliac joint denervation. (From Waldman SD: Interventional Pain Management, 2nd ed. Philadelphia, WB Saunders, 2001, p 256.)

the approximate position of the second sacral dorsal foraminal aperture, and a $1\frac{1}{4}$-inch, 16-gauge intravenous catheter is inserted to facilitate placement of the blunt-tipped electrode. Through this single skin entry site, the electrode may be serially repositioned to approach the posterior primary rami of L5, S1, S2, and, if necessary, S3.

Under anteroposterior fluoroscopic guidance, the electrode is introduced through the intravenous catheter and directed craniad, toward the superomedial aspect of the ipsilateral sacra ala. The electrode tip is rotated to overlap slightly the cranial and dorsal aspect of the sacral ala, and sensory stereotactic localization of the L5 posterior primary ramus is performed as described previously. In contrast to L5 posterior primary ramus denervation of the L5-S1 lumbar facet joint, the sensory branch innervating the proximal sacroiliac joint may lie 0.5 to 1.5 cm lateral to the most medial aspect of the sacral ala. The electrode is repositioned until the sacral contribution of the L5 posterior primary ramus is identified. If concordant pain is elicited with sensory stimulation, the electrode is gently manipulated until the minimum patient-blinded sensory stimulation voltage is obtained; ideally, this should be in the 0.2- to 0.3-V range (Fig. 169–16). Care is taken during the sacral posterior rhizotomy procedure to ensure that the elicited stimulation covers only the areas of concordant pain; unintentional lesioning of closely related cutaneous branches often leads to the discomfort of postrhizotomy dysesthesias, cutaneous hyperalgesia, or numbness. The elicitation of paresthesia covering areas of pain, but not reproducing concordant pain, indicates localization of asymptomatic sensory branches at the anatomic level examined. Only branches that cause symptoms should be denervated.

After the localization of any symptomatic branch has been confirmed with patient-blinded sensory stimulation, motor stimulation should be performed at 2 Hz at 0.8 to 1 V to minimize the likelihood that nearby motor branches to the gluteal musculature would be involved in the RF lesion. Before an RF lesion is generated, 1 mL of 2% lidocaine should be injected through the RF cannula to provide

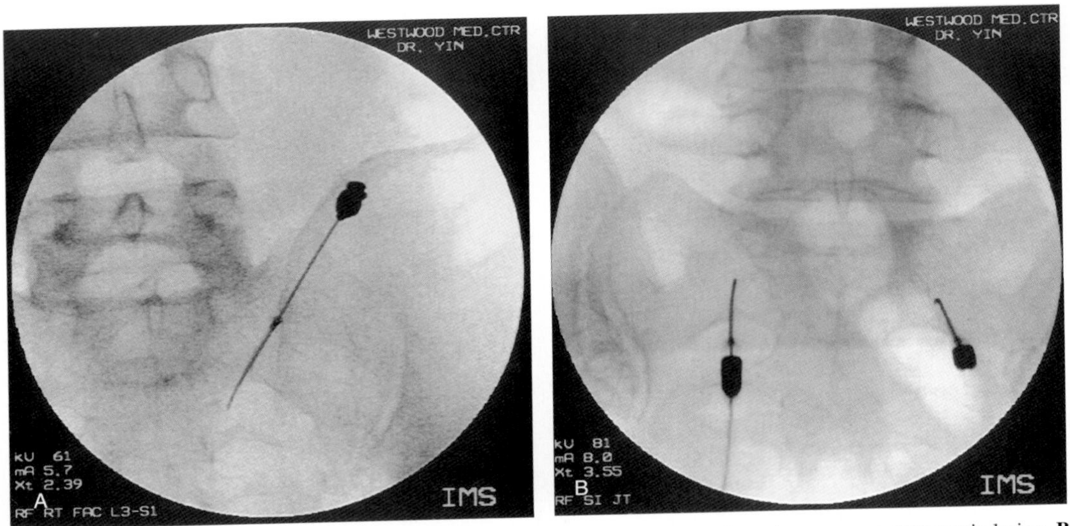

FIGURE 169–17 ■ **A,** Anteroposterior image illustrates position of electrode for right S1 posterior primary ramus stereotactic lesion. **B,** Anteroposterior image of different positions of S1 posterior primary ramus determined by sensory stereotaxy in bilateral sacroiliac joint denervation. (From Waldman SD: Interventional Pain Management, 2nd ed. Philadelphia, WB Saunders, 2001, p 257.)

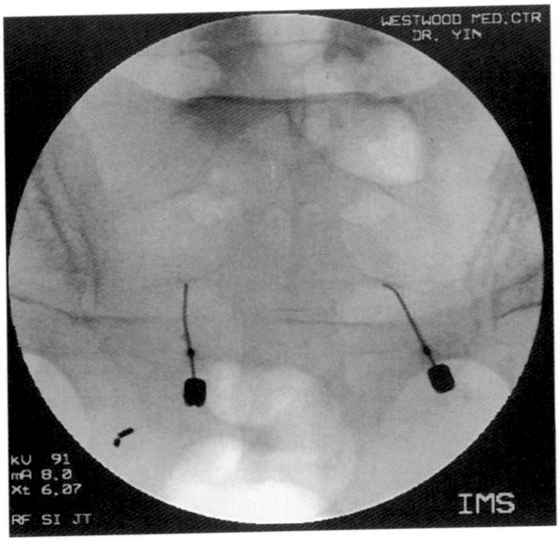

FIGURE 169–18 ■ Anteroposterior radiograph illustrates bilateral electrode placement for S2 posterior primary ramus stereotactic lesion. (From Waldman SD: Interventional Pain Management, 2nd ed. Philadelphia, WB Saunders, 2001, p 257.)

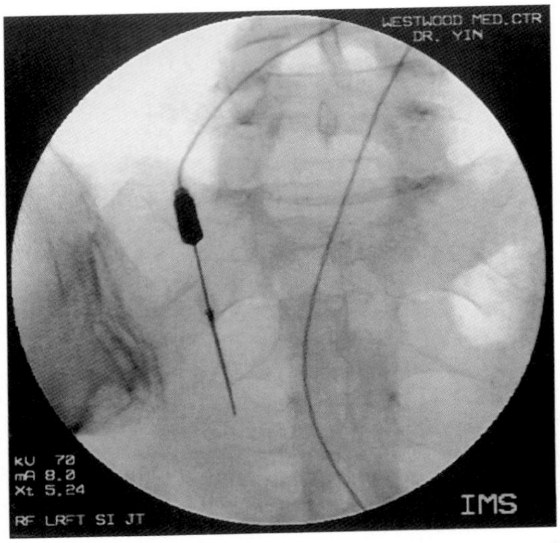

FIGURE 169–19 ■ Anteroposterior radiograph illustrates electrode placement for S3 posterior primary ramus stereotactic lesion. (From Waldman SD: Interventional Pain Management, 2nd ed. Philadelphia, WB Saunders, 2001, p 257.)

adequate local anesthesia during the lesioning process. Typically, RF lesioning applies 80°C to 85°C for 60 seconds.

The sensory branches at the levels of S1 (Fig. 169–17), S2 (Fig. 169–18), and S3 (Fig. 169–19) are approached in the following fashion. Under anteroposterior fluoroscopic imaging, the lateral aspect of the dorsal sacral foraminal apertures is visualized. Occasionally, slight oblique projections with craniad angulation of the imaging system may be required to visualize these faint structures. Initially, the blunt-tipped RF cannulas should be placed along the lateral aspect of the dorsal sacral foraminal aperture of interest, with the tip of the electrode just barely sliding into the foramen itself. Sensory stereotactic localization of the posterior primary rami branches innervating the posterior sacroiliac structures is performed, the tip of the electrode being manipulated along the lateral arc of the dorsal sacral foraminal aperture until regional paresthesias are elicited or concordant pain is reproduced. The electrode is manipulated further until the sensory stimulation voltage required to reproduce concordant pain is at its minimum (0.2 to 0.4 V).

The stimulation is performed with the patient blinded, to eliminate bias. Motor stimulation is kept within the range of 0.8 to 1 V to ensure that no motor branches to the gluteal musculature would be involved in the lesion. The electrode *must not* rest within the dorsal foraminal apertures proper, lest unintentional lesioning of the sacral nerve roots or branches to the perineal, genital, or perianal regions results. When performing bilateral procedures, the location of symptomatic posterior primary rami branches often is not symmetric, a finding that has been implicated in the wide variety of referred somatic pain patterns that accompany sacroiliac joint pain.[86] The posterior primary rami branches of S2 and S3 are similarly examined. Of patients with symptomatic sacroiliac joint complex pain, 90% to 100% have identifiable symptomatic L5 and S1 posterior primary rami contributions. Approximately 60% to 70% have an identifiable contribution from S2, and approximately 30% to 40% have a significant S3 contribution.

Lumbar Diskogenic Pain

Diskogenic pain can occur in the absence of disk herniation or even obvious disk injury. Internal disruptions of a disk can appear entirely normal when studied by imaging methods.[87-89] Electromyography studies frequently do not provide any specific diagnosis for an internally disrupted disk. Patients with an internally disrupted disk can present with low back pain and referred lower extremity symptoms and may have normal findings on neurologic examination. Patients with lumbar diskogenic pain frequently have a painful and biphasic deflexion maneuver, and the sitting, straight leg raising examination produces low back pain. Sometimes, the only way to identify a diskogenic pain syndrome accurately is with diagnostic disk injections. The sources of innervation within the disk anulus include the sinuvertebral nerves, branches of the lumbar ventral rami, the gray ramus communicans, and branches of the sympathetic chain. The gray ramus communicans (ramus communicans nerve) is a target for RF lesions. RF lesions of the ramus communicans nerve are particularly useful for treating pain emanating from the anterior and lateral aspects of the disk anulus.

Currently, RF techniques developed for the treatment of lumbar diskogenic pain include RF lesions of the ramus communicans nerves and intradiscal RF lesions.[37,90] More recently, intradiscal electrothermal (IDET) annuloplasty has been developed as a specific means for treating lumbar diskogenic pain.

Lesioning of the Ramus Communicans Nerve

Anatomic studies suggest that the ramus communicans nerve sends fibers to more than one level. If diskography has shown that the L4-5 disk is the painful level, lesions of the ramus communicans nerves should be performed at L4 and L5.

The patient first is placed prone on the fluoroscopy table. The newer "curved-blunt" RF cannula should be considered for this procedure. It allows easier and more precise placement with less chance for trauma to the segmental nerves. Electrodes 150 mm long with 10-mm active tips are used. Alternatively, 22-gauge, 150-mm SMK electrodes with 5-mm active tips may be used if the blunt electrodes are unavailable. The patient is monitored and given intravenous sedation, but is kept awake enough to provide accurate verbal responses during the stimulation portion of the procedure.

At each level to be lesioned, the fluoroscopy unit should be directed craniad or caudad so that the disk is clearly visualized. The end plates of the disk and the vertebral body should be clearly visualized. Oblique angulation at 15 to 25 degrees is used so that the body of the vertebra just covers the lateral tip of the transverse process. The ramus communicans nerve tends to run at the lower third of the vertebral body.

The skin and subcutaneous tissues overlying the entry points are anesthetized with 0.5% lidocaine. The RF cannula is introduced parallel to the fluoroscopy beam and is advanced until the periosteum at the lower third of the vertebral body is contacted. At this point, a lateral fluoroscopic view is taken, and the cannula is advanced until it is halfway between the anterior and posterior borders of the vertebral body. Direct contact with the periosteum should be maintained at all times. When the cannula is properly positioned, electrical stimulation is applied; proper stimulation of the ramus communicans nerve produces a deep aching sensation in the back with 50-Hz stimulation at 1 V. Stimulation with 2 Hz at 2.5 V should fail to produce lower extremity motor stimulation. If motor stimulation is seen, the tip of the RF cannula is too close to the lumbar nerve roots. A lesion should not be produced when the cannula tip is in such a position. The cannula should be moved slightly craniad, caudad, anteriorly, or posteriorly, until stimulation of the ramus communicans nerve can be done without stimulating the motor portion of the lumbar nerves. This usually requires only a small change in position. A 1-mL dose of 2% lidocaine is passed through the RF cannula, and a 60-second delay is allowed for it to take effect. A thermal lesion is created for 60 seconds at 80°C. Lesions at the L4 and L5 ramus communicans nerves are made in similar fashion. Angulation of the fluoroscopy tube differs according to what level is being lesioned. The same theory applies at all levels, however. If the diskogenic pain is unilateral, the ramus communicans lesions should be made only on the symptomatic side. If the pain is bilateral, ramus communicans lesions need to be made on both sides.

Lumbar Disk Procedure

Because the nerves within the disk anulus serve as the messengers for the pain signal leaving the disk, interruption of these fibers can lessen the symptoms of diskogenic pain. Selective provocational or analgesic diskography is crucial for accurate diagnosis of lumbar diskogenic pain. Diskography must be done as a staging procedure before lesioning of the ramus communicans or the RF lumbar disk procedure. The RF lumbar disk procedure calls for the placement of a 150-mm cannula with a 10-mm active tip into the nucleus of the affected disk. A 6-minute 85°C lesion is performed.

The patient is given preoperative antibiotics as prophylaxis against disk infection. The patient is placed prone on the fluoroscopy table, and the fluoroscopy unit is angled at 15 to 20 degrees from an oblique approach to image the painful disk correctly. The skin and subcutaneous tissues are anesthetized with lidocaine, and the RF cannula is advanced in a percutaneous manner until it contacts the disk anulus (just lateral to the inferior aspect of the superior articulating process). The cannula is passed into the disk and advanced until it enters the central aspect of the nucleus as seen by posteroanterior and lateral views. Electrical stimulation is checked at 2 Hz. If lower extremity motor fasciculations are negative at 2.5 V, it is safe to perform the lesion. No intradiscal local anesthetic is used. Reproduction of pain usually is noted, but does not begin until 90 seconds has passed. It peaks between 3 and 4 minutes of the lesion process. Thermal equilibrium for this lesion requires at least 4 minutes, in contrast to other types of RF lesions (Fig. 169–20).[91]

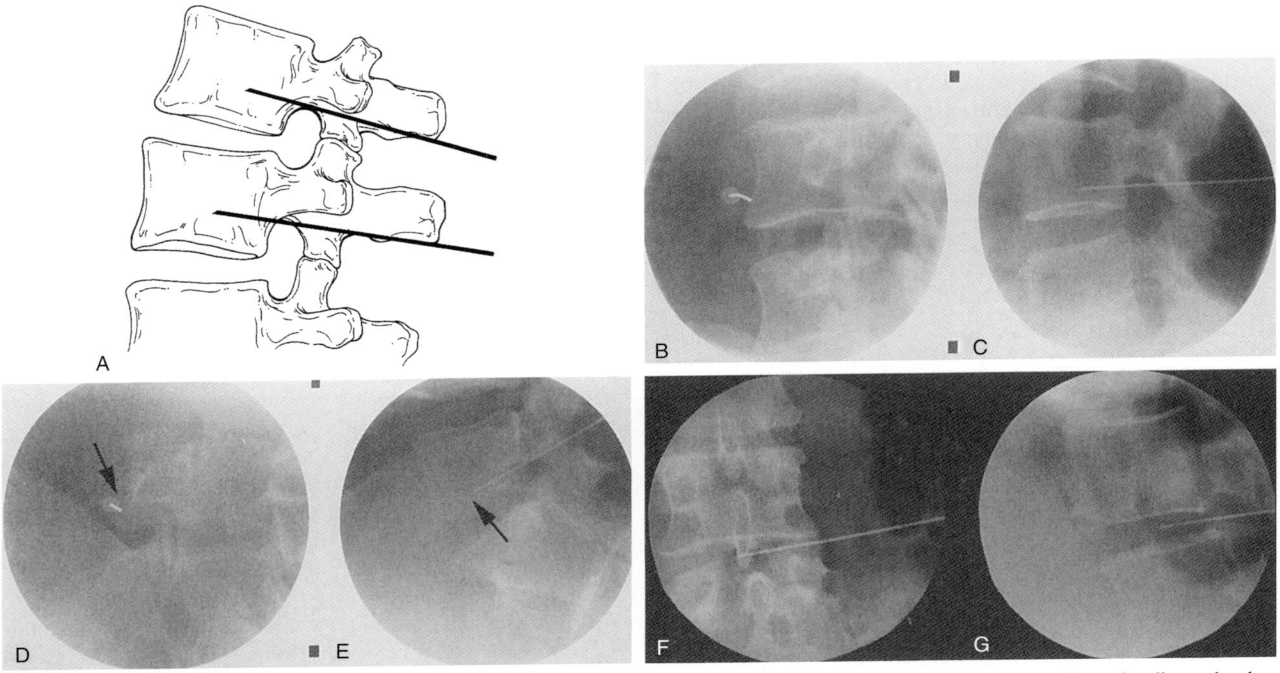

FIGURE 169–20 ■ **A,** Drawing of the cannula positions for lesions of the ramus communicans nerves. **B** and **C,** Oblique and lateral radiographs show RF cannula position for lesioning of the L4 ramus communicans nerve. **D** and **E,** Oblique and lateral views show the RF cannula position *(arrows)* for lesioning the L5 ramus communicans nerve. **F** and **G,** Posteroanterior and lateral radiographs show the RF cannula position for an intradiskal RF lesion. (**B-G** from Waldman SD: Interventional Pain Management, 2nd ed. Philadelphia, WB Saunders, 2001, p 259.)

Sequelae and Complications

Patients tend to have postoperative pain for 1 to 2 weeks after RF lesioning of the ramus communicans nerve or intradiskal RF lesioning. It is not unusual to develop mild dysesthesias that last 7 to 10 days. Most such dysesthesias resolve without complication within 3 weeks. In most patients, 2 to 4 weeks must pass before the full efficacy of the procedure can be determined.

Risks of the procedure include injury to the lumbar nerve roots with sensory or motor changes. The intradiscal RF lesion has the potential complication of postoperative disk infection; use of prophylactic antibiotics is recommended. Occasionally, patients have significant postoperative pain and dysesthesias, and when disk space infection has been ruled out, a 5- to 7-day course of oral steroid therapy is required. Disk infection is uncommon, but strict aseptic technique, including surgical scrub before the surgical skin preparation, plus preoperative antibiotic therapy, should be part of any intradiscal procedure.

Intradiskal Electrothermal Annuloplasty

A novel application of RF technology has been developed specifically for lumbar intradiskal lesioning. This system (SpineCATH Intradiscal Catheter; Oratec Interventions, Menlo Park, Calif) differs significantly from existing intradiscal RF technologies. The length of the active lesioning thermocouple is nearly 6 cm, and the diameter is nearly 18 gauge. The system does not rely on ionic heating of the surrounding tissue; RF energy is used to generate heat through a resistive coil, heating an insulating coating covering the thermocouple. Transfer of heat to surrounding tissue occurs through conduction rather than ionic heating. This mechanism of tissue heating is fundamentally different from traditional RF lesioning, in which the electrode actually absorbs heat from the surrounding tissue. The heat lesion is controlled through a feedback bimetal thermistor at the end of the thermocouple. The thermocouple also is flexible and to a certain extent "steerable" within the nucleus of the disk. The thermocouple is introduced into the disk through an introducer needle, which is not insulated. The advantages of this system over a rigid electrode include a significantly larger thermal lesion (the combination of larger thermocouple radius and length), the ability to direct the flexible thermocouple over a relatively large portion of the nuclear-annular boundary, and more consistent transannular heating.[32] Conductive intradiskal thermal lesioning also may be less dependent on the homogeneity of disk nuclear water content.

The Oratec SpineCATH system also differs fundamentally from traditional RF methods in that it has been designed for the single purpose of intradiskal heating. No sensory or motor stimulation is possible because the system is internally grounded. The impedance measured by the system (120 to 200 Ω) is independent of surrounding tissue properties and is used to verify the electrical integrity of the resistive coil and surrounding insulation. The SpineCATH may be used only with an Oratec lesion generator and is not cross-compatible with other RF generators.

Mechanism of Action

In vitro and in vivo studies have shown that outer annular temperatures of 40°C to 45°C can be produced with the

SpineCATH system. This temperature range should be sufficient to denervate annular nociceptive fibers, although permanent cell death may not follow axonal injury. Exposure of collagen to temperatures between 60°C and 75°C results in disruption of intermolecular hydrogen bonds; this finding has been correlated with demonstrable shrinking of collagen molecules on electron microscopy. Intradiskal heating has been shown in vitro to result in a 7% reduction in overall disk volume, although no in vivo studies have validated a long-term reduction in disk volume after IDET annuloplasty.

Theoretically, reduction in chronic diskogenic pain by IDET annuloplasty may result from thermal denervation of annular nociceptive fibers (including chemically sensitized fibers), thermal remodeling of annular collagen, and possibly reduction in disk volume. The precise mechanism of action is unclear, however. Maximum reduction in pain after IDET annuloplasty may not occur until 3 to 4 months after the procedure. A combination of varied physiologic processes in response to intradiscal thermal injury is most likely involved, including the inflammatory, proliferative, and fibrotic phases of normal wound healing.

Efficacy

Several clinical studies examining IDET annuloplasty have shown promising results in patients with diskogenic pain without radiculopathy. As with other interventional or surgical procedures, proper patient selection seems to be crucial for success, in conjunction with a methodical, prolonged, graduated, postprocedure home-based rehabilitation and back exercise program. Patients with preserved intradiskal height seem more likely to benefit than patients with severe degenerative disease, and patients with previously operated disks and diskogenic pain in levels adjacent to previous fusion may have poorer prognoses.[92] In one controlled study, 32 of 36 patients reported improvement in pain after IDET annuloplasty. Significant mean reductions in Visual Analog Scale pain scores were reported in this group (8/10 to 2.7/10), with concomitant reductions in supplemental opioid analgesic requirements and improvements in disability scores compared with conservative care.[93] Long-term follow-up studies are in progress, and the duration of benefit in early-phase long-term follow-up studies is promising.[94] For patients with diskogenic pain without radiculopathy, IDET annuloplasty may represent an attractive, less invasive alternative to lumbar diskectomy and fusion.

Lumbar Lesioning

The patient is placed in the prone position on the fluoroscopy table. The back is prepared with antiseptic solution as for diskography; it is recommended that a formal surgical preparation be performed. Preoperative antibiotics may be administered intravenously. The patient may be lightly sedated, but must be easily aroused, responsive to voice, and able to report pain during the procedure. The physician dons a sterile gown and gloves, and meticulous aseptic technique is observed throughout.

Posterior lateral oblique fluoroscopic images are obtained, and the target disk is identified. Oblique projections, with cephalad angulation as required, are obtained so that the lateral border of the superior articular process overlaps the middle of the target disk in anteroposterior and lateral dimensions (35 to 50 degrees), and the inferior and superior end plates of the adjoining vertebral bodies are distinct. A skin entry site is marked over the lateral aspect of the superior articular process overlying the target disk and anesthetized with buffered lidocaine. A 1¼-inch, 14-gauge intravenous catheter introduced through the skin and Scarpa's fascia greatly facilitates the subsequent introduction of the styleted SpineCATH 17-gauge introducer needle and preserves a modified two-needle approach to the disk. Before the 17-gauge needle is introduced, a 5-inch, 22-gauge spinal needle may be used to inject a small amount (0.5 mL) of lidocaine over the sensitive periosteum of the superior articular process.

The 17-gauge introducer needle may be gently curved to facilitate steering, although this may be necessary only at the L5-S1 level in most patients. The introducer needle is advanced through the 14-gauge intravenous catheter under posterior oblique fluoroscopic guidance toward the lateral aspect of the superior articular process overlapping the target disk. Care is taken to remain close to the lateral aspect of the superior articular process, medial to the ipsilateral exiting nerve root at that level (Fig. 169–21). The disk is entered along its posterolateral margin, and the needle is advanced slightly ventrally. In contrast to diskography, the ideal introducer needle position is not in the center of the disk. The introducer needle should lie in the posterolateral quadrant of the disk, ipsilateral to the annular entry site (Fig. 169–22). Multiplanar fluoroscopic images are taken throughout the needle insertion process. The bevel of the introducer needle is turned toward the center of the disk, and the stylet is removed. The SpineCATH heating element is introduced through the introducer needle; placing a gentle curve in the catheter may facilitate intradiskal placement along the nuclear-annular boundary. A small volume of local anesthetic with antibiotic may be injected into the nucleus of the disk before placing the heating element (e.g., 0.5 mL of 0.5% bupivacaine with 4 to 30 mg/mL of cefazolin).

Under anteroposterior and lateral fluoroscopic imaging, the heating element is directed carefully across the midline of

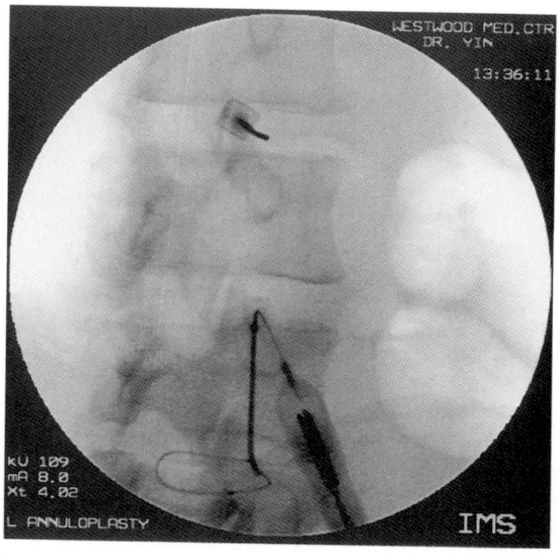

FIGURE 169–21 ■ Oblique radiograph shows intradiskal placement of introducer needle in L2-3 disk. Note presence of SpineCATH in L4-5 disk, ready for intradiskal lesion. (From Waldman SD: Interventional Pain Management, 2nd ed. Philadelphia, WB Saunders, 2001, p 260.)

the disk and around the periphery of the posterior lateral and posterior inner anulus (Fig. 169–23). Care is taken to ensure that the heating element does not penetrate the disk anulus; extradiskal positioning of the element may result in thermal lesioning or other injury to the spinal cord or nerve roots, with catastrophic consequences. In severely disrupted disks, the heating element may be passed through the anulus without significant resistance, underscoring the importance of obtaining frequent multiplanar fluoroscopic views during catheter advancement (Fig. 169–24A). Ideally positioned, the active portion of the heating element spans the posterolateral disk from pedicle to pedicle (Fig. 169–24B).

When proper placement of the intradiskal heating element has been verified with multiplanar fluoroscopy, the radiopaque markers denoting the length of the active tip of the heating element should span the target lesion zone, ideally from pedicle to pedicle. Incomplete coverage of the posterior disk anulus has prompted some clinicians to advocate a bilateral approach with a second lesion performed if necessary. Repositioning of the catheter has been associated with kinking of the catheter and with damage to its insulation; either situation requires that the catheter be removed and replaced. Before heat lesioning, the proximal portion of the active heating element must *not* be in contact with the distal end of the introducer needle.

When the SpineCATH is acceptably positioned, and correct system impedance and thermistor function are verified, intradiskal heating is performed. Temperature guidelines

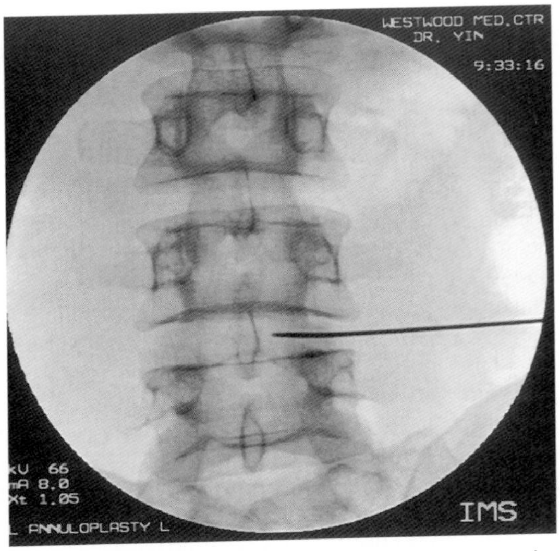

FIGURE 169–22 ■ Anteroposterior radiograph shows introducer needle placed in superolateral quadrant of L4-5 disk. (From Waldman SD: Interventional Pain Management, 2nd ed. Philadelphia, WB Saunders, 2001, p 260.)

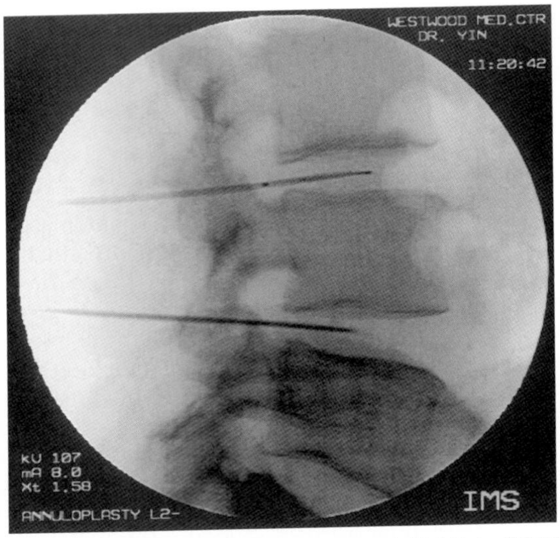

FIGURE 169–23 ■ Lateral radiograph shows initial SpineCATH insertion. Proximal heating element marker is visible within the introducer needle. (From Waldman SD: Interventional Pain Management, 2nd ed. Philadelphia, WB Saunders, 2001, p 261.)

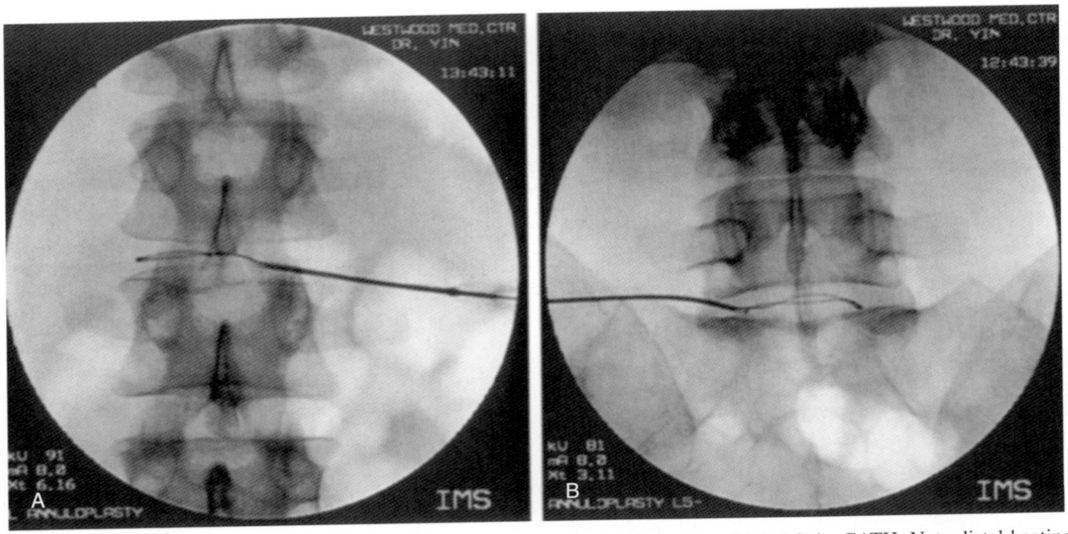

FIGURE 169–24 ■ **A,** Anteroposterior radiograph shows nearly complete intradiskal placement of L3-4 SpineCATH. Note distal heating element marker is only at midline; in its final position, the active portion of the heating element extends from pedicle to pedicle. **B,** Final positioning of SpineCATH heating element within L5-S1 disk. Note pedicle-to-pedicle placement of active element of catheter spanning the posterior nuclear-annular boundary. (From Waldman SD: Interventional Pain Management, 2nd ed. Philadelphia, WB Saunders, 2001, p 261.)

have been recommended by the manufacturer and involve incremental (1°C) increases from 65°C to 80°C or 90°C over 14 to 17 minutes. The procedure is generally tolerated well; complaints of severe back pain or lower extremity pain should prompt cessation of heating and reevaluation of catheter position and catheter integrity. Occasional complaints of leg pain, sometimes extending below the knee, may reflect referred pain of disk origin (as opposed to direct thermal stimulation of the nerve root) and have been correlated with increasing intradiskal thermal stimulation intensity.[93] Before intradiskal catheter placement, 0.5 mL of 0.5% bupivacaine may be injected through the introducer needle into the disk to enhance the patient's comfort.

Sequelae and Complications

Reported complications from IDET annuloplasty have been rare. In skilled hands, complications likely would be few, but the number of technical and infectious complications may increase as the technology is more variously applied. Many patients experience exacerbation of back pain, and some may experience radicular symptoms after IDET annuloplasty. Putatively, this pain corresponds with the inflammatory phase of thermal injury and may represent sterile diskitis. Most cases respond to activity limitations, nonsteroidal antiinflammatory drug therapy, and opioid analgesia. In the case of severe exacerbation of back or leg pain after the procedure, a careful evaluation should be done for epidural hematoma, abscess, and infectious diskitis. If no infectious cause is suspected, and no other complication is evident, intravenous or oral "pulse dose" steroid therapy may be effective. Persistent pain may be treated with lesion-specific epidural or transforaminal steroid injection.

Thoracic Lesioning

Treatment of thoracic diskogenic pain remains problematic. Results of open or thoracoscopic video-assisted thoracic diskectomy and fusion are discouraging. Intradiskal thermal lesioning may be a tantalizing, minimally invasive alternative to surgical thoracic diskectomy and fusion. Although no clinical studies have addressed the efficacy or safety of IDET annuloplasty or other intradiscal RF lesioning techniques for the treatment of thoracic diskogenic pain, a case report is presented in the hope of stimulating further research in this area.

Case Report: Thoracic Intradiscal Electrothermal Lesion for Intractable Thoracic Diskogenic Pain with Thoracic Radiculopathy (W.Y.)

A 49-year-old man with a 20-year history of intractable and progressively disabling midthoracic pain radiating to the left flank with torsional movement of the trunk had failed to derive benefit from a comprehensive array of conventional, noninterventional modalities of therapy over the past 2 decades. An exhaustive evaluation revealed no intra-abdominal or thoracic visceral abnormalities. Cardiology and gastroenterology evaluations revealed no disease. Plain films of the thoracic spine were unremarkable, and MRI of the dorsal spine revealed central and right-sided disk protrusion without extruded fragment at T7-8. Two separate sets of thoracic epidural and foraminal low-volume steroid injections provided reproducible, nearly complete (85% to 90%) relief of the patient's midthoracic and radiating flank pain, but of limited duration (3 weeks), without incremental improvement. Selective provocative thoracic diskography revealed multiple morphologic derangements of the thoracic disks at all levels from T6 to T10. Left-sided contrast extravasation through an annular tear outlining the left T6 nerve root was visualized at T6-7, but no pain was reproduced with contrast injection (peak 60 psi). The disk protrusion at T7-8 seen on MRI was not observed on diskography, and no symptoms were reproduced with intradiscal injection, although a left lateral annular tear was present with extravasation of contrast material outlining the left T7 nerve root (peak 120 psi). At T8-9, a clear posterior lateral annular tear was visualized during injection (120 peak psi), with extravasation of contrast circumferentially outlining the left-sided nerve roots of T8 and T9 (Fig. 169–25). Precise reproduction of the patient's

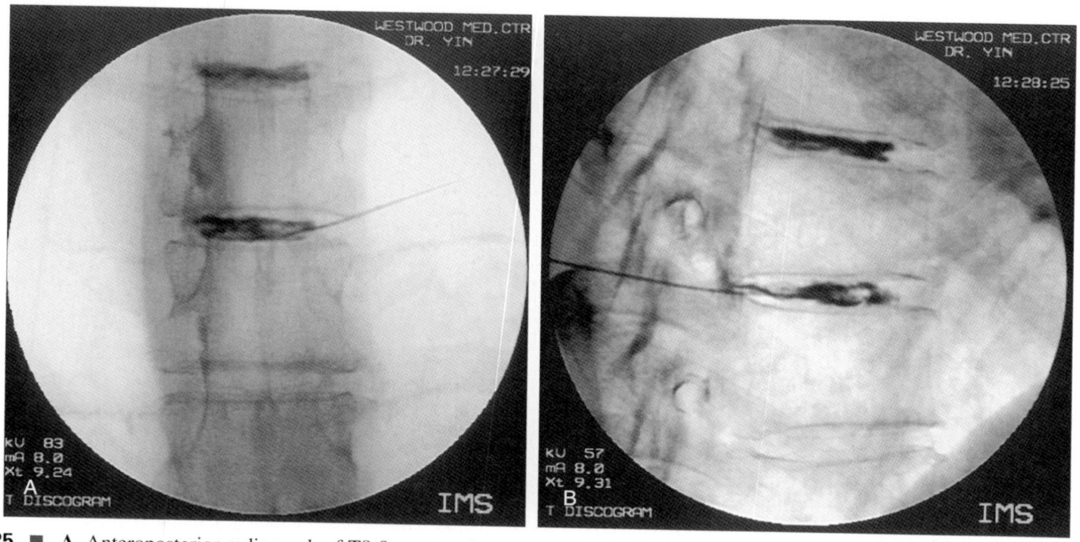

FIGURE 169–25 ■ **A,** Anteroposterior radiograph of T8-9 provocative diskography. **B,** Lateral radiographs of T8-9 provocative diskography. Note clearly visible left posterior lateral annular fissure and extravasation of contrast material outlining left T8 and T9 nerve roots and lateral epidural space. (From Waldman SD: Interventional Pain Management, 2nd ed. Philadelphia, WB Saunders, 2001, p 262.)

concordant pain was achieved despite the lack of clear disk protrusion or herniation. Epidural extravasation of contrast material through a clearly defined right posterolateral disk bulge was visualized on injection of the T9-10 disk (peak 60 psi); however, this injection did not elicit any pain.

The patient was referred for surgical consultation. After discussing the risks and potential benefits of open and thoracoscopic thoracic diskectomy and fusion with the surgeon, the patient declined surgical intervention. He continued to work full-time as the president of his own oil exploration services company.

Alternative options were discussed in detail with the patient. The possibility of performing a thoracic intradiscal annuloplasty procedure was discussed, along with the experimental nature of this particular application of the technology. A detailed discussion of the potential known and unknown risks associated with the procedure ensued. After thorough consideration of his available options, the patient elected to proceed with IDET annuloplasty at the T8-9 level.

A right-sided modified posterior parasagittal curved cannula technique was employed, and entry was gained into the target disk without pain or technical difficulty. A precurved SpineCATH catheter was inserted into the T8-9 disk without difficulty, and the active tip was oriented to cover the area of the annular tear completely. A 90°C intradiskal lesion was created without intraoperative complications (Fig. 169–26). (Owing to the smaller size of the thoracic disk, the needle was withdrawn 3 mm to gain adequate clearance from the active proximal portion of the heating element.) The patient tolerated the procedure well, had no evidence of pneumothorax or other complication on postoperative chest films, and was discharged home the same day.

On postoperative follow-up, the patient reported mild worsening of pain after the procedure. Two weeks after the procedure, he felt that his pain had been reduced approximately 50% and reported complete resolution of thoracic radicular symptoms. He complained of mild burning pain in the midback region. His subsequent recovery was unremarkable, with

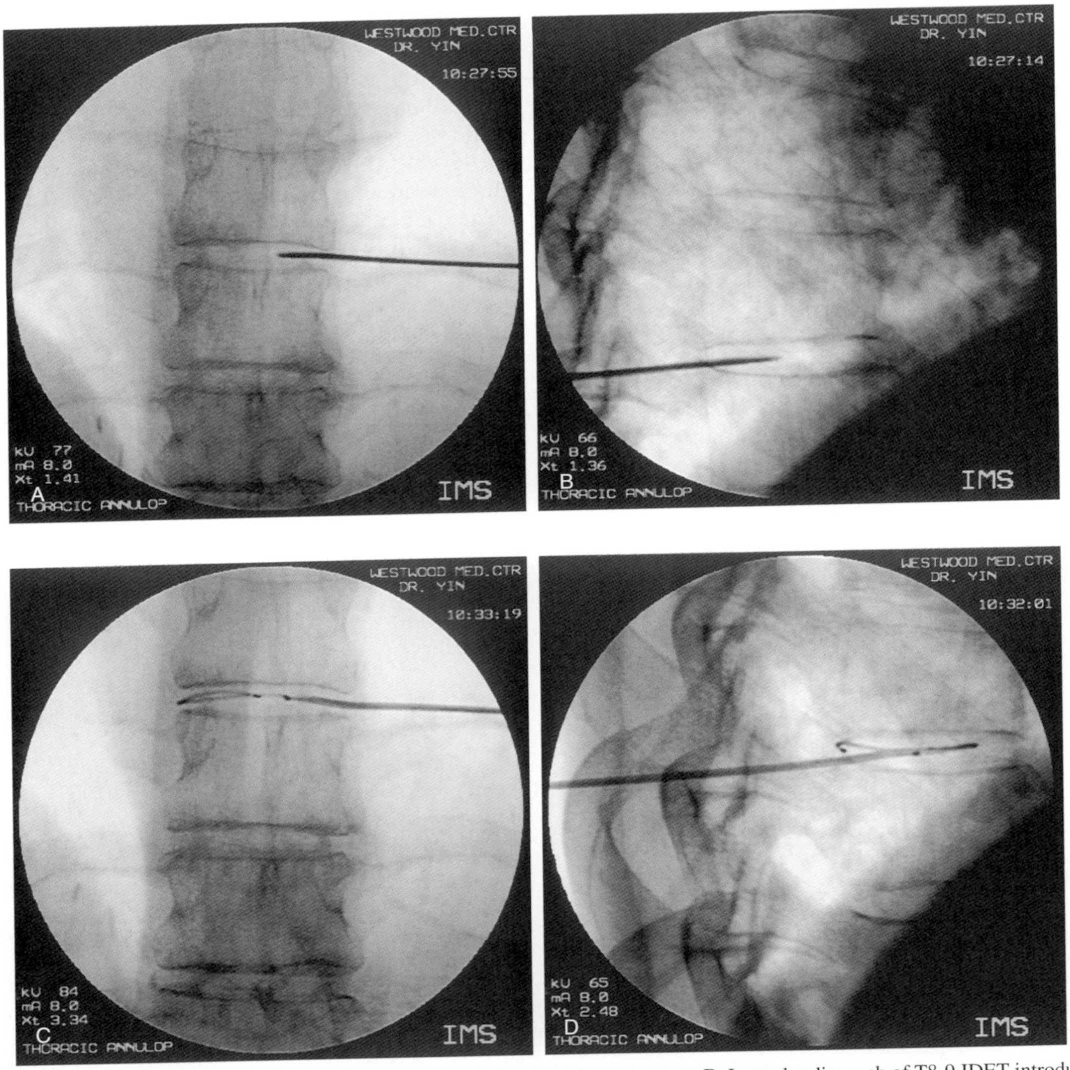

FIGURE 169–26 ■ **A,** Anteroposterior radiograph of T8-9 IDET introducer needle placement. **B,** Lateral radiograph of T8-9 IDET introducer needle placement. **C,** Anteroposterior radiograph shows SpineCATH placement for T8-9 intradiskal thermal lesion. **D,** Lateral radiograph shows final SpineCATH placement for thermal lesion of left posterior lateral T8-9 annular fissure. Introducer needle has been withdrawn 3 mm to clear proximal marker of heating electrode. (From Waldman SD: Interventional Pain Management, 2nd ed. Philadelphia, WB Saunders, 2001, p 263.)

incremental improvement reported at 6-week postprocedure follow-up. Four months after thoracic IDET annuloplasty, the patient reported greater than 75% subjective improvement in thoracic pain, with a corresponding decrease in his Visual Analog score from 8/10 to 2/10. Although not completely eliminated, the patient's back pain was markedly improved, and he was extremely pleased with the outcome.

Dorsal Root Ganglionotomy

RF dorsal root ganglion lesioning is useful for pain emanating from the lumbar spinal nerves.[33,37,38,58,95] This procedure is reserved for patients who have failed more conservative interventional treatments and for whom open surgical intervention is not an option. If prognostic blocks of the posterior column (facet joints) and the anterior column (disk) are negative, and if the pain predominantly involves the lower extremity, diagnostic sleeve blocks of the segmental nerve roots are indicated. Although disease of the segmental lumbar nerves does not cause back pain per se, injuries to the segmental nerves commonly are associated with other injuries in the lumbar spine. Back pain is usually a direct result of mechanical abnormalities of the lumbar spine, but patients commonly have combined mechanical symptoms and radiculopathy. Under these circumstances, it is important to determine whether the practitioner is dealing with a problem that represents mechanical pain with referred mechanical symptoms or lower extremity symptoms secondary to disease of the spinal nerves.

When the diagnosis of referred mechanical pain in the lower extremities has been excluded, the practitioner needs to explore the role of the segmental spinal nerves and the sympathetic nervous system. Diagnostic blocks of the spinal nerves and the sympathetic nerves must be performed to distinguish between radiculopathy and sympathetically maintained pain. The distinction is important because the treatments differ. When the appropriate diagnostic blocks have been performed, however, the practitioner is in a position to treat the segmental nerve problems with a dorsal root ganglion lesion.

Lumbar Ganglionotomy

Lumbar ganglionotomy is usually performed using a 150-mm cannula with a 5-mm active tip. The cannula is passed percutaneously toward the vertebral body (just inferior to the transverse process). As the cannula approaches the vertebral body, a lateral fluoroscopic view is taken to ensure that the foramen is clearly visualized. The cannula is directed toward the dorsal and superior quadrant of the foramen and is advanced until it passes beneath the transverse process into the superior, dorsal quadrant of the foramen. A direct posteroanterior view is taken, and the cannula is advanced until it reaches the midpoint of the respective facet joint line. A repeat lateral view is taken to ensure that the cannula still resides within the superior, dorsal quadrant of the foramen. With the cannula in this position, stimulation is performed, and satisfactory paresthesia into the leg (along the dermatome that is affected) should be noted at less than 1 V with 50-Hz stimulation. If stimulation is noted at less than 0.3 V, the cannula should be repositioned because it is too close to the ganglion, and postoperative neuritis could result. Ideal stimulation is between 0.4 V and 0.7 V at 50-Hz stimulation. Sensory stimulation should be done in increments of 0.1 V to avoid unnecessary pain. Stimulation is performed at 2 Hz. There should be a clear dissociation between motor and sensory stimulation; that is, the voltage required to see motor fasciculations in the lower extremity at 2 Hz should be at least twice the voltage that produces sensory stimulation in the lower extremity at 50 Hz. If good sensory stimulation at 50 Hz was noted at 0.5 V, motor fasciculations at 2 Hz should not be seen at voltages less than 1 V. The point of dissociation defines the position of the dorsal root ganglion. If dissociation between sensory and motor stimulation cannot be obtained, the cannula is not aligned with the dorsal root ganglion, and lesioning is not advisable.

When correct dissociation has been obtained, 1 mL of 2% lidocaine is passed onto the ganglion. A 10-minute delay is allowed for the anesthetic to work, and a thermal lesion is created at a temperature between 60°C and 65°C, depending on the stimulation threshold. The lower the stimulation threshold, the lower the temperature should be. The lesion is maintained for 60 seconds (Fig. 169–27).

Sacral Dorsal Root Ganglionotomy

After the prognostic blocks have been performed, and the painful level has been identified, the patient is brought back for a dorsal root ganglion lesion. It is useful to give the patient a bowel preparation the day before because bowel gas sometimes obscures the sacral foraminal openings. This practice is particularly useful for clinicians who are relatively new at performing these procedures.

The S1 and S2 nerves are commonly affected. The S5 ganglionotomy is useful for the treatment of chronic coccygeal pain. The S1 and S2 ganglionotomy procedures are performed in a similar fashion. The S1 technique is performed by passing a needle through the S1 foraminal opening

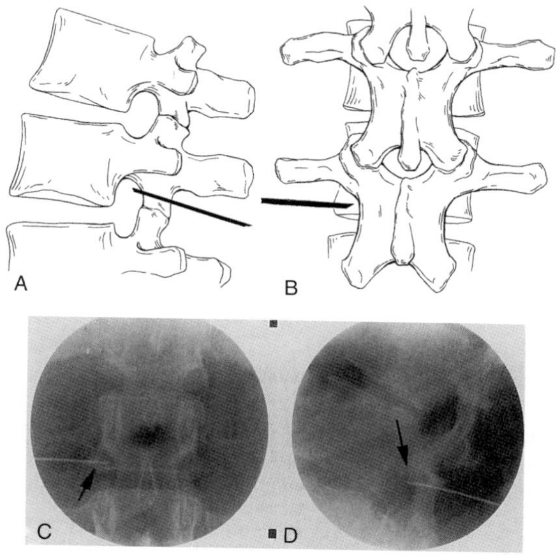

FIGURE 169–27 ■ Lumbar ganglionotomy. **A** and **B,** Lateral and posteroanterior views of the cannula position for a lumbar ganglionotomy procedure. **C** and **D,** Posteroanterior and lateral views show the RF cannula position *(arrows)* for a lumbar ganglionotomy procedure. (**B-D** from Waldman SD: Interventional Pain Management, 2nd ed. Philadelphia, WB Saunders, 2001, p 264.)

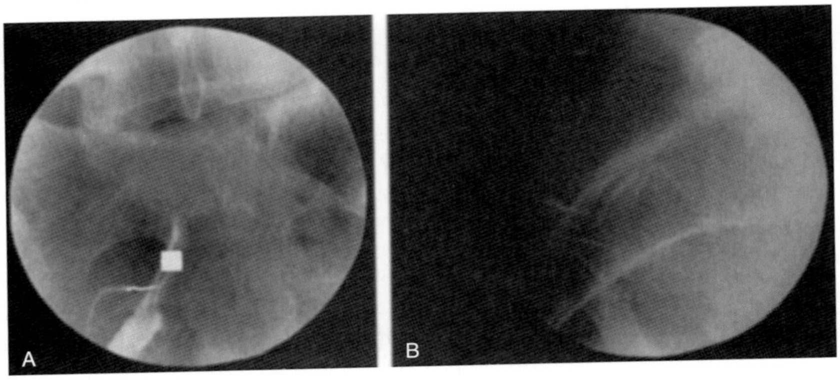

FIGURE 169–28 ■ S2 ganglionotomy procedure. **A,** Posteroanterior radiograph. The introducer cannula overlies the outline of the S2 root sleeve. The introducer cannula is seen in the middle of the root sleeve. The fine needle is the introducer needle used to inject the root sleeve with contrast material. **B,** Lateral view through the sacrum. The lower needle has been passed through the sacral foramina onto the peripheral aspect of the nerve for injection of contrast material. The upper needle is the RF cannula, which has been passed through the burr hole to rest over the S2 ganglion. (From Waldman SD: Interventional Pain Management, 2nd ed. Philadelphia, WB Saunders, 2001, p 265.)

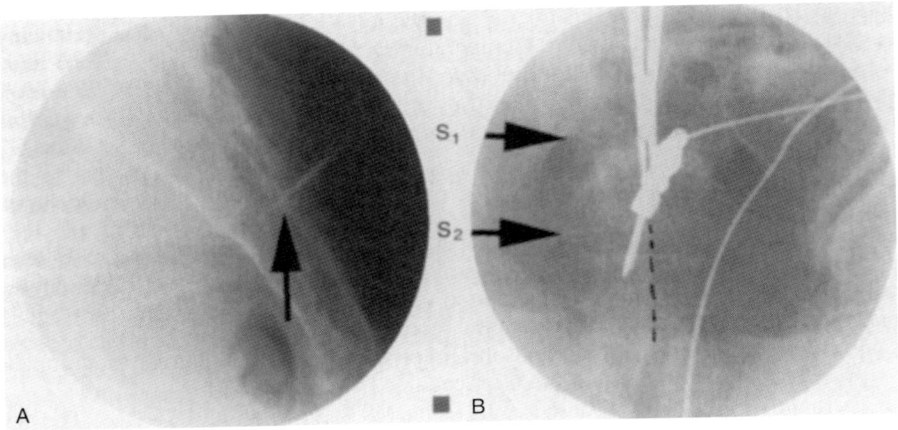

FIGURE 169–29 ■ Radiographs of S5 ganglionotomy procedure. **A,** Lateral view through the sacrum. The tip of the RF cannula *(arrow)* has been passed through the posterior aspect of the sacrum via a burr hole. **B,** Posteroanterior view. The introducer cannula is just lateral to the medial border of the sacrum *(dashed line)* and 1 cm inferior to the S2 foraminal opening. (The foramina are marked S1 and S2.) (From Waldman SD: Interventional Pain Management, 2nd ed. Philadelphia, WB Saunders, 2001, p 265.)

adjacent to the nerve. Contrast material is injected to outline the S1 root sleeve. We prefer to use Omnipaque 240 water-soluble contrast material for all procedures. A point halfway between the S1 foraminal opening and the craniad border of the sacrum, which intersects the sacral root sleeve, is chosen, and a burr hole is made through the plates of the posterior sacrum. The burr hole is created with a Kirschner wire and a small pneumatic drill.

The S2 dorsal root ganglion resides halfway between the S1 and S2 foraminal openings, where the halfway point intersects the S2 nerve. It is mandatory that an accurate outline of the respective root sleeve be seen so that the Kirschner wire can be passed through the sacrum directly over the dorsal root ganglion.

After the burr hole has been created, and the RF cannula has been passed into the sacral canal (directly over the dorsal root ganglion), stimulation can be performed. The cannula should have a 5-mm active tip. Dissociation between sensory and motor stimulation should be obtained. The stimulation and dissociation parameters are identical to the parameters described earlier for lumbar ganglionotomy. It is desirable to have good stimulation at 50 Hz between 0.4 V and 0.7 V. Lesioning temperatures are 60°C to 65°C, and the duration is 60 seconds. After lesioning, 40 mg of triamcinolone is injected through the cannula to lessen the postoperative pain (Fig. 169–28).

S5 Dorsal Root Ganglionotomy

Dorsal root ganglion lesioning of the S5 nerves can be useful in the management of coccygodynia. Coccygodynia may or may not be associated with trauma and is commonly difficult to treat. Many patients continue to experience pain even if the coccyx is removed. Because the coccyx is innervated by the S5 nerves, lesions of the S5 ganglia can be useful in treating this difficult problem. If a patient is experiencing pain on both sides of the coccyx, bilateral S5 lesions must be made. The S5 ganglion lies behind the sacrum at a level 1 cm inferior to the S2 foraminal opening, along the *midline* of the sacrum. A point approximately 1 cm caudal to the S2 foraminal opening and approximately 2 mm lateral to the midline of the sacrum is chosen as the entry site. No contrast material is used for this procedure.

The skin and subcutaneous tissues are anesthetized over the entry point. An introducer is passed through the tissues until it touches the periosteum 1 cm caudal to the S2 foraminal opening and 2 mm lateral to the midline of the sacrum. A Kirschner wire is passed through the introducer, and a burr hole is created through the posterior sacrum under direct fluoroscopic guidance. An RF cannula with a 5-mm active tip is passed through the introducer into the canal over the S5 ganglion (Fig. 169–29). Stimulation is performed, and response should be noted between 0.4 V and 1 V at 50 Hz. It should be felt *directly* in the area of the coccyx. To check for motor fasciculations, the clinician should place a finger gently in the external sphincter of the patient's anus. When motor stimulation is performed at 2 Hz, contractions of the external sphincter of the anus should not be noted at twice the sensory stimulation. If motor stimulation of the external sphincter is noted at lower thresholds, the cannula is too close to the S4 ganglion and needs to be repositioned in a more *medial* direction because the S4 ganglion is just a few millimeters lateral to the S5 ganglion. After proper dissociation between S5 and S4 stimulation has been shown, 1 mL of 2% lidocaine is passed onto the ganglion, and 5 minutes is allowed to pass. A thermal lesion is created at a temperature between 60°C and 65°C, depending on the level of stimulation. The duration of the lesion is 60 seconds. After the lesion has been created, 40 mg of triamcinolone is passed onto the lesion site. If the patient has bilateral coccygeal pain, the contralateral S5 dorsal root ganglion lesion should be performed 4 weeks later, if no complications are apparent after the initial lesion.

Curved Cannula Approach for Sacral Dorsal Root Ganglion Lesioning

A curved electrode approach toward RF sacral dorsal root ganglion lesioning may be performed as an alternative to the burr hole rhizotomy. The curved cannula technique is technically more demanding than the burr hole approach, but is particularly applicable to the S1 and S2 levels. A theoretical advantage of the curved cannula technique is that it places a relatively larger section of the active electrode (2 to 5 mm) adjacent to the target nerve tissue. The curved electrode approach also is associated with less postoperative discomfort than the burr hole approach. A more pronounced continuous curve is placed over the distal 2 to 2.5 cm of the electrode at an angle of approximately 20 to 30 degrees. The patient is placed in the prone position on the fluoroscopic table. A posterior oblique approach is made under fluoroscopic guidance through the dorsal sacral foraminal aperture, with the electrode guided along the dorsal aspect of the foramen until the tip lies over the region of the dorsal root ganglion. A high-quality contrast study is mandatory to outline the silhouette of the selected nerve root and the swelling of the dorsal root ganglion using nonionic contrast medium (e.g., iohexol, 240 mg/mL). Visualization of the dorsal root ganglion is essential to facilitate placement of the electrode adjacent to it. Sensory stereotactic stimulation at 0.15 to 0.2 V is performed until concordant pain or paresthesias are reproduced over the target somatic region. At these sensory stimulation thresholds, motor stimulation should be absent at 0.5 to 0.7 V (2 Hz, 1 msec pulse duration). It is important to maintain sensory and motor dissociation to minimize the risk of motor nerve injury.

Advances in RF generator design have permitted the delivery of RF energy with a high concentration of heat. These design modifications allow the delivery of lower temperature RF lesions while maintaining a relatively high current and voltage. The precise relationships between these variables and their effects on the ultimate clinical outcome are unclear. In our experience, the creation of lower temperature lesions for sensitive procedures, such as dorsal root ganglion and gasserian rhizotomy, seems to decrease significantly the risk of postprocedure neuritis, while preserving the desired beneficial clinical outcome.

For selective partial dorsal root ganglion rhizotomy, a high verniation lesion at a temperature of 50°C to 54°C is performed for 120 to 240 seconds. Selective sensory stereotaxy and subsequent sacral dorsal root ganglion lesioning has been invaluable for the treatment of rare intractable buttock region pain (S2) and the elimination of acetabular pain after total hip arthroplasty (S1) (Fig. 169–30).

Risks of this procedure include postoperative neuritis, motor dysfunction, and sensory loss over the superficial cutaneous distributions of the targeted nerve root. Owing to the potential for these sequelae, meticulous attention must be paid to radiologic, stereotactic stimulation, and technical parameters.

Thoracic Dorsal Root Ganglionotomy

In the thoracic region, a dorsal root ganglionotomy can be performed in a manner similar to that for the ganglionotomy technique in the lumbar region. The dorsal root ganglion in the thoracic region lies in the superior dorsal quadrant of the foramina (at a point halfway across the line of the pedicle). At the lower levels, it is possible to use an approach identical to that described for the lumbar region. The cannula position, stimulation, and lesion parameters are the same.

In the higher thoracic regions, the pleura can be injured when an oblique approach is used. In the upper thoracic

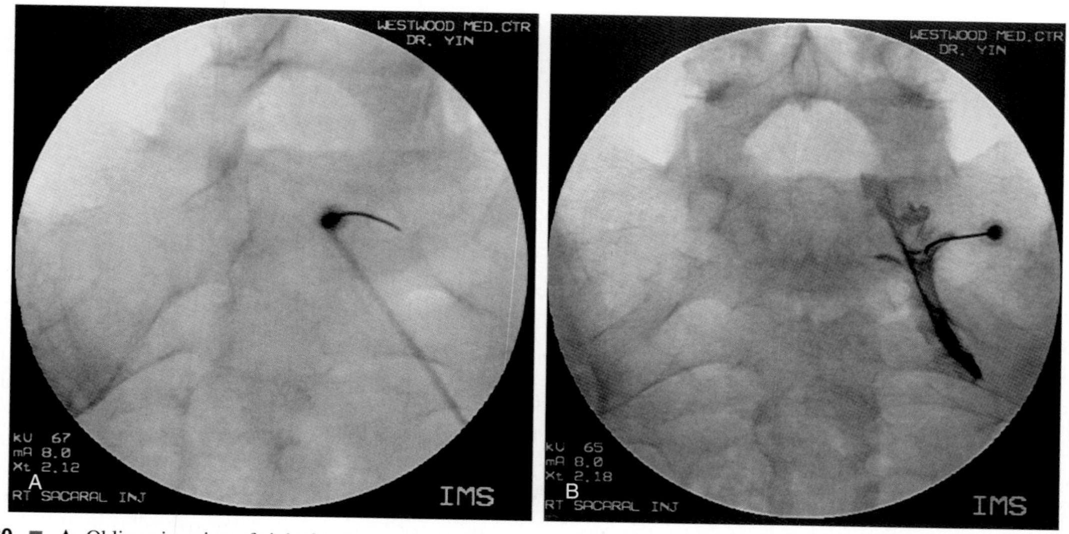

FIGURE 169–30 ■ **A,** Oblique imaging of right S1 curved electrode approach for dorsal root ganglion lesion. **B,** Right S1 contrast study outlining distal dorsal root ganglion at initiation of sensory stereotaxy. (From Waldman SD: Interventional Pain Management, 2nd ed. Philadelphia, WB Saunders, 2001, p 266.)

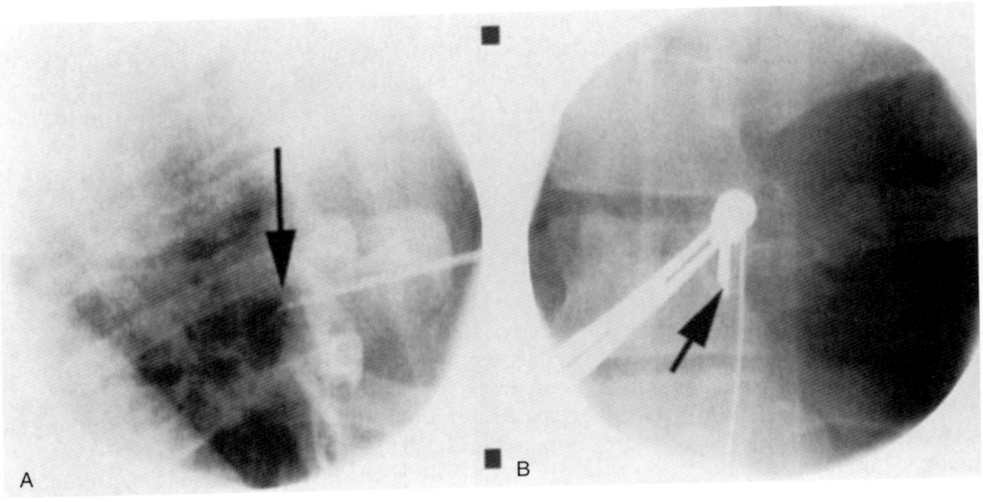

FIGURE 169–31 ■ **A,** Lateral radiograph shows cannula position *(arrow)* for a thoracic ganglionotomy. **B,** A burr hole through the thoracic lamina *(arrow)* allows the RF cannula to be passed into the thoracic foramen. (From Waldman SD: Interventional Pain Management, 2nd ed. Philadelphia, WB Saunders, 2001, p 267.)

regions, it is recommended that a burr hole be placed through the lamina at a point directly over the midpoint of the pedicle as seen on a posteroanterior view and over the dorsal and superior foramina as seen on a lateral view. Proper mediolateral orientation is rechecked with a posteroanterior view. This approach allows access through the burr hole to the dorsal and superior foraminal quadrant where the ganglion resides.

A repeat lateral fluoroscopic view is checked to ensure that the cannula lies within the superior dorsal quadrant of the foramina. An RF cannula with a 5-mm active tip is used and is passed through the burr hole into proper position. Stimulation is identical to that for the lumbar ganglionotomy procedure. When appropriate stimulation with dissociation between sensory and motor function has been obtained, the dorsal root ganglion is anesthetized, and a lesion is made in a manner identical to that described for the lumbar ganglionotomy (Fig. 169–31).

Parasagittal Approach

A modification of a posterior parasagittal curved-electrode approach may be used as an alternative to the burr hole technique for thoracic dorsal root ganglion lesioning. *Both approaches, similar to other procedures outlined in this chapter, carry significant potential for morbidity in inexperienced hands. The risks of the burr hole laminotomy approach parallel those of an open procedure performed with an operating microscope, without allowing direct visualization of relevant anatomic structures. The curved-electrode approach carries the additional potential for pneumothorax and other visceral, vascular, or neural injuries.*

For the sacral curved-electrode approach, the patient is placed in the prone position on the fluoroscopy table. A pronounced curve is placed over the distal 2 to 2.5 cm of the electrode; typically a 100-mm, 2-mm active tip SMK electrode is chosen. A skin entry site is marked approximately 2 cm lateral to the junction between the inferior medial aspect of the thoracic transverse process and the lamina of the target spinal level. Under anteroposterior fluoroscopic imaging, the electrode is advanced in such a manner that the tip contacts the lateral aspect of the lamina at its junction with the inferior

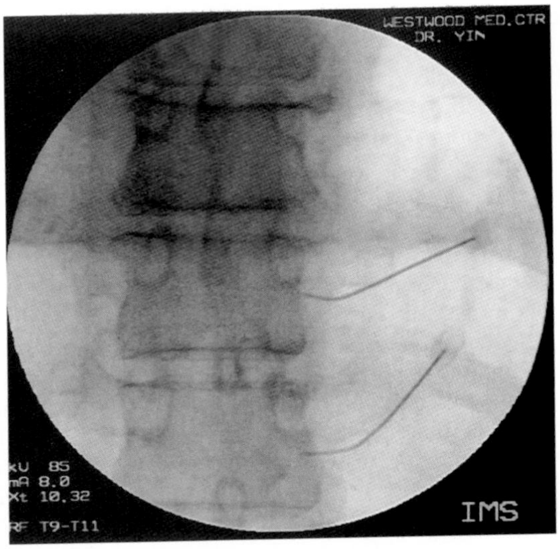

FIGURE 169–32 ■ Anteroposterior image shows posterior parasagittal curved electrode approach toward right T8 and T9 dorsal root ganglia. (From Waldman SD: Interventional Pain Management, 2nd ed. Philadelphia, WB Saunders, 2001, p 267.)

medial border of the transverse process. The electrode is advanced carefully just deep to the lateral border of the lamina, toward the region overlying the exiting thoracic nerve root, ensuring that the tip of the electrode remains dorsal to the exiting nerve root (Fig. 169–32). When the electrode has been advanced into the midsuperior dorsal aspect of the intervertebral neural foramen, a contrast study is performed to outline the exiting nerve root (Fig. 169–33). A lateral fluoroscopic image is taken to confirm proper electrode tip position (Fig. 169–34).

Sensory stereotactic localization of the dorsal root ganglion is performed using sensory stimulation at 0.15 to 0.2 V (50 Hz, 1 msec pulse duration) (Fig. 169–35). Motor dissociation is confirmed with 2-Hz stimulation at 0.5 to 0.7 V. When patient-blinded precise reproduction of concordant pain or paresthetic coverage of the desired somatic region is obtained,

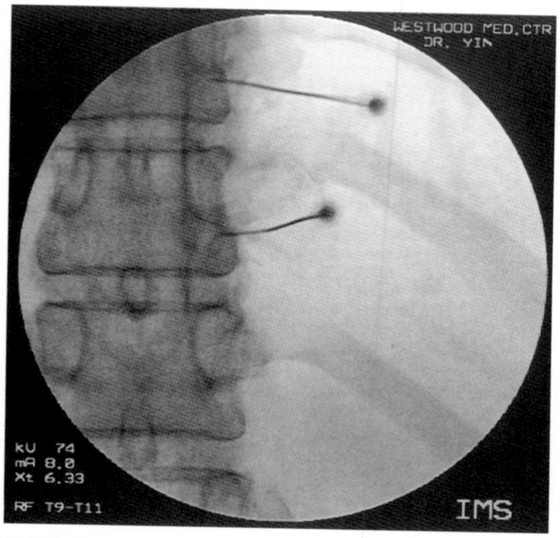

FIGURE 169–33 ■ Anteroposterior image of contrast study outlining the right thoracic dorsal root ganglion and adjacent electrode placement. (From Waldman SD: Interventional Pain Management, 2nd ed. Philadelphia, WB Saunders, 2001, p 268.)

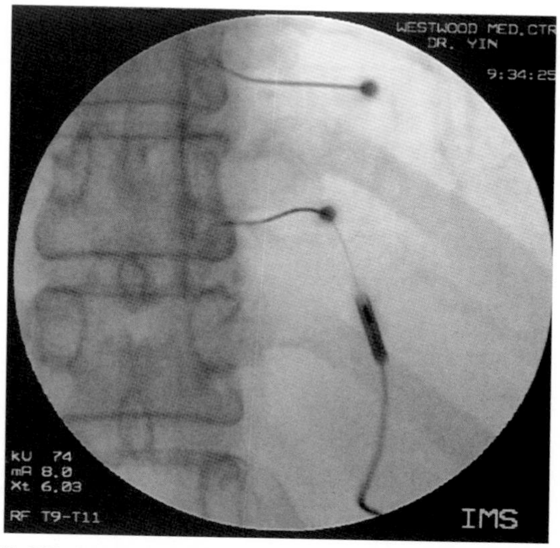

FIGURE 169–35 ■ Anteroposterior image of sensory stereotactic localization of right T8 and T9 dorsal root ganglia. (From Waldman SD: Interventional Pain Management, 2nd ed. Philadelphia, WB Saunders, 2001, p 268.)

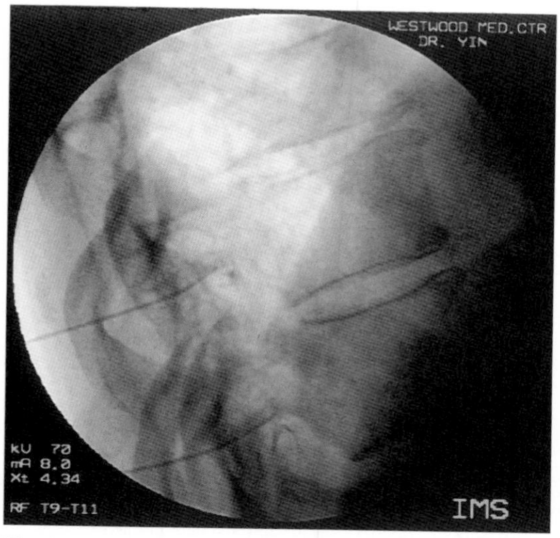

FIGURE 169–34 ■ Lateral image with contrast enhancement shows initial placement of RF electrodes before T8 and T9 dorsal root ganglion sensory stereotaxy. (From Waldman SD: Interventional Pain Management, 2nd ed. Philadelphia, WB Saunders, 2001, p 268.)

a small amount of local anesthetic (0.5 mL of 2% lidocaine) is injected before lesioning. For this type of selective thoracic dorsal root ganglion lesion, a high verniation lesion at a temperature of 50°C to 54°C is performed for 120 to 240 seconds.

General Use of Sacral, Lumbar, and Thoracic Ganglionotomy Procedures

In general, ganglionotomies should *not* be used to treat deafferentation pain. The dorsal root ganglion lesion usually should be reserved for radiculopathy or pain related to a specific, well-defined dermatome. Deafferentation pain (e.g., postherpetic neuralgia, poststroke syndromes, and multiple sclerosis) and sympathetically maintained pain are not commonly treated with a dorsal root ganglion lesion, owing to the risk of exacerbating the deafferentation pain. The purpose of this technique is to produce a well-defined lesion in the dorsal root ganglion, while maintaining an adequate afferent input. It is *not* desirable to produce numbness in the area that is lesioned. A lesion that produces numbness on a long-term basis can be associated with deafferentation pain as a postoperative complication. Because the dorsal root ganglion cells are more sensitive to heat than other structures within the mixed nerve, the clinician is using a differential heat lesion to affect pain pathways preferentially, while leaving the motor, proprioceptive, and afferent pathways relatively intact. It would be unwise to use higher temperatures in an attempt to produce longer acting pain relief because higher temperatures have a greater chance of decreasing afferent input and of producing deafferentation pain as a postoperative complication. If more than one level is involved, it is best to wait 4 weeks between lesions. The greater the number of levels lesioned, the greater is the chance of producing deafferentation pain as a complication.

Lesions in the Cervical Region

RF lesions can be useful to treat pain in the cervical spine, but the operator must appreciate the complex anatomic relationships.[33,38,58,68-70,95-99] Distinct structures that are dense with pain receptors can cause localized and referred pain (Table 169–1). Similar to lumbar disks, cervical disks have nerve fibers in the outer portion of the anulus.[100] Diskogenic irritation in the cervical spine can produce neck pain with headaches and symptoms referred to the shoulder and upper extremities. The cervical disk is a joint that maintains a distinct relationship with its associated facet joints. In the cervical region, the disk and the associated facet joints at each level form a three-joint complex (as they do in the lumbar

Table 169–1

Cervical Pain Generators

Structure	***Implications***
Cervical disks	May cause neck pain, chronic headaches, and symptoms referred to facial region. Facial pain requires exploration of relationship between cervical disks and facial pathways. Arm or hand pain may be radiculopathy or a referred mechanical symptom from abnormal cervical disk
Cervical facet joints	Can cause chronic mechanical symptoms in neck, shoulder, and intracapsular region. Upper and midcervical facet joint abnormalities may cause headaches. Do not usually cause referred facial pain. C0-1 and C1-2 joints are included here and are associated with occipital headaches
Cervical nerve roots	Can cause upper extremity pain, especially if isolated; such isolated pain also may be sympathetically maintained
Myofascial tissues in neck and suboccipital region	May cause mechanical symptoms in neck, referred symptoms in shoulders, and chronic headaches. May also cause facial pain. Should be examined for increased muscle tension, trigger points, and tight bands. Myofascial abnormalities owing to underlying mechanical trauma also are common

spine). Combined diskogenic and facet joint pain commonly develops.[101]

Pain related to these areas can be associated with degenerative disease or acute injury, as from whiplash or other trauma.[102-110] There is often poor correlation between imaging findings and the actual site of the mechanical pain pathway.[89] A normal-looking cervical disk can be disrupted and painful, and an abnormal-looking disk can be asymptomatic.[88] Facet joints may appear normal, yet still be painful. As in the lumbar spine, it is important to perform prognostic blocks of the suspect structures to determine whether they are painful. The most common sources of symptoms are the cervical disks, facet joints, nerve roots, and supporting cervical musculature. The importance of cervical myofascial symptoms (tight bands, trigger points, and asymmetric muscle tissues) should not be underestimated. RF lesions in the neck can be useful in the treatment of diskogenic pain, facet joint problems, and irritated nerve roots.

Disease of the cervical spine can produce referred symptoms in the face and chronic headaches. For patients with headaches or facial pain, it is important to evaluate the cervical spine thoroughly as a potential source of the problem. The upper cervical nerve roots (C2-4) have connections with the superior cervical ganglion. The superior cervical ganglion has connections with the deep petrosal nerve, which has connections with the vidian nerve. The vidian nerve leads directly to the sphenopalatine ganglion, which has connections with branches of the trigeminal nerve. Pain from the upper cervical spine can cause symptoms referred into the frontal and maxillary region. The caudal nucleus of the trigeminal nerve can descend to the C3 or C4 level. Constant stimuli in the upper cervical region from irritated pathways can cause stimulation of the lower portion of the caudal nucleus of the trigeminal nerve; this phenomenon can produce referred facial pain. The sphenopalatine ganglion, which may act as a central pathway between the cervical spine and the facial region, is a complicated structure with multiple types of afferent fibers and ganglion cells (Figs. 169–36 and 169–37).

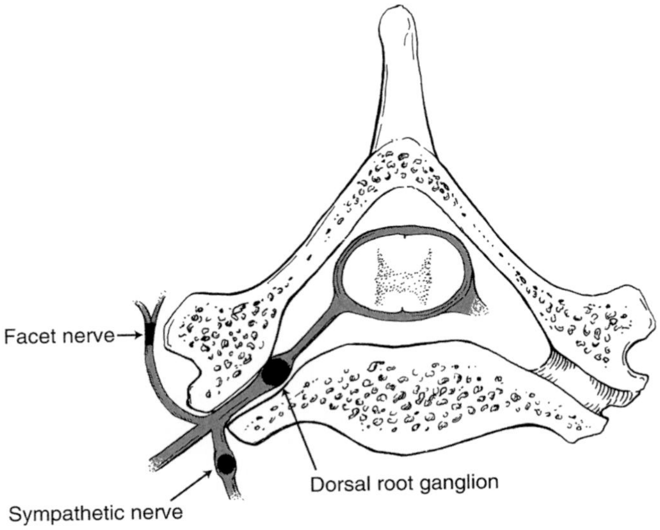

FIGURE 169–36 ■ Cross section through the cervical spine. The relationships among the facet joint nerves, sympathetic nerves, and dorsal root ganglion are shown. Each of these nerves can be lesioned with an RF procedure.

Cervical Facet Joints

When a patient presents with well-circumscribed pain overlying the cervical facet joints, there is a good possibility that the joints are involved in the problem.[110] Affected patients commonly report pain in the neck and shoulder girdle with associated headaches and even ear pain.[111,112] Diagnostic injections of the facet joints are important and can help to make the diagnosis, but false-positive results sometimes occur.[113] A careful history and detailed manual examination should be done.[110]

Anatomy

The medial branch wraps around the posterior aspect and sends branches along the waist of the cervical facet column

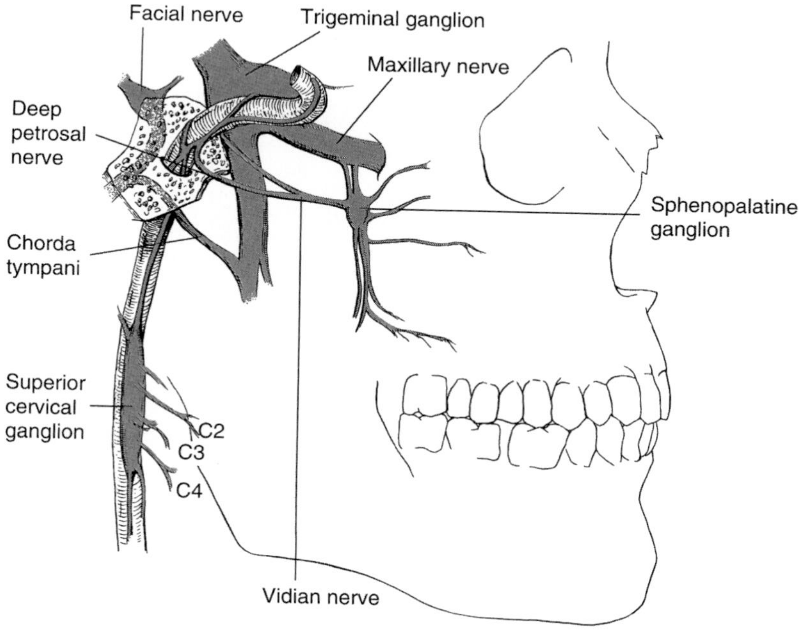

FIGURE 169–37 ■ The complex anatomic relationship between the cervical nerves and the trigeminal system is shown.

at two levels for each joint. The C2-3 facet joint is supplied by part of the third occipital nerve as it crosses the midportion of the C2-3 joint and a communicating branch of C2 just adjacent and craniad to the midportion of the C2-3 joint, on the arch of C2.

Lesions

To denervate the facet joints at any level from C2 to C6, the patient is placed in a supine position, and an oblique approach is used.[38,68,69,98] For the C7 medial branch, the patient is placed in the prone position, and an approach similar to that for the lumbar facet joint denervation is used; the cannula is passed onto the superomedial aspect of the transverse process of C7 and "walked off" the leading edge (approximately 2 mm anteriorly) until the facet joint nerve can be stimulated. For the C8 medial branch, a similar approach may be taken at the superomedial aspect of the T1 transverse process for the articular branches of this nerve; however, the main trunk of the C8 medial branch is located at the inflection point of the (superior lateral) T1 transverse process.[79,85] Sometimes the C5-6 joint requires a posterior approach when the patient has a short, thick neck. Positioning for the C2 communicating nerve contribution is different. The posterior primary ramus of C2, which is larger than the anterior ramus, continues as the greater occipital nerve. It is not prudent to lesion that nerve. There are, however, communicating branches from the posterior primary ramus of C2 that supply the C2-3 facet joint. To denervate these branches, the cannula is placed on the C2 arch at a point 3 to 5 mm craniad to the midportion of the C2-3 facet joint. The C3 contribution (third occipital nerve) to the C2-3 facet joint is lesioned as it crosses the midpoint of the joint. Lesions are first made at the middle of the joint and then 3 to 5 mm craniad, to lesion the C2 communicating branch (exact distances depend on stimulation).

A 50-mm cannula with a 4-mm active tip is used for the lesions. The cannulas all are placed so that the bare metal tip comes to rest on the waist of the facet joint column. An oblique approach is used at first. The cannula enters from a point posterior to the spine and is moved anteriorly until it is aligned with the waist of the facet joint column. This point is just posterior to the associated transverse process and is well posterior to the associated foraminal opening. It is important to avoid the segmental nerve. On a lateral view, the electrode is seen at the "centroid" of the articular pillar. Stimulation at 50 Hz should be felt in the neck and shoulder region at 1 V or less. Absence of upper extremity motor fasciculations should be noted with 2 V at 2-Hz stimulation. Motor fasciculations in the paracervical musculature are common. After proper stimulation, 0.5 mL of 2% lidocaine is passed through each cannula to anesthetize the lesion site. Lesioning is performed at 80°C for 60 seconds (Fig. 169–38).

Lesions of the lower facet joint nerves are made through a posterior approach with the patient in the prone position. For the medial branch of C7 and the articular branches of C8 and T1, the fluoroscopy unit is set up for a posterior view with some craniad angulation so that the appropriate transverse process can be distinguished. A 50-mm or 100-mm cannula with a 5-mm active tip is passed until it touches the superomedial border of the transverse process. The cannula is advanced 2 mm over the leading edge of the transverse process. Stimulation is performed as previously described, and absence of upper extremity motor fasciculations should be noted. Lesion parameters are the same as those described for the upper cervical spine. For cervical facet lesioning, it is prudent to take at least two different views (anteroposterior, lateral, and, when necessary, oblique) to confirm correct needle placement. Anteroposterior views should show the cannula lying next to the lateral aspect of the midportion (waist) of the lamina. Lateral views should show that the cannula tip is posterior to the foraminal opening and level with the "centroid" of the articular pillar. The C8 and T1 lateral views are not seen clearly because of the overlying

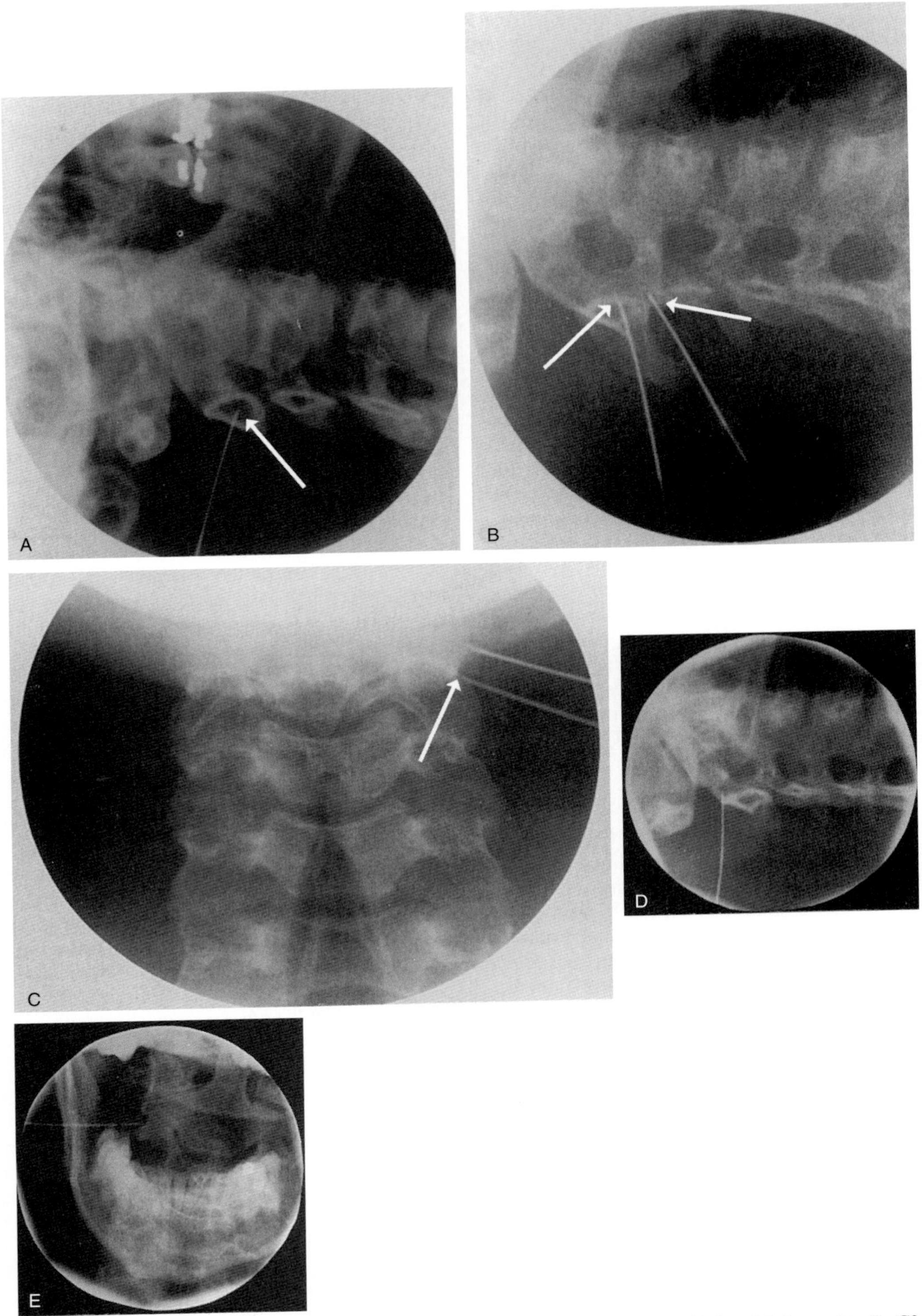

FIGURE 169–38 ■ **A,** Radiograph shows the RF cannula position for lesioning of the C3 contribution (third occipital nerve) to the C2-3 facet joint. **B** and **C,** Oblique and posteroanterior radiographs show RF cannula position *(arrows)* for lesioning of the C3 facet joint nerves to the C2-3 joint (left cannula in **B**) and the C3-4 joint (right cannula in **B**). In **C,** the lower C3 cannula is resting directly along the waist of the cervical facet joint line *(arrow)*. **D,** RF cannula position for lesion of the C2 communicating branch, oblique view. **E,** Anteroposterior view (through the mouth) of the RF cannula position for lesioning of the C2 communicating branch. (From Waldman SD: Interventional Pain Management, 2nd ed. Philadelphia, WB Saunders, 2001, p 271.)

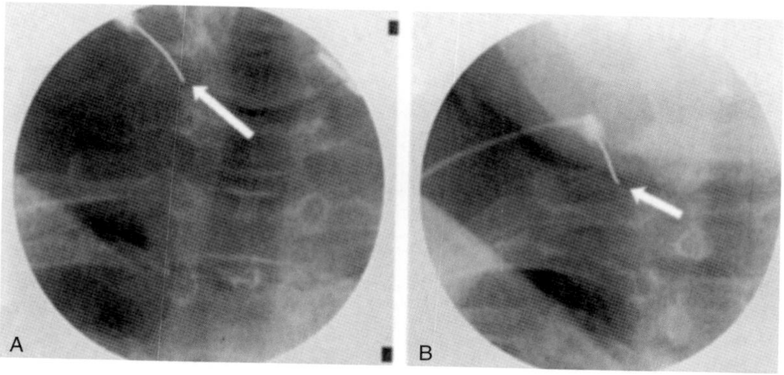

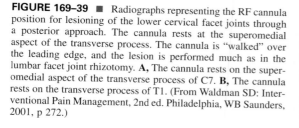

FIGURE 169–39 ■ Radiographs representing the RF cannula position for lesioning of the lower cervical facet joints through a posterior approach. The cannula rests at the superomedial aspect of the transverse process. The cannula is "walked" over the leading edge, and the lesion is performed much as in the lumbar facet joint rhizotomy. **A,** The cannula rests on the superomedial aspect of the transverse process of C7. **B,** The cannula rests on the transverse process of T1. (From Waldman SD: Interventional Pain Management, 2nd ed. Philadelphia, WB Saunders, 2001, p 272.)

scapula. The most important criterion for the facet joint lesion is to *combine* correct stimulation parameters with correct radiographic placement whenever possible. If the cannula appears to have correct anatomic alignment but the proper stimulation parameters are not obtained, RF lesioning should not be performed. When parameters are in doubt, it is best to abandon the procedure (Fig. 169–39).

Recovery from a cervical facet joint denervation is fairly rapid, and most patients show signs of good relief within 10 days. Minor dysesthesias and patchy numbness can occur, but are not dangerous complications. Occasionally, painful hypersensitivity of the neck or shoulder necessitates a brief course of steroids. Lesions of a C2-3 joint sometimes produce short-term vertigo, which is treated with meclizine for a few days. Such complications usually resolve within 2 to 4 weeks after the procedure.

Cervical Facet Joints: Alternate Posterior Parasagittal Approach with Curved-tip Electrodes

An alternative to the oblique approach that facilitates access to the lower cervical medial branch nerves is posterior parasagittal entry. The patient is placed in the prone position with the neck flexed slightly forward. The region from the nuchal crest to the upper dorsal spine is cleansed with antiseptic solution. The fluoroscopy unit is brought in from the head of the table.

Anteroposterior images are obtained to visualize the waist of the lamina (medial indentations of the cervical lamina just caudal to the superior articulating processes) from C3 through C6. At the level of C7 and T1, the transverse processes are identified. At C2, the lateral aspect of the lamina just cephalad to the inferior articular process of C2 is identified.

The aforementioned bony landmarks are identified, and skin entry sites are marked directly overlying the bony targets, coaxial with the x-ray beam. An electrode 100 mm in length with an active 22-gauge tip is used, with a slight (10 to 15 degrees) smooth curve placed in the distal 5 to 7 mm. The C2 communicating branch of the posterior primary ramus supplying the superior portion of the C2-3 joint is approached under anteroposterior fluoroscopic imaging. The electrode is guided down to the C2 dorsal lamina in a posterior parasagittal plane, coaxial with the x-ray image. When bony contact is made (generally near the midpoint of the junction of the caudal and middle thirds of the C2 lamina, 3 to 5 mm craniad

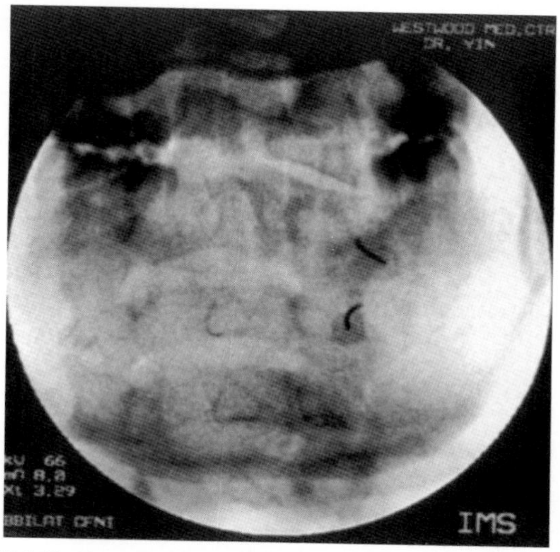

FIGURE 169–40 ■ Anteroposterior image shows placement of C2 and C3 medial branch electrodes. (From Waldman SD: Interventional Pain Management, 2nd ed. Philadelphia, WB Saunders, 2001, p 272.)

to the lesion point of the third occipital nerve at the level of the C2-3 facet joint), the electrode is rotated laterally and advanced 1 to 2 mm around the lateral aspect of the C2 lamina, then redirected medially so that the electrode tip hugs the lateral lamina (Fig. 169–40). Lateral images are taken, verifying placement of the electrode's active tip overlying the midportion of the C2 lamina but well dorsal of the exiting C3 nerve root (Fig. 169–41).

The C3-6 medial branch nerves are approached at the level of the waist of the lamina, in a posterior parasagittal plane, under anteroposterior imaging. The goal of the posterior approach is to approximate the active electrode tips parallel and adjacent to the medial branch nerves as they wrap around the waist of the lamina before decussating into individual superior and inferior articular branches. The electrodes are advanced to contact the dorsal lateral cervical lamina, then rotated so that the curve of the electrode tip is directed laterally. The electrode is advanced fractionally around the lateral border of the lamina. The electrode tip is redirected medially, and lateral fluoroscopic images are used to guide further

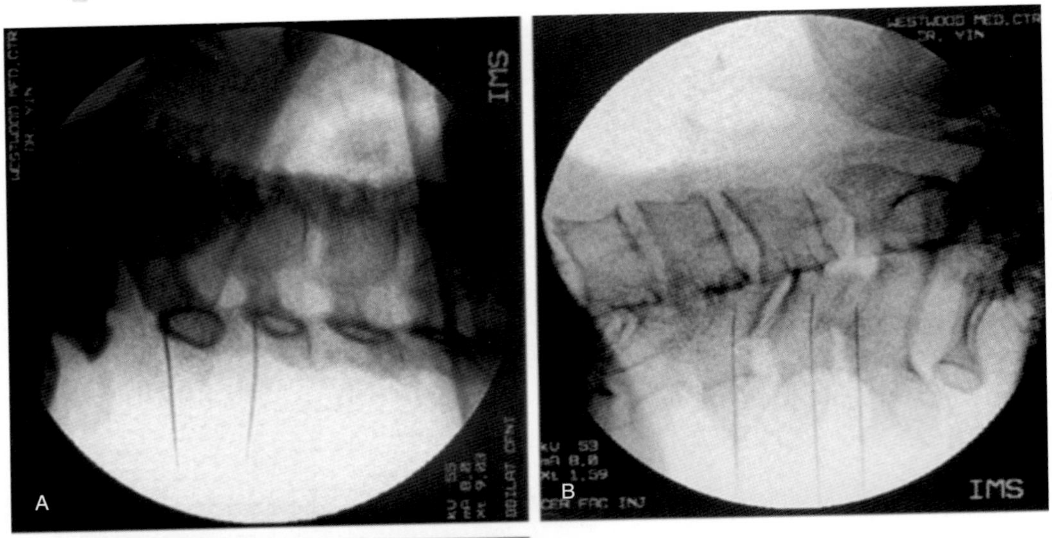

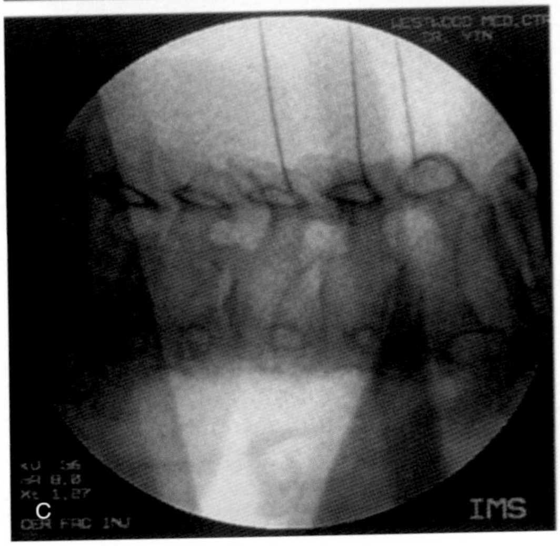

FIGURE 169–41 ■ **A,** Oblique radiograph of electrode placement for C2 and C3 medial branch lesion. **B,** Lateral radiograph shows electrode placement for C2-4 medial branch denervation. **C,** Oblique radiograph shows electrode positioning for third occipital nerve denervation. (From Waldman SD: Interventional Pain Management, 2nd ed. Philadelphia, WB Saunders, 2001, p 273.)

advancement of the electrode (approaching the "centroid" of the articular pillar). The electrode is held close to the lateral lamina, parallel to the dorsally directed medial branch nerves (Fig. 169–42).

At the levels of C7, C8, and T1, the transverse processes of C7 and T1 are used as radiographic landmarks. The C7 medial branch nerve is approached at the level of the superior medial aspect of the transverse process of C7; the electrode tip is maneuvered to overlap slightly this portion of the process. The C8 medial branch nerve is approached at the superior lateral aspect of the T1 transverse process, but articular branches often are found at the superior medial aspect of the T1 transverse process (Fig. 169–43). The T1 medial branch nerve crosses the superior lateral aspect of the T2 transverse process,[79] although specific articular branches may be found medially along the dorsal aspect of the lamina adjacent to the superior and inferior articular processes.

After the RF electrodes have been placed in positions approximating the location of the medial branch nerves or their articular branches, sensory and motor stereotaxy is performed to guide or "fine-tune" final electrode placement. Patient-blinded sensory stimulation that reproduces concordant pain (at 0.2 to 0.3 V, 50 Hz), in conjunction with segmental multifidus contraction, verifies placement of the electrode tip over symptomatic levels. Observed multifidus contraction without concordant pain or the development of nonpainful paresthesias indicates localization of an asymptomatic branch. Only the symptomatic levels are lesioned, as with the oblique approach.

Diagnosis and Treatment of Cervical Symptoms

Lesions of the cervical dorsal root ganglion can be useful for diskogenic pain or segmental pain related to disease of the spinal nerve.[33,34,56] C2 and C3 ganglion lesions can be useful for treating "resistant" C2-3 facet pain. Prognostic blocks are important for correctly isolating the painful segment before lesioning. Lesions of the dorsal root ganglion have the potential to produce deafferentation pain; careful prognostic blocks should be performed as a staging procedure. If cervical diskogenic pain is suspected, diskography can be performed to isolate the specific segment causing the problems. If a radiculopathy is considered the source of the upper extremity pain, electromyography studies and prognostic sleeve blocks are helpful for determining the involved level.

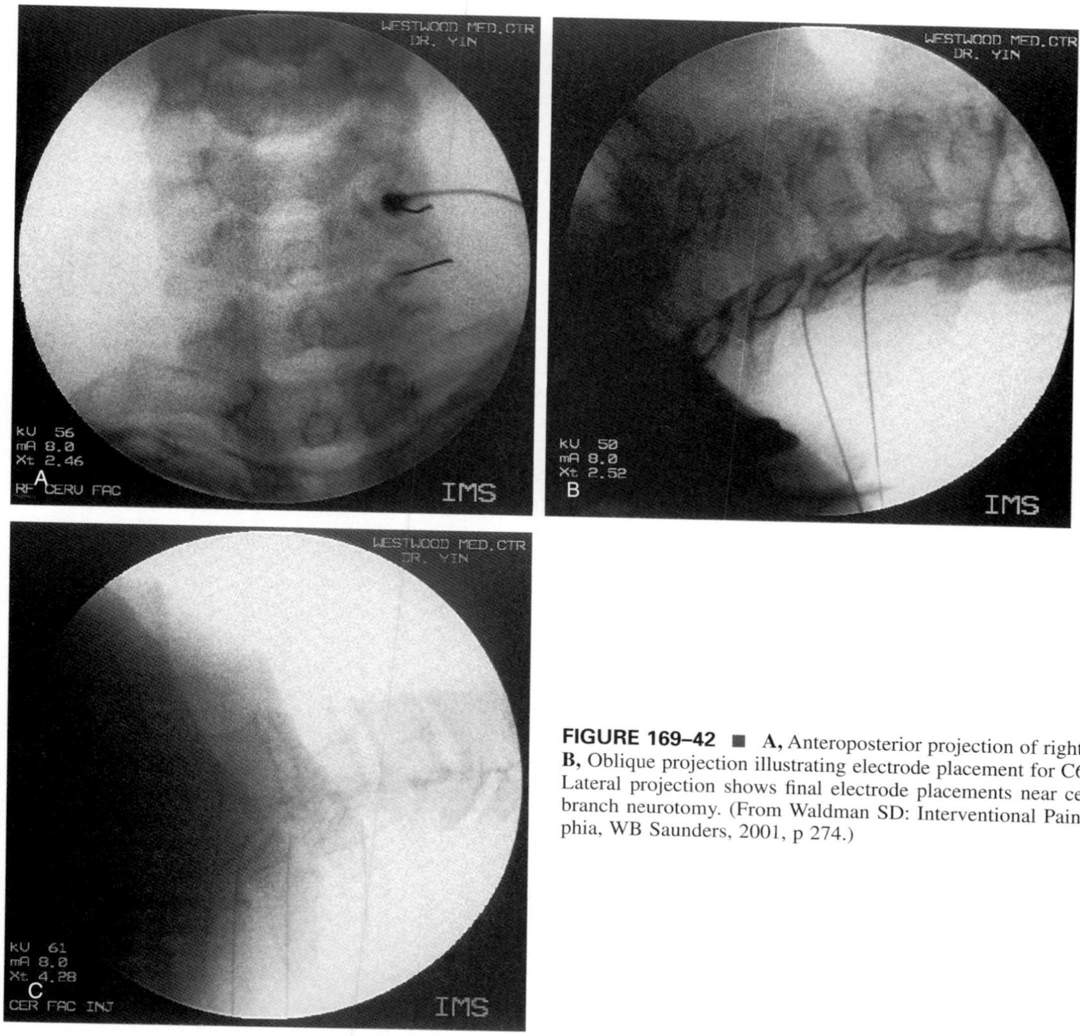

FIGURE 169–42 ■ **A,** Anteroposterior projection of right C6-7 medial branch neurotomy. **B,** Oblique projection illustrating electrode placement for C6-7 medial branch neurotomy. **C,** Lateral projection shows final electrode placements near centroid of C5-7 for C5-7 medial branch neurotomy. (From Waldman SD: Interventional Pain Management, 2nd ed. Philadelphia, WB Saunders, 2001, p 274.)

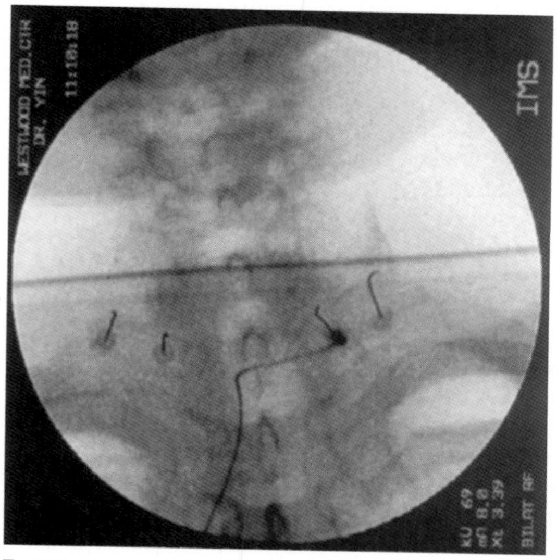

FIGURE 169–43 ■ Anteroposterior radiograph illustrates placement of electrodes for bilateral C8 medial branch denervation. Note placement of electrode for C8 medial branch at superolateral aspect of T1 transverse process and placement of electrode at superomedial aspect of T1 transverse process for C8 articular branch localized with sensory stereotaxy. (From Waldman SD: Interventional Pain Management, 2nd ed. Philadelphia, WB Saunders, 2001, p 275.)

Cervical Ganglionotomy

RF lesions of the cervical dorsal root ganglion are made in a similar manner at C3-7. C8 should be avoided, owing to its tendency to develop neuritis and deafferentation pain. The RF cannula is advanced from an oblique approach until it touches the 6 o'clock position of the posterior foraminal canal. The cannula is advanced along the floor of the canal and halfway across the facet joint line. It is closely applied to the floor (posterior aspect) of the foraminal canal to maintain a safe distance from the vertebral artery.

Stimulation parameters are similar to the parameters described for the lumbar ganglionotomy. At 50 Hz, good paresthesia in the upper extremity should be noted between 0.4 V and 0.7 V. At 2 Hz, motor fasciculations should be seen at twice the voltage needed for the sensory stimulation. Then 1 mL of 2% lidocaine is passed through the cannula, and a 10-minute delay is allowed for it to take effect. Thermal lesions are made between 60°C and 65°C, depending on the stimulation threshold, for 60 seconds. The correct cannula to use for this lesion is the SMK 50 mm with a 4-mm active tip or the SMK 100 mm with a 5-mm active tip. The goal of this procedure is to produce a discrete injury to the pain pathways while preserving normal proprioception, touch, and motor function. Numbness is not a desirable outcome. Some sensory changes may be noted during the first days to weeks after the procedure. Most patients have normal sensory function after 4 weeks. It takes 4 weeks to determine the full effects of the procedure because inflammation of the ganglion follows lesioning. Patients commonly experience increasing pain for days to weeks, until all postoperative pain resolves.

Ganglionotomy at the C2 level is different. Under lateral fluoroscopic guidance, a 50-mm electrode with a 4-mm active tip is advanced perpendicular to a point at the upper two thirds of the arch of C2 (junction of posterior two thirds with the ventral third of the arch). The cannula is advanced (under anteroposterior fluoroscopic viewing) halfway across (and posterior to) the C1-2 joint using a through-the-mouth view. Because motor function from the C2 level is not a significant concern, sensory stimulation is the only parameter that needs to be checked. At 50-Hz stimulation, paresthesia to the suboccipital region should be noted between 0.4 and 0.7 V. Then 1 mL of 2% lidocaine is passed onto the ganglion to anesthetize the lesion site. A thermal lesion is created between 55°C and 60°C, depending on the stimulation threshold. Lesions at the C2 level more often tend to be associated with postoperative neuritis. We recommend performing cooler, high-verniation lesions at C2. Ganglionotomy at the C2 and C3 levels can be helpful in the treatment of C2 and C3 "pattern" headaches. Mechanical problems of *any* aspect of the motion segment anywhere from C0 through C4 can cause occipital neck pain with associated headaches; cervical disk lesions even farther caudad also can cause headaches (Fig. 169–44). Indications for cervical ganglionotomy include pain from the cervical disk, radiculopathy, and headaches. Patients generally are discharged 2 hours after the procedure.

Cervical Disk Procedure

Cervical diskogenic pain is an important and underdiagnosed cause of chronic headaches and neck pain. Injury to *any* cervical disk can be associated with headaches. Provocational or analgesic diskography (or both) is the key for diagnosing a painful cervical disk. If a painful level is discovered, the clinician should consider the RF cervical disk procedure.

The patient is placed in the supine position. An oblique approach from the *right* side is used for the procedure. The patient is given preoperative antibiotics 45 minutes beforehand. After sterile preparation, fluoroscopy is used to visualize the painful disk.

A 100-mm cannula with a 5-mm active tip is used. The cannula is placed into the disk from a right oblique approach, just anterior to the uncovertebral joint. A curved cannula is advanced into the center of the disk as seen by lateral and anteroposterior views. Stimulation with 2 V at 50 Hz and 2 Hz should be negative. No local anesthetic is used for the lesion. Pain is common during the lesion process, beginning at about 90 seconds and peaking at 3.5 minutes. The lesion temperature is increased over 20 to 30 seconds to 80°C and maintained for 4 minutes.

Pain relief is sometimes immediate. Other patients achieve maximal relief 2 to 4 weeks after the procedure. Disk infection is a risk, but it is minimized with preoperative antibiotics and a right-sided approach (to avoid the esophagus). Nerve root injury is another potential risk, but should be quite rare when proper technique is used. If clear-cut radicular symptoms occur during the lesion process, the procedure should be stopped immediately (see Fig. 169–44I and J).

Lesions of the Stellate Ganglion

The stellate ganglion is a combination of the inferior cervical and the first thoracic sympathetic ganglia. RF lesions of the stellate ganglion can be useful in managing sympathetically maintained pain.[114] The ganglion lies just anterior to the longus colli muscle at the anterior and lateral borders of the C7 vertebral body. It is a diffuse structure. Partial lesions of the stellate ganglion can produce long-term, high-quality pain relief.

Under fluoroscopic guidance, an RF cannula with a 5-mm active tip is advanced from an anterior approach until the superolateral aspect of C7 is encountered. The cannula is pulled back anteriorly approximately 2 mm to ensure that the active tip is anterior to the longus colli. The final position is on the vertebral body at its junction with the transverse process. Proper stimulation technique is crucial to avoid injury to the phrenic or recurrent laryngeal nerves. Anteroposterior and lateral views are checked before each lesion. Three lesions are made; these include the point just described, a point just lateral and caudal (on the medial aspect of the transverse process), and a point 5 mm caudal (on the anterolateral aspect of the vertebral body). These three lesions create a triangular zone of thermal interruption to the cervical sympathetic fibers.

Before each lesion, the following stimulation technique should be used. At 2 Hz, the patient is asked to say "E" while stimulation is applied at 2.5 V. The patient's ability to articulate should not be at all impaired. If it is, the cannula is too close to the recurrent laryngeal nerve (which is anterior and medial to the proper lesion zone). At the same time, the operator's hand is placed just under the rib cage to feel for movement of the diaphragm. Although the phrenic nerve should be well lateral to the lesion site, any movement of the diaphragm with 2.5 V at 2 Hz warrants immediate investigation of the cannula position. After proper stimulation parameters have been met, 0.5 mL of 0.25% bupivacaine is passed through the cannula, and a lesion is made at 80°C for 30 seconds. The cannula is moved immediately, and the entire process is repeated for the second and third lesions. Bupivacaine is chosen for its slow onset, which makes inadvertent anesthetizing of the phrenic or recurrent laryngeal nerves less likely before the lesion process.

If a cannula with a 7-mm active tip is used, the cannula can be applied directly to bone and does not need to be pulled back in an anterior fashion. The longus colli muscle is approximately 5 mm thick at its thickest point. The lesion, at least 2 mm, is made anterior to the muscle while using this variation. It is preferable to have the cannula firmly anchored—hence the appeal of this approach.

Careful stimulation technique is crucial for safe performance of this procedure. The lesion on the medial aspect of the transverse process must be made with extreme care. The anterior portion of the transverse process is quite narrow at this point, and the RF cannula *must* stay in the same plane as for the ventral aspect of the vertebral body, to prevent injury to the segmental nerves or vertebral artery (Fig. 169–45).

Last, the clinician may wish to direct the RF cannula caudad, to the "groove" where the head of the first rib meets the ventrolateral aspect of the body of T1. At this ventrolateral

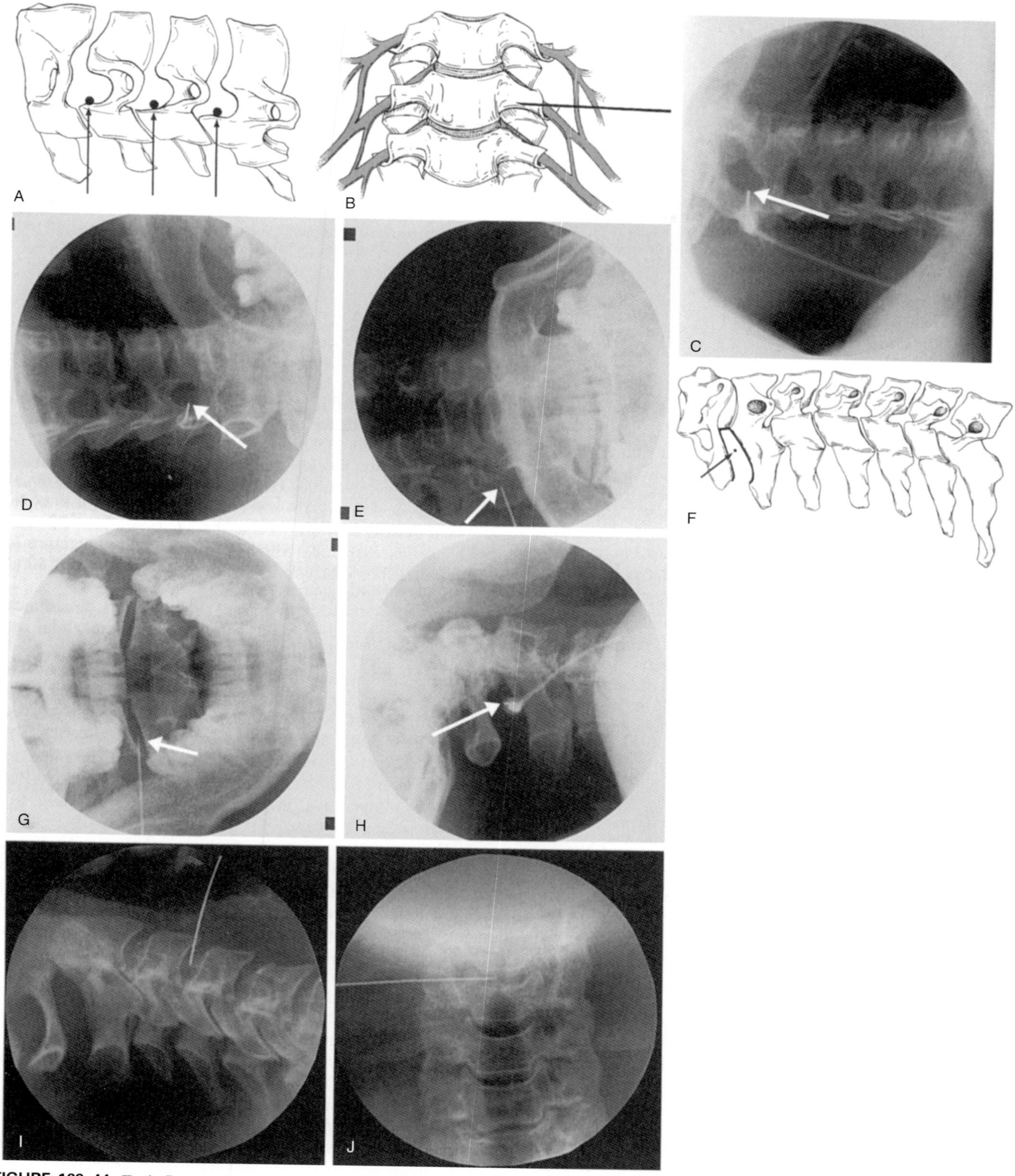

FIGURE 169–44 ■ **A,** Drawing of the entry points *(solid circles)* for a cervical dorsal root ganglionotomy procedure. Each point is on the floor of the foraminal canal at the 6 o'clock position *(arrows)*. **B,** Posteroanterior view of the cervical spine. The RF cannula tip *(arrow)* is in the correct position for a cervical dorsal root ganglionotomy. The tip of the cannula has passed halfway across the cervical facet joint line. **C,** Oblique radiograph of a cervical spine. The RF cannula has entered the 6 o'clock position along the floor of the C3 foraminal canal *(arrow)*. **D,** Oblique radiograph shows the RF cannula position *(arrow)* for a C4 ganglionotomy. **E,** Posteroanterior radiograph shows the cannula position for a C4 dorsal root ganglionotomy procedure. The RF cannula tip has passed halfway across the cervical facet joint line *(arrow)*. **F,** Drawing of a lateral view of the cervical spine. The dot in the arch of the C2 *(arrow)* represents the entry point for a C2 dorsal root ganglionotomy procedure. **G** and **H,** The correct cannula position for a C2 dorsal root ganglionotomy. The lateral view through the arch of C2. **H,** RF cannula *(arrow)* is entering the arch of C2. **G,** On the posteroanterior view through the mouth, the RF cannula is passing halfway across the C1-2 joint *(arrow)*. **I,** Lateral view of RF cannula position for a C3-4 disk procedure. **J,** Anteroposterior view of RF cannula position for a C3-4 disk procedure. (**C-E**, **G-J** from Waldman SD: Interventional Pain Management, 2nd ed. Philadelphia, WB Saunders, 2001, p 276.)

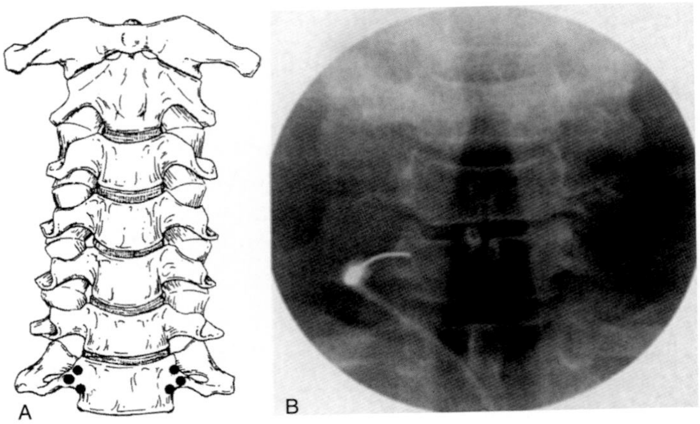

FIGURE 169–45 ■ **A,** Drawing of posteroanterior view of the cervical spine. Dots mark the target points for RF lesioning of the cervical sympathetic nerves. These are at the junction of the medial aspect of the transverse process with the lateral aspect of its respective vertebral body. **B,** Posteroanterior radiograph of the cervical spine. At the C7 level, the RF cannula rests at the junction of the lateral aspect of the vertebral body with the medial aspect of the transverse process. This represents the correct cannula position for lesioning of the C7 sympathetic fibers. (**B** from Waldman SD: Interventional Pain Management, 2nd ed. Philadelphia, WB Saunders, 2001, p 277.)

position, a fourth lesion can be done to interrupt some of the thoracic sympathetic fibers. Care must be taken to stay on the ventral aspect of the vertebral body at the junction of the rib and vertebral body. Alternatively, one may wish to proceed instead to the T2 and T3 sympathectomy (described later). If hand pain is the predominant symptom, the T2-3 technique should be considered because a significant amount of sympathetic outflow to the hand comes from these two levels.

This is a discrete lesion that does not interrupt the entire ganglion. Impressive results can be seen, however, and the technique can be repeated if necessary. Lesions of the stellate ganglion can be useful for the treatment of sympathetically maintained pain, including reflex sympathetic dystrophy, causalgia, posttraumatic dystrophies, and Raynaud phenomenon. This technique usually does not produce Horner syndrome (superior cervical ganglion) as can other sympatholytic procedures.

Lesions Used to Treat Chronic Headaches

The use of RF procedures to manage chronic occipital pain and headaches has been reported by several authors.[97,115-118] It is important to determine whether the mechanical components of the cervical spine are contributing to the headache. A thorough neurologic evaluation is mandatory for any patient with chronic headaches. Appropriate studies, as indicated by the clinical history, are important. Even if a patient does have mechanical findings in the cervical spine, other more serious problems that could be contributing to the headache must be ruled out. A careful neurologic evaluation is needed to rule out problems such as chronic inflammatory disease, vasculitis, vascular anomalies, and neoplasms. Migraine headaches, although considered a vascular phenomenon, can be triggered by abnormalities in the cervical spine. A patient with a true migraine headache may respond to appropriate RF lesions in the cervical spine. Although the headache may not be cured, the frequency and duration of the headache can be improved if the mechanical problem is treated. Some individuals who have been diagnosed with migraine headaches have pure mechanical problems. They show significant decreases in frequency and intensity of their headaches when the cervical abnormalities are treated.

Cluster headaches also can respond favorably to RF lesions. Some patients with cluster headaches have concomitant mechanical problems in the cervical spine. Many of these patients have evidence of cervical disease on physical examination, and many have functional abnormalities.

If prognostic blocks show that the facet joints are causing or contributing to the headaches, RF cervical facet rhizotomy should be performed. If diagnostic root sleeve injections or cervical diskography shows that the headaches are related to an abnormal disk, an RF cervical disk procedure or ganglionotomy should be considered, but only after careful prognostic blocks have been performed.

Upper Cervicogenic Headache

Cervicogenic headaches involving the upper cervical and suboccipital region are common and can be caused by various bony, articular, and soft tissue lesions. Secondary myofascial tension may make definitive clinical diagnosis, based solely on detailed history and careful physical examination, even more difficult, and a methodical, systematic diagnostic approach is imperative for success in dealing with these frequently challenging cases.

The general evaluation of suboccipital, occipital, and upper cervical headaches begins with a careful history and meticulous physical examination. A history of cervical or cranial trauma may be relevant, and symptoms suggesting nerve root involvement (greater or lesser occipital neuralgia, cervical radicular pain) may steer the investigation toward evaluation of the cervical disks and related nerve root structures. Before consideration of interventional diagnostic or therapeutic procedures, conservative and pharmacologic modalities must be exhausted, and diagnostic evaluations must be performed, including plain films and MRI of the cervical and cranial regions. Identifying treatable sources of cervicogenic or suboccipital headache is often complex and time-consuming, and most patients have seen several specialists. Nonetheless, treatable sources of cervicogenic and suboccipital headache often are identifiable with a careful and methodical approach.

A history of radiating scalp pain in the distribution of the occipital nerves, coupled with exacerbation and reproduction of pain on palpation of these structures at or proximal to the nuchal crest, should prompt consideration of occipital neuralgia. Differential diagnostic injections of the greater and lesser occipital nerves definitively diagnose primary occipital neuralgia (C2 or C3 dorsal root ganglion involvement).

Affected patients generally respond well to steroid injections over the dorsal root ganglia of C2 or C3, and in refractory cases, excellent results have been obtained with percutaneous functional stereotactic RF dorsal root ganglion lesioning with high verniation at 50°C to 54°C, 45 to 55 V, for 120 to 240 seconds. Severe refractory cases also have been managed with open exploration of the occipital nerve just proximal to the nuchal crest and cryolesioning of the greater occipital nerve and its branches under direct vision. Implanted quadripolar occipital nerve stimulation devices also have been effective as a rescue intervention.

Suboccipital pain without nerve root involvement may be secondary to upper cervical facet capsular pain or degenerative disease; upper cervical diskogenic pain (most commonly C2-3 and C3-4); pain secondary to bony lesions, including metastases and rare ligamentous instability of the C1-2 or C2-3 vertebral joint complexes; atlanto-occipital joint/capsular pain; and atlantoaxial joint/capsular pain. Advanced diagnostic procedures, such as C2, C3, or C4 medial branch injection, provocative cervical diskography, and atlanto-occipital and atlantoaxial joint injection, may provide definitive diagnosis of the predominant source of pain in the suboccipital and upper cervical regions. Definitive therapeutic interventions exist for medial branch–mediated pain (see section on cervical facet rhizotomy), and many patients with cervical diskogenic pain of C2-3 or C3-4 origin respond to intradiskal steroid or intradiskal RF lesion.

C2 Ramus Communicans Lesion

Pain of atlantoaxial and atlanto-occipital joint origin is more difficult to treat because the sensory innervation of these joints and joint capsules is poorly understood. Sluijter[119] advocated a lower-temperature high-verniation lesioning of the C1 nerve as effective treatment for suboccipital headaches presumed to be of atlanto-occipital or atlantoaxial joint origin.

One of the authors (W.Y.) has developed an approach targeting the ramus communicans nerves at the C2 level, located adjacent to the ventral lateral aspect of the vertebral body of C2 at its junction with the ventral inferior medial transverse process. A small sulcus, or groove, exists in this region of the C2 vertebra, directed lateral to medial at an angle of approximately 45 to 60 degrees from horizontal, pointing to the dens.

Although a comparative study examining the possible correlation of atlantoaxial and atlanto-occipital joint pain with C1 dorsal root ganglion or C2 ramus communicans origin has yet to be performed, we believe that, based on sensory stereotactic findings, the C2 ramus communicans may provide a source for some treatable atlantoaxial, and possibly atlanto-occipital, joint-mediated pain. Deep suboccipital pain without occipital radiation and unresponsive to diagnostic occipital nerve block, exacerbated by palpation over the C1-2 arch, seems to correlate well with C2 ramus communicans–mediated pain. Patients also occasionally complain of coexisting nonradiating pain over the crown or vertex. This clinical impression has led one of the authors (W.Y.) to abandon diagnostic atlanto-occipital and atlantoaxial joint injections in favor of C2 ramus communicans injection and, if required, RF lesion.

The confirmation of C2 gray rami–mediated suboccipital headache is made with fluoroscopically confirmed small-volume injection of local anesthetic and depot corticosteroid (bupivacaine, 0.5 to 0.7 mL, with triamcinolone, 8 mg/mL). Approximately 20% to 25% of patients benefit dramatically from local anesthetic with steroid injection alone, obviating more aggressive therapy. Patients with recurrent, refractory pain who have experienced reproducible high-grade temporary improvement with local anesthetic and steroid injection over the C2 ramus communicans may benefit from a percutaneous sensory stereotactic RF C2 ramus communicans lesion. The long-term results are frequently stunning.

Technique

Similar to C2 cervical dorsal root ganglion lesioning and percutaneous cordotomy, the technique of C2 ramus communicans lesion is technically demanding. Considerable potential for patient morbidity exists if the technique is performed by inexperienced practitioners unfamiliar with advanced fluoroscopy-guided procedures and upper cervical bony and soft tissue anatomy.

The patient is placed supine on the fluoroscopy table with the head and neck slightly extended. The neck, submandibular, and retroauricular regions are prepared. The fluoroscopic unit is brought in from the head. Lateral fluoroscopic images are obtained, and the "lateral mass" of C2 (including the C2 transverse process and inferior articular pillar) and the ventral aspect of the C2 vertebral body are identified. Parallax is eliminated with rotation and cephalad or caudad angulation of the x-ray beam as needed. A skin entry site is marked and anesthetized below the angle of the mandible, lateral to the carotid sheath, similar to that which would be used for C3 or C4 ganglionotomy. (Anterior oblique angulation of the fluoroscopic unit is used initially; after the electrode has been introduced through the skin, lateral images are used to guide placement because no clear radiographic landmarks are present on anterior oblique fluoroscopic images. A coaxial, or "tunnel vision," approach is not feasible.) A 100-mm, 2-mm active tip 22-gauge RF electrode with a small distal curve (10 to 15 degrees) is introduced under lateral fluoroscopic guidance and directed medially and cephalad under lateral fluoroscopic imaging toward the ventral lateral aspect of the C2 vertebral body at its junction with the ipsilateral ventral inferior medial C2 transverse process. The path of the electrode passes lateral and dorsal to the carotid sheath. Care is taken to stay ventral to the exiting C3 nerve root and ventral to the vertebral artery yet dorsal to the pharyngeal structures. Bony contact may be made at the ventrolateral aspect of the lateral inferior end plate of the C2 vertebral body at its junction with the C2-3 intervertebral disk. The electrode is rotated and directed cephalad, hugging bone, into the sulcus along the ventral lateral aspect of the C2 vertebral body, medial to the ventral aspect of the C2 transverse process (Fig. 169–46).

Careful aspiration is performed; no blood or other body fluid should be aspirated. A small-volume contrast study is performed, using 0.2 to 0.4 mL of nonionic contrast medium, such as iohexol, 240 mg/mL. Contrast spread should be limited to the immediate perivertebral region, outlining the sulcus on anteroposterior fluoroscopic imaging. In lateral radiographs, the contrast material should appear to silhouette the ventral aspect of the transverse process of C2 (Fig. 169–47).

Sensory stereotaxy is performed next, using 0.15 to 0.2 V at 50 Hz, 1 msec pulse duration. The electrode is manipulated with very small movements along the ventral sulcus of C2

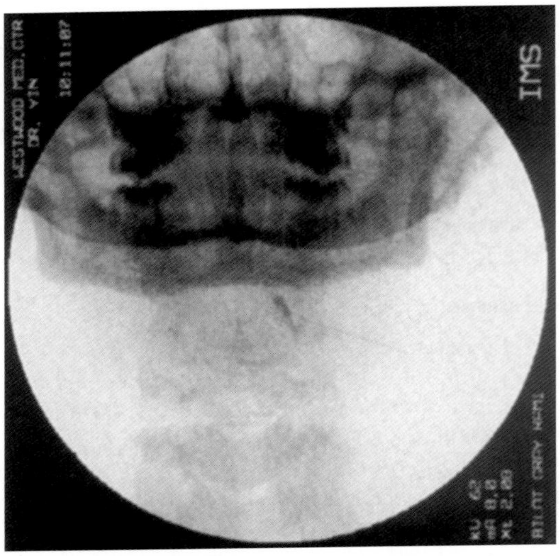

FIGURE 169–46 ■ Anteroposterior radiograph shows the ventral sulcus (filled with contrast material) at C2 with the electrode positioned for a ramus communicans RF lesion. (From Waldman SD: Interventional Pain Management, 2nd ed. Philadelphia, WB Saunders, 2001, p 279.)

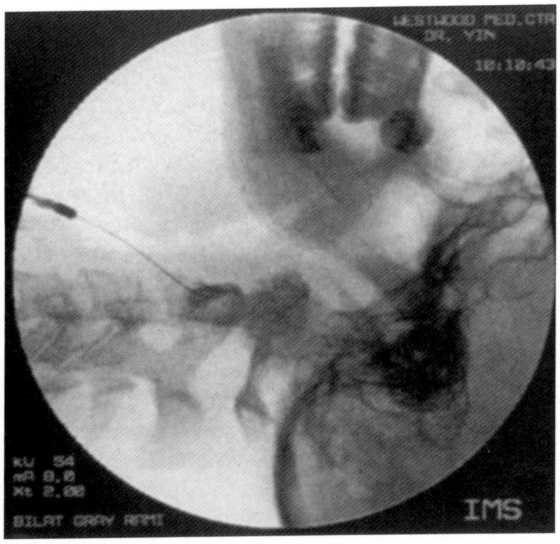

FIGURE 169–47 ■ Lateral radiograph shows contrast medium ventral to C2 "lateral mass" and electrode positioned for a ramus communicans RF lesion. (From Waldman SD: Interventional Pain Management, 2nd ed. Philadelphia, WB Saunders, 2001, p 279.)

until concordant suboccipital pain is reproduced in a patient-blinded fashion. Elicitation of sharp radiating infra-auricular/neck pain indicates stimulation of the ventral C3 nerve root and is unacceptable. Elicitation of deep or superficial infra-auricular pain or anterior cervical/submandibular pain may indicate possible stimulation of the chorda tympani and is unacceptable. There are no motor branches associated with the ramus communicans nerve; motor stimulation generally is not performed. After concordant suboccipital pain has been elicited in a reproducible, patient-blinded fashion, 0.5 to 1 mL of 2% lidocaine is injected before RF lesioning.

The RF lesion is performed at 80°C for 60 seconds and repeated when the electrode tip has returned to ambient body temperature. The size of the lesion created by the 2-mm active tip is small, but this approach reduces the risk of inadvertent C3 or chorda tympani lesion that could occur with a 5-mm active tip. After the lesioning, a small amount of corticosteroid, with or without local anesthetic, may be injected, and the electrode may be removed. The patient may be discharged after a 1- to 2-hour postprocedure observation period. Patients frequently complain of some deep neck soreness, which may last 2 to 3 days, and occasionally of pain with swallowing, which is similarly self-limited. Occasionally, despite negative stimulation, patients may complain of some temporary radiating pain in the infra-auricular region radiating down the ipsilateral neck. This pain may be a result of localized inflammation irritating the chorda tympani or ventral C3 nerve root after the thermal lesion and is generally self-limited.

Lesions of the Sphenopalatine Ganglion

Lesions of the sphenopalatine ganglion can be useful in the treatment of patients with cluster headaches, certain types of migraine headaches, and neuritis of the sphenopalatine ganglion. On lateral fluoroscopic view, the sphenopalatine fossa sits at the tip of the petrous bone, just beneath the sphenoid sinus. This ganglion lies in the sphenopalatine "groove," which connects the fossa with the nasal cavity. The sphenopalatine ganglion lies medial to the maxillary nerve, and its fossa can be recognized on a lateral radiograph as a wedge-shaped structure situated at the tip of the petrous mass and just inferior to the anterior aspect of the sphenoid sinus.

If a prognostic block provides good relief, an RF lesion of the sphenopalatine ganglion is performed as follows. The patient is placed in the supine position on the fluoroscopy table. Preoperative antibiotics are given 45 minutes beforehand. The head should be fixed in neutral position with a strip of tape. The fluoroscopy unit is set up to produce a lateral projection. An opaque marker is held over the sphenopalatine fossa, and a mark is placed on the skin at that point. After the patient has been prepared and draped, the skin and subcutaneous tissues are anesthetized with local anesthetic. The entry point is usually just superior to the mandibular arch. A 100-mm cannula with 2-mm active tip is used for the procedure. The cannula is advanced perpendicular to and between the prominences of the mandible, usually in the center of the sphenopalatine fossa as seen on fluoroscopy. A curved cannula tip facilitates movement around the bony structures. The cannula is advanced slowly medially until it enters the sphenopalatine fossa. Intermittent anteroposterior views are taken to ensure that the cannula is on course and well caudad to the orbit. As the cannula is advanced farther, it makes contact with the maxillary nerve. A paresthesia to the maxilla is noted at that point. The fluoroscopy unit is changed to an anteroposterior projection. The cannula is advanced farther medially until it is just adjacent to the lateral wall of the nasal cavity. It is advanced 1 to 2 mm at a time until it slips into the groove in the nasal cavity. If the cannula contacts bone instead of the groove, its position should be changed slightly until it is felt to move into the groove.

As the cannula slips into proper position, stimulation should begin at 50 Hz. If the cannula is in correct position, a tingling sensation in the nose is noted at approximately 1 V. Frequently, tingling is noted in the soft palate, in which case the cannula should be advanced in a slightly more medial direction. Stimulation should be performed again, and if the cannula is in correct position, most of the stimulation is noted in the nasal region. If only a small amount of paresthesia is felt in the soft palate and most in the nasal cavity, the cannula is in correct position, and 1 mL of 2% lidocaine can be injected through the cannula to anesthetize the sphenopalatine ganglion. The thermal lesion is created for 60 seconds at 80°C, and the cannula is advanced 1 mm medially. A second lesion is made in an identical manner, and the cannula is advanced 1 mm again, where the third and final lesion is then created.

The cannula is withdrawn after the third lesion, and the patient is observed for 2 hours. Approximately 10% to 20% of patients experience epistaxis after the procedure. This is not a dangerous problem, but the patient should not be discharged until it has fully resolved. Postoperative discomfort can last 2 weeks. A small percentage of patients develop some sensory loss in the soft palate after this procedure (Fig. 169–48).

Lesions of the Trigeminal Ganglion

The first descriptions of RF thermal lesions of the trigeminal ganglion were published by Sweet and Wepsic,[120] who confirmed its efficacy. Reports of trigeminal thermal lesions in more than 1000 cases over a 10-year period were published in 1990 by Broggi and colleagues.[121] The value of RF procedures in the treatment of trigeminal neuralgia has been confirmed by numerous series over 15 years. Initially, analgesia or hypalgesia was believed to be a normal component of the procedure. Over time, it has been shown that use of lower temperatures can control the paroxysmal pain, while minimizing sensory loss.

Other techniques, such as glycerol rhizolysis and microcompression injury to the gasserian ganglion, have been used to treat trigeminal neuralgia. RF procedures have the most long-term follow-up data, however. Interventional treatment should be reserved for patients whose disease is not controlled by medications and for patients who are unable to use medications because of intolerable side effects.

In one large study, almost 95% of patients had dramatic reductions in paroxysmal pain after RF lesion of the trigeminal ganglion.[121] The mortality rate in this series was 0%, and the morbidity was approximately 35%. Complications included masseter weakness (10.5%), parasthesias requiring medical management (5.2%), painful anesthesia (1.5%), ocular palsies (0.5%), corneal reflex impairment without keratitis (1.7%), corneal reflex impairment with keratitis (0.6%), and vasomotor rhinorrhea (0.1%). Despite a fairly high incidence of manageable complications, most patients were satisfied with the procedure; that is, the relief of pain was so significant that the morbidity was considered relatively minor in comparison.

No long-term prospective studies have compared the efficacy, morbidity, and mortality of RF thermal lesions of the trigeminal ganglion and open decompression of the posterior fossa. Percutaneous procedures might be safer in elderly patients and in patients with serious underlying medical problems. For young, healthy patients with trigeminal neuralgia, many neurosurgeons believe that open decompression is the treatment of choice.

The advantage of the RF procedure is that the lesion can be well controlled. A disadvantage of techniques that use liquid neurolytic agents is possible spread into the subarachnoid space with harm to the central nervous system. A higher incidence of neuropathy is associated with the use of liquid neurolytic agents. Whether or not glycerol produces the same incidence of neuropathy as phenol or alcohol has yet to be shown. Even with glycerol, control of the solution is not as precise as control of a thermal lesion. With a thin, insulated RF cannula and 2-mm active tip, it is possible to produce lesions to individual branches of the trigeminal ganglion without affecting the remaining branches. It is not possible to do this with neurolytic solutions. The technique of percutaneous microcompression of the trigeminal ganglion shows some early promising results, but, as yet, no long-term follow-up has been performed with a sufficient number of patients.

Trigeminal Neuralgia: Symptom Complex

Trigeminal neuralgia is a disease of intermittent facial pain seen commonly in middle-aged and older patients. The pain is usually unilateral and is most commonly associated with the lower divisions of the trigeminal nerve. There are usually pain-free intervals between attacks, and the pain tends to come in paroxysms. It is not unusual for the pain to be provoked by stimulation of trigger points, points on the face, jaw, or neck where the pain can be triggered. Usually, no sensory loss is associated with this disease. The disorder can be associated with other diseases, such as multiple sclerosis, posterior fossa tumors, posterior fossa vascular anomalies, and herpes zoster. For most cases, the cause is unknown.

Patients with trigeminal neuralgia require a comprehensive neurologic evaluation. Appropriate evoked potential and spinal fluid analyses are necessary to rule out the possibility of multiple sclerosis (prevalence 2% to 3%). Most patients with trigeminal neuralgia can be managed medically, most often with carbamazepine. Some patients who are unable to tolerate therapeutic doses of these medications or whose symptoms do not respond may be candidates for interventional management (Fig. 169–49).

Located in the medial aspect of the middle cranial fossa, the gasserian ganglion is surrounded by dura within Meckel's cavern. On the medial aspect of the gasserian ganglion lie the cavernous sinus and internal carotid artery. The ganglion sits posterior and superior to the foramen ovale. Entrance to it is via the foramen ovale, which measures 5 to 10 mm in diameter and 5 to 7 mm in depth. The most important part of the technique of RF ablation of the gasserian ganglion is proper fluoroscopic imaging of the foramen ovale. The most medial aspect of the foramen ovale leads to the first division, the central portion leads to the second division, and the lateral aspect leads to the third division of the gasserian ganglion. The third division is most superficial; the second, intermediate; and the first, the deepest.

Technique of Gasserian Ganglionotomy

Prophylactic antibiotics should be given 1 hour before the operative procedure. The patient is placed in the supine position with the neck extended. A steep subzygomatic fluoroscopic view is taken with 10 to 15 degrees of lateral rotation. The foramen ovale can be directly visualized "just medial" to the mandibular arch. To perform this technique smoothly, the needle should be passed in a line parallel to the fluoroscopic

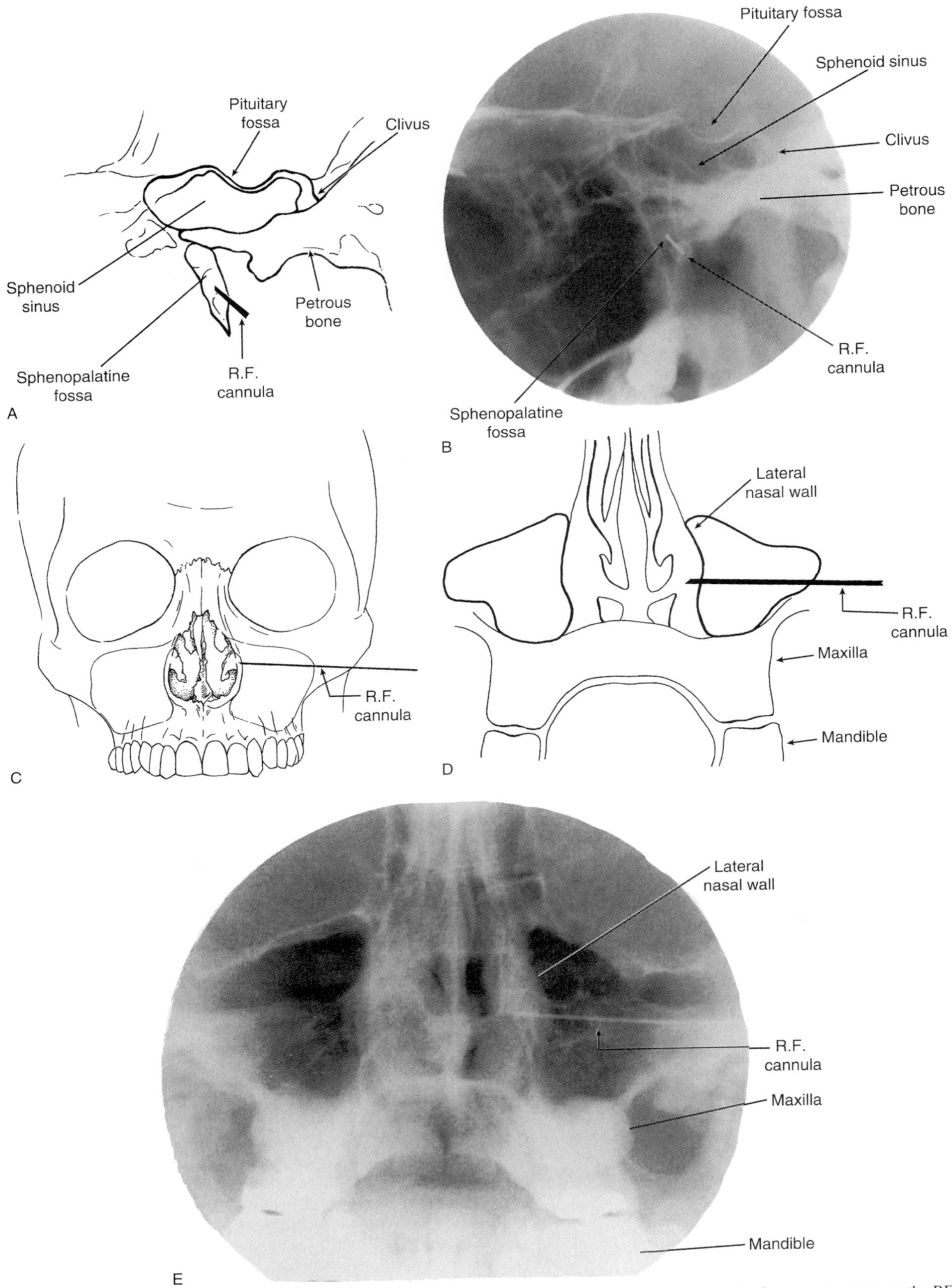

FIGURE 169–48 ■ **A** and **B,** Drawing and radiograph are lateral views of the base of the skull as it is seen on the fluoroscopy screen as the RF cannula passes through the sphenopalatine fossa toward the sphenopalatine ganglion. Note the relative positions of the identified structures. **C,** Drawing of a posteroanterior view through the nasal and maxillary region. The RF cannula is shown entering the lateral wall of the nasal cavity. The sphenopalatine ganglion resides within the lateral wall of the nasal cavity (middle turbinate). **D** and **E,** Drawing and radiograph show a closer view of the lateral walls of the nasal cavity and the maxilla. Note the relative positions of the lateral wall of the nasal cavity and the RF cannula. (**B** and **E** from Waldman SD: Interventional Pain Management, 2nd ed. Philadelphia, WB Saunders, 2001, p 281.)

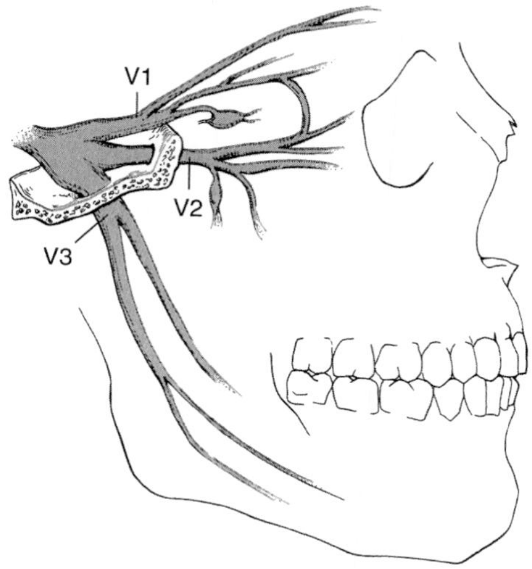

FIGURE 169–49 ■ Drawing of the distribution of the trigeminal nerves. V1 is the first division; V2, the second; and V3, the third division of the trigeminal system.

beam. Doing this enables the electrode to follow the beam directly into the foramen ovale, eliminating all guesswork and allowing precise positioning of the cannula. With this technique, superficial landmarks are no longer needed because the operator simply follows the beam directly to the target site.

The technique of RF lesioning of the gasserian ganglion is described here as it is performed in a patient with trigeminal neuralgia of the first division. The patient is positioned as previously described. The x-ray beam should be directly beneath the zygoma with 10 to 15 degrees of lateral rotation, to bring the foramen ovale clearly into view. A mark is placed on the skin overlying the foramen ovale as seen under fluoroscopy (usually 1 to 2 cm lateral and 1 cm inferior to the corner of the mouth). In this example, the electrode tip is directed toward the most medial aspect of the foramen ovale.

After the patient's face has been prepared and draped, an anesthetic dose of propofol (isopropyl phenol) is given intravenously by the monitoring anesthesiologist. The physician performing the procedure should not be involved in giving the anesthetic. After the patient has lost consciousness but is breathing spontaneously, the physician places one finger in the patient's mouth and advances the RF cannula percutaneously. The finger is in the mouth to detect penetration of the oral cavity. If this occurs, the cannula should be removed, and a new cannula should be used. As the cannula is advanced subcutaneously beneath the zygoma, it is directed parallel to the fluoroscopic beam and toward the foramen ovale. The cannula is advanced to the medial aspect of the foramen ovale, then approximately 2 mm farther after it has entered the canal (Fig. 169–50). A lateral view is obtained through the region of the petrous bone and clivus. The cannula is advanced farther, until it reaches the junction of the petrous mass and the clivus. At this point, the stylet of the cannula is removed, and slow leakage of CSF should be seen, indicating that the dura within Meckel's cavern has been punctured.

After the patient has emerged from the anesthetic, stimulation is performed. At 50-Hz stimulation, good paresthesia along the first division of the fifth nerve should be noted at less than 0.5 V. At 2-Hz stimulation, one should fail to see masseter muscle contraction with 0.7 to 1 V. For lesioning of the third division, it may not be possible to avoid masseter stimulation, and some mild masseter weakness may be an unavoidable result. It is best to give additional doses of propofol if the cannula is advanced or withdrawn because such maneuvers can be quite painful. After proper paresthesia has been obtained, the first lesion can be created.

The physician can never go wrong choosing a thermal lesion that is too cool. Significant perioperative problems can result, however, from a needle that is too hot. It is best to start with thermal lesions at 60°C for 60 seconds. If the patient has multiple sclerosis, using less heat should be considered. Excessively hot lesioning temperatures can cause deafferentation pain after the procedure.

After appropriate stimulation parameters are identified, the patient is given an additional dose of propofol until consciousness is lost again. At that point, a lesion is made. *Profound anesthesia should be avoided.* Such a lesion can lead to deafferentation pain and loss of the corneal reflex. Done properly, however, most patients achieve excellent pain relief and maintain an adequate corneal reflex. This technique need not be painful or unpleasant for the patient. With modern short-acting intravenous anesthetics, patients can be fully anesthetized for the placement of the cannula and the creation of the lesion.

Thermal lesions of the gasserian ganglion can be useful in the management of intractable cluster headaches that fail to respond to the sphenopalatine lesion. This technique also is useful for treating pain secondary to cancer.

Patients are admitted for overnight observation after the procedure. Dexamethasone should be given immediately after the procedure and for the first 48 hours. This regimen decreases edema and the chances of corneal insensitivity. If there is any drying of the cornea, saline eye drops should be used to lubricate it. Discomfort can last 2 to 4 weeks after the procedure, and appropriate analgesics may be necessary during this period. Some patients also have unpleasant dysesthesias. If patients were taking medications such as carbamazepine preoperatively, the therapy should not be stopped abruptly. All such medications should be tapered in dose over 2 weeks after the procedure. At least 80% of patients can be anticipated to experience high-grade pain relief. In the first year, approximately 15% to 20% of patients have a partial recurrence of pain; for these patients, a second ganglionotomy can be done.

SYMPATHECTOMY IN THE LUMBAR AND THORACIC REGIONS

The use of neurodestructive techniques in the sympathetic nervous system was first described in 1924.[122] The technique was later refined and used to promote improved blood flow in patients with peripheral vascular disease.[123] Over the years, lumbar sympathectomy has been shown to be useful in the treatment of certain patients with reflex sympathetic dystrophy, vascular occlusive diseases, vasospastic diseases (Raynaud syndrome), and other types of sympathetically maintained pain. Sympathectomy, with resultant vasodilation, improved blood flow, and higher temperatures in the arm and leg, can be achieved readily and safely with percutaneous RF lesions of the thoracic or lumbar sympathetic chain. The tech-

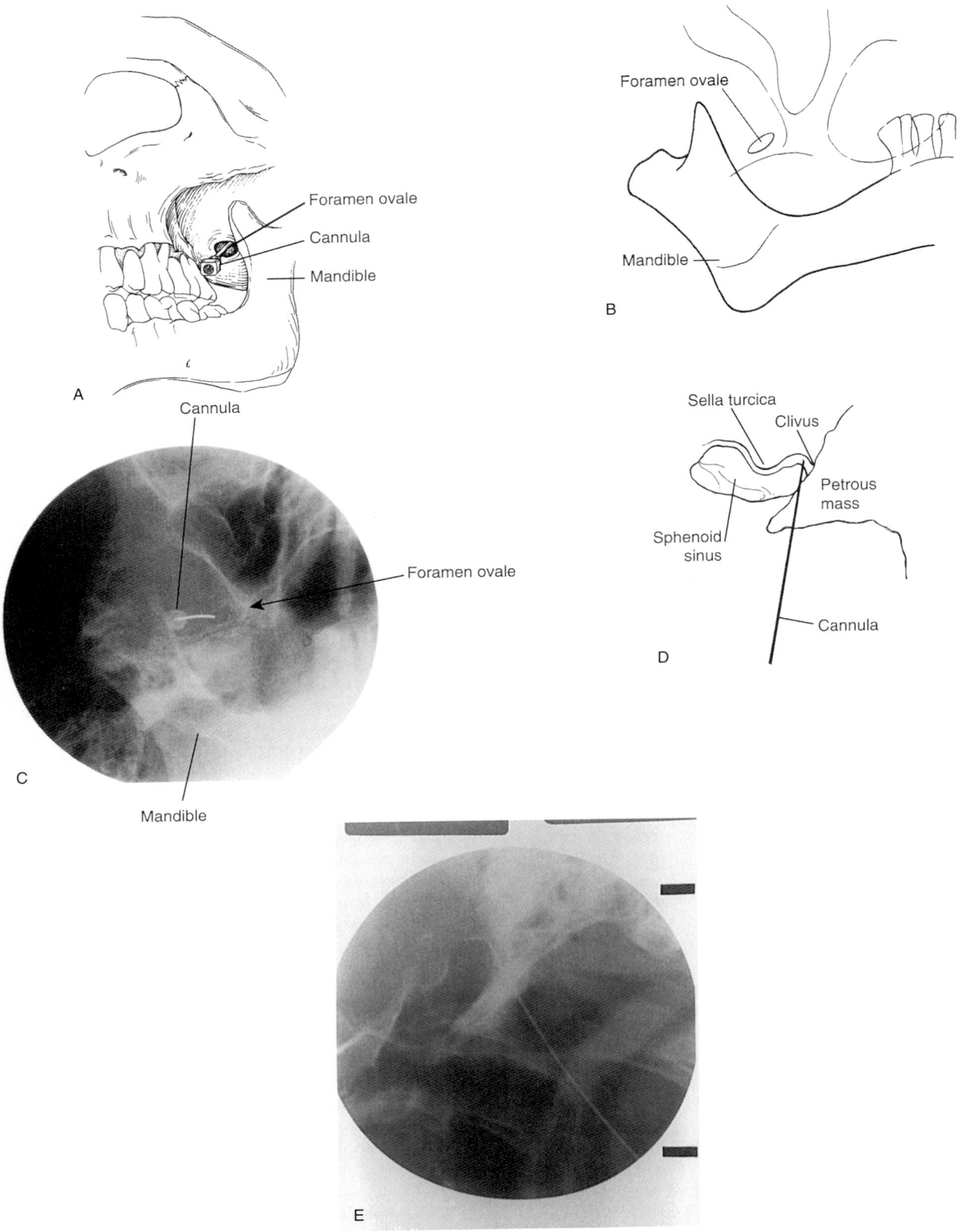

FIGURE 169–50 ■ **A,** Drawing shows the entry of an RF cannula into the foramen ovale. The cannula passes beneath the zygoma to enter the foramen ovale at the base of the skull. **B** and **C,** Drawing and radiograph of the steep subzygomatic view as seen on the fluoroscopy screen. With approximately 15 degrees of lateral angulation, the foramen ovale is seen just inside the upper aspect of the mandible. **C,** The RF cannula has entered the lateralmost aspect of the foramen ovale. **D,** Drawing of the lateral view through the base of the skull as it appears during placement of an RF cannula through the foramen ovale. Note the relationships between the identified structures. The RF cannula tip is just at the junction of the clivus with the sphenoid sinus. **E,** Lateral radiograph through the base of the skull shows the RF cannula passing through the junction of the sphenoid sinus and the clivus. (**C** and **E** from Waldman SD: Interventional Pain Management, 2nd ed. Philadelphia, WB Saunders, 2001, p 284.)

nique of RF lumbar sympathectomy has been well-described in the literature.[124-126]

Anatomy of Lumbar Sympathetic Chain

In the lumbar region, the sympathetic chain and ganglia extend from L1 to L5. These chains are continuous with the thoracic sympathetic chain above and the pelvic sympathetic fibers below. In the lumbar region, the sympathetic chain and its ganglia lie near the anterolateral surface of the vertebral body. There is variability in the position, but the chain always lies anterior to the psoas sheath. The sympathetic chain and ganglia are separated from the somatic nerves, and if the RF cannula is placed properly, precise lesions of the sympathetic chain and ganglia can be performed without producing injury to the somatic nerves. RF lesioning of the sympathetic nerves should not be performed until fluoroscopy-directed test blocks with local anesthetic have shown a desired clinical effect.

The aorta and inferior vena cava sit just anterior to the body of the vertebra, and puncture of these structures should be avoided. The ureters and somatic nerves are close to the sympathetic chain, and injury to these structures must be avoided. At L2-3, the genitofemoral nerve lies close to the sympathetic chain, and injury to this structure can cause severe postoperative groin pain.

The test block should be performed using only 2 mL of combination local anesthetic with a final concentration of 1% lidocaine and 0.25% bupivacaine at each level. The test block should be done at L2-4 or, if the foot is involved, at L3-5. The purpose of a small volume of local anesthetic is to avoid extravasation onto the somatic nerves (which would invalidate the test block). A proper sympathetic test block produces sympathetic blockade with no loss of sensory or motor function. If sensory or motor dysfunction is noted after the test block, the results are invalid, and the test must be repeated. If possible, sedation should not be used during sympathetic test blocks because it can prevent proper interpretation of the clinical results. If absolutely necessary, only short-acting agents, such as propofol, should be given.

Technique of Lesioning of the Lumbar Sympathetic Chain and Ganglia

The patient is placed in the prone position on the fluoroscopy table and is sedated and monitored. A C-arm fluoroscopic device is used to identify the vertebral bodies at L2-4. If the foot is involved, L5 needs to be lesioned as well. The sympathetic ganglia at L2 and L3 can vary, sometimes being 15 mm posterior to the anterior aspect of the vertebral body (depending on the level). The ganglion at L2 rests near the junction of the lower third with the upper two thirds of the vertebral body. The ganglion at L3 lies near the junction of the upper third with the lower two thirds of the vertebral body. It is preferable to lesion these levels to include the sympathetic chain and its associated ganglia to produce a longer-lasting lesion. The position of the L4 ganglion is more variable than that of the L2 and L3 ganglia.

The new curved-blunt RF cannula (discussed earlier) should be considered for RF lumbar sympathectomy procedures. An electrode 150 mm in length with a curved 10-mm active tip is used. A posterior view under fluoroscopic guidance is used to identify the second, third, and fourth vertebral bodies. An oblique view is taken with craniad or caudad rotation so that the disk space is sharply visualized. With the fluoroscopic device obliquely rotated to approximately 20 degrees (so that the vertebral bodies "cover" the transverse processes), the cannulas are inserted and directed toward the target points described earlier. The cannulas should be directed parallel to the fluoroscopy beam until the lateral aspect of the vertebra is contacted.

Small amounts of intravenous sedation are given to enable the patient to lie comfortably during placement of the RF cannulas. After contact with the vertebral bodies has been made, a lateral view is taken. The cannulas are advanced so that they touch the periosteum of the vertebral body, and they are moved anteriorly until they contact the anterior aspect. The fluoroscopy unit is moved to produce a posteroanterior view. The cannulas are in correct position when their tips are directly behind the middle of the facet joint line while in contact with the vertebral body.

At 50-Hz stimulation, the patient should develop a deep pain in the back at approximately 1 V. Lower extremity motor fasciculations should be negative with 3 V at 2-Hz stimulation. If sensory stimulation at L2 or L3 provokes parasthesias in the groin, the cannula should be repositioned because it is too close to the genitofemoral nerve. When the radiologic criteria have been met, and the stimulation parameters are correct, the lesions can be made.

The lesions are made after 1 mL of 2% lidocaine is injected through the cannula. A thermal lesion is created for 60 seconds at 80°C. At the L2 level, one lesion is adequate to produce a 10-mm lesion from the anterior aspect of the vertebral body posteriorly. The cannulas at L3 and L4 should be positioned initially at a point 5 mm posterior to the anterior aspect of the vertebral body. Stimulation and lesioning should be done at this position. The cannulas should be moved 5 mm anterior for the second stimulation and lesion at each of these levels. With this technique, the cannulas are moved away from the segmental nerves when the second lesion is done. A 15-mm "strip" lesion is made at L3 and L4, and a 10-mm lesion is made at L2. If the foot is involved, another 15-mm lesion must be made at L5. The lesions at each level are made between the anterior aspect of the vertebral body and the anteromedial aspect of the psoas sheath (Fig. 169–51).

Injury to the genitofemoral nerve (which could produce neuropathic pain in the groin) is a potential complication. Injury to the somatic nerves, with subsequent sensory or motor loss, is possible, but can be avoided with proper stimulation. Retrograde ejaculation can occur in men and is seen more often after bilateral lumbar sympathectomy. Postoperative discomfort lasts approximately 5 days, but pain relief should be immediate if the lesions have been targeted correctly.

The incidence of injury to the lumbar spinal and genitofemoral nerves is higher with liquid neurolytic techniques than with the RF procedure, which also produces a better-controlled lesion. Vascular uptake of neurolytic solutions can lead to complications. Ureteral injuries also may occur with neurolytic agents.

The low morbidity and almost zero mortality with the RF technique speak well for its safety. The technique can be repeated if necessary, and the repeat procedure carries no higher risk of morbidity than the first one. The RF technique is an outpatient procedure and is safer and more

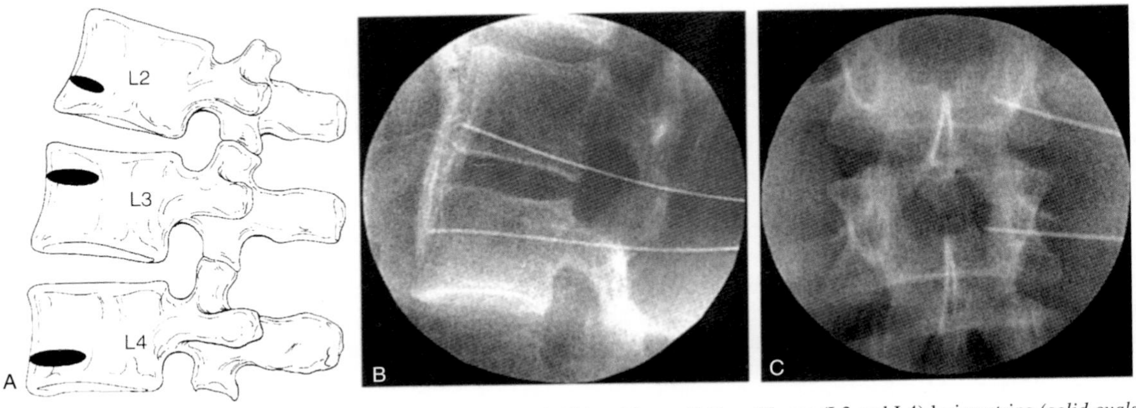

FIGURE 169–51 ■ **A,** Drawing of the vertebral bodies of L2, L3, and L4. Either 10-mm (L2) or 15-mm (L3 and L4) lesion strips *(solid ovals)* are used to interrupt the lumbar sympathetic chain. Note the positions of the lesion strips relative to the anterior aspect of the vertebral bodies. The lumbar sympathetic chain is always anterior to the psosas muscle, but the relative positions of the sympathetic chain with the anterior aspect of the vertebral body can vary. Using lesion strips increases the probability of interrupting the sympathetic chain with an RF lesion. **B,** Lateral radiograph shows the RF cannula positions at the L2 and L3 levels for lesioning of the lumbar sympathetic chain. **C,** Posteroanterior radiograph shows the RF cannula positions during lesioning of the lumbar sympathetic chain. The tips of the RF cannulas are directly behind the facet joint line. (**B** and **C** from Waldman SD: Interventional Pain Management, 2nd ed. Philadelphia, WB Saunders, 2001, p 285.)

cost-effective than open surgical sympathectomy. Given the low morbidity, almost zero mortality, cost-effectiveness, and ability to repeat the technique if necessary, RF ablation of the lumbar sympathetic chain seems to be the procedure of choice for producing long-term lumbar sympatholysis.

Lesioning of Thoracic Sympathetic Structures

Anatomy and Test Blocks

The upper thoracic sympathetic chain is an extension of the cervical sympathetic chain and continues caudad. It lies along the periosteum of the vertebral body farther posterior than the lumbar sympathetic chain (Fig. 169–52A).[127] The technique of upper thoracic RF sympathectomy has been thoroughly discussed in the literature.[128-131]

The technique of thoracic sympathectomy usually involves lesions of the sympathetic chain at T2 and T3. These levels have significant outflow to the upper extremity and can be involved in sympathetically maintained upper extremity pain. A small amount of local anesthetic placed on the stellate ganglion tends to produce physiologic effects similar to those seen when a small amount of local anesthetic is placed on the thoracic sympathetic chain at T2 and T3 (i.e., a warm, dry, vasodilated upper extremity). The T2 and T3 levels probably have even more outflow to the hand than does C7, however. Test blocks should be performed with local anesthetic before the RF procedure and should be performed under direct fluoroscopic guidance. The volume of local anesthetic solution should be limited to 2 mL to produce precise and highly reproducible results. If the patient obtains greater relief when the cervical sympathetic fibers are anesthetized, it is prudent to perform an RF lesion of those fibers (see section on lesioning of the stellate ganglion). If test blocks of the T2 and T3 sympathetic chain show more favorable results, an RF lesion of the T2 and T3 sympathetic fibers should be performed. In some instances, lesions to the cervical and the thoracic outflow are needed to control symptoms.

Posterior Parasagittal Approach

The thoracic nerve root, dorsal root ganglia, sympathetic ganglia, and splanchnic structures may be reached by a novel posterior parasagittal approach using curved electrodes. This approach provides access to the thoracic paravertebral sympathetic structures at any level from T2 through T12, decreases the risk of inadvertent pneumothorax, and allows access to the midthoracic levels, which were previously difficult to approach safely using a traditional posterolateral approach. The use of blunt-tipped electrodes greatly improves the safety of thoracic posterior parasagittal techniques, especially when applied toward lesions of the thoracic sympathetic and splanchnic structures. This "posterior parasagittal curved-needle approach" developed by one of the authors (W.Y.) has been used in more than 500 individual thoracic segmental procedures, with no pneumothorax to date.

The technique takes advantage of the fact that the thoracic paravertebral ganglionic structures generally lie directly ventral and medial to the junction of the inferior medial border of the transverse processes with the superior lateral thoracic lamina at the same level when viewed in the anteroposterior fluoroscopic plane. This bony landmark is constant throughout the thoracic region from T1 to T11; at the level of T12, radiographically, the transverse process is essentially vestigial. The necessity to steer the tip of the electrode during fluoroscopically guided placement demands a curved-tip electrode. Blunt-tipped and cutting-tip 20-gauge RF electrodes with 10-mm active tips are commercially available (Radionics, Inc, Burlington, Mass) in 100-mm lengths. The blunt-tipped ones are recommended for thoracic paravertebral sympathetic ganglionic and splanchnic RF procedures. For discrete selective thoracic dorsal root ganglion RF procedures, 22-gauge, 100-mm, short-beveled electrodes with 2- to 5-mm active tips are preferred (see earlier sections).

All percutaneous thoracic procedures carry the risk of pneumothorax, even in skilled hands. Paravertebral procedures carry the risk of vascular, visceral (e.g., esophagus, bronchi), and nerve (e.g., spinal cord, vagus, phrenic,

A

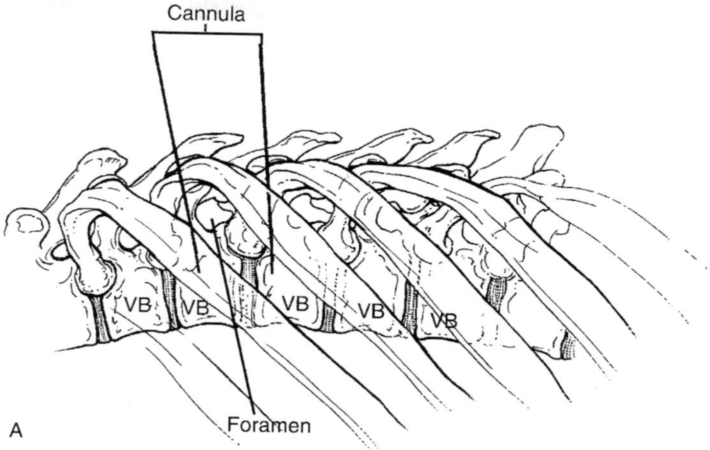

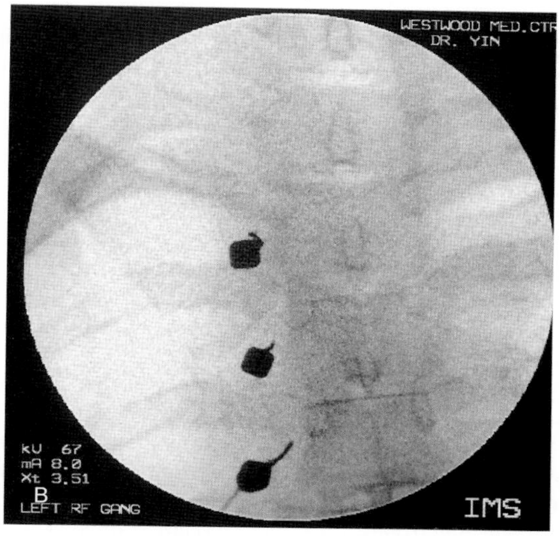

FIGURE 169–52 ■ **A,** Drawing of a lateral view through the thoracic spine. Note the relative positions of the thoracic foramina, the vertebral bodies (VB), and the tips of the RF cannulas. This is the correct position for RF lesions of the thoracic sympathetic chain at the T2 and T3 levels. **B,** Anteroposterior image of electrode placement for left T2-4 posterior parasagittal sympathetic ganglia RF lesion. Note medial orientation of electrode tips toward the costovertebral junction approaching the posterolateral aspect of vertebral bodies, beneath lamina. (**B** from Waldman SD: Interventional Pain Management, 2nd ed. Philadelphia, WB Saunders, 2001, p 286.)

intercostal) injury and the potential to injure other anatomically proximal structures (e.g., lymphatic vessels). These procedures should be performed only by skilled physicians who are experts in percutaneous stereotactic RF interventions under fluoroscopic guidance.

In the upper thoracic region (T1-6), the thoracic sympathetic ganglia lie just ventral to the level of the heads of the ribs, approximately at the junction of the dorsal and middle thirds of the vertebral body as visualized in lateral projections and just deep to the thoracic parietal pleura. In the lower thoracic region (T7-12), the sympathetic ganglia may lie slightly more ventral, approaching the midpoint of the vertebral body in lateral projections. In contrast to the corresponding ganglia in the lumbar regions, the thoracic sympathetic ganglia *do not* lie along the anterolateral aspect of the vertebral bodies.

A common posterior parasagittal fluoroscopically guided approach may be made toward the thoracic nerve root, dorsal root ganglia, sympathetic ganglia, and, in the lower thoracic region, splanchnic nerves. The patient is placed prone on the fluoroscopy table, and the skin of the back is prepared in the standard fashion. Anteroposterior fluoroscopic images are obtained, and the imaging system is tilted cephalad or caudad to "square off" the vertebral end plates of the area of interest. The inferomedial border of the transverse process at its junction with the superior lateral lamina of the level desired is identified, and a skin entry site is marked and anesthetized directly overlying this mark. If the recommended blunt-tipped electrodes are used, a $1\frac{1}{4}$-inch, 16-gauge intravenous catheter is introduced percutaneously at a depth just sufficient to penetrate the dermis and underlying thoracic paravertebral fascia. (Overvigorous insertion of this introducer cannula may result in inadvertent lung injury.)

The blunt, curved-tip electrode is inserted through the introducer cannula and directed under anteroposterior fluoroscopic guidance to contact the bony landmark previously described. After contact is made with bone, the electrode tip is rotated laterally, and the electrode is advanced just past the lateral lamina. When past the lamina, the electrode tip is immediately rotated medially and directed toward the superior lateral vertebral body (Fig. 169–52B). Lateral fluoroscopic images are obtained to ascertain the depth of electrode placement. Maintaining medial electrode tip direction, the electrode may be advanced to the desired level before sensory stereotactic localization of the target structure. In the upper thoracic spine (levels T1-4), the transverse processes are relatively prominent, and care must be taken to ensure that the tip of the electrode is directed medially when it is past the level of the lateral lamina.

When past the lamina, the electrodes are advanced until contact is made with the superolateral aspect of the vertebral body. (The operator takes care to avoid transfixing the exiting thoracic nerve root; if radiating paresthesias are encountered at this stage, the electrode is withdrawn and redirected, with the approach adjusted slightly caudal, aiming to traverse medial and caudal to the exiting nerve root.) The blunt-tipped electrodes are advanced along the periosteum of the thoracic vertebral body, with the depth of placement guided by lateral fluoroscopic imaging. When the active tip of the electrode has bisected the imaginary junction between the dorsal and middle thirds of the vertebral body, further advance is halted, and anteroposterior images are obtained to verify electrode placement directly adjacent to the vertebral body. Because there may be only 2 to 3 mm of potential space between the lateral thoracic vertebral periosteum and the pleura, meticulous attention to multiplanar fluoroscopic technique and use of blunt-tipped RF cannulas are imperative to minimize risk of pneumothorax or collateral tissue injury. The distal tips of the electrodes are oriented cephalad. Lateral fluoroscopic images are obtained to verify that the electrode tip does not venture near the ventral aspect of the vertebral body; thermal lesioning of the esophagus might result, with disastrous consequence (Fig. 169–53). Anteroposterior fluoroscopic images are obtained again to verify juxtaposition of the electrode to the vertebral body. Careful aspiration is performed, and a confirmatory contrast study is performed to verify electrode placement in the paravertebral potential space. In the upper thoracic region, oblique fluoroscopic projections may be useful if the scapulae and humeri compromise adequate visualization (Fig. 169–54).

Sensory stereotactic stimulation is performed at 0.5 to 0.7 V at 50 Hz, 1-msec pulse duration. Reproduction of concordant pain is sought with sequential sensory stimulation of the sympathetic ganglia. Elicitation of radiating somatic dermatomal pain indicates stimulation of the thoracic nerve roots, and the electrodes must be repositioned ventrally or angled more cephalad and ventral to the exiting nerve root. After concordant pain is reproduced, signifying successful stereotactic localization of symptomatic sympathetic ganglia, fine manipulation of the electrode tip is performed under real-time fluoroscopic imaging to maximize stimulation, while the stimulation threshold is decreased to 0.3 to 0.5 V. In our experience, reproduction of sympathetic-mediated pain with ganglionic stimulation may require higher stimulation voltages than reproduction of somatic pain.

After the symptomatic sympathetic ganglia levels have been localized with sensory stereotaxy, motor stimulation is performed to verify adequate electrode distance from the exiting thoracic nerve roots and to verify that other motor nerves (e.g., phrenic nerve) would not be involved in the ensuing thermal lesion. Before RF lesioning, 1 to 1.5 mL of 2% lidocaine is injected. The lesion generally is made at 80°C for 60 seconds.

The positioning of even blunt-tipped electrodes in the thoracic paravertebral region is often accompanied by significant patient discomfort. The judicious application of small amounts of reversible intravenous benzodiazepine and opioid analgesia may be required. The services of a qualified anesthesiologist administering intravenous analgesia may be invaluable. Bolus infusions of short-acting induction agents (e.g., isopropyl phenol or thiopental) are discouraged because of concerns of involuntary patient movement and concerns of providing adequate airway management should overzealous sedation result in respiratory depression or airway obstruction. As with other functional stereotactic procedures, the patient must be fully awake and capable of fine sensory discrimination before sensory stereotactic localization of the sympathetic ganglia is undertaken.

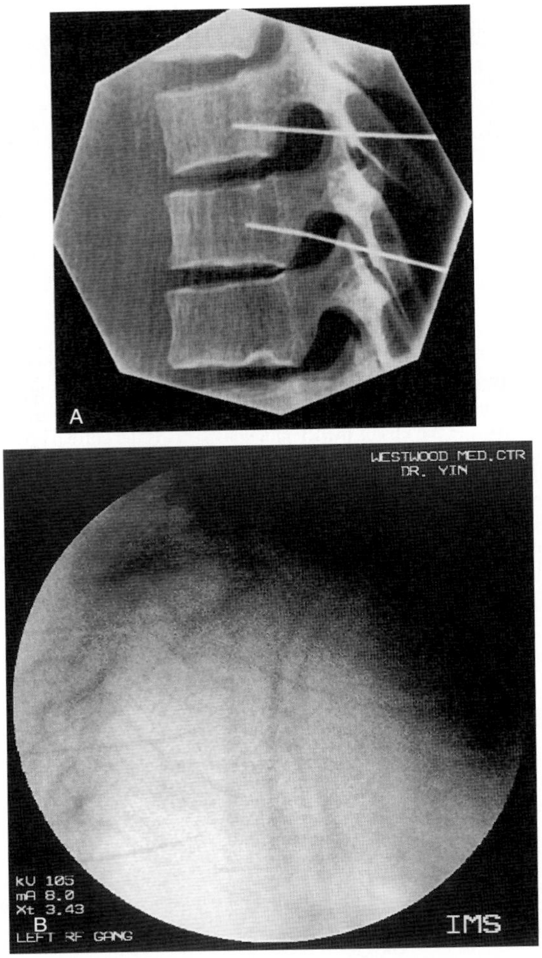

FIGURE 169–53 ■ **A,** Lateral view through skeleton shows T2-3 sympathetic lesion. **B,** Lateral radiograph of electrode placement for T2-4 sympathetic ganglion RF lesion. Note active tips of electrodes overlapping the junction of posterior and middle thirds of vertebral bodies. (From Waldman SD: Interventional Pain Management, 2nd ed. Philadelphia, WB Saunders, 2001, p 288.)

Thoracic Splanchnic Denervation

Thoracic splanchnic denervation provides a lesion-specific alternative to lytic celiac plexus injection and chemical splanchnectomy for the management of chronic celiac plexus–mediated pain. The thoracic splanchnic nerves provide afferent and efferent autonomic (primarily sympathetic) and sensory innervation to many of the retroperitoneal viscera of the upper abdominal area. Afferent sensory fibers may conduct sensation from the capsule of the spleen, liver (Glisson capsule), biliary tree, kidneys, and pancreas,[132] and they have been surgically ablated for the treatment of suprarenal and essential hypertension (Pende and Peet procedures).[133] Chemical splanchnectomy has been shown to equal lytic celiac plexus injection in efficacy.[134] Percutaneous

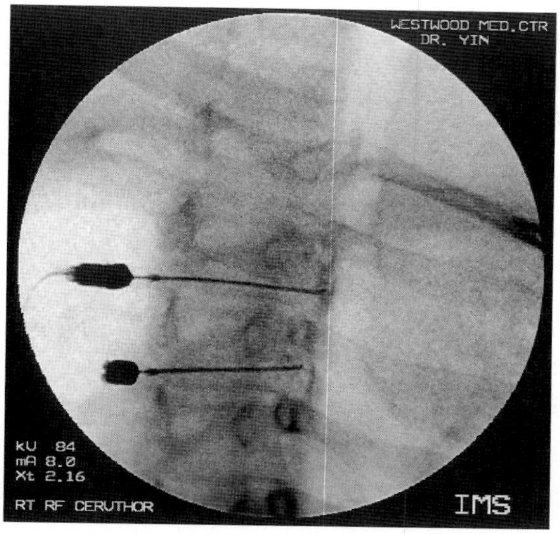

FIGURE 169–54 ■ Oblique projection illustrates electrode placement and contrast study for right T2 and T3 sympathetic ganglia RF lesion. Contrast medium is limited to the paravertebral region at the junction of rib heads and vertebral bodies. (From Waldman SD: Interventional Pain Management, 2nd ed. Philadelphia, WB Saunders, 2001, p 288.)

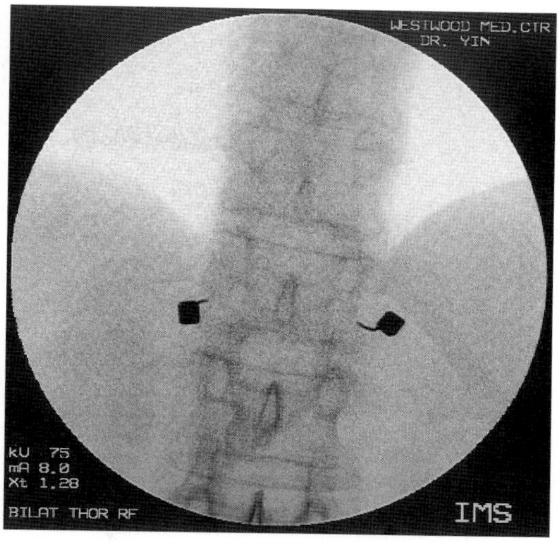

FIGURE 169–55 ■ Anteroposterior image of RF electrode placement for bilateral thoracic stereotactic splanchnic lesion. Note position of electrodes close to the lateral aspect of T12 vertebral body. (From Waldman SD: Interventional Pain Management, 2nd ed. Philadelphia, WB Saunders, 2001, p 288.)

stereotactic RF thoracic splanchnic lesions may be used for the control of celiac plexus–mediated retroperitoneal visceral pain and, in contrast to other techniques of neurolysis, provide advantages of definitive identification of pain-conducting structures and generation of a controlled neurolytic lesion of predictable size. Before consideration of thoracic RF splanchnic lesioning, confirmatory low-volume thoracic splanchnic injections must be performed.

Three splanchnic nerves have been identified in adults. The greater splanchnic nerve, composed of myelinated preganglionic and visceral afferent fibers, typically is thought to provide primary sensory innervation to the pancreas and proximal retroperitoneal visceral structures and generally arises from the thoracic sympathetic ganglia of T5-9. The lesser splanchnic nerve (approximately 95% of adults have one) arises from filaments from the sympathetic ganglia of T9-12, and the least splanchnic nerve (55% of adults have one) may be related to the thoracic splanchnic ganglion at T12.[135] The splanchnic nerves course over the anterior lateral and lateral thoracic vertebral bodies ventral to the thoracic sympathetic chain.

A common stereotactic RF lesion of the splanchnic nerves is made with a posterior parasagittal approach at the level of T12. Because of the relative proximity of the individual splanchnic nerves (greater, lesser, least), it may be impossible to lesion any one of these particular nerves definitively and differentially. Sensory stereotaxy is invaluable in establishing the location of symptomatic splanchnic fibers before RF lesioning.

In contrast to other thoracic levels, the transverse process of T12 is generally small and may not be visible on anteroposterior radiographs. The skin entry site is marked over the lateral aspect of the vertebral body at T12, at the junction of the caudal (inferior) and middle thirds of the vertebral body, caudad to the exiting T12 nerve root (Fig. 169–55). A 16-gauge intravenous introducer catheter is introduced as previously described, and a 100-mm, 10-mm active tip, blunt, curved-tip electrode is inserted through the introducer cannulas. The electrodes are directed under anteroposterior fluoroscopic imaging to contact the posterolateral aspect of the T12 vertebral body. Lateral images are obtained to guide initial depth of electrode placement. The electrodes are advanced along the periosteum of the lateral aspect of the T12 vertebral body until the distal tip of the electrode approaches the junction of the middle and ventral (anterior) thirds of the vertebral body on lateral radiographs (Fig. 169–56). The procedure is repeated on the contralateral side. It is imperative that the distal extent of the electrodes does not approach the ventral

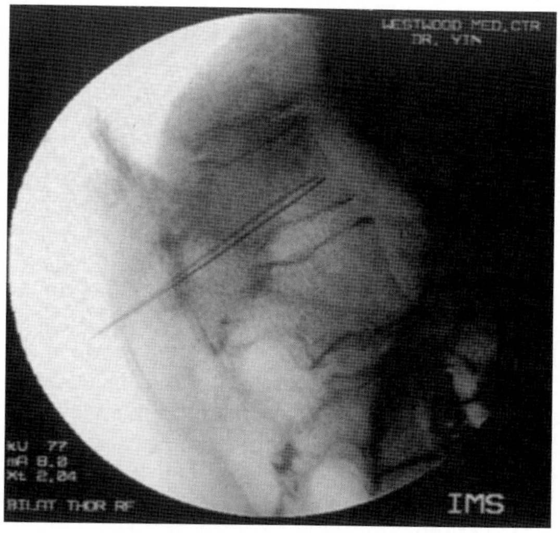

FIGURE 169–56 ■ Lateral image illustrates absolutely farthest ventral placement of RF electrodes for thoracic stereotactic splanchnic lesion. (From Waldman SD: Interventional Pain Management, 2nd ed. Philadelphia, WB Saunders, 2001, p 289.)

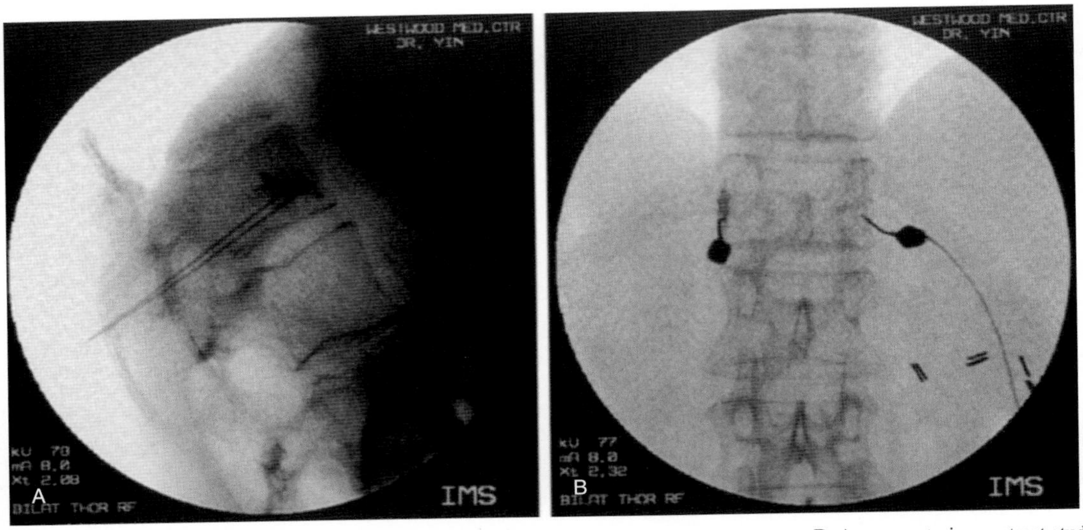

FIGURE 169–57 ■ **A,** Lateral contrast study before stereotactic localization of thoracic splanchnic nerves. **B,** Anteroposterior contrast study during stereotactic splanchnic lesion. (From Waldman SD: Interventional Pain Management, 2nd ed. Philadelphia, WB Saunders, 2001, p 290.)

aspect of the vertebral body; esophageal injury might result, with devastating consequences. Careful aspiration tests and contrast studies are performed, and confirmatory anteroposterior and lateral radiographs are taken. The spread of contrast material should remain in the immediate paravertebral region; some caudal spread of contrast material may be seen if the electrodes rest ventral and medial to the crus of the diaphragm (Fig. 169–57).

Sensory stereotactic localization of the splanchnic nerves is performed; initial stimulation may require 0.7 to 1 V. Subjective localized back pain is common in the higher range of stimulating voltages. The electrodes are maneuvered incrementally along the lateral aspect of the T12 vertebral body until the patient's visceral pain is reproduced. The stimulating voltage is decreased to the target range of 0.3 to 0.5 V with further fine manipulation of the electrode. As with thoracic sympathetic stereotaxy, radiating paresthesias along the flank indicate stimulation of the T12 nerve root. Should they occur, the electrode must be repositioned before RF lesioning, to avoid unintentional thermal injury to the nerve root. Motor stimulation is performed at 2 Hz, 1 to 1.5 V to verify that the distal electrode is not in the immediate vicinity of the phrenic nerve. If sensory stereotaxy does not reproduce concordant pain, lesions may be performed, although with a correspondingly lower expectation of success. RF lesions are performed at 80°C for 60 seconds. Secondary and tertiary lesions are performed overlapping the 50°C to 55°C isotherm of previous lesions to ensure adequate splanchnic denervation.

As with all thoracic percutaneous paravertebral procedures, the patient is observed in the recovery area for signs of respiratory compromise or other complication, and postprocedure chest films are mandatory before discharge. Typically, splanchnic denervation is tolerated well; a predominant complaint is back pain that subsides within the first several postoperative days and generally responds to mild opioid analgesics or nonsteroidal antiinflammatory drug. The relief of visceral pain is typically immediate when the procedure is successful. Postoperative complaints of worsening abdominal pain or chest pain must be evaluated promptly because potential complications could include visceral (pancreatic, esophageal, pulmonary) or major vascular injury (hemorrhagic complications).

Acknowledgments

The authors thank William Rittman III and Eric Cosman, PhD, for technical and historical data provided; Wolfram Klawitter from Ziehm International, for his technical support and assistance in the capture and reproduction of the fluoroscopic images contained herein; Don Garlotta and Beverly Sanchez, for their technical assistance in the operating rooms in the capture and reproduction of the fluoroscopic images contained herein; and Barbara Urmston, for her support and preparation of the manuscript.

References

1. Onik GM, Porterfield B, Rubinsky B, Cohen J: Percutaneous transperineal prostate cryosurgery using transrectal ultrasound guidance: Animal model. Urology 37:277, 1991.
2. Onik GM, Cohen JK, Reyes GD, et al: Transrectal ultrasound-guided percutaneous radical cryosurgical ablation of the prostate. Cancer 72:1291, 1993.
3. Mundinger F, Weigel K: Long-term results of stereotactic interstitial curietherapy. Acta Neurochir Suppl (Wien) 33:367, 1984.
4. Ostertag CB, Groothius D, Kleihue P: Experimental data on early and late morphologic effects on permanently implanted gamma and beta sources (iridium 1692, iodine 125, and yttrium 90) in the brain. Acta Neurochir Suppl (Wien) 33:271, 1984.
5. Ostertag CB, Weigel K, Birg W: CT after long-standing implantation of cerebral gliomas. In Szikla G (ed): Stereotactic Cerebral Irradiation. Amsterdam, Elsevier/North Holland, 1979.
6. Gutin PH, Bernstein M, Sanyo Y, et al: Combination therapy with BCNU and low dose rate radiation in the 9L rat brain tumor and spheroid models: Implications for brain tumor brachytherapy. Neurosurgery 15:781, 1984.
7. Gutin PH, Dormandy RH: A coaxial catheter system for afterloading radioactive sources for the interstitial irradiation of brain tumors. J Neurosurg 56:734, 1982.
8. Gutin PH, Phillips TL, Hosobuchi Y, et al: Permanent and removable sources for the brachytherapy of brain tumors. Int J Radiat Oncol Biol Phys 7:1371, 1981.

9. Gutin PH, Phillips TL, Wara WM, et al: Brachytherapy of recurrent malignant brain tumors with removable high-activity iodine-125 sources. J Neurosurg 60:61, 1984.
10. Gutin PH, Phillips TL, Wara WM, et al: Brachytherapy with removable ^{125}I sources for the treatment of recurrent malignant brain tumors. Acta Neurochir Suppl (Wien) 33:363, 1984.
11. Gutin PH, Leibel SA, Wara WM, et al: Recurrent malignant gliomas: Survival following interstitial brachytherapy with high-activity iodine-125 sources. J Neurosurg 67:864, 1987.
12. Kooy HM, Nedzi LA, Loeffler JS, et al: Treatment planning for stereotactic radiosurgery of intracranial lesions. Int J Radiat Oncol Biol Phys 21:683, 1991.
13. Tsai JS, Buck BA, Svensson GK, et al: Quality assurance in stereotactic radiosurgery using a standard linear accelerator. Int J Radiat Oncol Biol Phys 21:737, 1991.
14. Alexander E III, Loeffler JS, Lunsford LD: Stereotactic Radiosurgery. New York, McGraw-Hill, 1993.
15. Young RF: Clinical experience with radiofrequency and laser DREZ lesions. J Neurosurg 72:715, 1990.
16. Sweet WH, Mark VH: Unipolar anodal electrolyte lesions in the brain of man and cat: Report of five human cases with electrically produced bulbar or mesencephalic tractotomies. AMA Arch Neurol Psychiatry 70:224, 1953.
17. Hunsperger RW, Wyss OAM: Production of localized lesions in nervous tissue by coagulation with high frequency current. Helv Physiol Pharmacol Acta 11:283, 1953.
18. Mundinger F, Reichert T, Gabriel E: Untersuchungen zu den physikalischen und technischen Voranssetzungeneiner dosierten Hochfrequenzkoagulation bei stereptaktischen Hirnoperation. Zeitsch Chir 169:1051, 1960.
19. Rosomoff HL, Carroll F, Brown J, Sheptak T: Percutaneous radiofrequency cervical cordotomy: Technique. J Neurosurg 23:639, 1965.
20. Brodkey J, Miyazaki Y, et al: Reversible heat lesions: A method of stereotactic localization. J Neurosurg 21:49, 1964.
21. Cosman ER, Nashold BS, Ovelan-Levitt J: Theoretical aspects of radiofrequency lesions in the dorsal root entry zone. Neurosurgery 156:945, 1984.
22. Fox JL: Experimental relationship of radio-frequency electrical current and lesion size for application to percutaneous cordotomy. J Neurosurg 33:415, 1970.
23. Lin PM, Gildenberg PL, Polakoff PP: An anterior approach to percutaneous lower cervical cordotomy. J Neurosurg 25:553, 1966.
24. Mullan S: Percutaneous cordotomy. J Neurosurg 35:360, 1971.
25. Levin AB, Cosman ER: Thermocouple-monitored cordotomy electrode: Technical note. J Neurosurg 53:266, 1980.
26. Bogduk N, Twomey LT: Clinical Anatomy of the Lumbar Spine. Edinburgh, Churchill Livingstone, 1987.
27. Bogduk N: The innervation of the lumbar spine. Spine 8:286, 1983.
28. Schwarzer AC, Aprill CN, Derby R, et al: The relative contributions of the disc and zygapophysial joint in chronic low back pain. Spine 169:801, 1994.
29. Schwarzer AC, Aprill CN, Derby R, et al: The roles of the zygapophysial joint and intervertebral disc in chronic low back pain: Results of a multicenter study. ISIS Newsletter 2:59, 1994.
30. Travel JG, Simons DG: Myofascial Pain and Dysfunction—the Trigger Point Manual. Baltimore, Williams & Wilkins, 1983.
31. Schwarzer AC, Aprill CN, Bogduk N: The sacroiliac joint in chronic low back pain. Spine 20:31, 1995.
32. Gharpuray V, Clemson S, et al: Intervertebral disc temperature distribution comparison: Radiofrequency needle versus thermal catheter. North American Spine Society, 14th Annual Meeting, Chicago, 1999.
33. Nash TP: Clinical note percutaneous radiofrequency lesioning of dorsal root ganglia for intractable pain. Pain 24:67, 1986.
34. North RB, Kidd DH, Campbell JN, Long DM: Dorsal root ganglionectomy for failed back surgery syndrome: A 5-year follow-up study. J Neurosurg 74:236, 1991.
35. North RB, Zahurak M, Kidd D: Radiofrequency lumbar facet denervation: Analysis of prognostic factors. Pain 57:77, 1994.
36. Ray CD: Percutaneous Radiofrequency Facet Nerve Block. Radionics Procedure Technique Series. Burlington, MA, Radionics Corp, 1982.
37. Sluijter ME: The use of radiofrequency lesions for pain relief in failed back patients. Int Disabil Studies 10:37, 1988.
38. Kline MT: Stereotactic Radiofrequency Lesions as Part of the Management of Chronic Pain. Orlando, Paul M Deutsch, 1992.
39. Goldthwait JE: The lumbosacral articulation: An explanation of many cases of "lumbago," "sciatica" and paraplegia. Boston Med Surg J 64:365, 1911.
40. Putti V: New conceptions in the pathogenesis of sciatic pain. Lancet 2:53, 1927.
41. Williams PC, Yglesias L: Lumbosacral facetectomy for post fusion persistent sciatica. J Bone Joint Surg 15:579, 1933.
42. Ghormely RK: Low back pain with special reference to articular facet with presentation of an operative procedure. JAMA 101:1773, 1933.
43. Helbig T, Lee CK: The lumbar facet syndrome. Spine 13:61, 1988.
44. Anderson KH, Mosel C, Varnet K: Percutaneous facet denervation in low-back and extremity pain. Acta Neurochir (Wien) 87:48, 1987.
45. Arbit E, Krol G: Percutaneous radiofrequency neurolysis guided by computed tomography for the treatment. Neurosurgery 29:580, 1991.
46. Banerjee T, Pittman HH: Facet rhizotomy: Another armamentarium for treatment of low backache. NC Med J 37:354, 1976.
47. Bogduk N, Long DM: Lumbar medical branch neurotomy: A modification of facet denervation. Spine 5:1693, 1980.
48. Burton CV: Percutaneous radiofrequency facet denervation. Appl Neurophysiol 39:80, 1977.
49. Hickey RFJ, Tregonning GD: Denervation of spinal facet joints for treatment of chronic low back pain. NZ Med J 85:96, 1976.
50. Ignelzi RJ, Cummings TW: A statistical analysis of percutaneous radiofrequency lesions in the treatment of chronic low back pain and sciatica. Pain 8:181, 1980.
51. Ignelzi RJ: Radiofrequency lesions in the treatment of lumbar spinal pain. Contemp Neurosurg 12:1, 1990.
52. McCulloch JA: Percutaneous radiofrequency lumbar rhizolysis (rhizotomy). Appl Neurophysiol 39:87, 1976.
53. McCulloch JA, Organ LW: Percutaneous radiofrequency lumbar rhizolysis. Can Med Assoc J 116:300, 1977.
54. Mehta M, Sluijter ME: The treatment of chronic back pain: A preliminary survey of the effect of radiofrequency denervation of the posterior vertebral joints. Anaesthesia 34:768, 1979.
55. Ogbury JS, Simons H, Lehrman RAW: Facet "denervation" in treatment of low back syndrome. Pain 2:257, 1977.
56. Oudenhoven RC: Articular rhizotomy. Surg Neurol 2:275, 1974.
57. Oudenhoven RC: Results of facet denervation. Presented at the International Society for the Study of the Lumbar Spine, Paris, 1981.
58. Pagura JR: Percutaneous radiofrequency spinal rhizotomy. Proceedings of the American Society of Stereotactic and Functional Neurosurgery, Durham, NC. Appl Neurophysiol 46:138, 1983.
59. Pawl RP: Results in the treatment of low back syndrome from sensory neurolysis of the lumbar facets (facet rhizotomy) by thermal coagulation. Proc Inst Med Chicago 30:150, 1974.
60. Pierron D, Robine D, Cornejo M, Dubeaux P: Chronic low back pain and lumbar rhizotomy. Agressologie 32:263, 1991.
61. Rashbaum RF: Radiofrequency facet denervation. Orthop Clin North Am 14:569, 1983.
62. Savitz MH: Percutaneous radiofrequency rhizotomy of the lumbar facets: Ten years' experience. Mt Sinai J Med 58:177, 1991.
63. Schaerer JP: Radiofrequency facet rhizotomy in the treatment of chronic neck and low back pain. Int Surg 63:53, 1978.
64. Schaerer JP: Treatment of prolonged neck pain by radiofrequency facet rhizotomy. Neurol Orthop Med Surg 72:74, 1988.
65. Shealy CN: Percutaneous radiofrequency denervation of spinal facets: Treatment for chronic back pain of sciatica. Neurosurgery 43:448, 1975.
66. Shealy CN: Technique for Percutaneous Spinal Facet Rhizotomy. Radionics Procedure Technique Series. Burlington, MA, Radionics Corp, 1975.
67. Shealy N: Facet denervations in the management of back and sciatic pain. Clin Orthop 115:157, 1976.
68. Sluijiter ME, Mehta M: Recent developments in radiofrequency denervation for chronic back and neck pain (abstract). Pain Suppl 1:290, 1981.
69. Sluijiter ME, Mehta M: Treatment of chronic back and neck pain by percutaneous thermal lesions. In Lipton S, Miles J (eds): Modern Methods of Treatment, vol 3: Persistent Pain. London, Academic Press, 1981, p 141.
70. Sluijiter ME: Percutaneous Thermal Lesions in the Treatment of Back and Neck Pain. Radionics Procedure Techniques Series. Burlington, MA, Radionics Corp, 1981.
71. Stolker RJ, Vervest ACM, Groen GJ: Percutaneous facet denervation in chronic thoracic spinal pain. Acta Neurochir (Wien) 122:82, 1993.

72. Gallagher J, Vadi PLP, Wedley JR, et al: Radiofrequency facet joint denervation in the treatment of low back pain: A prospective controlled double-blind study to assess its efficacy. Pain Clin 7:1693, 1994.
73. Koning HM, Mackie DP: Percutaneous radiofrequency facet denervation in low back pain. Pain Clin 7:1699, 1994.
74. Dreyfuss P, Halbrook B, Pauza K, et al: Lumbar radiofrequency neurotomy for chronic zygaphophysial joint pain. North American Spine Society, 14th Annual Meeting, Chicago, 1999.
75. Taylor JR, Twomey LT, Corker M: Bone and soft tissue injuries in post-mortem lumbar spines. Paraplegia 28:1169, 1990.
76. Twomey LT, Taylor JR, Taylor MM: Unsuspected damage to lumbar zygapophysial joints after motor-vehicle accidents. Med J Aust 151:210, 1989.
77. Schwarzer AC, Wang S-C, O'Driscoll D, et al: The ability of computed tomography to identify a painful zygapophysial joint in patients with chronic low back pain. Spine 20:907, 1991.
78. Schwarzer AC, April CN, Derby R, et al: The false-positive rate of uncontrolled diagnostic blocks of the lumbar zygapophysial joints. Pain 58:1695, 1994.
79. Chua W, Bogduk N: The surgical anatomy of thoracic facet denervation. Acta Neurochir 136:140, 1995.
80. Stolker RJ, Vervest ACM, Ramos LMP, Groen GJ: Electrode positioning in thoracic percutaneous partial rhizotomy: An anatomical study. Pain 57:241, 1994.
81. Bogduk N: Clinical Anatomy of the Lumbar Spine and Sacrum. New York, Churchill Livingstone, 1997.
82. Laslett M, Williams M: The reliability of selected pain provocation tests for sacroiliac joint pathology. Spine 169:1243, 1994.
83. Schwarzer A, Aprill C, et al: The sacroiliac joint in chronic low back pain. Spine 20:31, 1995.
84. Dreyfuss P, Cole A, et al: Sacroiliac joint injection techniques. In: Injection Techniques: Principles and Practice. Philadelphia, WB Saunders, 1995, p 785.
85. Chua WH: Clinical anatomy of the thoracic dorsal rami. Presented at the Second Annual Scientific Meeting of the International Spinal Injection Society (ISIS), Minneapolis, 1994.
86. Bernard T, Cassidy J: The sacroiliac joint syndrome: Pathophysiology, diagnosis, and management. In Frymoyer J (ed): The Adult Spine: Principles and Practice. New York, Raven, 1991, p 2017.
86a. van Kleef M, Barendse G, Dingemans W, et al: Effects of producing a radiofrequency lesion adjacent to the dorsal root ganglion in patients with thoracic segmental pain. Clin J Pain 11:325, 1995.
87. Bernard TN Jr: Lumbar discography followed by computed tomography—refining the diagnosis of low-back pain. Spine 15:690, 1990.
88. Kornberg M: Discography and magnetic resonance imaging in the diagnosis of lumbar disc disruption. Spine 14:1363, 1989.
88a. Sluijter ME, Koesveld-Baart CC: Interruption of pain pathways in the treatment of the cervical syndrome. Anaesthesia 35:302, 1980.
89. Aprill C: Diagnostic disc injection. In Frymoyer JW (ed): The Adult Spine: Principles and Practice. New York, Raven, 1991, p 403.
90. Sluijter ME: The use of radiofrequency lesions of the communicating ramus in the treatment of low back pain. In Gabor R (ed): Techniques of Neurolysis. Boston, Kluwer, 1989.
91. Troussier B, Lebus JF, Chirossel JP, et al: Percutaneous intradiscal radio-frequency thermocoagulation: A cadaveric study. Spine:1713, 1995.
92. Maurer P: Thermal lumbar disc annuloplasty: Initial clinical results. North American Spine Society, 14th Annual Meeting, Chicago, 1999.
93. Karasek M, Karasek D, et al: A controlled trial of the efficacy of intradiscal electrothermal treatment for internal disc disruption. North American Spine Society, 14th Annual Meeting, Chicago, 1999.
94. Saal J, Saal J: Intradiscal electrothermal annuloplasty (IDET) for chronic disc disease: Outcome assessment with minimum one year follow-up. North American Spine Society, 14th Annual Meeting, Chicago, 1999.
95. Sluijter ME: Interruption of nerve pathways in the treatment of nonmalignant pain. Appl Neurophysiol 47:1695, 1984.
96. Bogduk N, Barnsely L: Radiofrequency neurotomy of the medial branches of the cervical dorsal rami (abstract). Aust NZ J Med 22:736, 1992.
97. Sluijter ME, Vercruysse PR: Radiofrequency Lesions in the Treatment of Cervical Headache. Amsterdam, Pain Relief Clinic, Lutherse Diakoneesen Ziekenhuis, 1987.
98. Sluijter ME: Radiofrequency Lesions in the Treatment of Cervical Pain Syndromes. Radionics Procedure Technique Series. Burlington, Mass, Radionics, 1990.
99. Lord SM, Barnsley L, Wallis BJ, et al: Percutaneous radio-frequency neurotomy for chronic cervical zygapophysial-joint pain. N Engl J Med 335:1721, 1996.
100. Bogduk N, Windsor M, Inglis A: The innervation of the cervical intervertebral discs. Spine 13:2, 1988.
101. Bogduk N, Aprill C: On the nature of neck pain, discography and cervical zygapophysial joint blocks. Pain 54:213, 1993.
102. Taylor J, Twomey L: Disc injuries in cervical trauma. Lancet 44:1318, 1990.
103. Taylor JP, Twomey LT: Acute injuries to cervical joints: An autopsy study of neck sprain. Spine 18:1115, 1993.
104. Taylor JR, Finch P: Acute injury of the neck: Anatomical and pathological basis of pain. Ann Acad Med 22:187, 1993.
105. Aprill C, Bogduk N: The prevalance of cervical zygapophysial joint pain. Spine 17:744, 1991.
106. Barnsley L, Lord SM, Wallis BJ, Bogduk N: The prevalence of chronic cervical zygapophysial joint pain after whiplash. Spine 20:20, 1995.
107. Bogduk N: Mechanisms of neck injuries. Aust Dr Weekly 24:38, 1989.
108. Bogduk N: The anatomy and pathophysiology of whiplash. Clin Biomech 1:92, 1986.
109. Bogduk N, Marsland A: The cervical zygapophysial joints as a source of neck pain. Spine 13:610, 1986.
110. Jull G, Bogduk N, Marshall A: The accuracy of manual diagnosis for cervical zygapophysial joint pain syndromes. Med J Aust 148:233, 1988.
111. Bovim G, Berg R, Dale LG: Cervicogenic headache: Anesthetic blockades of cervical nerves (C2-C5) and facet joint (C2-C3). Pain 49:315, 1992.
112. Lamer TJ: Ear pain due to cervical spine arthritis: Treatment with cervical facet injection. Headache 31:682, 1991.
113. Barnsley L, Lord S, Wallis B, Bogduk N: False-positive rates of cervical zygapophysial joint blocks. Clin J Pain 9:124, 1993.
114. Geurts JWM, Stolker RJ: Percutaneous radiofrequency lesion of the stellate ganglion in the treatment of pain in upper extremity reflex sympathetic dystrophy. Pain Clin 6:17, 1993.
115. Chambers WR: Posterior rhizotomy of the second and third cervical nerves for occipital pain. JAMA 155:431, 1954.
116. Blume H, Kakolewski J, Richardson R, Rojas C: Radiofrequency denaturation in occipital pain: Results in 450 cases. Appl Neurophysiol 45:541, 1981.
117. Kleef MV, et al: Effects and side effects of a percutaneous thermal lesion of the dorsal root ganglion in patients with cervical pain syndrome. Pain 52:49, 1993.
118. Koch D, Wakhloo AK: CT-guided chemical rhizotomy of the C1 root for occipital neuralgia. Neuroradiology 34:451, 1992.
119. Sluijter M: C1 dorsal nerve root lesion in the treatment of suboccipital headache. Personal communication, 1998.
120. Sweet WH, Wepsic JG: Controlled thermocoagulation of trigeminal ganglion and rootlets for differential destruction of pain fibers. J Neurosurg 40:143, 1974.
121. Broggi G, Franzini A, Lasio G, et al: Long-term results of percutaneous retrogasserian thermorhizotomy for "essential" trigeminal neuralgia: Considerations in 1000 consecutive patients. Neurosurgery 26:783, 1990.
122. Adson AW, Brown GE: Treatment of Raynaud's disease by lumbar ramisection and ganglionostomy and perivascular sympathetic neurectomy of the common iliac. JAMA 84:16908, 1924.
123. DeBakey ME, Creech O, Woodhall JP: Evaluation of sympathectomy in arteriosclerotic peripheral vascular disease. JAMA 144:1227, 1950.
124. Pernak J: Percutaneous radiofrequency thermal lumbar sympathectomy. Pain Clin 80:99, 1995.
125. Noe CE, Haynesworth RF: Lumbar radiofrequency sympatholysis. J Vasc Surg 17:801, 1993.
126. Haynesworth RF, Noe CE: Percutaneous lumbar sympathectomy: A comparison of radiofrequency denervation versus phenol neurolysis. Anaesthesiology 74:459, 1991.
127. Yarzebski JL, Wilkinson HA: T2 and T3 sympathetic ganglia in the adult human: A cadaver and clinical-radiologic study and its clinical application. Neurosurgery 21:339, 1987.

128. Wilkinson HA: Radiofrequency percutaneous upper thoracic sympathectomy. N Engl J Med 311:34, 1984.
129. Wilkinson HA: Percutaneous radiofrequency upper thoracic sympathectomy: A new technique. Neurosurgery 15:811, 1984.
130. Wilkinson HA: Percutaneous radiofrequency upper thoracic sympathectomy. Neurosurgery 38:715, 1996.
131. Wilkinson HA: Stereotactic radiofrequency sympathectomy. Pain Clin 8:107.
132. Raj P: Visceral pain (tutorial review). Pain Dig 9:1697, 1999.
133. Banerjee T, Domingues da Silva A: Signs, Syndromes and Eponyms: Our Legacy. Lebanon, NH, American Association of Neurological Surgeons, 1999.
134. Ischia S, Ischia A, Polati E, Finco G: Three posterior celiac plexus block techniques: A prospective, randomized study in 61 patients with pancreatic cancer pain. Anesthesiology 76:4, 1992.
135. Williams P, Warwick R (eds): Gray's Anatomy. Philadelphia, WB Saunders, 1980.

chapter 170

Cryoneurolysis

Lloyd R. Saberski

Cryoanalgesic therapy has widespread and diverse applications in the fields of pain management and neurosurgery. This chapter introduces the practitioner to the proper use and limitations of this relatively new technology so that appropriate clinical decisions can be made. Examples of applications are presented, but it is not my intent to address all potential uses of cryoanalgesia.

HISTORICAL CONSIDERATIONS

Cryoanalgesia is a technique in which cold is applied to produce pain relief. The analgesic effect of cold has been known to humans for more than a millennium.[1] Hippocrates (460-377 BC) provided the first written record of the use of ice and snow packs applied before surgery as a local pain-relieving technique.[2] Early physicians, such as Avicenna of Persia (980-1070 AD) and Severino of Naples (1580-1656) recorded using cold for preoperative analgesia.[3,4] In 1712, Napoleon's surgeon general, Baron Dominique Jean Larre, recognized that the limbs of soldiers frozen in the Prussian snow could be amputated relatively painlessly.[5] In 1751, Arnott described using an ice-salt mixture to produce tumor regression and to obtain an anesthetic and hemostatic effect.[6] Richardson introduced ether spray in 1766 to produce local analgesia by refrigeration; this was superseded in 1790 by ethyl chloride spray.

Contemporary interest in cryoanalgesia was sparked in 1961, after Cooper described a cryotherapy unit in which liquid nitrogen was circulated through a hollow metal probe that was vacuum-insulated except at the tip. With this equipment, it was possible to control the temperature of the tip by interrupting the flow of liquid nitrogen at temperatures within the range of room temperature and −196°C. Because it was a totally enclosed system, cold could be applied to any part of the body accessible to the probe. The first clinical application of this technique was in neurosurgery for treatment of parkinsonism.[7,8] In 1967, Amoils[9] developed a simpler hand-held unit that used carbon dioxide or nitrous oxide. These devices were the prototypes for the current generation of cryoprobes used in cryoanalgesia (Figs. 170–1 and 170–2). The coldest temperature is approximately −70°C.

PHYSICS AND CELLULAR BASICS FOR CRYOANALGESIA

The working principle of a cryoprobe is that compressed gas (nitrous oxide or carbon dioxide) expands. The cryoprobe consists of an outer tube and a smaller inner tube that terminates in a fine nozzle (Fig. 170–3). High-pressure gas (650 to 800 psi) is passed between the two tubes and is released via a small orifice into a chamber at the tip of the probe. In the chamber, the gas expands, and the substantial reduction in pressure (80 to 100 psi) results in a rapid decrease in temperature and cooling of the probe tip. (Absorption of heat from surrounding tissues accompanies expansion of any gas, according to the principles of the general gas law; this is the adiabatic principle of gas cooling and heat extraction, also known as the Joule-Thomson effect.) The low-pressure gas flows back through the center of the inner tube and back to the console, where it is vented. The sealed construction of the cryoprobe ensures that no gas escapes from the probe tip, handle, or hose.

The rapid cooling of the cryoprobe produces a tip surface temperature of approximately −70°C. Tissue in contact with the tip cools rapidly and forms an ice ball. The ice ball varies in size, depending on probe size, freeze time, tissue permeability to water, and presence of vascular structures (heat sink). The ice ball typically measures 3.5 to 5.5 mm in diameter. Further increase in size is prevented when thermal equilibrium is attained.

Precise levels of gas flow through the cryoprobe are essential for maximum efficiency. Inadequate gas flow does not freeze tissue. Excessive gas flow results in freezing down the stem of the probe and the associated risk of cold skin burns. The cryoprobe console is fitted with a regulator and indicator that are adjusted for optimal performance.

The application of cold to peripheral nerves, whether by direct cooling of localized segments or complete immersion of tissue in a cold medium, induces reversible conduction block. The extent and duration of the effect depend on the temperature attained in the tissues and the duration of exposure.[1] When nerve fibers are progressively cooled, a conduction block similar to that produced by local anesthetic develops. At 10°C, larger myelinated fibers cease conduction before unmyelinated fibers, but at 0°C, all nerve fibers entrapped in the ice ball stop conduction. Some fibers resume conduction on rewarming. To obtain a prolonged effect from

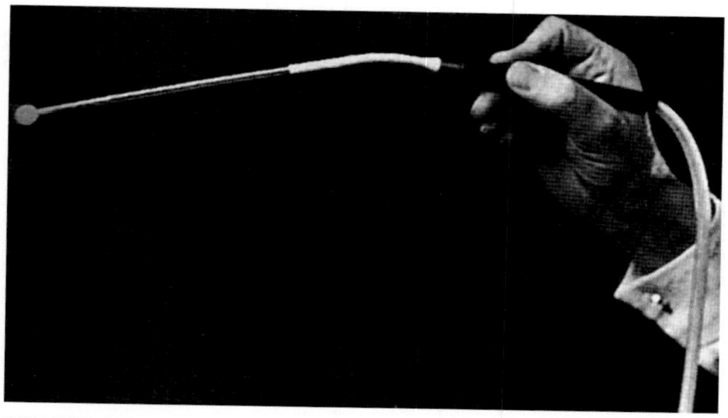

FIGURE 170–1 ■ An early hand-held cryoprobe with ice ball. (From Holden HB: Practical Cryosurgery. London, Pitman Medical, 1975.)

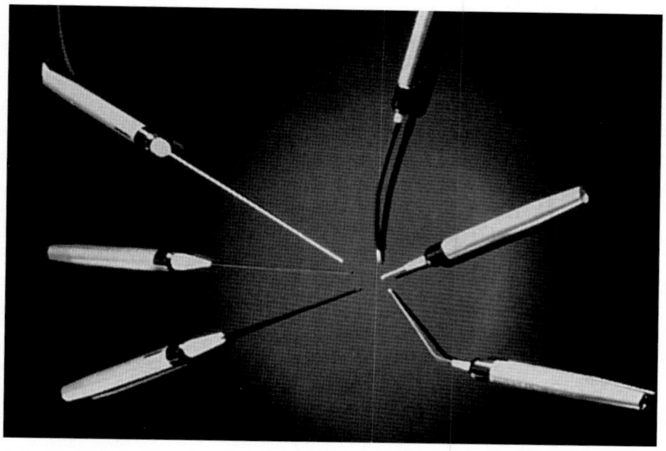

FIGURE 170–2 ■ Contemporary hand-held Lloyd cryoprobes. (Courtesy of Westco Medical Corporation, San Diego, CA.)

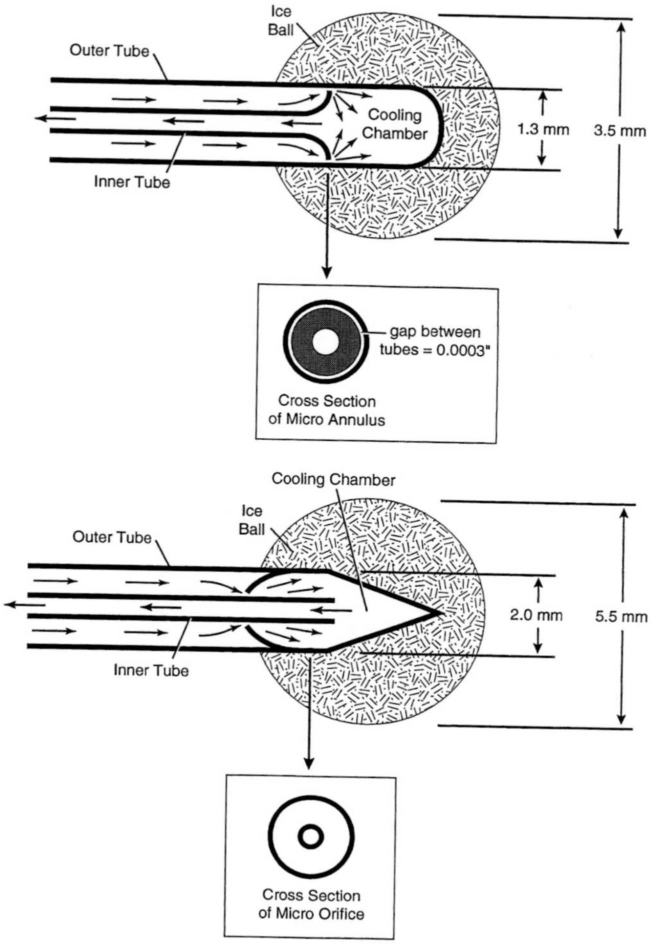

FIGURE 170–3 ■ **A** and **B,** Cross sections of two commonly used cryoprobe designs. High-pressure gas goes in through the outer tube at 650 to 800 psi. Low-pressure gas is vented out at 80 to 100 psi. Gas flow is at 7 to 9 L/min. Test conditions: Tip is inserted into water at 36°C ± 1°C. An ice ball is formed within 60 seconds.

a cryolesion, the intracellular contents of the nerve must be turned into ice crystals. There is little clinical difference as long as the temperature is less than −20°C for 1 minute.[10] When the nerve is frozen amidst other tissues, the duration of exposure becomes more important. Within the limitations of a specific cryoprobe and its steady state of thermal equilibrium, prolonging application of the cryoprobe increases the size of the ice ball and the likelihood of the nerve's being entrapped by a cryolesion. In practice, a freeze of 2 to 3 minutes' duration produces a good result. Prolonged exposure and repeated freeze-thaw cycles likely are beneficial with percutaneous techniques, especially when abundant surrounding soft tissue and nerve localization are poor.[1]

Histologically, the axons and myelin sheaths degenerate after cryolesioning (wallerian degeneration), but the epineurium and perineurium remain intact, allowing subsequent nerve regeneration. The duration of the block is a function of the rate of axonal regeneration after cryolesioning, which is reported to be 1 to 3 mm/day.[10] Because axonal regrowth is constant, the return of sensory and motor activity is a function of the distance between the cryolesion and the end organ.[1] The absence of external damage to the nerve and the minimal inflammatory reaction to freezing ensure that regeneration is exact. The regenerating axons are unlikely to form painful neuromas. (Surgical and thermal lesions interrupt perineurium and epineurium.) Other neurolytic techniques (alcohol, phenol) potentially can produce painful neuromas because the epineurium and perineurium are disrupted.

A cryolesion provides a temporary anesthetic block. Clinically, a cryoblock lasts weeks to months. The result depends on numerous variables, including operator technique and clinical circumstances. The analgesia often lasts longer than the time required for axons to regenerate.[16] The reasons are still a matter of speculation, but it is obvious that there is more to cryoanalgesia than just temporary disruption of axons. It is possible that sustained blockade of afferent input to the CNS has an effect on CNS windup. A report suggested that cryolesions release sequestered tissue protein or facilitate changes in protein antigenic properties.[11] The result is an autoimmune response targeted at cryolesioned tissue. The first report of such a response was from Gander and colleagues,[12] who showed tissue-specific autoantibodies after cryocoagulation of male rabbit accessory glands. This report was followed by a parallel clinical report of regression of metastatic deposits from prostatic adenocarcinoma after cryocoagulation of the primary tumor.[13] The significance for pain management is unclear; however, it does indicate that tumor growth and regression are affected by immune function. Perhaps immune mechanisms play a role in the analgesic response after cryoablation.

INDICATIONS AND CONTRAINDICATIONS

Cryoanalgesia is best suited for clinical situations when analgesia is required for weeks or months. Permanent blockade does not usually occur because the cryoinjured axons regenerate. The median duration of pain relief is 2 weeks to 5 months.[14,15] Cryoanalgesia is suited for painful conditions that originate from small, well-localized lesions of peripheral nerves (e.g., neuromas, entrapment neuropathies, and postoperative pain).[16] Longer than expected periods of analgesia have been reported and may result from the patient's ability to participate more fully in physical therapy or from an effect of prolonged analgesia on central processing of pain (preemptive analgesic effect). Sustained blockade of afferent impulses[17-20] with cryoanalgesia may reduce plasticity (windup) in the CNS and decrease pain permanently.[21]

Cryoablative procedures can be performed open or closed (percutaneous), depending on the clinical setting. Most often, open procedures are performed as part of postoperative analgesia. Under direct visualization, the operator identifies the neural structure of concern, and the cryoprobe is applied for 1 to 4 minutes, depending on tissue heat, which is a function of blood supply and distance of the probe from the nerve. Care is taken not to freeze adjacent vascular structures. The cryoprobe is withdrawn only after the tissue thaws because removing it earlier can tear tissue.

Percutaneous (closed) cryoablation is the technique of choice for outpatient chronic pain management. It has the advantage of easy application and few complications. Percutaneous (closed) cryoablative procedures have been used successfully for many benign and malignant pain syndromes, but few scientific studies have been published, in part because there was little interest until more recently in pain management techniques and because of lack of industry funding for advanced research.

Patients must give informed consent. The consent form should describe the risk-to-benefit ratios of cryoanalgesia and of regional anesthesia. Patients should be fully aware that a cryoanalgesia procedure usually is not a permanent solution. It can ameliorate symptoms, however, and allow the patient to participate better in physiotherapy. In some cases when there has been CNS windup, it may serve as a form of preemptive anesthetic and facilitate prolonged relief. Cryoanalgesia for chronic pain syndromes always should be preceded by diagnostic/prognostic local anesthetic injections. After a test block with local anesthetic, the examiner should inquire about the patient's tolerance to the numbness and the extent of pain reduction. If response to the test injections is inadequate, the patient will not have a good response to cryodenervation. Patients also should be aware that numbness can replace pain, and small areas of skin depigmentation can occur if the ice ball frosts skin because the probe is not deep enough or is inadequately insulated from tissues. All procedures are done with appropriate sterile preparation. As a general rule, infected areas are avoided.

CLINICALLY RELEVANT ANATOMY

For any given procedure, it is essential that the provider of cryoanalgesia be aware of the regional anatomy of interest. Because cryoanalgesia has widespread applications, thorough knowledge of neuroanatomy and regional anesthesia is required. In the next section, detailed descriptions and illustrations are provided for numerous procedures. The reader is referred to standard anatomy textbooks for more detailed discussion.

CLINICAL PEARLS AND TRICKS OF THE TRADE

Postoperative Pain Management

Postoperative use of cryoanalgesia should be widespread, but in the United States, it is used routinely for postoperative analgesia in only a few centers. The reasons are several, among them a lack of controlled studies and physicians' reluctance to add time and costs to procedures, especially when they believe patients already are receiving adequate care. At many institutions, cryoanalgesia is reserved for patients with special analgesia needs and patients at high risk who cannot receive standard postoperative treatment. Of the handful of studies that have been done,[22-26] most indicate significant reductions in pain and medication requirements. It is likely that use of postoperative cryoanalgesia will increase if it can be shown that cost savings and improved long-term outcomes are the results.

Cryoanalgesia procedures are provided intraoperatively by surgeons who have access to involved peripheral nerve and pain management specialists participating in the operative procedure. At times, pain specialists are called on to provide cryoanalgesia postoperatively, in which case they must decide whether some alternative is more suitable than open or closed cryodenervation.

Popular Cryodenervation Techniques for Postoperative Pain Management

Post-thoracotomy Pain

Intraoperative intercostal cryoneurolysis was first described by Nelson and associates in 1974.[27] Since that time, a large body of literature has been published that supports use of cryoderavation as a component of a postoperative analgesia plan.[22-24,28] Post-thoracotomy cryoanalgesia is most effective for treating incisional pain, but it is ineffective for pain from visceral pleura supplied by autonomic fibers or for ligament pain of the chest secondary to rib retraction. Post-thoracotomy cryoanalgesia often has little effect on chest tube pain, for the same reasons. Patients treated with cryotherapy during thoracotomy have relatively less postoperative discomfort and opioid requirements in the immediate postoperative period and over subsequent weeks. There has been only one documented report of neuritis as a complication of cryoneurolysis.[29] Sensory anesthesia lasts longer than 6 months along the sensory field of treated intercostal nerves.

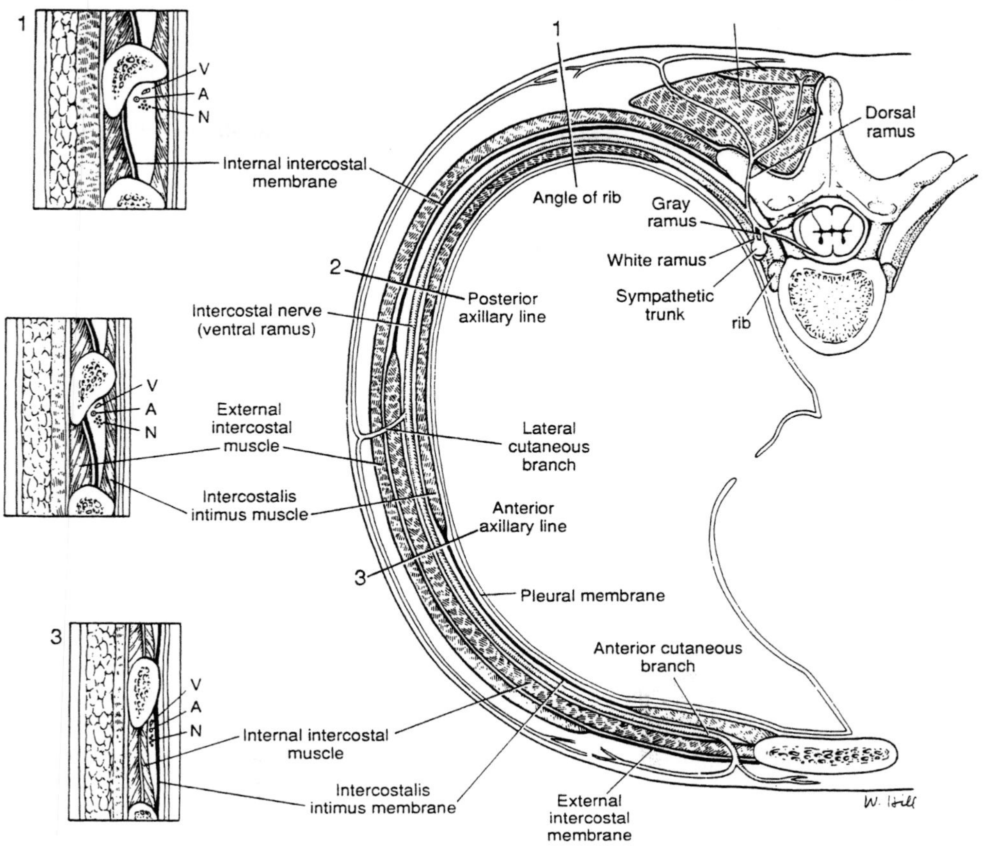

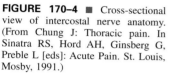

FIGURE 170–4 ■ Cross-sectional view of intercostal nerve anatomy. (From Chung J: Thoracic pain. In Sinatra RS, Hord AH, Ginsberg G, Preble L [eds]: Acute Pain. St. Louis, Mosby, 1991.)

For effective intraoperative cryoneurolysis, intercostal nerves on each side of the thoracotomy incision are lesioned. If a rib is removed, that intercostal nerve also is cryolesioned. The intercostal nerves are best cryoablated just lateral to the transverse process, before the collateral intercostal nerve branches (Fig. 170–4). Only a small area of skin innervated by the dorsal primary ramus is missed. Care is taken to separate the intercostal nerves from the intercostal vessels, removing a large heat sink that would be counterproductive to cryotherapy. The vessels also are protected from cold-induced thrombosis. A cryolesion sufficient to produce visible evidence of freezing is required. In general, such a lesion takes 1 to 2 minutes. A second lesion can be placed after tissue thaws, but whether that is necessary when freezing of the first lesion is complete remains to be determined.

Postherniorrhaphy Pain.

Cryoneurolysis after herniorrhaphy was first described by Wood and coworkers in 1979.[30] A cryolesion of the ilioinguinal nerve reduces analgesic requirements during the postoperative period. The follow-up study in 1981 compared recovery from herniorrhaphy among three study groups: patients treated with oral analgesics, cryoanalgesia, and paravertebral blockade (the last two treatments supplemented with oral analgesics as needed). The study indicated that the cryoanalgesic group not only had less pain in the postoperative period, but also used less opioid, resumed a regular diet earlier, were mobilized faster, and returned to work sooner.[25] Despite these successes, the technique is not widely used. Given its effectiveness and freedom from side effects, it is ideal for ambulatory surgery. After repair of the internal ring, posterior wall of the inguinal canal, and internal oblique muscle, the ilioinguinal nerve on the surface of the muscle is identified and mobilized. The surgeon elevates the nerve above the muscle, and an assistant performs the cryoablation.

Chronic Pain Management

For management of chronic pain, open cryoablation is avoided whenever the procedure can be performed effectively percutaneously. Before committing to cryoablation, the provider must perform a series of test blocks to determine presence of a consistent analgesic response. A favorable response before cryoablation is when the local anesthetic injection decreases pain, and the numbness that replaces the pain is tolerated by the patient. Care always must be taken to ensure correct positioning of the needles. When necessary, fluoroscopic guidance should be used. The smallest amount of local anesthetic required to achieve blockade must be used. A tuberculin syringe that injects 0.1 mm at a time ensures that the anesthetic does not contaminate other structures, which otherwise would make interpretation of the block difficult. This contributes to accurate localization of the primary pain generator. If the block is successful, an appropriate dermatomal representation of the analgesia is present. Subsequently, the patient is assessed for subjective changes in pain; however, this alone is insufficient to determine suitability for cryoablation. Many pain patients have suffered for a long time and are hopeful that the next procedure is going to be the long-awaited successful treatment. They are responsive to suggestion and placebo effect. To identify such effects, the first test injection is done with lidocaine and the second with bupivacaine. In appropriate responders, a significantly longer duration of analgesia can be found with bupivacaine, assuming that all other variables remain the same. The effects of peripheral blockade on windup and chronic pain are not clearly understood. To responsive patients, a cryoablative procedure can be offered. For patients who do not have the desired response to bupivacaine or lidocaine, further testing is necessary, including differential blockade with local anesthetics and normal saline and consideration of consultation with a clinical psychologist.

To perform percutaneous cryoablation successfully, it is essential that the cryoprobe be placed properly. This is a disadvantage compared with open cryoablative techniques used for postoperative pain management. The operator must ensure proper cryoprobe placement by using a combination of techniques (see later) that improve the chances that the ice ball would be made precisely on the pain generator. In addition, special care must be taken when using the cryoprobe for percutaneous procedures. Bending the probe during percutaneous introduction can distort the lumen of the low-pressure outer tube, increase the resistance pressure to the expanding nitrous oxide gas, and convert a low-pressure exhaust system to one of higher pressure. That eventuality would impede gas expansion, inhibit ice ball formation, and limit cooling of the probe. To maintain the integrity of the cryoprobe, the probe should be placed through an introducer. The preferred introducers are large-bore intravenous catheters: 12-gauge, 14-gauge, or 16-gauge, depending on the size of the cryoprobe. The operator always should check to see that the cryoprobe fits through the lumen of the catheter. The depth at which the probe emerges from the distal tip of the catheter should be marked on the proximal shaft of the cryoprobe to ensure that the cryoprobe tip extends far enough beyond the catheter to create a full-sized ice ball.

Several techniques are used to enhance precise placement of the cryoprobe, as follows:

1. Careful palpation with a small blunt instrument, such as a felt-tipped pen, can help to localize a soft tissue neuroma or another palpable pain generator.
2. An image intensifier (fluoroscopy) can identify bony landmarks.
3. Contrast medium improves definition of tissue planes, capsules, and spaces. (Nonionic contrast medium should be used in areas close to neural tissue.)
4. The nerve stimulator at the tip of the cryoprobe is used to produce a muscle twitch in a mixed nerve. The stimulator is set at 5 Hz for recruitment of motor fibers. The probe is closest to the nerve when the lowest output produces a twitch response. In general, we like to see twitches at 0.5 to 1.5 V. Small sensory branches contain no motor component and do not twitch with electrical stimulation. These fibers are localized by using higher frequency (100 Hz) stimulation, which produces overlapping dysesthesia in the distribution of the small sensory nerve. This may reproduce the patient's pain. Use of low-output (<0.5 to 1.5 V) stimulation ensures closer placement of the cryoprobe to the nerve in question.

The operator freezes the nerve for 2 to 3 minutes. Often there is discomfort initially as cooling begins, but it should dissipate quickly. If significant pain persists beyond 30 seconds, the operator should investigate whether the ice ball is in the proper position. (If the ice ball is not sufficiently close to the nerve, and there is only partial freezing, mostly of larger myelinated fibers, unchecked unmyelinated fiber input is left. This theoretically accounts for increased pain.) The brief cooling already may have altered nerve function, in which case, if positioning of the probe depends on feedback from the patient, it could be impeded. Before moving the probe, the operator must be sure to thaw the tip to prevent tissue damage from an ice ball sticking to the tissues. In general, with closed procedures, two freeze cycles of 2 minutes each followed by thaw cycles are sufficient. In areas where there is a large vascular heat sink, longer periods of cryotherapy are necessary. Pain relief should be immediate and should be assessed subjectively and by physical examination while the patient is on the procedure table. All relevant clinical information should be recorded in the medical record. A hard-copy radiograph should be obtained for most procedures when a fluoroscope is used.

Applied Cryoanalgesia for Chronic Pain

This section provides the reader with the skills necessary to make proper clinical decisions regarding cryoanalgesia. Listing every procedure is beyond the scope of this chapter. This section reviews many of the pain syndromes that are amenable to cryodenervation and describes in detail the techniques that are requested most often. To perform cryolytic treatments correctly, the provider must be familiar with the regional anatomy and the principles of localizing pain generators described earlier.

Intercostal Neuralgia

Percutaneous cryolesions of the intercostal nerves can be offered for a variety of pain syndromes, including post-thoracotomy pain, traumatic intercostal neuralgia, rib fracture pain, and occasionally postherpetic neuropathy. For each of these conditions, a meticulous series of local anesthetic blocks is performed before consideration is given to cryoablation. The volume of local anesthetic should be kept to less than 3 to 4 mL to prevent tracking back into the epidural space. In addition, only two or three levels should be injected at any one time because systemic absorption could confound interpretation of the patient's response. Because the intercostal nerve runs with a large arterial and venous heat source, two 4-minute cryolesions at each level is suggested. The lesions should be made proximal to the pain at the inferior border of the rib (Fig. 170–5). After the procedure, a chest film is obtained to check for pneumothorax. Effective blockade of some patients with postherpetic neuropathy suggests that this pain is sometimes related to peripheral afferent input, as opposed to being strictly a central neuropathy.

Neuromas

Typically, painful neuromas are associated with lancinating or shooting pain that is aggravated by movement or deformation of nearby soft tissues. Neurophysiologically, this phenomenon is thought to reflect lower neural thresholds and ephatic transmission. First-line therapy should include empirical trials of anticonvulsants, tricyclic antidepressants, steroids, and local anesthetics, including topical local anesthetic cream or patch. These agents are thought to play a role in modulating

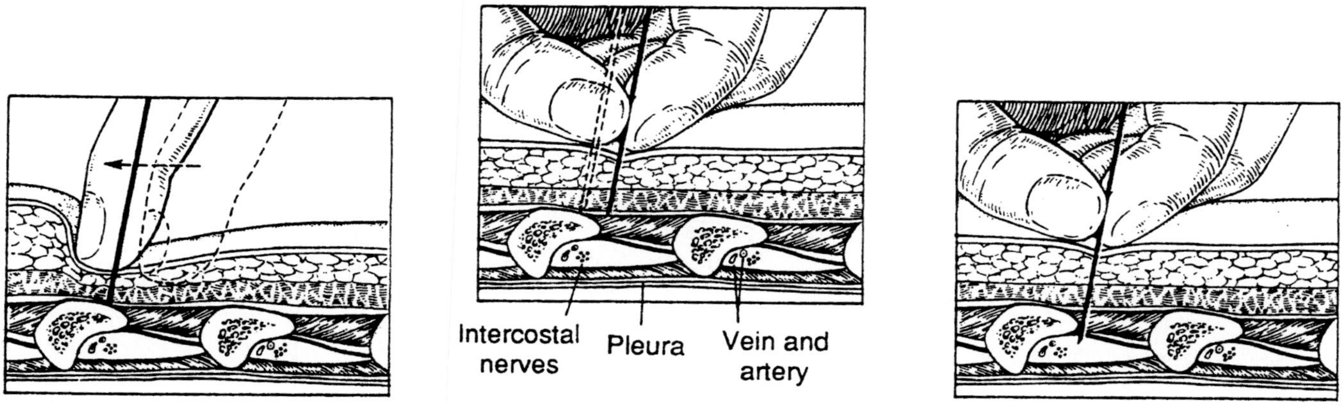

FIGURE 170–5 ■ Percutaneous placement of a needle (introducer) onto an intercostal nerve at the inferior border of a rib. (From Chung J: Thoracic pain. In Sinatra RS, Hord AH, Ginsberg G, Preble L [eds]: Acute Pain. St. Louis, Mosby, 1991.)

neural thresholds. Cryoablation is considered only after careful mapping has isolated a very discrete pain generator (i.e., a neuroma). The initial injection can use a relatively larger volume of local anesthetic, but subsequent blocks should deliver small increments from a tuberculin syringe to ensure accurate interpretation. Cryoablation seems most effective when the volume of local anesthetic necessary to produce analgesia is 1 mL or less. After the block with lidocaine, the patient's response and its duration are recorded. If initial blockade is successful in decreasing the patient's symptoms, it should be followed by at least one more injection with bupivacaine. A response of longer duration might be expected with the longer-acting local anesthetic.

Iliac Crest Bone Harvest

The pain associated with the harvest of iliac crest bone for fusion often responds to cryoablation when more conservative therapies have failed. Such pain often is associated with deep, lancinating pain and often is attributed to periosteal neuromas. The surface area is often large, and careful diagnostic mapping is required to localize the primary pain generator as precisely as possible. When no single pain generator is found, and the periosteal surface that is the source of the pain remains large and unresponsive to other therapies (e.g., steroid injections and nonsteroidal antiinflammatory drugs [NSAIDs]), multiple cryoablations may be necessary during one session (Fig. 170–6).

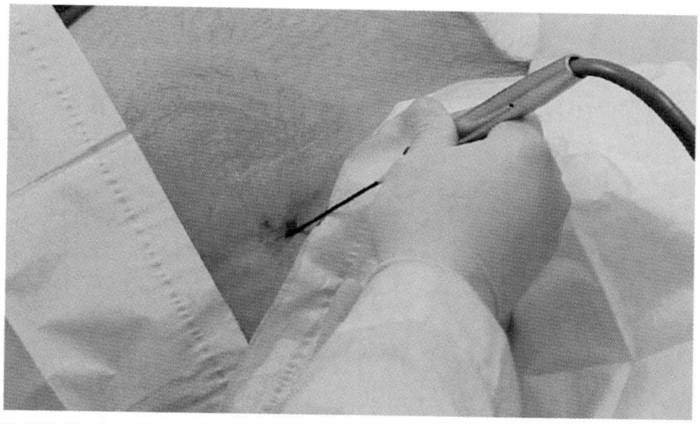

FIGURE 170–6 ■ Cryoablation of an anterior iliac crest bone harvest site. (From Waldman SD: Cryoneurolysis in clinical practice. In Interventional Pain Management, 2nd ed. Philadelphia, WB Saunders, 2001.)

Biomechanical Spine Pain

Typically, biomechanical spine pain is exacerbated with movement, so physiotherapy often is futile. In general, there are no neurologic deficits, and the pain is ascribed to numerous structures, including the articular facet nerves, the meningeal nerves, the anterior communicating ramus, and other branches of the posterior primary ramus (Figs. 170–7 and 170–8). Cryolesions have been used effectively for cervical and lumbar facet syndromes[31] and for pain from the interspinous ligaments.[32] The success of cryolesioning is a function of patient selection, accurate probe placement, and follow-up rehabilitation program. For biomechanical pain of lumbar facet origin, the patient typically has pain that is exacerbated by hyperextension of the lumbar spine. The pain localizes to the lumbosacral junction and often radiates into the buttocks and the posterior aspect of the thigh, generally never below the knee. These patients have significant muscle spasm, at times extending cephalad and caudad. They complain that movement is uncomfortable and are unable to participate in lumbar physiotherapy. Palpation reveals exquisite tenderness along the lumbar paravertebral margin. There are no significant neurologic changes, but typically other biomechanical problems are present, such as pelvic obliquity, functional leg-length discrepancy, and sacroiliac joint dysfunction.

Before an isolated facet arthropathy is addressed, attention should be directed to the associated biomechanical disorders. If a patient has a leg-length discrepancy and pelvic shift, a shoe orthosis should be prescribed. When a patient has severe pain from the facet arthropathy, little is gained from prescribing physiotherapy. In such circumstances (which are common), denervation of the facet may enable the patient to participate in physiotherapy. A fluoroscopically guided diagnostic intra-articular facet block can be performed on patients who fulfill the aforementioned criteria. The levels chosen for injection are determined by bone scan, CT, plain films, and, most important, physical examination findings.

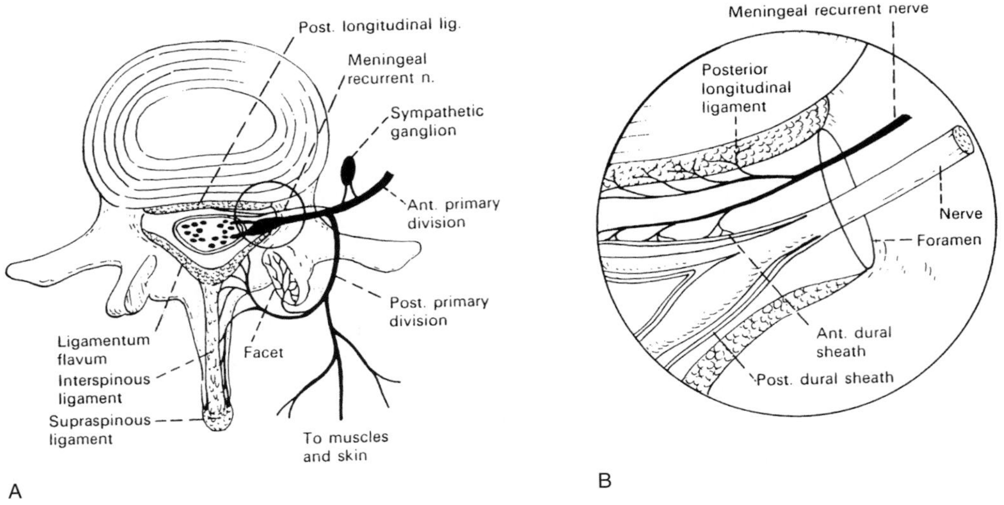

FIGURE 170–7 ■ Cross-sectional view of innervation of the posterior motion segment, including the facet. (From Bonica J: The Management of Pain. Philadelphia, Lea & Febiger, 1990.)

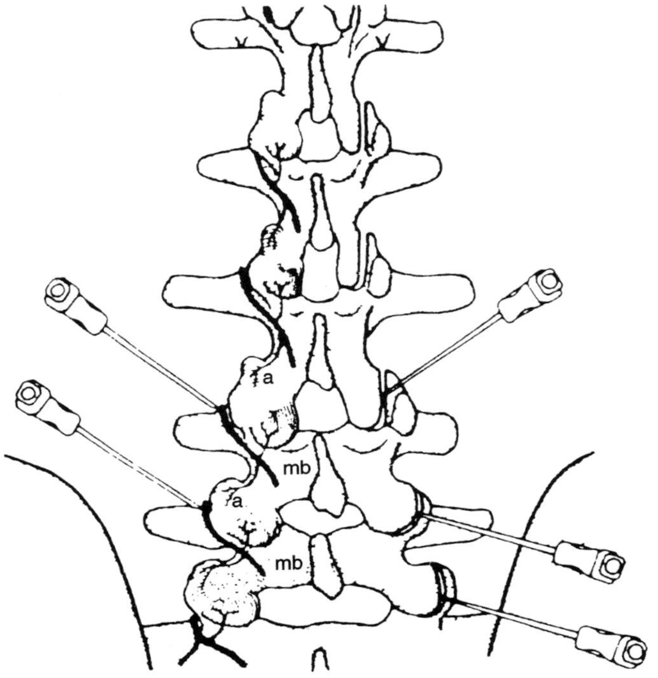

FIGURE 170–8 ■ Dorsum of lumbar spine. Needles placed into lumbar facet joints and onto medial branches. a, articular branch of facet; mb, medial branch of the posterior primary division. (From Cousins M, Bridenbaugh P [eds]: Neural Blockade in Clinical Anesthesia and Management of Pain, 2nd ed. Philadelphia, JB Lippincott, 1994.)

Initial needle placement into the facet is guided by anteroposterior fluoroscopic visualization (Fig. 170–9A-C) after a small skin wheal is made. Correct intra-articular placement is confirmed with oblique imaging; the needle should be in the ear of the Scottie dog (Fig. 170–9D). (Often, as the needle enters the joint space, the operator feels as though the needle is being pushed through an orange peel; that is, he feels the loss of resistance.) When the needle is within the joint, 1 mL of nonionic contrast medium is injected. With facet arthropathy, this is often very painful. A fluoroscopic review of the area of interest of the contrast study shows the facet capsule filled with radiodense contrast medium. In some circumstances, the capsule is deformed or leaky. At times, the capsule is large and cystic and projects into the canal. At this point, the patient is asked to consider carefully whether this is the usual pain or a different pain and to rate it on the visual analog scale (VAS). If the pain reproduced is representative of the usual pain, 1 mL of 1% lidocaine is injected. The needle is manipulated further, and the patient is asked how he or she feels and to arch the back. If the patient has a dramatic decrease in pain and improved movement, it is likely that a facet pain generator is present. If there is little change in symptoms, an additional 4 mL of lidocaine can be injected incrementally. If there is no change in symptoms at the level under study, it is unlikely to be a primary pain generator. In patients who respond, a set of flexion-extension films should be made before discharge because the analgesia provided by the block should allow better motion and help to reveal occult posterior elemental movement. If such movement is found, the patient would benefit from an orthopedic evaluation and consideration of fusion.

To confirm a facet pain generator, repeat blockade of the facet nerves can be done next. If the result is similar, it is reasonable to consider ablation. Each facet has at least dual innervation and requires at least two local anesthetic injections. A needle is placed at the junction of the transverse process and the pedicle (the Scottie dog's eye on the oblique projection; see Fig. 170–9D) at the level previously studied and the level above. A 100-Hz nerve stimulator is used to locate the sensory nerve. Subsequently, 2 mL of 0.25% bupivacaine is injected. Ten minutes later, the patient is reexamined. In patients who continue to be responsive, improvement is observed on physical examination, especially with lumbar hyperextension. For these patients, a cryoablative procedure can be considered.

For the cryoablative procedure, the patient is positioned prone in the fluoroscopy suite. The lumbar spine is prepared and draped in standard sterile fashion. Superficial skin wheals are raised at the levels where cryoablations are to be performed. There is, however, a clinical suggestion that there also are contributions to facet innovation from the level below. For this reason, lumbar facet cryodenervations often are done at three levels, a technique popularized by Thomas. A 12-gauge

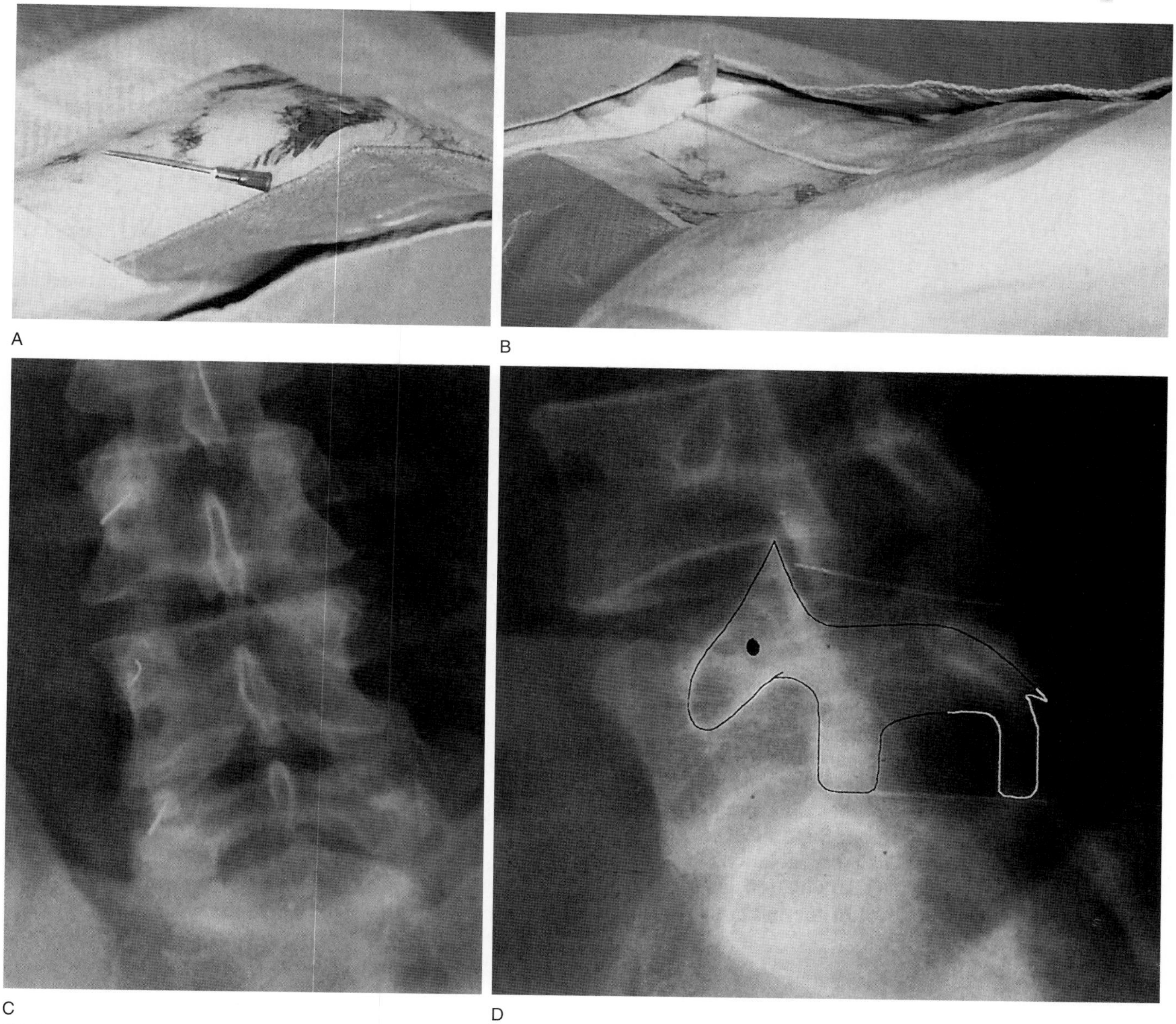

FIGURE 170–9 ■ **A,** Using fluoroscopy, the point of a needle is placed over the lumbar facet of interest. This corresponds to the junction of the transverse process and the pedicle. **B,** A 22-gauge finder (spinal) needle is inserted through the skin at the point of the needle down to bone. **C,** Anteroposterior x-ray projection shows the needle at the junction of the transverse process and the pedicle near the facet joint. **D,** Using an oblique projection, the needle is manipulated into the Scotty dog's ear for intra-articular placement or into the Scottie dog's eye for the articular nerve (medial branch). (From Waldman SD: Cryoneurolysis in clinical practice. In Interventional Pain Management, 2nd ed. Philadelphia, WB Saunders, 2001, p 233.)

introducer catheter (Fig. 170–10A) is introduced to the junction of the transverse process and the pedicle, the Scottie dog's eye. At this point, the cryoprobe is inserted into the introducer catheter (Fig. 170–10B). The nerve stimulator is used to locate the sensory branch. When pain is reproduced or the patient feels a dysesthesia overlapping the region of the pain, motor testing is in order to ensure that the ice ball is not near a motor nerve. Two cryolesions are made, each of 2 minutes' duration.

The patient is expected to have some postprocedure discomfort, but should notice improvement. In the recovery room, ice can be applied to the operative site for 30 minutes for local postoperative irritation and swelling. Application of ice may decrease swelling and facilitate mobilization. The patient should continue with lumbar strengthening programs as an outpatient. If the musculature is significantly deconditioned, it may be better to restart the program in water. After muscle condition improves, the patient should begin a supervised industrial rehabilitation program that offers vocational retraining and job placement.

Cervical Facet Syndrome

Patients with cervical facet syndrome typically present with severe posterior neck pain and muscle spasm. Palpation elicits

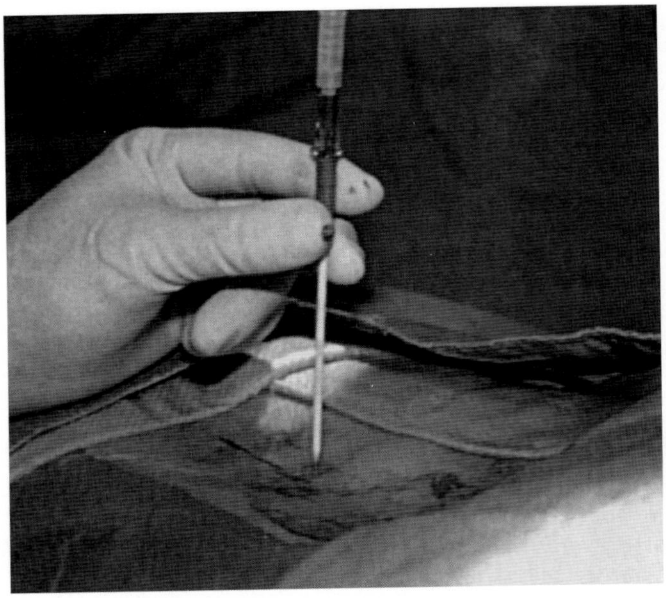

A

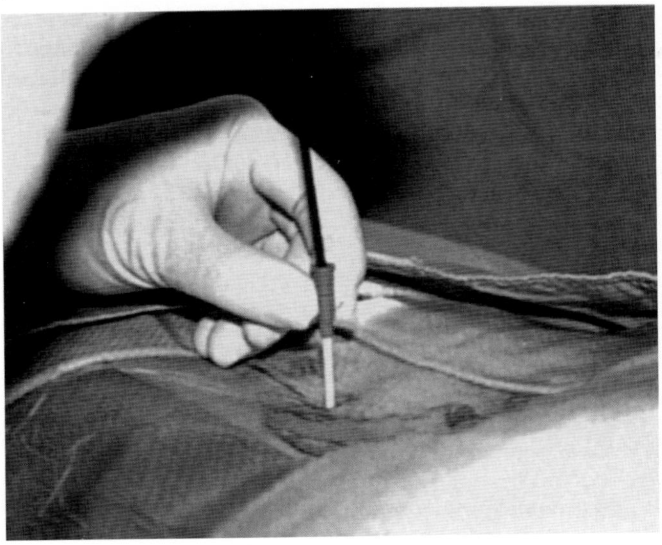

B

FIGURE 170–10 ■ For facet cryodenervation a 12-gauge introducer catheter is placed percutaneously along the tract of the finder needle. **B**, The cryoprobe is then placed through the introducer catheter. The final position of the probe is determined by the patient's response to 100 Hz stimulation. There should be no motor response to 5 Hz stimulation. (From Waldman SD: Cryoneurolysis in clinical practice. In Interventional Pain Management, 2nd ed. Philadelphia, WB Saunders, 2001, p 234.)

pain over cervical facets and at the midline. The pain becomes considerably worse with hyperextension and loading of the cervical spine. Cervical facet syndromes generally are not associated with long tract neurologic findings. A radionuclide bone scan and a plain film may show evidence of posterior elemental arthritic disease. Spondylolisthesis should be sought with flexion-extension films. Significant movement might be better addressed with fusion.

If these patients fail to respond to conservative therapy, a diagnostic series of injections with fluoroscopic guidance is considered. To patients who respond to local anesthetic injections with reduction in pain, cryodenervations can be offered as an adjunct to comprehensive physical therapy and rehabilitation. For patients with apparent biomechanical neck pain that does not respond to local anesthetic injection, further workup is necessary to identify pain generators.

Interspinous Ligament Pain

Interspinous ligament pain is common after a spine operation (lumbar, thoracic, or cervical). Pain impulses from interspinous ligaments are carried by the medial branch of the posterior ramus (see Fig. 170–8). Patients report severe movement-related spine pain, identified to midline, which is worsened with hyperextension and relieved by small volumes of local anesthetic injected into the intraspinous ligament. When cervical interspinous ligaments are involved, the patient frequently complains of posterior cervical headache. This headache often is mistaken for occipital neuralgia. Cryodenervation can be considered in local anesthetic–responsive patients. The pain relief helps the patient to complete the necessary course of physical therapy.

Mechanical Spine Pain

Anterior mechanical (diskogenic) spine pain is transmitted via different nerves, depending on the location of the injury—the sinuvertebral nerve (recurrent meningeal), small rami of the segmental nerve, rami of the communicating ramus, or sympathetic fibers.[33] Cryolesions have been placed successfully on rami communicantes after diagnostic local anesthetic injections have reduced the pain. Pain of sympathetic origin is not likely to respond to cryodenervation because the heat carried by the major blood vessels interferes with ice-ball formation. Percutaneous sympathectomy is best performed with radiofrequency thermal ablation or with phenol.

Coccygodynia

When coccygodynia has failed to respond to conservative therapy, including the patient's using a donut pillow, NSAIDs, and local steroid injections, consideration can be given to coccygeal neural blockade as the coccygeal nerve exits from the sacral canal at the level of the cornu. Bilateral test injections should produce short-term analgesia before cryoablation is considered. For cryoablation of the coccygeal nerve, the probe must be inserted into the canal to make contact with the nerve. Accurate placement of the ice ball is facilitated by using the 100-Hz stimulator and gauging the patient's response. Care should be taken to prevent bending the relatively large cryoprobe while inserting it into the canal.

Perineal Pain

Pain over the dorsal surface of the scrotum, perineum, and anus that has not responded to conservative management at times can be managed effectively with cryodenervation from inside the sacral canal with bilateral S4 lesions. Test local anesthetic injections should produce a positive response before cryoablations are performed bilaterally at S4. Inserting the cryoprobe through the sacral hiatus up to the level of the fourth sacral foramen for placement of a series of cryolesions can give good analgesia. Bladder dysfunction usually is not encountered, and analgesia lasts 6 to 8 weeks.[34] Perineal pain is difficult to treat with intrathecal neurolytic agents without risking bladder and bowel dysfunction.

Ilioinguinal, Iliohypogastric, and Genitofemoral Neuropathies

Ilioinguinal, iliohypogastric, and genitofemoral neuropathies often complicate herniorrhapy, general abdominal surgery, and cesarean section. Patients present with sharp, lancinating to dull pain radiating into the lower abdomen or groin. The pain is exacerbated by lifting and defecating. If the patient is responsive to a series of low-volume test injections, consideration can be given to cryodenervation of the appropriate nerve. Significant care and time must be spent localizing the nerve with the sensory nerve stimulator. The patient may help to localize the pain generator by pointing with one finger to the point of maximum tenderness. These nerves are difficult to localize percutaneously, and that difficulty has led to frequent misdiagnosis of the pain generator. In an effort to improve accuracy of diagnosis, Saberski and Rosser[35] developed the *conscious pain mapping* technique. In a lightly sedated patient, a general surgeon working with a pain management specialist performs laparoscopic evaluation of the abdomen in an operating suite. The genitofemoral nerve, lateral femoral cutaneous nerve, and other structures are easily visualized (Fig. 170–11). Blunt probing and patient feedback help to direct the physician to the area of pain. At times, objects such as ligatures and staples are found wrapped around the nerve, in which case they should be removed. If direct mechanical or electrical stimulation to the nerve reproduces the pain, cryoablation can be performed under direct vision. (Cryoablation is chosen as the appropriate test because duration of bupivacaine does not outlast discomfort of the perioperative period. The cryoblockade provides weeks to months of reliable analgesia and helps physicians and patients determine if that structure under surveillance carried the pain information.) Pain usually returns. A repeat cryoablation is possible when analgesia is long or an open surgical procedure with sectioning and burying can be performed.

Lower Extremity Pain

Many cutaneous nerve branches are responsive to cryodenervation. The clinician always must perform a complete physical examination, touching the painful area carefully. After the primary pain generator is localized, a series of low-volume local anesthetic injections can be given. If the patient has a consistent response, cryodenervations, as outlined earlier, can be employed. Some common lower extremity nerve pain syndromes that are often amenable to cryodenervation are described next.

Neuralgia resulting from irritation of the *infrapatellar branch of the saphenous nerve* develops weeks to years after blunt injury to the tibial plateau or after knee replacement. The nerve is vulnerable as it passes superficial to the tibial collateral ligament, piercing the sartorious tendon and fascia lata and running inferior and medial to the tibial condyle. The clinical presentation consists of dull pain in the knee joint and achiness below the knee. Patients tend to adopt an antalgic gait. Pain with digital pressure is diagnostic. Patients are considered candidates for cryodenervation when they respond consistently to local anesthetic blocks. A 12-gauge intravenous catheter is used as the introducer, to prevent cold injury to the skin. Because prodding with a felt-tipped pen alone is sufficient to localize the pain generator, the sensory nerve stimulator does not have to be used.

Neuralgia secondary to irritation of the *deep and superficial peroneal and intermediate dorsal cutaneous nerves* can be seen weeks to years after injury to the foot and ankle. These superficial sensory nerves pass through strong ligamentous structures and are vulnerable to stretch injury with inversion of the ankle, compression injury owing to edema, and penetrating trauma from bone fragments. The intermediate dorsal cutaneous nerve runs superficial and medial to the lateral malleolus and continues superficial to the inferior extensor retinaculum, terminating in the fourth and fifth toes. This nerve is particularly vulnerable to injury after sprains of the lateral ankle. The clinical presentation consists of dull ankle pain that is worse with passive inversion of the ankle. Disproportionate swelling, vasomotor instability, and allodynia are remarkably common. Patients tend to adjust their gait to minimize weight bearing on the lateral aspect of the foot. Pain with digital pressure in the area between the lateral malleolus and extensor retinaculum is diagnostic.

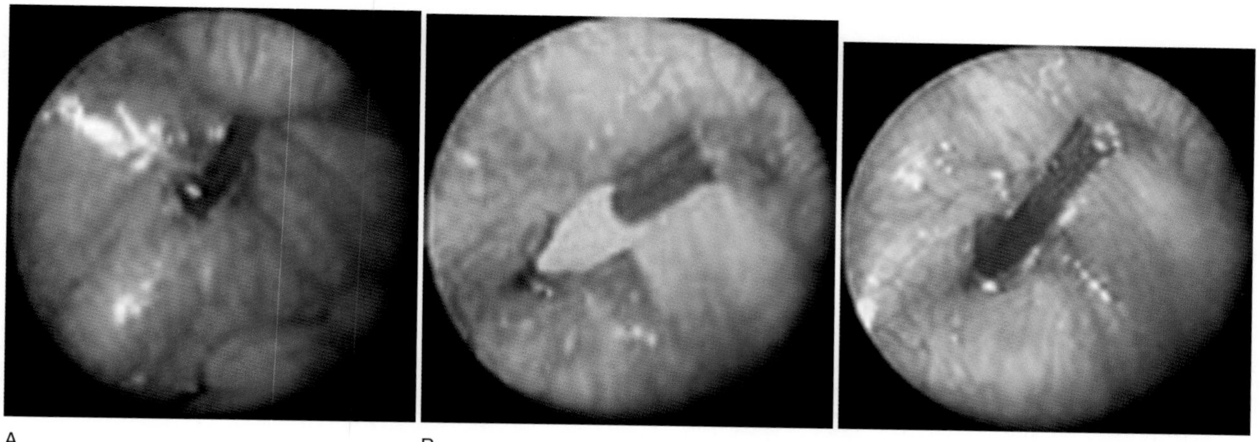

A B C

FIGURE 170–11 ■ **A,** Insertion of the Lloyd cryoprobe through the abdominal wall and fascia onto the genitofemoral nerve. **B,** Ice-ball formation for cryodenervation of the genitofemoral nerve. **C,** Lloyd cryoprobe immediately after defrost. (From Waldman SD: Cryoneurolysis in clinical practice. In Interventional Pain Management, 2nd ed. Philadelphia, WB Saunders, 2001.)

Peroneal Nerve

Superficial and deep peroneal nerve injury often occurs in diabetics, who are vulnerable to compression injury from tight-fitting shoes, and is less common after blunt injury to the dorsum of the foot. The clinical presentation consists of dull pain in the great toe that is often worse after prolonged standing. Patients tend to adjust their gait to minimize weight bearing on the anterior portion of the foot. Pain with digital pressure in the area between the first and second metatarsal heads is often diagnostic.

Superior Gluteal Nerve

Neuralgia resulting from irritation of the superior gluteal branch of the sciatic nerve is common after injury to the lower back and hip sustained while lifting. After exiting the sciatic notch, the superior gluteal nerve passes caudal to the inferior border of the gluteus minimus and penetrates the gluteus medius. Vulnerable as it passes in the fascial plane between the gluteus medius and gluteus minimus musculature, the superior gluteal nerve is injured as a result of shearing between the gluteal muscles on forced external rotation of the leg and with extension of the hip under mechanical load. Rarely, it is injured by forced extension of the hip, an injury that might occur in a head-on automobile collision when the foot is pressed against the floorboards with the knee in extension as the patient braces for impact. The clinical presentation consists of sharp pain in the lower back, dull pain in the buttock, and vague pain to the popliteal fossa. Pain below the knee is unusual. Patients generally experience pain with prolonged sitting, leaning forward, or twisting to the contralateral side. Often, patients describe "giving way" of the leg. They usually sit with the weight on the contralateral buttock or cross their legs to minimize pressure on the involved side. With the patient in the prone position, the medial border of the ilium is palpated. The nerve is located 5 cm lateral and inferior to the attachment of the gluteus medius. The peripheral nerve stimulator is employed to ensure that motor units are not inadvertently blocked.

Craniofacial Pain

Craniofacial nerves can be cryolesioned with a percutaneous or open technique.[36] Entrapment neuropathies and neuromas are more responsive to local anesthetic and cryodenervations than are neuropathies of medical causes. Meticulous diagnostic injection ensures the best outcome with cryoablation.[15] If there is good analgesic response to a series of local anesthetic injections, cryodenervation is an option. The technique of cryodenervations of cranial and facial nerves is the same as that for other peripheral nerves. A nerve stimulator is used to localize the nerve. Because these areas are relatively densely vascular, injecting a few milliliters of saline containing 1:100,000 epinephrine is recommended before inserting the cryoprobe introducer cannula. A postprocedural ice pack applied for 30 minutes reduces pain and swelling.

An irritative neuropathy of the *supraorbital nerve* (Fig. 170–12) often occurs at the supraorbital notch.[37] Vulnerable

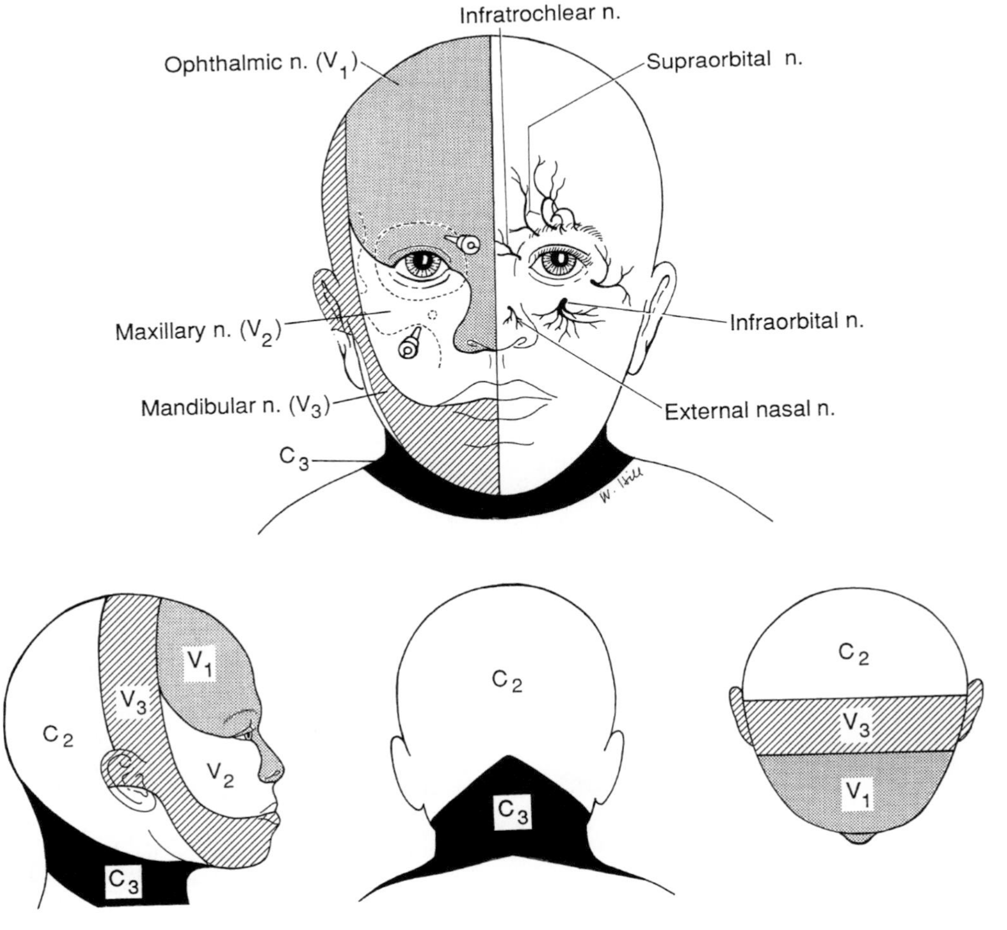

FIGURE 170–12 ■ Dermatome man showing commonly blocked cutaneous branches of the trigeminal nerve.

to blunt trauma, this nerve often is injured by deceleration against an automobile windshield. Commonly confused with migraine and frontal sinusitis, the pain of supraorbital neuralgia often manifests as a throbbing frontal headache. At times, many of the hallmarks of vascular headache are present, including blurred vision, nausea, and photophobia. This neuralgia often worsens over time, perhaps owing to scar formation around the nerve.

Neuropathic pain in the distribution of the supraorbital nerve can be addressed with an open or closed cryoablative procedure as long as appropriate conservative therapy has failed and the pain responds to a series of test local anesthetic injections. For an open procedure, the incision is buried beneath the eyebrow, so there is no obvious scar. For the percutaneous technique, the introducer catheter should be inserted at the eyebrow line to avoid damage to hair follicles.

The *infraorbital nerve* (see Fig. 170–12) is the termination of the second division of the trigeminal nerve. An irritative neuropathy can occur at the infraorbital foramen secondary to blunt trauma or fracture of the zygoma with entrapment of the nerve in the bony callus. Commonly confused with maxillary sinusitis, the pain of infraorbital neuralgia most often is exacerbated with smiling and laughing. Referred pain to teeth is common, and a history of dental pain and dental procedures is typical. Cryoablation can be accomplished via open or closed technique. The closed technique can be done from inside the mouth through the superior buccolabial fold. In both operations, the probe is advanced until it lies over the infraorbital foramen. The intraoral approach has cosmetic advantages only.

The *mandibular nerve* can be irritated at many locations along its path. It is often injured as the result of hypertrophy of the pterygoids secondary to chronic bruxism, but it also can be irritated if the vertical dimension of the oral cavity is reduced owing to tooth loss or altered dentition. Pain is often referred to the lower teeth, and patients frequently undergo dental evaluations and procedures.

Injury to the *mental nerve,* the terminal portion of the mandibular nerve, frequently occurs in edentulous patients. Pain can be reproduced easily with palpation.

The *auriculotemporal nerve* can be irritated at many sites, including immediately proximal to the parietal ridge at the attachment of the temporalis muscle and, less commonly, at the ramus of the mandible. Patients often present with temporal pain associated with retro-orbital pain. Pain often is referred to the teeth. Patients frequently awaken at night with temporal headache. The pain, described as throbbing, aching, and pounding, can be bilateral, and it is commonly associated with bruxism and functional abnormalities of the temporomandibular joint, maxilla, and mandible. The clinician must rule out other medical causes for this form of headache, including temporal arteritis, before considering treatments for auriculotemporal neuralgia. Posterior auricular neuralgia often follows blunt injury to the mastoid area. It is common in abused women and usually involves the left side owing to the preponderance of right-handed abusers. The clinical presentation consists of pain in the ear associated with a feeling of "fullness" and tenderness. This syndrome often is misdiagnosed as a chronic ear infection. The posterior auricular nerve runs along the posterior border of the sternocleidomastoid muscle, superficially and immediately posterior to the mastoid.

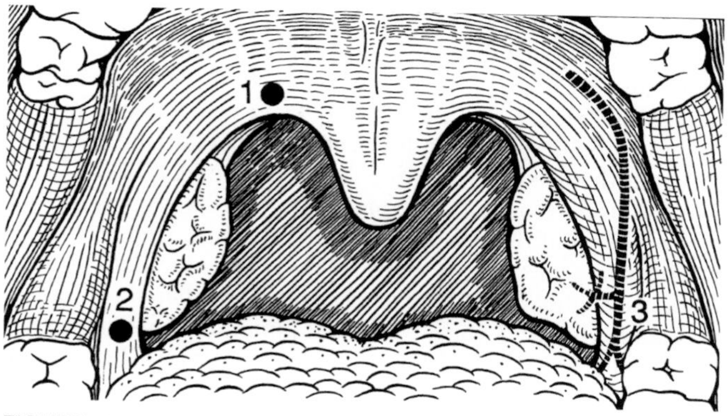

FIGURE 170–13 ■ The distal glossopharyngeal nerve subjacent to the tonsillar fossa. *1, 2,* Locations for local anesthetic and cryodenervation. *3,* The pathway of the glossopharyngeal nerve is superficial at this site. Care must be taken to avoid entering the artery.

The *glossopharyngeal nerve* lies immediately subjacent to the tonsillar fossa (Fig. 170–13). This painful condition can be treated by applying the cryoprobe for two cycles of 2 minutes each after local anesthetic injections have produced the appropriate responses. This is essentially a simple procedure, but it has distinct advantages over injection of this cranial nerve at the tip of the mastoid, where injection could block the vagus in addition to the spinal accessory nerves.[36]

Many other common peripheral nerve injuries are amenable to cryodenervation, including most cutaneous branches and the occipital, suprascapular, superficial radial, and anterior penetrating branches of the intercostal nerves. Applied carefully, the techniques outlined in this chapter would help to achieve the safest and best possible outcome.

■ CASE REPORT

A 58-year-old woman sustained a traumatic spondylolisthesis at L4-5 for which a spinal fusion was performed.[38] Autogenous bone graft for the vertebral fusion was obtained from the left posterior iliac crest. Postoperatively, the patient continued to experience wrenching and searing pain at the iliac crest donor site (pain score 7 on the 10-point VAS). Treatment with NSAIDs for 3 weeks and transcutaneous electrical nerve stimulation for 2 weeks did not alleviate the pain (VAS = 5). The patient was referred to the pain medicine center for additional evaluation and treatment. The initial clinical assessment indicated the primary painful locus (7.5 cm × 5 cm) to be within the defect of the posterior iliac bone harvest site. The patient's symptoms—a constant, wrenching, and searing pain with radiation into the calf—were aggravated by walking and assuming the standing or sitting position and were partially relieved with rest.

A diagnosis of postoperative iliac crest pain syndrome (a new name for this symptom complex) was made. Inflammation and a posttraumatic neuroexcitatory state induced by the surgical trauma were posited to be responsible for the pain. For these reasons, the iliac crest donor site was infiltrated with a series of local anesthetic injections (10 mL of 0.5% bupivacaine), NSAID (60 mg of ketorolac), and steroid (20 mg of triamcinolone) at 2- to 3-week intervals. The first four injections contained 10 mL of 0.5% bupivacaine and 60 mg of ketorolac. The first injection relieved the patient's pain completely (VAS = 0). The pain gradually returned to pretreatment levels (VAS = 7) during the next 2 weeks, with the notable difference that the locus of pain was reduced in size (5 cm × 2.5 cm). The pain locus corresponded to the center of the graft donor site. The three subsequent injections of bupivacaine and ketorolac had minimal effect on pain scores or size of the painful locus. For the fifth injection, 10 mL of 0.5% bupivacaine was mixed with 20 mg of triamcinolone. The response to this injection was dramatic—further shrinking of the painful locus (3 cm × 2 cm) and diminution in pain scores (VAS = 1). A sixth (and final) injection at week 12 produced further diminution of the painful locus to two discrete (1 cm × 1 cm) foci. The patient nevertheless described this pain as sharp and excruciating (VAS = 7). The relatively smaller size of the painful loci prompted selection of cryodenervation as a second step of treatment. A cryoprobe that produced 0.5-cm ice balls at thermal equilibrium was selected. A grid was visualized over the area, and seven cryodenervations were performed, each of 3 minutes' duration. The patient experienced postprocedure discomfort, but it disappeared over the first week (VAS = 0) (Table 170–1), and the patient resumed all previous preoperative activities after 1 month. One year after the procedure, the patient continued to have complete mobility and activity.

DISCUSSION

The harvesting of bone has been used frequently in orthopedic surgery since 1901, when Von Eiselberg first reported autogenous cancellous bone transplantation.[39,40] The sites frequently used to harvest donor bone include the iliac crests, ribs, and calvaria.[41-45] There is no consensus about one preferred site.[42-46] The posterior iliac crest is used for bone harvesting in many orthopedic and reconstructive procedures owing to its suitability as a donor site.[41,46] The complications associated with bone graft harvesting from the posterior iliac crest include chronic pain, altered sensation at the harvest site, superior gluteal arteriovenous fistula, ureteral injury, sacroiliac joint dislocation, osteomyelitis, gluteal weakness, lumbar hernia, and injury to the sciatic and gluteal nerves.[47-52] Chronic pain is the most common postharvest complication (reported incidence 25% to 38%).[47,49,52] The persistence of iliac crest donor site pain is thought to be a complication of total or partial injury to the cutaneous continuations of the lateral branches of the dorsal rami of L1-3, collectively called the *superior cluneal nerves.*[48,53] Modifying the surgical technique to avoid this complication has not altered significantly the incidence and characteristics of donor site pain.[47,54-57] Findings of a few studies suggest the benefit of perioperative infiltration of the donor site with a local anesthetic (bupivacaine).[58-60] Others suggest giving bupivacaine via an indwelling epidural catheter for postharvest pain.[60,61] Perioperative infiltration of the donor site with a local anesthetic may alleviate the acute pain, but, considering the incidence of chronic pain at donor site (25% to 38%),[47,49,52] approximately 62% to 75% of patients receive local donor site anesthetic infiltration or intraoperative catheter treatment without any long-term benefit. It increases direct and indirect hospital costs because of the additional procedure, longer hospital stay, and increased risk of complications.

The pathophysiologic mechanisms of persistent pain at the donor site are likely to be multiple and may involve various biochemical pathways. Injury, regeneration, and remodeling of cancellous bone are thought to be associated with marked increases in osteoclastic activity that is affected by prostaglandins via many different pathways.[62,63] Harvey and coworkers[64] used a dental model to show significant concentrations of prostaglandins in alveolar bone cysts. Inflammatory cells, macrophages, lymphocytes, and monocytes initiate degradation of connective tissue[65] presumably through increased prostaglandin E_2 production. The plasma level of prostaglandins is of little clinical use because there is 95% clearance by the pulmonary vascular bed within 3 to 6 seconds.[66-68] Shindell and coworkers[69] showed that injections

Table 170–1

Overview of Patient History

Treatment Category	*VAS Reduction* (%)*	*Reduction in Area of Painful Locus†‡ (%)*
Pretreatment (postoperative)	7 (N/A)	7.5 × 5 (N/A)
Symptomatic treatment (NSAID and TENS)	5 (28.6)	7.5 × 5 (0)
Injection Therapy		
Bupivacaine and ketorolac		
First injection	0 (100)	0 (100)
Second injection	5 (28.6)	5 × 3 (60)
Third injection	4 (42.9)	5 × 2 (73.3)
Fourth injection	5 (28.6)	4.5 × 3 (64)
Bupivacaine and triamcinolone		
Fifth injection	1 (85.7)	3 × 2 (84)
Sixth injection	6 (14.3)	1 × 1 and 1 × 1 (94.7)
Cryodenervation	1 (100)	0 (100)

*Reduction is expressed as % of baseline values at pretreatment (postoperative) stage.
†Measured by same physician using same amount of pressure for deep palpation and recorded in centimeters.
‡One week after cryodenervation.
TENS, transcutaneous electrical nerve stimulation; VAS, visual analog score.

of steroid into bone cysts reduced prostaglandin E_2 concentrations by 52% to 93%. The reduction in prostaglandin E_2 concentration has been proposed as one of the biochemical mechanisms responsible for the effectiveness of intralesional steroid therapy.[69] Also, ketorolac, a direct inhibitor of cyclooxygenase, decreases prostaglandin biosynthesis and likely increases neural threshold. Prostaglandins, in addition to causing bone destruction, increase the sensitivity of peripheral nociceptors to pain mediators, including bradykinin.[70] The local anesthetic may affect the outcome by attenuating afferent input[71] and diminishing the plasticity of the CNS.

The reduction in the size of the patient's pain locus to only two discrete points most likely resulted from attenuation of afferent sensory input. This decrease in size of the painful locus made it possible to consider cryodenervation of the underlying periosteum. Cryodenervation has been used successfully for postoperative and chronic pain relief. Few long-term outcome studies on the effectiveness of cryodenervation are available. A 10-year audit of cryodenervation for trigeminal neuralgia indicated a 6 months' median duration of relief and comparable pain-free intervals after repeated cryodenervations.[72] Cryoanalgesia relieves pain by producing long-lasting neurolysis combined with axonal regeneration. Freezing of nerve results in axonal disintegration and degeneration of the myelin sheaths. The perineurium and epineurium are preserved, however, and regrowth of axons occurs in the original supporting structures at the rate of 1 to 3 mm/day.[73] This obviates growth of painful neuromas, a problem associated with other neurolytic and surgical techniques, but also limits the duration of effective analgesia.[72,74,75] At present, there is no conclusive physiologic explanation for the sometimes prolonged analgesic effect because regeneration of axons seems to be completed in a matter of weeks after the procedure.[73,76] It is possible that cryoanalgesia affects the plasticity of the CNS and diminishes pain overall. The complications associated with cryotherapy are relatively minor, but include cold injury, skin discoloration, and numbness in the distribution of the treated peripheral nerve. An important limitation is that it can be applied only to sensory nerves because ablation of mixed nerves would produce temporary paralysis of the corresponding muscles. Improvement can be attributed to additive analgesic effects of ketorolac, steroid, local anesthetic, and cryotherapy on several different nociceptive pathways. This combination may produce a balanced analgesia that is likely to be more effective and to have fewer side effects than any other approach. This two-step therapeutic approach may prove to be the treatment of choice for prolonged relief of chronic iliac crest harvest pain.

FUTURE DIRECTIONS

Cryotechnology offers promise for a wide variety of pain management needs. Its unparalleled track record for safety is remarkable. Its effective and safe use on sensory and mixed nerves contrasts with radiofrequency technology, which has the potential to produce deafferentation when applied to peripheral nerves. The lack of controlled studies, lack of uniform training, and poor communication between providers has impeded widespread use of the technology. To address these issues better, WESTCO Medical Corporation (San Diego, CA), a major supplier of cryotechnology, has set up a cryotechnology users club whose primary objective is exchange of information and development of studies.

References

1. Evans P: Cryo-analgesia: The application of low temperatures to nerves to produce anesthesia or analgesia. Anaesthesia 36:1003, 1981.
2. Hippocrates: Aphorisms. vol 4. Heracleitus on the Universe. London, Heinemann, 1931.
3. Gruner O: A Treatise on the Canon of Medicine of Avicenna. London, Luzac, 1930.
4. Bartholini T: De Nivis usu Medico Observationes Variae, Hafniae. Copenhagen, P. Haubold, 1661.
5. Larre D: Surgical Memoirs of the Campaigns of Russia, Germany and France. Philadelphia, Carey & Lea, 1732.
6. Arnott J: On severe cold or congelation as a remedy of disease. London, Medical Gazette, 1748, p 936.
7. Holden HB: Practical Cryosurgery. London, Pitman, 1975, 2.
8. Cooper IS: Cryosurgery in modern medicine. J Neurol Sci 2:493, 1965.
9. Amoils SP: The Joule-Thomson cryoprobe. Arch Ophthalmol 78:201, 1978.
10. Evans P, Lloyd J, Green C: Cryo-analgesia: The response to alterations in freeze cycle temperature. Br J Anaesth 53:1121, 1981.
11. Holden HB: Practical Cryosurgery. London, Pitman, 1975, p 9.
12. Gander MJ, Soanes WA, Smith V: Experimental prostate surgery. Invest Urol 1:610, 1964.
13. Soanes WA, Ablin RJ, Gander MJ: Remission of metastatic lesions following cryosurgery in prostatic cancer: Immunologic considerations. J Urol 104:154, 1970.
14. Lloyd J, Barnard J, Glynn C: Cryo-analgesia: A new approach to pain relief. Lancet 2:932, 1976.
15. Barnard J, Lloyd J, Glynn C: Cryosurgery in the management of intractable facial pain. Br J Oral Surg 16:135, 1978.
16. Peuria M, Krmpotic-Nemanic J, Markiewitz A: Tunnel Syndromes. Boca Raton, FL, CRC Press, 1991.
17. Wall PD: The prevention of postoperative pain. Pain 33:289, 1988.
18. Armitage EN: Postoperative pain-prevention or relief? Br J Anaesth 63:136, 1989.
19. Cousins MJ: Acute pain and injury response, immediate and prolonged effects. Reg Anaesth 14:162, 1989.
20. McQuay HJ, Carroll D, Moore RA: Postoperative orthopedic pain—the effect of opiate premedication and local anesthetic blocks. Pain 33:291, 1988.
21. Woolf CJ, Wall PD: Morphine sensitive and insensitive actions of C-fibre input on the rat spinal cords. Neurosci Lett 64:221, 1986.
22. Glynn C, Lloyd J, Barnard J: Cryo-analgesia in the management of pain after thoracotomy, Thorax 35:325, 1980.
23. Katz J, Nelson W, Forest R, Bruce D: Cryo-analgesia for postthoracotomy pain. Lancet 1:512, 1980.
24. Orr I, Keenan D, Dundee J: Improved pain relief after thoracotomy: Use of cryoprobe and morphine infusion. BMJ 283:88, 1981.
25. Wood G, Lloyd J, Bullingham R, et al: Postoperative analgesia for day case herniorrhaphy patients: A comparison of cryo-analgesia, paravertebral blockade and oral analgesia. Anesthesia 36:603, 1981.
26. Gough JD, Williams AB, Vaughan RS: The control of post-thoracotomy pain: A comparative evaluation of thoracic epidural fentanyl infusions and cryo-analgesia. Anesthesia 43:780, 1988.
27. Nelson K, Vincent R, Bourke R: Interoperative intercostal nerve freezing to prevent postthoracotomy pain. Ann Thorac Surg 170:280, 1974.
28. Maiwand O, Makey AR: Cryo-analgesia for relief of pain after thoracotomy. BMJ 282:49, 1981.
29. Conacher ID, Locke T, Hilton ML: Neuralgia after cryo-analgesia for thoracotomy. Lancet 1:277, 1986.
30. Wood G, Lloyd J, Evans P, et al: Cryo-analgesia and day case herniorrhaphy (letter). Lancet 2:479, 1979.
31. Brechner T: Percutaneous cryogenic neurolysis of the articular nerve of Lushka. Reg Anesthesiol 6:170, 1981.
32. Trescott A: Workshop for Cryotherapy. 6th International Congress on Pain, Atlanta, April 20, 1994.
33. Sluijter ME: Radiofrequency lesions of the communicating ramus in the treatment of low back pain. In Racz G (ed): Techniques of Neurolysis. Boston, Kluwer, 1989.
34. Raj P: Practical Management of Pain. Chicago, Year Book Medical Publishers, 1986, 779.

35. Saberski L, Rosser J: Laparoscopic concious pain mapping.
36. Raj P: Practical Management of Pain. Chicago, Year Book Medical Publishers, 1986, p 777.
37. Klein DS, Schmidt RE: Chronic headache resulting from postoperative supraorbital neuralgia. Anesth Analg 73:490, 1991.
38. Saberski LR, Ahmad M, Munir A, Brull S: Identification of a new therapeutic approach for iliac crest donor site chronic pain: A case report. Anesth Analg 89:1538-1540, 1999.
39. Witsenburg B: The reconstruction of anterior residual bone defects in patients with cleft lip, alveolus and palate: A review. J Maxillofac Surg 13:197, 1985.
40. Canady JW, Zeitler DP, Thompson SA, Nicholas CD: Suitability of the iliac crest as a site for harvest of autogenous bone grafts. Cleft Palate Craniofac 30:579, 1993.
41. Citardi MJ, Friedman CD: Nonvascularized autogenous bone grafts for craniofacial skeletal augmentation and replacement. Otolaryngol Clin North Am 27:891, 1994.
42. Laurie SW, Kaban LB, Mulliken JB, Murray JE: Donor-site morbidity after harvesting rib and iliac bone. Plast Reconstr Surg 73:933, 1984.
43. Raulo Y, Baruch J: Utilisation de la voute cranienne comme site de greffes osseuses en chirurgie cranio-maxillo-faciale. Chirurgie 116:359, 1990.
44. Motoki DS, Mulliken JB: The healing of bone and cartilage. Clin Plast Surg 17:527, 1990.
45. Gerbino G, Berrone S, De Gioanni PP, Appendino P: Valutazione clinica degli esiti di prelievo osseo da cresta iliaca. Minerva Stomatol 41:57, 1992.
46. Fernyhough JC, Schimandle JJ, Weigel MC, et al: Chronic donor site pain complicating bone graft harvesting from the posterior iliac crest for spinal fusion. Spine 17:1474, 1992.
47. Kurz LT, Garfin SR, Booth RE Jr: Harvesting autogenous iliac bone grafts: A review of complications and techniques. Spine 14:1324, 1989.
48. Goulet JA, Senunas LE, DeSilva GL, Greenfield ML: Autogenous iliac crest bone graft: Complications and functional assessment. Clin Orthop 83:76, 1997.
49. Arrington ED, Smith WJ, Chambers HG, et al: Complications of iliac crest bone graft harvesting. Clin Orthop 82:300, 1996.
50. Younger EM, Chapman MW: Morbidity at bone graft donor sites. J Orthop Trauma 3:192, 1989.
51. Summers BN, Eisenstein SM: Donor site pain from the ilium: A complication of lumbar spine fusion. J Bone Joint Surg Br 71:677, 1989.
52. Kurz LT, Garfin SR, Booth RE: Iliac bone grafting: Techniques and complications of harvesting. In: Garfin SR (ed): Complications of Spine Surgery. Baltimore, Williams & Wilkins, 1989, p 323.
53. Tanishima T, Yoshimasu N, Ogai M: A technique for prevention of donor site pain associated with harvesting iliac bone grafts. Surg Neurol 44:131, 1995.
54. Schnee CL, Freese A, Weil RJ, Marcotte PJ: Analysis of harvest morbidity and radiographic outcome using autograft for anterior cervical fusion. Spine 22:2222, 1997.
55. Fernandes HM, Mendelow AD, Choksey MS: Anterior cervical discectomy: An improvement in donor site operative technique. Br J Neurosurg 8:201, 1994.
56. David DJ, Tan E, Katsaros J, Sheen R: Mandibular reconstruction with vascularized iliac crest: A 10-year experience. Plast Reconstr Surg 82:792, 1988.
57. Brull SJ, Lieponis JV, Murphy MJ, et al: Acute and long-term benefits of iliac crest donor site perfusion with local anesthetics. Anesth Analg 74:145, 1992.
58. Hahn M, Dover MS, Whear NM, Moule I: Local bupivacaine infusion following bone graft harvest from the iliac crest. Int J Oral Maxillofac Surg 25:400, 1996.
59. Wilkes RA, Thomas WG: Bupivacaine infusion for iliac crest donor sites. J Bone Joint Surg Br 76:503, 1994.
60. Dunstan SP, Korczak PK: Use of epidural catheter for postoperative pain relief for bone harvesting from iliac crest. Br J Oral Maxillofac Surg 34:436, 1996.
61. Kennedy BD, Hiranaka DK: Use of a modified epidural catheter for analgesia after iliac crest bone procurement. J Oral Maxillofac Surg 53:342, 1995.
62. Dietrich JW, Goodson JM, Raisz LG: Stimulation of bone resorption by various prostaglandins in organ culture. Prostaglandins 10:231, 1975.
63. Vaes G: Cell-to-cell interactions in the secretion of enzymes of connective tissue breakdown, collagenase and proteoglycan-degrading neutral proteases: A review. Agents Actions 10:474, 1980.
64. Harvey W, Guat-Chen F, Gordon D, et al: Evidence for fibroblasts as the major source of prostacyclin and prostaglandin synthesis in dental cysts in man. Arch Oral Biol 29:223, 1984.
65. Vaes G, Huybrechts-Godin G, Hauser P: Lymphocyte-macrophage-fibroblast co-operation in the inflammatory degradation of cartilage and connective tissue. Agents Actions Suppl 7:100, 1980.
66. Clyman RI, Mauray F, Heymann MA, Roman C: Effect of gestational age on pulmonary metabolism of prostaglandin E1 and E2. Prostaglandins 21:505, 1981.
67. Weiss M, Forster W: Pharmacokinetics of prostaglandins: Prediction of steady-state concentrations during intravenous infusion. Int J Clin Pharmacol Ther Toxicol 170:344, 1980.
68. Vane JR: The release and fate of vaso-active hormones in the circulation. Br J Pharmacol 35:209, 1969.
69. Shindell R, Huurman WW, Lippiello L, Connolly JF: Prostaglandin levels in unicameral bone cysts treated by intralesional steroid injection. J Pediatr Orthop 9:516, 1989.
70. Buckley MM, Brogden RN: Ketorolac: A review of its pharmacodynamic and pharmacokinetic properties, and therapeutic potential. Drugs 39:86, 1990.
71. Young ER, MacKenzie TA: The pharmacology of local anesthetics—a review of the literature. J Can Dent Assoc 58:34, 1992.
72. Zakrzewska JM: Cryotherapy for trigeminal neuralgia: A 10-year audit. Br J Oral Maxillofac Surg 29:1, 1991.
73. Evans PJ: Cryo-analgesia: The application of low temperatures to nerves to produce anaesthesia or analgesia. Anaesthesia 36:1003, 1981.
74. Lloyd JW, Barnard JD, Glynn CJ: Cryo-analgesia: A new approach to pain relief. Lancet 2:932, 1976.
75. Barnard D, Lloyd J, Evans J: Cryo-analgesia in the management of chronic facial pain. J Maxillofac Surg 9:101, 1981.
76. Saberski L: Cryo-neurolysis in clinical practice. In Waldman S, Winnie A (eds): The Textbook of Interventional Pain Management. Philadelphia, WB Saunders, 1994, pp 172-184.

chapter 171

Vertebroplasty and Kyphoplasty

Ronald A. Alberico and Ahmed Nabil Abdelhalim

Vertebral compression fractures are affecting an increasing number of people in the United States as the population ages. These fractures may be due to primary or secondary osteoporosis or to malignancy. In the past, vertebral compression fractures have been treated conservatively with bed rest, pain medications, and back bracing to decrease the patient's pain, but the spine was left in its deformed state. Open surgical treatment can address the deformity but is usually reserved for patients with a neurologic deficit. Vertebroplasty and kyphoplasty have been developed as alternatives to surgery for the treatment of painful vertebral compression fractures whether caused by osteoporosis or malignancy.

It is well documented that malignant disease frequently metastasizes to bones. The length of time that a patient suffers with metastatic disease increases the likelihood of bony involvement. As we become better at treating patients with malignancy, bony involvement will therefore become more prevalent. Between 30% and 70% of bone metastases involve the vertebrae.[1] The result is chronic back pain secondary to bone involvement in the majority of patients with metastatic disease and in those with marrow-infiltrating diseases such as multiple myeloma and leukemia. Most bony metastases compromise the strength of the involved bone. In the vertebral bodies this decreased bone strength leads to pathologic compression fractures in 8% to 30% of patients, frequently without trauma.[2,3] It would appear that that the physiologic load on the spine acting in isolation is sufficient to fracture a pathologically involved vertebral body. Other causes of vertebral compression fractures in patients with malignant disease include secondary osteoporosis from malnutrition, radiation treatment, and chronic steroid administration.

The consequences of pathologic compression fractures of the vertebral bodies are well documented in the osteoporotic population.[4] These complications include an acceleration of bone mineral loss as a result of inactivity perpetuating the likelihood of additional fractures. Inactivity also conveys a risk for embolic and thrombotic complications in the lungs, as well as the lower extremities. The biomechanical effects of kyphosis secondary to vertebral body fractures include an increased risk of falling, a shift of biomechanical forces anteriorly, thereby increasing the risk for additional fractures, and physiologic decreases in lung capacity and appetite.[5,6] These processes describe a downward spiral that is known to significantly decrease the lifespan of patients after their first compression fracture. One study correlated a person's first vertebral compression fracture with a significant increase in 1-year mortality.[7] This study revealed that the 1-year mortality of osteoporotic patients suffering one compression fracture is 23% higher than that of age-matched controls. This number increases to >30% for patients with multiple fractures.

Historically, medicine has had little to offer cancer patients with painful vertebral compression fractures that did not respond well to analgesic therapy. Frequently, surgical options are not possible in this population because of the overall suboptimal health of the patients and their relatively long recovery time. Surgeons also avoid patients with multilevel disease.[8] As a result, surgery is reserved for those with anatomic compression of the spinal canal contents by retropulsion of bone. Therapeutic and palliative radiation therapy is an alternative to surgery for malignant bone pain and spinal canal compromise caused by epidural extension of tumor. Palliative radiation can be ineffective in up to 30% of patients, however, and cannot be given if maximal doses to the spine were already delivered for tumor treatment of the spine or adjacent structures. Radiation may also contribute to secondary osteoporosis and thereby increase the risk for compression fracture, particularly after therapeutic doses. In recent years, the intravenous administration of bisphosphonates has shown some efficacy in those with chronic bone pain and may help prevent pathologic fractures, but their efficacy in pain relief for patients who have already suffered fractures is not established.[9] With the exception of surgery, none of the treatments listed addresses the issue of altered biomechanical forces in the spine and the other consequences of kyphosis.

In recent years, interventional techniques have significantly improved our ability to perform minimally invasive procedures. The advantage of these procedures is that they can often be performed on patients who are otherwise too sick to endure more extensive techniques while providing a significant improvement in response over that of medical therapy alone. The remainder of this chapter describes the two minimally invasive procedures that are designed to address vertebral compression fractures and the associated chronic back pain. Both procedures have advantages and disadvantages, which will be discussed, as well as indications, contraindications, and risks. This chapter will not serve as a tutorial for performing the techniques because that would require formal training in an established course with the guidance of experienced instructors.

VERTEBROPLASTY

Percutaneous vertebroplasty was first described by Galibert and Deramond in France in 1987.[10] The initial procedure was designed for the treatment of a painful vertebral body hemangioma. The procedure itself can be summarized as percutaneous fixation of pathologic vertebral compression fractures by injection of polymethylmethacrylate (PMMA) through a needle inserted into the vertebral body. Most procedures use a transpediculate approach for needle insertion to avoid the segmental arteries that extend along the side of the vertebral body. Vertebroplasty is usually performed with the patient in the prone position and the use of strict sterile technique, conscious sedation, local anesthesia, and fluoroscopic guidance. Approaches using one or two pediculate needles have been described with similar results.[11,12] The fluoroscopic target is well defined anatomically, and success at accessing the pedicle with proper fluoroscopic technique and knowledge of patient anatomy is dependent on adequate visualization of the target during the procedure (Fig. 171–1).

Indications and Contraindications

Two main groups of patients may benefit from vertebroplasty, those with pathologic fractures and associated pain and those with progressive vertebral compression from pathologic fractures. All patients must have a vertebral compression fracture that is related to a pathologic process to qualify for treatment at this time. Trauma-associated fracture without pathologic bone is not treated because more definitive surgical options are available. It is also thought that the small amount of space available in the trabecular network of normal bone increases the likelihood of cement extravasation during the injection process. For patients with painful compression fractures, the pain should be directly related to the vertebral fracture on clinical examination, limit patient mobility or quality of life, and require chronic medication for control. Some patients who are more difficult to assess in terms of pain localization can benefit from imaging with MRI or a bone scan.[13] Patients with increased uptake on bone scan or demonstrable edema within the bone on MRI are more likely to obtain pain relief than those without imaging abnormalities beyond simple compression. For patients with progressive vertebral compression deformity over time demonstrated on radiography, MRI, or CT, vertebroplasty is indicated to arrest the progress of the deformity. Contraindications to vertebroplasty include active osteomyelitis, all contraindications to conscious sedation, severe (>30%) preexisting stenosis of the spinal canal, existing coagulopathy or thrombocytopenia (platelet count <80,000), pregnancy, and hypersensitivity to PMMA or other implanted devices. Coagulopathy and thrombocytopenia can, of course, be corrected before the procedure. Epidural or intradural neoplastic disease compressing or encasing the thecal sac or nerve roots is also a contraindication to treatment. Relative contraindications include a dehiscent posterior cortical wall in the

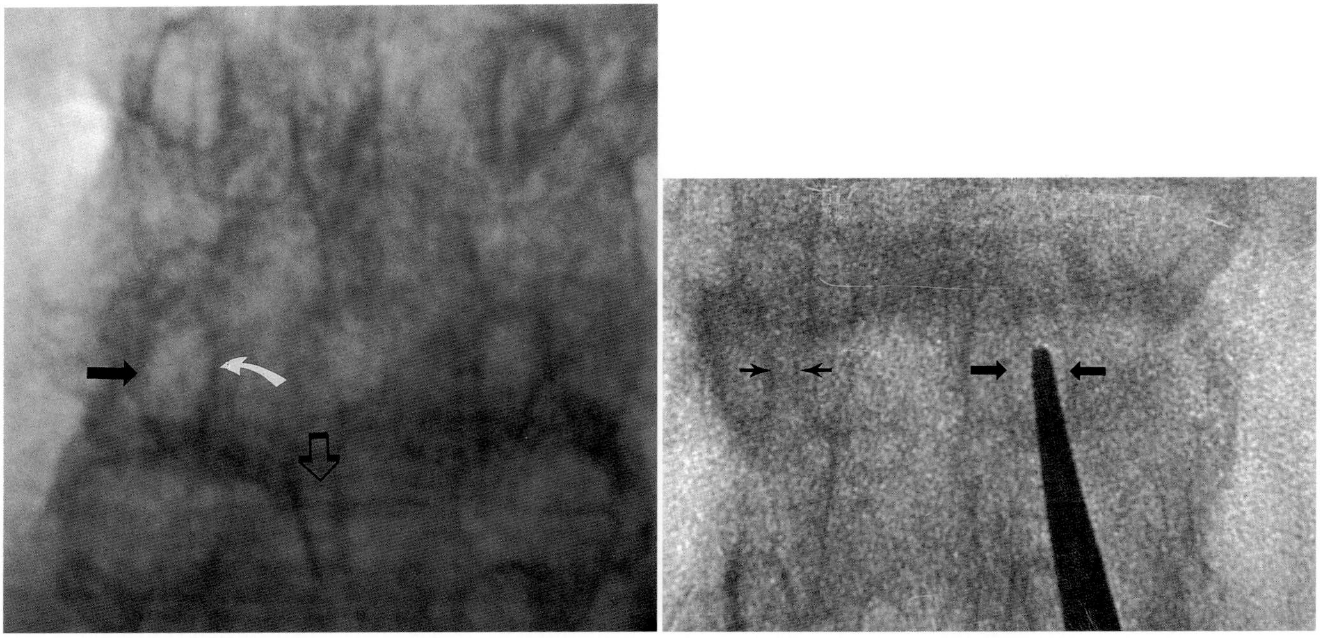

A B

FIGURE 171–1 ■ **A,** An anteroposterior view of the spine shows the lateral wall (*black arrow*) and medial wall (*curved white arrow*) of the pedicle. Note that the spinous process projects in the midline (*open arrow*). **B,** This oblique view of the spine shows a clamp projected over the midline of the pedicle. The *large arrows* point to the lateral and medial wall of the pedicle. The *small arrows* demonstrate the proximity of the lateral wall of the spinous process and the medial wall of the other pedicle when the obliquity is optimized for a two-needle approach (*small arrows*). A single-needle approach would project the spinous process on top of the pedicle.

affected vertebral body, inability of the patient to assume the prone position, and difficulty visualizing the vertebral structures at fluoroscopy. Ongoing or future radiation therapy is not a contraindication to vertebroplasty. PMMA has been shown to be unaffected by radiation at therapeutic doses in vitro.[14]

Efficacy

The literature on vertebroplasty is extensive and has evaluated both osteoporotic fractures and fractures secondary to solid and marrow-based malignancy.[15-18] Rates of pain relief after treatment vary somewhat among the reports but usually range from 80% to 85%. Pain relief is generally realized within 5 days of treatment and is maximal within 2 weeks. Pain relief is usually assessed with a visual analog scale and reported as complete, improved, unchanged, or worse. Reported relief is less frequent for cancer patients than for those with osteoporosis, but it is still significant at 50% to 80% in most series. Lack of equivalent efficacy in cancer patients is undoubtedly due to multifactorial sources of pain in that population. Durability of pain relief after vertebroplasty is also demonstrated in some studies with follow-up assessment extending to 2 to 5 years. Despite the success with vertebroplasty, the procedure does not attempt to correct kyphotic deformity or reestablish normal vertebral body height.

The exact mechanism of pain relief in vertebroplasty and kyphoplasty is not yet established. A potential source of pain relief is fixation of chronically mobile bone fragments. Another possibility includes thermal neurolysis. PMMA polymerization is an exothermic process that can produce temperatures close to 70° C. It is theorized that this may damage nerve endings in the affected bone and thereby decrease the pain response.

Procedure

In our institution, vertebroplasty is performed by neuroradiology and is almost exclusively done as an outpatient procedure. Patients are initially evaluated regarding the source of pain and appropriate level or levels to treat by the neuroradiologist through a clinic appointment and are scheduled for an ambulatory surgery appointment on the day of treatment. Patients are instructed to take nothing orally after midnight on the day of treatment and are confirmed to have a normal coagulation profile and platelet count before proceeding. Almost all vertebroplasties are performed successfully with conscious sedation administered by the operating physician in cooperation with a nurse. The nurse performs appropriate monitoring and documentation during the procedure. The majority of cases require 2 to 4 mg of intravenous midazolam (Versed) and 150 to 250 mg of fentanyl for patient comfort over the course of 1 to 2 hours. Lidocaine, 1%, is used over each access point for anesthesia, and care is taken to infiltrate the region directly over the entry site into bone. All patients receive a dose of antibiotics and 100 mg of hydrocortisone (Solu-Cortef) intravenously during the procedure. Some centers mix tobramycin powder with the PMMA before injection for prophylaxis as well. No more than three levels are treated at one setting, primarily because of the negative effects of prolonged prone positioning, but also to avoid injecting high volumes of PMMA and the associated potential toxicity of unpolymerized monomer. Vertebroplasty can usually be performed with one needle for each treated level (Fig. 171–2). The large majority of patients are discharged the afternoon of the procedure. Instructions given to the patient include restrictions on heavy lifting (>5 lb) for 1 week, restrictions on submerging the wounds for 1 week (showers are allowed), and instructions regarding signs and symptoms of infection. Patients are told to expect discomfort from the needle tracks for 5 to 7 days and that their existing pain medicine can be taken as directed for this pain. The patient is contacted by telephone 2 days after the procedure either by the operating physician or by a nurse. Follow-up visits are arranged at 2 weeks and 3 months after the procedure in the vertebroplasty clinic.

Though minimally invasive, vertebroplasty is not without risk. Complications have been shown to include fracture (of the vertebral body being treated and of ribs related to prone positioning), infection, major vessel or nerve injury, epidural hematoma, cerebrospinal fluid leak, and cement extravasation. Cement extravasation is the most frequent and occasionally the most serious complication and can result in cord compression (<0.5%), nerve root compression (1% to 2%), and pulmonary emboli (<1%). The complication rate has been demonstrated to be directly related to the volume of injected PMMA.[15-19] Fortunately, pain relief is not related to the volume of injection and seems to occur with relatively small amounts of injected PMMA (2 to 4 mL).[20,21] Proper technique is critical in avoiding complications. To successfully perform vertebroplasty procedures, optimal visualization of the PMMA during the injection process is required. This is best done in a fully functional angiography suite with biplane or single-plane high-quality fluoroscopy. Alternatively, similar safety can be achieved with high-quality portable fluoroscopy in an operating room setting, but poor-quality portable fluoroscopy opens the door for major undetected extravasation of PMMA. We should note that the great majority of patients with cement extravasation are asymptomatic (Fig. 171–3).

KYPHOPLASTY

Although it has been demonstrated to be effective for painful vertebral compression fractures, several concerns about vertebroplasty exist in the medical community. The fact that kyphotic deformity has been shown in the literature to significantly affect the biomechanics of the spine has led some physicians to question the wisdom of stabilizing a compressed vertebral body without reduction of the deformity. Other concerns about the use of vertebroplasty center on the injection process itself. Vertebroplasty involves an injection of relatively low-viscosity PMMA into a collapsed vertebral body. The result is stabilization of the bone fragments without reduction of the deformity and a relatively high rate of cement extravasation (30% to 60%).[19-21] Although extravasation is asymptomatic in most cases, there is a definite risk for neurologic compression and associated severe deficits. Because vertebroplasty does not address the issue of deformity,

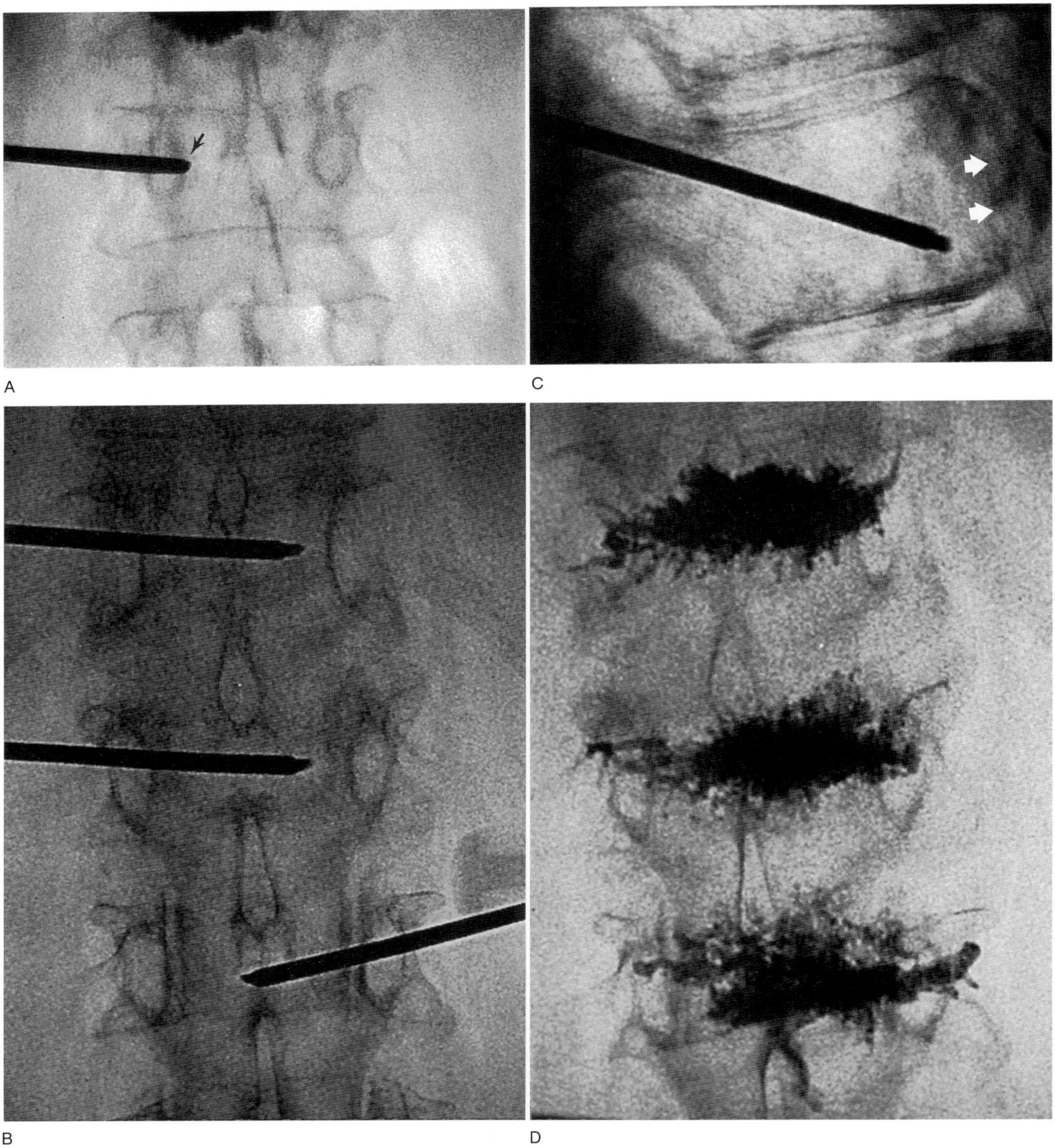

FIGURE 171–2 ■ The images show stages of a vertebroplasty from start to finish. **A,** The pedicle needle (*arrow*) in the anteroposterior (AP) projection appears to extend beyond the medial wall of the pedicle, but this is an artifact of projection. The true needle position can be seen only with a combination of two orthogonal views or with a view down the needle barrel. **B,** The needle is advanced until the tip crosses the midline in the AP projection as seen here in these three levels. **C,** The lateral projection shows the optimal position of the needle tip relative to the anterior vertebral body wall (*arrows*). **D,** The AP view after completion reveals excellent bilateral filling of all three levels.

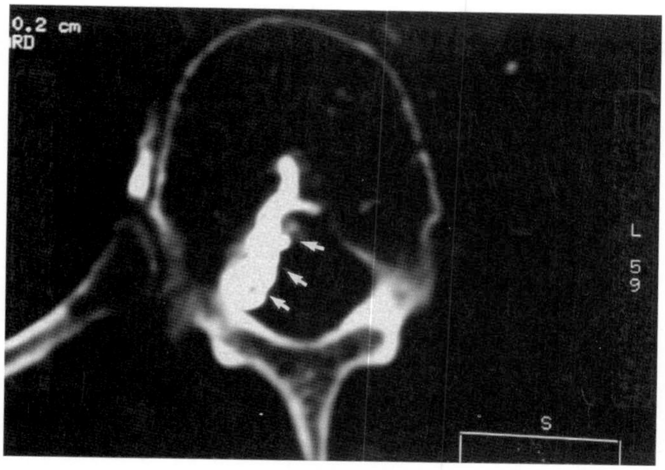

A

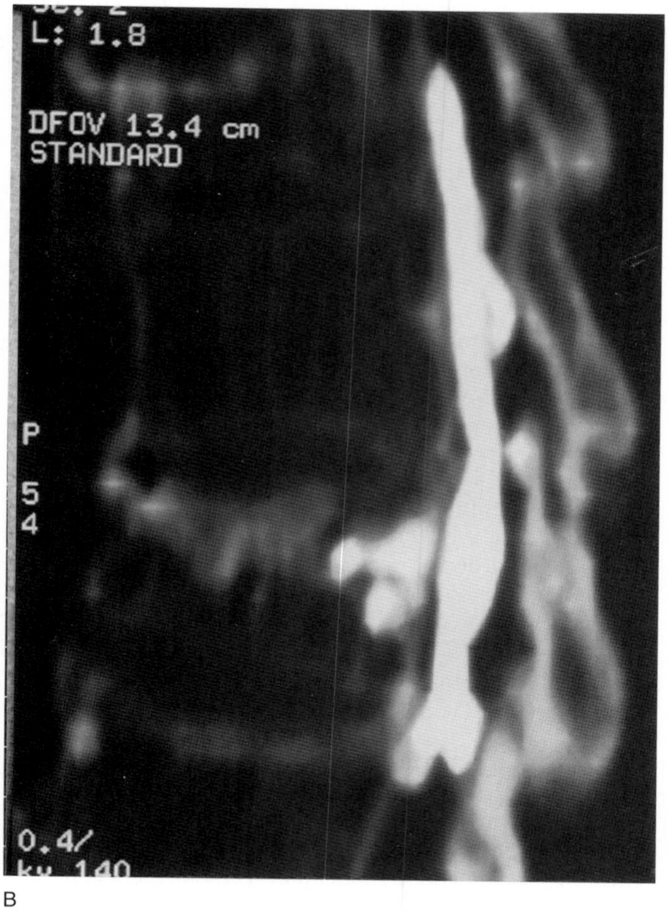

B

FIGURE 171–3 ■ **A,** An axial post-vertebroplasty CT section reveals significant epidural extravasation of polymethylmethacrylate (*arrows*). **B,** A sagittal reformatted image from the CT image reveals that extravasation of cement extended for three levels. This patient was asymptomatic from the extravasation but complained of persistent unchanged pain after the procedure.

techniques were advanced to correct that deficiency, and kyphoplasty was conceived.

Balloon kyphoplasty is a recently developed, minimally invasive surgical treatment of vertebral compression fractures. This procedure addresses pain related to both the fracture and the spinal deformity. Regardless of whether vertebral fractures are acutely painful, they are associated with loss of vertebral height, spinal deformity, decreased quality of life, and sometimes chronic pain. Pain is usually the main symptom that brings a fracture to clinical attention.

Pathologic compression fractures can be either benign or malignant. Benign fractures are due to osteoporosis, whereas malignant fractures are due to multiple myeloma or metastatic tumor. Kyphoplasty has resulted in improvement in clinical symptoms in patients with vertebral compression fractures whether caused by osteoporosis or neoplastic disease. This technique was first performed in 1998 and involves fracture reduction with an inflatable bone tamp (IBT) to restore vertebral anatomy.[22] After initial success, more structured evaluation of the technique was undertaken as part of the FDA approval process for the IBT. The IBT is a balloon similar to an angioplasty balloon that is inserted into the compressed vertebral body and inflated to reduce the fracture and create a cavity that can be filled under fine manual control and low pressure with bone cement.

Good clinical outcomes and restoration of vertebral body height have been reported with kyphoplasty.[23,24] A retrospective study by Ledlie and Renfro[25] demonstrated that kyphoplasty markedly improves pain and function and results in significant restoration of vertebral height and normalization of morphologic shape indices that remain stable for at least 2 years after treatment. In their study of 117 patients (151 fractures), vertebral height significantly increased at all postoperative intervals. Asymptomatic cement extravasation occurred in 11.3% of fractures. There were no kyphoplasty-related complications.

Another cadaveric study by Hiwatashi et al.[26] compared the restoration of vertebral height achieved with kyphoplasty and vertebroplasty in fresh cadavers by using CT. The results showed that the increase in vertebral height was greater with kyphoplasty than with vertebroplasty. The original vertebral height was restored in 93% of vertebrae with kyphoplasty and in 82% with vertebroplasty. There was a greater decrease in the wedge angle with kyphoplasty than with vertebroplasty; however, this difference was not significant. They concluded that kyphoplasty increased vertebral body height more than vertebroplasty did in this model of acutely created fractures in fresh cadaver specimens. Phillips et al.[27] conducted a detailed analysis of the sagittal plane and evaluated the efficiency of the kyphoplasty procedure in correction of kyphosis. They demonstrated a significant improvement in the kyphotic angle.

Although the kyphoplasty technique presented an attractive alternative to vertebroplasty in the osteoporotic population, its use for malignant compression fractures, mainly multiple myeloma, is well established now. When considering solid tumors, there are concerns centered on the potential asymmetric strength of these pathologic bones. If sclerotic bone was present anteriorly in the vertebral body with osteolytic foci present posteriorly, it is conceivable that the IBT would cause retropulsion of the posterior vertebral wall and subsequent neuronal compression. Liquid- or marrow-based malignancy such as multiple myeloma was considered similar to osteoporotic bone in that the weakness of the bone was more likely diffuse.

In 2002 a report on 55 kyphoplasty procedures performed on patients with multiple myeloma established the technique as safe and effective in this population.[28] The series demonstrated restoration of 34% of lost vertebral height in approximately 70% of treated levels. Cement extravasation occurred in 4% based on review of post-procedure radiographs. Pain relief was significant in all patients treated based on Short Form 36 Health Survey data completed before and after treatment. In 2003 a report of vertebroplasty and kyphoplasty for malignant compression fractures included kyphoplasty performed at nine levels involved with solid tumor processes. No complications occurred in this study, and pain relief was achieved in 84% of patients. Cement extravasation did not occur in the kyphoplasty group.[29] Although more work needs to be done with regard to kyphoplasty in patients with solid tumor metastases, the initial results are promising.

Kyphoplasty requires a dual-needle approach, followed by insertion of IBTs bilaterally into the fractured vertebral body. The balloons are inflated to elevate the end plates and create a cavity. The balloons are deflated and withdrawn, and the resulting cavity is filled with bone cement (Fig. 171–4).

A recent study by de Falco et al.[30] looked at the effectiveness and safety of kyphoplasty as a new treatment method for traumatic fracture of the thoracolumbar junction. They treated 12 patients. In patients older than 50 years, they used PMMA as the filling material, whereas in younger patients, they used either Calcibon (Biomet, Inc., Warsaw, IN) or KyphOs (Kyphon Inc., Sunnyvale, CA). These last two types are made up of tricalcium phosphate, which despite being less manageable than PMMA and less resistant to fracture initially, will in time be reabsorbed and osteointegrated. All patients experienced swift pain relief, and they concluded that kyphoplasty is an effective, simple, and safe treatment of traumatic fracture of the thoracolumbar junction.

The incidence of cement leakage with kyphoplasty is significantly lower than with vertebroplasty. The explanation for the different leakage rates is that kyphoplasty creates a cavity in the bone that allows for lower-pressure, more controlled cement injection. Phillips et al.[31] have shown that rates of epidural, inferior vena cava, and transcortical extravasation are significantly lower for kyphoplasty than for vertebroplasty. A recent study of vertebroplasty demonstrated cement leakage in 258 of 363 (71%) fractures treated.[32] This group also reported 10 patients with PMMA emboli. Fortunately, they were all asymptomatic. More recent studies have indicated that radiculopathy or pedicle fractures are more common complications of PMMA extravasation than symptomatic emboli or neurologic deficits are.[33-36] These complications are likely to be encountered much less frequently in kyphoplasty because of the lower rate of cement extravasation inherent in that procedure.

Kyphoplasty markedly improves the quality of life for patients with vertebral fractures and results in significant restoration of vertebral height. Whether restoration of the height of the vertebral body results in long-term improved outcomes remains to be determined. A question still unanswered is whether kyphoplasty increases the risk for subsequent fractures at adjacent vertebrae. A retrospective study conducted in 2004 included 38 patients in whom 47 levels were treated initially.[37] Over the follow-up period, 10 patients sustained 17 subsequent fractures. There were nine at adjacent-above levels, four at adjacent-below levels, and four at remote levels. Most of those at an adjacent level occurred within 2 months of the procedure. A similar risk is seen with vertebroplasty, especially when cement extravasates into the disk. This study suggests that cement augmentation places additional stress on adjacent levels, but others suggest that extravasation into the disk is the main reason for the added fracture risk. Nevertheless, patients with increasing back pain after kyphoplasty or vertebroplasty should be evaluated carefully for possible subsequent adjacent fractures, especially during the first 2 months after the procedure. Although no randomized trials comparing vertebroplasty with kyphoplasty head to head have been published, several studies are under way.

Finally, there is a clear cost difference between vertebroplasty and kyphoplasty, with kyphoplasty costing several thousand dollars more than vertebroplasty. Many sites admit kyphoplasty patients overnight for recovery. In our experience this has not been necessary in most cases. Sedation requirements for kyphoplasty have averaged higher than those for vertebroplasty but rarely exceed the standard for conscious sedation.

The preoperative evaluation and clinic appointments for kyphoplasty and vertebroplasty are identical. The interventionalist should decide, based on the patient's health, pain severity, and location of compressed levels, which procedure or combination of procedures is most appropriate for each individual patient. The selection process itself is evolving as the technology and indications continue to expand.

CONCLUSION

As with all invasive techniques, maximal safety for vertebroplasty and kyphoplasty is achieved with maximal information. Efficacy is dependent on meticulous technique and appropriate patient selection. This is optimally achieved through a multidisciplinary approach with cooperation of the interventionalist, the neurosurgeon or orthopedic surgeon, the radia-

FIGURE 171–4 ■ Images **A** to **I** demonstrate the steps involved in kyphoplasty. **A,** The guide needle is typically 11 gauge and here is positioned before advance along the pedicle. **B,** After the needle is positioned, a guide pin is advanced through the needle to maintain an access corridor for advancing the larger working needle. **C,** The lateral view reveals that the guide pin is inserted to within a few millimeters of the anterior cortex. Note that the needle remains only a few millimeters deep to the pedicle. **D,** The lateral view reveals the position of the working cannula after exchange over the guide pin. The distal markers of the inflatable balloon tamp (IBT) are visible in the cannula lumen (*arrows*). **E,** The IBT has been advanced into the vertebral body after a hand drill was used to clear away a cavity for it. **F,** After placement of the second working cannula and IBT, this anteroposterior (AP) view shows good central position of the IBTs within the bone.

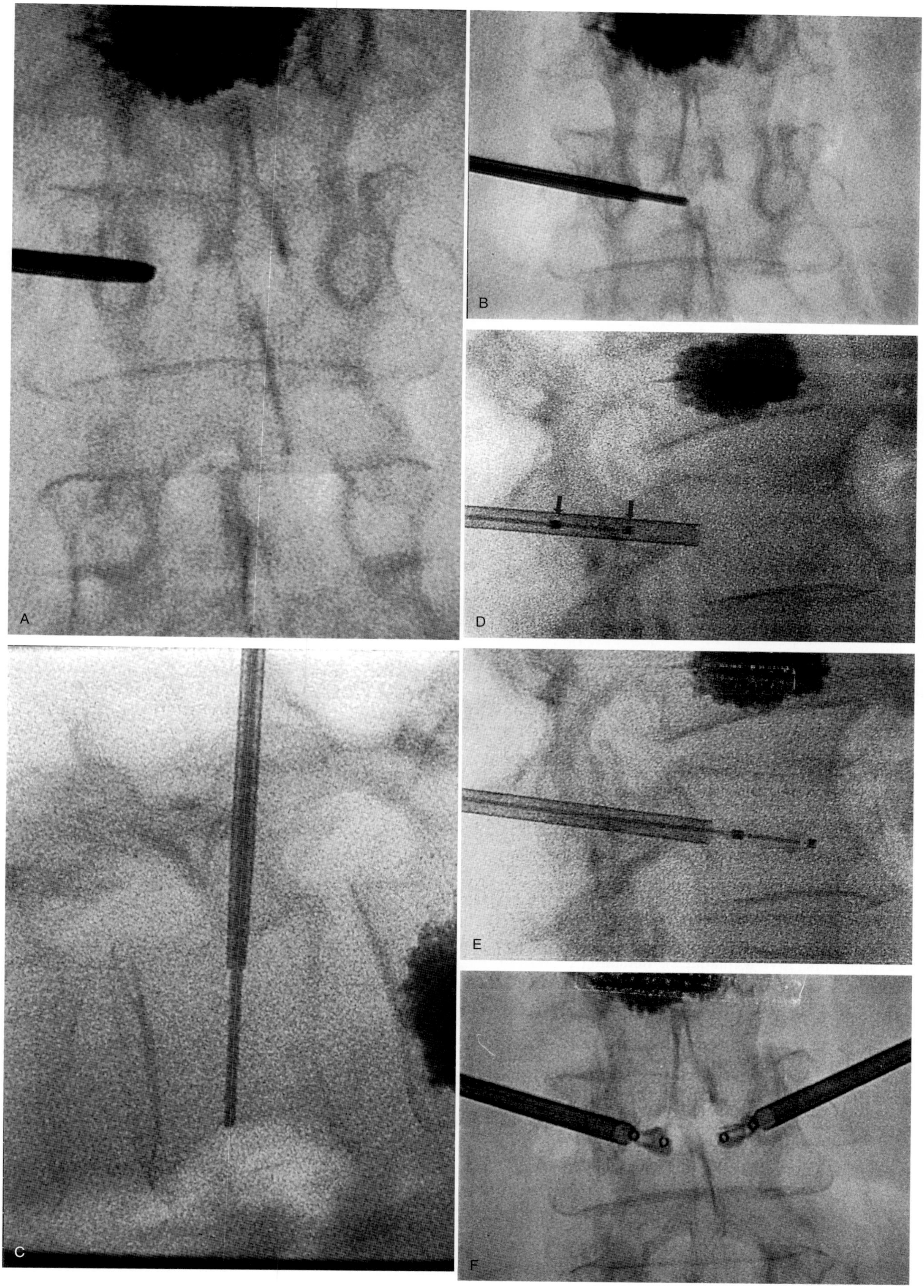
A
B
C
D
E
F

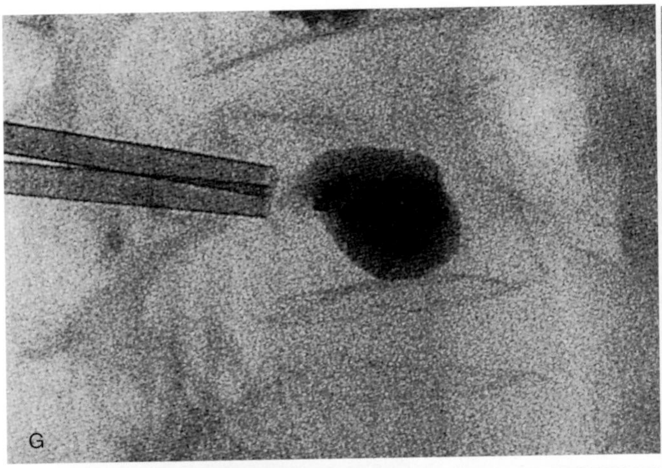
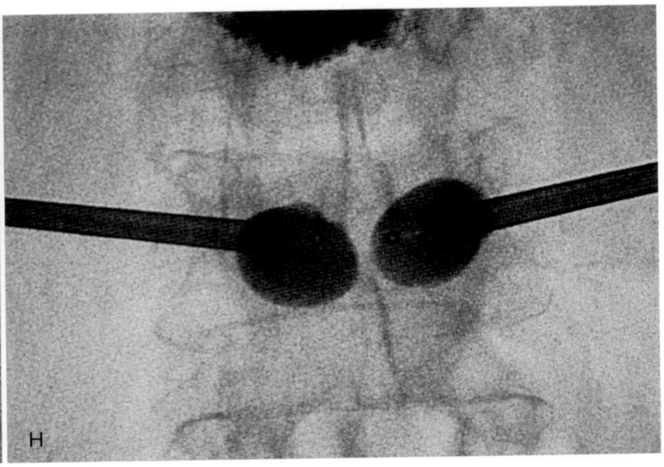
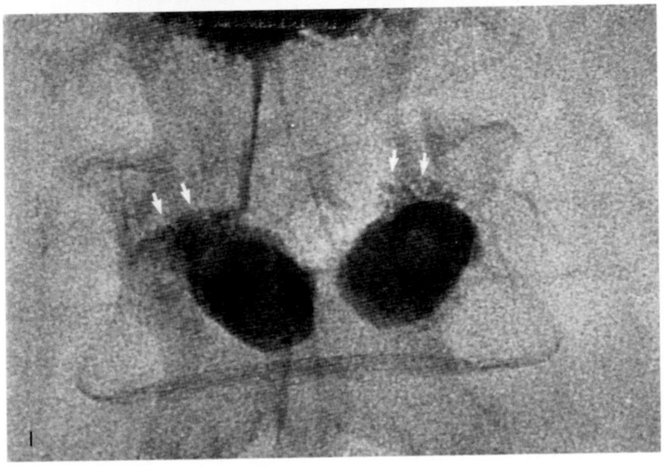

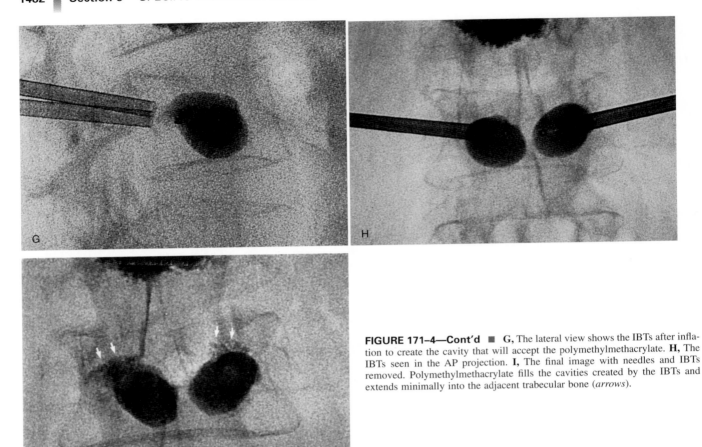

FIGURE 171–4—Cont'd ■ **G,** The lateral view shows the IBTs after inflation to create the cavity that will accept the polymethylmethacrylate. **H,** The IBTs seen in the AP projection. **I,** The final image with needles and IBTs removed. Polymethylmethacrylate fills the cavities created by the IBTs and extends minimally into the adjacent trabecular bone (*arrows*).

tion oncologist/oncologist, and the pain management team. The preoperative evaluation must include a complete physical examination together with a detailed neurologic assessment, appropriate imaging, and blood work, including a platelet count and coagulation profile. The interventionalist should have adequate support in the form of available surgical options and medical management in the treatment center in the event of a complication. Anyone performing these techniques should undergo dedicated training under the direct supervision of an experienced instructor. High-quality fluoroscopic equipment is required, as is knowledge of fluoroscopic landmarks and operative techniques. Attempting to perform these procedures with any one of these components missing could potentially lead to serious complications such as paralysis or death. When done properly, these procedures result in the rapid onset of significant durable pain relief with few complications in a population that has historically been difficult to treat.

References

1. Janjan N: Bone metastases: Approaches to management. Semin Oncol 28(Suppl 11):28, 2001.
2. Patel B, DeGroot H: Evaluation of the risk of pathologic fractures secondary to metastatic bone disease. Orthopedics 24:612, 2001.
3. Bunting R, Lamont-Havers W, Schweon D, et al: Pathological fracture risk in rehabilitation of patients with bony metastases. Clin Orthop 249:256, 1985.
4. Riggs LR, Melton LJ: The worldwide problem of osteoporosis: Lessons from epidemiology. Bone 17:505s, 1995.
5. Schlaich C, Minne HW, Bruckner T, et al: Reduced pulmonary function in patients with spinal osteoporotic fractures. Osteoporos Int 8:261, 1998.
6. Silverman S: The clinical consequences of vertebral compression fracture. Bone 13:27, 1992.
7. Kado DM, Browner WS, Palermo L, et al: Vertebral fractures and mortality in older women: A prospective study. Study of Osteoporotic Fractures Research Group. Arch Intern Med 159:1215, 1999.
8. Greenberg MS: Handbook of Neurosurgery, 5th ed. New York, Theime, 2001.
9. Body JJ: Effectiveness and cost of bisphosphonates therapy in tumor bone disease. Cancer 97(Suppl):859, 2003.
10. Galibert P, Deramond H, Rosat P, et al: Note preliminaire sur le traitment des angiomes vertebraux par vertebroplastie acrylique percutanee. Neurochirurgie 33:166, 1987.
11. Evans AJ, Jensen ME, Kip KE, et al: Vertebral compression fractures: Pain reduction and improvement in functional mobility after percutaneous polymethylmethacrylate vertebroplasty—retrospective report of 245 cases. Radiology 226:366, 2003.
12. Deramond H, Depriester C, Galibert P, et al: Percutaneous vertebroplasty with polymethylmethacrylate. Techniques, indications, and results. Radiol Clin North Am 36:533, 1998.
13. Baur A, Stabler A, Arbogast S, et al: Acute osteoporotic and neoplastic vertebral compression fractures: Fluid sign at MR imaging. Radiology 225:730, 2002.
14. Murray JA, Bruels MC, Lindberg RD: Irradiation of polymethylmethacrylate: In vitro gamma radiation effect. J Bone Joint Surg Am 56:311, 1974.
15. Garfin SR, Yuan HA, Reiley MA: Kyphoplasty and vertebroplasty for the treatment of painful osteoporotic compression fractures. Spine 26:1511, 2001.

16. Lane JM, Johnson CE, Khan SN, et al: Minimally invasive options for the treatment of osteoporotic vertebral compression fractures. Orthop Clin North Am 33:431, 2002.
17. Lin JT, Lane JM: Nonmedical management of osteoporosis. Curr Opin Rheumatol 14:441, 2002.
18. Fourney DR, Schomer DF, Nader R, et al: Percutaneous vertebroplasty and kyphoplasty for painful vertebral compression fractures in cancer patients. J Neurosurg 98(Suppl):21, 2003.
19. Moreland DB, Landi MK, Grand W: Vertebroplasty: Techniques to avoid complications. Spine J 1:66, 2001.
20. Cotton A, Dewatre F, Cortet B, et al: Percutaneous vertebroplasty for osteolytic metastases and myeloma: Effects of the percentage of lesion filling and the leakage of methyl methacrylate at clinical follow-up. Radiology 200:525, 1996.
21. Tomeh AG, Mathis JM, Fenton DC, et al: Biomechanical efficacy of antipedicular versus bipedicular vertebroplasty for the management of osteoporotic compression fractures. Spine 24:1772, 1999.
22. Wong W, Reilly MA, Garfin S: Vertebroplasty/kyphoplasty. J Womens Imaging 2:117, 2000.
23. Garfin SR, Yuan HA, Reiley MA: New technologies in spine: Kyphoplasty and vertebroplasty for the treatment of painful osteoporotic compression fractures. Spine 26:1511, 2001.
24. Lieberman IH, Dudeney S, Reinhardt MK, et al: Initial outcome of "kyphoplasty" in the treatment of painful osteoporotic vertebral compression fractures. Spine 26:1631, 2001.
25. Ledlie JT, Renfro MB: Kyphoplasty treatment of vertebral fractures: 2-year outcomes show sustained benefits. Spine 31:57, 2006.
26. Hiwatashi A, Sidhu R, Lee RK, et al: Kyphoplasty versus vertebroplasty to increase vertebral body height: A cadaveric study. Radiology 237:1115, 2005.
27. Phillips F, Ho E, Campbell-Hupp M, et al: Early radiographic and clinical results of balloon kyphoplasty for the treatment of osteoporotic vertebral compression fractures. Spine 28:2260, 2003.
28. Dudeney S, Lieberman IH, Reinhardt MK, et al: Kyphoplasty in the treatment of osteolytic vertebral compression fractures from multiple myeloma. J Clin Oncol 20:2382, 2002.
29. Ledlie JT, Renfro M: Balloon kyphoplasty: One-year outcomes in vertebral body height restoration, chronic pain, and activity levels. J Neurosurg 98(Suppl):36, 2003.
30. de Falco R, Scarano E, Di Celmo D, et al: Balloon kyphoplasty in traumatic fractures of the thoracolumbar junction. Preliminary experience in 12 cases. J Neurosurg Sci 49:147, 2005.
31. Phillips FM, Wetzel FT, Lieberman I, et al: An in vivo comparison of the potential for extravertebral cement leak after vertebroplasty and kyphoplasty. Spine 27:2173, 2002.
32. Hodler J, Peck D, Gilula LA: Midterm outcome after vertebroplasty: Predictive value of technical and patient-related factors. Radiology 227:662, 2003.
33. Evans AJ, Jensen ME, Kip KE, et al: Vertebral compression fractures: Pain reduction and improvement in functional mobility after percutaneous polymethylmethacrylate vertebroplasty: Retrospective report of 245 cases. Radiology 226:366, 2003.
34. Perez-Higueras A, Alvarez L, Rossi RE, et al: Percutaneous vertebroplasty: Long-term clinical and radiological outcome. Neuroradiology 44:950, 2002.
35. Cohen JE, Lylyk P, Ceratto R, et al: Percutaneous vertebroplasty: Technique and results in 192 procedures. Neurol Res 26:41, 2004.
36. Diamond TH, Champion B, Clark WA: Management of acute osteoporotic vertebral fractures: A randomized trial comparing percutaneous vertebroplasty with conservative therapy. Am J Med 114:257, 2003.
37. Fribourg D, Tang C, Sra P, et al: Incidence of subsequent vertebral fracture after kyphoplasty. Spine 29:2270, 2004.

chapter 172

Intradiskal Electrothermal Annuloplasty

Michael L. Whitworth

■ HISTORICAL CONSIDERATIONS

Since the mid-1990s, intradiskal radiofrequency heating was being considered as a method of treatment for diskogenic pain. Cadaver studies demonstrated that placement of a bipolar probe did not result in end plate or vertebral body damage and was associated with a temperature change at the edges of the disk of 3° to 4° C.[1] Later experiments evaluated the thermal diffusion capacity of the intervertebral disks. It was determined that there is an age-related differential in thermal dissipation with the disk of a 32-year-old person having 250% the thermal diffusion capability as a 61-year-old person.[2] Ostensibly, this is due to the relatively greater aqueous content of the younger disk. Interest in diskogenic disease—and the etiology of such—heightened after the seminal 1997 paper demonstrating the presence of neural ingrowth into the inner annulus and nucleus 0% of the time in diskogram negative disks but 57% of the time in diskogram positive disks.[3] Additional sources of potential nociception transmission were also found in the vertebral end plate in patients with severe disk degeneration. The end plate in such cases was associated with an increased sensory nerve innervation and neoangiogenesis adjacent to the end plates.[4]

Tony Yeung, a pioneer in endoscopic spine surgery attempted to use a prototype intradiskal radiofrequency probe during endoscopic spine surgery but found the temperatures produced in tissues were erratic. He later developed endoscopic laser annuloplasty. Interest in the radiofrequency intradiskal approach continued with subsequent clinical studies, but with disappointing results. A prospective randomized human trial using a 90-second intradiskal radiofrequency lesion at 70° C did not produce any differences from controls.[5] A later study comparing two heating protocols of 120 and 360 seconds at 80° C failed to produce long-term positive results. At 6 months post procedure, the Visual Analog Scale (VAS) scores had returned to baseline, although there was a statistically significant short-term response to the procedure.[6]

The Saals selected a thermoresistive heating element as a means of producing sufficient heat to cause interruption in intradiskal neural transmission—if not overt intradiskal neural destruction. Although their energy source remained a radiofrequency generator, the energy was not directly imparted to the nucleus pulposus or the annulus fibrosus because the "spine wand" was insulated. Instead, unlike intradiskal radiofrequency application of energy, the radiofrequency current was used to heat a resistive coil inside the insulated intradiskal portion of the device that secondarily heated the surrounding tissues with thermal energy. An initial report on the procedure termed *intradiskal electrothermal* (IDET) annuloplasty was published in 1999.[7] In early 2000, a preliminary report on a 20-patient study was published with the results that 72% of patients received 50% relief.[8] A 1-year outcome study using the IDET device was published in October 2000. The study had 62 participants with chronic low back pain, diskogram positive; some improvement was found at 1 year in 71% of the patients.[9] Unfortunately, this was not a controlled trial, and although the authors cautioned that the results should be verified by placebo-controlled randomized trials, these follow-up studies were not forthcoming for several years.

A company was formed very early to aggressively market the device to physicians through training courses for physicians and, subsequently, there were tens of thousands of uses before the first validated clinical trials were released. The company manufacturing the device at that time reported to this writer in one training conference in 1999 that reimbursement for the procedure was in the range of $3,500 to $7,000, and the company had a reimbursement department for physician use. Eventually insurers became increasingly reluctant to pay for an expensive procedure with so little clinical data and with marginal results. Insurers subsequently began to block payment for the procedure in their medical policies. At the time of this writing, in the United States, very few major insurers will cover the IDET procedure because it is considered to be "investigational."

Other alternatives to IDET began to appear around the turn of the millennium, such as endoscopic annuloplasty, discTRODE intra-annular radiofrequency procedure, bipolar annuloplasty, and so on. However, there are few studies on these procedures and these have only marginal results.

■ INDICATIONS

The indications and contraindications for annuloplasty are summarized in Table 172–1. The International Spine

Table 172–1

Indications and Contraindications for Annuloplasty

- No evidence of emergency spinal intervention indicators
- No medical contraindications
- Absence of radiculopathy and myelopathy
- Negative Lasègue sign
- MRI with no other pathologies correlating to the pain production
- No evidence for spinal instability or spondylolisthesis at the level of interest
- No significant untreated or uncontrolled psychiatric issues
- Motivated patient with realistic outcome expectations
- No greater than 25% loss of disk height
- Criteria for intradiskal disease (IDD) satisfied:
  - Disk stimulation is positive at low pressures (<50 psi)
  - Disk stimulation reproduces pain of intensity (>6/10)
  - Disk stimulation reproduces concordant pain
  - CT diskography reveals a grade 3 or greater annular tear
  - Control disk stimulation is negative in at least one adjacent disk

Intervention Society (ISIS) publishes *Practice Guidelines: Spinal Diagnostic & Treatment Procedures*, which represents the only validated operating guidelines for this and many other spinal procedures. These guidelines detail IDET theory, practice, and controversy.

ANATOMY AND PATHOLOGY

Painful annular radial fissures as seen during diskography are evidence for internal disk disruption, which is the sole indication for IDET.[10] It is known these fissures are associated with vascular and neural ingrowth from the outer annulus, that there may be leakage of diskal enzymes that are toxic to extradiskal materials, and that there are mechanical changes in the disk that occur with disk degeneration. The mechanism by which IDET actually works is not known but is thought to be by sealing off the fissures with thermal energy, destruction of the nociceptor nerve ingrowth, and stabilization of the collagen and biomechanics of the disk. There have been some studies of these mechanisms in cadavers,[11-13] but clearly this model has little to do with the dynamic human intervertebral disk, and the processes of tissue healing. The annular fissures are both radial and circumferential, splitting the laminar layers of the annulus. Provocative manometric diskography with a negative control disk and post-diskography CT or MRI are the absolute minimum requirements for proper selection of patients for IDET. Fluoroscopic diskography may demonstrate annular fissures, but the three-dimensional location of the radial tears cannot be determined accurately with fluoroscopy. Both circumferential and radial annular tears may be

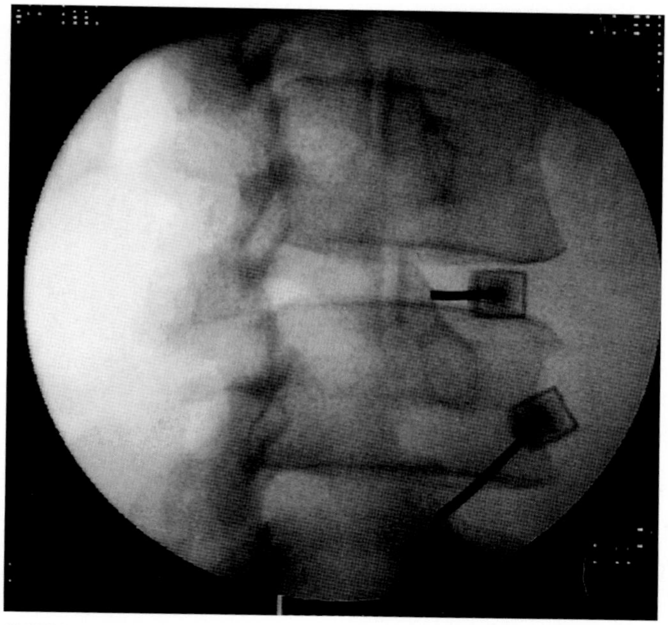

FIGURE 172–1 ■ X-ray showing positioning of the intradiskal electrothermal (IDET) needle.

visualized on post-diskography CT. The fissures are thought to begin peripherally and gradually expand as the degree of internal disk disruption expands to involve increasing amounts of the nucleus pulposus by cavitation.

TECHNIQUE

In the United States, the acquisition cost of the SpineCath is more than $1200, so it is prudent to select the patients carefully. At times, it will be impossible to advance the SpineCath into the area containing the annular tear as demonstrated on CT diskography. Other times, the SpineCath will fold over on itself, making it utterly useless from that point on in the procedure. In such cases, a new SpineCath will be required, thereby making the IDET an extremely expensive procedure to the entity purchasing the SpineCath. Fundamentally, a posterolateral approach is used, targeting the superior articular process with a 17-gauge IDET needle with a relatively smooth beveled edge to avoid shearing of the catheter (Fig. 172–1). The trajectory of the needle is usually between 25 and 40 degrees to the sagittal plane with an entry point on the contralateral side from the CT-demonstrated radial tears. The target for the needle tip is halfway between the end plates and just medial to the medial pedicular line, at the inner aspect of the annulus fibrosus (Fig. 172–2). Once the needle is placed into the inner annular fibers/outer nucleus pulposus, the SpineCath is slowly inserted and, as much as possible, is "guided" into place via the flexible bent tip. However, frequently the catheter will lodge in irregularities in the inner annulus or travel in a circumferential annular tear or even create its own separation of the lamina of the annulus fibrosus (Fig. 172–4). In any case, the final resting place for the SpineCath tip is across the posterior annulus to cover the CT-demonstrated location of the radial tear. Frequent manipulations of the catheter may be necessary, and in some cases

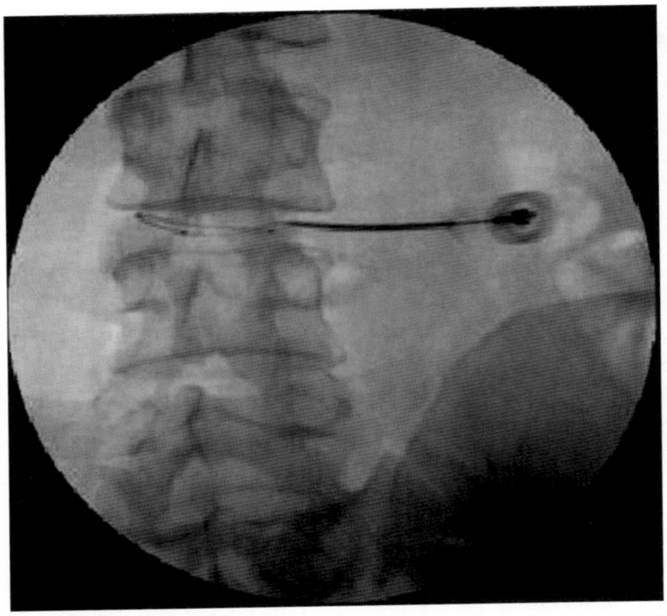

FIGURE 172–2 ■ The target for the needle tip is halfway between the end plates and just medial to the medial pedicular line, at the inner aspect of the annulus fibrosus.

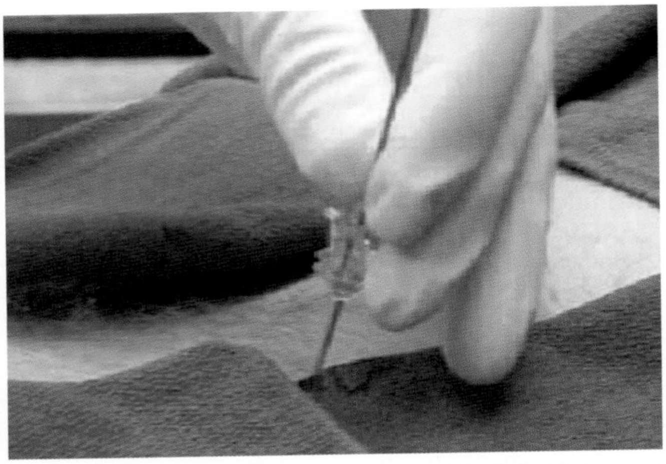

FIGURE 172–3 ■ Technique for threading the SpineCath catheter.

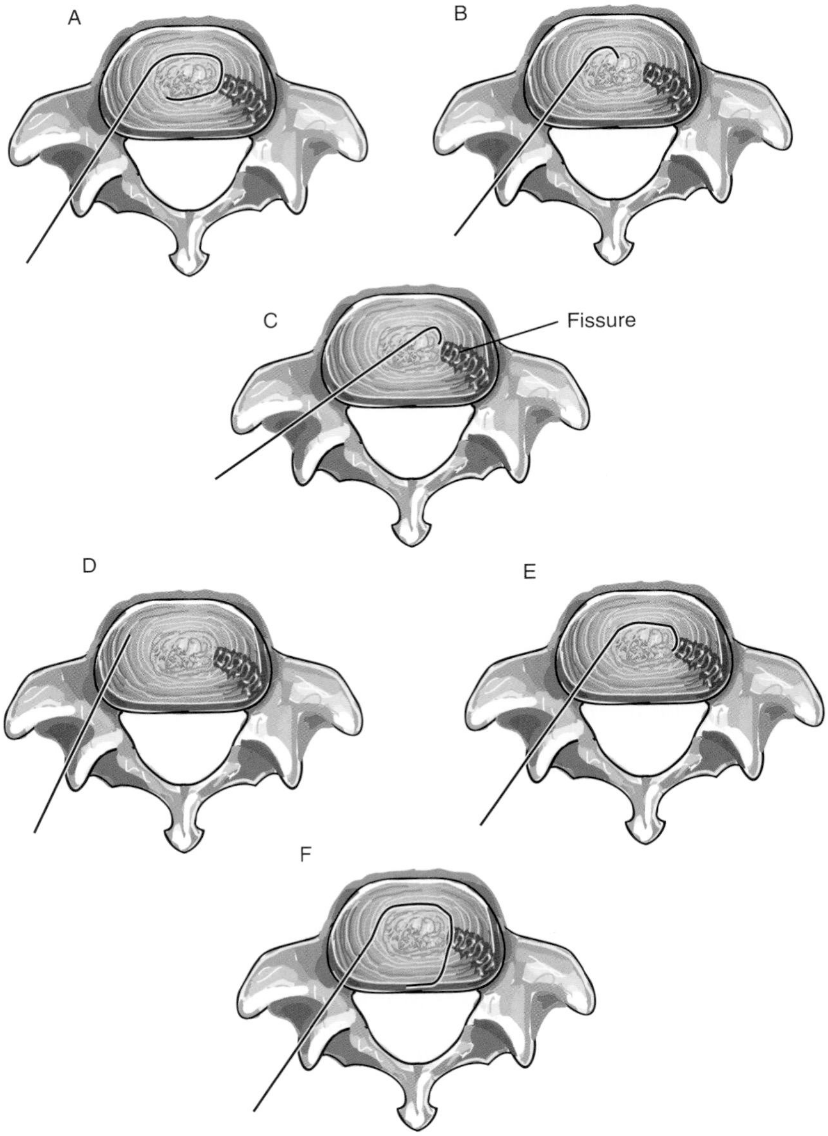

FIGURE 172–4 ■ Problems with catheter advancement. **A,** Desired catheter position. **B,** Needle is advanced too far, causing acute deflection. **C,** Deflection angle is too acute and the catheter does not follow annulus. **D,** Needle is intra-annular and the catheter cannot be advanced. **E,** Catheter tip enters annual tear and the catheter cannot be advanced. **F,** Intracanal catheter placement.

where excessive force would bend the catheter, a contralateral or bilateral approach will be necessary with dual heatings. The SpineCath has two markings—one at the tip and one more proximal—that denote the location of the thermoresistive coil, which is the active heating element. The patient must be awake enough to render feedback regarding potential nerve root heating, although this is uncommon. A manufacturer heating protocol is usually incorporated in which the temperature is gradually ramped up to 90° C for 16.5 minutes. The safest method of catheter removal is *en bloc* with the needle and catheter removed as a unit. If antibiotic is to be given in the disk, this should be done prior to introducing the catheter into the needle or if the catheter can easily be removed through the needle, after the heating.

Controversy continues regarding the location of the catheter with respect to any circumferential fissures. It is the philosophy of some that the SpineCath should be placed deep into the annulus fibrosus within the circumferential tear, whereas others use the more traditional approach of the annulus/nucleus junction. Manipulation may, at times, be very time consuming, requiring up to an hour of manipulation of the catheter. However, experienced physicians will usually be able to carefully place the catheter/needle within several minutes.

COMPLICATIONS

Shortly after the first published reports of IDET, several serious complications were described in the literature. The first noted complication was that of cauda equina syndrome.[14] Post-procedure pain flare-ups are relatively common, and they seem to be temperature dependent.[15] Intradural migration from a broken SpineCath that ultimately required surgery for the resultant radiculopathy has been reported.[16] Osteonecrosis of the vertebral body after IDET has also been reported in the literature.[17,18] I personally have observed during subsequent endoscopic disk surgery charring of the diskal tissues from IDET.

The complications from the procedure are divided into access issues and heating issues. Those not versed in diskography may not understand the anatomic barriers to the disk, such as furcal nerves, iliac crest overriding the disk space in the oblique fluoroscopic rotation, safe access zone shape and size, the potential for end plate damage, and the risk of diskitis (septic and aseptic). The IDET catheter may travel outside the posterior annulus fibrosus into the epidural space or even into the dura or nerve roots. Heating may cause radicular type pain that cannot be readily explained in the absence of proximity to nerve roots.

OUTCOME STUDIES

Many of the IDET studies group their results effectively into nonresponders and responders. Patients who do respond are then given an average VAS reduction citation. The adoption of this methodology appears to connect failure to respond with poor patient selection, inadequate technical placement of the SpineCath, or disease that was so severe that IDET with its 2-mm thermal excursion could not help. Such methodology also calls into question the validity of the technique as an effective treatment. Bogduk[19] has published an excellent review of the IDET literature and methodology. The first placebo-controlled trial demonstrated a powerful placebo effect on pain relief that suggests caution in the adaptation of IDET.[20] However, the entire effect of pain relief cannot be entirely explained by placebo; therefore, IDET was believed to have a positive but modest effect. Other studies generally reveal modest reduction in pain in the 50% responders (usually 3 points on a 10-point VAS scale) with no relief in the other 50%.

SUMMARY

Electrothermal annuloplasty is only occasionally practiced in the United States today owing to lack of financial reimbursement. The elevation of physician and corporate avarice to a level that superseded scientific demonstration of the effectiveness of the technique has cast a pall on future use of this technique. Hopefully, interventional pain practitioners will learn from this tragic episode and become more acutely aware of our role as stewards of monetary resources and available for the treatment of pain and as gatekeepers against wholesale acceptance of experimental techniques. The technique actually did work in the treatment of some patients, and we should build on that knowledge to advance the potential modifications necessary to enhance effectiveness. There are, perhaps, improvements on the IDET model that may be employed in the future—such as a bipolar radiofrequency electrode energy applied across the posterior annulus; a more expansive heating device; or consideration of neuromodulation of the posterior annulus. There are now outcome studies for both discTRODE (a flexible radiofrequency catheter that splits the lamellae of the annulus circumferentially)[21,22] and intradiskal endoscopic laser annuloplasty with modest improvements in pain.[23] Future of the development of techniques to treat annular fissures will be partially predicated on fiscal responsibility to the medical system by demonstrating effectiveness before massive release and promotion of a product. As our understanding of the pathology of internal disk disruption increases, we may be able to develop enhanced therapies that may include intradiskal injections along with structural support methods.

References

1. Troussier B, Lebas JF, Chirossel JP, et al: Percutaneous intradiscal radio-frequency thermocoagulation. A cadaveric study. Spine 20:1713, 1995.
2. Houpt JC, Conner ES, McFarland EW: Experimental study of temperature distributions and thermal transport during radiofrequency current therapy of the intervertebral disc. Spine 21:1808, 1996.
3. Freemont AJ, Peacock TE, Goupille P, et al: Nerve ingrowth into diseased intervertebral disc in chronic back pain. Lancet 350:178, 1997.
4. Brown MF, Hukkanen MV, McCarthy ID, et al: Sensory and sympathetic innervation of the vertebral end plate in patients with degenerative disc disease. J Bone Joint Surg Br. 79:147, 1997.
5. Barendse GA, van Den Berg SG, Kessels AH, et al: Randomized controlled trial of percutaneous intradiscal radiofrequency thermocoagulation for chronic discogenic back pain: Lack of effect from a 90-second 70° C lesion. Spine 26:287, 2001.
6. Ercelen O, Bulutcu E, Oktenoglu T, et al: Radiofrequency lesioning using two different time modalities for the treatment of lumbar discogenic pain: A randomized trial. Spine 28:1922, 2003.
7. Kennedy M: IDET: A new approach to treating lower back pain. Wis Med J 98:18, 1999.

8. Saal JS, Saal JA: Management of chronic discogenic low back pain with a thermal intradiscal catheter. A preliminary report. Spine 25:382, 2000.
9. Saal JA, Saal JS: Intradiscal electrothermal treatment for chronic discogenic low back pain: A prospective outcome study with minimum 1-year follow-up. Spine 25:2622, 2000.
10. Bogduk N: The lumbar disc and low back pain. Neurosurg Clin North Am 2:791, 1991.
11. Kleinstueck FS, Diedrich CJ, Nau WH: Acute biomechanical and histological effects of intradiscal electrothermal therapy on human lumbar discs. Spine 26:2198, 2000.
12. Shah RV, Lutz GE, Lee J: Intradiskal electrothermal therapy: A preliminary histologic study. Arch Phys Med Rehabil 82:1230, 2001.
13. Lee J, Lutz GE, Campbell D: Stability of the lumbar spine after intradiscal electrothermal therapy. Arch Phys Med Rehabil 82:120, 2001.
14. Hsia AW, Isaac K, Katz JS: Cauda equina syndrome from intradiscal electrothermal therapy. Neurology 55:320, 2000.
15. Derby R, Seo KS, Kazala K, et al: A factor analysis of lumbar intradiscal electrothermal annuloplasty outcomes. Spine J 5:256, 2005.
16. Orr RD, Thomas SA: Intradural migration of broken IDET catheter causing a radiculopathy. J Spinal Disord Tech 18:185, 2005.
17. Djurasovic M, Glassman SD, Dimar JR 2nd, Johnson JR: Vertebral osteonecrosis associated with the use of intradiscal electrothermal therapy: A case report. Spine 27:E325, 2002.
18. Scholl BM, Theiss SM, Lopez-Ben R, Kraft M: Vertebral osteonecrosis related to intradiscal electrothermal therapy: A case report. Spine 28(9):E161, 2003.
19. Bogduk N: Review of intradiscal electrothermal annuloplasty techniques. Reg Anesth Pain Med 9:1, 2005.
20. Pauza KJ, Howell S, Dreyfuss P: A randomized, placebo-controlled trial of intradiscal electrothermal therapy (IDET) for discogenic low back pain. Spine J 4:27, 2004.
21. Finch PM, Price LM, Drummond PD: Radiofrequency heating of painful annular disruptions: One-year outcomes. J Spinal Disord Tech 18:6, 2005.
22. Erdine S, Yucel A, Celik M: Percutaneous annuloplasty in the treatment of discogenic pain: Retrospective evaluation of one year follow-up. Agri 16:41, 2004.
23. Tsou PM, Alan Yeung C, Yeung AT: Posterolateral transforaminal selective endoscopic discectomy and thermal annuloplasty for chronic lumbar discogenic pain: A minimal access visualized intradiscal surgical procedure. Spine J 4:564, 2004.

chapter 173

Percutaneous Laser Diskectomy

Michael L. Whitworth

HISTORICAL CONSIDERATIONS

Since 1934, when open diskectomy was first introduced at Massachusetts General Hospital, millions of diskectomies have been performed in the United States, with the rate now approaching 500,000 operations per year. The search for a less invasive approach to laminectomy/diskectomy began in the 1960s with chymopapain—Lyman Smith 1964,[1] microdiskectomy by Yasargil in 1968, percutaneous diskectomy introduced by Hijikata in 1975, endoscopic monitoring of disk removal by Leu in 1982, endoscopic diskectomy first used by Schreiber and Suezawa in 1986 and improved by Mayer, Brock, and Mathews, arthroscopic diskectomy by Kambin in 1983, nucleotome introduction by Onik in 1984, percutaneous non-endoscopic laser diskectomy by Ascher in 1986,[1] and Choy[2] in 1987 and endoscopic laser diskectomy by Mayer[3] in 1992 and Savitz[4] in 1994, and the subsequent refinement of endoscopic laser methods by Yeung. In 2000 to 2001, newer minimally invasive methods of diskectomy were introduced, such as coblation nucleoplasty followed by disk decompression.

Lasers were first reported to be clinically used in the intervertebral disk in 1977[5] as part of an open thoracic diskectomy using a CO_2 laser (Fig. 173–1). Animal models for use of the same laser during canine anterior cervical open diskectomy did not occur until 1984.[6] In the 1980s, several lasers were available for treatment of ocular disorders including the argon, carbon dioxide, and excimer (XeCl) laser. The road to published science behind percutaneous diskectomy with a laser began in 1989 when an excimer laser was used on cadaveric disk tissue[7] even though the first percutaneous diskectomy had occurred several years earlier in 1986. The neodymium:yttrium/aluminum/garnet (Nd:YAG) laser was applied in laboratory applications and clinically from 1986 to 1990 and was first introduced to the scientific literature by Yonezawa in 1990.[8] The KTP laser (green) was used at least as far back as 1990 for diskectomy.[9] The early 1990s saw a proliferation of other laser development with the introduction of Ho:YAG, Er:YAG, and excimer lasers for widespread use in medicine and dentistry. Because of practical considerations, the Ho:YAG (Fig. 173–2) became the tool of choice for most physicians performing laser diskectomy.[10] This is largely due to the fact that a fiberoptic waveguide can be employed instead of a mirror system, the penetration depth into tissue is very low giving fine control of tissue modulation and ablation, and the laser output power available is very high—up to 100 watts.

Much of the history of development of lasers for diskectomy was not published until many years later, partially due to financial considerations tied to patent and technique development. The most expansive description of one author's quest to develop laser for intradiskal therapy is found in Choy's book *Percutaneous Laser Decompression.*[11] Choy pioneered the development of laser coronary angioplasty with an argon laser, having performed the first such surgery in September, 1983.[12] From 1984 to 1986 Choy and his colleagues worked on the basic science and animal models before introducing the laser for human diskectomy. The initial experiments, published much later, included proving the hypothesis that a minimal volumetric decompression of a pressurized disk using a laser would result in a disproportionately greater reduction in intradiskal pressure.[13] An Nd:YAG laser at 1064 nm was used to deliver 1000 J energy to create 20-mm by 6-mm elliptical tracks in the nucleus of fresh cadaver disks loaded to 260 to 410 kPa (37 to 59 psi). Control disks were used in which the laser was not turned on. The results are presented in Figure 173–3. Next, different lasers were examined as to their capability of disk ablation. At 900 J energy, the mass of disk ablated ranged from 120 to nearly 200 mg disk tissue. Er:YAG, Nd:YAG (1318 and 1064 nm, respectively), CO_2, argon, excimer, and Ho:YAG lasers were evaluated. The most effective in disk ablation was the pulsed CO_2 laser and erbium laser, but all other lasers were nearly as effective. However, the Ho:YAG lasers of that time were very weak compared to later lasers. For practical purposes, the Nd:YAG 1064 nm was chosen by Choy for percutaneous laser disk decompression (PLDD) owing to the availability of fiberoptic waveguides and the high powers available with the Nd:YAG. Other experiments were conducted using bovine disks demonstrating temperature rises of less than 2°C in the neural foramina, the anterior surface of the spinal canal, and 1 cm away from the laser tip directly in the line of fire of the laser. Next, experiments with mongrel dogs where employed under IRB approval. PLDD was performed through an 18-gauge needle with 1000 J energy delivered. The dogs were subsequently sacrificed and on autopsy, there were no extradiskal injuries. Clinical use in humans began in February 1986 in Austria, when Choy performed the first PLDD successfully. Because of bureaucratic obstacles in obtaining IRB approval, it was

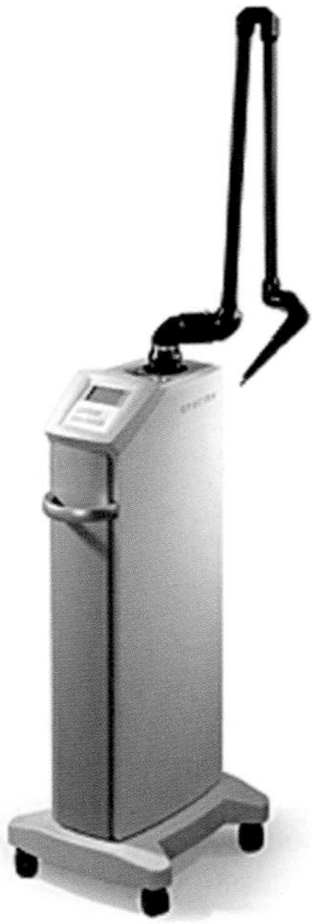

FIGURE 173–1 ■ Carbon dioxide laser.

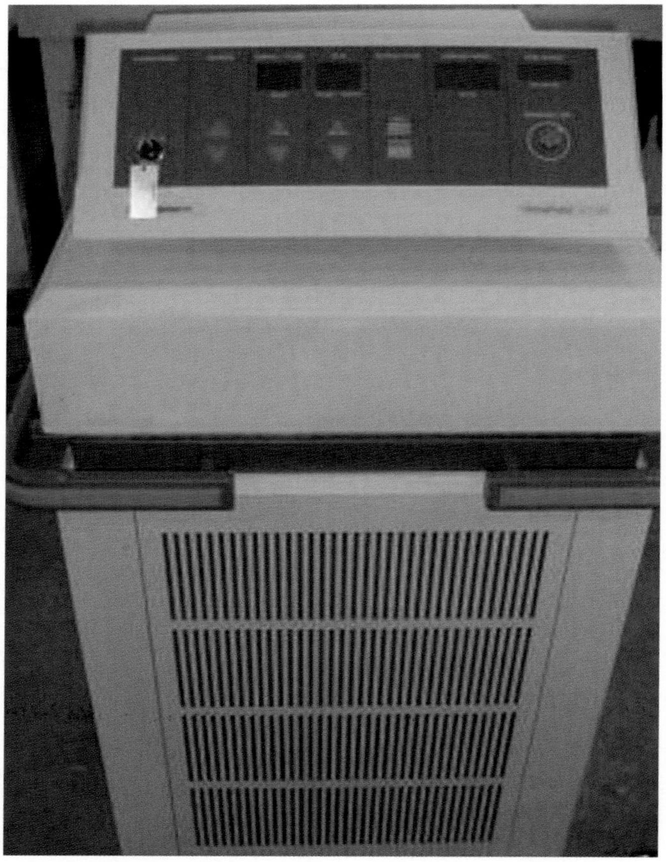

FIGURE 173–2 ■ Ho:YAG laser.

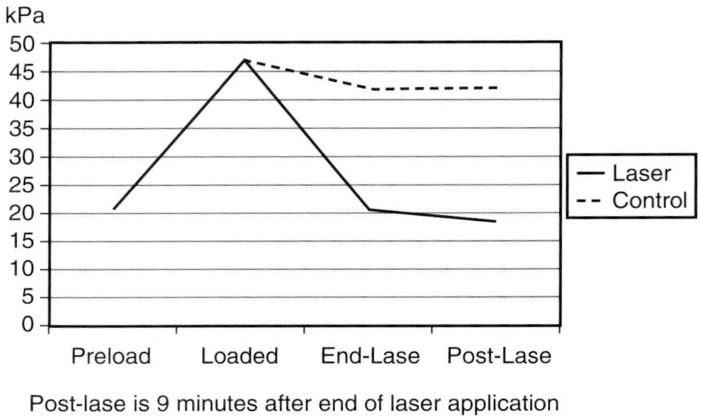

FIGURE 173–3 ■ Decrease in intradiskal pressure after Nd:YAG laser at 1000 J. (From Choy DS, Altman P: Fall of intradiskal pressure with laser ablation. J Clin Laser Med Surg 13[3]:149, 1995.)

not until September 1988, when the first U.S. use occurred. FDA approval of PLDD was received in 1991, and since that time it is estimated there have been over 100,000 users worldwide of intradiskal laser for intervertebral disk decompression.

INDICATIONS

Relative indications for this technique depend partially on the technologies employed and partially on the specific targeted pathology. In general, the major indication is the presence of a contained intervertebral disk herniation (confirmed by an MRI, CT scan, or CT myelogram) in addition to a clinical presentation of radicular pain with or without neurologic deficits, and a minimum of 6 weeks of conservative treatment without significant improvement. Exclusion criteria are patients with foraminal or central canal stenosis, symptoms of facet syndrome, previous spinal surgery in the same region, bony deformities—such as congenital abnormalities, spondylolisthesis, and hemivertebrae—cauda equina syndrome, other symptoms of myelopathy, and pregnancy. It should be noted a contained disk herniation is not simply a diffuse bulge, but should be less than 25% of the circumference of the annulus fibrosus and usually contacts the nerve roots or cord (for cervical or thoracic presentations). Technically, a contained disk herniation is one in which there is displaced disk tissue that is wholly within an outer perimeter of uninterrupted outer annulus or capsule. Extruded disk fragments are not treatable by this technique because there is no continuity with the central nucleus pulposus.

Using the selection criteria (leg pain, positive physical findings such as motor/sensory/reflex deficits and/or straight leg raise, contained disk herniation confirmed by diskography) and exclusion criteria (normal physical examination, presence of stenosis, spondylolisthesis, extruded disk fragment, leakage of diskographic dye from the outer annulus, multiple prior lumbar surgeries), the performance of laser disk decompression resulted in a success rate of 71%, whereas those who did not meet all the section criteria were successful only 29% of the time.[14] Some authors advocate the use of disk decompression for the treatment of spinal stenosis that is primarily caused by a significant disk bulge. Intradiskal and extradiskal endoscopic diskectomy with laser assistance can be performed in the hands of experts using a posterior or posterolateral approach (foraminal).

TECHNICAL ASPECTS OF LASERS

Laser stands for *l*ight *a*mplification through *s*timulation of *e*mitted *r*adiation and is used universally as an acronym for obvious reasons. The original equations describing its operation were developed by Albert Einstein in 1917.[15] The first optical laser was developed by Gordon Gould in 1958. Theodore Maiman developed the first solid-state laser, the ruby laser, in 1960 and was followed shortly thereafter by Ali Javan with the first gas laser (He Ne) in 1960, and the CO_2 laser by Kumar Patel in 1964. Now there are more than 100 known lasing media. Lasers produce an extremely focused monochromatic light that is virtually uniform in wavelength. The mechanism of laser function is presented in Figure 173–4. There is usually a primary wavelength and several secondary wavelengths of lesser amplitude produced from each laser. A resonating chamber is used (cylindrical tube) containing a lasing medium (gas, liquid, crystal) and a full mirror on one end of the tube with the other end partially mirrored. External energy is applied to the tube through the application of electricity, a flash lamp, or another laser and this causes the electrons in the lasing medium to become excited to a higher orbit. When they fall back to their baseline orbit, the electrons give off monochromatic photons which are reflected back and forth internally until the energy of the photons is sufficient to break through the semi-mirrored end. These photons are collected in a fiberoptic or mirrored waveguide and are transmitted to the target. Different lasing media produce different wavelengths of light. The CO_2 laser generates an infrared light of 10,600 nm, whereas the Er:YAG generates 2940 nm; Ho:YAG produces 2150 nm; Nd:YAG produces wavelengths of 1318 nm and 1064 nm; KTP generates 532 nm; and the excimer laser produces 193 nm. More recently diode lasers, especially in parallel arrays, have been shown to give wavelengths up to 2100 nm. The lasing medium is often a crystal that is doped with a rare earth impurity (holmium, neodymium, erbium) during the growth of the crystal. In reality, most lasers generate more than one wavelength of light, and in fact some, such as the CO_2 laser, generate dozens. But in most lasers, the light generated at each wavelength is *coherent* (i.e., the waves generated are all in phase with each other). Lasers are very inefficient, with usually less than 1% of the input energy being converted to the laser beam. The

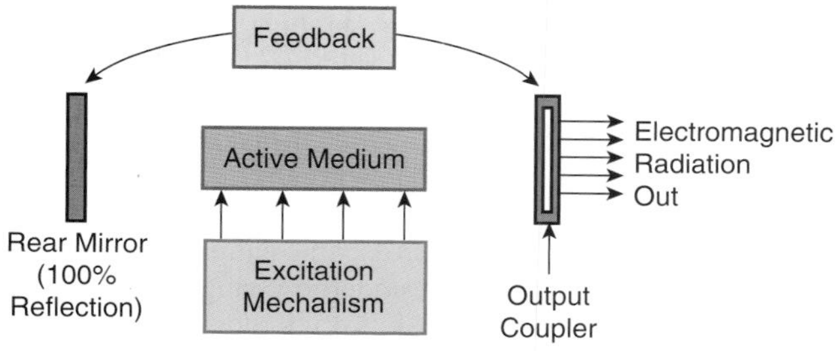

FIGURE 173–4 ■ Schematic representation of the mechanism of laser function.

remainder is emitted as heat.[16] With a laser that operates at an efficiency of 2% and has an output of 80 watts, the excess heat produced is about 4000 watts. When the heat generation is excessive and cannot be diffused, the laser crystal medium may fracture. Therefore, in larger lasers, forced air or circulating water is used to dissipate heat. The efficiency of the typical YAG laser is 0.1% to 1%; the excimer laser is 2%; and CO_2 lasers have an efficiency up to 20%. Laser output power is measured in watts, whereas the tissue effect is measured in joules (watts times seconds). Pulsed lasers deliver small pulses of energy with time for thermal dissipation to occur in tissues when the pulses are far enough apart and the pulse width is narrow enough. Double-pulsed lasers can result in summation effects of thermal energy rather than permitting dissipation, thereby approximating the effect of a continuous-wave laser.

Because not all lasers are visible (e.g., Ho:YAG, Nd:YAG, Er:YAG), a second laser is used as an aiming laser through the same fiberoptic waveguide. Usually a low-power helium laser is employed (bright red) and the intensity of the aiming laser may be varied. If the aiming laser is interfering with visualization of tissue vaporization from the primary laser, the aiming laser can often be turned off.

LASER SAFETY

It is imperative to consider the hazards of a laser beam before engaging in laser use. Most manufacturers have laser courses designed to educate both the staff and physician about radiation hazards from the powerful laser beams. Hospitals and surgery centers usually have a "laser safety officer" who should be well versed in laser safety. Nd:YAG lasers can cause permanent retinal damage and absolutely require safety glasses. All lasers with wavelengths in the UV (excimer) or visible spectrum (KTP), and below 1.55 microns in wavelength (Nd:YAG) can seriously damage the retina by causing punctate lesions, thereby permanently reducing vision. The effect of a milliwatt laser in this wavelength range striking the eye is similar to that of staring into the sun. Laser beam energy can enter the orbit from direct beam (e.g., end of the laser fiber, disconnect in the coupling, and so on) or indirectly (reflective surfaces from needles, cannulas, instrumentation), both with devastating effects on the retina. Lasers with wavelengths longer than 1.55 μ (Ho:YAG, Er:YAG) cannot reach the retina but can do damage to the cornea and skin. CO_2 lasers can be so powerful that they can cut through any tissue because they are available in output powers up to 15,000 watts. Laser glasses are designed to be specific for different laser wavelengths, and certainly for wavelengths below 1.55 microns (1550 nm). They are mandatory for everyone in the room, including the patient. The laser beam must *never ever* be pointed at a person, and when removing the laser from the patient, the laser operator must switch to standby mode. The laser may never be fired toward a paper drape or gown.

INTERACTIONS OF LASERS WITH INTERVERTEBRAL DISKS

Almost immediately after the introduction of lasers, the concern regarding tissue interactions was of research interest.[17-18]

Cadaver and Animal Disk Laser Research

The search for the optimal laser for use in the intervertebral disk began in the 1980s with surveys of absorption of laser energy by intervertebral disk material.[19] It was found that the higher wavelengths such as Nd:YAG 1320-nm and mid-infrared lasers had a higher absorption than the lower-wavelength Nd:YAG 1064-nm or argon lasers. A higher amount of absorbed energy would theoretically be advantageous. However, control of the degree of heating of the disk is also necessary because with Nd:YAG 1320-nm powers above 20 W, instead of tissue shrinkage, a thermal bubble develops that ruptures tissues.[20] When intradiskal tissues reach 65° C, permanent changes are introduced to the disk—resulting in both morphology changes in the disk and also a permanently increased tension in the disk with a volume loss of 20% to 70% of the nucleus pulposus. Using an Ho:YAG laser, radial bulging is increased with low-energy level laser application whereas after 1500 J, the radial bulge and transverse disk diameter decrease.[21] One group claims Ho:YAG lasers without cooling (as is the case with nonarthroscopic applications) cause immediate tissue damage to surrounding tissues, whereas in the case of arthroscopy there is irrigation cooling—thereby avoiding damage to surrounding tissues. The same group found that Nd:YAG lasers were much more dependent on the color of the tissue for ablation, with the highly colored tissue causing an increased absorption of energy, thereby concluding the Nd:YAG is the superior laser for intradiskal ablation.[22] Of course, the disk material that is herniated is usually not highly colored, therefore it is perplexing why these conclusions were reached. A study of power and energy from an Ho:YAG laser with respect to ablated disk material mass and time demonstrated temperature does not rise any more after the application of 500 J to the disk, and that the mass of ablated material was related to energy, but not to power.[23] Similarly, in another cadaver study, it was discovered that energy, not time, power, or pulse frequency best determined the rate of disk ablation, and the rate of ablation was enhanced through suction application.[24] The same group determined that end plate damage and adjacent tissue damage is avoided if the laser remains in the middle of the disk, and that there is little tissue damage 1 cm from the tip of the laser. The amount of disk material removed with a Ho:YAG laser was determined via experiment on human cadaver spines to be 104 mg/kJ.[25] MRI correlation with histology in cadaver disks subjected to different energy pulses of Ho:YAG radiation demonstrated cavitation with end plate involvement at high pulse energies of 1 to 2 J/pulse, whereas low pulse energy of <1 J/pulse produced tissue modulation with end plate sparing. The overall loss of mass was determined by total energy applied rather than pulse energy.[26] Tissue absorption and ablation of an Ho:YAG laser is limited to approximately 500 microns, which makes aggressive ablation of the disk difficult, but also reduces the likelihood of the laser contacting dura or nerve roots.

In summary we may conclude the following from the above research:

- There are different mechanisms of laser-tissue interaction at low power and high power. Low-power laser application (<20 watts) results in tissue modulation and shrinkage, whereas high power results in thermal bubble formation and tissue rupture/ablation.
- Low-energy versus high-energy application results in different responses of the disk. Low energy (<1500 J) results in an increased radial bulge and transverse disk diameter, whereas a higher energy application results in a reduction in the radial bulge, transverse diameter of the disk, and a substantially increased disk tension with a permanently altered nucleus pulposus.
- Disk ablation is influenced more by total energy than the power selected for multiple IR lasers.
- Temperature increases do not extend more than 1 cm beyond the tip of the Nd:YAG or Ho:YAG laser and do not cause end plate damage if the tip is aimed in the center of the disk parallel to the end plates. However, with Nd:YAG lasers, high cannula temperatures may sometimes be measured, and if the laser is not moved during lasing, tissue ablation extends to 2 cm beyond the tip.
- Suction markedly increases the ablation rate.
- Ho:YAG laser ablates disk at the rate of 0.1 g/kJ disk 0.1 g of energy applied.

Live Animal Laser Research

A dog study examined the disk at several points in time after laser diskectomy and found initially a cavity was formed, followed by growth of fibrous tissue 2 to 4 weeks later, then replacement by cartilage 12 weeks later. At no time up to 40 weeks was there any evidence of new bone formation.[27] Another dog study using a CO_2 laser demonstrated erratic amounts of nucleus pulposus ablated with 300 J total energy and with significant damage to the end plates.[28] This implies the CO_2 laser may not be the best choice for diskectomy. Several dog studies have been performed using Ho:YAG disk decompression prophylactically in dogs exhibiting signs of back pain, with the outcomes demonstrating good results and with relatively few complications.[29,30] One mechanism of decreased pain after laser diskectomy involves the reduction in inflammatory agents phospholipase A_2 and prostaglandin E_2,[31] which is similar to the response demonstrated with coblation nucleoplasty.

ANATOMY AND PATHOLOGY OF HERNIATED DISKS

The pathology of the disk herniation has been studied continuously since 1934, yet there is still much to be known about the process and initiating factors. The posterior lamellar annular layers are thinner in the posterior spine than in the anterior spine, which assists in spinal flexion and extension, but also predisposes the posterior annulus to disruption. Both trauma and internal disk derangement can lead to disk herniation, which consists of rupture of the nucleus pulposus through the annulus fibrosus. To add confusion to the picture, a disrupted outer annulus fibrosus without herniation can also be painful.[32]

The morphology of the macroscopic annulus fibrosus and the microscopic anatomy both undergo changes in disk herniation. The concavity of the disk is often reduced or inverted, whereas the cellular structure itself in the annulus fibrosus undergoes a transformation from spindle-shaped cells to rounded chondrocytes at the area of disk herniation. There are chemical changes in the wall of the herniated disks that may produce a chemical cascade from degeneration to herniation. Specifically, fibroblast growth factor-beta immunoreactivity is found in degenerative but not control disks.[33] There is a soup of inflammatory mediators that can induce neurologic symptoms of pain inside the herniated disks. These include tumor necrosis factor-alpha (TNF-α), phospholipase A_2, and interleukin 1-beta (IL1-β), that exist in a complex and not yet completely defined interrelationship. IL1-β induces neurologic symptoms, yet sets up a feedback loop to produce increased concentrations of cyclooxygenase-2 (induces production of inflammatory agents prostaglandin, prostacyclin, thromboxane); matrix metalloproteinase-1 (MMP1) that degrades the disk matrix, cleaves collagen type IV; dissolves the basement membrane protein fibronectin matrix metalloproteinase (MMP3) that degrades numerous extracellular matrix (ECM) substrates—including collagens III, IV, V, IX, X, and XI, laminin, elastin, entactin, fibronectin, fibrin, fibulin, link protein, osteonectin, vitronectin, and ECM proteoglycans; releases cell surface molecules such as TNF-α, EGF growth factor, and so on.[34]

Some of these agents, specifically TNF-α, are present in high concentrations in disk herniation patients[35] but they are also present in lesser quantities in both asymptomatic juvenile and elderly disks, but not disks in middle adulthood. It has been shown that the herniated disk has the ability to disrupt the elastic capsule around the dorsal root ganglion (DRG) and permit large molecules, such as albumin, to enter the DRG within a few hours after herniation[36] with the potential to cause endoneural edema and scarring. TNF-α has been demonstrated to have an extreme inflammatory effect on the DRG.[37] Indeed, early application of intravenous infliximab (a TNF inhibitor) has been demonstrated in human studies to produce sustained pain resolution after disk herniation.[38] Animal studies with TNF inhibitors given at the time of disk herniation demonstrate a significant reduction in damage to the DRG histologically.[39] But the TNF-α is only one of many inflammatory factors that are produced, and TNF-α does not reduce the disk herniation size, but only the inflammatory effect of TNF-α on the nerve root. Worsening of the herniation could potentially occur without depressurization of the nucleus pulposus in such situations. In a pilot study, intradiskal injection of TNF-α inhibitors into the disk did not reduce pain from disk degeneration nor did it reduce back pain associated with disk herniation. However, application of the TNF-α inhibitors on the nerve root did substantially reduce leg pain by virtually 100%.

The pathology of disk herniation is often a narrow neck of disk protruding through the annular fibers with a "mushroom" head of the nucleus pulposus compressing the nerve roots, posterior longitudinal ligament (PLL), or dura. Because the sinuvertebral nerve innervates the dura and PLL, inflammatory cytokines exuding from the exposed nucleus pulposus have the potential to cause back pain without leg pain. Compression of the nerve root by the disk herniation often produces dermatomal numbness, dysesthesias, reflex changes, and weakness. If the nerve root is not directly mechanically compressed, there may be radicular pain from the inflammatory response of the DRG to the chemicals and enzymes from the nucleus pulposus, but without the other signs of a radiculopathy. Those with neurologic deficits demonstrated a 500% increase in blood flow after diskectomy compared to those who did not have neurologic deficits.[40] This suggests the mechanism of neurologic deficit is partially related to vascular ischemia from compression of the nerve root. Rat studies demonstrate that application of herniated nucleus pulposus placed proximal to the DRG develops a significant decrease in blood flow compared to the control group that had muscle placed proximal to the DRG.[41] This suggests that an inflammatory response with nerve root edema is at least partially responsible for the neurologic symptoms. It has also been shown that human patients with disk herniation exhibit a marked reduction in the gliding motion of the nerve root during intraoperative straight leg raising tests with an associated significant decrease in nerve root blood flow.[42] After decompression, there is improvement in both the gliding motion and in the blood flow to the nerve.

The predisposing factors have been examined for disk herniation both in humans and in cadaver models. It appears the sequence begins peripherally with tears in the outer annulus, which is predisposed to disruption from repeated loads plus bending and twisting.[43] A strong familial predisposition in juvenile disk herniation with an odds ratio of 5.61, suggests a genetic influence may be operant.[44]

Anatomic considerations for laser disk decompression include patient size, location of the disk herniation, neuroforaminal size, presence of furcal nerves, presence of an overlying annular inflammatory membrane, disk height, anatomic impediments to access (osteophytes in the neuroforamen, iliac crest morphology), and applicability to the technique selected. Using the standard foraminal posterolateral approach, the morbidly obese patient presents anatomic limitations to treatment of disk herniations. The straight anteroposterior skin-to-disk measurement may be 15 cm or more. Using a 45-degree angled insertion of a needle for laser access in a standard extrapedicular approach (as used in diskography) would require a needle length of 21 cm or more (>8 inches). Therefore depending on the access needles or cannulas available and the length of the laser wand, obese patients may not be candidates for laser diskectomy. Disk herniation location is less likely to be a significant determinant of success when most laser disk decompression techniques (intradiskal) are used. But some systems such as the Wolf YESS system utilize lasers to enlarge the cavity directly beneath the disk herniation with subsequent intradiskal removal of the herniation with mechanical articulating tools. A small neuroforamen predisposes to injury during disk access with large needles because of the exiting nerve root being displaced inferiorly in the neuroforamen. The safe triangle for disk access is smaller when there is significant apical foraminal impingement. The presence of osteophytes also causes some difficulties when there is zygapophyseal hypertrophy or vertebral body osteochondrosis. A calcified annulus fibrosus also causes some difficulty with disk access. The presence of a high iliac crest poses significant problems with rigid cannula or needle systems at L5-S1 because the trajectory of the disk entry will predispose to damage to the superior S1 end plate, in addition to posing problems when nonflexible instruments or lasers are used through the cannula. Curved needle systems may be advantageous in accessing the L5-S1 disk for laser decompression. A transiliac approach has been possible in cadavers[45] but this requires drilling holes through the ilium for access. Furcal nerves are accessory nerves present in approximately

15% of the population,[46] and are found primarily at L4-L5 93% of the time.[47] They traverse the foramen quite laterally, have their own separate DRG, then exit with the L5 nerve root. Compression of the furcal nerves with a lateral disk herniation can cause both L4 and L5 symptoms. The nerves are primarily sensory nerves and because of their anatomic location, can be injured by a needle placed across the neuroforamen into the disk. Inflammatory membranes have been described clinically by Tony Yeung during endoscopic diskectomy as a beefy red, angry membrane over the surface of the annulus fibrosus. These membranes are exquisitely sensitive to pressure, which may make posterolateral needle placement quite painful. However, they are an infrequent finding in disk herniations.

TECHNIQUES OF LASER DISK DECOMPRESSION

Different techniques of laser disk decompression are available, some of which have elaborate systems of instrumentation. The basic approach to all laser disk decompression is through placement of a needle or cannula via a posterior-lateral transforaminal entry into the intervertebral disk. Once the needle or cannula has entered the inner annular fibers, a laser is advanced into the disk and activated to decompress the nucleus pulposus. This may be achieved with fluoroscopic guidance, rigid endoscopic guidance, or flexible endoscopic guidance. The laser tip may be a rigid end-firing laser wand, a rigid side-firing laser wand, or a fiberoptic waveguide laser tip (polished or cross-cut). Laser choices include Ho:YAG, Nd:YAG (two wavelengths), KTP, Er:YAG, multidiode, and tunable diode. Generally, a Ho:YAG laser is preferred, although the new multidiode laser is much less expensive. After laser disk decompression, generally the needle is withdrawn, but the cannula often remains for further mechanical dissection of the disk using long instrumentation through an endoscope.

Stepwise Laser Disk Decompression

Access to the intervertebral disk is achieved by horizontal fluoroscopy beam through the intervertebral disk, then a standard posterolateral approach is used with a needle placed onto the lateral border of the superior articular process (Fig. 173–5). Because the safe zone for needle placement is much larger at the superior end plate of the lower disk, it is strongly preferred to take an approach that will bring the needle tip low in the intervertebral disk. One study revealed the tolerances for error may be much less than previously thought;[48] therefore, it is prudent to avoid needle placement in the mid to upper disk. The angle chosen for needle entry partially depends on the location of the disk herniation and the importance in targeting the exact area. Greater than 55 degrees oblique from the sagittal plane can cause bowel injury or dural entry. Too shallow an angle places the laser too far anterior in the disk. Therefore, if anatomically possible, the needle angle chosen is usually between 40 and 55 degrees in the lumbar spine or 30 to 40 degrees in the upper lumbar and thoracic spine. While cervical endoscopic systems do exist, the entry is at the anterior right side at approximately 20 to 30 degrees to the sagittal plane.

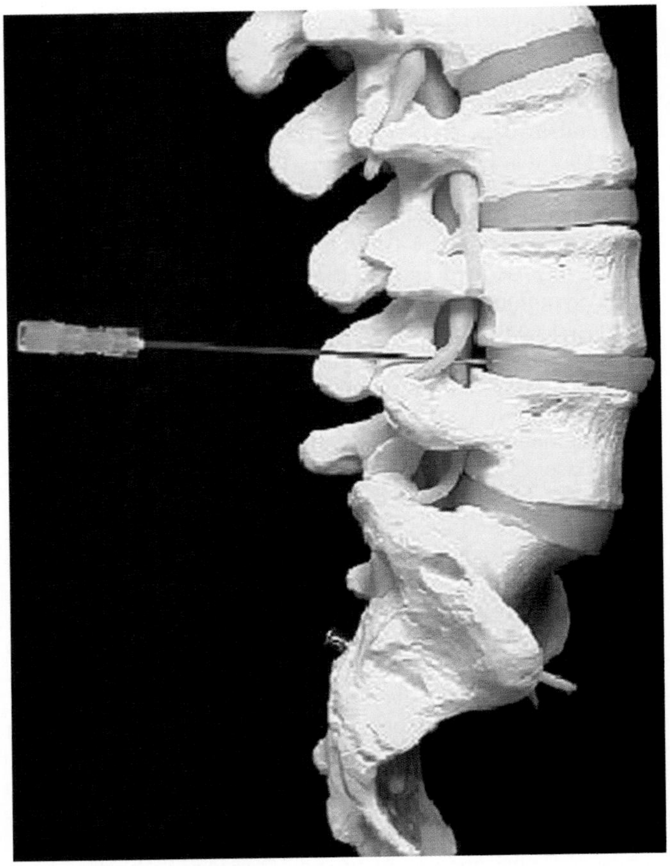

FIGURE 173–5 ■ Stepwise laser disk decompression.

LASER DISKECTOMY TECHNIQUES

LASE System

The LASE disk access needle system consists of a straight (2.8-mm, 12 gauge) and curved needle (3.0-mm for L5-S1) (Fig. 173–6). The needle is inserted into the safe zone as described earlier. When the disk is contacted, a small trephine may be placed through the needle to assist with annulotomy. If the angle of the straight needle placed at L5-S1 is too acute to the sagittal plane (15 to 30 degrees), the straight needle will have its final placement too far lateral in the disk. In such cases, the beam is angled more cephalad (no longer in a direct plane with the disk) then more lateral oblique to permit use of the 3.0-mm curved cannula. The curved cannula is advanced over the superior iliac crest; then a steep inferior angle is selected to guide the needle tip to the lateral-anterior border of the SAP of S1. The needle is subsequently advanced over the trephine into the inner annular fibers and a needle-stop set screw is tightened to fix the maximum needle ingress. With the 1.7-mm diameter endoscope connected to a light source and camera (preferably CCD 3 chip), white balancing is performed. Rotor pump pressurized irrigation is turned on with an irrigant of normal saline or normal saline mixed with bacitracin 50,000 U per 3 L is infused through the irrigation port of the wand.

A Ho:YAG laser fiber (400 microns) is inserted through the flexible scope and locked into place with the tip of the

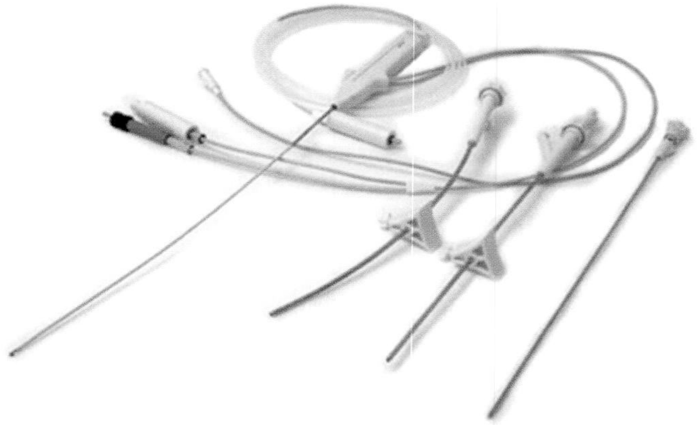

FIGURE 173–6 ■ LASE endoscope and access needles.

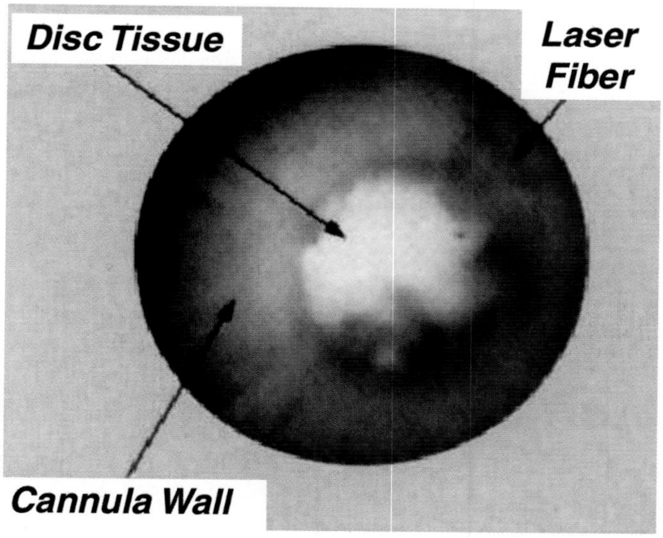

FIGURE 173–7 ■ Approach to herniated disk using the LASE wand.

fiber protruding 1 mm beyond the end of the laser. The wand is inserted through the LASE needle until white disk material is seen. Grasping forceps or pituitary forceps are used to remove disk material in the needle and at the tip of the needle in order to advance the LASE wand just beyond the tip. It is prudent not to fire the laser inside the needle due to the potential for flashback and thermal damage to the LASE wand. The LASE wand is slowly advanced across the disk and may be curved into an area immediately anterior to the disk herniation if desired owing to the flexible guidable endoscope feature (Fig. 173–7).

Fluoroscopic and endoscopic guidance are used simultaneously for confirmation of intra-nucleus pulposus placement. Typically about 10,000 to 15,000 J per disk are delivered with a double-pulsed setting of 20 watts. The optics of the fiberoptic scope produce modestly good visualization of tissues, and one can usually discern differences in the nucleus pulposus versus annulus fibrosus. If there is insufficient irrigation, too high a power setting (>20 W), inadequate outflow of the irrigation, or excessive lasing in one location without laser tip

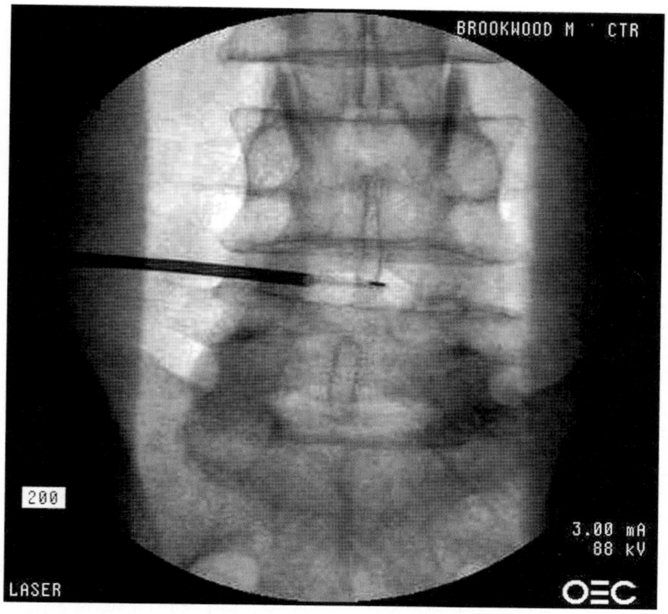

FIGURE 173–8 ■ Fluoroscopic view with LASE system.

movement (Fig. 173–8), carbonization will occur and the disk tissues will become blackened; visualization will degrade with blackened fragments floating in the field of view.

It is preferred to lase for 5 seconds on, then 5 seconds off because during lasing, the cavitation obscures the optical resolution of the tissues being lased. If the tip approaches the end plate, a bright flashback can occur with reflection of the laser beam off the bone and back through the waveguide toward the laser source. This can damage the end plate (very undesirable) and potentially the laser itself if there is inadequate flashback protection built into the laser. Typically one to two disks may be treated with a single laser wand. The optics of the fiberoptic system can degrade with extended use and the tip of the laser fiber itself may degrade. If the laser fiber is not polished, it is possible to cut the laser fiber back with a special laser fiber knife and resume the LASE procedure.

After termination of the procedure, the laser wand and needles are withdrawn with local anesthetic injected in the needle track outside the neuroforamen. It is not desirable to inject local anesthesia near the DRG or exiting nerve root because if there exists a rare neurologic deficit after the termination of the procedure, the effect of the local anesthetic could muddle the diagnosis and result in significant diagnostic delay.

Nonendoscopic Laser Fiber Diskectomy (Modified Choy Technique)

The original Choy procedure used lateral decubitus patient positioning and did not employ targeting the safe operating zone of the neuroforamen. Choy used a fixed 10-cm lateral entry from the midline and an initial 45-degree angulation. Of course, in obese patients a fixed distance from the midline skin needle entry will result in a trajectory that is less than 45 degrees to the sagittal plane and potential entry into the disk at the site of exiting nerve root owing to deflection of the needle by the superior articular process (SAP). Very thin patients have the opposite issue with a fixed needle skin entry site and it may result in excessively posterior needle placement if the SAP is targeted and potential pithing of the exiting nerve root if a 45-degree entry angle is selected. Therefore, the technique has been modified to use the standard precision "down the barrel" pain medicine method.

With the patient in the prone position, for central disk targeting the fluoroscopy beam is used to provide a horizontal trajectory across the end plates, then the beam is rotated obliquely approximately 45 degrees at L3-L4 and L4-L5, 35 to 40 degrees at L1-L2 and L2-L3. The angle at L5-S1 is as far oblique as possible until the iliac crest overrides the superior articular process. At each level the lateral-inferior border of the SAP is targeted at the junction between the superior end plate and the disk. An aliquot of local anesthetic is infiltrated in the skin at the selected entry site, then a 6-inch spinal needle is passed in the selected trajectory to, but not beyond, the SAP—during which time local anesthetic is infiltrated. A 20-cm, 18-gauge needle is subsequently advanced in the anesthetized track and the SAP is contacted. On advancement across the neuroforamen (*slowly*), the patient may experience some intense back pain but should not experience any radicular pain. Repositioning is necessary if there is radicular pain, which can be due to a hypersensitized DRG, furcal nerve contact, or overt contact with a displaced exiting nerve root. When annular cannulation has occurred, the end point of needle advancement is on AP projection, halfway between the lateral border of the spinous process and the medial border of the pedicle. On lateral fluoroscopic projection, the needle tip should reside at the junction of the posterior quarter of the disk with the anterior three quarters. An Nd:YAG fiber is inserted through the needle to the tip and 1 cm beyond. The needle is subsequently not moved. Lesioning at 20 W with 5 seconds between 1-second pulses is used. If a flashback is observed, the laser tip is retracted and inspected for damage. If the tip is damaged, the tip is cut and the laser reinserted. The total energy applied is 1000 J or up to 1500 J if the patient is >165 cm in height. (Note: The energy used with this technique incorporating an Nd:YAG laser is only 1/10 of that required with the Ho:YAG laser). If the disks have a narrowed height, the amount of energy applied is reduced by 25%. During lasing, the patient should alert the physician of any new radicular pain. (Note: This method is completely blind and is incapable of guiding the laser tip. It also does not employ any aqueous irrigation, which can lead to charring and end plate damage. However, numerous publications attest to the safety of this procedure.)

An alternative laser source is an Ho:YAG fiber or multidiode laser but the same limitations apply. With an Nd:YAG laser, the lesion produced is 2 cm long and 6 mm wide. An Ho:YAG laser produces a much smaller lesion in the disk tissue unless the laser fiber is moved; this system is not desirable because of potential laser fiber fracture within the disk.

Rigid-Scope Endoscopic Laser Diskectomy

This technique of endoscopic laser diskectomy uses a rigid scope in contrast to the LASE (flexible, steerable fiberoptic scope). The optics and visualization are much better than the fiberoptic scope and the working channels in the scope permit introduction of dissection and probing instruments. The two systems used in pain medicine are the PercScope by Clarus and the YESS scope by Wolf. The PercScope uses a 30,000-pixel fiberoptic bundle housed in a 5.2-mm rigid scope housing and contains a large 3.1-mm working channel. This size of working channel will permit the introduction of a variety of instruments, as depicted subsequently, that permit laser-assisted dissection. The lasers may be either a non-steerable bare fiber, fiberoptic steerable laser, or a rigid laser housing for side-firing or end-firing laser output. The Wolf system uses a 7-mm OD cannula for a 6-mm OD scope. The working channel is 2.7 mm, but there are several irrigation ports. The optical system uses a rigid rod system with crystal-clear non-pixelated viewing. There is a European scope with a much larger working channel (Fig. 173–9), up to 4 mm, that will permit introduction of large dissection instruments and automated rotating dissectors and burrs.

Fundamentally, both systems incorporate the same basic technique of disk access and dissection. The cannula systems are so large that primary introduction is not possible without a guidewire (Fig. 173–10). An initial posterolateral placement of an intradiskal needle is the first step. When the disk has been entered, an injection of indigo carmine blue/iodinated contrast is rendered into the nucleus pulposus. Indigo carmine has been shown to selectively stain the degenerative/herniated parts of intervertebral disks blue.[49] A guidewire is then inserted through the needle, and the needle is removed. Next,

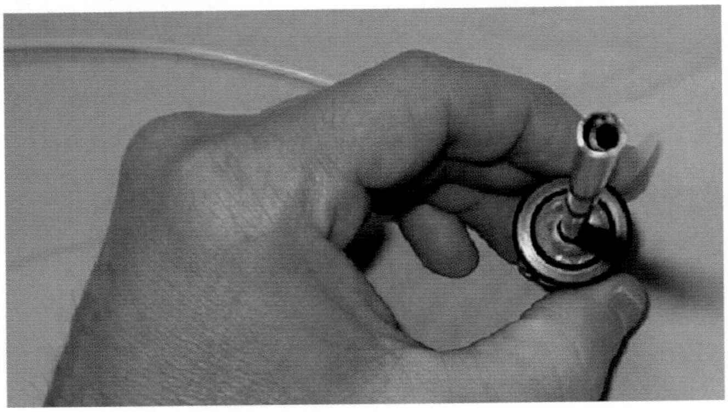

FIGURE 173–9 ■ PercScope working channel.

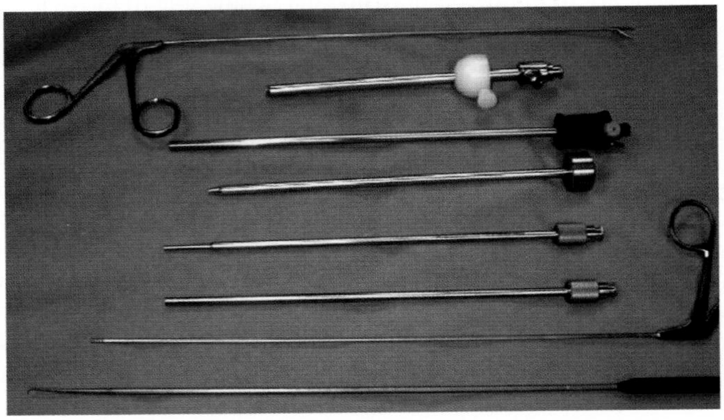

FIGURE 173–10 ■ PercScope access cannulas and surgical instruments.

a dilator is placed over the guidewire under fluoroscopic guidance to avert bending the guidewire. A cannula is placed over the dilator which is advanced to the external annulus fibrosus. With the cannula held in place, the external annulus is probed with the dilator for underlying nerve roots. If none are discovered, the dilator is removed and the cannula is held firmly in place; a trephine or annulotome is advanced to the annulus. If the trephine is used, the cannula is simply advanced into the intervertebral disk. However, if the annulotome is used, the dilator is replaced through the cruciate incision of the annulus, and subsequently is advanced into the nucleus pulposus. The cannula is then slid off the dilator into the nucleus pulposus. Following removal of the dilator, the endoscope is inserted with continuous saline or bacitracin containing saline irrigation flowing into the nucleus pulposus. Pituitary forceps are inserted through the endoscope to clear disk tissue from the end of the cannula. The blue-stained material is targeted with the forceps and then the laser, as this represents the herniated and severely degenerative portion of the disk (Fig. 173–11). An end-firing or side-firing laser wand may be placed through the working channel, and the Ho:YAG laser at 20 to 40 W is used to clear the area under the disk herniation. The usual laser energy applied is between 5000 and 25,000 J. A side-firing laser has a mirror placed at a 45-degree angle near the tip of the scope, deflecting the laser at right angles to the wand. This has several advantages, including that a more posterior laser diskectomy may be performed. Care must be taken not to excessively weaken the posterior annulus fibrosus by firing the laser in one location onto the annulus. With the PercScope system, the procedure is terminated at this point, whereas with the Wolf system, the laser dissection is usually followed by an aggressive articulating forceps used to grasp the neck of the herniation, pulling the hernia back inside the disk and out through the cannula. At the termination of the procedure, the cannula is removed and the patient may receive steroids along the nerve root to help control postoperative periradicular edema.

Non-Lumbar Systems

The cervical and thoracic areas can be approached with a laser technique for diskectomy. The lower three thoracic disks can often be accessed inferior to the transverse process, whereas the mid and upper thoracic levels may require obtuse angulations. The LASE system is ideal for these applications.

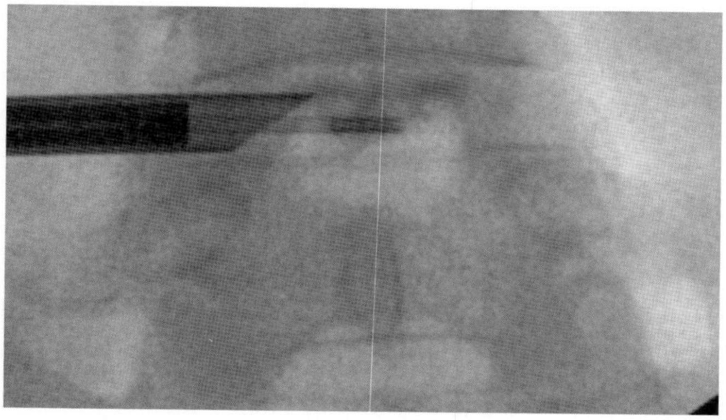

FIGURE 173–11 ■ Laser through YESS endoscope.

Cervical diskectomy may be performed with a special cervical LASE system or a 2.5-mm cannulated system such as a Blackstone or other access system. Usually the cervical disk is approached very much like cervical diskography, except extreme care must be used in the anterior cervical spine owing to the carotid and jugular systems' being in the line of the needle trajectory. It is suggested that cervical diskectomy not be performed unless the physician has immense experience with both lumbar and thoracic diskectomy and with cervical diskography.

OUTCOME STUDIES

Ho:YAG

Using 1500 J energy at 15 watts through an 18-gauge needle, one group had a 91% successful outcome rate at 18 months' follow-up.[50] Using a laser-assisted disk decompression with a side-firing laser placed through an endoscope, success was achieved on the 1 year's follow-up at a 90% level[51] and at 87% at 2 years' follow-up.[52]

Nd:YAG

The results for non-endoscopic lumbar disk decompression with an Nd:YAG laser are variable, but generally range from 70% to 90% good to excellent results. A 4-year follow-up study of 200 patients with Nd:YAG 1064-nm nonendoscopic laser diskectomy produced a 74% success rate.[53] Another study used non-endoscopic Nd:YAG diskectomy in 42 patients with *thoracic* disk extrusions and protrusions, with improvement in all clinical parameters in 41 out of the 42 patients.[54] Choy's experience with 389 patients using a non-endoscopic laser diskectomy with the Nd:YAG laser demonstrated a 75% success rate according to good and excellent results by the modified MacNab criteria,[55] although in his book *Percutaneous Laser Disc Decompression* he states the success rate in later cases rose to 89%.

COMPLICATIONS

Generally the complication rate for laser diskectomy is relatively low, around 1%. The specific complication profile for cervical, thoracic, and lumbar diskectomy are different due to anatomic considerations, and are listed in Table 173–1.

Most complications are relatively mild and involve transient increases in pain due to prone patient positioning when the patient may not have assumed that position in years, muscle spasm from the needle/cannula, and subcutaneous or intramuscular hematomas. However, on rare occasions serious complications will occur. This author has had one case of a Brown Séquard syndrome when an access cannula displaced a protruding disk herniation fragment into the cervical spinal cord, with only partial long-term neurologic recovery. Poor patient selection can lead to severe complications such as cauda equina syndrome in very rare cases.[56]

When larger cannulas are used to access the disk, a finite percentage (about 5% to 7%) will develop a transient CRPS II syndrome,[57] but this does not seem to occur as frequently with a needle access system. Both osteomyelitis and diskitis have been reported after laser diskectomy[58,59] although these

Table 173–1

Potential Complications of Laser Diskectomy

	Cervical Complications	*Thoracic Complications*	*Lumbar Complications*
Disk access complications	Perforation of carotid, jugular, thyroid, esophagus, trachea	Pneumothorax, cord or nerve root penetration, chylothorax, hemothorax, CSF leak	CSF leak, nerve root injury, bowel penetration, epidural hematoma, epidural abscess, cord injury (above L2)
Laser/needle complications	Needle perforation of the end plates, cord with Brown Séquard syndrome, nerve root penetration, diskitis, CSF leak, PLL destruction, lasing the cord or nerve roots, late disk space collapse or degeneration, pseudodiskitis, epidural hematoma from lasing of epidural vessels	Lasing the cord, nerve root thermal injury, aortic/caval injury, diskitis, epidural hematoma, epidural abscess, end plate damage/pseudodiskitis	Iliac penetration, sympathetic chain injury, end plate damage/pseudodiskitis, diskitis, bowel injury, genitofemoral nerve injury, late disk degeneration, disk space collapse with increased disk bulge

PLL, posterior longitudinal ligament.

are rare, and most are aseptic. It is highly probable that most instances of aseptic diskitis are caused by over-reading postoperative MRIs or mistaking end plate laser damage for diskitis. The potential for long-term disk degeneration acceleration is a very real concern when using the larger cannulas for disk access because the sheep model for long-term degeneration is coring the annulus fibrosus The use of slit lesions with a 2.5-mm device caused much less disk degeneration and instability than did the use of a box window excision of the disk,[60] which implies that if the larger cannulae are to be used, they should be preceded by an annulotome incision. Excessive removal of disk is also potentially deleterious owing to the removal of the central nucleus pulposus support with a biomechanical weight transfer to the annulus fibrosus. The annulus is not designed to hold significant weight and undergoes progressive collapse with annular bulging.

Another significant concern is the damage to the end plates that are the nutrient conduits to the avascular nucleus pulposus. The cartilaginous end plates gradually become sclerotic with subchondral bone formation because there is increased force affecting the trabecular bone when the disk is no longer serving as a hydraulic shock absorber. Additionally, Ito has demonstrated a direct correlation between calcification of the nutrient canaliculi and MRI grade of disk degeneration.[61] Adams demonstrated that even minor damage to the vertebral end plates may lead to progressive structural changes in the adjacent disk.[62] One study demonstrated after endoscopic laser diskectomy, that there were subchondral marrow abnormalities identified in 41 out of 109 patients. However in a subset of patients examined 5 to 7 years after laser diskectomy, both back pain and marrow abnormalities improved on MRI.[63] The nature of such subchondral osteonecrosis was examined on MRI imaging and was found to include a wedge-shaped area of low signal intensity on T1 images, of high and low signal intensity on T2-weighted images, and of gadolinium-enhanced high signal intensity on T2-weighted images respectively. The speculative causes of such changes were thought to include thermal energy and photoacoustic shock.[64] An experimental animal model of Nd:YAG laser injury to the end plates revealed an early decrease in vascularization at 1 month post laser application, however by 2 months post laser application, the vascularization of the end plate had effectively doubled.[65] Using an experimental guinea pig model with a carbon dioxide laser fired at the end plates, as little as 300 J of energy was required to damage the end plates.[66] However, it was demonstrated by Hoogland that curettage of the end plates of severely degenerative disks may later reverse some of the MRI changes of disk degeneration including that of disk desiccation.[67] But the latter was based on limited clinical evidence; therefore, the *modus operandi* at this juncture would invoke end plate preservation.

SUMMARY

Laser diskectomy is an alternative to open or microdiskectomy for selected patients at a small fraction of the costs. Least expensive is the Choy technique but it has the theoretical disadvantage of increased risks of end plate damage because the laser fiber angle cannot be controlled when the laser waveguide is inserted through the needle. Although the other techniques are more expensive, they provide steerability of the laser that is useful in avoiding the end plates. The Nd:YAG laser is much more aggressive than the Ho:YAG; therefore, tissue ablation will occur at a much more rapid rate. The advantage of the Ho:YAG is the safety imparted through a 500-micron controlled tissue penetration, especially when operating in a continuously irrigated field.

The major barriers to more widespread use of laser disk decompression include high cost of a laser ($50,000 to $180,000); reluctance of hospital medical staff to open laser use to pain medicine due to infrequent use by the specialty; equipment costs (endoscopes, light sources, cannula systems, video system, and flexible laser wands); lack of double-blind controlled studies; alternative more simple solutions (coblation nucleoplasty, disk decompression), and global skill level deficits of most pain physicians in endoscopy of the spine. However, most hospitals and some surgery centers have acquired lasers (e.g., Ho:YAG lasers are often used to perform laser lithotripsy of kidney stones) and already own the video towers and cameras necessary to perform video procedures. PLDD is effective 75% to 90% of the time in selected patients at a fraction of the cost of microdiskectomy or open diskectomy.

References

1. Maroon JC: Current concepts in minimally invasive discectomy (5 Suppl). Neurosurgery. 51:S137, 2002.
2. Choy DSJ, Case RB, Fielding JW, et al: Percutaneous laser nucleolysis of the lumbar disc. N Engl J Med 317:771, 1987.
3. Mayer HM, Brock M, Berlien HP, Weber B: Percutaneous endoscopic laser discectomy (PELD). A new surgical technique for non-sequestrated lumbar discs. Acta Neurochir Suppl (Wien) 54:53, 1992.
4. Savitz MH: Same-day microsurgical arthroscopic lateral-approach laser-assisted (SMALL) fluoroscopic discectomy. J Neurosurg 80(6):1039, 1994.
5. Heppner F, Ascher PW: First experience with laser beams in the treatment of neurosurgical diseases. Zentralbl Neurochir 38(1):77, 1977.
6. Gropper GR, Robertson JH, McClellan G: Comparative histological and radiographic effects of CO_2 laser versus standard surgical anterior cervical discectomy in the dog. Neurosurgery 14(1):42, 1984.
7. Wolgin M, Finkenberg J, Papaioannou T, et al: Excimer ablation of human intervertebral disc at 308 nanometers. Lasers Surg Med 9(2):124, 1989.
8. Yonezawa T, Onomura T, Kosaka R, et al: The system and procedures of percutaneous intradiscal laser nucleotomy. Spine 15(11):1175, 1990.
9. Davis JK: Early experience with laser disc decompression. A percutaneous method. J Fla Med Assoc 79(1):37, 1992.
10. Siebert WE: Use of lasers in arthroscopy. Orthopade 21(4):273, 1992.
11. Choy DSJ: Percutaneous Laser Disc Decompression. New York, Springer-Verlag, 2003.
12. Choy DSJ, Stertzer SH, Myler RF, et al: Human coronary laser recanalization. Clin Cardiol 7:377, 1984.
13. Choy DS, Altman P: Fall of intradiscal pressure with laser ablation. J Clin Laser Med Surg 13(3):149, 1995.
14. Ohnmeiss DD, Guyer RD, Hochschuler SH: Laser disc decompression. The importance of proper patient selection. Spine 19(18):2054, 1994.
15. Wright VC: Laser surgery: Using the carbon dioxide laser. Can Med Assoc J 126(9):1035, 1982.
16. Hecht J: Understanding Lasers. New York, IEEE Press, 1992, p 127.
17. Solon LR, Aronson R, Gould G: Physiological implications of laser beams. Science 134:1506, 1961.
18. Zaret MM, Breinin GM, Schmidt H, et al: Ocular lesions produced by an optical maser (laser). Science 134:1525, 1961.
19. Vorwerk D, Husemann T, Blazek V, et al: Laser ablation of the nucleus pulposus: Optical properties of degenerated intervertebral disk tissue in the wavelength range 200 to 2200 nm. Rofo Fortschr Geb Rontgenstr Neuen Bildgeb Verfahr 151(6):725, 1989.
20. Choi JY, Tanenbaum BS, Milner TE, et al: Thermal, mechanical, optical, and morphologic changes in bovine nucleus pulposus induced by Nd:YAG (lambda = 1.32 micron) laser irradiation. Lasers Surg Med 28(3):248, 2001.
21. Castro WH, Halm H, Jerosch J, et al. Changes in the lumbar intervertebral disk following use of the Ho:YAG laser—a biomechanical study. Z Orthop Ihre Grenzgeb 131(6):610, 1993.
22. Anders JO, Pietsch S, Staupendahl G: Critical evaluation of indications for the Ho:YAG laser and the neodymium:YAG laser in orthopedic surgery based on an in vitro study. Biomed Tech (Berl) 44(4):83, 1999.
23. Buchelt M, Schlangmann B, Schmolke S, Siebert W: High power Ho:YAG laser ablation of intervertebral discs: Effects on ablation rates and temperature profile. Lasers Surg Med 16(2):179, 1995.
24. Schlangmann BA, Schmolke S, Siebert WE: Temperature and ablation measurements in laser therapy of intervertebral disk tissue. Orthopade 25(1):3, 1996.
25. Min K, Leu H, Zweifel K: Quantitative determination of ablation in weight of lumbar intervertebral discs with Ho:YAG laser. Lasers Surg Med 18(2):187, 1996.
26. Phillips JJ, Kopchok GE, Peng SK, et al: MR imaging of Ho:YAG laser diskectomy with histologic correlation. J Magn Reson Imaging 3(3):515, 1993.
27. Qi Q, Dang GD, Cai QL: Laser ablation of intervertebral disc: Animal experiment. Zhonghua Wai Ke Za Zhi 32(3):187, 1994.
28. Nerubay J, Caspi I, Levinkopf M, et al: Percutaneous laser nucleolysis of the intervertebral lumbar disc. An experimental study. J Clin Orthop (337):42, 1997.
29. Bartels KE, Higbee RG, Bahr RJ, et al: Outcome of and complications associated with prophylactic percutaneous laser disk ablation in dogs with thoracolumbar disk disease: 277 cases (1992-2001). J Am Vet Med Assoc 222(12):1733, 2003.
30. Dickey DT, Bartels KE, Henry GA, et al: Use of the holmium yttrium aluminum garnet laser for percutaneous thoracolumbar intervertebral disk ablation in dogs. J Am Vet Med Assoc 208(8):1263, 1996.
31. Iwatsuki K, Yoshimine T, Sasaki M, et al: The effect of laser irradiation for nucleus pulposus: An experimental study. Neurol Res 27(3):319, 2005.
32. Peng B, Hou S, Wu W, et al: The pathogenesis and clinical significance of a high-intensity zone (HIZ) of lumbar intervertebral disc on MR imaging in the patient with discogenic low back pain. Eur Spine J Online Jul 27, 2005.
33. Tolonen J, Gronblad M, Vanharanta H, et al: Growth factor expression in degenerated intervertebral disc tissue: An immunohistochemical analysis of transforming growth factor-beta, fibroblast growth factor and platelet-derived growth factor. Eur Spine J Online Jun 25, 2005.
34. Jimbo K, Park JS, Yokosuka K, et al: Positive feedback loop of interleukin-1 beta upregulating production of inflammatory mediators in human intervertebral disc cells in vitro. J Neurosurg Spine 2(5):589, 2005.
35. Weiler C, Nerlich AG, Bachmeier BE, Boos N: Expression and distribution of tumor necrosis factor alpha in human lumbar intervertebral discs: A study in surgical specimen and autopsy controls. Spine 30(1):44, 2005.
36. Murata Y, Rydevik B, Takahashi K, et al: Incision of the intervertebral disc induces disintegration and increases permeability of the dorsal root ganglion capsule. Spine 30(15):1712, 2005.
37. Cuellar JM, Montesano PX, Carstens E: Role of TNF-alpha in sensitization of nociceptive dorsal horn neurons induced by application of nucleus pulposus to L5 dorsal root ganglion in rats. Pain 110(3):578, 2004.
38. Korhonen T, Karppinen J, Malmivaara A, et al: Efficacy of infliximab for disc herniation-induced sciatica: One-year follow-up. Spine 29(19): 2115, 2004.
39. Murata Y, Onda A, Rydevik B, et al: Selective inhibition of tumor necrosis factor-alpha prevents nucleus pulposus-induced histologic changes in the dorsal root ganglion. Spine 29(22):2477, 2004.
40. Hida S, Naito M, Kubo M: Intraoperative measurements of nerve root blood flow during discectomy for lumbar disc herniation. Spine 28(1):85, 2003.
41. Yabuki S, Igarashi T, Kikuchi S: Application of nucleus pulposus to the nerve root simultaneously reduces blood flow in dorsal root ganglion and corresponding hind paw in the rat. Spine 25(12):1471, 2000.
42. Kobayashi S, Shizu N, Suzuki Y, et al: Changes in nerve root motion and intra-radicular blood flow during an intraoperative straight-leg-raising test. Spine 28(13):1427, 2003.
43. Gordon SJ, Yang KH, Mayer PJ, et al: Mechanism of disc rupture. A preliminary report. Spine 16(4):450, 1991.
44. Matsui H, Terahata N, Tsuji H, et al: Familial predisposition and clustering for juvenile lumbar disc herniation. Spine 17(11):1323, 1992.
45. Osman SG, Marsolais EB: Endoscopic transiliac approach to L5-S1 disc and foramen. A cadaver study. Spine 22(11):1259, 1997.
46. Haijiao W, Koti M, Smith FW, et al: Diagnosis of lumbosacral nerve root anomalies by magnetic resonance imaging. J Spinal Disord 14(2): 143, 2001.
47. Kikuchi S, Hasue M, Nishiyama K, Ito T: Anatomic features of the furcal nerve and its clinical significance. Spine 11(10):1002, 1986.
48. Min JH, Kang SH, Lee JB, et al: Morphometric analysis of the working zone for endoscopic lumbar discectomy. J Spinal Disord Tech 18(2):132, 2005.

49. Kim IS, Kim KH, Shin SW, et al: Indigo carmine for the selective endoscopic intervertebral nuclectomy. J Korean Med Sci 20(4):702, 2005.
50. Agarwal S, Bhagwat AS: Ho:YAG laser-assisted lumbar disc decompression: A minimally invasive procedure under local anesthesia. Neurol India 51(1):35, 2003.
51. Casper GD, Mullins LL, Hartman VL: Laser-assisted disc decompression: A clinical trial of the Ho:YAG laser with side-firing fiber. J Clin Laser Med Surg 13(1):27, 1995.
52. Casper GD, Hartman VL, Mullins LL: Results of a clinical trial of the Ho:YAG laser in disc decompression utilizing a side-firing fiber: A two-year follow-up. Lasers Surg Med 19(1):90, 1996.
53. Gronemeyer DH, Buschkamp H, Braun M, et al: Image-guided percutaneous laser disk decompression for herniated lumbar disks: A 4-year follow-up in 200 patients. J Clin Laser Med Surg 21(3):131, 2003.
54. Hellinger J, Stern S, Hellinger S: Nonendoscopic Nd:YAG 1064 nm PLDN in the treatment of thoracic discogenic pain syndromes. J Clin Laser Med Surg 21(2):61, 2003.
55. Choy DS: Clinical experience and results with 389 PLDD procedures with the Nd:YAG laser,1986 to 1995. J Clin Laser Med Surg 13(3):209, 1995.
56. Epstein NE: Laser-assisted diskectomy performed by an internist resulting in cauda equina syndrome. J Spinal Disord 12(1):77, 1999.
57. Casper GD: Case report: Complex regional pain syndrome type 2 (causalgia) after automated laser discectomy. Spine 23(4):508, 1998.
58. Farrar MJ, Walker A, Cowling P: Possible *Salmonella* osteomyelitis of spine following laser disc decompression. Eur Spine J 7(6):509, 1998.
59. Naim-ur-Rahman N, Khan FA, Jamjoom A, Jamjoom ZA: Lumbar discitis complicating percutaneous laser disc decomposition: Case report and review of literature. J Pak Med Assoc 46(3):62-4, 1996.
60. Ahlgren BD, Vasavada A, Brower RS, et al: Annular incision technique on the strength and multidirectional flexibility of the healing intervertebral disc. Spine 19(8):948, 1994.
61. Benneker LM, Heini PF, Alini M, et al: 2004 Young Investigator Award Winner: Vertebral endplate marrow contact channel occlusions and intervertebral disc degeneration. Spine 30(2):167, 2005.
62. Adams MA, Freeman BJ, Morrison HP, et al: Mechanical initiation of intervertebral disc degeneration. Spine 25(13):1625, 2000.
63. Cvitanic OA, Schimandle J, Casper GD, Tirman PF: Subchondral marrow changes after laser diskectomy in the lumbar spine: MR imaging findings and clinical correlation. AJR Am J Roentgenol 174(5):1363; 175(6):1748, 2000.
64. Tonami H, Kuginuki M, Kuginuki Y, et al: MR imaging of subchondral osteonecrosis of the vertebral body after percutaneous laser diskectomy. AJR Am J Roentgenol 173(5):1383, 1999.
65. Turgut M, Sargin H, Onol B, Acikgoz B: Changes in end-plate vascularity after Nd:YAG laser application to the guinea pig intervertebral disc. Acta Neurochir (Wien) 140(8):819, 1998.
66. Nerubay J, Caspi I, Levinkopf M, et al: Percutaneous laser nucleolysis of the intervertebral lumbar disc. An experimental study. J Clin Orthop 337:42, 1997.
67. Hoogland T: Presented at the AAMISMS Conference, Las Vegas, Nev, 2002.

chapter 174

Percutaneous Cordotomy

Steven Rosen

Percutaneous cordotomy is an extraordinary technique useful primarily for cancer pain management. A radiofrequency lesion is made in the anterolateral quadrant of the spinal cord to interrupt pain transmission through the spinothalamic fibers. Good to excellent results generally are achieved in almost 90% of patients, with minimal morbidity. The use of percutaneous cordotomy has declined for two reasons. First, knowledge and skill in the use of systemic and spinal narcotics are increasing. Narcotics are least effective, however, in patients with neuropathic or incident pain. Cordotomy offers such patients dramatic, sustained relief. Second, skilled practitioners are few. The technique must be performed by a practitioner skilled in percutaneous interventional work. The operator must be comfortable with the use of fluoroscopy and radiofrequency lesioning. It is hoped that, as interventional pain management is popularized and the number of skilled practitioners increases, percutaneous cordotomy will become a standard technique in comprehensive cancer care. When used in such a manner, percutaneous cordotomy is a gratifying procedure that helps cancer patients live out their lives pain-free and with as much dignity as possible.

HISTORICAL CONSIDERATIONS

The development of cordotomy mirrors progress in medicine. *Cordotomy* refers to creating a lesion in the spinothalamic tracts by a surgical scalpel or a radiofrequency generator. The first surgical cordotomy was reported by Spiller and Martin[1] in 1912. It had been noted that patients with pathologic lesions in the anterolateral quadrants of the spinal cord developed contralateral loss of pain and temperature discrimination, yet retained the sensation of light touch. Spiller and Martin[1] performed cordotomy in the midthoracic spine to relieve lower limb pain. Only high cervical cordotomy could relieve pain from below the middle cervical segments, however.[2,3] Despite gratifying pain relief, considerable morbidity was associated with high cervical cordotomy.[4] This morbidity was attributed to the surgical resection itself and to interference with automatic respiratory function. Patients would breathe on command, but developed sleep apnea. The complication was especially common after bilateral high cervical lesions. Severinghaus and Mitchell[5] called this complication *Ondine's curse,* a reference to the water nymph Ondine, who, having been jilted by her husband, took away his automatic respiratory functions so that he had to remember to breathe. When he fell asleep, he died. The mortality rate from high cervical cordotomy was cited as 4% to 25%.[6,7]

The first percutaneous cordotomies were described by Millan and colleagues[6] in 1963, who placed a radioisotope-tipped probe near the anterolateral quadrant of the cord at C1-2. The lesions were inconsistent, however, and radioisotope-tipped needles were not generally available. In 1965, Millan and associates[8] described percutaneous cordotomy using direct current. Lesions took 10 to 30 minutes to take effect as compared with 2 to 3 months after radioisotope-tipped needles were removed. Percutaneous radiofrequency cordotomy was first described by Rosomoff and associates[9] in 1965. With minor modifications, theirs is the technique used today. Lesions were reproducible and could be performed in less than 1 minute. The technique was relatively simple and allowed patients who might not have been acceptable surgical risks for the more extensive open operation to enjoy pain relief.

It was hoped that respiratory mortality would be less with the percutaneous approach, but this turned out not to be the case. To minimize the risk of respiratory trespass, Lin and coworkers[10,11] developed the anterior approach. Needles were placed through either the C5-6 or the C6-7 disk and then into the anterolateral quadrant of the cord, which is below the exit of the respiratory fibers with the phrenic nerve. It was difficult to realign poorly positioned needles embedded in disk material, however, and today the anterior approach is rarely used. Crue and associates[12] and Hitchcock[13] developed a posterior approach. The probe was placed through the posterior columns and into the final position in the anterolateral quadrant. The high lateral cervical approach at C1-2 is relatively simple to perform, is easy to conceptualize, and has withstood the test of time.

Since 1965, modifications have been directed toward improving target visualization. For stereotactic surgery, the target must be identified radiologically and physiologically. After the target has been identified, it must be destroyed in a precise and reproducible manner.

In percutaneous cordotomy, the target is the anterolateral quadrant of the spinal cord. The dentate ligament separates the anterior from the posterior quadrant. Identification of the dentate ligament greatly aids electrode placement. Millan and colleagues[6] and Rosomoff and associates[9] simply injected air to outline the anterior surface of the cord. The electrode was placed just below the anterior surface, and incremental lesions were made until either contralateral analgesia was obtained or motor weakness occurred. Onofrio[14] used an emulsion of iophendylate (Pantopaque) in air to outline the anterior surface of the cord and the dentate ligament. This step significantly reduced the time needed to search for the anterolateral quadrant. CT-guided placement of electrodes has been described by Kanpolat and coworkers.[15,16] More precise lesioning may decrease postoperative complications by increasing the selectivity of the procedure. Gildenberg and coworkers[17] emphasized impedance monitoring to identify penetration of the spinal cord. Physiologic identification of the spinothalamic fibers was emphasized by Taren and associates.[18] Different areas of the spinal cord exhibit characteristic responses to motor and sensory stimulation.[19,20] Evoked potentials were recorded from the anterolateral quadrant in 1983 by Campbell and Lipton.[21] Impedance monitoring to detect the subarachnoid space also has been described.[22]

After the target is identified, it must be destroyed in a precise and reproducible manner. Principles of radiofrequency lesioning have been reviewed by Cosman and colleagues.[23] A comprehensive review of radiofrequency techniques is now available.[24] A significant development has been the thermocoupled electrode.[25] Cordotomy lesions had been performed by gradually increasing the current and lesioning time, while carefully observing for pain relief and monitoring for neurologic deficits. The thermocoupled electrode allows direct temperature monitoring to guide lesion making. The tissue temperature, not the current, causes neural destruction, and it now could be precisely controlled. The active tip of the Levin thermocoupled electrode was 2 mm in length and 0.5 mm in diameter, ensuring easy placement through a 20-gauge spinal needle. The resulting 4-mm oval-shaped lesion is ideal to denervate the anterolateral quadrant of the cord adequately.

More recent efforts have been devoted to defining the role of percutaneous cordotomy in comprehensive pain care. Tasker and associates[26] described the role of cordotomy in patients with noncancer pain of spinal cord origin. Ischia and associates[27-30] published several excellent articles detailing the risks and benefits of percutaneous cordotomy in cancer patients. They described results of cordotomy for pain of vertebral body lesions[27] and pain of Pancoast tumor and upper thoracic lesions.[28] These investigators also reported on the complementary roles of cordotomy and subarachnoid neurolysis in patients with pelvic malignancy.[29] Ischia and associates[30] discussed the benefits and the respiratory risks involved in bilateral lesioning.

Histologic correlation with clinical results after cordotomy has been used to define the functional neuroanatomy of the spine. Nathan and Smith[31,32] and Lahuerta and coworkers[33] used histologic evidence to identify respiratory pathways in the spinal cord. In a similar manner, the location of the sympathetic fibers[34] and the pathways involved in voiding and defecation[35] have been ascertained. Histologic evidence has shown that lesions 5 mm deep to the surface that destroy about 20% of the hemicord give optimal analgesia.[36] A fascinating phenomenon is the development of reference of sensation after cordotomy.[37] Mirror-image pain may develop, or noxious sensations may be referred to the side of the body opposite to the cordotomy target. New subsidiary pain pathways have been postulated.[38] This observation has led to new theories about the roles of inhibitory pain pathways. Further research will continue to expand knowledge of the intricacy of nerve transmission in humans.

INDICATIONS AND CONTRAINDICATIONS

Percutaneous cervical cordotomy is best used for unilateral cancer pain below the shoulder in patients with life expectancy less than 1 year. A lesion is created in the spinothalamic tract. Complications develop from extension of the lesion to adjoining tracts or to development of a zone of edema that temporarily interferes with transmission by adjacent fibers. This section reviews the indications and contraindications to percutaneous cordotomy and published results.

It cannot be emphasized enough that pain-relieving procedures are part of comprehensive cancer care and cannot be viewed in isolation. Cancer is a complex, multifactorial disease, and it is unlikely that one procedure, no matter how well performed, would result in sustained lifelong pain relief. A percutaneous cordotomy is just one part of a comprehensive treatment plan that includes surgery, radiation therapy, medications, pain-relieving procedures, and psychological support. Review of the literature is disappointing because few attempts have been made to define indications or to stratify results according to location of disease and type of pain. As spinal narcotic techniques have evolved, the role of cordotomy has decreased, but we can hope that it soon will be better defined.

From January 1990 to December 1998, I performed 54 percutaneous cordotomies. The patients all had experienced failure of aggressive medical pain therapy. During the same interval, 58 subarachnoid pumps and 31 permanently tunneled epidural catheters were implanted in cancer patients. Depending on the study, 30% of cancer patients are candidates for pain-relieving procedures or surgeries. Some of these patients can benefit from invasive but opioid-sparing techniques, such as percutaneous cordotomy. More than 100 celiac ablations, hypogastric ablations, and spinal neurolyses were performed.

Indications

As mentioned, the best indication for cordotomy is unilateral cancer pain below the shoulder. Percutaneous cordotomy generally is performed at C1-2. At this level, the spinothalamic tract is in the anterolateral quadrant of the cord. Pain fibers enter the cord through the dorsal horn and may ascend several levels before crossing over and taking their final position in the spinothalamic tract. A lesion at C1-2 is almost guaranteed to produce analgesia below C4 or C5, the levels that innervate the shoulder. An open surgical cordotomy at T1-2 does not produce analgesia in the upper extremity, but does produce analgesia in the lower chest, abdomen, and lower extremity. It does not affect respiratory fibers because they already have exited the spinal cord via the phrenic nerve. As will become clearer later, this point is important in the consideration of bilateral lesioning.

A percutaneous cordotomy is especially useful for neuropathic or incident pain. Although neuropathic pain exhibits some narcotic responsiveness,[39] brachial or sacral plexopathy generally responds poorly to medical pain therapy. Better responses can be obtained with spinal narcotic techniques, especially when local anesthetics or clonidine or both[40-43] are added. Even with these measures, however, pain relief may be unsatisfactory or barely acceptable. Patients with brachial plexopathy from Pancoast tumor or sacral plexopathy from pelvic malignant disease are excellent candidates for cordotomy.

Incident pain is when the patient is comfortable at rest, but develops severe pain with weight bearing. Examples are pelvic, hip, femur, and humeral lesions or fractures. Incident pain also may arise from a vertebral body fracture. If affected patients are not candidates for surgical stabilization, they may be good candidates for cordotomy. Patients with incident pain who are comfortable while standing with analgesics invariably are oversedated at rest. Incident pain is extraordinarily difficult to treat with medical management. It is remarkable to see a patient with a hip fracture walk pain-free after a cordotomy.

The ideal indications for cordotomy are incident pain and neuropathic pain of the lower extremity. In my series, 26 of 54 patients had incident pain, and another 15 had neuropathic pain of the lower extremity. Six patients underwent cordotomy for upper extremity pain secondary to Pancoast tumor. Seven had cordotomies for cancer-related chest wall pain. Patients with incident pain and lower extremity plexopathies are the most difficult to treat with medical or procedural interventions and are excellent candidates for percutaneous cordotomy.

Neuropathic pain must be distinguished from deafferentation pain, which would not be relieved by cordotomy. Examples of deafferentation pain are postherpetic neuralgia, thalamic pain, and many cases of pain secondary to spinal cord lesions or reflex sympathetic dystrophy. The pain usually is described as dysesthetic or causalgic. Patients complain of burning pain and show hyperpathia and allodynia. Deafferentation pain is related to the loss of afferent sensory input and usually occurs in the setting of at least partial sensory loss in the affected distribution. In a cancer patient, pain would be caused not by tumor pressing on a nerve, but from actual damage to the nerve itself. Deafferentation pain is uncommon in terminal cancer patients, but considerably more common in patients with noncancer, or "benign," pain. Deafferentation pain accounts for the relatively poor results of cordotomy in noncancer patients and is probably responsible for most postcordotomy dysesthesias.

Tasker and associates[26] elucidated the role of percutaneous cordotomy in patients with spinal cord lesions. Destructive surgery, predominantly cordotomy, was most effective in patients with intermittent or evoked pain. Cordotomy was marginally effective in patients with steady pain, which was usually causalgic or dysesthetic. The point is that quality and origin of pain are crucial in determining whether cordotomy is indicated, especially in a patient with noncancer pain.

The benefit of cordotomy tends to decrease with time. Although nerve regeneration has not been shown, cordotomies can wear off over time. Pain can recur years later, and lesioning sometimes can be repeated, with renewed long-term benefit.[44,45] In 1974, Rosomoff[46] reported on 1279 cordotomies performed in 789 patients. Immediately after cordotomy, more than 90% of patients were pain-free. By the end of 1 year, almost 40% of patients no longer had absolute pain relief. Sixteen percent of patients developed postcordotomy dysesthesia of varying degrees. Nagaro and colleagues[47] classified pain recurrence as deafferentation pain or pain secondary to recovery of nerve function. Deafferentation could be secondary to increasing tumor-related peripheral nerve injury or destruction of second-order neurons by the cordotomy. Because of pain recurrence and the development of postcordotomy dysesthesias, cordotomies are not generally recommended for patients whose life expectancy is longer than 1 year. The procedure is mostly limited to terminal cancer patients. As the indications for the technique become better defined, it is expected that more longer term survivors and noncancer patients will be candidates for this powerful pain-relieving technique. At this time, patients with relatively long life expectancy should be preferentially considered for neuroaugmentation or a spinal narcotic infusion.

Because cancer is a systemic disease, unmasking of contralateral pain after a successful cordotomy is common. Most cancer pain can be treated satisfactorily with medications, and it is likely that newly unmasked pain would be relieved with analgesics alone and would be easier to treat than the pain relieved by the cordotomy. Macaluso and colleagues[48] reported the results of cordotomies in 20 patients with lumbosacral, pelvic, and lower extremity pain. Contralateral pain was unmasked in 18 patients and responded to opioids in 15, to intrathecal phenol in 1, and to contralateral cordotomy in 2. In my practice, contralateral pain was unmasked postoperatively in 5 patients, and 30 of 54 patients developed contralateral pain before death; 27 of these patients were treated with medical management. Two patients required bilateral cordotomies, and one required local anesthetic and narcotic infusion through a tunneled epidural catheter.

Contraindications

The major contraindication to cordotomy is preexisting respiratory dysfunction; this condition is discussed more fully in the section on complications. In short, the automatic respiratory fibers course through the reticulospinal tract. The reticulospinal tract is adjacent to the spinothalamic tract. Reticulospinal fibers may mingle with fibers of the spinothalamic tract. It is easy to see how lesions in the spinothalamic tract could interfere with automatic respiratory function. Voluntary respiratory control fibers are in the corticospinal tract located in the posterior quadrant of the cord and so are unlikely to be affected by a percutaneous cordotomy. Many respiratory fibers exit the cord via the phrenic nerve, which contains fibers from C3, C4, and C5. A C1-2 cordotomy can cause ipsilateral respiratory dysfunction along with contralateral pain relief. Cordotomy decreases the forced expiratory volume (FEV_1) by an average of 20%,[49] but it is impossible to predict beforehand who will and who will not be affected.

When does respiratory function become a concern? A patient with a lung tumor and ipsilateral pain may depend on the function of the contralateral lung to stay alive. This would be the side on which respiratory function is affected by the contralateral cordotomy. What parameters can be used to predict the safety of the procedural intervention? At this time, no good guidelines are available. I obtain pulmonary function tests and a sniff test to check diaphragm function. An estimate also is made of the relative pulmonary function of each lung. FEV_1 greater than 1.2 L would allow a small margin of safety, even after a 20% decrease. As a rough guideline, a patient who is able to lie supine without difficulty is probably a good candidate for a cordotomy. This is a practical screening test because patients who could not perform this maneuver in any case would not be able to cooperate sufficiently during the procedure itself to ensure a successful outcome.

Respiratory function is an even more serious issue when bilateral cordotomy is contemplated. Bilateral procedures should be staged at least several weeks apart to allow cord edema from the first lesion to dissipate. Bilateral lesions of the reticulospinal tract have disastrous consequences. As I describe in the discussion of clinical anatomy in the next section, the spinothalamic fibers from the cervical segments are closest to the reticulospinal fibers. If the first cordotomy produces cervical analgesia, it is likely that the reticulospinal fibers were damaged. The patient is at increased risk from contralateral cordotomy. If the second cordotomy also damages the automatic respiratory fibers, the patient is likely to develop sleep apnea syndrome and possibly respiratory death.

In a patient considered for bilateral cordotomy, when the first cordotomy produces a high level of cervical analgesia, the surgeon has three options. Tasker[50] suggested tailoring the lesion. The spinothalamic fibers serving the lumbar dermatomes are relatively far from the reticulospinal tract. Stimulation preferentially should be sought from the lumbar segments so that the resulting lesion would be less likely to include the automatic respiratory fibers. A second option is cordotomy at or below C6. The percutaneous anterior approach is theoretically possible, but in practice difficult to perform. If a contralateral cordotomy is necessary, the best option would be an open surgical procedure in the lower cervical or upper thoracic region. This procedure would not be appropriate for a patient who needs bilateral analgesia extending to the cervical dermatomes.

At this time, there are two indications for open surgical cordotomy. The first is the situation just described. The second is unavailability of the expertise or equipment needed to perform percutaneous cordotomy. If bilateral cervical analgesia is needed, a spinal narcotic technique would be more appropriate.

There is risk of urinary retention and sexual dysfunction after unilateral cordotomy, and that risk increases significantly with bilateral lesioning. Although the risks and benefits of cordotomy should be discussed in detail, it is unlikely that the need for permanent catheterization or risk of sexual dysfunction would contraindicate the procedure in a terminally ill patient with severe pain that is unresponsive to conventional pain therapy.

RESULTS

Since the 1990s, much work has been devoted to defining the role of cordotomy in comprehensive cancer pain. The most important work has been published by Ischia's group.[28] They analyzed the results of unilateral percutaneous cervical cordotomies in patients with Pancoast tumor or thoracic malignant pain. Of patients, 92% obtained excellent results, as evidenced by analgesia to pinprick in the middle cervical dermatomes. As a result of the cordotomy alone, 44% of patients with Pancoast syndrome were pain-free until death. Only 22% of patients with thoracic pain were pain-free as a result of the cordotomy alone, owing to a 70% incidence of mirror pain in this group (mirror pain is discussed fully in the section on pitfalls). Cordotomy plus aggressive medical pain therapy afforded complete pain control in 75% of patients with Pancoast syndrome and in 86% of patients with thoracic pain. Nagaro and associates[51] and Orlandini[52] compared percutaneous cordotomy with subarachnoid phenol in patients with chest pain secondary to cancer. Subarachnoid phenol gave excellent but short-term relief. Cordotomy resulted in excellent long-term relief at the expense of generalized weakness, mirror pain, and temporary hemiparesis.

Ischia and associates[27] studied the role of unilateral cordotomy in the treatment of patients with vertebral metastatic lesions. The pain was either unilateral or bilateral. Seventy-one percent of patients obtained substantial benefit from the combination of cordotomy and appropriately used analgesics. These investigators also compared the roles of cordotomy and subarachnoid neurolytic block in patients with pelvic cancer.[29] The issue is important because the sacral segments tend to be missed by cordotomy, either because they are farthest from the lesion or because of the higher incidence of deafferentation pain in patients with rectal lesions. Ischia and associates[29] obtained excellent relief using cordotomy for predominantly unilateral pain, subarachnoid phenol for perineal pain, and pharmacologic therapy in all cases.

Ischia's group also reported the results of bilateral percutaneous cordotomies.[31] The electrode was positioned just anterior to the dentate ligament so that the lesion was more likely to affect the lumbar segments and less likely to damage the reticulospinal tract. Bilateral lesions were created in one session. There were no respiratory deaths in the 36 patients treated, 60% of whom substantially benefited from the procedure. Sanders and Zuurmond[53] reported on patients after unilateral and then staged bilateral cordotomies. Excellent relief was noted for the unilateral procedure. Bilateral lesioning gave only 50% total pain relief at the expense of a high incidence of urinary retention and mirror-image pain.

Other authors have reported series of cancer pain patients who have undergone cordotomy. Meglio and Cioni[54] performed 53 cordotomies; excellent surgical results were noted in 63% of patients 15 weeks postoperatively. Eleven of these patients had Pancoast syndrome, and 31 had lower extremity pain secondary to pelvic or abdominal cancer. Lahuerta and colleagues[55] reported on 100 cordotomies, 95% of which were performed in cancer patients. Complete pain relief was obtained in 64% of patients, and partial relief was obtained in 23%. Only one of the five patients with nonmalignant pain obtained complete relief via cordotomy. Macaluso and colleagues[48] performed 20 cordotomies for lumbosacral, pelvic, and lower extremity pain of malignant origin. Their patients' opioid requirements were reduced by 80% at 4 weeks; the opioid reduction generally lasted 12 weeks. Amano and coworkers[56] described the results of 281 cordotomies. Unilateral cordotomy gave good or excellent results in 82% of patients. The rate was 95% for bilateral lesions. Jackson and colleagues[57] described results in patients with mesothelioma after the procedure; 83% were able to decrease opioid dosage by at least half.

White and Sweet[58] compared the results of large series of open and percutaneous cordotomies in a 1979 study and found that results with the two were comparable. Eighty-five percent of patients obtained good initial analgesia after open or percutaneous procedures. Mortality and morbidity rates were lower, however, with the percutaneous technique (see section on complications).

Summary

Percutaneous cordotomy is an excellent technique for cancer pain management. The best indication is unilateral pain below the shoulder in a patient with a life expectancy of less than 1 year. The major contraindication to a percutaneous cordotomy is preexisting respiratory dysfunction on the side opposite the one to be rendered analgesic. Because cancer is a systemic disease, it is unlikely that cordotomy alone would ensure complete pain relief. The rate of good to excellent results of cordotomy should approach 90% when the procedure is combined with aggressive pharmacologic and other appropriate procedural therapies.

CLINICALLY RELEVANT ANATOMY

During percutaneous cordotomy, a lesion is created in the spinothalamic tract. This tract is located in the anterolateral quadrant of the spinal cord. Results and side effects depend on the size and location of the lesion. Thorough knowledge of the applied anatomy is essential to guide electrode placement and radiofrequency lesioning. The clinically relevant anatomy at C1-2 is described here because virtually all procedures are performed at this level.

The lateral approach to C1-2 is optimal. Because of anterior migration of the interarticular facets, there are no bony obstacles to the anterolateral quadrant. The C1-2 level has the largest intervertebral opening. Also, vertebral artery injury is unlikely there because the vertebral artery generally lies well anterior to the cord. The artery enters the dura mater at the atlanto-occipital space, so a lateral approach would be riskier at C0-1. Variations in the course of the vertebral artery have been documented by Katoh and associates.[59] The vertebral artery is anterior to the cord in 95% of cases at C1-2. In 5% of cases, however, the artery passes over the middle to the posterior third of the cord. Vertebral artery injury is possible.

The other vascular structure of interest is the anterior spinal artery (Fig. 174–1), which is generally located in the anterior commissure. Perese and Fracasso[60] report almost 50% incidence of bilateral anterior spinal arteries in the cervical region. A more laterally placed anterior spinal artery could be affected by the radiofrequency lesion, and thrombosis with cord infarction is theoretically a complication.

In addition to the vascular structures, the C2 nerve root must be considered. It exits the spinal canal at C1-2 and continues as the greater occipital nerve. There is a high likelihood that the cordotomy needle could impinge on the C2 nerve root, and C2 paresthesias could occur during the performance of percutaneous cordotomy. Greater occipital nerve headaches can last 1 week postoperatively. The last reason to perform cordotomy at C1-2 already has been mentioned. Because of variable crossover of spinothalamic fibers, only high lateral cordotomies reliably produce analgesia up to C5 so that pain from brachial plexopathies may be relieved.

Figure 174–2 shows a cross section of the spinal cord at C1-2. Correlation of histologic staining after open and percutaneous lesions with the resulting sensory and motor deficits has allowed functional identification of spinal cord tracts.

The spinothalamic tract contains ascending fibers that transmit pain and temperature sensation. These neurons ascend from the dorsal root ganglion and cross through the anterior commissure to the contralateral anterolateral

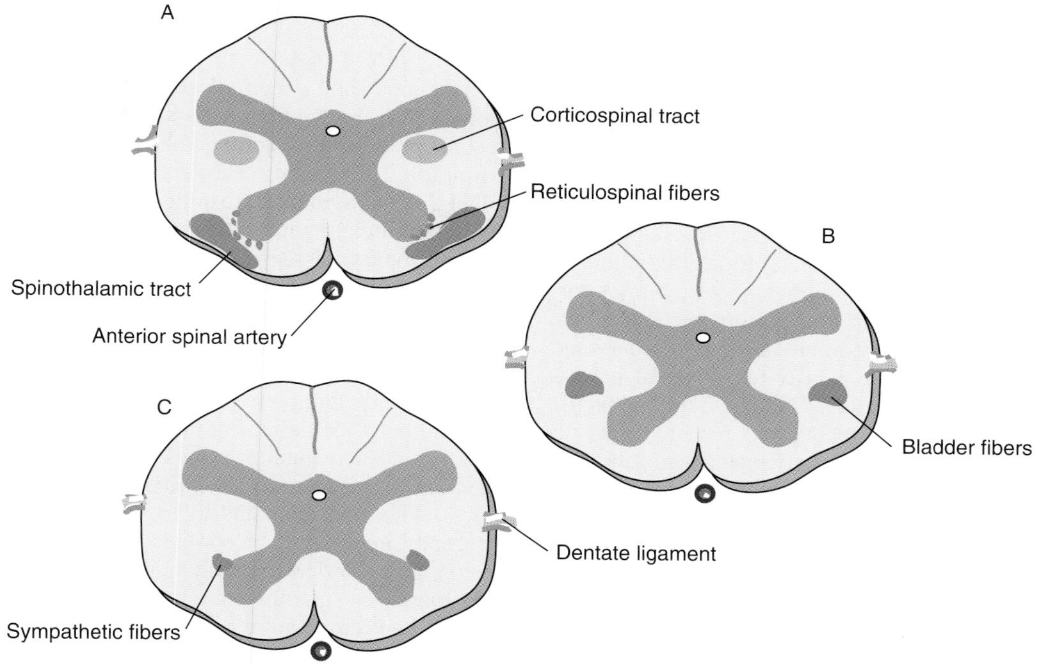

FIGURE 174–1 ■ **A-C,** Axial section of the spinal cord at C1-2 shows the anterior spinal artery, dentate ligament, and anterolateral quadrant.

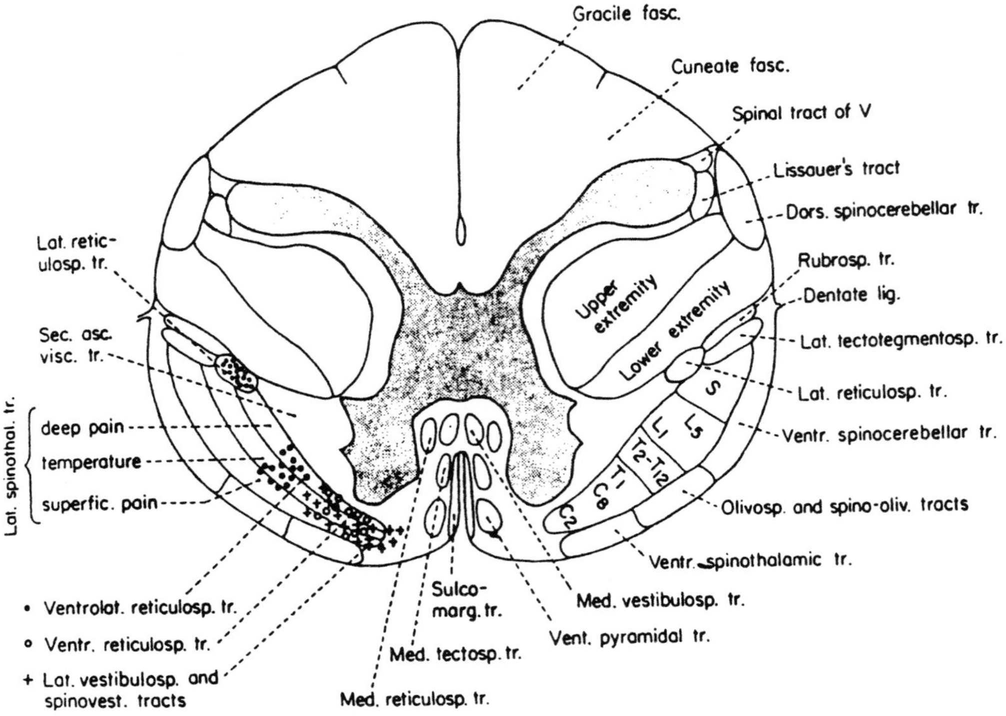

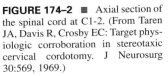

FIGURE 174–2 ■ Axial section of the spinal cord at C1-2. (From Taren JA, Davis R, Crosby EC: Target physiologic corroboration in stereotaxic cervical cordotomy. J Neurosurg 30:569, 1969.)

quadrant. The crossover[61] may be delayed by several segments so that only a high cervical lesion reliably gives pain relief below C5. These neurons terminate at various levels in the brain. That spinothalamic fibers terminate in the nucleus ventralis posterolateralis of the thalamus was shown by dissection in monkeys.[62] In humans, the same anatomic configuration was shown by DiPiero and colleagues[63] using positron emission tomography. These researchers also found that patients with cancer pain had decreased blood flow to the contralateral thalamus that normalized after percutaneous cordotomy.

The spinothalamic tracts are organized in a somatotropic manner (see Fig. 174–2). Fibers transmitting impulses from cervical levels are more anterior, and fibers from the lumbar and sacral segment are more posterior. This arrangement has clinical implications, which are discussed later. Some authors stratify the spinothalamic fibers; the more superficial fibers transmit superficial pain, and deeper fibers transmit temperature and deep pain.[18] The spinothalamic tract relays pain and temperature from the periphery to the contralateral thalamus. Contralateral stimulation to deep pinprick is not felt after cordotomy in most cases.[64] Similarly, deep somatic sensations, such as pressure, are reduced by anterolateral cordotomy and are best correlated with cancer pain relief. Visceral pain is relieved by anterolateral cordotomy.[65] Nathan[66] studied tactile sensitivity in postcordotomy patients and reported the following results: Senses of position, movement, and vibration were normal after cordotomy; graphesthesia was unaltered; light touch was unaffected; itching sensations were removed by cordotomy, but tickle sensation was unaffected. White and Sweet[65] wrote that patients who have undergone cordotomy "will be able to detect a mosquito when he alights, although they will not be able to feel him bite nor be annoyed by the subsequent itch." Temperature discrimination is generally lost after cordotomy, so patients must learn to pick up hot or cold objects with the hand in which temperature discrimination is intact. Friehs and colleagues[67] reported that pain and temperature may be conducted by adjacent but separate pathways. They noted different dermatomal levels for pain as opposed to temperature sensations after cordotomy. Usually pain discrimination and temperature discrimination are lost. White and Sweet[65] wrote, "The patient walking barefoot in the dark can tell whether he is walking on a stone or wooden floor, on a carpet or on linoleum. He must only beware that he does not step on a tack and in particular that he does not burn himself."

Figure 174–3 shows the respiratory pathways as outlined by Hitchcock and Leece.[68] Nathan[31] first worked out the location of the descending respiratory tracts. He realized that lesions of the anterolateral quadrant interfered with automatic respiration, but lesions of the corticospinal tract had no effect. Fibers of the automatic respiratory tract have been found to be intermingled with reticulospinal fibers.[33] There is also somatotropic division of fibers: Fibers controlling automatic diaphragmatic function are more anterior, and fibers controlling intercostal and abdominal musculature are more posterior. The voluntary respiratory fibers are in the corticospinal tract. The concept of at least two distinctive respiratory tracts, one automatic and one voluntary, explains why patients have died in their sleep after high bilateral cervical cordotomy.

The corticospinal tract lies posterior to the dentate ligament. It is posterior to the spinothalamic and spinoreticular fibers. This tract contains fibers involving motor control. It descends uncrossed, in contrast to spinothalamic fibers. A lesion in the corticospinal tract produces ipsilateral weakness; a lesion in the spinothalamic tract results in contralateral loss of pain and temperature discrimination.

The concept of somatotropy in the reticulospinal and spinothalamic tracts explains why high cervical lesions are

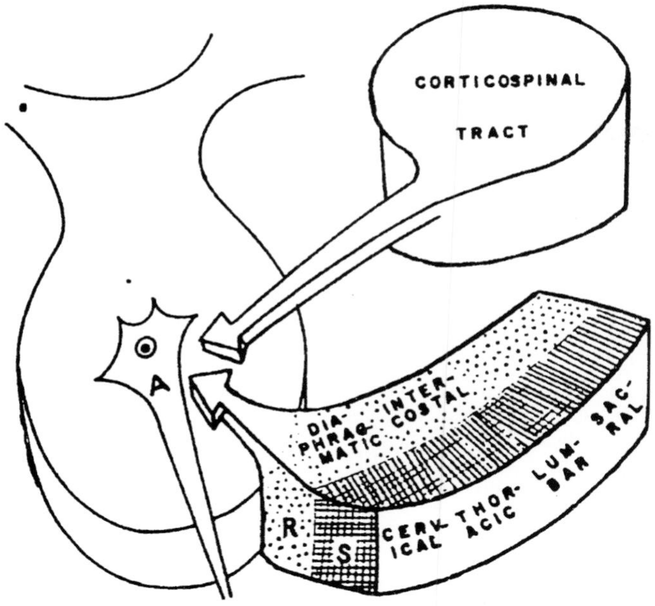

FIGURE 174–3 ■ Somatotropic division of spinothalamic (S) and reticulospinal (R) tracts. A, axon. (From Hitchcock E, Leece B: Somatic representation of the respiratory pathways in the cervical cord of man. J Neurosurg 27:320, 1967.)

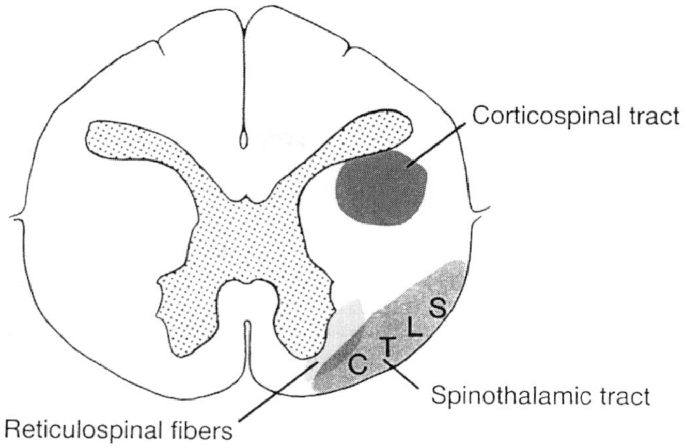

FIGURE 174–4 ■ Interrelationship of spinothalamic and reticulospinal fibers. (From Waldman SD: Interventional Pain Management, 2nd ed. Philadelphia, WB Saunders, 2001, p 688.)

more likely to result in respiratory dysfunction. The spinoreticular fibers serving automatic diaphragmatic respirations are adjacent to, and in many cases intertwined with, the spinothalamic fibers that transmit pain and temperature sensation from the cervical segments (Fig. 174–4). Lesions involving cervical pain transmission are likely also to result in ipsilateral automatic respiratory dysfunction. This condition is of minimal importance when contralateral lung function is acceptable. Bilateral lesions are more dangerous. This concept also explains why a lesion centered in the lumbar or sacral pain fibers would be more likely to result in ipsilateral paresis secondary to cord edema affecting the nearby corticospinal tract.

The location of sympathetic preganglionic fibers has been described by Nathan and Smith.[34] These fibers lie close to the posterior portion of the anterior horn (Fig. 174–5). Transient Horner syndrome develops after many percutaneous cordotomies. Unilateral cordotomies do not upset vasomotor function, however, because crossing and mixing of sympathetic fibers probably starts no higher than T1.

Nathan and Smith[36] also worked out the location of pathways implicated in voiding and defecation. These fibers are situated lateral to the lateral horn of the gray matter (Fig. 174–6). Bilateral damage to these fibers leads to impairment of these functions. Transient impairment of bladder function can occur after percutaneous cordotomy. Such impairment is more likely in patients with preexisting disease or with bilateral lesions.

The dentate ligament is the external landmark that separates the anterior from the posterior tract (Fig. 174–7). This is an important landmark for surgical and percutaneous cordotomies, and much effort has been devoted to visualizing it during the procedure.[14,69,70] The spinothalamic tract is anterior to the dentate ligament, whereas the corticospinal tract lies

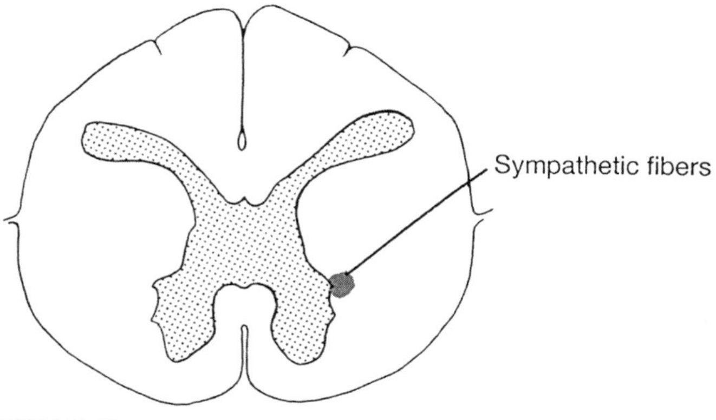

FIGURE 174–5 ■ Location of sympathetic fibers. (From Waldman SD: Interventional Pain Management, 2nd ed. Philadelphia, WB Saunders, 2001, p 688.)

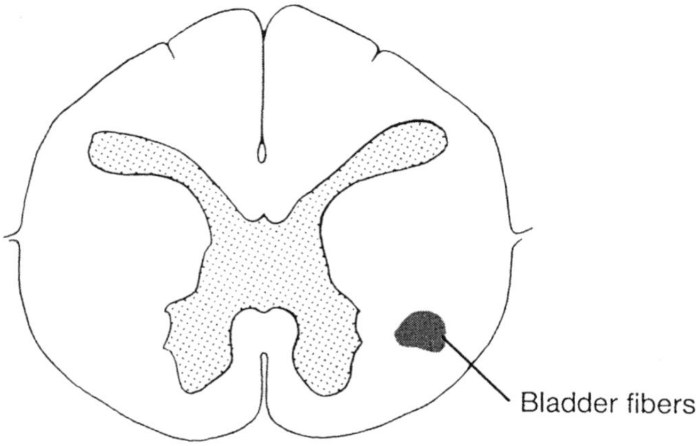

FIGURE 174–6 ■ Location of fibers involved in micturition. (From Waldman SD: Interventional Pain Management, 2nd ed. Philadelphia, WB Saunders, 2001, p 688.)

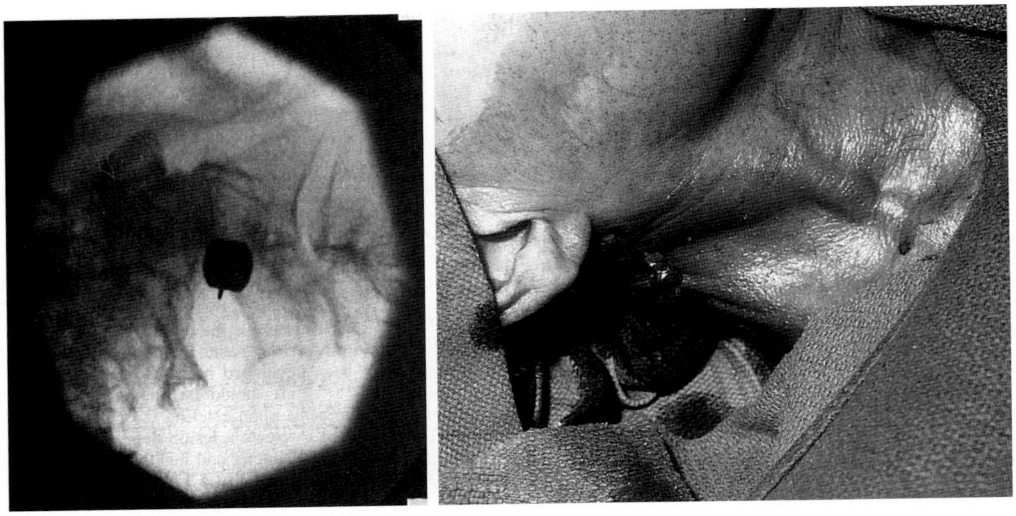

A B

FIGURE 174–7 ■ **A,** Fluoroscopic view of initial needle placement into subarachnoid space. **B,** Photograph of needle shown in **A.** (From Waldman SD: Interventional Pain Management, 2nd ed. Philadelphia, WB Saunders, 2001, p 689.)

posterior. As Sweet[71] pointed out, however, the position of the dentate ligament varies, so before a lesion can be safely made, physiologic corroboration is needed to confirm that the electrode is actually in the spinothalamic tract.

Summary

Percutaneous cordotomy is an elegant demonstration of the correlation between neuroanatomy and clinical outcome. A lesion is made in the spinothalamic tract. Pain and temperature discrimination are interrupted on the contralateral side. This tract is somatotropically organized. Fibers from the cervical region are interrelated with fibers in the reticulospinal tract that serve automatic diaphragm functions. Fibers that transmit lumbar information are adjacent to the corticospinal tract. Fibers that transmit sympathetic and bladder function also are in the anterolateral quadrant of the cord. Pain relief and side effects correlate with the size and location of the lesion.

CLINICAL PEARLS AND TRICKS OF THE TRADE

The percutaneous cordotomy is described next. With rare exceptions, percutaneous cordotomy should be performed with the patient minimally sedated. The physician should conduct a thorough physical examination beforehand so that changes during and after the cordotomy may be appreciated. Millan[72] emphasized that considerable time should be invested in the preoperative visit. As in all radiofrequency procedures, patient cooperation is essential. Overdependence on anesthetic drugs is no substitute for adequate patient preparation.

Preoperative Preparation

Certain points must be emphasized during the preoperative interview. Patients should understand that the procedure can take 1 hour, and that they will have to remain supine during the procedure. As the spinal needle is inserted, the C2 nerve root can be irritated, resulting in occipital and scalp pain until the local anesthetic takes effect. Needle puncture of the dura can be uncomfortable and difficult to anesthetize. Electrical stimulation and radiofrequency lesioning generally are tolerated well. Postoperatively, patients may develop a spinal headache. Greater occipital nerve headaches can last 1 week. Patients may need intermittent bladder catheterization, especially during the first several days. Ipsilateral paresis may develop, and the patient may need a walker, possibly for several weeks. Mirror pain develops in 10% of patients and is more common when the cordotomy is performed to relieve thoracic pain.

Over the longer term, patients lose temperature discrimination as they gain pain relief. They must be cautioned to pick up hot or cold objects first with the hand whose temperature discrimination is intact. Sexual stimulation and function may be decreased by the cordotomy. Patients must understand that, depending on the course of the disease, contralateral pain may develop, and that lifelong pain relief is unlikely.

If narcotic dosage can be reduced, and mental faculties improve, patients may begin to focus on issues of death and dying. Postoperative depression can occur, so appropriate support for the patient and family should be provided for before the pain-relieving procedure. The patient must have confidence that, no matter what the postoperative course, the pain management team will continue to optimize symptom control as long as necessary.

Operative Technique

Percutaneous cordotomy should be performed with intravenous sedation. The patient should be maximally sedated during insertion of the spinal needle from skin to the dura and during the lesioning. The patient must be alert during electrophysiologic testing. There are many variations of the operative technique, but they all follow the same general theme.[45,73,74] Different techniques have been developed to visualize the cord and the dentate ligament.[14,69,70] The impedance measurements on entering the cord and the amperage needed to create a lesion depend on several factors,[75] including the diameter and length of the active tip and the tissue conductivity. I use a Levin cordotomy electrode[25] with a Radionics (Burlington, MA) lesion generator. Other excellent electrode[22,76] and radiofrequency generators are available (Owl

Instruments, Willowdale, Ontario, Canada, and Stryker-Leibinger, Dallas, TX).

As in many precision percutaneous techniques, proper patient positioning is essential. The patient is supine with the neck slightly flexed to enlarge the C1-2 opening. The fluoroscope C-arm is positioned so that a true lateral view is obtained; this is essential to minimize errors from parallax and to identify best the proper radiologic targets. After the best image is visualized, the head is fixed in position. The technique is to reposition the needle continuously until the fixed target is identified.

After the patient is prepared, local anesthetic is infiltrated. It should not be injected too deep, lest the epidural or subarachnoid space inadvertently be anesthetized. A 20-gauge spinal needle is inserted toward the apex of the C1-2 space. Paresthesia generally is noted as the needle contracts the C2 nerve root. To anesthetize the nerve root, 1 mL of 2% lidocaine is sufficient. Because this is a large nerve, it takes several minutes for the anesthetic to become effective. The spinal needle is advanced to the epidural space and then through the dura and into the CSF (see Fig. 174–7). CSF flow can be slow, and the surgeon should not insert the needle too aggressively. This spinal needle should be inserted anterior to the dentate ligament so that the anterior border of the cord and the dentate ligament are outlined by falling contrast emulsion (see later). The depth at which the dura is punctured should be noted. If any doubt exists as to correct needle position, it may be checked with an anteroposterior projection, which should show the needle medial to the midfacet line and lateral to the odontoid.

At this point, contrast emulsion is prepared. It is used to outline the important landmarks—the anterior surface of the spinal cord, the dentate ligament, and the posterior dura. The spinothalamic tract is located between the anterior border of the dura and the dentate ligament. The best emulsion is a combination of oil-based contrast agent, such as iophendylate (Pantopaque) and air. Pantopaque is no longer available, however. Alternative techniques[69,70] may not outline the dentate ligament as effectively. An excellent emulsion consists of 3 mL of Ethiodol (ethiodized oil) mixed with 7 mL of preservative-free saline and 10 mL of air. Ethiodol is iodine based, so allergic reactions can occur. The emulsion is mixed vigorously for 3 minutes, excess air is evacuated, and 1 mL of the emulsion is injected through a syringe with an eccentric nipple located in the dependent position.

The contrast emulsion should outline the anterior border of the cord, the dentate ligament, and the posterior dura (Fig. 174–8). If it does not, the emulsion may have been

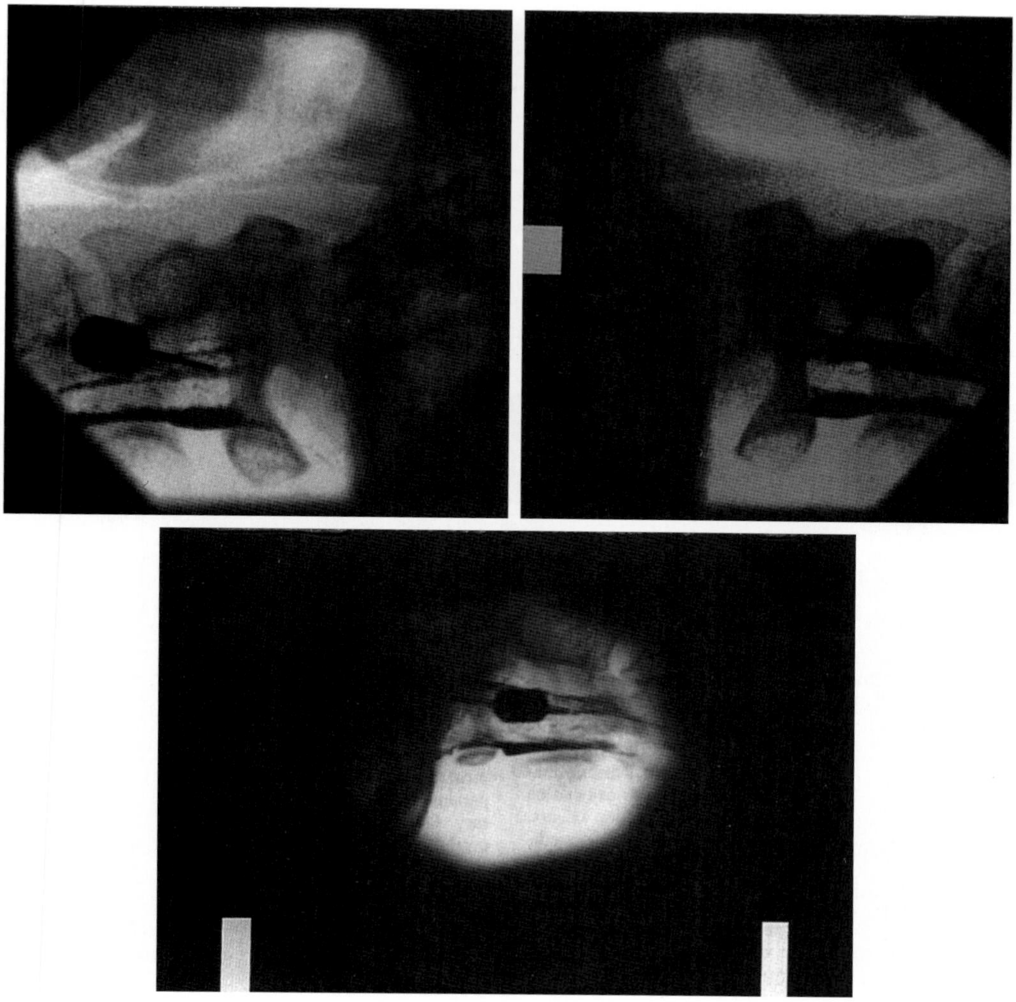

FIGURE 174–8 ■ Three views of contrast emulsions, all outlining the anterior border of the cord, dentate ligament, and posterior border of cord. (From Waldman SD: Interventional Pain Management, 2nd ed. Philadelphia, WB Saunders, 2001, p 691.)

incompletely mixed, or the needle could have been posterior to the dentate ligament. Multiple lines of contrast emulsion indicate that a true lateral view was not obtained. A dual-screen C-arm fluoroscope with memory capability is recommended because the contrast emulsion can quickly pulsate away. The image should be saved for use as a reference.

The first needle is now removed, and a second is inserted at right angles to the correct area of the cord between the anterior border and the dentate ligament. This step should be performed accurately and efficiently before the contrast emulsion pulsates away. The depth of the subarachnoid space was noted during the placement of the first needle. After the needle enters the CSF, the thermocoupled probe is inserted (Fig. 174–9).

Impedance measurements depend on which electrode system is being used. When the Levin cordotomy electrode is in the CSF, the impedance nears 200 Ω. It increases to greater than 1000 Ω as the probe enters the cord. At 1000 to 1500 Ω, the probe is deep enough to begin electrical stimulation.

Stimulation is first performed at 50 Hz. Spinothalamic tract stimulation generally produces contralateral thermic sensations, which patients have described variously as heat, cold, and blowing wind. These sensations occur at less than 0.4 V. If thermic stimulation occurs in the upper extremity, the patient usually obtains analgesia over the entire half of the body below C5. Thermic stimulation in the lower extremity tends to produce analgesia only over the extremity. Occasionally, pain or paresthesia is produced over a particular area of the body. If this area overlaps the painful area, lesioning is likely to have a good result. Otherwise, the probe should be repositioned until thermic stimulation to the upper extremity is obtained or the pain or paresthesias cover the appropriate area.

Electrical stimulation is performed at 2 Hz. If the electrode is in the spinothalamic tract, no motor stimulation occurs with less than 1 V. If ipsilateral stimulation is noted below the neck at 2 Hz and 50 Hz, the electrode is probably in the corticospinal tract and should be repositioned anterior to the dentate ligament. Patients occasionally note ipsilateral sensations from the neck in addition to contralateral sensory stimulation. Such sensations imply that the probe is near the anterior horn cells. Similarly, stimulation of ipsilateral cervical musculature at 2 Hz and less than 1 V also indicates that the probe is near the anterior horn. This does not contraindicate lesioning if contralateral sensory stimulation is obtained at less than 0.4 volt. If stimulation is produced only in the neck, however, caution should be exercised because the electrode may be too near the anterior horn cells, and a lesion made here might be ineffective. High stimulation thresholds may be noted from scarring secondary to previous cervical radiation or a previous cordotomy. Stimulation parameters are summarized in Table 174–1.

Table 174–1

Stimulation Parameters at C1-2

Location of Electrode	*Results of Stimulation*	
	At 50 Hz	*At 2 Hz*
Spinothalamic tract	Contralateral thermic stimulation at <0.4 V	No motor stimulation at <1 V
Corticospinal tract	Ipsilateral paresthesias and tetanization below neck	Ipsilateral motor stimulation below neck at <1 V
Anterior horn	Ipsilateral paresthesias and tetanization in neck	Ipsilateral motor stimulation in neck

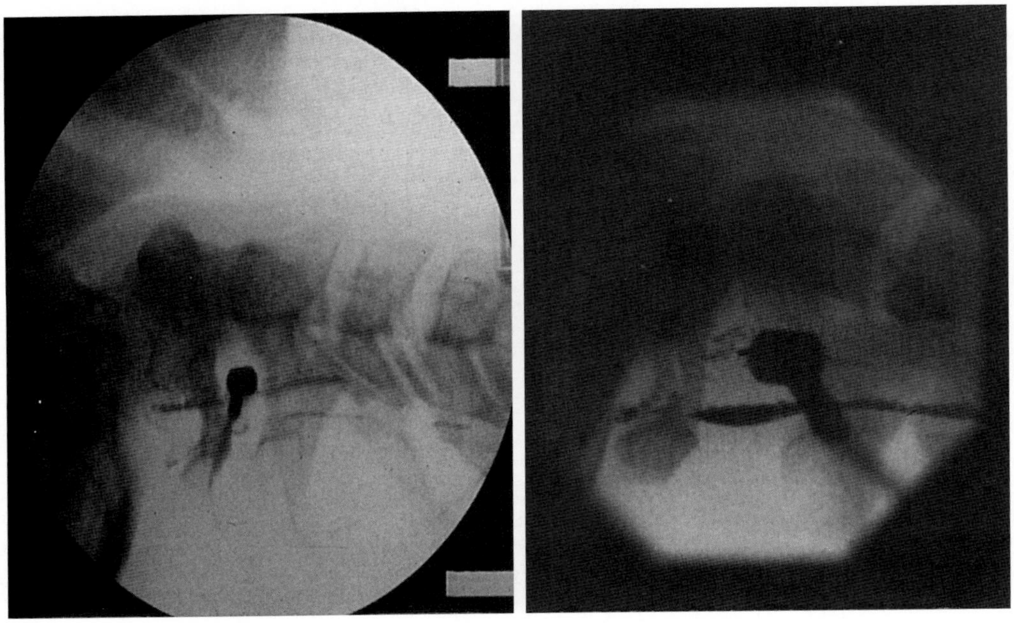

FIGURE 174–9 ■ Two views of the thermocoupled electrode inserted into the anterolateral quadrant. The contrast emulsion has dissipated. (From Waldman SD: Interventional Pain Management, 2nd ed. Philadelphia, WB Saunders, 2001, p 692.)

Electrophysiologic monitoring[77] by somatosensory evoked potentials has not been shown to improve outcome or decrease complications.

A lesion is created only after proper stimulation is obtained. Similar to any other radiofrequency techniques, the procedure should be abandoned if proper stimulation cannot be achieved. (This happened in 1 of my 54 cases.) Lesioning causes a mild headache that disappears after several seconds. Lesioning may be performed by either of two techniques. One uses a constant current, and lesioning time is increased incrementally until either analgesia to pinprick is shown or side effects occur. I use a thermocoupled electrode. Lesions are made at not more than 98°C for 15-second intervals. After each lesion, analgesia to pinprick and loss of thermal discrimination are tested for on the contralateral side. Lesion times can be increased up to 30 seconds. If boiling or cavitation occurs, the voltage jumps, and the lesioning should be terminated immediately. Otherwise, an uncontrolled lesion will have been created.

Before the needle is withdrawn, it is prudent to deposit steroids directly onto the C2 nerve root sleeve. The needle is withdrawn just lateral to the midfacet line, and 0.5 mL of contrast dye is injected to outline the C2 root sleeve. To decrease the frequency and severity of any resulting C2 headache, 20 mg of triamcinolone or methylprednisolone acetate can be deposited.

Kanpolat and colleagues[16] described CT-guided cordotomy. The advantage may be ease in tailoring the lesions to the painful area. There is good correlation between CT and actual cord measurements.[78] Another advantage is fewer attempts at needle positioning in difficult cases because the anterolateral quadrant of the spinal cord can be visualized in all cases. The longer duration of the procedure is a drawback.

Postoperative Course

The postoperative course after percutaneous cordotomy is generally benign. Initially, patients are given high doses of steroids, which are tapered over the next week. This regimen decreases cord edema and the risk of complications. If a spinal headache occurs, bed rest is encouraged for at least 1 day. For discomfort at the needle insertion site, mild analgesics only are necessary. The patient should be monitored for urine output. Occasionally, bladder catheterization is necessary; this is more likely for patients with a history of prostatism or bladder dysfunction. Approximately 10% of patients develop ipsilateral paresis, which is temporary. Occasionally, patients are discharged with a walker until their motor strength returns to baseline.

Patients should be weaned from narcotics. If their pain was unilateral, they should be given 25% of preoperative doses to prevent withdrawal symptoms. When the dose is reduced, contralateral pain may be unmasked. It must be differentiated from mirror pain (discussed later). If contralateral pain is discovered, radiation therapy, chemotherapy, or surgery may be appropriate in addition to medical or procedural pain treatments.

A patient whose preoperative respiratory status was unstable should be monitored for 3 days for signs of respiratory decompensation. By day 3, cord edema decreases, along with the risk of complications. If respiratory status is problematic, I recommend intensive care monitoring with frequent checks of respiration and serial blood gas measurements to check for evidence of carbon dioxide retention. The patients' and families' wishes concerning intubation and ventilatory support should have been discussed before the cordotomy. One of my patients died from respiratory failure after bilateral staged cordotomy while being monitored in an intensive care setting.

Summary

Visualization of the bony landmarks is crucial to accurate cordotomy, and time spent positioning the patient and C-arm fluoroscopic device before the procedure is time well spent. Visualization of the dentate ligament and anterior surface of the cord helps to guide the needle toward the spinothalamic tract. Impedance values and thresholds for electrical stimulation depend on the electrode being used. If the patient is adequately prepared, and the technique is executed meticulously, gratifying results are achieved.

PITFALLS

Recurrence of pain is a common problem after cordotomy. The mechanisms for recurrence are discussed here. Treatment options depend on the mechanism of the recurrent pain.

Inadequate Lesioning

Short-term pain relief before recurrence is probably secondary to an inadequate lesion. A misplaced lesion can cause cord edema that temporarily interferes with pain transmission through the spinothalamic tract. As cord edema resolves, normal transmission returns, and pain recurs. Tasker[45] repeated 2.6% of cordotomy lesions within a few weeks because of fading or falling levels of analgesia; most of the second procedures gave satisfactory results. Lahuerta and coworkers[36] showed that approximately 20% of the hemicord must be destroyed to produce the most satisfactory pain relief (Fig. 174–10). Nagaro and colleagues[79] showed oval-shaped lesions in the anterolateral cord correlating with pain relief. Ischia and colleagues[28] emphasized that results definitely vary according to the ability of the surgeon, and Gybels and Sweet[74] warned, "This is not an easy procedure." It should be performed by someone skilled in the use of fluoroscopy and radiofrequency lesioning. A major source of difficulty is working from views of C1-2 that are not true lateral views. I optimize the view of the "cathedral window" at C1-2 before fixing the fluoroscope and the patient's head in position. Only then is the patient prepared and draped. If a true lateral view is not obtained, multiple contrast lines can appear so that identification of the anterolateral quadrant becomes problematic. In these cases, the size of the C1-2 opening is not optimal. Even if only the nearest dentate ligament is outlined, parallax errors confound identification of the true size and location of the anterolateral quadrant. To obviate frustration that occurs when contrast dye rapidly pulsates away from the operative site, a dual-screen fluoroscope with memory is essential. It cannot be overemphasized that this procedure should be performed only by an operator skilled in precision percutaneous techniques.

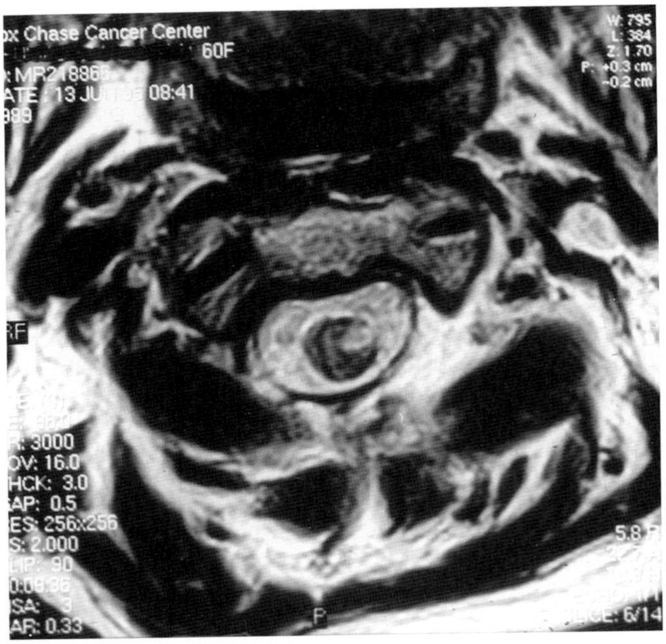

FIGURE 174–10 ■ Postoperative MRI shows lesion in the anterolateral cord. (From Waldman SD: Interventional Pain Management, 2nd ed. Philadelphia, WB Saunders, 2001, p 693.)

New and Unmasked Pain

Pain can recur even after a successful lesion.[80] A common cause is unmasking of contralateral pain as narcotic doses are tapered postoperatively. Macaluso and associates[48] reported unmasked contralateral pain in 18 of 20 patients treated by cordotomy for pain from lumbosacral or pelvic cancer. This complication occurred in 5 of my 54 patients during the first postoperative week; 25 other patients developed contralateral pain before death. Most cancer patients obtain satisfactory pain control with oral medications. Only a few such patients need invasive procedures to relieve new or unmasked pain.

I cannot overemphasize that pain-relieving procedures are only part of an overall cancer pain treatment program. Cancer is a dynamic, progressive disease, and it is likely that bilateral pain eventually will develop opposite or above the areas rendered analgesic by the cordotomy. Any new pain should be treated according to standard cancer pain protocols. If possible, therapy should be directed toward the underlying disease. If this is impossible, palliative radiation or surgery should be considered, complemented by adequate analgesics and pain-relieving procedures.

Complete lifelong pain relief after cordotomy is the exception rather than the rule. Tasker[45] reported that only 33.7% of his patients were totally pain-free at the latest follow-up. Forty percent developed pain opposite the side of original pain, owing to undiagnosed or new disease or to the development of mirror pain (discussed later). Of their patients with pelvic malignant disease, Ischia and colleagues[29] reported that 36% obtained complete pain relief from cordotomy alone. Another 40% obtained relief when narcotic and non-narcotic analgesics were added to therapy. Similar results were observed in patients with cervicothoracic pain.[28] Of patients with Pancoast tumor, 75% obtained complete pain control through cordotomy and analgesics, and 86% of patients with thoracic pain obtained excellent relief. Fewer than one third of these patients obtained complete relief, however, with the procedural intervention alone. Similar results have been noted after celiac plexus ablation.[81] Only 10% to 24% of patients obtain lifelong pain relief from this block. Pain recurs as the block wears off or as tumor extends outward from the celiac plexus.

Postcordotomy Dysesthesias

When postcordotomy dysesthesia occurs, it is difficult to treat. Dysesthesias probably constitute previously undiagnosed deafferentation pain or new deafferentation pain that developed after the cordotomy. Deafferentation pain occurs in the absence of normal afferent sensory input. In a cancer patient, the cause of the pain no longer would be pressure on neural tissue from the tumor itself, but rather the damaged neural tissue. Tasker[45] believed that almost 40% of his patients developed deafferentation pain below a level of adequate analgesia. It occurred immediately postoperatively in 6.7% of patients, indicating that the syndrome had been present preoperatively. Another 33.7% of Tasker's patients developed dysesthesia pain postoperatively that differed in character from the pain that had been present previously. It is unclear why this situation was so frequent. Nathan and Smith[82] noted only three cases of postcordotomy dysesthesia after 74 unilateral procedures and no cases after 40 bilateral procedures. Nagaro and coworkers[47] described postcordotomy dysesthesias in 15.2% of 66 patients. They believed that 2 out of 10 patients had recurrence of pain secondary to recovery of pain sensitivity, 8 had deafferentated pain, and 6 had deafferentating peripheral nerve damage caused by tumor invasion after a successful cordotomy. Two patents had diffuse dysesthesia, presumably secondary to destruction of additional second-order neurons by the cordotomy. Regardless of the exact frequency, cordotomies should be avoided in patients with dysesthetic sensations in areas of preexisting sensory loss.

References of Sensation

Another form of pain recurrence is known as *mirror pain* or *reference of sensation.* The pain occurs in a distribution that mirrors the pain present before the cordotomy. *Mirror pain* is a misnomer because the pain occurs horizontally and cranially from the preoperative location. The phenomenon also has been referred to as *allachesthesia* (*allesthesia*).[65] Painful sensations are referred from the side of the body previously rendered analgesic to the contralateral side. Reference of sensation was first described in a postcordotomy patient by Ray and Wolff[83] in 1945. Nathan[37] reported the phenomenon in 15 patients in 1956; 13 of the cases occurred after cordotomy. Another patient had a thrombosed anterior spinal artery, and one developed the syndrome after an upper limb amputation. Nathan noted reference of sensation after 17 of 61 surgical cordotomies.[84] Nagaro and colleagues[38] counted it in 7 of their 66 patients. Ischia and associates[28] noted mirror pain in 73% of patients who had thoracic pain secondary to lung cancer or metastatic disease. This high frequency in association with chest wall lesions has been noted by many operators. Mirror pain occurred after four of seven cordotomies I performed for chest wall pain.

A typical case is as follows: A patient presents with right chest wall pain from lung cancer unresponsive to conventional analgesics. The right-sided pain is eliminated by the cordotomy. Three days later, as analgesics are tapered, however, the patient develops similar left-sided pain. The right side of the body below the shoulder is still analgesic to pinprick. A workup for a new cancerous lesion is negative. The new pain is bothersome, but can be controlled partially with analgesics until the patient dies (which happened 2 months later).

Nathan[37] described reference of sensation in a patient who underwent cordotomy for right-sided chest pain. Forty hours postoperatively, reference of sensation developed so that, "When a pin was applied to the analgesic right side, the patient immediately put up his hand and covered an analogous place on the left side of the chest. When asked why he did this, he replied that he did not know…. Eventually he said that he could hardly believe his senses but it seemed to him that he felt the pinprick applied to the right side of the chest as if it were on the left."[37] Bowsher[85] noted that naloxone increases the severity of the referred pain, indicating that the newly opened fibers were opioidergic.

If reference of pain occurs, bilateral lesioning eliminates it. Pain tends to decrease as cordotomy-induced analgesia turns to hypalgesia. Nagaro and associates[86] theorized that subsidiary pathways connect dorsal horns longitudinally and laterally, which connect to the intact spinothalamic tract. Usually, the subsidiary pathways are inhibited by a feedback loop involving the spinothalamic tracts. Reference of pain results as release of feedback inhibition allows transmission through the intact spinothalamic tract.

Consider a patient whose left leg pain is relieved by a right-sided cordotomy. Reference of sensation develops, and the pain is referred to the right leg. Noxious stimuli are transmitted from the left leg through the right spinothalamic tract, but are blocked by the cordotomy at C1-2. The loss of feedback inhibition allows the signal to cross through subsidiary pathways to the intact left spinothalamic tract. The brain perceives the signal as emanating from the right side of the body. Nagaro and associates[86] described referral of left groin and thigh pain to the right chest after a right C1-2 cordotomy. The chest pain was eliminated by an epidural block below T10, proving that the new pain was referred from the originally painful region. In another article, Nagaro and associates[87] reported having relieved referred pain with thoracic intrathecal phenol applied to the side of the original cancer pain.

Summary

Recurrence of pain can be due to technical errors in the performance of the procedure. Pain may recur even after successful cordotomy, however, sometimes because of unmasking of pain during tapering of narcotics. It also can be due to spread of new tumor ipsilateral to the lesion or above the area rendered analgesic by cordotomy. Postcordotomy pain can be either a deafferentation phenomenon or secondary to reference of sensation. Treatment options depend on proper characterization of the recurrent pain.

COMPLICATIONS

Mortality after percutaneous cordotomy is due to rapid unexpected progression of the underlying disease or to respiratory decompensation. Morbidity includes ipsilateral paresis and urinary retention. Horner syndrome can occur, but is usually temporary. Sexual sensitivity decreases after cordotomy. Postcordotomy dysesthesias were discussed in an earlier section. Other than progression of disease and postcordotomy dysesthesias, the mortality and morbidity after percutaneous cordotomy are due entirely to the size and location of the lesion created in the anterolateral quadrant.

Respiratory Complications

Respiratory complications were first noted in the 1930s,[4] soon after the introduction of high cervical cordotomy. It was thought that the smaller, more accurate lesions made by the percutaneous technique would decrease the incidence of respiratory embarrassment, but this turned out not to be the case.

As discussed previously, the reticulospinal tract controls involuntary function of the intercostal, abdominal, and diaphragmatic muscles and is just behind or intermingled with the spinothalamic tract. The location of the reticulospinal fibers was first diagrammed by Hitchcock and Leece.[68] Lahuerta and colleagues[33] studied histologic sections at C1-2 taken from patients who died of respiratory complications after cordotomy. They showed that all cases involved the region of the anterolateral funiculus, which contains spinothalamic fibers from the second to the fifth thoracic dermatomes. They postulated that this region may be the afferent pathway that transmits signals from the periphery to the brain stem respiratory centers. Much effort has been devoted to differentiating the afferent spinoreticular tract from the efferent reticulospinal tract. From a practical point of view, it is clear that involuntary control of respiration is transmitted through the anterolateral quadrant, and Ischia and colleagues[28] remarked that bilateral cervical lesions cannot be made without "running the risk of killing the patient." Tasker[50] emphasized "tailoring" the lesion. Ischia and colleagues[30] performed one-stage bilateral cervical cordotomy, taking care to align the electrode with the dentate ligament or at most 1 mm anterior to it, to avoid lesioning the anterior part of the anterolateral quadrant.

Belmusto and associates[88] were the first to note an intraoperative reduction in tidal volume immediately after section of the cord. This occurred in every case when the lesion was deep enough to produce pain relief. Nathan[31] observed similar changes and noted that respiratory movements on the affected side were not eliminated. Rosomoff and coworkers[89] observed that unilateral cordotomy resulted in little change in vital capacity, but a significant reduction in tidal volume and a compensatory increase in respiratory rate. Bilateral cordotomy resulted in a significant reduction in minute ventilation. In patients with high levels of analgesia, the increase in respiratory rate was insufficient to compensate for the reduction in tidal volume. In patients who developed respiratory embarrassment, the most consistent alteration was a reduction in carbon dioxide sensitivity.

Krieger and Rosomoff[90] found that respiratory dysfunction could begin 6 days after cordotomy. Subjective signs of respiratory dysfunction appeared before clinical impairment could be shown. Characteristically, patients manifested the subjective sensation of panic, and respirations were interrupted with frequent sighing. Signs were similar to those of an anxiety reaction. Afterward, patients exhibited the classic syndrome: They would hypoventilate when awake, but became apneic when asleep. When awakened, they would resume breathing, but hypoventilation persisted. The most common syndrome showed a decrease in carbon dioxide response and vital capacity. Occasionally, patients manifested no change in vital capacity and an attenuated carbon dioxide response.

Lema and Hitchcock[49] measured FEV_1 after percutaneous and open cordotomies. Eleven of 15 patients showed a decrease in FEV_1 after percutaneous cordotomy, the average decrease being 20%. The average decrease after open cordotomy was 25%. Decrease in FEV_1 was more marked with deeper incisions. Although this observation was not quantified, the authors agreed that respiratory decompensation is more likely in patients who have preexisting respiratory disease or bilateral cordotomies with high cervical levels of analgesia.

Ondine's curse was named by Severinghaus and Mitchell,[5] who observed it in three patients after cordotomy. Polatty and Cooper[91] described a patient who survived with Ondine's curse for 14 months. Nocturnal mechanical ventilation through a tracheostomy was necessary, and eventually phrenic nerve pacemakers were implanted. Rosomoff and coworkers[89] counseled against using pharmacologic depressants in patients with postcordotomy pulmonary dysfunction. The need to titrate narcotics downward after cordotomy was emphasized by Wells and colleagues,[92] who observed respiratory depression after cordotomy in patients who took long-acting morphine preparations. Sleep apnea may disappear as postcordotomy edema subsides, and reticulospinal fibers return to normal.

Patients with bilateral cordotomies are most at risk for sleep apnea. Although Ischia and associates[30] performed bilateral cordotomies in a single session, most authors recommend staging the procedures and delaying the second cordotomy at least 2 weeks, to allow cord edema to subside. If the remaining pain is centered in the trunk or lower extremities, high open thoracic cordotomy is an option. If the pain is in the upper chest or upper extremity, contralateral cordotomy is an option if good analgesia was not obtained with the first procedure. If high levels of analgesia were achieved, performing the second cordotomy carries considerable risk.

Patients at risk for respiratory failure should be monitored in the intensive care unit. Spirometry, arterial blood gases, and vital signs should be used to guide therapy. Shortness of breath, confusion, and anxiety may herald the onset of sleep apnea. Apnea alarms may be useful. Physician, patient, and family should have a thorough discussion of the respiratory risks before the procedure. The decision to provide or withhold aggressive ventilatory support should be made at that time. The sleep apnea syndrome is generally self-limiting, and patients can be weaned off the ventilator within 2 weeks.

The incidence of postoperative respiratory failure is impossible to estimate, owing to the varying skills and experience of the operators and the lack of standardized indications for the procedure. Rosomoff and associates[93] reported a 3% incidence of major respiratory complications in 1279 cordotomies, including one death from sleep apnea.[93] Tasker[45] observed a 0.5% incidence of respiratory death and an additional 0.5% incidence of temporary respiratory failure after 380 cordotomies. Among 103 patients with cervicothoracic cancer, the incidence of respiratory failure was 4.2%; this was clearly a high-risk group.[28] White and Sweet[58] compared open and percutaneous cordotomy. Mortality after percutaneous cordotomy was 1% in 3357 cases and was primarily due to respiratory failure. The incidence was 8% after the open procedure. The difference was attributed to the longer hospitalization needed after the open procedure and to the fact that some of the patients who underwent open cordotomy would have been chosen for the percutaneous procedure after the authors had gained experience with the technique.

Paresis

As previously discussed, paresis can occur ipsilateral to the lesion, secondary to the effect of cord edema on the corticospinal tracts. Motor function should return to the preoperative level as cord edema subsides. The risk of ipsilateral hemiparesis increases if stimulation is obtained only to the contralateral lower extremity because those fibers are closest to the corticospinal tracts. With proper electrical stimulation and a lightly sedated patient, permanent paresis should occur rarely, if at all.

Ipsilateral limb weakness was reported in 69% of patients by Lahuerta and colleagues.[55] The condition was present in only 4% of patients after 1 month. White and Sweet[58] noted transient weakness in 6.5% of patients. Tasker[45] reported transient paresis after 8% of unilateral cordotomies and 16% of bilateral procedures. Paresis persisted in 0.8% of the unilateral cordotomy group and in 1.6% of the bilateral group. Rosomoff and coworkers[93] noted a 5% incidence of temporary ipsilateral paresis; in 3% of patients, the paresis proved to be permanent.

Urinary Complications

The fibers involved in micturition run near the spinothalamic fibers from the sacral segments of the body. Reported rates of permanent catheterization vary greatly, depending on surgical technique and patient selection criteria. The risk increases with bilateral lesions and in patients with preexisting bladder dysfunction, prostatism, or pelvic cancer. Tasker[45] noted deterioration of bladder function after 2.9% of unilateral procedures and after 18.8% of bilateral procedures. Catheterization was needed in 10% of patients in the series reported by Rosomoff and coworkers.[93] Two percent were left with permanent catheters, mainly for nursing convenience. Ischia and associates[28] noted permanent urinary retention in 9 of 103 patients treated with cordotomy for cervicothoracic pain, and a 7.2% catheterization rate in patients treated for neoplastic vertebral pain.[27] Urinary retention after cordotomy developed in 11.1% of the patients who underwent cordotomy for malignant pelvic disease.[29] This group was at high risk. Palma and associates[94] reported transient bladder dysfunction in 10 of 163 patients after cordotomy.

Horner Syndrome

Horner syndrome also may develop after cordotomy. Referring to open procedures, Gybels and Sweet[74] stated that

Horner syndrome is "almost the rule following high cervical cordotomy." After percutaneous procedures, transient self-limited Horner syndrome can occur. The incidence of Horner syndrome depends on the site and location of the radiofrequency lesion. I have noted Horner syndrome in approximately half of 29 cases, which generally disappeared within a day or so. When the sympathetic fibers are lesioned, transient hypotension can occur. This seems to be more of a problem after open cordotomies, and the risk increases with bilateral lesioning.

Sexual Dysfunction

Loss of sexual sensitivity occurs on the side rendered analgesic by cordotomy.[65] Bilateral lesions eliminate orgasm in women. Loss of erection and ejaculation can occur in men in the presence of preexisting urinary tract dysfunction or pelvic malignancy. Otherwise, libido and potency are not affected. Lahuerta and associates[64] observed that "unlike alcohol, cordotomy takes away (some of) the pleasure but not the performance."

Summary

The major risk of percutaneous cordotomy is respiratory decompensation. A sleep apnea syndrome may develop. The risk is difficult to estimate, but increases with preexisting pulmonary disease and bilateral lesions producing high levels of cervical analgesia. Less serious complications include ipsilateral paresis and urinary retention. Transient Horner syndrome also may occur. The lesser complications are generally transient. Sexual sensitivity may decrease. The risk of urinary retention increases in patients with preexisting urinary tract disease, pelvic disease, or bilateral cordotomy.

FUTURE DIRECTIONS

The use of cordotomy has declined. It is hoped that publications such as this one will stimulate interest in precision percutaneous techniques and reverse this trend. Although aggressive narcotic-based cancer pain management is an immense improvement over what was available 10 to 15 years ago, many patients are living out their lives with mediocre pain relief and significant medication side effects. This large group of patients could benefit immensely from techniques such as percutaneous cordotomy. Cordotomy is complementary to other pain control techniques. Cordotomy is most valuable for patients with neuropathic or incident pain. Literature on the treatment of neuropathic pain is accumulating. New publications describe subcutaneous lidocaine,[95] systemic local anesthetics,[96] intravenous narcotics,[39] and local anesthetic epidural[41] and subarachnoid[42] infusions. Epidural and intrathecal clonidine[43,97] may be useful for opioid-resistant neuropathic pain; ziconotide[43] also may be specific to neuropathic pain. Many patients with neuropathic pain would be excellent cordotomy candidates, were the procedure available to them.

There are too few outcome studies of interventional pain management. Ischia and colleagues[27-30] have published excellent studies describing the risks, benefits, and outcomes of percutaneous cordotomy in selected cancer patients, but much work still needs to be done. Most of the studies of percutaneous cordotomy were published before use of spinal narcotics was widespread, and no studies have yet prospectively compared spinal narcotic and local anesthetic infusions with percutaneous cordotomy for cancer patients with neuropathic or incident pain. Similarly, with the exception of Tasker's[26] article on cordotomy for pain of spinal cord origin, there is no good information on how cordotomy fits into the management of pain not related to cancer.[26]

CONCLUSION

Percutaneous cordotomy is useful principally for cancer patients with unilateral pain below the shoulder and life expectancy of less than 1 year. No other procedure available to the interventional pain management specialist offers such dramatic, immediate, and long-term benefits. The goal is to integrate percutaneous cordotomy into comprehensive pain care so that the maximum number of patients may benefit from this extraordinary technique.

References

1. Spiller WG, Martin E: The treatment of persistent pain of organic origin in the lower part of the body by division of the anterolateral column of the spinal cord. JAMA 58:1489, 1912.
2. Foerster O: Uber die Vorderseiten Strangdurchschneidung. Arch Psychiatr Nerv Krankh 81:707, 1927.
3. Stookey B: Chordotomy of the second cervical segment for relief from pain due to recurrent carcinoma of the breast. Arch Neurol 26:443, 1931.
4. Peet M, Kahn EA, Allen SS: Bilateral cervical chordotomy for relief of pain in chronic infectious arthritis. JAMA 100:488, 1933.
5. Severinghaus JW, Mitchell RA: Ondine's curse: Failure of respiratory center automaticity while awake. Clin Res 10:122, 1992.
6. Millan S, Harper PV, Hekmatpanah J, et al: Percutaneous interruption of spinal pain tracts by means of a strontium needle. J Neurosurg 20:931, 1963.
7. Belmusto L, Owens G: Surgical control of pain in the elderly patient with cancer. Am J Surg 103:709, 1962.
8. Millan S, Hekmatpanah J, Dobben G, et al: Percutaneous, intramedullary cordotomy utilizing the unipolar anodal electrolytic lesion. J Neurosurg 22:548, 1965.
9. Rosomoff H, Carroll F, Brown F, et al: Percutaneous radiofrequency cervical cordotomy: Technique. J Neurosurg 23:639, 1965.
10. Lin PM, Gildenberg PL, Polakoff PP: An anterior approach to percutaneous lower cervical cordotomy. J Neurosurg 25:533, 1966.
11. Gildenberg PL, Lin PM, Polakoff PP, et al: Anterior percutaneous cervical cordotomy: Determination of target point and calculation of angle of insertion. J Neurosurg 28:173, 1968.
12. Crue EL, Todd EM, Carregal EJA: Posterior approach for high cervical percutaneous radiofrequency cordotomy. Contemp Neurol 30:41, 1968.
13. Hitchcock E: Stereotaxic spinal surgery: A preliminary report. J Neurosurg 31:386, 1969.
14. Onofrio EM: Cervical spinal cord and dentate delineation in percutaneous radiofrequency cordotomy at the level of the first to second cervical vertebrae. Surg Gynecol Obstet 133:30, 1971.
15. Kanpolat Y, Akyar S, Caglar S, et al: CT-guided percutaneous selective cordotomy. Acta Neurochir (Wien) 123:92, 1993.
16. Kanpolat Y, Caglar S, Akyar S, Temiz C: CT-guided procedures for intractable pain in malignancy. Acta Neurochir Suppl (Wien) 64:88, 1995.
17. Gildenberg PL, Zanes C, Flitter M, et al: Impedance-measuring device for detection of penetration of the spinal cord in anterior percutaneous cervical cordotomy (technical note). J Neurosurg 30:87, 1969.
18. Taren JA, Davis R, Crosby EC: Target physiologic corroboration in stereotaxic cervical cordotomy. J Neurosurg 30:569, 1969.
19. Tasker RR, Organ LW: Percutaneous cordotomy: Physiological identification of target site. Contemp Neurol 35:110, 1973.

20. Tasker RR, Organ LW, Smith KC: Physiological guidelines for the localization of lesions by percutaneous cordotomy. Acta Neurochir Suppl (Wien) 21:111, 1974.
21. Campbell JA, Lipton S: Somatosensory evoked potentials recorded from within the anterolateral quadrant of the human spinal cord. Adv Pain Res Ther 5:23, 1983.
22. Myerson BA, von Holst H: Extramedullary impedance monitoring and stimulation of the spinal cord surface in percutaneous cordotomy. Acta Neurochir (Wien) 107:63, 1990.
23. Cosman ER, Nashold BS, Bedenbaugh P: Stereotactic radiofrequency lesion making. Appl Neurophysiol 46:160, 1983.
24. Kline MT: Stereotactic Radiofrequency Lesions as Part of the Management of Pain. Orlando, Paul M. Deutsch, 1992.
25. Levin AB, Cosman ER: Thermocouple-monitored cordotomy electrode (technical note). J Neurosurg 53:266, 1980.
26. Tasker RR, DeCarvalho GTC, Dolan EJ: Intractable pain of spinal cord origin: Clinical features and implications for surgery. J Neurosurg 77:373, 1992.
27. Ischia S, Luzzani A, Ischia A, et al: Role of unilateral percutaneous cervical cordotomy in the treatment of neoplastic vertebral pain. Pain 19:123, 1984.
28. Ischia S, Ischia A, Luzzani A, et al: Results up to death in the treatment of persistent cervicothoracic (Pancoast) and thoracic malignant pain by unilateral percutaneous cervical cordotomy. Pain 21:339, 1985.
29. Ischia S, Luzzani A, Ischia A, et al: Subarachnoid neurolytic block (L5-S1) and unilateral percutaneous cervical cordotomy in the treatment of pain secondary to pelvic malignant disease. Pain 20:139, 1984.
30. Ischia S, Luzzani A, Ischia A, et al: Bilateral percutaneous cervical cordotomy: Immediate and long-term results in 36 patients with neoplastic disease. J Neurol Neurosurg Psychiatry 20:129, 1984.
31. Nathan PW: The descending respiratory pathway in man. J Neurol Neurosurg Psychiatry 26:487, 1963.
32. Nathan PW, Smith MC: Clinicoanatomical correlation in anterolateral cordotomy. Adv Pain Res Ther 3:71, 1979.
33. Lahuerta J, Buxton P, Lipton S, et al: The location and function of respiratory fibers in the second cervical spinal cord segment: Respiratory dysfunction syndrome after cervical cordotomy. J Neurol Neurosurg Psychiatry 55:1142, 1992.
34. Nathan PW, Smith MC: The location of descending fibres to sympathetic preganglionic vasomotor and sudomotor neurons in men. J Neurol Neurosurg Psychiatry 50:1253, 1987.
35. Nathan PW, Smith MC: The centrifugal pathway for micturition within the spinal cord. J Neurol Neurosurg Psychiatry 21:177, 1958.
36. Lahuerta J, Bowsher D, Lipton S, Buxton P: Percutaneous cervical cordotomy: A review of 181 operations on 146 patients with a study on the location of "pain fibers" in the C-2 spinal cord segment of 29 cases. J Neurosurg 80:975, 1994.
37. Nathan PW: Reference of sensation at the spinal level. J Neurol Neurosurg Psychiatry 19:88, 1956.
38. Nagaro T, Amakawa K, Kimura S, et al: Reference of pain following percutaneous cervical cordotomy. Pain 53:205, 1993.
39. Portenoy RK, Foley KM, Inturrisi CE: The nature of opioid responsiveness and its implications for neuropathic pain: New hypotheses derived from studies of opioid infusions. Pain 43:273, 1990.
40. Hogan Q, Haddox JD, Abram S, et al: Epidural opiates and local anesthetics for the management of cancer pain. Pain 46:271, 1991.
41. DuPen S, Kharasch ED, Williams A, et al: Chronic epidural bupivacaine-opioid infusion in intractable cancer pain. Pain 49:293, 1992.
42. Van Dangen RIM, Crul BJP, DeBock M: Long-term intrathecal infusion of morphine and morphine/bupivacaine mixtures in the treatment of cancer pain: A retrospective analysis of 51 cases. Pain 55:119, 1993.
43. Hassenbush SJ, et al: Alternative intrathecal agents for the treatment of pain. Neuromodulation 2:85, 1999.
44. Lipton S: Percutaneous cervical cordotomy. Acta Anaesthesiol Belg 1:81, 1981.
45. Tasker RR: Percutaneous cordotomy: The lateral high cervical technique. In Schmidek HH, Sweet WH (eds): Operative Neurosurgical Techniques: Indications, Methods, and Results, 2nd ed. New York, Grune & Stratton, 1988, p 1191.
46. Rosomoff HL: Percutaneous radiofrequency cervical cordotomy for intractable pain. Adv Neurol 4:683, 1974.
47. Nagaro T, Oka S, Amakawa K, et al: Classification of post-cordotomy dysesthesia. Masui 43:1356-1361, 1994.
48. Macaluso C, Foley KM, Arbit E: Cordotomy for lumbosacral, pelvic and lower extremity pain of malignant origin: Safety and efficacy. Neurology 38:51, 1988.
49. Lema JA, Hitchcock E: Respiratory changes after stereotactic high cervical cord lesions for pain. Appl Neurophysiol 49:62, 1986.
50. Tasker RR: Percutaneous cordotomy: Neurosurgical and neuroaugmentative intervention. In: Cancer Pain. Philadelphia, JB Lippincott, 1993, p 482.
51. Nagaro T, Amakawa K, Yamacuchi Y, et al: Percutaneous cervical cordotomy and subarachnoid phenol block using fluoroscopy in pain control of costopleural syndrome. Pain 60(3):355-356, 1994.
52. Orlandini G: Evaluation of life expectancy in selection of patients undergoing percutaneous cervical cordotomy or subarachnoid phenol block for pain control of costopleural syndrome. Pain 61:492, 1995.
53. Sanders M, Zuurniond W: Safety of unilateral and bilateral percutaneous cordotomy in 80 terminally ill cancer patients. J Clin Oncol 13:1509, 1955.
54. Meglio M, Cioni B: The role of percutaneous cordotomy in the treatment of chronic cancer pain. Acta Neurochir (Wien) 59:111, 1981.
55. Lahuerta J, Lipton S, Wells J: Percutaneous cervical cordotomy: Results and complications in a recent series of 100 patients. Ann R Coll Surg Engl 174:41, 1985.
56. Amano K, Kawamura H, Tanikawa T, et al: Bilateral versus unilateral percutaneous high cervical cordotomy as a surgical method of pain relief. Acta Neurochir Suppl (Wien) 52:143, 1991.
57. Jackson MB, Pounder D, Price C, et al: Percutaneous cervical cordotomy for the control of pain in patients with pleural mesothelioma. Thorax 54:238, 1999.
58. White JC, Sweet WH: Anterolateral cordotomy: Open versus closed: Comparison of end results. Adv Pain Res Ther 3:47, 1979.
59. Katoh Y, Itoh T, Tsuji H, et al: Complications of lateral C1-C2 puncture myelography. Spine 15:1085, 1990.
60. Perese IM, Fracasso JB: Anatomical considerations in surgery of the spinal cord: A study of vessels and measurements of the cord. J Neurosurg 16:314, 1959.
61. Sweet WH, Poletti CE: Operations in the brain stem and spinal canal, with an appendix on open cordotomy. In Wall PD, Melzack R (eds): Textbook of Pain, 2nd ed. Edinburgh, Churchill Livingstone, 1984, p 624.
62. Mehler WR, Feferman ME, Nauta WJH: Ascending axon degeneration following anterolateral cordotomy: An experimental study in the monkey. Brain 83:718, 1960.
63. DiPiero V, Jones AKP, Iannotti F, et al: Chronic pain: A PET study of the central effects of percutaneous high cervical cordotomy. Pain 46:9, 1991.
64. Lahuerta J, Bowsher D, Campbell J, et al: Clinical and instrumental evaluation of sensory function before and after percutaneous anterolateral cordotomy at cervical level in man. Pain 4:23, 1990.
65. White JC, Sweet WH: Pain and the Neurosurgeon: A Forty-Year Experience. Springfield, IL, Charles C Thomas, 1983.
66. Nathan PW: Touch and surgical division of the anterior quadrant of the spinal cord. J Neurosurg 53:935, 1990.
67. Friehs GM, Schrottner O, Pendl G: Evidence for segregated pain and temperature conduction within the spinothalamic tract. J Neurosurg 83:8, 1995.
68. Hitchcock E, Leece B: Somatotopic representation of the respiratory pathways in the cervical cord of men. J Neurosurg 27:320, 19174.
69. Krol G, Arbit E: Percutaneous lateral cervical cordotomy: Target localization with water-soluble contrast medium. J Neurosurg 79:390, 1993.
70. Lipton S: Neurolytic blocks around the head. In Raez GB (ed): Techniques of Neurolysis. Boston, Kluwer Academic, 1989, p 99.
71. Sweet WH: Recent observations pertinent to improving anterolateral cordotomy. Clin Neurosurg 23:80, 1975.
72. Millan S: Percutaneous cordotomy. J Neurosurg 35:360, 1971.
73. Rosomoff HL: Percutaneous spinothalamic cordotomy. In Wilkens RH, Rengachary SS (eds): Neurosurgery. New York, McGraw-Hill, 1985, p 2446.
74. Gybels JM, Sweet WH: Percutaneous anterolateral cordotomy. In Gildenberg PL (ed): Neurosurgical Treatment of Persistent Pain. Basel, Karger, 1989, p 173.
75. Fox JL: Experimental relationship of radiofrequency electrical current and lesion size for application to percutaneous cordotomy. J Neurosurg 33:415, 1970.
76. Kanpolat Y, Cosman ER: Special radiofrequency electrode system for computed tomography-guided pain-relieving procedures. Neurosurgery 38:602, 1996.

77. Zileli M, Coskun E, Yegul I, Oyar M: Electrophysiological monitoring during CT-guided percutaneous cordotomy. Acta Neurochir Suppl (Wien) 64:92, 1995.
78. Kanpolat Y, Akyar S, Caglar S: Diametral measurements of the upper spinal cord for stereotactic pain procedures: Experimental and clinical. Surg Neurol 43:478, 1995.
79. Nagaro T, Tabo E, Koju H, et al: The histological changes in the spinal cord following percutaneous cervical cordotomy (PCC) and correlation of these changes with the efficacy of PCC. Masui 44:325, 1995.
80. Mooij JJA, Bosch DA, Beks JWF: The cause of failure in high cervical percutaneous cordotomy: An analysis. Acta Neurochir (Wien) 72:1, 1984.
81. Ischia S, Ischia A, Polati E, et al: Three posterior percutaneous celiac plexus block techniques. Anesthesiology 76:534, 1992.
82. Nathan PW, Smith MC: Dysesthesie après cordotomie. Med Hyg 42:1788, 1984.
83. Ray BS, Wolff SG: Studies on pain, "spread of pain," evidence on site of spread within the neuraxis of effects of painful stimulation. Arch Neurol Psychiatry 53:257, 1945.
84. Nathan PW: Results of anterolateral cordotomy for pain in cancer. J Neurol Neurosurg Psychiatry 26:353, 1963.
85. Bowsher D: Contralateral mirror-image pain following anterolateral cordotomy. Pain 88:63, 1988.
86. Nagaro T, Amakawa K, Arai T, et al: Ipsilateral referral of pain following cordotomy. Pain 55:275, 1993.
87. Nagaro T, Kimura S, Arai T: A mechanism of new pain following cordotomy: Reference of sensation. Pain 30:89, 1987.
88. Belmusto L, Brown E, Owens G: Clinical observations on respiratory and vasomotor disturbance as related to cervical cordotomies. J Neurosurg 20:225, 1963.
89. Rosomoff HL, Krieger AJ, Kuperman AS: Effects of percutaneous cervical cordotomy on pulmonary function. J Neurosurg 31:620, 1969.
90. Krieger AJ, Rosomoff HL: Sleep-induced apnea: Part I. A respiratory and autonomic dysfunction syndrome following bilateral percutaneous cervical cordotomy. J Neurosurg 39:168, 1974.
91. Polatty RC, Cooper KR: Respiratory failure after percutaneous cordotomy. South Med J 79:897, 1986.
92. Wells CJ, Lipton S, Lahuerta J: Respiratory depression after percutaneous cervical anterolateral cordotomy in patients on slow-release oral morphine. Lancet 1:739, 1984.
93. Rosomoff HL, Papo I, Loeser J, et al: Neurosurgical operations on the spinal cord. In Bonica JJ (ed): Management of Pain. Philadelphia, Lea & Febiger, 1990, p 2067.
94. Palma A, Holzer J, Cuadra O, et al: Lateral percutaneous spinothalamic tractotomy. Acta Neurochir (Wien) 93:100, 1988.
95. Brose WG, Cousins MJ: Subcutaneous lidocaine for treatment of neuropathic cancer pain. Pain 45:145, 1991.
96. Glazer S, Portenoy RK: Systemic local anesthetics in pain control. J Pain Symptom Manage 6:30, 1991.
97. Eisenreich J, DuPen S, Dubois M, et al: Epidural clonidine analgesia for intractable cancer pain. Pain 61:391, 1995.

Index

Note: Page numbers followed by f indicate figures; those followed by t indicate tables.